The IASGO Textbook of Multi-Disciplinary Management of Hepato-Pancreato-Biliary Diseases

Masatoshi Makuuchi · Norihiro Kokudo
Irinel Popescu · Jacques Belghiti
Ho-Seong Han · Kyoichi Takaori · Dan G. Duda
Editors

The IASGO Textbook of Multi-Disciplinary Management of Hepato-Pancreato-Biliary Diseases

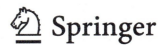

Editors
Masatoshi Makuuchi
Emeritus Professor
The University of Tokyo
Tokyo, Japan

Irinel Popescu
"Dan Setlacec" Center of General Surgery
and Liver Transplantation
Fundeni Clinical Institute
Bucharest, Romania

Ho-Seong Han
Department of Surgery
Seoul National University College of Medicine
Seoul National University Bundang Hospital
Seoul, Korea

Dan G. Duda
Massachusetts General Hospital
Harvard Medical School
Boston, USA

Norihiro Kokudo
National Center for Global Health and Medicine
The University of Tokyo
Tokyo, Japan

Jacques Belghiti
Emeritus Professor University Paris Cité
Paris, France

Kyoichi Takaori
Nagahama City Hospital Network
Shiga, Japan

Asahi University
Gifu, Japan

ISBN 978-981-19-0062-4   ISBN 978-981-19-0063-1   (eBook)
https://doi.org/10.1007/978-981-19-0063-1

© International Association of Surgeons, Gastroenterologists and Oncologists 2022
This work is subject to copyright. All rights are solely and exclusively licensed by the Publisher, whether the whole or part of the material is concerned, specifically the rights of translation, reprinting, reuse of illustrations, recitation, broadcasting, reproduction on microfilms or in any other physical way, and transmission or information storage and retrieval, electronic adaptation, computer software, or by similar or dissimilar methodology now known or hereafter developed.
The use of general descriptive names, registered names, trademarks, service marks, etc. in this publication does not imply, even in the absence of a specific statement, that such names are exempt from the relevant protective laws and regulations and therefore free for general use.
The publisher, the authors and the editors are safe to assume that the advice and information in this book are believed to be true and accurate at the date of publication. Neither the publisher nor the authors or the editors give a warranty, expressed or implied, with respect to the material contained herein or for any errors or omissions that may have been made. The publisher remains neutral with regard to jurisdictional claims in published maps and institutional affiliations.

This Springer imprint is published by the registered company Springer Nature Singapore Pte Ltd.
The registered company address is: 152 Beach Road, #21-01/04 Gateway East, Singapore 189721, Singapore

Foreword

It is with great emotion and satisfaction that I write this foreword to the International Association of Surgeons, Gastroenterologists, and Oncologists (IASGO) Textbook of Multi-Disciplinary Management of Hepato-Pancreato-Biliary Diseases.

When Professor Nikolaos Lygidakis founded the Association in 1988, he had a vision: to put together in the same meeting doctors from all over the world, experts and non-experts, the ones who teach and the ones who learn, exchanging knowledge in all fields of GI diseases, and in all specialties: surgeons, gastroenterologists and then oncologists. When I participated for the first time at the meeting, I was surprised to meet people coming from countries that are not represented in usual meetings, keen to learn and bringing their own experience.

When later on I was asked to be President after Professors Thomas Starzl, Meinhard Classen, and Enrique Moreno-Gonzalez, it was a great pleasure and honor to accept. The young small society called at that time Gastro Surgical Club had grown to a large association of thousands of surgeons, gastroenterologists, and oncologists and it was time to transform the visionary project of Professor Nick Lygidakis into the unique worldwide organization that the present IASGO has become.

This first edition of the IASGO Textbook reflects well the history of IASGO and the breadth and depth of our organization, as well as its worldwide outreach. Edited by Professor Masatoshi Makuuchi, the IASGO President, and by Professor Kyoichi Takaori, the General Secretary, and other expert surgeons and oncologists, the IASGO Textbook offers an outstanding overview of current approaches and future directions in the multi-disciplinary treatment of challenging hepato-biliary-pancreatic diseases.

I am sure that, beyond its historical significance, this Textbook will certainly inspire a new generation of medical professionals in the spirit and vision of our organization.

Paris, France

Henri Bismuth
Honorary President, IASGO

Preface

The International Association of Surgeons, Gastroenterologists, and Oncologists (IASGO) was founded in Amsterdam in 1988. Today, we are privileged to have strong IASGO sections in more than 70 countries, which greatly assists in assessing educational needs. The main goal of this organization has been and remains globalization of medical knowledge and expertise through a well-structured and precisely organized system of continued medical education. This visionary approach has impacted medical communities and the career of young specialists from all continents.

It is my pleasure to introduce you to our new landmark project, the first edition of the IASGO Textbook of Multi-Disciplinary Management of Hepato-Pancreato-Biliary Diseases. Along with Drs. Norihiro Kokudo, Irinel Popescu, Jacques Belghiti, Ho-Seong Han, Kyoichi Takaori, and Dan G. Duda, I hereby thank all contributors for their excellent chapters on behalf of the editors. The diverse display of multi-disciplinary, innovative, and creative approaches to treatment of these complex diseases is a perfect representation of our organization's mission and vision. I take this opportunity to express my sincere thanks to my former President of IASGO, Professor Henri Bismuth for his continuous support. I would like to dedicate this textbook to the loving memory of IASGO founder, the late Professor Nikolaos Lygidakis.

Tokyo, Japan   Masatoshi Makuuchi
                                                                                                                       President, IASGO

Introduction

To address the complexity and aggressiveness of hepato-pancreato-biliary diseases, surgeons, gastroenterologists, and oncologists have made great efforts to improve their treatment for many decades. Despite these efforts, management of these diseases has remained a challenge for medical professionals and largely an unmet need in medicine. What's worse, the incidence of these cancers is increasing worldwide at alarming rates. Treating the diseases in hepato-pancreato-biliary regions is particularly difficult due to the complex anatomy, aggressive biological behavior, and poor prognosis.

We think that the key to success in this ongoing crusade is a multi-disciplinary approach to the treatment. IASGO was founded on this principle by late Professor Nikolaos Lygidakis more than 30 years ago. In keeping with this unique vision, we have been organizing, apart from Annual World Congresses, a number of Advanced Post-Graduate Training Courses all over the world. The main characteristics of this program have been the multi-disciplinary structure and global reach. These courses are always organized in close cooperation with national Academic Centers or local Governmental authorities, aiming to update the participants in the field of Surgery, Gastroenterology, Oncology, Radiology, Pathology, and Tumor Biology as well as in the newest developments in Radiological and Endoscopic Interventions.

Here, we are expanding our efforts with this first edition of the IASGO Textbook of Multi-Disciplinary Management of Hepato-Pancreato-Biliary Diseases. Edited by Drs. Masatoshi Makuuchi, Norihiro Kokudo, Irinel Popescu, Jacques Belghiti, Ho-Seong Han, Kyoichi Takaori, and Dan G. Duda, the textbook includes 70 chapters from an exceptional group of experts in all areas of hepato-pancreato-biliary diseases. We are so fortunate to have these leading experts as our IASGO colleagues and friends.

We would like to extend our gratitude to Professor Irinel Popescu and Doctor Florin Botea, whose efforts have been essential for the development of this project and the publication of this textbook. Last but not least, we would like to dedicate this textbook to all of our colleagues and patients around the globe.

Kyoto, Japan Kyoichi Takaori
Secretary General, IASGO

Boston, USA Dan G. Duda
Secretary General, IASGO

Contents

1. **Surgical Anatomy of the Liver** 1
   Kenji Yoshino, Kojiro Taura, Kyoichi Takaori, Yosuke Kasai, and Etsuro Hatano

2. **Surgical Anatomy of the Pancreas** 7
   Akihiko Horiguchi, Masahiro Ito, Yukio Asano, Satoshi Arakawa, Hiroyuki Kato, and Masahiro Shimura

3. **Surgical Anatomy of the Biliary Tract** 15
   Eduardo Olivera Pertusso, Joaquin Garcia, and Luis Ruso Martinez

4. **Liver Function and Posthepatectomy Liver Failure** 23
   Takanobu Hara and Susumu Eguchi

5. **Surgical Approach to Pancreas, Liver, Biliary Physiologic Impairment** 31
   Alexandra W. Acher, Amir A. Rahnemai-Azar, Sharon M. Weber, and Timothy M. Pawlik

6. **Biliary Tract Functions and Impairment** 51
   Hideo Ohtsuka and Michiaki Unno

7. **Preinvasive Intraductal Biliary Neoplasm: Biliary Intraepithelial Neoplasm and Intraductal Papillary Neoplasm of Bile Duct** 57
   Yasuni Nakanuma, Katsuhiko Uesaka, and Takuro Terada

8. **Pathology of Biliary Tract Cancers** 65
   Claudio Luchini, Michele Simbolo, and Aldo Scarpa

9. **Multifocal Hepatocellular Carcinoma: Genomic and Transcriptional Heterogeneity** 71
   Ming Kuang, Lixia Xu, Sui Peng, Manling Huang, Xin Liu, and Guanrui Liao

10. **Intraductal Neoplasms of the Pancreas** 77
    Toru Furukawa

11. **Mucinous Cystic Neoplasms** 85
    Noriyoshi Fukushima

12. **Pathology of Pancreatic Cancer** 91
    Ralph H. Hruban and Elizabeth Thompson

13. **CT in Hepato-Bilio-Pancreatic Surgical Pathology** 99
    Ioana G. Lupescu and Mugur C. Grasu

14. **Magnetic Resonance Elastography (MRE) to Assess Hepatic Fibrosis** 113
    Aliya Qayyum

15. **FDG-PET for Management on Hepato-Pancreato-Biliary Disease** 123
    Koji Murakami

16	**Endoscopic Ultrasound for Hepato-Pancreato-Biliary Diseases** 135
	Yasunobu Yamashita and Masayuki Kitano
17	**Intraoperative Imaging Techniques in Liver Surgery** 145
	Florin Botea, Alexandru Barcu, and Irinel Popescu
18	**Use of Radiotherapy Alone and in Combination with Other Therapies for Hepatocellular Carcinoma: Rationale and Future Directions** 153
	Dan G. Duda and Franziska D. Hauth
19	**Recent Update in Chemotherapy of Cholangiocarcinoma** 165
	Jung Hyun Jo, Seungmin Bang, and Si Young Song
20	**Chemotherapy in Pancreatic Ductal Adenocarcinoma** 171
	Hee Seung Lee, Seung Woo Park, and Si Young Song
21	**Immune-Checkpoint Inhibitors in Hepatocellular Carcinoma** 177
	Rubens Copia Sperandio, Roberto Carmagnani Pestana, and Ahmed O. Kaseb
22	**Molecularly Targeted Therapy in Cholangiocarcinoma** 185
	Aakash Desai and Mitesh J. Borad
23	**Systemic Therapies for Pancreatic Cancer** 193
	Faysal Dane and Nazim Can Demircan
24	**Endoscopic Biliary Drainage and Associated Procedures Required for Patients with Malignant Biliary Strictures** 201
	Hiroyuki Isayama, Toshio Fujisawa, Shigeto Ishii, Ko Tomishima, Muneo Ikemura, Hiroto Ota, Daishi Kabemura, Mako Ushio, Sho Takahashi, Yusuke Takasaki, Akinori Suzuki, Koichi Ito, Kazushige Ochiai, and Hiroaki Saito
25	**Endoscopic Management of Peripancreatic Fluid Collection** 209
	Yukitoshi Matsunami, Shuntaro Mukai, and Takao Itoi
26	**Endoscopic Ultrasound and Fine Needle Tissue Acquisition for Pancreatic Tumors** 215
	Razvan Iacob and Cristian Gheorghe
27	**Enhanced Recovery After Surgery (ERAS): Concept and Purpose** 225
	Gregg Nelson and Olle Ljungqvist
28	**Multidisciplinary Enhanced Recovery After Surgery (ERAS) Pathway for Hepatobiliary and Pancreatic Surgery** 229
	Didier Roulin and Nicolas Demartines
29	**ERAS in Pancreatic Surgery** 235
	Julie Perinel and Mustapha Adham
30	**Ultrasound-Guided Anatomic Resection of the Liver** 241
	Junichi Shindoh, Kiyoshi Hasegawa, and Masatoshi Makuuchi
31	**Parenchyma-sparing Hepatic Resection for Multiple Metastatic Tumors** 247
	Bruno Branciforte, Flavio Milana, and Guido Torzilli
32	**Open and Laparoscopic Liver Hanging Maneuver** 257
	Jacques Belghiti and Safi Dokmak
33	**The Glissonean Pedicle Approach: The Takasaki Technique** 265
	Shun-ichi Ariizumi and Masakazu Yamamoto

34	**Laparoscopic Major Hepatectomy and Parenchymal-Sparing Anatomical Hepatectomy**	271
	Kohei Mishima, Go Wakabayashi, Kazuharu Igarashi, and Takahiro Ozaki	
35	**Laparoscopic Anatomical Resection of the Liver: Segmentectomy and Sub-segmentectomy**	279
	Boram Lee and Ho-Seong Han	
36	**Modified ALPPS Procedure**	285
	Nobuyuki Takemura, Kyouji Ito, and Norihiro Kokudo	
37	**Artery-First Approach in Pancreaticoduodenectomy**	289
	Daisuke Ban and Minoru Tanabe	
38	**Organ- and Parenchyma-sparing Pancreatic Surgery**	297
	Calogero Iacono, Mario De Bellis, Andrea Ruzzenente, and Alfredo Guglielmi	
39	**Isolated Pancreatoduodenectomy with Portal Vein Resection Using the Nakao Mesenteric Approach**	307
	Akimasa Nakao	
40	**Pancreaticoduodenectomy with Hepatic Artery Resection**	313
	Atsushi Oba, Tomotaka Kato, Marco Del Chiaro, Y. H. Andrew Wu, Yosuke Inoue, and Yu Takahashi	
41	**Pancreaticoduodenectomy with Splenic Artery Resection for Tumors of the Pancreatic Head and/or Body Invading the Splenic Artery**	319
	Shugo Mizuno, Kazuyuki Gyoten, and Motonori Nagata	
42	**Pancreaticoduodenectomy with Superior Mesenteric Resection and Reconstruction for Locally Advanced Tumors**	327
	Philippe Bachellier and Pietro Addeo	
43	**Robotic Pancreaticoduodenectomy**	335
	Thilo Hackert	
44	**Duodenum-Preserving Pancreatic Head Resection**	341
	Elena Usova	
45	**Artery-First Approaches to Distal Pancreatectomy**	347
	Kyoichi Takaori, Yosuke Kasai, and Kenji Yoshino	
46	**Spleen-Preserving Distal Pancreatectomy**	353
	Kohei Nakata and Masafumi Nakamura	
47	**Distal Pancreatectomy with *En Bloc* Celiac Axis Resection**	361
	Satoshi Hirano, Toru Nakamura, and Toshimichi Asano	
48	**Modified Distal Pancreatectomy with Celiac Axis En-bloc Resection**	365
	Ken-ichi Okada and Hiroki Yamaue	
49	**Robotic Distal Pancreatectomy**	373
	Marco Vito Marino, Marco Ramera, and Alessandro Esposito	
50	**Total Pancreatectomy**	377
	Aleksandar Karamarkovic, Jovan Juloski, and Vladica Cuk	
51	**Pancreatic Resection for Solid Pseudopapillary Neoplasms**	385
	Wenming Wu, Qiang Xu, and Rui Jiang	

52 Pancreatic Resection for Neuroendocrine Neoplasms of the Pancreas 389
Yosuke Kasai, Toshihiko Masui, Kyoichi Takaori, Kenji Yoshino, and
Eric K. Nakakura

**53 International Consensus Guidelines for the Management of Intraductal
Papillary Mucinous Neoplasms** 395
Brian K. P. Goh

54 Remnant Pancreatic Cancer After Surgical Resection for Pancreatic Cancer ... 401
Yoshihiro Miyasaka and Masafumi Nakamura

55 Benign Biliary Diseases 407
Abdel Hadi S. Al Breizat, Salam S. Daradkeh, and Ali A. Al-Sarira

56 Major Hepatic Resection for Peri-hilar Biliary Cancers 413
Fabio Bagante, Marzia Tripepi, Alfredo Guglielmi, Calogero Iacono, and
Andrea Ruzzenente

57 Surgical Management of Intrahepatic Cholangiocarcinoma 421
Mohamed Abdel-Wahab and Ahmed Shehta

58 Hepatopancreatoduodenectomy (HPD) for Biliary Tract Cancers 429
Tomoki Ebata, Takashi Mizuno, and Shunsuke Onoe

59 Hepato-biliary Injuries 435
Ender Dulundu

60 Surgical Treatment for Severe Liver Injuries 441
Florin Botea, Alexandru Barcu, and Irinel Popescu

**61 Indications for Liver Transplantation in Adults: Selection of Patients
with End Stage Liver Diseases** 451
Speranta Iacob and Liana Gheorghe

62 Indications for Liver Transplantation in Acute Liver Failure 461
Dana Tomescu and Mihai Popescu

63 Liver Graft Retrieval in Deceased Donors 473
Florin Botea, Genadyi Vatachki Roumenov, Radu Zamfir, Vladislav
Brasoveanu, and Irinel Popescu

64 Deceased Donor Liver Transplantation: The Pendulum of Visions and Ideas ... 487
Jan Lerut and Quirino Lai

65 Living Donor Liver Transplantation 501
Nobuhisa Akamatsu, Kiyoshi Hasegawa, Norihiro Kokudo, and Masatoshi
Makuuchi

66 Pyogenic Liver Abscess 509
Kai Siang Chan and Vishal Shelat

**67 Liver Transplantation for Colorectal and Neuroendocrine Liver Metastases
and Hepatoblastoma** 521
Taizo Hibi

**68 Technical Variant Liver Transplantation: Split, Dual Graft, and Auxiliary
Transplantation** 527
Vladislav Brasoveanu, Doina Hrehoret, Florin Botea, Florin Ichim, and
Irinel Popescu

69	**Domino Liver Transplantation**	535
	Irinel Popescu, Vladislav Brasoveanu, Doina Hrehoret, Florin Botea, Simona Dima, and Florin Ichim	
70	**Cell Transplantation**	541
	Takayuki Anazawa, Takashi Ito, Koichiro Hata, Toshihiko Masui, and Kojiro Taura	

Contributors

Mohamed Abdel-Wahab Department of Surgery, Liver Transplantation Unit, Gastrointestinal Surgery Center, Mansoura University, Mansoura, Egypt

Alexandra W. Acher Department of Surgery, Division of Surgical Oncology, University of Wisconsin School of Medicine and Public Health, Madison, WI, USA

Pietro Addeo Hepato-Pancreato-Biliary Surgery and Liver Transplantation, Pôle des Pathologies Digestives, Hépatiques et de la Transplantation, Hôpital de Hautepierre-Hôpitaux Universitaires de Strasbourg, Université de Strasbourg, Strasbourg, France

Mustapha Adham Department of Digestive Surgery, Edouard Herriot Hospital, Hospices Civils de Lyon, UCBL1, Lyon, France

Nobuhisa Akamatsu Artificial Organ and Transplantation Division, Department of Surgery, Graduate School of Medicine, The University of Tokyo, Tokyo, Japan

Abdel Hadi S. Al Breizat HPB Unit-Surgical Department-AL Bashir Hospital MOH, Amman, Jordan

Ali A. Al-Sarira Royal Hospital, Amman, Jordan

Takayuki Anazawa Division of Hepato-Biliary-Pancreatic Surgery and Transplantation, Department of Surgery, Graduate School of Medicine, Kyoto University, Kyoto, Japan

Satoshi Arakawa Department of Gastroenterological Surgery, Fujita Health University School of Medicine Bantane Hospital, Nagoya, Japan

Shun-ichi Ariizumi Department of Surgery, Institute of Gastroenterology, Tokyo, Japan

Toshimichi Asano Department of Gastroenterological Surgery II, Hokkaido University Faculty of Medicine, Sapporo, Japan

Yukio Asano Department of Gastroenterological Surgery, Fujita Health University School of Medicine Bantane Hospital, Nagoya, Japan

Philippe Bachellier Hepato-Pancreato-Biliary Surgery and Liver Transplantation, Pôle des Pathologies Digestives, Hépatiques et de la Transplantation, Hôpital de Hautepierre-Hôpitaux Universitaires de Strasbourg, Université de Strasbourg, Strasbourg, France

Fabio Bagante Department of Surgery, Dentistry, Gynecology and Pediatrics, Division of General and Hepato-Biliary Surgery, University of Verona, Verona, Italy

Daisuke Ban Department of Hepatobiliary and Pancreatic Surgery, National Cancer Center Hospital, Tokyo, Japan

Seungmin Bang Division of Gastroenterology, Department of Internal Medicine, Yonsei University College of Medicine, Seoul, South Korea

Alexandru Barcu Center of General Surgery and Liver Transplantation, Fundeni Clinical Institute, Bucharest, Romania

Jacques Belghiti APHP Paris, Paris, France

Mitesh J. Borad Mayo Clinic Cancer Center, Phoenix, AZ, USA
Center for Individualized Medicine, Mayo Clinic, Rochester, MN, USA
Department of Molecular Medicine, Mayo Clinic, Rochester, MN, USA
Division of Hematology/Oncology, Mayo Clinic, Phoenix, AZ, USA

Florin Botea Fundeni Clinical Institute, Bucharest, Romania
Center of General Surgery and Liver Transplantation, Fundeni Clinical Institute, Bucharest, Romania
"Dan Setlacec" Center of General Surgery and Liver Transplantation, Fundeni Clinical Institute, Bucharest, Romania
"Titu Maiorescu" University, Bucharest, Romania

Bruno Branciforte Division of Hepatobiliary and General Surgery, Humanitas Clinical and Research Center IRCCS, Milan, Italy

Vladislav Brasoveanu Center of General Surgery and Liver Transplantation, Fundeni Clinical Institute, Bucharest, Romania
"Dan Setlacec" Center of General Surgery and Liver Transplantation, Fundeni Clinical Institute, Bucharest, Romania
"Titu Maiorescu" University, Bucharest, Romania

Vladica Cuk Department of HPB Surgery, Surgical Clinic "Nikola Spasic", University Clinical Center Zvezdara, Belgrade, Serbia
Faculty of Medicine University of Belgrade, Belgrade, Serbia

Faysal Dane Division of Medical Oncology, Department of Internal Medicine, Altunizade Acibadem Hospital, Istanbul, Turkey

Salam S. Daradkeh The University of Jordan, Amman, Jordan

Mario De Bellis Department of Surgery, Unit of HPB Surgery, University of Verona Medical School, Verona, Italy

Marco Del Chiaro Division of Surgical Oncology, Department of Surgery, University of Colorado, Denver, CO, USA

Nicolas Demartines Department of Visceral Surgery, Lausanne University Hospital, University of Lausanne, Lausanne, Switzerland

Nazim Can Demircan Division of Medical Oncology, Department of Internal Medicine, Marmara University School of Medicine, Istanbul, Turkey

Aakash Desai Department of Oncology, Mayo Clinic, Rochester, MN, USA

Simona Dima "Dan Setlacec" Center of General Surgery and Liver Transplantation, Fundeni Clinical Institute, Bucharest, Romania

Safi Dokmak Department of HPB Surgery and Liver Transplantation, Beaujon Hospital, Clichy, France
France University Paris VII, Paris, France

Dan G. Duda Department of Radiation Oncology, Massachusetts General Hospital Research Institute, Boston, MA, USA
Harvard Medical School, Boston, MA, USA

Contributors

Ender Dulundu Department of General Surgery, HPB Unit, Director of Liver Transplantation Unit, Istanbul University-Cerrahpasa, Cerrahpasa Medical School, Istanbul, Turkey

Tomoki Ebata Division of Surgical Oncology, Department of Surgery, Nagoya University Graduate School of Medicine, Nagoya, Japan

Susumu Eguchi Department of Surgery, Nagasaki University Graduate School of Biomedical Sciences, Nagasaki, Japan

Alessandro Esposito General and Pancreatic Surgery Department, University and Hospital Trust of Verona, Verona, Italy

Toshio Fujisawa Department of Gastroenterology, Graduate School of Medicine, Juntendo University, Tokyo, Japan

Noriyoshi Fukushima Department of Pathology, Jichi Medical University, Shimotsuke, Tochigi, Japan

Toru Furukawa Department of Investigative Pathology, Tohoku University Graduate School of Medicine, Sendai, Japan

Joaquin Garcia School of Medicine, University of Republic (UdeLar), Montevideo, Uruguay

Cristian Gheorghe University of Medicine and Pharmacy "Carol Davila", Bucharest, Romania

Fundeni Clinical Institute, Digestive Diseases and Liver Transplantation Center, Bucharest, Romania

Liana Gheorghe Digestive Diseases and Liver Transplantation Center, Fundeni Clinical Institute, Bucharest, Romania

"Carol Davila" University of Medicine and Pharmacy, Bucharest, Romania

Brian K. P. Goh Department of Hepatopancreatobiliary and Transplant Surgery, Singapore General Hospital, Singapore, Singapore

Duke-National University of Singapore Medical School, Singapore, Singapore

Mugur C. Grasu Radiology, Medical Imaging and Interventional Imaging Department of Fundeni Clinical Institute, University of Medicine and Pharmacy "Carol Davila", Bucharest, Romania

Alfredo Guglielmi Department of Surgery, Unit of HPB Surgery, University of Verona Medical School, Verona, Italy

Department of Surgery, Dentistry, Gynecology and Pediatrics, Division of General and Hepato-Biliary Surgery, University of Verona, Verona, Italy

Kazuyuki Gyoten Department of Hepatobiliary Pancreatic and Transplant Surgery, Mie University Graduate School of Medicine, Tsu, Mie, Japan

Thilo Hackert Department of General, Visceral and Transplantation Surgery, University of Heidelberg, Heidelberg, Germany

Ho-Seong Han Department of Surgery, Seoul National University College of Medicine, Seoul National University Bundang Hospital, Seoul, Korea

Takanobu Hara Department of Surgery, Nagasaki University Graduate School of Biomedical Sciences, Nagasaki, Japan

Kiyoshi Hasegawa Hepatobiliary-Pancreatic Surgery Division, Department of Surgery, Graduate School of Medicine, The University of Tokyo, Tokyo, Japan

Artificial Organ and Transplantation Division, Department of Surgery, Graduate School of Medicine, The University of Tokyo, Tokyo, Japan

Koichiro Hata Division of Hepato-Biliary-Pancreatic Surgery and Transplantation, Department of Surgery, Graduate School of Medicine, Kyoto University, Kyoto, Japan

Etsuro Hatano Division of Hepato-Biliary-Pancreatic Surgery and Transplantation, Department of Surgery, Graduate School of Medicine, Kyoto University, Kyoto, Japan

Franziska D. Hauth Department of Radiation Oncology, Massachusetts General Hospital Research Institute, Boston, MA, USA

Harvard Medical School, Boston, MA, USA

Department of Radiation Oncology, University of Tübingen, Tübingen, Germany

Taizo Hibi Department of Pediatric Surgery and Transplantation, Kumamoto University Graduate School of Medical Sciences, Kumamoto, Japan

Satoshi Hirano Department of Gastroenterological Surgery II, Hokkaido University Faculty of Medicine, Sapporo, Japan

Akihiko Horiguchi Department of Gastroenterological Surgery, Fujita Health University School of Medicine Bantane Hospital, Nagoya, Japan

Doina Hrehoret "Dan Setlacec" Center of General Surgery and Liver Transplantation, Fundeni Clinical Institute, Bucharest, Romania

Ralph H. Hruban Department of Pathology, The Sol Goldman Pancreatic Cancer Research Center, Baltimore, MD, USA

Department of Oncology, The Johns Hopkins University School of Medicine, Baltimore, MD, USA

Manling Huang Cancer Center, The First Affiliated Hospital, Sun Yat-sen University, Guangzhou, Guangdong Province, China

Razvan Iacob University of Medicine and Pharmacy "Carol Davila", Bucharest, Romania

Fundeni Clinical Institute, Digestive Diseases and Liver Transplantation Center, Bucharest, Romania

Speranta Iacob Digestive Diseases and Liver Transplantation Center, Fundeni Clinical Institute, Bucharest, Romania

"Carol Davila" University of Medicine and Pharmacy, Bucharest, Romania

Calogero Iacono Department of Surgery, Unit of HPB Surgery, University of Verona Medical School, Verona, Italy

Department of Surgery, Dentistry, Gynecology and Pediatrics, Division of General and Hepato-Biliary Surgery, University of Verona, Verona, Italy

Florin Ichim "Dan Setlacec" Center of General Surgery and Liver Transplantation, Fundeni Clinical Institute, Bucharest, Romania

Kazuharu Igarashi Center for Advanced Treatment of HBP Diseases, Ageo Central General Hospital, Saitama, Japan

Muneo Ikemura Department of Gastroenterology, Graduate School of Medicine, Juntendo University, Tokyo, Japan

Yosuke Inoue Division of Hepatobiliary and Pancreatic Surgery, Cancer Institute Hospital, Japanese Foundation for Cancer Research, Tokyo, Japan

Hiroyuki Isayama Department of Gastroenterology, Graduate School of Medicine, Juntendo University, Tokyo, Japan

Shigeto Ishii Department of Gastroenterology, Graduate School of Medicine, Juntendo University, Tokyo, Japan

Koichi Ito Department of Gastroenterology, Graduate School of Medicine, Juntendo University, Tokyo, Japan

Kyouji Ito Department of Surgery, Hepato-Biliary Pancreatic Surgery Division, National Center for Global Health and Medicine, Tokyo, Japan

Masahiro Ito Department of Gastroenterological Surgery, Fujita Health University School of Medicine Bantane Hospital, Nagoya, Japan

Takashi Ito Division of Hepato-Biliary-Pancreatic Surgery and Transplantation, Department of Surgery, Graduate School of Medicine, Kyoto University, Kyoto, Japan

Takao Itoi Department of Gastroenterology and Hepatology, Tokyo Medical University, Tokyo, Japan

Rui Jiang Department of General Surgery, State Key Laboratory of Complex Severe and Rare Diseases, Peking Union Medical College Hospital, Chinese Academy of Medical Science and Peking Union Medical College, Beijing, China

Jung Hyun Jo Division of Gastroenterology, Department of Internal Medicine, Yonsei University College of Medicine, Seoul, South Korea

Jovan Juloski Department of HPB Surgery, Surgical Clinic "Nikola Spasic", University Clinical Center Zvezdara, Belgrade, Serbia

Faculty of Medicine University of Belgrade, Belgrade, Serbia

Daishi Kabemura Department of Gastroenterology, Graduate School of Medicine, Juntendo University, Tokyo, Japan

Aleksandar Karamarkovic Department of HPB Surgery, Surgical Clinic "Nikola Spasic", University Clinical Center Zvezdara, Belgrade, Serbia

Faculty of Medicine University of Belgrade, Belgrade, Serbia

Yosuke Kasai Department of Surgery, Nagahama City Hospital, Nagahama, Shiga, Japan

Department of Surgery, Graduate School of Medicine, Kyoto University, Kyoto, Japan

Department of Surgery, University of California, San Francisco, CA, USA

Ahmed O. Kaseb Department of Gastrointestinal Medical Oncology, The University of Texas MD Anderson Cancer Center, Houston, TX, USA

Hiroyuki Kato Department of Gastroenterological Surgery, Fujita Health University School of Medicine Bantane Hospital, Nagoya, Japan

Tomotaka Kato Division of Hepatobiliary and Pancreatic Surgery, Cancer Institute Hospital, Tokyo, Japan

Masayuki Kitano Second Department of Internal Medicine, Wakayama Medical University, Wakayama, Japan

Norihiro Kokudo Department of Surgery, Hepato-Biliary Pancreatic Surgery Division, National Center for Global Health and Medicine, Tokyo, Japan

Department of Surgery, National Center for Global Health and Medicine, Tokyo, Japan

Ming Kuang Center of Hepatopancreatobiliary Surgery, The First Affiliated Hospital, Sun Yat-sen University, Guangzhou, Guangdong Province, China

Cancer Center, The First Affiliated Hospital, Sun Yat-sen University, Guangzhou, Guangdong Province, China

Institute of Precision Medicine, The First Affiliated Hospital, Sun Yat-sen University, Guangzhou, Guangdong Province, China

Quirino Lai General Surgery and Organ Transplantation Unit, Sapienza University of Rome, Rome, Italy

Boram Lee Department of Surgery, Seoul National University, Bundang Hospital, Seoul National University College of Medicine, Seoul, South Korea

Hee Seung Lee Division of Gastroenterology, Department of Internal Medicine, Institute of Gastroenterology, Yonsei University College of Medicine, Seoul, South Korea

Jan Lerut Institute for Experimental and Clinical Research [IREC], Université catholique Louvain (UCL), Brussels, Belgium

Guanrui Liao Center of Hepatopancreatobiliary Surgery, The First Affiliated Hospital, Sun Yat-sen University, Guangzhou, Guangdong Province, China

Xin Liu Center of Hepatopancreatobiliary Surgery, The First Affiliated Hospital, Sun Yat-sen University, Guangzhou, Guangdong Province, China

Olle Ljungqvist Örebro University, Örebro, Sweden

Claudio Luchini Department of Pathology, University of Verona, Verona, Italy

Ioana G. Lupescu Radiology, Medical Imaging and Interventional Imaging Department of Fundeni Clinical Institute, University of Medicine and Pharmacy "Carol Davila", Bucharest, Romania

Masatoshi Makuuchi Koto Hospital, Tokyo, Japan

The University of Tokyo, Tokyo, Japan

Marco Vito Marino General Surgery Department, Policlinico di Abano Terme, Padova, Italy

General and Emergency Surgery Department, Azienda Ospedaliera, Ospedali Riuniti Villa Sofia-Cervello, Palermo, Italy

General Surgery Department, Hospital Universitario Marques de Valdecilla, Santander, Cantabria, Spain

General and Pancreatic Surgery Department, University and Hospital Trust of Verona, Verona, Italy

Luis Ruso Martinez School of Medicine, University of Republic (UdeLar), Montevideo, Uruguay

Toshihiko Masui Division of Hepato-Biliary-Pancreatic Surgery and Transplantation, Department of Surgery, Graduate School of Medicine, Kyoto University, Kyoto, Japan

Yukitoshi Matsunami Department of Gastroenterology and Hepatology, Tokyo Medical University, Tokyo, Japan

Flavio Milana Division of Hepatobiliary and General Surgery, Humanitas Clinical and Research Center IRCCS, Milan, Italy

Kohei Mishima Center for Advanced Treatment of HBP Diseases, Ageo Central General Hospital, Saitama, Japan

Yoshihiro Miyasaka Department of Surgery, Fukuoka University Chikushi Hospital, Chikushino, Fukuoka, Japan

Department of Surgery and Oncology, Graduate School of Medical Sciences, Kyushu University, Higashi-ku, Fukuoka, Japan

Shugo Mizuno Department of Hepatobiliary Pancreatic and Transplant Surgery, Mie University Graduate School of Medicine, Tsu, Mie, Japan

Takashi Mizuno Division of Surgical Oncology, Department of Surgery, Nagoya University Graduate School of Medicine, Nagoya, Japan

Shuntaro Mukai Department of Gastroenterology and Hepatology, Tokyo Medical University, Tokyo, Japan

Koji Murakami Department of Radiology, Graduate School of Medicine, Juntendo University, Tokyo, Japan

Motonori Nagata Department of Radiology, Mie University Graduate School of Medicine, Tsu, Mie, Japan

Eric K. Nakakura Department of Surgery, University of California, San Francisco, CA, USA

Masafumi Nakamura Department of Surgery and Oncology, Graduate School of Medical Sciences, Kyushu University, Higashi-ku, Fukuoka, Japan

Toru Nakamura Department of Gastroenterological Surgery II, Hokkaido University Faculty of Medicine, Sapporo, Japan

Yasuni Nakanuma Department of Diagnostic Pathology, Shizuoka Cancer Center, Shizuoka, Japan

Department of Diagnostic Pathology, Fukui Prefecture Saiseikai Hospital, Fukui, Japan

Akimasa Nakao Professor Emeritus, Nagoya University, Nagoya, Japan

Department of Surgery, Nagoya Central Hospital, Nagoya, Japan

Kohei Nakata Department of Surgery and Oncology, Graduate School of Medical Sciences, Kyushu University, Fukuoka, Japan

Gregg Nelson University of Calgary, Calgary, AB, Canada

Atsushi Oba Division of Hepatobiliary and Pancreatic Surgery, Cancer Institute Hospital, Japanese Foundation for Cancer Research, Tokyo, Japan

Division of Surgical Oncology, Department of Surgery, University of Colorado, Anschutz Medical Campus, Denver, CO, USA

Kazushige Ochiai Department of Gastroenterology, Graduate School of Medicine, Juntendo University, Tokyo, Japan

Hideo Ohtsuka Department of Surgery, Tohoku University, Sendai, Miyagi, Japan

Ken-ichi Okada Second Department of Surgery, Wakayama Medical University, Wakayama, Japan

Shunsuke Onoe Division of Surgical Oncology, Department of Surgery, Nagoya University Graduate School of Medicine, Nagoya, Japan

Hiroto Ota Department of Gastroenterology, Graduate School of Medicine, Juntendo University, Tokyo, Japan

Takahiro Ozaki Center for Advanced Treatment of HBP Diseases, Ageo Central General Hospital, Saitama, Japan

Seung Woo Park Division of Gastroenterology, Department of Internal Medicine, Institute of Gastroenterology, Yonsei University College of Medicine, Seoul, South Korea

Timothy M. Pawlik Department of General Surgery, Division of Surgical Oncology, The Ohio State University College of Medicine, Columbus, OH, USA

Sui Peng Institute of Precision Medicine, The First Affiliated Hospital, Sun Yat-sen University, Guangzhou, Guangdong Province, China

Department of Gastroenterology and Hepatology, The First Affiliated Hospital, Sun Yat-sen University, Guangzhou, Guangdong Province, China

Clinical Trials Unit, The First Affiliated Hospital, Sun Yat-sen University, Guangzhou, Guangdong Province, China

Julie Perinel Department of Digestive Surgery, Edouard Herriot Hospital, Hospices Civils de Lyon, UCBL1, Lyon, France

Eduardo Olivera Pertusso School of Medicine, University of Republic (UdeLar), Montevideo, Uruguay

Roberto Carmagnani Pestana Centro de Oncologia e Hematologia Einstein Familia Dayan-Daycoval, Hospital Israelita Albert Einstein, São Paulo, Brazil

Irinel Popescu Center of General Surgery and Liver Transplantation, Fundeni Clinical Institute, Bucharest, Romania

"Dan Setlacec" Center of General Surgery and Liver Transplantation, Fundeni Clinical Institute, Bucharest, Romania

"Titu Maiorescu" University, Bucharest, Romania

Mihai Popescu Department of Anaesthesia and Critical Care, "Carol Davila" University of Medicine and Pharmacy, Bucharest, Romania

Department of Anaesthesia and Critical Care, Fundeni Clinical Institute, Bucharest, Romania

Aliya Qayyum, MD Anderson Cancer Center, Houston, TX, USA

Amir A. Rahnemai-Azar Department of Surgery, Division of Surgical Oncology, California University of Science and Medicine, Colton, CA, USA

Marco Ramera General and Pancreatic Surgery Department, University and Hospital Trust of Verona, Verona, Italy

Didier Roulin Department of Visceral Surgery, Lausanne University Hospital, University of Lausanne, Lausanne, Switzerland

Genadyi Vatachki Roumenov Center of General Surgery and Liver Transplantation, Fundeni Clinical Institute, Bucharest, Romania

Andrea Ruzzenente Department of Surgery, Unit of HPB Surgery, University of Verona Medical School, Verona, Italy

Department of Surgery, Dentistry, Gynecology and Pediatrics, Division of General and Hepato-Biliary Surgery, University of Verona, Verona, Italy

Hiroaki Saito Department of Gastroenterology, Graduate School of Medicine, Juntendo University, Tokyo, Japan

Aldo Scarpa Department of Pathology, University of Verona, Verona, Italy

Ahmed Shehta Department of Surgery, Liver Transplantation Unit, Gastrointestinal Surgery Center, Mansoura University, Mansoura, Egypt

G. Shelat Vishal Department of General Surgery, Tan Tock Seng Hospital, Singapore, Singapore

Lee Kong Chian School of Medicine, Nanyang Technological University, Singapore, Singapore

Masahiro Shimura Department of Gastroenterological Surgery, Fujita Health University School of Medicine Bantane Hospital, Nagoya, Japan

Junichi Shindoh Hepatobiliary-Pancreatic Surgery Division, Department of Gastroenterological Surgery, Toranomon Hospital, Tokyo, Japan

Chan Kai Siang Ministry of Health Holdings Limited, Singapore, Singapore

Department of General Surgery, Tan Tock Seng Hospital, Singapore, Singapore

Michele Simbolo Department of Pathology, University of Verona, Verona, Italy

Si Young Song Division of Gastroenterology, Department of Internal Medicine, Institute of Gastroenterology, Yonsei University College of Medicine, Seoul, South Korea

Rubens Copia Sperandio Centro de Oncologia e Hematologia Einstein Familia Dayan-Daycoval, Hospital Israelita Albert Einstein, São Paulo, Brazil

Akinori Suzuki Department of Gastroenterology, Graduate School of Medicine, Juntendo University, Tokyo, Japan

Sho Takahashi Department of Gastroenterology, Graduate School of Medicine, Juntendo University, Tokyo, Japan

Yu Takahashi Division of Hepatobiliary and Pancreatic Surgery, Cancer Institute Hospital, Tokyo, Japan

Kyoichi Takaori Department of Surgery, Nagahama City Hospital, Nagahama, Japan

Department of Surgery, Kyoto University Graduate School of Medicine, Kyoto, Japan

Yusuke Takasaki Department of Gastroenterology, Graduate School of Medicine, Juntendo University, Tokyo, Japan

Nobuyuki Takemura Department of Surgery, Hepato-Biliary Pancreatic Surgery Division, National Center for Global Health and Medicine, Tokyo, Japan

Minoru Tanabe Department of Hepatobiliary and Pancreatic Surgery, Graduate School of Medicine, Tokyo Medical and Dental University, Tokyo, Japan

Kojiro Taura Division of Hepato-Biliary-Pancreatic Surgery and Transplantation, Department of Surgery, Graduate School of Medicine, Kyoto University, Kyoto, Japan

Takuro Terada Department of Gastrointestinal Surgery, Fukui Prefecture Saiseikai Hospital, Fukui, Japan

Elizabeth Thompson Department of Pathology, The Sol Goldman Pancreatic Cancer Research Center, Baltimore, MD, USA

Department of Oncology, The Johns Hopkins University School of Medicine, Baltimore, MD, USA

Dana Tomescu Department of Anaesthesia and Critical Care, "Carol Davila" University of Medicine and Pharmacy, Bucharest, Romania

Department of Anaesthesia and Critical Care, Fundeni Clinical Institute, Bucharest, Romania

Ko Tomishima Department of Gastroenterology, Graduate School of Medicine, Juntendo University, Tokyo, Japan

Guido Torzilli Division of Hepatobiliary and General Surgery, Humanitas Clinical and Research Center IRCCS, Milan, Italy

Department of Biomedical Sciences, Humanitas University, Milan, Italy

Marzia Tripepi Department of Surgery, Dentistry, Gynecology and Pediatrics, Division of General and Hepato-Biliary Surgery, University of Verona, Verona, Italy

Katsuhiko Uesaka Department of Hepatobiliary Pancreatic Surgery, Shizuoka Cancer Center, Shizuoka, Japan

Michiaki Unno Department of Surgery, Tohoku University, Sendai, Miyagi, Japan

Mako Ushio Department of Gastroenterology, Graduate School of Medicine, Juntendo University, Tokyo, Japan

Elena Usova International Association of Surgeons, Gastroenterologists and Oncologists, Kyoto, Japan

Go Wakabayashi Center for Advanced Treatment of HBP Diseases, Ageo Central General Hospital, Saitama, Japan

Sharon M. Weber Department of Surgery, Division of Surgical Oncology, University of Wisconsin School of Medicine and Public Health, Madison, WI, USA

Y. H. Andrew Wu Division of Surgical Oncology, Department of Surgery, University of Colorado, Denver, CO, USA

Wenming Wu Department of General Surgery, State Key Laboratory of Complex Severe and Rare Diseases, Peking Union Medical College Hospital, Chinese Academy of Medical Science and Peking Union Medical College, Beijing, China

Lixia Xu Cancer Center, The First Affiliated Hospital, Sun Yat-sen University, Guangzhou, Guangdong Province, China

Department of Gastroenterology and Hepatology, The First Affiliated Hospital, Sun Yat-sen University, Guangzhou, Guangdong Province, China

Qiang Xu Department of General Surgery, State Key Laboratory of Complex Severe and Rare Diseases, Peking Union Medical College Hospital, Chinese Academy of Medical Science and Peking Union Medical College, Beijing, China

Masakazu Yamamoto Department of Surgery, Institute of Gastroenterology, Tokyo Women's Medical University, Tokyo, Japan

Yasunobu Yamashita Second Department of Internal Medicine, Wakayama Medical University, Wakayama, Japan

Hiroki Yamaue Second Department of Surgery, Wakayama Medical University, Wakayama, Japan

Kenji Yoshino Department of Surgery, Nagahama City Hospital, Nagahama, Japan

Department of Surgery, Graduate School of Medicine, Kyoto University, Kyoto, Japan

Radu Zamfir Center of General Surgery and Liver Transplantation, Fundeni Clinical Institute, Bucharest, Romania

Surgical Anatomy of the Liver

Kenji Yoshino, Kojiro Taura, Kyoichi Takaori, Yosuke Kasai, and Etsuro Hatano

Abstract

Liver is the largest internal organ in the body, occupying 2.5% of the total body weight, characterized by the complex anatomy of the internal vascular and the ductal system. Despite the recent advances in the understanding of the physiology and pathology of the liver, the anatomy of this organ still remains not fully defined. The detailed anatomy of the liver described by Couinaud has been the basis both in surgical techniques and in diagnostics and for decades. However, the anatomic variation of the liver is not rare, and the frequencies of variant hepatic artery, portal vein, and bile duct have been reported to be approximately 45%, 14%, and 43%, respectively. Currently, owing to advances in diagnostic imaging, we can predict the anatomy of individual cases in detail before surgery. However, not all anomalies can be reliably detected even with the modern diagnostic tools. Hence, knowledge of the basic anatomy and anatomical variation of the liver is essential to ensure safe and successful hepatic surgery.

K. Yoshino (✉) · Y. Kasai
Department of Surgery, Nagahama City Hospital, Nagahama, Japan

Department of Surgery, Graduate School of Medicine, Kyoto University, Kyoto, Japan

K. Takaori
Department of Surgery, Nagahama City Hospital, Nagahama, Japan

Department of Surgery, Graduate School of Medicine, Kyoto University, Kyoto, Japan

K. Taura · E. Hatano
Division of Hepato-Biliary-Pancreatic Surgery and Transplantation, Department of Surgery, Graduate School of Medicine, Kyoto University, Kyoto, Japan

1.1 Introduction

Many anatomists and surgeons have contributed to our current understanding of liver anatomy. The French anatomist and surgeon Couinaud has described the anatomy of the liver in detail and demonstrated that liver functional anatomy is based on vascular and biliary relationships rather than external surface morphology [1]. Bismuth further improved the concept of functional anatomy of the liver by meticulous analysis on the distribution of the portal pedicles and the location of the hepatic veins with the aim to improve the feasibility and safety of hepatobiliary surgery [2]. Furthermore, there is a demand for more advanced hepatobiliary surgery with increasing complexity, and it became mandatory for us to carry out precise anatomical evaluation of the hepatic vasculature and biliary system preoperatively. The vascular anatomy of the liver intricately consists of the hepatic arteries, portal veins, bile ducts, and hepatic veins. The recent advances in hepatic surgery as well as those in endoscopic and radiological interventions necessitate comprehensive knowledge of the complex anatomy of the liver in order to avoid possible complications and to achieve the most effective results. The development of imaging technologies such as multidetector computed tomography with reconstruction of three-dimensional angiography and high-resolution magnetic resonance cholangiopancreatography has enabled us to carry out the anatomical evaluation of high precision [3, 4]. In this chapter, taking advantage of the next-generation imaging technologies, we describe the surgical anatomy of the liver with special reference to hepatic arteries, portal veins, bile ducts, and hepatic veins.

1.2 Arterial Anatomy

Arterial supply of the liver from the common hepatic artery (CHA) contributes 20–25% of hepatic blood inflow. The CHA proceeds laterally and branches into the proper hepatic

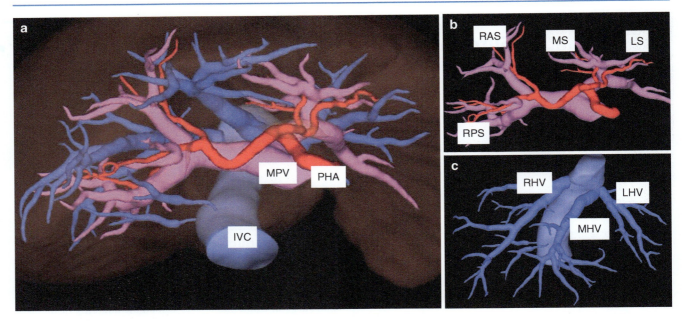

Fig. 1.1 CT imaging anatomy of the liver. (**a**) Typical vascular anatomy of the liver; (**b**) portal veins and hepatic arteries and segments; (**c**) hepatic veins. *IVC* inferior vena cava, *LHV* left hepatic vein, *LS* lateral segment, *MHV* middle hepatic vein, *MPV* main portal vein, *MS* median segment, *PHA* proper hepatic artery, *RAS* right anterior segment, *RPS* right posterior segment

artery (PHA) and the gastroduodenal artery. The PHA turns upward to ascend into the hepatoduodenal ligament. In the typical hepatic arterial anatomy, the PHA is divided into right (RHA) and left hepatic arteries (LHA) [3, 5, 6]. The LHA is located in front of and below the transverse part of the left portal branch in 80% and behind the left portal branch in 20% of cases [7, 8]. The middle hepatic artery (MHA) originates from LHA in 54%, from RHA in 34%, from trifurcation with LHA and RHA from PHA in 8%, and from CHA in 4% [8]. The cystic artery branches off the RHA in the hepatocystic triangle located between the cystic duct (CD) and the common bile duct (CBD). However, the extra-hepatic arterial anatomies are especially complex, showing many anatomic variations. The typical vascular anatomy of the liver is shown in Fig. 1.1 and the anatomical variation of the hepatic arteries according to the Michel's classification is described in Table 1.1 [9]. A replaced RHA may most commonly originate from the superior mesenteric artery (SMA) in 10–21% of individuals (Fig. 1.2) while a replaced left gastric artery (LGA) may arise from the LHA in 3–10% [5, 10, 11]. Also, an accessory LHA and RHA may exist in 1–8%. Another variant to this anatomy is a CHA which may come off the SMA in about 1.5% of the population [5, 10, 11].

The intrahepatic arteries harbor relatively less anatomical variation as compared to the extrahepatic artery. Within the liver or extra-hepatically, the RHA divides into anterior and posterior segmental arteries, which further divide to supply the respective subsegments in almost all cases [2, 7]. The anatomic variations, such as LHA running to the right side of the umbilical portion of the portal vein and the posterior segmental artery running to the cranial side of the RPV, are potentially very important, as they may alter the surgical procedure of a hepatectomy for biliary tract cancer. The arterial tributary toward the caudate lobe also originates from the RHA and supplies the caudate process and the right side of

Table 1.1 Anatomical variations in branching patterns of the hepatic arteries according to Michel's classification

Type	Pattern	Population (%)
1	Normal (RHA, MHA, LHA)	55
2	Replaced LHA from LGA	10
3	Replaced RHA from SMA	11
4	Replaced MHA from SMA Replaced LHA from LGA	1
5	Small LHA and an accessory LHA from LGA	8
6	Small RHA and an accessory RHA from SMA	7
7	RHA and an accessory RHA from SMA LHA and an accessory LHA from LGA	1
8	Replaced RHA from SMA and an accessory LHA from LGA or Replaced LHA from LGA and an accessory RHA from SMA	2
9	CHA absent—the entire hepatic trunk derived from SMA	2.5
10	CHA absent—the entire hepatic trunk derived from LGA	0.5

CHA common hepatic artery, *LGA* left gastric artery, *LHA* left hepatic artery, *MHA* middle hepatic artery, *RHA* right hepatic artery, *SMA* superior mesenteric artery

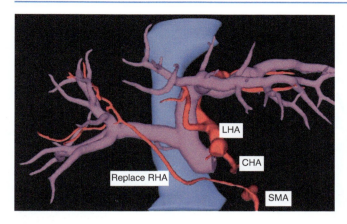

Fig. 1.2 CT imaging of the replaced right hepatic artery arising from the superior mesenteric artery. The right hepatic artery arising from the superior mesenteric artery (type 3 according to Michel's classification) is one of the most common anomalies. *CHA* common hepatic artery, *LHA* left hepatic artery, *RHA* right hepatic artery, *SMA* superior mesenteric artery

Table 1.2 Anatomical variations in blanching patterns of the portal veins according to Akgul's classification

Type	Pattern	Population (%)
I	Bifurcation of MPV (classical)	86.2
II	Trifurcation of MPV	12.3
III	RPPV from MPV + LPV and RAPV as a common trunk	0.3
IV	RPPV from MPV + RAPV from LPV	0.9
V	LPV absent	0
VI	RPV with branches absent	0
VII	LPV from RAPV, horizontal segment of LPV absent	0
VIII	MPV divides into RAPV and RPPV, LPV from RAPV	0.3

LPV left portal vein, *MPV* main portal vein, *RAPV* right anterior portal vein, *RPPV* right posterior portal vein, *RPV* right portal vein

the caudate lobe. The medial segmental artery supplies the quadrate lobe. The lateral segmental artery divides into superior and inferior arteries for the respective subsegments. Furthermore, the left hepatic artery gives off a branch for the caudate lobe, supplying its left side.

1.3 Portal Venous Anatomy

The majority of the hepatic blood inflow (75–80%) comes from the portal vein. The portal vein bifurcates into the right and left branches before entering the liver. In general, portal veins are found posterior to the hepatic arteries and bile ducts in their lobar and segmental distribution.

The left branch of the portal vein runs horizontally with a long extrahepatic course and commonly gives off a small branch to the caudate lobe. However, the branch to the caudate lobe may arise from the main or right portal vein, since the caudate portal vein inflow is variable. The left branch of the portal vein crosses the umbilical segment, where it gives rise to branches for segment II prior to the division into branches to segment III and segment IV.

The right branch of the portal vein is located anterior to the caudate process, and it gives off a branch to the caudate lobe and then an anterior branch and a posterior one. Eventually, the anterior and posterior branches divide into branches for the segments V and VIII, and those for VI and VII, respectively.

The branching patterns of the portal vein according to Akgul's classification are shown in Table 1.2 [12]. So-called classical portal anatomy (Type I) is present in 65–99% of the population. In 15% of individuals, the portal vein trifurcates into right anterior, right posterior, and left portal vein at a common place [12]. Also, the right posterior portal vein may arise from the portal vein trunk instead of the right portal vein in 7% of individuals [13]. In previous reports, types 5, 6, and 7 are also present in less than 0.3% [13, 14]. Depending on whether these anatomical abnormalities are present or not, alteration of the surgical procedure may be considered. Furthermore, anatomical variation may not be limited to the portal vein but may also coexist in the artery and bile ducts. For example, in a donor hepatectomy for living donor liver transplantation, a left trisegmental resection is required instead of a right hepatectomy in cases of type III anatomical variation with arterial variation (Fig. 1.3) [15]. Hence, surgeons need to plan their operative procedures in advance with possible anatomical variations in mind.

1.4 Biliary Anatomy

The segmental biliary branches accompany the arterial and venous portals surrounded by the Glissonian sheath. Generally, bile ducts II, III, and IV constitute the left hepatic duct (LHD), and V, VI, VII, and VIII form the right hepatic duct (RHD). Segment I is commonly drained by several ducts into the RHD and LHD (80%), and therefore, surgeons should be mindful of the variable anatomy of bile ducts when operating at the hilum of the liver. LHD and RHD are located superior to the primary branches of portal vein, and they join in front of and right of the portal vein trunk. As the common hepatic duct (CHD) courses caudally, it is joined by the CD to form the CBD which empties into the duodenum.

The anatomical pattern of the bile ducts consists of six types according to Smadja and Blumgart's classification (Table 1.3) [16]. The classic biliary anatomy appears in about 60% of the population [17]. The most common anatomic variation of the bile duct is trifurcation in 11–14% of the

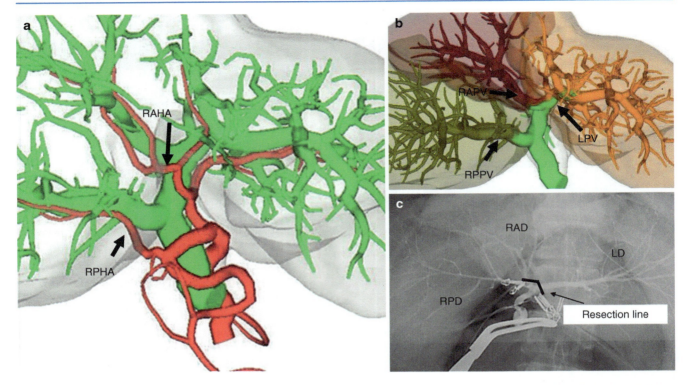

Fig. 1.3 Anatomical variation of the hepatic vasculature in a donor who underwent a left trisegmental resection of the liver for living donor liver transplantation. (**a**) The right anterior hepatic artery arises from the left hepatic artery. (**b**) The right anterior portal vein branches off from the umbilical portion. (**c**) The common hepatic duct trifurcated into the left, anterior, and posterior ducts. *LD* left bile duct, *LPV* left portal vein, *RAD* right anterior bile duct, *RAHA* right anterior hepatic artery, *RAPV* right anterior portal vein, *RPD* right posterior bile duct, *RPHA* right posterior hepatic artery, *RPPV* right posterior portal vein

Table 1.3 Anatomical variations in drainage patterns of the bile ducts according to Smadja and Blumgart's classification

Type	Pattern	Population (%)
I	Normal	57
II	Triple confluence of RASD, RPSD, and LHD	12
III	Lower drainage of	
	RPSD into CHD	16
	RASD into CHD	4
IV	Aberrant drainage of	
	RPSD into LHD	5
	RASD into LHD	1
V	CHD is formed by union of two or more ducts from either lobe	3
VI	RPSD into CD	2

CD cystic duct, *CHD* common hepatic duct, *LHD* left hepatic duct, *RASD* right anterior sectoral duct, *RPSD* right posterior sectoral duct

cases. The right posterior superior duct (RPSD) draining into the CHD is present in 7–16% and right anterior superior duct (RASD) draining into the CHD is observed in 1–4% [18, 19]. When performing a left hepatectomy in a liver transplant donor, positive recognition of this aberration is necessary to prevent bile leakage and obstruction.

1.5 Venous Anatomy

Blood from the liver is drained into the inferior vena cava (IVC) by three major hepatic veins and a series of dorsal hepatic veins. In 60% of the cases, the middle (MHV) and left hepatic veins (LHV) merge to form a common trunk before draining into the IVC [20].

The LHV lies in the upper part of the left fissure. It drains segment II, III and IV. The middle hepatic vein lies in the median fissure and drains segments IV, V, and VIII. The right hepatic vein (RHV) is typically larger, with a short extrahepatic course, and drains segments V–VII and a part of the segment VIII. The variations of three major hepatic veins described by Sureka are shown in Table 1.4 [21].

The minor hepatic veins including the short hepatic, middle right hepatic, and right inferior hepatic vein emerge in the lower portions of the retrohilar space and immediately drain into the IVC, draining the territories immediately adjacent to it. The liver volume drained by these minor hepatic veins and three major hepatic veins is shown Table 1.5 [22]. The area drained by these minor veins is not small. When mobilizing

Table 1.4 Anatomical variations in the number and branching patterns of hepatic vein described by Sureka

Pattern	Population (%)
RHV variations	
Single RHV	92
Early branching of RHV	40
2 RHV:	
Common trunk	5.4
Independent drainage	1.8
3 RHV:	
Common trunk	0.6
Independent drainage	0
Accessory inferior RHV	37
Small RHV with well-developed MHV	1.2
MHV and LHV variations	
Common trunk of MHV and LHV	81
Independent drainage of LHV and MHV into IVC	19

IVC inferior vena cava, *LHV* left hepatic vein, *MHV* middle hepatic vein, *RHV* right hepatic vein

Table 1.5 Volume of venous drainage areas from each drainage vein

Drainage vein	Volume (ml)	% of total liver volume
Major hepatic vein		
LHV	234.2 ± 61.6	20.7 ± 4
MHV	369.3 ± 96.6	32.7 ± 7
RHV	456.7 ± 188.1	39.6 ± 12
Minor hepatic vein		
Middle right hepatic vein	88.4 ± 53.7	8.0 ± 4
Inferior right hepatic vein	117.3 ± 75.6	10.6 ± 6

LHV left hepatic vein, *MHV* middle hepatic vein, *RHV* right hepatic vein

the liver, especially during major hepatectomies, it is imperative to maintain awareness of vascular tributaries from the IVC at all times.

1.6 Conclusion

Both intra and extrahepatic vasculobiliary anatomies are complex with the existence of many common and uncommon anatomic variations. Preoperative identification of these anatomies is mandatory for us to create the optimal surgical plan and to reduce postoperative complications. Moreover, advances in intraoperative mapping and parenchymal resection techniques have made and are making liver surgery safer and more effective [23]. Surgeons as well as gastroenterologists, oncologists, radiologists, and other specialists should respect the complexity and nuances of the anatomical structure of the liver, which require lifelong learning.

Acknowledgments The authors have no conflicts of interest to disclose.

References

1. Couinaud C. Liver lobes and segments: notes on the anatomical architecture and surgery of the liver. Presse Med. 1954;62(33):709–12.
2. Bismuth H. Surgical anatomy and anatomical surgery of the liver. World J Surg. 1982;6(1):3–9.
3. Arifuzzaman M, Nasim Naqvi SS, Adel H, Adil SO, Rasool M, Hussain M. Anatomical variants of celiac trunk, hepatic and renal arteries in a population of developing country using multidetector computed tomography angiography. J Ayub Med Coll Abbottabad. 2017;29(3):450–4.
4. Reinbold C, Bret PM, Guibaud L, Barkun AN, Genin G, Atri M. MR cholangiopancreatography: potential clinical applications. Radiographics. 1996;16(2):309–20.
5. Noussios G, Dimitriou I, Chatzis I, Katsourakis A. The main anatomic variations of the hepatic artery and their importance in surgical practice: review of the literature. J Clin Med Res. 2017;9(4):248–52.
6. Sahani D, Mehta A, Blake M, Prasad S, Harris G, Saini S. Preoperative hepatic vascular evaluation with CT and MR angiography: implications for surgery. Radiographics. 2004;24(5):1367–80.
7. López D. Anatomy of the Liver (A05.8.01.001). Worldwide review, 2019. New findings, concepts and definitions support a division of the liver into seven portal segments. Int J Morphol. 2019;37(3):1179–86.
8. Suzuki H. Correlation and anomalies of the vascular structure in Glisson's area around the hepatic hilum, from the standpoint of hepatobiliary surgery. Nihon Geka Hokan. 1982;51(5):713–31.
9. Michels NA. Newer anatomy of the liver and its variant blood supply and collateral circulation. Am J Surg. 1966;112(3):337–47.
10. Shukla PJ, Barreto SG, Kulkarni A, Nagarajan G, Fingerhut A. Vascular anomalies encountered during pancreatoduodenectomy: do they influence outcomes? Ann Surg Oncol. 2010;17(1):186–93.
11. Hiatt JR, Gabbay J, Busuttil RW. Surgical anatomy of the hepatic arteries in 1000 cases. Ann Surg. 1994;220(1):50–2.
12. Akgul E, Inal M, Soyupak S, Binokay F, Aksungur E, Oguz M. Portal venous variations. Prevalence with contrast-enhanced helical CT. Acta Radiol. 2002;43(3):315–9.
13. Cheng YF, Huang TL, Lee TY, Chen TY, Chen CL. Variation of the intrahepatic portal vein; angiographic demonstration and application in living-related hepatic transplantation. Transplant Proc. 1996;28(3):1667–8.
14. Fraser-Hill MA, Atri M, Bret PM, Aldis AE, Illescas FF, Herschorn SD. Intrahepatic portal venous system: variations demonstrated with duplex and color Doppler US. Radiology. 1990;177(2):523–6.
15. Taura K, Kaido T, Anazawa T, Yagi S, Okajima H, Uemoto S. Living donor liver transplantation with a left trisegmental graft from a donor with anomalous branching of the portal vein. Liver Transpl. 2017;23(6):853–6.
16. Smadja C, Blumgart LH. The biliary tract and the anatomy of biliary exposure. In: Blumgart LH, editor. Surgery of the liver and biliary tract, vol. 1. 3rd ed. Edinburgh: Churchill Livingstone; 2000. p. 19.
17. Cucchetti A, Peri E, Cescon M, Zanello M, Ercolani G, Zanfi C, et al. Anatomic variations of intrahepatic bile ducts in a European series and meta-analysis of the literature. J Gastrointest Surg. 2011;15(4):623–30.
18. Cucchetti A, Ercolani G, Cescon M, Ravaioli M, Zanello M, Del Gaudio M, et al. Recovery from liver failure after hepatectomy for hepatocellular carcinoma in cirrhosis: meaning of the model for end-stage liver disease. J Am Coll Surg. 2006;203(5):670–6.

19. Garga S, Kumarb KH, Sahnia D, Yadavb TD, Aggarwala A, Guptaa T. Surgical anatomy of the vasculobiliary apparatus at the hepatic hilum as applied to liver transplantations and major liver resections. J Anat Soc India. 2018;67:61–9.
20. Alonso-Torres A, Fernández-Cuadrado J, Pinilla I, Parrón M, de Vicente E, López-Santamaría M. Multidetector CT in the evaluation of potential living donors for liver transplantation. Radiographics. 2005;25(4):1017–30.
21. Sureka B, Sharma N, Khera PS, Garg PK, Yadav T. Hepatic vein variations in 500 patients: surgical and radiological significance. Br J Radiol. 2019;92(1102):20190487.
22. Tani K, Shindoh J, Akamatsu N, Arita J, Kaneko J, Sakamoto Y, et al. Venous drainage map of the liver for complex hepatobiliary surgery and liver transplantation. HPB (Oxford). 2016;18(12):1031–8.
23. Nishino H, Hatano E, Seo S, Nitta T, Saito T, Nakamura M, et al. Real-time navigation for liver surgery using projection mapping with indocyanine green fluorescence: development of the novel medical imaging projection system. Ann Surg. 2018;267(6):1134–40.

Surgical Anatomy of the Pancreas

Akihiko Horiguchi, Masahiro Ito, Yukio Asano, Satoshi Arakawa, Hiroyuki Kato, and Masahiro Shimura

Abstract

In gastroenterological surgery, pancreatoduodenectomy is a difficult operation and requires solid anatomical knowledge and skill to perform the procedure itself and be safely completed. Venous bleeding because of the venous congestion of the pancreatic head and duodenum may be encountered when the vein that flows from the pancreatic head to the superior mesenteric vein is cut when performing a pancreatoduodenectomy, and this may hinder subsequent procedures. It is possible to prevent the congestion of the pancreatic head and duodenum by dealing with the incoming artery from the pancreatic head early in the operation. This incoming artery is the inferior pancreatic duodenal artery. Although the bifurcation of the inferior pancreatic duodenal artery takes multiple forms, an artery-first approach is a useful method for safely performing surgery because it allows confirmation prior to surgery. Using this method, not only can the amount of intraoperative bleeding be reduced but dissection of the lymph nodes and nerve plexus around the superior mesenteric artery can also be safely and reliably performed for the cancer of the pancreatic head. In this study, we report our results on the anatomy of the veins and arteries of the pancreatic head and duodenum based on multidetector computed tomography imaging, which is useful when performing a pancreatoduodenectomy.

2.1 Introduction

In gastroenterological surgery, pancreatoduodenectomy (PD) is a difficult operation that requires a solid anatomical knowledge and skill in the procedure itself to be safely com-

A. Horiguchi (✉) · M. Ito · Y. Asano · S. Arakawa · H. Kato
M. Shimura
Department of Gastroenterological Surgery, Fujita Health University School of Medicine Bantane Hospital, Nagoya, Japan
e-mail: akihori@fujita-hu.ac.jp

pleted. When performing a PD, venous bleeding because of the venous congestion of the pancreatic head and duodenum may be encountered when the vein that flows from the pancreatic head to the superior mesenteric vein (SMV) is cut. This bleeding may hinder subsequent procedures. It is possible to prevent the congestion of the pancreatic head and duodenum by dealing with the incoming artery from the pancreatic head, the inferior pancreatic duodenal artery (IPDA), early in the operation. This is referred to as an artery-first PD [1] or an IPDA-approached PD [2–4]. Not only can the amount of intraoperative bleeding be reduced using such methods, but dissection of the lymph nodes and nerve plexus around the superior mesenteric artery (SMA) can be safely and reliably performed. In recent years, laparoscopic PD has been increasingly utilized, making it all the more important to determine the anatomical structure of the pancreatic head. In this study, we will report our results on performing the dissection of veins and arteries of the pancreatic head and duodenum primarily using multidetector computed tomography (MDCT) imaging.

2.1.1 Arteries of the Pancreatic Head/Duodenum

The pancreatic head is controlled by blood flow from the gastroduodenal artery (GDA) and SMA, and the arteries of the pancreatic head form arcades on the anterior and posterior surfaces. The branching patterns and hemodynamics of these arteries can vary.

2.1.1.1 IPDA
The IPDA normally bifurcates from the first jejunal artery, running from the dorsal side of the SMA to the left, across to the right dorsal side and branching into the posterior inferior pancreaticoduodenal artery (PIPDA) and the anterior inferior pancreaticoduodenal artery (AIPDA). A report by researchers regarding the morphology of the IPDA prior to

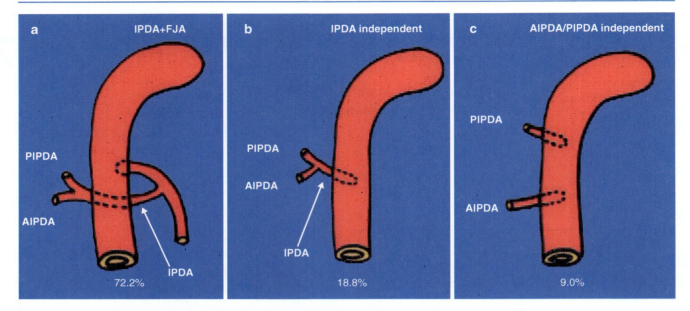

Fig. 2.1 Variation in the origin of the inferior pancreaticoduodenal artery (referred from Ref. 4). (**a**) A type in which the IPDA formed a common vessel with the first jejunal branch. *IPDA* inferior pancreaticoduodenal artery, *FJA* first jejunal artery. (**b**) A type in which the IPDA branched directly from the superior mesenteric artery. *IPDA* inferior pancreaticoduodenal artery. (**c**) A type in which the PIPDA and AIPDA branched separately. *PIPDA* posterior inferior pancreaticoduodenal artery, *AIPDA* anterior inferior pancreaticoduodenal artery, *IPDA* inferior pancreaticoduodenal artery, *FJA* first jejunal artery, *PIPDA* posterior inferior pancreaticoduodenal artery, *AIPDA* anterior inferior pancreaticoduodenal artery, *IPDA+FJA* a type in which the IPDA formed a common vessel with the first jejunal branch, *IPDA* independent, a type in which the IPDA branched directly from the superior mesenteric artery, *AIPDA/PIPDA* independent, a type in which the AIPDA and PIPDA branched separately

and after surgery based on MDCT images showing artery structure [3] revealed three different types: the type that forms a common trunk with the first jejunal artery (72%) (Fig. 2.1a), the type that directly bifurcates from the SMA (18.7%) (Fig. 2.1b), and the type that bifurcates separately before the SMA and after the IPDA (9.3%) (Fig. 2.1c) [4]. Moreover, when performing a PD as mentioned above, bleeding because of congestion from the PD side may be encountered during the operation. Dealing first with the arteries that flow into the head of the pancreas, namely GDA and IPDA, can prevent PD-related venous bleeding and reduce the overall amount of bleeding. In terms of the approaches of easily confirming the IPDA using MDCT, we reported that observing a common trunk with the first jejunal artery or independent branching directly from the SMA can confirm the beginning of the middle colic artery (MCA). From there the first jejunal artery can be confirmed on the dorsal side within 2 cm on the central side along the SMA [4]. With the independently branching type, the AIPDA can be confirmed within 2 cm of the MCA origin to the central side, and the PIPDA can be confirmed within 2 cm of the beginning of the SMA on the downstream side [5]. Furthermore, with the type where the right hepatic artery branches from the SMA, many cases have branching of the PIPDA from the right hepatic artery. Therefore, an easy way of confirming the IPDA is to cranially lift the transverse colon to confirm MCA branching on the ventral side from the SMA, release the Treitz ligament, and verify the IPDA from the left side of the SMA (Treitz ligament approach).

2.1.1.2 Posterior Superior Pancreatoduodenal Artery (PSPDA)

PSPDA is the first branch of GDA that bifurcates from the common hepatic artery (CHA) and normally passes from the left side of the anterior surface of the common bile duct from a point 1–2 cm from the origin of the GDA. After this point, it passes from the posterior surface of the common bile duct to the pancreatic parenchyma. In rare cases, there is branching from the proper hepatic artery (PHA). Moreover, the PSPDA has a branch that nourishes the main papilla from the lower bile duct around the dorsal side along the common bile duct.

2.1.1.3 Anterior Superior Pancreaticoduodenal Artery (ASPDA)

After the GDA branches into the PSPDA, it branches into the right gastroepiploic artery, which runs to the greater curvature of the gastric pyloric antrum, and the ASPDA, which runs between the pancreatic parenchyma and the duodenum from the anterior to the posterior surface of the pancreas. The ASPDA has fine branches that reach into the duodenum and pancreatic parenchyma and forms an anterior arcade from the duodenum on the anterior surface of the papilla of Vater. The arteries of the papilla of Vater are nourished by the

PSPDA; however, as there is a branch leading to the papilla of Vater can be confirmed while preserving ASPDA, it is nourished by ASPDA.

Posterior Inferior Pancreatoduodenal Artery (PIPDA) and Anterior Inferior Pancreatoduodenal Artery (AIPDA)

Normally, IPDA branches into PIPDA and AIPDA, and the PIPDA runs from the posterior fascia of the pancreas to the upper right side of the pancreatic parenchyma to join the PSPDA. Both PSPDA and PIPDA run through the posterior fascia of the pancreas on the posterior surface of the pancreas. The AIPDA shallowly runs through the pancreatic parenchyma in the pancreatic uncinate.

2.1.1.4 Dorsal Pancreatic Artery (DPA)

In a PD, when the pancreatic head is transected in front of the portal vein, the DPA is present in the residual pancreas. However, if a PD is performed when a tumor is present near the SMA because of the cancer of the pancreatic head, in some cases, the pancreatic head may be resected in front of SMA. In such cases, it is necessary to pay attention to where DPA runs through. In an examination of DPA branch morphology using MDCT (Fig. 2.2), 40% of cases were reported

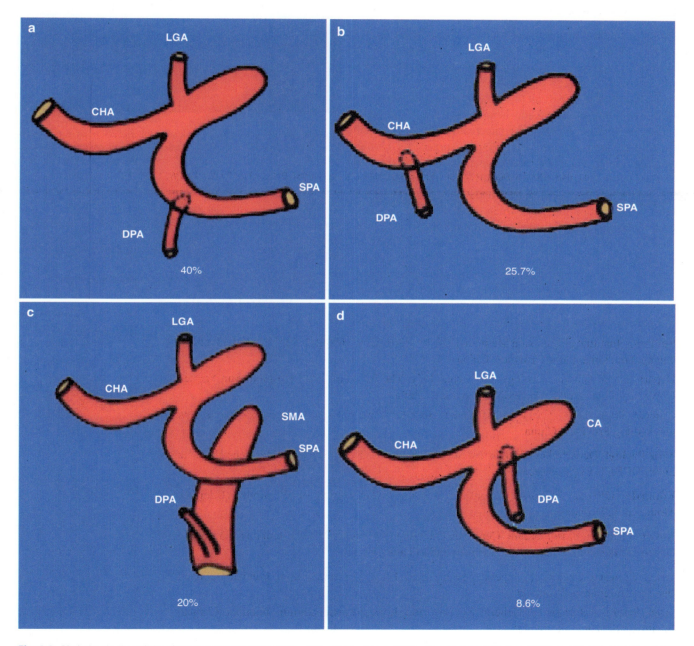

Fig. 2.2 Variation in the origin of the dorsal pancreatic artery. *SPA* splenic artery, *CHA* common hepatic artery, *SMA* superior mesenteric artery, *LGA* left gastric artery, *CA* celiac artery, *DPA* dorsal pancreatic artery. Inferior pancreaticoduodenal artery (referred from Ref. 4)

to branch from the splenic artery, 25.7% from the common hepatic artery, and 20.0% from the SMA [3]. After ligation of the IPDA and GDA, which are inflow arteries, arterial bleeding may be observed from the cranial stump of the pancreas during pancreatic dissection. In such cases, an arcade is considered to be formed between the DPA and GDA. Therefore, it is important to determine branch morphology in situations where it is necessary to deal with DPA in advance.

2.2 The Veins of the Pancreatic Head

During PD, the duodenum may become congested. If the outflow veins are ligated before the pancreatic head inflow arteries are ligated, the pancreatic head and duodenum will become congested and the amount of intraoperative bleeding will increase.

Therefore, it is important to have complete understanding of the anatomy of pancreatic head veins. The gastrocolic trunk is an important vein in the pancreatic head that is often encountered by surgeons during PD and surgery for gastric or colon cancer, and it is difficult to perform subsequent procedures if bleeding occurs. Henle [6] reported in 1868 that the right anterior colonic vein and the right gastroepiploic vein formed a common duct, which is referred to as Henle's gastrocolic trunk and flows into the superior mesenteric vein (SMV). The common trunk that flows into the SMV is referred to as Henle's venous trunk, and the trunk that flows from that area into the ileocolic vein is called the surgical trunk. When performing a right hemicolectomy, it is important to bear this venous anatomy in mind. The anterior superior pancreatoduodenal vein (ASPDV), which flows into the right colonic vein and the right gastroepiploic vein, runs across the anterior surface of the pancreas, becomes the anterior inferior pancreaticoduodenal vein (AIPDV), forms an arcade, and finally flows into the SMV. The posterior superior pancreatoduodenal vein (PSPDV) is a vein of the second part of the duodenum and the pancreatic bile duct that runs through the bile duct or the posterior surface of the pancreas and into the primary duct of the portal vein. The posterior inferior pancreatoduodenal vein (PIPDV) is a vein of the duodenal papilla and is downstream from the duodenum. It directly flows in the first jejunal vein or the SMV (Fig. 2.3). In certain cases, PSPDV and PIPDV can form arcades. Takamuro et al. [7] mentioned that PSPDV and PIPDV in certain cases form arcades while in others they do not.

The inferior mesenteric vein (IMV) most commonly merges with the SMV; however, the second most common type merges with the splenic vein. Other types flow into the confluence of the SMV and the splenic vein. If pancreatic cancer invades the confluence of the SMV and the splenic vein, splenic vein dissection is required. Although in most

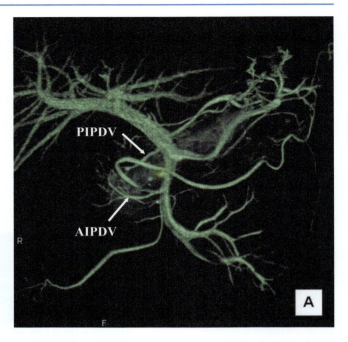

Fig. 2.3 Inferior pancreaticoduodenal vein. *PIPDV* posterior inferior pancreaticoduodenal vein, *AIPDV* anterior inferior pancreaticoduodenal vein

cases it is not necessary to reconstruct the splenic vein, in some rare cases, splenomegaly may occur because of intraoperative spleen congestion. Therefore, it is extremely important to ascertain the IMV inflow site using preoperative MDCT.

2.3 Surgical Techniques

2.3.1 Treitz Ligament Approach for Artery-First PD

Using this approach, the transverse colon is cranially lifted while the retroperitoneum, which is just above the Treitz ligament, is incised to identify the first jejunal artery and the middle colic artery as well as expose the SMA trunk. Releasing the Treitz ligament as much as possible will facilitate IPDA ligation. Passing a tape attached to the origin of the SMA from the right hand side of the opening of the Treitz ligament to the left hand side facilitates the identification of SMA and IPDA orientation. The inferior mesenteric vein (IMV) is often reported on the left side of the SMA trunk (the left cranial side of the Treitz ligament), which can limit the identification of the IPDA and is dissected in such cases. When dissecting the inferior margin of the pancreatic head toward the origin of the SMA, the IPDA can be identified in the origin of the middle colic artery (MCA) on the central dorsal side. It is ligated twice after identification. Although an approach from the left side offers a good field of view, it is possible to approach from the right side in cases with less adipose tissue. Because there are multiple variations, such as cases in which the IPDA branches from the first jejunal branch (Fig. 2.4a, b), directly bifurcates from the SMA (Fig. 2.5a, b), and bifurcates separately before the SMA (Fig. 2.6a, b), preoperative identification is important. After dealing with inflowing arteries of the head of pancreas to prevent the congestion of the pancreatic head and the duode-

num, and associated persistent bleeding, the upper jejunum is dissected and pulled to the right. Tunneling of the portal vein is performed and the pancreas is sharply dissected with a scalpel. The vein flowing from the excised side of the pancreas to the SMV is ligated and dissected, and then PD is performed. Although with conventional PD, the pancreatic duodenum becomes congested during the procedure and becomes swollen in certain cases, which increases the

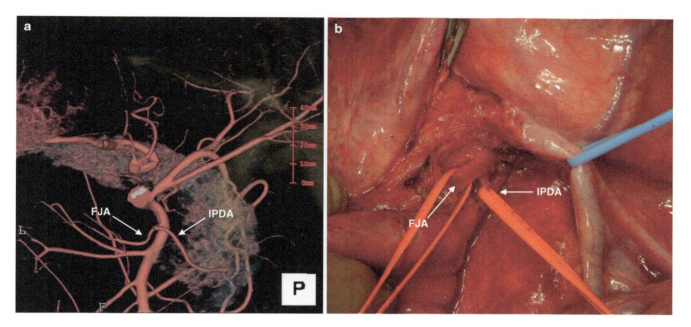

Fig. 2.4 IPDA+FJA type (**a**: 3D angiogram of MD-CT, **b**: the intraoperative photograph). *IPDA* inferior pancreaticoduodenal artery, *FJA* first jejunal artery, *IPDA* inferior pancreaticoduodenal artery

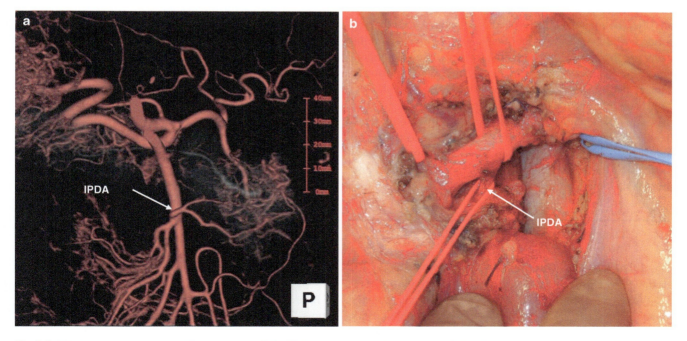

Fig. 2.5 IPDA independent type (**a**: 3D angiogram of MD-CT, **b**: the intraoperative photograph). *IPDA* inferior pancreaticoduodenal artery

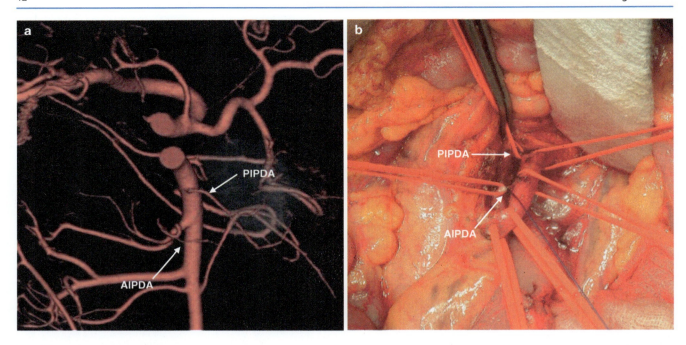

Fig. 2.6 AIPDA/PIPDA independent type (**a**: 3D angiogram of MD-CT, **b**: the intraoperative photograph). *PIPDA* posterior inferior pancreaticoduodenal artery, *AIPDA* anterior inferior pancreaticoduodenal artery

amount of bleeding. With an IPDA-approached PD, bleeding at this point is reduced and the procedure can be performed with peace of mind. For laparoscopic surgery, the caudal field of view is extremely good, indicating that procedures where it is usually difficult to obtain a good field of view when performed using laparotomy can be performed from the front. Furthermore, the magnifying effect facilitates the easy identification of SMA (Fig. 2.4).

As cases where the PIPDA and AIPDA branch separately are often complicated, the procedure must be carefully performed while confirming the location of arteries and veins using preoperative MDCT imaging. In each case, it is important to be familiar with the branching morphology prior to surgery. Horiguchi et al. confirmed the IPDA from the left hand side, carried out ligation and taped it, and then after dissecting the jejunum, they pulled out the IPDA to the right hand side past the posterior side of the SMA and the portal vein, and subsequently confirmed the IPDA again at the pancreatic hook before performing double ligation to thoroughly remove the lymph nodes around the SMA.

2.4 Discussion

The IPDA presents with various branching patterns [8]. Horiguchi et al. [3] roughly classified these into three different types based on MDCT imaging: a type that directly branches from the SMA, a type that forms a common trunk with the first jejunal artery, and a type that branches from the right hepatic artery of the SMA. Artery-first PD using the Treitz ligament approach is a useful method of reducing the amount of bleeding that makes it easy to detach veins that run from the pancreatic head to the SMV.

The artery-first approach was first reported by Sanjay et al. in 2012 [1]. There are multiple ways to approach SMA. In 1993, Nakao et al. [9] reported a mesenteric approach, which is considered to be the world's first artery-first PD. In 2007, Horiguchi et al. [2] reported that the left-sided approach from the SMA was useful for dealing with IPDA. However, the concept of artery-first PD is used in laparoscopic PD. In 2011, the authors reported on the first case of robot-assisted laparoscopic PD in Japan [10, 11]. Nagakawa et al. reported a method of dealing with the IPDA from the right side of the SMA during laparoscopic PD [12]. This is a useful method for safely dealing with the jejunal veins from the right side of the SMA. Sugiyama et al. reported an intestinal derotation procedure for easily dealing with IPDA, which involves performing complex pancreatic head and duodenal dissection by derotating the pancreatic head and duodenum [13].

The vascular anatomy of the pancreatic head is complex and gaining a preoperative understanding using MDCT is extremely useful.

2.5 Conclusion

In future, it is expected that the number of cases of laparoscopic PD as well as PD by laparotomy will increase and ascertaining the vascular structure of the pancreatic head is extremely important to safely perform PD.

References

1. Sanjay P, Takaori K, Govil S, Shrikhande SV, Windsor JA. 'Artery-first' approaches to pancreatoduodenectomy. Br J Surg. 2012;99:1027–35.
2. Horiguchi A, Ishihara S, Ito M, Nagata H, Shimizu T, Furusawa K, et al. Panceatoduodenectomy in which dissection of the efferent arteries of the head of the pancreas is performed first. J Hepato-Biliary-Pancreat Surg. 2007;14:575–8.
3. Horiguchi A, Ishihara S, Ito M, Nagata H, Asano Y, Yamamoto T, et al. Multislice CT study of pancreatic head arterial dominance. J Hepato-Biliary-Pancreat Surg. 2008;15:322–6.
4. Horiguchi A, Ishihara S, Ito M, Asano Y, Furusawa K, Tsuda K, et al. Vascular anatomy of the pancreas head region. Tan to Sui. 2011;32:1143–8.
5. Horiguchi A, Ishihara S, Ito M, Asano Y, Yamamoto T, Miyakawa S, et al. Three-dimensional models of arteries constructed using multidetector-row CT images to perform pancreatoduodenectomy safely following dissection of the inferior pancreaticoduodenal artery. J Hepato Biliary Pancreat Sci. 2010;17:523–6.
6. Henle J. Handbuch der systematischen Anatomie des Menschen. Druck und Verlag von Friedrich Vieweg und Sohn. 391. Braun schweig.1868. (cited by ref. 7 Gillot et al. 1964).
7. Takamuro T, Oikawa I, Murakami G, Hirata K. Venous drainage from the posterior aspect of the pancreatic head and duodenum. Okajimas Folia Anat Jpn. 1998;75:1–8.
8. Bertelli E, Di Gregorio F, Bertelli L, Civeli L, Mosca S. The arterial blood supply of the pancreas: a review. III. The inferior pancreaticoduodenal artery. An anatomical review and a radiological study. Surg ZRadiol Anat. 1996;18:67–74.
9. Nakao A, Takagi H. Isolated pancreatectomy for pancreatic head carcinoma using catheter bypass of the portal vein. Hepato-Gastroenterology. 1993;40:426–9.
10. Horiguchi A, Uyama I, Miyakawa S. Robot-assisted laparoscopic pancreaticoduodenectomy. J Hepatobiliary Pancreat Sci. 2011;18:287–91.
11. Horiguchi A, Uyama I, Ito M, Ishihara S, Asano Y, Yamamoto T, et al. Robot-assisted laparoscopic pancreatic surgery. J Hepatobiliary Pancreat Sci. 2011;18:488–92.
12. Nagakawa Y, Hosokawa Y, Sahara Y, Takishita C, Nakajima T, Hijikata Y, et al. A novel "artery first" approach allowing safe resection in laparoscopic pancreaticoduodenectomy: the uncinate process first approach. Hepato-Gastroenterology. 2015;62:1037–40.
13. Sugiyama M, Suzuki Y, Nakazato T, Yokoyama Y, Kogure M, Abe N, et al. Intestinal derotation procedure for facilitating pancreatoduodenectomy. Surgery. 2016;159:1325–32.

Surgical Anatomy of the Biliary Tract

Eduardo Olivera Pertusso, Joaquin Garcia, and Luis Ruso Martinez

Abstract

The anatomical aspects of the biliary tract and its vascularization are of special surgical interest. The area of Glisson's capsule (hilar plate) that surrounds the vasculobiliary structures of the hepatic hilum has a great importance, as well as the crossed arterial vascularization that allows the supply flow, during the injuries of the main hepatic arteries.

Anatomical variations in the origin of the superior biliary confluent, the cystic duct, and its relationship with the cystic artery are determinants of the aspect of the triangle of Calot and keys for safe cholecystectomy and avoiding surgical injuries to the bile duct.

The length of the left hepatic duct allows a wide exposure that facilitates to make of the hepatic jejunal anastomosis, associating the Hepp-Couinaud maneuver.

The so-called hepatic pedicle is formed by the common bile duct, the portal vein, with the hepatic artery. Its structure is practically constant, but in 15% of cases the right hepatic artery is located in front of the main bile duct.

This chapter describes the anatomical structure of the biliary tract, morphological patterns, most important variations, and the relevant aspects of its vascularization.

3.1 Introduction

Precise knowledge of the anatomy of the biliary tree is critical to obtain optimum results in hepatobiliary surgery and to avoid surgical lesions of its conducts.

In this chapter, we describe the anatomic structure of the biliary system, its morphologic patterns, the most important variants, and the most important aspects of its vascularization, based on current knowledge [1–13].

The biliary tree is formed by a system of ducts of progressively higher caliber that conduct the bile secreted by the liver to the duodenum. It originates in microscopic canaliculi in the hepatic parenchyma, in which the walls are formed by hepatocytes.

From a topographic point of view, the biliary tree can be divided into an intrahepatic biliary tract and an extrahepatic one. The latter is formed by the common hepatic and the choledochus, the main biliary tract, and an accessory biliary tract, namely the gallbladder and the cystic duct.

There are three fundamental aspects from the surgical point of view:

(a) The variations in the formation of the superior biliary confluent, key to perform a correct oncologic hepatic surgery.
(b) The anatomic variations related to the cystic duct and its relationship with the cystic artery are determinant of the position of the triangle of Calot and also very important for a safe cholecystectomy.
(c) The arterial vascularization at the level of the hilar plate allows to sustain a substitution flow, in case of lesions of the main hepatic arteries (right and left).

3.2 Intrahepatic Biliary Tract

The intrahepatic bile ducts are part of the portal triad and are surrounded by an invagination of the Glisson's capsule. Next, there are branches of the portal vein, whose nomenclature is based on the consensus of Brisbane in the year 2000.

The hepatic parenchyma is divided into two by the line of Cantlie which goes from the fossa vesicae to the right edge of the inferior vena cava. The bile of each hemiliver is drained by the right and left hepatic ducts that join at the level of the hilar plate to form the superior biliary confluent, from which the common hepatic duct originates.

E. O. Pertusso · J. Garcia · L. R. Martinez (✉)
School of Medicine, University of Republic (UdeLar), Montevideo, Uruguay

3.2.1 Right Hepatic Confluent and Its Anterior and Posterior Branches

The right hepatic duct is short (0–23 mm) and vertical, and its way is external to the hepatic parenchyma. It is formed by the confluence of the sectoral posterior and anterior right ducts, which drain bile of the segments 6–7 and 5–8, respectively.

The posterior sectoral duct has a horizontal and anterior-posterior direction. It is longer than the anterior sectoral duct, and it is located above it. It ends joining the posterior surface of this duct after crossing the superior surface of the anterior branch of the right portal vein, although in 20% of the cases, it may run under this portal branch.

The anterior sectoral duct is vertical, and it is located in front and to the left of the anterior branch of the right portal vein. In 20% of the cases, it is retroportal. It receives the canaliculi of the segments 5 and 8; however, these may present variations (segment 8 may drain in the posterior sectoral duct or segment 5 in the right hepatic duct, the posterior sectoral duct or the common hepatic duct).

3.2.2 Left Hepatic Confluent and Its Affluents

The left hepatic duct is longer than the right one (20–50 mm), and it has a horizontal pathway, running behind the posterior margin of the quadrate lobe. Initially located above and behind the left portal vein, it crosses its superior surface to locate itself in front of the transverse portion of that vein. It has a long path in the hepatic hilum, where it is located outside the parenchyma. This long extrahepatic path has surgical importance because it allows to have a better dominion and exposure of the left hepatic duct, key to the performance of a wide hepatic jejunal anastomosis by the maneuver of Hepp-Couinaud.

The left hepatic duct receives the bile from the segments 2, 3, and 4, which converge usually in stages in a common duct. The duct of the segment 2 is superior and oblique, while one of the segment 3 is wider and it has a concave pathway, its confluence is usually to the left of the round ligament.

The bile from segment 4 is usually collected by four ducts, two superior ones and two inferior, which drain in the left hepatic duct through a common duct, but they may drain all or some of them independently in the left hepatic duct.

3.2.3 Biliary Drainage of Segment 1

The caudate lobe drains through 1 to 6 ducts which are located underneath the portal branches. In most of them exist a bilateral drainage, and the ducts flow out in the posterior surface of the right and left hepatic ducts, next to the biliary confluence. In 15% of the cases, the drainage is exclusively to the left hepatic duct, while only 5% is exclusively to the right hepatic duct.

3.2.4 Accessory Biliary Ducts

Initially described by Luschka, they are thin ducts usually originating in the right lobe and drain subsegmentary areas of hepatic parenchyma and also drain in intrahepatic ducts, in the right hepatic duct or the common bile duct. The subvesical duct is the most frequent one (30–35%), and it runs between the visceral surface of the liver and the superior surface of the gallbladder. Sometimes there is a network of aberrant biliary canaliculi which ends in a cecum end point in the fossa vesicae, and they drain in the hepatic ducts. They are a frequent cause of bilirrhage post cholecystectomy, which justifies the clipping and ligation of the internal and inferior sector of the gallbladder bed.

Less frequent is the presence of an aberrant biliary duct that drains from the liver straight to the gallbladder.

3.2.5 Biliary Confluence and Its Variations

The right and left hepatic ducts converge in the hepatic hilum, where they are surrounded by the biliary plate, a thickening of the Glisson's capsule that wraps the vascular-biliary structures, adhering to the walls of the biliary tract and making its dissection difficult. There are three sectors: the gallbladder plate (in front of the gallbladder), the umbilical plate, in relation to the left biliary tree, and the hilar plate in front of the superior biliary confluence. Its knowledge is key to the surgical approach of the hepatic hilum. The tissue of the hilar plate gets in the hepatic parenchyma surrounding the elements of the portal triad, while downwards it is in continuity with the hepatoduodenal ligament and the minor omentum (Photo 3.1).

In its usual configuration (68%), the common bile duct is formed by the confluence of the right and left hepatic ducts outside the hepatic parenchyma, in front and slightly to the right of the right branch of the portal vein. The anatomic variations of the superior biliary confluence are not rare and are dominated by the high incidence of variations in the outlet of the right sectoral posterior duct.

In 18% of the cases, the right sectoral ducts converge jointly in the left hepatic duct giving place to the triple confluence or trifurcation of the biliary tract. When this happens, the right posterior sectoral branch is usually located above the anterior sectoral branch, and there is not a hepatic duct as such.

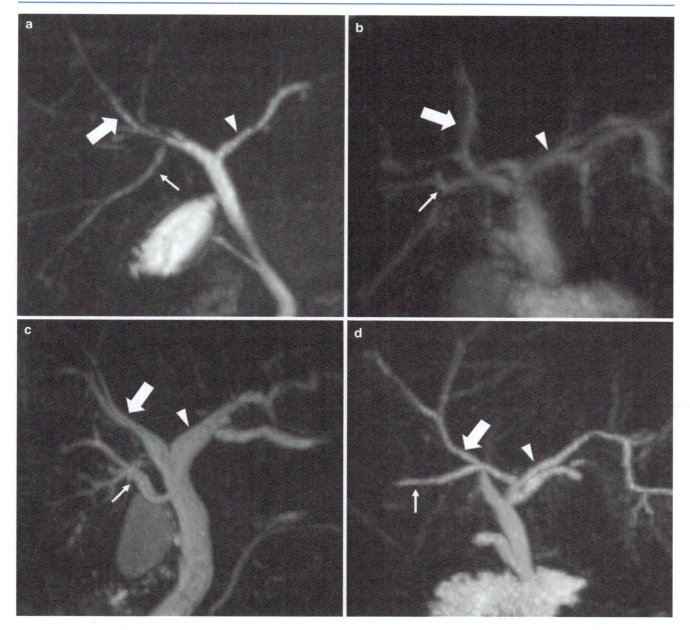

Photo 3.1 Biliary confluence and its variations. (**a**) Modal configuration. (**b**) Triple confluence or trifurcation of the biliary tract. (**c**) Aberrant right posterior duct. (**d**) Right posterior duct drains in the left hepatic duct. Arrow head: left hepatic duct. Fine Arrow: Right posterior duct. Thick arrow: Right anterior duct.

In 8% of the cases, one of the right sectoral branches, usually the posterior one, drains in the posterior surface of the left hepatic duct, forming an acute triangle. In these cases, the left hepatic duct drains the bile of the left hemiliver and the anterior sector of the right one.

In 6% of the cases, the right posterior sectoral duct has an aberrant pathway and can converge in the right hepatic duct, the common biliary duct at a variable distance of the superior biliary convergence, and even in the superior edge of the cystic duct. This morphologic variation is an important risk factor for biliary surgical lesion during cholecystectomy.

The segmentary canaliculi of both lobes may drain in the common biliary duct independently, a fact that is known as "convergence étagée" or staggered confluence.

3.3 Extrahepatic Biliary Tract

The hepatic hilum originates the common hepatic duct, and it is called, arbitrarily, choledochus after receiving the mouth of the cystic duct. The cystic choledochus union or inferior biliary confluent takes place at a variable distance of the convergence of the hepatic ducts, so is better to call common biliary duct at the continuity of the common hepatic duct and the choledochus duct.

From a topographic point of view, the common bile duct may be divided into three portions: a supraduodenal portion, where it is part of the hepatic pedicle, a retroduodenopancreatic portion located behind the first portion of the duodenum and the head of the pancreas, and an intramural portion where it transits in the duodenum wall to debouch in the major duodenal papilla.

3.3.1 Supraduodenal Portion: Hepatic Pedicle

This portion runs from the origin of the common biliary duct to the crossing of the superior margin of the first portion of the duodenum. This sector becomes evident during the dissection of the hepatic hilum when descending to the superior and elevating the visceral surface of the liver, since both the organs are in touch in their anatomic position (Photo 3.2).

At its origin, the common biliary duct transits in the free margin or "pars flacida" of the minor omentum, between two visceral peritoneal sheets and surrounded by an independent fascia that allows its individualization during the surgical exploration.

It is located upfront the portal vein, slightly to the right, with the proper hepatic artery at its left. The relation to the portal vein is practically constant, although there are reports of cases where the main biliary tract was retroperitoneal.

Usually the proper hepatic artery is divided into its two terminal branches next to the inferior edge of the liver, and its right branch goes behind the common bile duct, between this and the portal vein. In 15% of the cases, the right hepatic artery is located upfront the main biliary tract.

In case of the existence of an aberrant right hepatic artery or a common hepatic artery originated from the superior mesenteric artery, these arteries may have a retroportal pathway and be located in the right margin of the bile duct.

3.3.2 Retroduodenopancreatic Portion

The retroduodenopancreatic portion extends from the crossing with the superior margin of the first portion of the duodenum to the duodenal wall. In this segment, the common bile duct becomes a retroperitoneal organ, separated from the anterior surface of the inferior vena cava by the fascia of Treitz. The maneuver of Kocher-Vautrin allows the decollation of this fascia and access the posterior surface of the duodenum–pancreas to approach the retropancreatic choledochus.

As it descends, the common bile duct relates to the posterior surface of the first portion of the duodenum and with the head of the pancreas, where most of the times, it is covered by a flap of pancreatic tissue or entirely surrounded by the glandular parenchyma. In 12% of the cases, its posterior surface is bare.

In its retropancreatic pathway, the common bile duct describes a double curvature backwards and to the right, to debouch in the second portion of the duodenum. At this point, it separates from the portal vein, which runs left where its origin is located, in the espleno-mesenteric confluence. The portocholedochal triangle is delimited at the origin of the gastroduodenal artery and its posterosuperior pancreatic-duodenal branch. This branch runs in front of the bile duct while its homonymous vein is located behind. Both of them originate multiple branches of fine caliber, branches that vascularize the biliary tract and the duodenum–pancreas.

3.3.3 Intramural Portion

In this portion, the common bile duct runs obliquely through the duodenum wall to debouch in the major duodenum papilla at the level of the second portion of the duodenum, in the union of the posterior wall, and medially in 80% of the cases. In the rest, the common bile duct may debouch in the third portion or in the second duodenal knee. As it runs through the duodenal wall, it runs by a fenestra in the proper muscle layer named duodenal window.

Usually, the bile duct and the main pancreatic duct join in one common duct of 1–12 mm in length and 4.4 mm in caliber, which opens in the vertex of the major duodenal papilla.

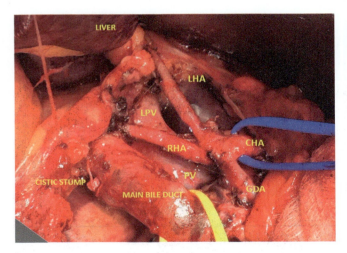

Photo 3.2 Hepatic pedicle. Supraduodenal portion. *CHA* common hepatic artery, *GDA* gastroduodenal artery, *RHA* right hepatic artery, *LHA* left hepatic artery, *PV* portal vein, *LPV* left portal vein

This morphology, named "anatomy of Opie" is what lets us explain the physiopathology of the acute lithiasic pancreatitis. In 70% of the cases, the common duct is dilated, and it is called ampulla of Vater.

Sometimes, both the ducts end independently in the major duodenal papilla after a short parallel pathway, with the orificium of the common bile duct located above and to the left of the main pancreatic duct. Less frequently, we can find an independent ending of both ducts in different places of the duodenum.

In the distal extreme of the main pancreatic duct and the bile duct, there is a complex sphincteral system described by Ruggero Oddi, formed by the circular and longitudinal smooth muscle fibers with a fine nerve and humoral regulation. Boyden described it more precisely, and nowadays, three main components are recognized: the choledochal and pancreatic sphincters, which surround the distal sector of each duct, and the ampullary sphincter that surrounds the common duct when this is present.

3.4 Vascularization of the Main Biliary Tract

Contrary to the hepatic parenchyma that receives a double vascularization, arterial and portal, the vascularization of the biliary tract depends exclusively of the arterial vascularization. The arterial vascularization of the biliary tract is very rich at the level of the hilum, retroduodenopancreatic and intramural, but it is poorer in its supraduodenal portion, which is the most vulnerable sector for ischemia and stenosis during the surgical manipulation.

3.4.1 Vascularization of the Biliary Confluence

The ducts of the biliary confluence receive their vascularization from a rich arterial plexus formed by branches of the right and left hepatic arteries and the cystic artery, which join forming an extrahepatic arterial arcade named caudate arcade. Apart from irrigating the bile ducts, this arterial network serves as a way of collateral interlobular arterial circulation from which the arterial substitution network is stablished when there is a unilateral lesion of the hepatic arteries.

3.4.2 Vascularization of the Common Bile Duct

The supraduodenal common bile duct is vascularized by 6–8 arteries of fine caliber of longitudinal disposition and an upward and downward pathway, which anastomose each other through transversal channels. Two thirds of the arterial vascular input comes from the upward branches originated in the posterosuperior pancreaticoduodenal, supraduodenal, gastroduodenal, and retroportal arteries, while the remaining third of the input comes from the downward branches originated in the right and left hepatic arteries, and the cystic one. Rarely, the proper hepatic artery gives direct branches to the common bile duct.

In the right and left margins of the common bile duct, the two predominant arteries are identified, named left and right marginal arteries or arteries of the hours 3 and 9, respectively, which justifies the longitudinal performance of the choledochotomy. In occasions, a third dominant artery may be found in the posterior surface or artery of the hour 6.

The retroduodenopancreatic segment of the common bile duct is vascularized by many branches of the posterosuperior pancreatic–duodenal artery, responsible for the vascularization of this segment, and the retroportal artery.

The venous drainage of the common bile duct originates in a epicholedochal plexus located in the surface of the common bile duct that drains in the veins of the paracholedochal plexus, formed by parallel vessels to the bile duct which organize themselves into two marginal veins known as the veins of the hours 3 and 9, existing in exceptional cases a marginal vein of the hour 6.

The marginal veins drain in the gastric veins, the posterosuperior pancreaticoduodenal ones, and in the gastrocolic trunk. Upwards, they communicate with the hilar venous plexus, which is tributary of the portal branches of the caudate lobe and segment 4. This complex venous system allows to develop a portal vicariant circulation, in cases of thrombosis of the portal vein, dilating and prompting the entity called portal cavernoma.

3.4.3 Vascularization of the Major Duodenal Papilla

The arterial vascularization of the major duodenal papilla is given by straight vessels which originate in the anterior and posterior pancreaticoduodenal arcades, formed by the anastomosis of the branches of the gastroduodenal and inferior mesenteric artery. Of these, the posterosuperior pancreaticoduodenal artery is the main input.

From both arcades, straight vessels originate that approach the papilla in a variable number, and two stand out: one artery of the hour 9 o'clock, originated in the posterior arcade, and one artery of the hour 3 o'clock originated in the anterior arcade. This determines a "safe area" of less vascularization between the hours 11 and 1 which is used to make the incision in the sphincterotomy.

3.5 Accessory Biliary Tract

3.5.1 Gallbladder and Cystic Duct

The gallbladder is a piriform sac located in the fossa vesicae in the inferior surface of the liver. When it is distended, its size is 40 mm wide and 70–100 mm long. The gallbladder can be divided into three sectors. The fundus is a blind extreme located under the inferior hepatic margin and projected in the intersection of the right costal margin with the midclavicular line at the level of the ninth costal cartilage. The body is its bigger portion, located between the visceral surface of the liver and the first knee of the duodenum. It decreases size while it goes backwards, forming the infundibulum which is continuous with the neck. On the right side of the gallbladder's neck, the patients with chronic obstruction a recess may be sometimes found, named Hartmann's pouch (Photo 3.3).

The visceral peritoneum covers the inferior surface of the gallbladder, but in some cases, it may cover its two surfaces and form the mesentery that joins it with the hepatic peritoneum (floating gallbladder). The superior gallbladder surface is separated from the hepatic parenchyma by the cystic plate, a thickening of the conjunctive tissue which is continuous with the hilar plate.

The anomalies of the gallbladder are rare; some cases are described with gallbladders in the left side of the liver or completely included in the hepatic parenchyma. Agenesia and the septated gallbladder, bilobed or duplicated, are extremely infrequent.

The cystic duct is continuous with the neck and its size is 4–65 mm long and an average diameter of 4 mm. The mucosa that covers it has 5–12 oblique folds that create a spiral valve known as the valve of Heister.

In most of the cases, the cystic-choledochal union is approximately at 20 mm from the superior biliary confluence, and it may be classified as angled, parallel, or spiral. When it debouches in the choledochus, it admits multiple variations, such as very caudal, next to the major duodenal papilla, which is known as low implantation of the cystic duct, and very close to the confluence of the right and left hepatic ducts.

The cystic duct joins the right lateral surface of the common bile duct in most of the cases. In 10% of the cases, it may join the posterior or anterior wall of the common bile duct or less frequently to the left wall. There are reports about aberrant cystic ducts that join in the right and left hepatic ducts or directly into the duodenum.

3.5.2 Vascularization

The arterial vascularization of the gallbladder is given by the cystic artery, which is a branch of the right hepatic artery; less frequently, its origin is in the left hepatic artery, gastroduodenal, or superior mesenteric. It runs by the superior margin of the cystic duct to the gallbladder neck, where it divides into two branches, a superficial one that follows the inferior surface of the gallbladder and a deep one located between the superior surface and the liver. The relation of the cystic artery with the triangle of Calot and the cystic duct is usually variable, which exposes it to lesion during cholecystectomy. In 65–85% of the cases, it crosses the Calot's triangle at some point, but 3% is parallel to the cystic and it even covers it.

The venous drainage is tributary of the intrahepatic veins, and there is not a satellite cystic vein of the artery.

3.5.3 Triangle of the Biliary Tract

At the level of the hepatic hilum, two triangles of great surgical importance are defined: The triangle of Calot is delimited by the cystic artery, the cystic duct, and the biliary tract. Frequently, the triangle of Calot is confused with another triangle defined between the inferior surface of the liver, the cystic duct, and the common bile duct, named hepatocystic triangle, of the biliary tract or triangle of Buddé. Inside this triangle are found the cystic artery and ganglion, the right hepatic artery and the lymphatic ducts. By this area also run right bile ducts or right accessory hepatic arteries or aberrant ones.

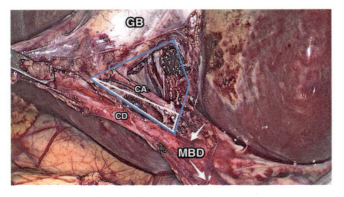

Photo 3.3 Triangles of the biliary tract. *MBD* main bile duct. Arrows: MBD path. *CD* cystic duct, *CA* cystic artery, *GB* gallbladder. White triangle: Calot's triangle. Blue triangle: hepatocystic triangle or Budde triangle

References

1. Babu C, Ramesh S, Sharma M. Biliary tract anatomy and its relationship with venous drainage. J Clin Exp Hepatol. 2014;4:S18–26.
2. Castaing D. Surgical anatomy of the biliary tract. HPB. 2008;10:72–6.

3. Catalano O, et al. Vascular and biliary variants in the liver: implications for liver surgery. Radiographics. 2008;28:359–78.
4. Cedrón H, Gutiérrez C, Ocaña J. Arteria cística: variantes anatómicas. In: Anales de la Facultad de Medicina, vol. 57. Universidad Nacional Mayor de San Marcos; 1996. p. 109–12.
5. Ding Y, Wang B, Wang W, Wang P, Yan J. New classification of the anatomic variations of cystic artery during laparoscopic cholecystectomy. World J Gastroenterol: WJG. 2007;2007(13):5629.
6. Belghiti J, Clavien P, Gadzijev E, Garden J, Lau W, Makuuchi M, Strong W. The Brisbane 2000 Terminology of Liver Anatomy and Resections Terminology Committee of the International Hepato-Pancreato-Biliary Association: Chairman, SM Strasberg (USA). HPB (Oxford). 2000;2:333–9.
7. Horiguchi S, Kamisawa T. Major duodenal papilla and its normal anatomy. Digest Surg. 2010;27:90–3.
8. Kawarada Y, Das B, Taoka H. Anatomy of the hepatic hilar area: the plate system. J Hepato-Biliary-Pancreat Surg. 2000;7:580–6.
9. Keplinger K, Bloomston M. Anatomy and embryology of the biliary tract. Surg Clin. 2014;94(2):203–17.
10. Lamah M, Karanjia N, Dickson G. Anatomical variations of the extrahepatic biliary tree: review of the world literature. Clin Anat. 2001;14:167–72.
11. Mirjalili S, Stringer M. The arterial supply of the major duodenal papilla and its relevance to endoscopic sphincterotomy. Endoscopy. 2011;43:307–11.
12. Vakili K, Pomfret E. Biliary anatomy and embryology. Surg Clin N Am. 2008;88:1159–74.
13. Couinaud C. Lobes et segments hépatiques. Presse Med. 1954;62:709.

Liver Function and Posthepatectomy Liver Failure

Takanobu Hara and Susumu Eguchi

Abstract

The possibility of liver resection is usually determined by the technical feasibility of radical surgery and the volumetric and functional capacity of the future liver remnant. With the addition of recent advances in surgical techniques and perioperative management, liver resection has become safer. Nevertheless, posthepatectomy liver failure (PHLF) is one of the most serious complications after liver resection, and PHLF remains the major cause of perioperative morbidity and mortality. The present article reviewed a definition of PHLF and the reported liver function assessment tools used for surgical decision-making. According to the safety criteria in the indocyanine green testing, morbidity and mortality after hepatic resection can be reduced. Recent advances in imaging studies enable precise preoperative surgical planning and calculating future liver remnant volume. Combining imaging studies and liver function testing will achieve more accurate preoperative surgical planning to avoid PHLF.

4.1 Introduction

Liver resection is an established method that is considered the only curative treatment option for patients with primary and metastatic liver tumors. As a result of recent advances in surgical techniques and perioperative management, liver resection has become safer; morbidity and mortality rates after surgery have decreased over the past 10 years [1–4]. The possibility of liver resection is usually determined by the technical feasibility of radical surgery and the volumetric and functional capacity of the future liver remnant (FLR). Recent reports indicated that a future liver remnant of 25% is sufficient in patients without parenchymal disease, and that an FLR of 40%–50% is necessary in patients with parenchymal liver disease [5–7]. In addition, three-dimensional volumetric analysis has contributed significantly to precise surgical planning [8–10]. Despite these developments, posthepatectomy liver failure (PHLF) is still one of the most serious complications after liver resection, and PHLF remains the major cause of perioperative morbidity and mortality. The incidence of PHLF varies between 1.2% and 32%; in the most recent literature, the incidence is up to 8% [11, 12]. This wide range in the frequency of PHLF can be attributed to the lack of a universal definition of PHLF. Predicting PHLF by evaluating preoperative liver function could help hepatobiliary surgeons decide whether hepatectomy can be performed safely or whether additional procedures are necessary prior to the planned hepatectomy.

This article provides a definition of PHLF and discusses recent topics regarding accurate and realistic evaluation of liver function testing to perform safe liver resection.

4.2 Posthepatectomy Liver Failure (PHLF)

A number of definitions of PHLF have been reported. PHLF has been most commonly defined quantitatively by postoperative laboratory tests using various cut-off values for serum bilirubin concentration and prothrombin time–international normalized ratio (PT–INR). In 2005, Balzan et al. analyzed the outcomes of 704 patients undergoing partial hepatectomy and proposed a definition of PHLF as the combination of PT < 50% and serum bilirubin >50 μmol/L (2.9 mg/dL) on postoperative day 5 ("50–50 criteria") [13]. This definition predicted in-hospital mortality with a sensitivity of 69.6% and specificity of 98.5%. Mullen et al. analyzed the outcomes of 1059 patients with normal preoperative liver function undergoing hepatectomy in 2007. The authors proposed a different criterion of peak postoperative bilirubin level > 7.0 mg/dL (120 μmol/L). The criterion predicted liver failure-related death with a sensitivity of 93.3% and specific-

T. Hara (✉) · S. Eguchi
Department of Surgery, Nagasaki University Graduate School of Biomedical Sciences, Nagasaki, Japan
e-mail: harataka@nagasaki-u.ac.jp

Table 4.1 IGLS Consensus definition and severity grading of posthepatectomy liver failure (From Rahbari et al. [12])

Definition of PHLF	A postoperatively acquired deterioration in the ability of the liver (in patients with normal and abnormal liver function) to maintain its synthetic, excretory, and detoxifying functions, characterized by an increased INR (or need of clotting factors to maintain normal INR) and hyperbilirubinemia (according to the normal cut-off levels defined by the local laboratory) on or after postoperative day 5. If INR or serum bilirubin concentration is increased preoperatively, PHLF is defined by an increasing INR (decreasing prothrombin time) and increasing serum bilirubin concentration on or after postoperative day 5 (compared with the values of the previous day). Other obvious causes for the observed biochemical and clinical alterations such as biliary obstruction should be ruled out
Grade	
A	PHLF resulting in abnormal laboratory parameters but requiring no change in the clinical management of the patient
B	PHLF resulting in a deviation from the regular clinical management but manageable without invasive treatment
C	PHLF resulting in a deviation from the regular clinical management and requiring invasive treatment

PHLF posthepatectomy liver failure, *INR* international normalized ratio

ity of 94.3% [14]. In 2011, the International Study Group of Liver Surgery (ISGLS) defined PHLF as postoperative deterioration in the ability of the liver to maintain its synthetic, excretory, and detoxifying functions, characterized by increased PT–INR and concomitant hyperbilirubinemia on or after postoperative day 5 (Table 4.1) [12]. A proposed grading system was based on a review of 1928 studies, including the above-mentioned references. Because the ISGLS definition is easily comparable, it can be used widely. The ISGLS also differentiated the severity of PHLF into three grades from A to C; grade B and C are generally considered to indicate clinically relevant PHLF [15].

4.3 Preoperative Evaluation of Liver Function

4.3.1 Portal Hypertension

Portal hypertension is considered a contraindication to liver resection according to the AASLD/BCLC guidelines [16]. Clinically relevant portal hypertension is defined as a hepatic vein pressure gradient greater than 10 mm Hg or the presence of esophageal varices or splenomegaly associated with a platelet count lower than 100×10^9/L [17]. Major hepatic resection increases portal venous pressure in both cirrhotic and non-cirrhotic livers. Although an association between portal hypertension and poor long-term outcomes after liver resection for HCC has been reported [18, 19], increased portal venous pressure does not appear to have a direct effect on early postoperative morbidity and mortality [20]. Recent reports indicated that limited resection in patients with preserved liver function and moderate portal hypertension yields competitive survival outcomes [21]. Therefore, the 2018 EASL Clinical Practice Guidelines do not consider portal hypertension a contraindication for minor liver resection [21].

4.3.2 Model for End-Stage Liver Disease (MELD) Score

The MELD score was initially reported to predict survival in patients with liver cirrhosis following a transjugular intrahepatic portosystemic shunt [22]. To improve the score's accuracy, pretransplant dialysis and serum sodium concentration have been added, and the MELD score is now widely used to allocate liver transplant candidates [23]. Since then, several studies have validated the score for predicting PHLF. Teh et al. retrospectively analyzed 82 patients with cirrhosis who underwent liver resection for HCC. The authors reported that a preoperative MELD score ≥ 9 was a significant risk factor for postoperative mortality [24]. In 2006, Cucchetti et al. analyzed 200 HCC patients with cirrhosis undergoing liver resection and demonstrated that preoperative MELD ≥11 and MELD score increases between postoperative day 3 and 5 were independent predictors of PHLF [25]. Citterio et al. reviewed data for 543 patients with chronic liver disease who underwent liver resection for HCC and reported that the combination of portal hypertension and MELD score was a useful predictor of PHLF [26]. In contrast, Schroeder et al. reported that preoperative MELD score was not an accurate predictor of morbidity or mortality [27]. MELD might not accurately predict mortality in patients without cirrhosis because the original formula was developed for patients with extremely poor liver function in whom liver resection is not indicated [28].

4.3.3 Blood Chemistry Tests

A number of studies have reported that a preoperative platelet count <10–15 × 10^4/μL was associated with PHLF or mortality [29–31]. In 2003, Wai et al. proposed the aspartate aminotransferase (AST) to platelet ratio index (APRI = AST level/upper normal limit of AST/platelet count [10^9/L] × 100) as a simple predictor of significant fibrosis and cirrhosis in patients with chronic hepatitis C [32]. Ichikawa et al. retrospectively evaluated 366 patients and reported the usefulness of APRI for predicting PHLF [33]. Likewise, Mai et al. evaluated 1044 patients with HCC who underwent liver resection and reported a sensitivity and specificity of the APRI score for predicting PHLF of 72.2% and 68.0%, respectively.

PHLF incidence and grade in patients with APRI scores >0.55 were significantly higher than in patients with lower scores [34].

In 2015, the albumin–bilirubin (ALBI) score was created to predict overall survival after hepatectomy in patients with HCC [35]. Zhang et al. analyzed 338 HCC patients undergoing liver resection and reported that ALBI predicted PHLF according to the ISGLS criteria. The rate of PHLF was 7.7% in the study, and higher ALBI grades correlated with higher PHLF grades. Notably, ALBI was a superior predictor compared with MELD and Child–Pugh–Turcotte (CP) scores using ROC analysis [35]. Zou et al. evaluated 229 HCC patients and reported that ALBI showed superior predictive value for PHLF over the CP score. In addition, the combination of standardized future liver remnant (sFLR) and ALBI scores was a stronger predictor of PHLF than either sFLR or ALBI score alone [36].

4.3.4 Indocyanine Green (ICG) Clearance Test

ICG is a highly plasma protein-bound, water-soluble anionic organic tricarbocyanine dye. Measuring ICG clearance is a dynamic method of studying liver functional reserve. After intravenous injection, ICG is taken up by organic anion transporting polypeptides (OATP) and Na^+-taurocholate co-transporting polypeptide, which are abundantly located in the basolateral membrane of hepatocytes [37]. ICG is almost exclusively extracted by the liver and excreted into the bile without intrahepatic biotransformation [38]. Its elimination is thought to be dependent on hepatocyte function, liver blood flow, and bile secretion [39].

The ICG retention ratio after 15 min (ICG R15) is the ratio between the ICG concentration 15 min after injection and the initial concentration. A surgical decision-making algorithm based on ICG R15 was reported by Makuuchi et al. in 1993 that includes ICG R15, presence of ascites, and serum total bilirubin concentration [40]. In cases of total bilirubin concentration < 1 mg/dl without ascites, major liver resections should only be performed in patients with ICG R15 lower than 20% [41] (Fig. 4.1). This algorithm has certainly contributed to a reduction in operative mortality in Japan [1].

Recently, Kokudo et al. proposed the albumin–indocyanine green evaluation (ALICE) grading system as a tool to assess the preoperative liver functional reserve of patients undergoing hepatectomy for HCC [42]. This score was superior for predicting postoperative long- and short-term out-

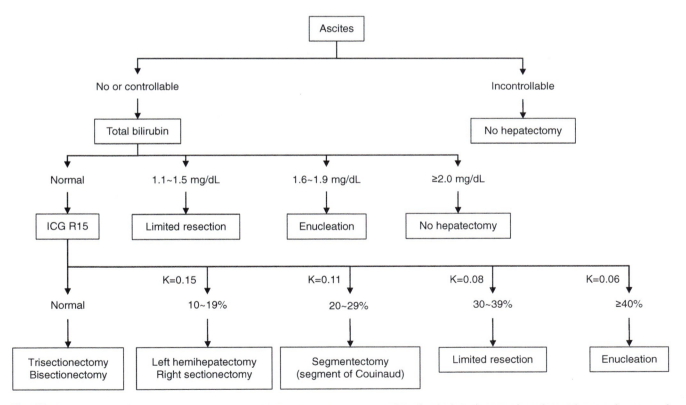

Fig. 4.1 A decision tree for hepatectomy proposed by Makuuchi et al. which involves the presence or absence of uncontrollable ascites, the serum bilirubin level, and the ICG R15. Because the ICG R15 is not a linear quantitative parameter, only the surgical procedure, and not the exact numbers for the hepatic parenchymal resection rate, is presented for each ICG category. The designations of the hepatectomy have changed according to the Brisbane 2000 Terminology of Liver Anatomy and Resections

comes compared with the risk class according to the presence/absence of portal hypertension. In 2018, the same group analyzed 1025 consecutive patients undergoing liver resection for HCC to evaluate the role of liver function factors in predicting postoperative large-volume ascites and PHLF. The incidence of large-volume ascites was 13.9%, and PHLF was 3.7%. The authors reported that the ALICE score was the strongest predictor of large-volume ascites and PHLF [43]. Another study suggested the possibility of using the ALICE score to predict portal hypertension in HIV/HCV co-infected hemophilia patients [44].

The plasma disappearance rate of ICG (KICG) can be calculated using linear regression analysis and plasma ICG concentrations [45]. KICG has been thought to reflect the pharmacokinetics of ICG more accurately than ICG R15. Lower preoperative KICG is a predictive factor for PHLF as well as increased ICG R15 [46].

Although the ICG clearance test is a reliable dynamic liver function test, results should be interpreted carefully in patients with cholestasis because bilirubin and ICG competitively bind to the same OATP, such as 1B3 [37]. Decreased ICG clearance values are observed in patients with intrahepatic shunts or sinusoidal capillarization because the ICG clearance test depends on overall liver blood flow [47].

4.4 M2BPGi

Recent studies have reported the usefulness of Mac-2 binding protein glycosylation isomer (M2BPGi) as a predictor of hepatic decompensation and HCC development in patients with chronic liver diseases [48, 49]. In 2017, Okuda et al. evaluated PHLF in 138 HCC patients who underwent liver resection. The authors reported that M2BPGi, platelet count, and resection rate were associated with PHLF ≥ grade B. In patients with HCV infection, the predictive ability of M2BPGi for PHLF was higher than for the other parameters [50].

4.5 Scintigraphy

The asialoglycoprotein receptor is located on the sinusoidal surface of hepatocytes and is involved in clearing glycoproteins containing terminal galactose residues from the circulation [51]. Scintigraphy using ^{99m}Tc-labeled diethylenetriaminepentaacetic acid galactosyl human serum albumin (GSA), an analog of asialoglycoproteins has been widely performed to estimate function in damaged livers [52]. The development of ^{99m}Tc-GSA single-photon emission computed tomography (SPECT) allows the evaluation of regional GSA accumulation in the liver. Because the uptake of ^{99m}Tc-GSA is not affected by high bilirubin serum levels, ^{99m}Tc-GSA scintigraphy is applicable in patients with cholestatic liver diseases [53]. A receptor index parameter obtained from the liver and heart time-activity data as the ratio of radioactivity of the liver to that of the liver plus heart 15 min after intravenous injection of ^{99m}Tc-GSA (LHL15) is used to evaluate liver function because the ratio correlates with serum albumin level, serum bilirubin level, prothrombin time, ICG R15, or CT score [54, 55]. In our institute, surgical decisions regarding safe hepatic resection were made using ICG R15 and LHL15, which reflects the severity of portal hypertension and hepatocyte function in moderately damaged livers [56] (Fig. 4.2).

In Europe, ^{99m}Tc-labeled mebrofenin hepatobiliary scintigraphy is more popular than ^{99m}Tc-GSA. Mebrofenin enters hepatocytes and is excreted into the bile canaliculi unmetabolized; therefore, ^{99m}Tc-labeled mebrofenin hepatobiliary scintigraphy measures the kinetic process of uptake and excretion by hepatocytes [57].

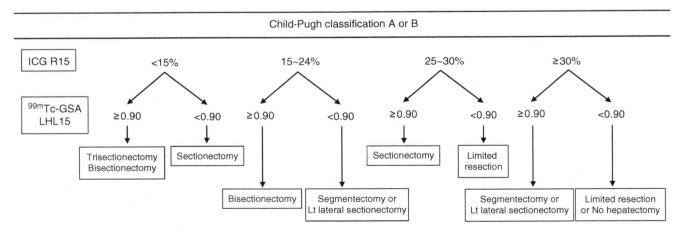

Fig. 4.2 A decision tree for hepatectomy currently used at Nagasaki University. This algorithm involves the ICG R15 and ^{99m}Tc-GSA scintigraphy LHL15. If the intraoperative portal venous pressure is higher than 20 cmH$_2$O, the resection area should be reduced by one step

These imaging studies have advantages in clarifying functional heterogeneity among the hepatic segments compared with the ICG clearance test.

4.6 Measuring Future Liver Remnant (FLR) Volume

Preoperative FLR volume calculation is the method of choice to evaluate the risk of PHLF. Several reports indicated the usefulness of FLR by calculating body surface area or body weight [58, 59]. Truant et al. suggested a cut-off value of remnant liver volume to body weight ratio of ≥0.5% to estimate PHLF [60]. Current consensus regarding the minimal safe FLR volume in patients with a normal liver is approximately 25%–30% of the total functional liver volume, with liver volume not including the volume occupied by the tumor [7, 61, 62]. However, remnant liver function estimated with CT volumetry is only completely reliable when liver function is assumed to be homogeneous throughout the whole liver [61].

4.7 Measuring FLR Function

To evaluate FLR function preoperatively, several methods combining liver volumetry and liver function testing have been reported. Nagino et al. evaluated the change in FLR volume and KICG in patients who underwent extended hepatectomy following portal vein embolization (PVE) for biliary cancer. This group proposed a KICG of the FLR defined by the formula KICG × FLR [ml]/total liver volume [ml] of ≥0.05 as a criterion for safe hepatectomy [63].

As functional heterogeneity among hepatic segments has been reported in damaged livers using ^{99m}Tc-GSA SPECT, the usefulness of this method for precisely predicting postoperative hepatic functional reserve in the damaged liver has been suggested [64–66]. Kwon et al. evaluated the maximal removal rate of ^{99m}Tc-GSA (GSA-Rmax) in the FLR measured from SPECT images. According to their analysis of 178 patients, 7 cases of postoperative hyperbilirubinemia occurred in the patients with GSA-Rmax in FLR of <0.15, and 2 patients died of postoperative failure with GSA-Rmax values in the FLR of <0.1. The authors concluded that GSA-Rmax in FLR should be maintained at >0.15 to avoid postoperative hyperbilirubinemia or hepatic failure and to consider preoperative PVE for cases with GSA-Rmax in the FLR of <0.15 [67].

Recent advances in 3D CT unable precise preoperative surgical planning. Therefore, fusion images combining ^{99m}Tc-GSA SPECT and X-ray CT could be critically helpful for preoperative surgical decision-making. Iimuro et al. evaluated fusion images combining ^{99m}Tc-GSA SPECT and X-ray CT to overcome the relatively poor anatomical resolution of SPECT for surgical simulation. The authors calculated the liver uptake ratio (liver radioactivity/injected radioactivity × 100%; LUR) and reported that estimated remnant LUR, but not the estimated remnant FLR volume, was significantly correlated with postoperative liver function parameters [68].

In European countries, hepatobiliary scintigraphy using ^{99m}Tc-mebrofenin is used to estimate functional distribution in the liver. de Graaf et al. proposed using the value of ≤2.69%/min/m^2 for the equation, 99mTc-labeled mebrofenin uptake rate in the FLR [%/min] divided by the body surface area [m^2], as a predictor of PHLF. The authors suggested that preoperative PVE be performed when FLR mebrofenin uptake is <2.69%/min/m^2 [69].

Another, simpler, method of evaluating FLR function is magnetic resonance imaging with intravenous injection of gadolinium ethoxybenzyl diethylenetriamine pentaacetic acid (Gd-EOB-DTPA), which is transported into hepatocytes. The increase in the signal intensity in the FLR in the hepatobiliary phase compared with the unenhanced phase might be an indicator of FLR function that could predict the risk of PHLF [70, 71]. Chuang et al. reported that the remnant contrast enhancement ratio measured using Gd-EOB-DPTA MRI strongly predicted postoperative liver failure [72]. Orimo et al. introduced the standardized remnant hepatocellular uptake index (SrHUI), which was calculated as FLR volume × [(signal intensity of the remnant liver in hepatobiliary phase images/signal intensity of the spleen in hepatobiliary phase images) − 1]/body surface area. The authors reported that the SrHUI cut-off value for predicting PHLF and PHLF grade ≥ B was 0.313 L/m^2 and 0.257 L/m^2, respectively [73].

4.8 Conclusions

The present article reviewed the reported liver function assessment tools used for surgical decision-making. According to the safety criteria in ICG R15 testing, morbidity and mortality after hepatic resection can be reduced. Recent advances in imaging studies enable precise preoperative surgical planning and calculating FLR volume. Combining imaging studies and liver function testing will achieve more accurate preoperative surgical planning to avoid PHLF.

References

1. Imamura H, Seyama Y, Kokudo N, Maema A, Sugawara Y, Sano K, et al. One thousand fifty-six hepatectomies without mortality in 8 years. Arch Surg (Chicago, IL: 1960). 2003;138(11):1198–1206; discussion 1206.
2. Virani S, Michaelson JS, Hutter MM, Lancaster RT, Warshaw AL, Henderson WG, et al. Morbidity and mortality after liver resec-

tion: results of the patient safety in surgery study. J Am Coll Surg. 2007;204(6):1284–92.
3. Dokmak S, Fteriche FS, Borscheid R, Cauchy F, Farges O, Belghiti J. 2012 Liver resections in the 21st century: we are far from zero mortality. HPB (Oxford). 2013;15(11):908–15.
4. Kenjo A, Miyata H, Gotoh M, Kitagawa Y, Shimada M, Baba H, et al. Risk stratification of 7,732 hepatectomy cases in 2011 from the National Clinical Database for Japan. J Am Coll Surg. 2014;218(3):412–22.
5. Adams RB, Aloia TA, Loyer E, Pawlik TM, Taouli B, Vauthey JN, et al. Selection for hepatic resection of colorectal liver metastases: expert consensus statement. HPB (Oxford). 2013;15(2):91–103.
6. Cieslak KP, Runge JH, Heger M, Stoker J, Bennink RJ, van Gulik TM. New perspectives in the assessment of future remnant liver. Dig Surg. 2014;31(4–5):255–68.
7. Shoup M, Gonen M, D'Angelica M, Jarnagin WR, DeMatteo RP, Schwartz LH, et al. Volumetric analysis predicts hepatic dysfunction in patients undergoing major liver resection. J Gastrointest Surg. 2003;7(3):325–30.
8. Wigmore SJ, Redhead DN, Yan XJ, Casey J, Madhavan K, Dejong CH, et al. Virtual hepatic resection using three-dimensional reconstruction of helical computed tomography angioportograms. Ann Surg. 2001;233(2):221–6.
9. Kokudo T, Hasegawa K, Uldry E, Matsuyama Y, Kaneko J, Akamatsu N, et al. A new formula for calculating standard liver volume for living donor liver transplantation without using body weight. J Hepatol. 2015;63(4):848–54.
10. Mise Y, Hasegawa K, Satou S, Shindoh J, Miki K, Akamatsu N, et al. How has virtual hepatectomy changed the practice of liver surgery?: Experience of 1194 virtual hepatectomy before liver resection and living donor liver transplantation. Ann Surg. 2018;268(1):127–33.
11. Paugam-Burtz C, Janny S, Delefosse D, Dahmani S, Dondero F, Mantz J, et al. Prospective validation of the "fifty-fifty" criteria as an early and accurate predictor of death after liver resection in intensive care unit patients. Ann Surg. 2009;249(1):124–8.
12. Rahbari NN, Garden OJ, Padbury R, Brooke-Smith M, Crawford M, Adam R, et al. Posthepatectomy liver failure: a definition and grading by the International Study Group of Liver Surgery (ISGLS). Surgery. 2011;149(5):713–24.
13. Balzan S, Belghiti J, Farges O, Ogata S, Sauvanet A, Delefosse D, et al. The "50–50 criteria" on postoperative day 5: an accurate predictor of liver failure and death after hepatectomy. Ann Surg. 2005;242(6):824–828, discussion 828–829.
14. Mullen JT, Ribero D, Reddy SK, Donadon M, Zorzi D, Gautam S, et al. Hepatic insufficiency and mortality in 1,059 noncirrhotic patients undergoing major hepatectomy. J Am Coll Surg. 2007;204(5):854–862; discussion 862–854.
15. Kishi Y, Vauthey JN. Issues to be considered to address the future liver remnant prior to major hepatectomy. Surg Today. 2020.
16. Bruix J, Reig M, Sherman M. Evidence-based diagnosis, staging, and treatment of patients with hepatocellular carcinoma. Gastroenterology. 2016;150(4):835–53.
17. Forner A, Llovet JM, Bruix J. Hepatocellular carcinoma. Lancet. 2012;379(9822):1245–55.
18. Hidaka M, Takatsuki M, Soyama A, Tanaka T, Muraoka I, Hara T, et al. Intraoperative portal venous pressure and long-term outcome after curative resection for hepatocellular carcinoma. Br J Surg. 2012;99(9):1284–9.
19. Berzigotti A, Reig M, Abraldes JG, Bosch J, Bruix J. Portal hypertension and the outcome of surgery for hepatocellular carcinoma in compensated cirrhosis: a systematic review and meta-analysis. Hepatology. 2015;61(2):526–36.
20. Kanematsu T, Furui J, Yanaga K, Okudaira S, Kamohara Y, Eguchi S. Measurement of portal venous pressure is useful for selecting the optimal type of resection in cirrhotic patients with hepatocellular carcinoma. Hepato-Gastroenterology. 2005;52(66):1828–31.
21. European Association for the Study of the Liver. Electronic address eee, European Association for the Study of the L. EASL Clinical Practice Guidelines: Management of hepatocellular carcinoma. J Hepatol. 2018;69(1):182–236.
22. Malinchoc M, Kamath PS, Gordon FD, Peine CJ, Rank J, ter Borg PC. A model to predict poor survival in patients undergoing transjugular intrahepatic portosystemic shunts. Hepatology. 2000;31(4):864–71.
23. Freeman RB Jr, Wiesner RH, Harper A, McDiarmid SV, Lake J, Edwards E, et al. The new liver allocation system: moving toward evidence-based transplantation policy. Liver Transpl. 2002;8(9):851–8.
24. Teh SH, Christein J, Donohue J, Que F, Kendrick M, Farnell M, et al. Hepatic resection of hepatocellular carcinoma in patients with cirrhosis: Model of End-Stage Liver Disease (MELD) score predicts perioperative mortality. J Gastrointest Surg. 2005;9(9):1207–1215; discussion 1215.
25. Cucchetti A, Ercolani G, Cescon M, Ravaioli M, Zanello M, Del Gaudio M, et al. Recovery from liver failure after hepatectomy for hepatocellular carcinoma in cirrhosis: meaning of the model for end-stage liver disease. J Am Coll Surg. 2006;203(5):670–6.
26. Citterio D, Facciorusso A, Sposito C, Rota R, Bhoori S, Mazzaferro V. Hierarchic interaction of factors associated with liver decompensation after resection for hepatocellular carcinoma. JAMA Surg. 2016;151(9):846–53.
27. Schroeder RA, Marroquin CE, Bute BP, Khuri S, Henderson WG, Kuo PC. Predictive indices of morbidity and mortality after liver resection. Ann Surg. 2006;243(3):373–9.
28. Kokudo T, Hasegawa K, Shirata C, Tanimoto M, Ishizawa T, Kaneko J, et al. Assessment of preoperative liver function for surgical decision making in patients with hepatocellular carcinoma. Liver Cancer. 2019;8(6):447–56.
29. Maithel SK, Kneuertz PJ, Kooby DA, Scoggins CR, Weber SM, Martin RC, 2nd, et al. Importance of low preoperative platelet count in selecting patients for resection of hepatocellular carcinoma: a multi-institutional analysis. J Am Coll Surg. 2011;212(4):638–648; discussion 648–650.
30. Tomimaru Y, Eguchi H, Gotoh K, Kawamoto K, Wada H, Asaoka T, et al. Platelet count is more useful for predicting posthepatectomy liver failure at surgery for hepatocellular carcinoma than indocyanine green clearance test. J Surg Oncol. 2016;113(5):565–9.
31. Golriz M, Ghamarnejad O, Khajeh E, Sabagh M, Mieth M, Hoffmann K, et al. Preoperative thrombocytopenia may predict poor surgical outcome after extended hepatectomy. Can J Gastroenterol Hepatol. 2018;2018:1275720.
32. Wai CT, Greenson JK, Fontana RJ, Kalbfleisch JD, Marrero JA, Conjeevaram HS, et al. A simple noninvasive index can predict both significant fibrosis and cirrhosis in patients with chronic hepatitis C. Hepatology. 2003;38(2):518–26.
33. Ichikawa T, Uenishi T, Takemura S, Oba K, Ogawa M, Kodai S, et al. A simple, noninvasively determined index predicting hepatic failure following liver resection for hepatocellular carcinoma. J Hepato-Biliary-Pancreat Surg. 2009;16(1):42–8.
34. Mai RY, Ye JZ, Long ZR, Shi XM, Bai Y, Chen J, et al. Preoperative aspartate aminotransferase-to-platelet-ratio index as a predictor of posthepatectomy liver failure for resectable hepatocellular carcinoma. Cancer Manag Res. 2019;11:1401–14.
35. Johnson PJ, Berhane S, Kagebayashi C, Satomura S, Teng M, Reeves HL, et al. Assessment of liver function in patients with hepatocellular carcinoma: a new evidence-based approach-the ALBI grade. J Clin Oncol. 2015;33(6):550–8.
36. Zou H, Wen Y, Yuan K, Miao XY, Xiong L, Liu KJ. Combining albumin-bilirubin score with future liver remnant predicts post-

hepatectomy liver failure in HBV-associated HCC patients. Liver Int. 2018;38(3):494–502.
37. de Graaf W, Hausler S, Heger M, van Ginhoven TM, van Cappellen G, Bennink RJ, et al. Transporters involved in the hepatic uptake of (99m)Tc-mebrofenin and indocyanine green. J Hepatol. 2011;54(4):738–45.
38. Paumgartner G. The handling of indocyanine green by the liver. Schweiz Med Wochenschr. 1975;105(17 Suppl):1–30.
39. Iimuro Y. ICG clearance test and 99mTc-GSA SPECT/CT fusion images. Visc Med. 2017;33(6):449–54.
40. Makuuchi M, Kosuge T, Takayama T, Yamazaki S, Kakazu T, Miyagawa S, et al. Surgery for small liver cancers. Semin Surg Oncol. 1993;9(4):298–304.
41. Seyama Y, Kokudo N. Assessment of liver function for safe hepatic resection. Hepatol Res. 2009;39(2):107–16.
42. Kokudo T, Hasegawa K, Amikura K, Uldry E, Shirata C, Yamaguchi T, et al. Assessment of preoperative liver function in patients with hepatocellular carcinoma – The Albumin-Indocyanine Green Evaluation (ALICE) grade. PLoS One. 2016;11(7):e0159530.
43. Shirata C, Kokudo T, Arita J, Akamatsu N, Kaneko J, Sakamoto Y, et al. Albumin-Indocyanine Green Evaluation (ALICE) grade combined with portal hypertension to predict post-hepatectomy liver failure. Hepatol Res. 2019;49(8):942–9.
44. Yoshimoto T, Eguchi S, Natsuda K, Hidaka M, Adachi T, Ono S, et al. Relationship between various hepatic function scores and the formation of esophageal varices in patients with HIV/hepatitis C virus co-infection due to contaminated blood products for hemophilia. Hepatol Res. 2019;49(2):147–52.
45. Uesaka K, Nimura Y, Nagino M. Changes in hepatic lobar function after right portal vein embolization. An appraisal by biliary indocyanine green excretion. Ann Surg. 1996;223(1):77–83.
46. Haegele S, Reiter S, Wanek D, Offensperger F, Pereyra D, Stremitzer S, et al. Perioperative non-invasive indocyanine green-clearance testing to predict postoperative outcome after liver resection. PLoS One. 2016;11(11):e0165481.
47. Imamura H, Sano K, Sugawara Y, Kokudo N, Makuuchi M. Assessment of hepatic reserve for indication of hepatic resection: decision tree incorporating indocyanine green test. J Hepato-Biliary-Pancreat Surg. 2005;12(1):16–22.
48. Hanai T, Shiraki M, Ohnishi S, Miyazaki T, Ideta T, Kochi T, et al. Impact of serum glycosylated Wisteria floribunda agglutinin positive Mac-2 binding protein levels on liver functional reserves and mortality in patients with liver cirrhosis. Hepatol Res. 2015;45(11):1083–90.
49. Yamasaki K, Tateyama M, Abiru S, Komori A, Nagaoka S, Saeki A, et al. Elevated serum levels of Wisteria floribunda agglutinin-positive human Mac-2 binding protein predict the development of hepatocellular carcinoma in hepatitis C patients. Hepatology. 2014;60(5):1563–70.
50. Okuda Y, Taura K, Yoshino K, Ikeno Y, Nishio T, Yamamoto G, et al. Usefulness of Mac-2 binding protein glycosylation isomer for prediction of posthepatectomy liver failure in patients with hepatocellular carcinoma. Ann Surg. 2017;265(6):1201–8.
51. Ashwell G, Morell A. The dual role of sialic acid in the hepatic recognition and catabolism of serum glycoproteins. Biochem Soc Symp. 1974;40:117–24.
52. Kudo M, Todo A, Ikekubo K, Yamamoto K, Vera DR, Stadalnik RC. Quantitative assessment of hepatocellular function through in vivo radioreceptor imaging with technetium 99m galactosyl human serum albumin. Hepatology. 1993;17(5):814–9.
53. Mimura T, Hamazaki K, Sakai H, Tanaka N, Mimura H. Evaluation of hepatic functional reserve in rats with obstructive jaundice by asyaloglycoprotein receptor. Hepato-Gastroenterology. 2001;48(39):777–82.
54. Kudo M, Todo A, Ikekubo K, Hino M, Yonekura Y, Yamamoto K, et al. Functional hepatic imaging with receptor-binding radiopharmaceutical: clinical potential as a measure of functioning hepatocyte mass. Gastroenterol Jpn. 1991;26(6):734–41.
55. Kudo M, Todo A, Ikekubo K, Hino M. Receptor index via hepatic asialoglycoprotein receptor imaging: correlation with chronic hepatocellular damage. Am J Gastroenterol. 1992;87(7):865–70.
56. Kamohara Y, Takatsuki M, Hidaka M, Soyama A, Kanematsu T, Eguchi S. 99mTc-Galactosyl sialyl albumin (GSA) scintigram adjusts hepatic resection range in ICG based estimation. Hepato-Gastroenterology. 2011;58(112):2058–61.
57. Krishnamurthy S, Krishnamurthy GT. Technetium-99m-iminodiacetic acid organic anions: review of biokinetics and clinical application in hepatology. Hepatology. 1989;9(1):139–53.
58. Kishi Y, Abdalla EK, Chun YS, Zorzi D, Madoff DC, Wallace MJ, et al. Three hundred and one consecutive extended right hepatectomies: evaluation of outcome based on systematic liver volumetry. Ann Surg. 2009;250(4):540–8.
59. Truant S, Boleslawski E, Sergent G, Leteurtre E, Duhamel A, Hebbar M, et al. Liver function following extended hepatectomy can be accurately predicted using remnant liver volume to body weight ratio. World J Surg. 2015;39(5):1193–201.
60. Truant S, Oberlin O, Sergent G, Lebuffe G, Gambiez L, Ernst O, et al. Remnant liver volume to body weight ratio > or =0.5%: a new cut-off to estimate postoperative risks after extended resection in noncirrhotic liver. J Am Coll Surg. 2007;204(1):22–33.
61. Schindl MJ, Redhead DN, Fearon KC, Garden OJ, Wigmore SJ, Edinburgh Liver S, et al. The value of residual liver volume as a predictor of hepatic dysfunction and infection after major liver resection. Gut. 2005;54(2):289–96.
62. Ferrero A, Vigano L, Polastri R, Muratore A, Eminefendic H, Regge D, et al. Postoperative liver dysfunction and future remnant liver: where is the limit? Results of a prospective study. World J Surg. 2007;31(8):1643–51.
63. Nagino M, Kamiya J, Nishio H, Ebata T, Arai T, Nimura Y. Two hundred forty consecutive portal vein embolizations before extended hepatectomy for biliary cancer: surgical outcome and long-term follow-up. Ann Surg. 2006;243(3):364–72.
64. Akaki S, Mitsumori A, Kanazawa S, Togami I, Takeda Y, Hiraki Y. Lobar decrease in 99mTc-GSA accumulation in hilar cholangiocarcinoma. J Nucl Med. 1999;40(3):394–8.
65. Sugahara K, Togashi H, Takahashi K, Onodera Y, Sanjo M, Misawa K, et al. Separate analysis of asialoglycoprotein receptors in the right and left hepatic lobes using Tc-GSA SPECT. Hepatology. 2003;38(6):1401–9.
66. Imaeda T, Kanematsu M, Asada S, Seki M, Doi H, Saji S. Utility of Tc-99m GSA SPECT imaging in estimation of functional volume of liver segments in health and liver diseases. Clin Nucl Med. 1995;20(4):322–8.
67. Kwon AH, Matsui Y, Kaibori M, Ha-Kawa SK. Preoperative regional maximal removal rate of technetium-99m-galactosyl human serum albumin (GSA-Rmax) is useful for judging the safety of hepatic resection. Surgery. 2006;140(3):379–86.
68. Iimuro Y, Kashiwagi T, Yamanaka J, Hirano T, Saito S, Sugimoto T, et al. Preoperative estimation of asialoglycoprotein receptor expression in the remnant liver from CT/99mTc-GSA SPECT fusion images correlates well with postoperative liver function parameters. J Hepatobiliary Pancreat Sci. 2010;17(5):673–81.
69. de Graaf W, van Lienden KP, Dinant S, Roelofs JJ, Busch OR, Gouma DJ, et al. Assessment of future remnant liver function using hepatobiliary scintigraphy in patients undergoing major liver resection. J Gastrointest Surg. 2010;14(2):369–78.
70. Asenbaum U, Kacirek K, Ba-Ssalamah A, Ringl H, Schwarz C, Waneck F, et al. Post-hepatectomy liver failure after major hepatic surgery: not only size matters. Eur Radiol. 2018;28(11):4748–56.
71. Kim DK, Choi JI, Choi MH, Park MY, Lee YJ, Rha SE, et al. Prediction of posthepatectomy liver failure: MRI with hepatocyte-

specific contrast agent versus indocyanine green clearance test. AJR Am J Roentgenol. 2018;211(3):580–7.

72. Chuang YH, Ou HY, Lazo MZ, Chen CL, Chen MH, Weng CC, et al. Predicting post-hepatectomy liver failure by combined volumetric, functional MR image and laboratory analysis. Liver Int. 2018;38(5):868–74.

73. Orimo T, Kamiyama T, Kamachi H, Shimada S, Nagatsu A, Asahi Y, et al. Predictive value of gadoxetic acid enhanced magnetic resonance imaging for posthepatectomy liver failure after a major hepatectomy. J Hepatobiliary Pancreat Sci. 2020;27(8):531–40.

Surgical Approach to Pancreas, Liver, Biliary Physiologic Impairment

Alexandra W. Acher, Amir A. Rahnemai-Azar, Sharon M. Weber, and Timothy M. Pawlik

Abstract

The multi-disciplinary management of hepato-pancreatobiliary diseases involves the treatment of both benign and malignant lesions. Benign liver lesions can be divided into non-infectious and infectious lesions. The most common infectious lesions include abscesses, parasitic lesions, fungal lesions, and granulomatous diseases. The most common non-infectious primary benign liver lesions include simple hepatic cysts, hepatic hemangiomas, focal nodular hyperplasia, hepatic adenoma, and biliary cystadenoma. The most common liver malignancies include metastatic disease from a non-hepatic primary followed by hepatocellular carcinoma, intrahepatic cholangiocarcinoma, and more rarely hepatic angiosarcoma. The treatment approach for liver malignancies should be rooted in a multidisciplinary collaboration between medical and radiation oncologists, interventional radiologists, pathologists, and hepatobiliary surgeons. Critically important to treatment planning is the ability to contextualize the surgical and medical options relative to a patient's disease burden, comorbidities, and underlying liver function. We herein review the pathophysiology and surgical management strategies of benign and malignant hepato-pancreatobiliary diseases.

A. W. Acher · S. M. Weber
Department of Surgery, Division of Surgical Oncology, University of Wisconsin School of Medicine and Public Health, Madison, WI, USA

A. A. Rahnemai-Azar
Department of Surgery, Division of Surgical Oncology, California University of Science and Medicine, Colton, CA, USA

T. M. Pawlik (✉)
Department of General Surgery, Division of Surgical Oncology, The Ohio State University College of Medicine, Columbus, OH, USA
e-mail: tim.pawlik@osumc.edu

5.1 Benign Liver Disease: Pathophysiology and Indications for Surgical Treatment

Benign liver lesions can be divided into non-infectious and infectious lesions. The most common infectious lesions include abscesses (pyogenic, amebic abscess), parasitic lesions (Echinococcus Granulosa or Hydatid cyst, Echinococcus Multilocularis, Schistosomiasis), fungal lesions (Candidiasis, Cryptococcus), and granulomatous diseases (Tuberculosis, Histoplasmosis) [1]. Depending on etiology and symptoms, the treatment of infectious lesions largely involves medical therapy, sometimes aided by percutaneous drainage, and only rarely surgical intervention [1]. This review therefore focuses on non-infectious lesion pathophysiology and surgical management strategies. The most common non-infectious primary benign liver lesions include simple hepatic cysts, hepatic hemangiomas, focal nodular hyperplasia, hepatic adenoma, and biliary cystadenoma.

5.1.1 Hemangioma

Hepatic hemangiomas are benign hepatic artery supplied vascular lesions that can contain thick fibrous septations and internal thromboses [2, 3]. Hepatic hemangiomas can be solitary or multifocal and range in size from a few millimeters to >20 cm in diameter. Although hemangiomas have been observed to grow in pregnancy and estrogen supplementation, targeted investigation has not demonstrated any association between estrogen-enhanced states and hemangioma incidence or growth [4, 5]. Hemangiomas are hypothesized to result from dysregulated congenital intrahepatic angiogenesis and although they rarely increase in size, enlargement occurs secondary to ectasia or dilation of the vessels rather than vessel hypertrophy or proliferation [2, 3].

Although hemangiomas are highly vascular lesions, the risk of spontaneous hemorrhage or rupture is very low due to the thick walls and internal septations; the majority remain asymptomatic over time [2, 3].

Management should be guided by the degree to which symptoms affect a patient's quality of life. Thorough evaluation should rule out other symptom etiology. There is no indication for surgical intervention or regular surveillance in asymptomatic or minimally symptomatic lesions. Significantly symptomatic lesions in healthy surgical candidates can be managed with either laparoscopic or open tumor enucleation, wedge resection, or formal liver resection depending on the tumor size and location. Giant hemangiomas and diffuse multifocal hepatic hemangiomatosis have also been treated with liver transplantation, although the data are limited to a few case reports [6]. In patients with symptomatic lesions who are not surgical candidates, radiotherapy and arterial embolization can be offered, although both have transient response and should only be considered as palliative treatments to improve quality of life [7–9].

5.1.2 Focal Nodular Hyperplasia

Focal Nodular Hyperplasia (FNH) arises from hepatocyte and cholangiocyte hyper-proliferation that represents a local cellular response to congenital arteriovenous malformation [4]. Although FNH lesions can be estrogen receptor positive, estrogen-enhanced states (pregnancy or estrogen use) do not increase the frequency or size of FNH lesions [10]. On axial imaging, FNH often present with a central stellate scar but this pathopneumonic characteristics can be absent (Fig. 5.1)

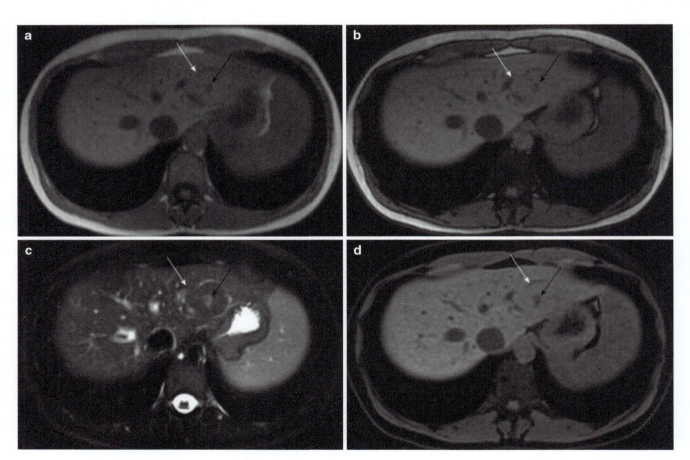

Fig. 5.1 Stellate scar in association with focal nodular hyperplasia. In- (**a**) and opposed-phase (**b**) GRE T1-WI, fat-suppressed FSE T2-WI (**c**), pre (**d**) and post hepatocyte-specific contrast agent (Eovist®) fat-suppressed 3D-GRE T1-WI at the arterial (**e**), portal venous (**f**), interstitial (**g**) and hepatobiliary (**h**) phases. There is a lesion on the left hepatic lobe (white arrow, **a–h**), showing isointense signal comparing to the surrounding liver on non-contrast T1-WI (**a**, **b** and **d**) and on T2-WI (**c**). The lesion also shows a central scar (black arrow, **a–h**), which is hypointense on T1-WI (**a**, **b** and **d**) and hyperintense on T2-WI (**c**). The lesion demonstrates homogeneous enhancement on early post-contrast images (**e**), becoming isointense to the underlying liver parenchyma (**f** and **g**). The progressive enhancement of the central scar is depicted on the delayed post-contrast images (**g**). On the hepatobiliary phase, 20 min after the administration the hepatocyte-specific contrast agent, the lesion shows uptake of the contrast agent, becoming minimally hyperintense comparing to the surrounding liver parenchyma. Since the central scar has no hepatocytes, there is no uptake of the contrast agent, becoming hypointense comparing to the liver and to the rest of the lesion. *GRE* Gradient-echo, *FSE* Fast spinecho, *T1-WI* T1-weighted images

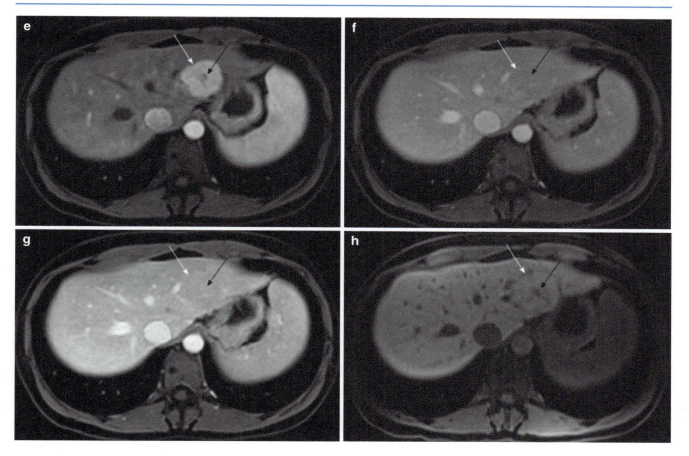

Fig. 5.1 (contnued)

[4]. Interestingly, the formation of the stellate scar is secondary to oxidative stress caused by an over-abundance of oxygenated blood inherent in the arteriovenous malformation, which activates stellate cells, the primary drivers of liver fibrosis [11].

Due to their benign, largely asymptomatic and non-progressive nature, management of FNH is observation-based with surgery rarely being indicated.

5.1.3 Simple Hepatic Cyst

Simple cysts are thin walled and lined by cuboidal epithelium that can contain septa. Simple hepatic cyst size can range from <1 cm to more than 20 cm in diameter, and are rarely symptomatic [12]. Simple cysts are thought to form congenitally when intrahepatic ductules fail to merge with the developing contiguous biliary system; over time, these cysts can dilate and fill with yellow serous fluid secondary to epithelial cyst wall secretion of fluid [12, 13].

Management options include observation, aspiration with or without sclerotherapy, cyst fenestration, or surgical resection [14, 15]. Aspiration (+/− sclerotherapy) has a high rate of recurrence and has largely been replaced by cyst fenestration in patients fit for surgery [14]. Although rare, hepatic cystadenoma (discussed subsequently) can appear indistinguishable from a simple hepatic cyst on axial imaging, but cystadenomas require resection due to associated risk of invasive cancer [16]. Cyst fenestration is therefore the definitive treatment for large peripheral or symptomatic cysts, as it allows for intraoperative biopsy/cytology and the ability to adjust the surgical plan if cystadenoma or cystadenocarcinoma is discovered. Cyst fenestration can be done safely with either a laparoscopic or open approach. Laparoscopic cyst fenestration has equivalent recurrence rates and less perioperative morbidity than an open approach, however, depending on the location of the cyst, an open approach may facilitate a more complete fenestration [17–19]. An open approach may also be preferred in the setting of a recurrent cyst.

5.1.4 Hepatic Adenoma

Hepatic adenomas are rare, soft, well-demarcated, hepatocyte-based tumors supplied by hepatic artery-derived arterioles, and occur as solitary or multifocal lesions. Hepatic adenomas are largely considered as benign lesions, yet can have malignant potential [20]. Solitary adenomas are associated with female gender, oral contraceptive use, obesity, alcohol use, and anabolic steroids [20, 21]. In contrast, hepatic adenomatosis (>10 lesions) can occur in association with glycogen storage diseases [20, 22]. Adenoma rupture and hemorrhage occurs in up to 20% of lesions and is associated with increasing tumor size (>4–5 cm), exophytic and peripheral tumor location, left lateral sector tumor location, and prominent supplying arteries on axial imaging [23]. The overall rate of malignant transformation is around 4% and is only associated with certain subtypes [24, 25]. Although hepatic adenomas are difficult to distinguish from FNH and hepatocellular carcinoma on routine imaging modalities, the use of gadoxetic acid enhanced MRI has increased diagnostic sensitivity from 50% to 96%, enabling more accurate risk stratification of these tumors [26, 27]. Small lesions (<2 cm) remain difficult, however, to distinguish; in turn, biopsy may be beneficial in some patients [28]. The clinical benefit of biopsy has increased with mutation-based subtyping of hepatic adenomas given that each subtype has varying degrees of malignant potential [28].

The most common hepatic adenoma subtype is associated with a mutation in TCF1, the gene responsible for hepatocyte nuclear factor-1 alpha (HNF-1a), a transcription factor involved in hepatic cell homeostasis, metabolism, and cell differentiation. This mutation inactivates HNF-1a, leading to non-regulated cell differentiation [25, 29]. HNF-1a subtype adenomas exhibit steatosis and have a frequency of malignant transformation of 7% [25, 30]. A second subtype results from an activation mutation in CTNNB1 gene that encodes beta-catenin, a transcriptional co-regulator protein that, when aberrantly activated, promotes the transcription of c-Myc and CycinD-1 oncogenes [25, 30, 31]. B-catenin subtype adenomas have pseudo-glandular cells with some cytological abnormalities and have a frequency of malignant transformation of 46% [25, 30]. A third subtype is associated with mutations in various oncogenes leading to uncontrolled activation of the IL-6 inflammatory pathway. Inflammatory hepatic adenomas are defined by inflammatory infiltrates and dystrophic vessels and have not demonstrated malignant potential [25, 30]. A fourth subtype, referred to as the unclassified subtype, is not associated with mutations or inflammation. The unclassified subtype does not have any marked steatosis, cytological abnormality, or inflammatory infiltration but is composed of stacked hepatocytes and has a 13% frequency of malignant transformation [25, 30]. A final subtype, referred to as the sonic hedgehog subtype, results from activation of the sonic hedgehog pathway that is involved in lipid metabolism and liver regeneration. This subtype is associated with obesity and while it does not have increased malignant potential, it is associated with a high risk of hemorrhage [25]. Independent of subtype, male gender and tumor size (> 5 cm) are associated with an increased risk of malignant transformation [32, 33].

Given the diversity of subtype and presentation, management strategies for hepatic adenomas must weigh patient sex and comorbidities, exogenous estrogen or androgen exposure, the genetic subtype, tumor size and the risks inherent in surgery. Given the increased risk of malignancy in male patients, discontinuation of androgen therapy and surgical resection is recommended as first line treatment [24, 25, 34]. For female patients with tumors <5 cm, initial conservative management may include discontinuation of any exogenous estrogen or androgen therapy, weight loss, and 6–12 months of surveillance imaging [34]. Tumor regression can occur in up to 79% of patients after discontinuation of OCPs [35]. In female patients with tumor progression after hormone cessation or with tumors >5 cm, surgical resection is the recommended first line treatment [34]. Microwave ablation is an alternative to surgical resection [36, 37]. With better understanding of malignant potential of certain hepatic adenoma subtypes, many clinicians advocate for surgical resection of B-catenin subtype tumors regardless of their size while inflammatory subtype or HFN1a subtype can be managed more conservatively [25, 34].

In the event that a patient presents with adenoma rupture and hemorrhage, transarterial embolization (TAE) of supplying vessels may be performed. Most patients who have continued bleeding will eventually tamponade the site of adenoma rupture and stabilize. The rate of complete tumor regression associated with TAE is 10% while partial regression can approach 75% [38]. However, eventual surgical resection is often necessary for definitive management [38].

5.1.5 Biliary Cystadenoma and the Potential for Cystadenocarcinoma

Biliary cystadenomas are rare multi-loculated cystic tumors composed of biliary columnar epithelial cells. Interestingly, spindle and ovarian stromal cells can also be present, which may offer insight into an otherwise obscure etiology [39]. These lesions are mostly associated with the intrahepatic biliary system and have a predominance in the left liver [39]. Biliary cystadenomas are slow growing lesions, which vary in size, and can be radiologically difficult to distinguish from simple hepatic cysts or biliary cystadenocarcinoma [39]. On final pathology, 10% of cystadenomas are found to have transformed to biliary cystadenocarcinoma [39].

Historically, the management options of cystadenoma varied from fenestration and wedge resection to formal hepatectomy. However, the current standard of care is to perform cyst enucleation or formal hepatic resection to mitigate the risk of recurrent disease and cystadenocarcinoma [40]. The rate of cystadenoma recurrence is 49% in cyst fenestrations versus 15% in partial hepatectomies/enucleations and 10% in formal hepatectomies [39]. Other factors associated with an increased risk of recurrence include an R1/R2 resection and the presence of ovarian stromal and spindle cells (present in up to 90% of biliary cystadenomas) [39]. If biliary cystadenocarcinoma is noted on final pathology, a formal hepatectomy may be considered as long as it is compatible with patient comorbidities, cyst location, and the future liver remnant (FLR). This is an especially relevant point as preoperative distinction of biliary cystadenoma from cystadenocarcinoma is limited by poor sensitivity (80%) and specificity (21%) using axial imaging modalities (CT or MRI) [39]. Surgeons who advocate for partial hepatectomy or cystadenoma enucleation should counsel patients that a formal hepatectomy may be required if cystadenocarcinoma is found on final pathology.

5.2 Malignant Liver Disease: Pathophysiology and Indications for Surgical Treatment

The most common liver malignancies include metastatic disease from a non-hepatic primary followed by hepatocellular carcinoma, intrahepatic cholangiocarcinoma, and more rarely hepatic angiosarcoma. The treatment approach for liver malignancies should be rooted in a multidisciplinary collaboration between medical and radiation oncologists, interventional radiologists, pathologists, and hepatobiliary surgeons. Critically important to treatment planning is the ability to contextualize the surgical and medical options relative to a patient's disease burden, comorbidities, underlying liver function, and FLR. Typically, the FLR should be >20% for patients with normal liver, $\geq$ 30% for patients with fibrosis or steatosis, and $\geq$ 40% for patients with cirrhosis [41]. The extent of resection, however, should also be assessed relative to patient age, functional status, and response to any neoadjuvant therapy exposure as these factors have been shown to influence post-hepatectomy outcome [41, 42]. Liver function can be assessed by the Child-Pugh scoring system or the Model for End Stage Liver Disease (MELD) scoring system [43, 44].

5.2.1 Hepatocellular Carcinoma

Hepatocellular carcinoma is the most common primary hepatic malignancy. Its incidence varies with geographic region, with a higher incidence in areas with endemic hepatitis B infection (i.e. sub-Saharan Africa, Eastern Asia, Mediterranean countries) [45]. Globally, the average 5-year cumulative risk of developing HCC is 0.1–0.3% in inactive HBV carriers, 0.6–2.4% in patients with chronic hepatitis B virus (HBV), and 10–15% in patients with chronic HBV and cirrhosis [46]. However, this risk is higher in areas with endemic HBV [46]. Other conditions that predispose to developing HCC include chronic hepatitis C infection with cirrhosis (the most common etiology in North and South America), alcohol liver disease with cirrhosis, non-alcoholic fatty liver disease, toxin exposure (aflatoxin, polyvinyl chloride, carbon chlorides), and non-alcoholic steatohepatitis with cirrhosis [45]. The common denominator underlying all these conditions is a state of chronic intrahepatic inflammation (largely mediated through IL-6 inflammatory pathway), which is thought to promote dysplasia and malignant transformation of hepatocytes [45]. Additionally, there is likely a synergistic and oncogenic relationship between underlying inflammation and genetic mutations that compound the risk of HCC [47]. Examples of the most common hepatocarcinogenic gene mutations include those in telomerase reverse transcriptase (TERT) promoter gene, CTNNB1 that encodes B-catenin, and TP53 that encodes the tumor suppressor protein p53 [47, 48].

Treatment of HCC is complex and requires a multidisciplinary approach with input from medical and radiation oncology, interventional radiology, pathologists, and hepatobiliary surgeons. Assessment of liver function and staging of disease are crucial to the preoperative work up and have very significant prognostic implications that should be weighed against the risks of surgery and the patient's goals. Liver function should be assessed by the Child-Pugh or the Model for End Stage Liver Disease (MELD) scoring system. The Barcelona Clinic Liver Cancer (BCLC) staging system is one of the most commonly used tools to guide treatment strategy by a summative assessment of tumor stage, liver function, and patient functional status and includes estimated prognosis of each treatment approach (Fig. 5.2) [49]. In general, very early stage and early stage HCC can be considered for tumor ablation, oncologic resection, or transplantation. According to institutional practice, the Milan or San Francisco Criteria may be used to guide transplant candidacy based on the number and size of tumors (Table 5.1) [50]. BCLC intermediate stage are recommended to undergo chemoembolization while patients with advanced stages can be enrolled in systemic therapy clinical trials [49]. Although

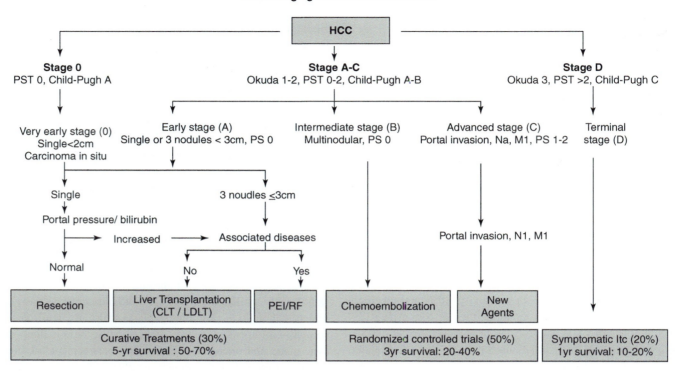

Fig. 5.2 Barcelona-Clinic Liver Cancer (BCLC) staging classification and treatment schedule. PST performance status; CLT/LDLT cadaver liver transplant/living donor liver transplant; RF/PEI radiofrequency ablation/percutaneous ethanol injection; TACE transarterial chemoembolization

Table 5.1 Milan and San Francisco criteria for liver transplantation in the setting of hepatocellular carcinoma

Milan Criteria	San Francisco Criteria
Single tumor <5 cm	Single tumor <6.5 cm
OR	OR
1–3 tumors, each <3 cm	1–3 tumors, each <4.5 cm
	OR
	Total combined tumor diameter < 8 cm

some patients with BCLC intermediate stage HCC may also be candidates for resection. Among surgical candidates, portal vein embolization can be used to induce contralateral liver hypertrophy prior to oncologic resection. Internal radiation therapy with Yttrium-90 can be used to treat the primary tumor as well as induce contralateral hypertrophy in support of eventual curative intent oncologic resection. Despite these treatment strategies, the 3 year survival for intermediate and advanced stage HCC is 20–40% [49].

5.2.2 Metastatic Disease

The liver is a common site of metastatic spread for multiple primary cancers. The majority of hepatic metastases originate from the gastrointestinal tract (70–75%) with nearly 50% originating from the colon or rectum [51]. However, other common origins include stomach, pancreas, biliary, breast, skin, and lung cancers [51]. The most common indication for hepatic metastectomy is for colorectal liver metastases. In surgically-fit patients with colorectal liver metastasis, complete oncologic resection of metastases is associated with a survival benefit [52–59]. Appropriately selected patients with hepatic metastases from primary pancreas or gastrointestinal neuroendocrine tumors may also benefit from metastectomy [60]. The data supporting hepatic resection of other metastatic lesions from a primary breast cancer, etc. are evolving; in turn, hepatectomy can be considered for appropriately selected patients [61].

5.2.3 Intrahepatic Cholangiocarcinoma

Intrahepatic cholangiocarcinoma (ICC) is rare and arises from malignant transformation of cholangiocytes lining the intrahepatic biliary tree (Fig. 5.3) [62]. Although biliary in nature, ICC is considered a primary liver cancer [62]. Primary sclerosing cholangitis, choledochal cyst disease, chronic hepatitis B or C infection, cirrhosis, fatty liver disease, toxin exposure (asbestos), parasitic infection, obesity, and diabetes are associated with increased risk of ICC development [63]. Similar to HCC, ICC is thought to result from a synergistic relationship between chronic inflammation and genetic aberrancies. Associated mutations include: KRAS

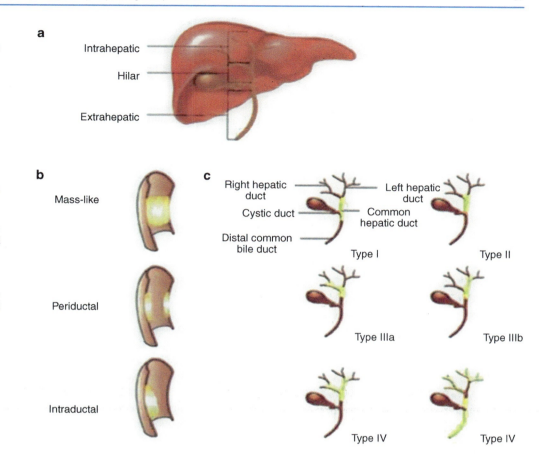

Fig. 5.3 Anatomic classification of cholangiocarcinoma. "**a**: The classification of cholangiocarcinoma can be based on anatomic location, intrahepatic, hilar or extrahepatic; **b**: Non-hilar lesions can be described as mass-like, periductal or intraductal; **c**: Bismuth classification for hilar lesions." Type I cholangiocarcinoma involves the common hepatic duct only; Type II cholangiocarcinoma involves the common hepatic duct and the confluence of the right and left hepatic ducts; Type IIIa and IIIb cholangiocarcinoma includes the common hepatic duct and either the right or left hepatic duct, respectively; and Type IV cholangiocarcinoma involves the biliary confluence and extends to both right and left hepatic ducts or refers to multifocal sites

gene which encodes K-Ras signaling protein of the RAS/MAPK pathway crucial to cell proliferation and differentiation; TP53 which encodes tumor suppressor protein, P53; IDH1 gene which encodes isocitrate dehydrogenase, an enzyme critical for NADPH-dependent cellular metabolism and sequestration of reactive oxygen species [64]. Other cell signaling pathways, including Hedgehog (previously referenced relation to hepatic adenoma subtypes) and WNT/B-catenin (previously referenced in relation to hepatic adenoma subtype malignant potential and HCC) are also altered [64]. As in HCC, IL-6 likely has a large role in linking a chronic inflammatory state and genetic alterations to facilitate malignant transformation of cholangiocytes [64].

Surgical resection provides the only option for potential cure in patients with ICC. Unfortunately, most patients present with advanced disease not amenable to curative resection. Contraindications to resection include extrahepatic disease, multiple bilobar or multicentric tumors, and lymph node metastases [65]. As in HCC, as markers of tumor biology are discovered, tumor biology may play an increasing role in helping to identify patients with the most potential to benefit from surgery; these advancements will undoubtedly change the surgical landscape for this disease [66].

5.2.4 Hepatic Angiosarcoma

Hepatic Angiosarcoma is a rare but aggressive vascular tumor that can present as a solitary lesion with satellite lesions or a diffuse infiltrative mass. These tumors are formed from malignant transformation of vascular endothelial cells and are prone to hemorrhage. The pathogenesis of these tumors is unclear, however, 25% may result from hemochromatosis or previous exposure to thorium dioxide, arsenic based insecticides, or vinyl chlorides [67]. Most patients present with metastatic disease and die within 6 months of presentation; unfortunately, even for patients who do undergo treatment, 3 year survival is only 3% [67].

Liver transplantation and liver resection have both been utilized as potential treatment options, however, liver transplantation has been redacted given the high rate of recurrence and mortality. Liver resection can be offered to patients with early stage disease, however, recurrence is exceedingly likely. Transcatheter arterial chemoembolization has also been employed as a palliative measure in patients who present with hemorrahge [67].

5.3 Benign Biliary Disease: Pathophysiology and Indications for Surgical Treatment

The most common extrahepatic benign biliary diseases include acute or chronic calculous cholecystitis, acalculous cholecystitis, biliary dyskinesia, choledocholithiasis, ascending cholangitis, gallstone pancreatitis, and Sphincter of Oddi dysfunction. Less common but potentially equally affecting pathologies include choledochal cysts and benign biliary strictures.

Calculous cholecystitis, choledocholithiasis, ascending cholangitis, gallstone pancreatitis are all potential complications from gallstones. Gallstones form secondary to imbalances in the three components of bile (phospholipids, bile salts, and cholesterols) and are either cholesterol stones (70%) or pigment stones (30%). Cholesterol stones form secondary to a relative abundance of cholesterol compared to solubilizing phospholipid and bile salts which leads to cholesterol crystallization [68]. Cholesterol stone precipitation is also catalyzed by mucus glycoprotein, secreted by gall bladder and biliary duct epithelial cells to bind lipids and bile pigments, and gall bladder hypomotility [68, 69]. Pigment stones can be either black or brown; black pigment stones precipitate in the gall bladder lumen and are produced in hemolytic disorders (sickle cell anemia, hereditary spherocytosis, Gilbert syndrome) when bilirubin polymers bind mucus glycoproteins [68, 70]. Brown stones precipitate in the bile ducts secondary to bacterial byproducts that increase the concentration of unconjugated bilirubin, which then complexes with calcium to form stones [68, 70].

5.3.1 Acute Calculous Cholecystitis

Acute calculous cholecystitis is an inflammation of the gallbladder that most commonly results from a stone-dependent outlet obstruction at either the infundibulum or cystic duct [71]. The outlet obstruction leads to gall bladder distension, wall edema and inflammation with resulting vascular congestion, that if left untreated progresses to wall necrosis and fundal perforation. Bactobilia occurs in 20% of patients with acute cholecystitis [72] while bacteremia develops in a minority of patients (<10%) but is associated with increased mortality [73]. In 87% of bacteremic patients, a single bacterial isolate is identified and is most often either Escherichia Coli or Klebsiella pneumonia [73].

The Tokyo Guidelines can be used to grade cholecystitis severity with predicted 30-day mortality rate, which can aid in guiding treatment options within the context of patient presentation, comorbidities, and goals [74]. For patients who are surgical candidates, standard of care treatment is urgent laparoscopic cholecystectomy with or without intraoperative cholangiogram to verify biliary anatomy and ensure common bile duct patency. Attaining a critical view of safety has been demonstrated to reduce the risk of bile duct injury [75]. This is accomplished by clearing the hepatocystic triangle of fat and fibrous tissue and dissecting the lower third of the gall bladder from the cystic plate to visualize *only* two structures, the cystic duct and cystic artery, entering the gall bladder [76]. If severe pericholecystic inflammation prevents safe definition of the critical view of safety, conversion to an open approach may be necessary [75, 77]. Risk factors for conversion to an open approach include male gender, obesity, leukocytosis and elevated serum bilirubin, and history of previous surgery [78–80]. Alternatively, if the critical view of safety is not attainable, a subtotal fenestrating or subtotal reconstituting cholecystectomy can be performed [81]. A subtotal *fenestrating* cholecystectomy involves excising the peritonealized gall bladder, leaving the posterior gall bladder wall in situ, and suture ligating the cystic duct [81]. A subtotal *reconstituting* cholecystectomy involves excising the peritonealized gall bladder and closing the inferior gallbladder (sewing or stapling) to recreate a small lumen with a patent cystic duct [81]. Fenestration is associated with a higher incidence of postoperative bile leak (18% vs 7%), wound infection (11% vs 3%), and longer hospitalization (5 vs 3 days); however, reconstitution is associated with a higher risk of recurrent biliary pathology (18% vs 9%) [82].

Non-operative management of acute calculous cholecystitis may be necessary for patients who are not surgical candidates or whose pericholecystic inflammation precludes safe dissection. Percutaneous cholecystostomy tube placement allows for immediate clinical improvement in >80% of patients and can be followed by interval cholecystectomy (performed at least 6 weeks after placement) in select patients [83–85].

A more recently developed management option for patients who are not surgical candidates (i.e. terminal cancer), includes internal drainage with lumen-apposing self-expandable metallic stents (LASEMS), placed between the stomach or duodenum and the gall bladder to facilitate enteric drainage [86]. Although preliminary observational studies report few complications and high rates of symptom resolution, outcomes data and randomized studies are still pending [86].

5.3.2 Chronic Cholecystitis

Chronic cholecystitis results from repeated transient gall bladder outlet obstruction, most commonly from intermittent stone impaction at the cystic duct or infundibulum. This pathology appears to be more common in obese female patients and is thought to be related to an increased biliary cholesterol concentration in this patient population [87].

Xanthogranulomatous cholecystitis is a form of chronic cholecystitis that can appear on ultrasound and axial imaging similarly to gall bladder cancer. It is defined by significant inflammation and fibrosis of the gall bladder wall with asymmetric wall thickening, mass formation, and bile extravasation into the gall bladder wall [88, 89]. Its exact pathogenesis is unknown, but it is associated with gallstones and geography (higher incidence in India) and may be associated with an increased risk of gall bladder cancer [89].

Management of chronic cholecystitis and xanthogranulomatous cholecystitis can be approached similarly to management of acute cholecystitis, however, given the chronicity of symptoms, cholecystectomy may be less urgently indicated.

5.3.3 Acalculous Cholecystitis

Acalculous cholecystitis occurs secondary to gall bladder aperistalsis in the context of concomitant major illness (i.e. sepsis, severe trauma or burns), severe vascular disease, or advanced diabetes [90–93]. In these physiologically compromised states, it is hypothesized that lack of gall bladder contraction promotes bile stasis and biliary sludge, eventually resulting in gall bladder wall edema, inflammation, and infection [94, 95].

Due to the concomitant severe illness, management of acalculous cholecystitis is non-operative. Gall bladder decompression is facilitated through percutaneous cholecystostomy tube placement with potential for interval cholecystectomy. Unfortunately, the mortality risk of patients who undergo percutaneous cholecystostomy placement for acalculous cholecystitis is almost 15%, which likely reflects the impact of severe systemic illness rather than cholecystitis-specific mortality alone [96, 97].

5.3.4 Biliary Dyskinesia

Biliary dyskinesia is a symptomatic functional disorder of the gall bladder with unclear etiology, but is hypothesized to result from metabolic disturbance of gastrointestinal and/or gall bladder motility. Patients have biliary symptoms (postprandial right upper quadrant pain with radiation to the right shoulder, nausea, anorexia) without any evidence of gallstones or gall bladder inflammation on ultrasound. Hepatobiliary diacetic acid scan (HIDA) with ejection fraction has been used to aid in the diagnosis of biliary dyskinesia. In the presence of biliary pain but the absence of stones or pericholecystic inflammation, an ejection fraction <35% may support a diagnosis of biliary dyskinesia [98, 99]. For patients with convincing clinical symptoms, elective laparoscopic cholecystectomy is indicated.

5.3.5 Choledocolithiasis

Symptomatic choledocolithiasis occurs when gallstones become impacted in the common bile duct. Choledocolithiasis may be transient and clinically occult; 4% of patients undergoing cholecystectomy for cholelithiasis with patent biliary ducts in preoperative workup have incidentally discovered choledocolithiasis [100]. However, choledocolithiasis may also present as biliary colic or more serious clinical sequelae such as obstructive jaundice with or without ascending cholangitis and gall stone pancreatitis. Primary choledocolithiasis refers to stones that form in the common bile duct and is more commonly seen with pigment stones [101]. In contrast, secondary choledocolithiasis refers to stones, more commonly cholesterol stones, that form in the gall bladder and then migrate via the cystic duct to the common bile duct [101].

Surgical management of symptomatic choledocolithiasis requires common bile duct clearance and cholecystectomy. Common bile duct clearance can be achieved with endoscopic retrograde cholangiopancreatography (ERCP) with sphincterotomy and ductal balloon dilation, laparoscopic transcystic common bile duct exploration with choledocoscopy, laparoscopic choledocotomy and common bile duct exploration, or less commonly, open cholecystectomy with duodenotomy and manual stone extraction. A two-stage approach consists of either pre- or post-cholecystectomy ERCP with sphincterotomy and balloon dilation, while a single stage approach refers to cholecystectomy with common bile duct exploration and stone clearance during the index operation. Both approaches are effective strategies with equivalent duct clearance success rates and morbidity [102].

A two stage approach, with ERCP prior to cholecystectomy, is preferred in patients who present with ascending cholangitis (with or without gallstone pancreatitis) both for source control and to increase safety of eventual cholecystectomy. However, for patients who present with obstructive jaundice or gallstone pancreatitis without sepsis, a period of observation may be beneficial as up to 75% of stones will pass spontaneously [103]. After symptom resolution, these patients may undergo laparoscopic cholecystectomy with intraoperative cholangiogram to ensure duct patency. This sequence is particularly important to consider, as it avoids ERCP and the potential for post-ERCP pancreatitis which occurs in 10–15% of patients and can result in severe systemic illness [104].

5.3.6 Sphincter of Oddi Dysfunction

Sphincter of Oddi dysfunction has an unclear etiology but is hypothesized to occur secondary to impaired contractility of the Sphincter of Oddi that results in recurrent biliary colic or pancreatitis. Sphincter of Oddi dysfunction is most commonly diagnosed in patients with post-cholecystectomy biliary colic. Treatment remains controversial, as does the diagnosis itself. In randomized trials of sphincterotomy versus sham procedure, patients with post-cholecystectomy biliary symptoms who underwent sphincterotomy did not have greater improvement in symptoms [105]. However, in randomized trials comparing symptom resolution in patients with manometry confirmed abnormal sphincter tone, greater symptom improvement was demonstrated in patients with abnormal sphincter who underwent sphincterotomy compared with individuals who underwent a sham procedure [106, 107].

5.3.7 Choledochal Cysts

Choledochal cysts (CC) are defined by dilation of the intra and/or extrahepatic biliary ductal system. While mainly considered benign lesions, certain subtypes of CC have significant potential for malignant transformation. There are 5 subtypes of CC, classified by location and extent of biliary involvement (Fig. 5.4). Type I CC are the most common subtype (50–80% of CC) with fusiform dilation of the common bile duct and lack of biliary mucosal cells [108, 109]. Type II

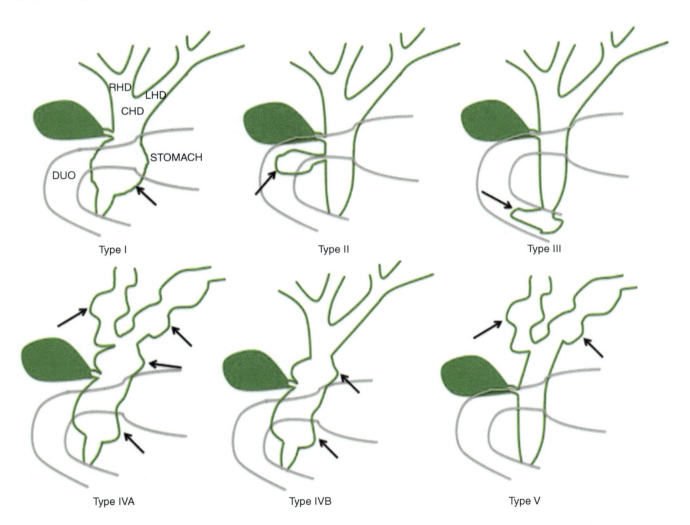

Fig. 5.4 Choledochal cyst classification. Type I cysts are fusiform dilatations of the common bile duct (CBD). Type II cysts are true diverticula of the CBD and type III CC (choledochoceles) are intraduodenal dilations of the common channel. Type IVA CC consist of multiple intrahepatic and extrahepatic biliary dilatations, while type IVB CC have extra-hepatic biliary dilatation with a normal intrahepatic biliary tree. Type V CC, or Caroli's disease, consist of cystic dilation of the intrahepatic biliary tree. *RHD* right hepatic duct, *LHD* left hepatic duct, *CHD* common hepatic duct, *DUO* duodenum

are rare (2% of CC) true biliary diverticula that project from the common bile duct and are histologically consistent with the gall bladder [108, 109]. Type III are rare (2–5% of CC) intra-duodenal dilations of the common pancreaticobiliary channel (choledochoceles) and are lined by duodenal mucosal cells [108, 109]. Type IV CC (15–25% of CC) are divided into two subtypes both of which lack biliary mucosal cells: Type IVA involves dilation of the common hepatic duct and intrahepatic biliary tree while Type IVB involves multiple areas of extrahepatic biliary dilation only ("string of beads") [108, 109]. Type V (20% of CC) involves diffuse dilation of the entire intrahepatic biliary system (Caroli's disease) and can be associated with hepatic fibrosis (Caroli's Syndrome) [108, 109]. There are many theories regarding the origins of CC, but most experts support the hypothesis that CC form secondary to a congenitally abnormal union of the pancreatic and biliary ducts (either extra-duodenally or > 15 mm distal to the ampulla of Vater) [109]. Such an aberrant anatomy allows for reflux of caustic pancreatic juice into the biliary system, predisposing to biliary cystic dilation [109]. While this hypothesis is generally supported Type I and Type IV CC, other pathogenic mechanisms may better explain the differences in location, histology, and malignant potential Types II, III, and V CC [109].

Malignant transformation occurs in 10–30% of Type I and Type IV CC and is thought to occur secondary to a synergistic relationship between caustic pancreatic enzyme exposure, bile stasis, and underlying K-Ras, p53, and DPC-4 mutations [109]. Associated cancers are most commonly extrahepatic cholangiocarcinoma (50–60% of associated cancers), gall bladder cancer (38–46% of associated cancers), and rarely intrahepatic cholangiocarcinoma (3% of associated cancers) [110]. Cancer can occur in the choledochal cyst or at sites of cyst-induced biliary stasis (i.e. the gall bladder) [110]. By subtype of CC, 68% of cancers occur in Type I CC, 5% in Type II, 2% in Type III, 21% in Type IV, and 6% in Type V [110, 111].

Surgical or endoscopic resection is generally recommended for Types I-IV to mitigate the risk of malignant transformation, however, the extent of surgery depends on the subtype. Management of Type I and IV CC require complete extrahepatic bile duct cyst excision down to the level of the pancreatic duct with cholecystectomy, followed by biliary reconstruction (hepaticoduodenostomy or roux-en-Y hepaticojejunostomy). Type IVA may require hepatectomy, however, if the intrahepatic component is minimal. Type II CC are typically treated with diverticulectomy. Large Type III CC are treated with transduodenal excision while small Type III CC can be treated with endoscopic sphincterotomy and drainage. Due to the intrahepatic nature of Type V CC, liver resection or orthotopic liver transplant is required for definitive management. Importantly, if diseased duct is not removed with hepatectomy for Type V CC, the patient remains at risk for continued biliary stasis and malignancy [109]. Patients who undergo cyst excision remain, however, at risk of biliary malignancy even after resection and therefore require routine laboratory and imaging surveillance [109].

5.3.8 Primary Sclerosing Cholangitis

Primary Sclerosing Cholangitis (PSC) is thought to represent an autoimmune process whereby repeated insult to the biliary tree results in inflammation, biliary stasis, eventual scarring, and predisposition to cancer. Additionally, this inflammatory cycle can lead to portal hypertension, cirrhosis, and liver failure. PSC is associated with inflammatory bowel disease (IBD) in 70% of cases but only 5% of people with IBD develop PSC [112]. It has also been hypothesized that PSC with colitis represents a disease process that is distinct from either isolated IBD or isolated PSC, as its patterns of colonic inflammation differ from those exhibited in IBD [112]. Cholangiocarcinoma is the most common PSC-associated cancer, which occurs in 10–15% of patients with PSC [113–115]. However, this may be an underestimation, as 10% of patients undergoing liver transplantation for PSC have clinically occult cholangiocarcinoma upon pathologic examination of the explanted liver [116]. Gallbladder cancer is also seen in 3–14% of patients with PSC and can occur independently from strictured areas [115]. Patients with PSC are also at increased risk of hepatocellular carcinoma [115].

Intervention to treat PSC-related biliary strictures depends on the extent and location of disease. For isolated extrahepatic strictures, ERCP with stricture biopsy and balloon dilation can be employed. Randomized trials have demonstrated that stenting across a dominant stricture has equivalent success and recurrence rates versus balloon dilation, but is associated with higher morbidity. Therefore stenting should not be routinely employed [117]. In the event that endoscopic approaches are unsuccessful or anatomically impossible, biliary tract resection with reconstruction may be considered in surgically-fit patients [118]. Of note, biliary reconstruction may technically complicate future liver transplantation, which is the standard of care treatment in advanced PSC. Previous biliary surgery is also associated with reduced survival in patients undergoing liver transplantation for PSC [119]. Indications for liver transplant in PSC include intractable/untreatable jaundice, severe recurrent cholangitis, cirrhosis with reduced liver function, concomitant small HCC or non-metastatic cholangiocarcinoma [119]. Unfortunately, 20–40% of patients who undergo liver transplantation for PSC will have recurrent disease [119].

5.3.9 Benign Biliary Stricture

Non-PSC benign biliary strictures may result from chronic pancreaticobiliary inflammation (recurrent pancreatitis, recurrent cholangitis), iatrogenic etiology (operative bile duct injury), postoperative scarring in biliary-biliary or biliary-enteric anastomosis, or scarring after repeated endoscopic sphincterotomy. An endoscopic approach with balloon dilation (preceded by biopsy to rule out malignancy) and sphincterotomy is the recommended initial treatment approach [120]. Temporary plastic stents may also be placed, but with risk of migration and necessity of replacement [120].

5.4 Malignant Biliary Disease: Pathophysiology and Indications for Surgical Treatment

The most common extrahepatic malignant biliary tumors include extrahepatic cholangiocarcinoma (ECC) and gall bladder cancer (GBC). The treatment approach for extrahepatic biliary malignancies should be based in multidisciplinary collaboration between medical and radiation oncologists, interventional radiologists, pathologists, and surgeons.

5.4.1 Extrahepatic Cholangiocarcinoma

ECC arises from biliary epithelial cells lining the extrahepatic biliary tract. ECC is classified as either distal or hilar (Fig. 5.3). Hilar cholangiocarcinomas are further categorized by their location relative to the confluence of the right and left hepatic ducts [121]. In the Bismuth-Corlette classification (Fig. 5.3), Type I tumors involve the common hepatic duct just inferior to the confluence of the right and left hepatic ducts and above the cystic duct origin. Type II tumors involve the confluence of the right and left hepatic ducts but do not extend superiorly. Type III tumors involve the hepatic duct confluence with extension to either the proximal right (Type IIIA) or left hepatic duct (Type IIIB). Type IV tumors extend from the confluence to bilateral hepatic ducts and may involve bilateral second-order biliary radical ducts. ECC is most commonly seen in association with PSC; in fact, 30% of cholangiocarcinomas are diagnosed in patients with PSC. ECC also occurs in up to 30% of patients with choledochal cysts [109]. Additionally, ECC is associated with toxin exposure (i.e. Thorotrast), biliary stone disease, and chronic pancreatitis [122, 123]. Although the exact pathogenic mechanism is unclear, ECC is thought to form secondary to biliary inflammation and stasis. In contrast, ICC is associated with chronic hepatitis B or C infection, cirrhosis, fatty liver disease, toxin exposure (asbestos), parasitic infection, obesity, and diabetes, in addition to PSC and CC [63].

Treatment of ECC should be approached from a multidisciplinary perspective. Long term survival is rare and only possible when a negative resection margin (R0) is achieved [124, 125]. Distal ECC can be approached with pancreaticoduodenectomy. Bismuth-Corlette Type I-III tumors require biliary duct resection, formal hepatectomy and caudate lobectomy, and biliary tract reconstrcution [124]. Historically, Bismuth-Corlette Type IV tumors have been considered unresectable due to their high perioperative morbidity (14–66%), mortality (19% in some series), and recurrence rates [125]. However, some centers have demonstrated improved 5 year survival (30–41% vs 11% in historical controls) when aggressive surgery (biliary resection with major hepatectomy, portal vein and hepatic artery reconstruction) is performed in select patients [126, 127]. General contraindications to resection include involvement of the portal vein trunk or bilobar involvement of portal vein branches, involvement of unilateral hepatic artery with contralateral hepatic duct involvement, or metastatic disease [124]. Portal vein embolization may be employed prior to surgery to increase FLR volume [124, 125]. Even with curative intent surgery and an R0 surgical margin, disease recurs in 65% of patients with a median time to recurrence of 12 to 43 months [125]. Because of these factors, orthotopic liver transplant has surfaced as a treatment option for patients with locally advanced hilar cholangiocarcinoma. Initial studies demonstrated prohibitively high recurrence and low 5 year survival (50% and 28% respectively) in patients who underwent liver transplantation for hilar cholangiocarcinoma [128]. However, the very stringently selected patients with early stage perihilar cholangiocarcinoma neoadjuvant radiation, brachytherapy, and chemotherapy (5-FU and oral capecitabine) have demonstrated a 5 year survival of 82% after transplant. The results of this study, however, may be heavily influenced by selection bias inherent in their stringent enrollment criteria [129]. Ultimately, despite a diversity of surgical approaches, prognosis associated with ECC remains poor.

5.4.2 Gall Bladder Cancer

Gall bladder cancer is the most common extrahepatic biliary tract cancer and is most commonly adenocarcinoma (80%) histologically. Gall bladder cancer results from chronic gallbladder inflammation that triggers malignant transformation of cholangiocytes [127]. Unfortunately, most gallbladder cancer is clinically occult until advanced stages that are not amenable to surgical resection [127].

Surgical approach depends on the T category of the tumor. Tumors that invade the inner most layer of the gallbladder, the lamina propria (T1a), are treated with cholecystectomy. Tumors that invade the muscularis propria (T1b) or perimuscular connective tissue (T2) are treated with radical cholecystectomy (cholecystectomy with segments 4b and 5 resection). T3 tumor stage (invasion to liver or other peritoneal organs) necessitates radical cholecystectomy and if the positive cystic duct margin is positive, bile duct resection with reconstruction is necessary [130]. Portal lymphadenectomy should always be performed during radical cholecystectomy. The all-stage post-resection 5 year survival is 40% and by T stage is 92% for T1a tumors, 87% for T1b tumors, 64% for T2 tumors, 19–27% for T3 tumors and < 10% for T4 tumors [131]. Unfortunately, first line systemic therapy offers only a small survival benefit (1 year) and is not associated with tumor response in all patients [127].

5.5 Benign Pancreas Disease: Pathophysiology and Indications for Surgical Treatment

Acute and chronic pancreatitis are common benign pathophysiologic derangements with potential for severe systemic implications. Pancreas neoplasms can be distinguished based on involvement of endocrine or exocrine function of the pancreas with varying degrees of malignant potential.

5.5.1 Acute Pancreatitis

Acute pancreatitis is an inflammatory process that occurs when injury or hyper-stimulation of the pancreas incites intra-acinar protease activation leading to auto-digestion of normal pancreas parenchyma. Pro-inflammatory cytokines (TNF-alpha, IL-1, IL-2, IL-6) are subsequently released and increase basolateral membrane permeability that further propagates this inflammatory cascade [132]. In western countries, gallstones and alcohol are the two most common causes of acute pancreatitis (80–90% of cases). However, < 7% of people with gallstones and < 10% of chronic alcohol users develop acute pancreatitis [132]. Less common causes include hypertriglyceridemia (both genetic and acquired), endoscopic retrograde cholangiography, trauma, medications, sphincter of Oddi dysfunction, congenital anomalies (pancreas divisum, annular pancreas), and hereditary predisposition [132].

The Atlanta Criteria can be used to diagnose acute pancreatitis, grade the severity of presentation, and guide treatment options (Table 5.2) [133]. Most sequelae from acute pancreatitis (sepsis, peripancreatic fluid collections, peripancreatic and pancreatic necrosis, pseudocyst, walled off necrosis) are treated medically and may involve percutaneous or endoscopic drainage procedures [134]. Historically,

Table 5.2 Revised Atlanta Criteria for the classification of acute pancreatitis

Mild acute pancreatitis
No organ failure
No local or systemic complications
Moderately severe acute pancreatitis
Organ failure that resolves within 48 hours
Local or systemic complications without persistent organ failure
Severe acute pancreatitis
Persistent organ failure >48 hours
Multiple organ failure

surgical necrosectomy was reserved for patients with infected necrotizing pancreatitis; however, endoscopic transgastric necrosectomy and retroperitoneal drainage is a more recent promising treatment strategy. Randomized trials comparing open necrosectomy with endoscopic transgastric necrosectomy and drainage for patients with infected necrotizing pancreatitis demonstrated faster normalization of IL-6 and lower rates of organ failure, bleeding, enterocutaneous fistula, and pancreatic fistula in the endoscopic arm [135].

5.5.2 Chronic Pancreatitis

Chronic pancreatitis occurs secondary to the cumulative impact of recurrent episodes of acute pancreatitis and is defined by permanent morphologic change, parenchymal atrophy, and reduced exocrine and endocrine function [136]. Chronic alcohol use, smoking, and hypertriglyceridemia are common etiologies associated with chronic pancreatitis. Additionally, chronic pancreatitis can result from a hereditary predisposition or autoimmune pancreatitis. Repeated episodes of acute pancreatitis predisposes to pancreatic duct strictures that unfortunately increase the likelihood of pancreatic duct obstruction and recurrent acute pancreatitis. Congenital anomalies (pancreas divisum, annular pancreas) usually manifest with recurrent pancreatitis during childhood [136].

Management of chronic pancreatitis is challenging and requires collaboration by gastroenterologists, hepatopancreatobiliary surgeons, interventional radiologists, and nutritionists. Surgical management is mainly reserved for patients who have failed medical and endoscopic management. Surgical management may involve pancreatic duct decompression (Puestow procedure), parenchymal resection with either biliary decompression or reconstruction (pancreaticoduodenectomy, distal pancreatectomy, Beger procedure, Frey procedure), or total pancreatectomy with islet cell autotransplantation in highly selected patients. The optimal approach is dictated by duct size, location and extent of pancreatic duct obstruction, degree of gland atrophy, and the patient's goals and comorbidities [137].

5.5.3 Pancreas Neuroendocrine Tumors

Pancreatic neuroendocrine tumors (PNETs) arise from endocrine cells within the pancreas, with varying degrees of malignant potential. These tumors likely arise from altered pluripotent stem cell differentiation resulting in hyper-proliferation of mature pancreatic endocrine cells (i.e. alpha, beta, delta, enterochromaffin, G, and pancreatic polypeptide cells) [138]. PNETs can manifest as specific clinical syndromes according to the type of cells that are involved. Although most PNETs occur sporadically, they are sometimes associated with other genetic disorders; PNETS occur in 80–100% of patients with multiple endocrine neoplasia Type I (MEN1), 10–20% of patients with von Hippel-Lindau syndrome, and 10% of patients with neurofibromatosis-1 [138]. Interestingly, Kras and p53 oncogene mutations are uncommon in PNETs [138]. About 10–30% of PNETS are functional tumors, while the majority are considered as non-functional tumors (60–90%) [138, 139]. The most common functional PNET syndromes is Insulinoma, followed by gastrinoma (Zollinger-Ellison syndrome) [138, 139]. Rare functional PNETs are associated with secretion of vasoactive intestinal peptide, glucagon, somatostatin, growth hormone, ACTH, and serotonin [139]. Even more rare functional PNETs are associated with secretion of renin, luteinizing hormone, erythropoietin, insulin-like growth factor, cholecystokinin, and glucagon-like peptide [139]. Tumor type, grade, Ki-67 index, and mitotic count are critical to staging and prognosis. The PNETs with the most malignant potential are gastrinomas (60–90%), VIPoma (40–70%), glucagonoma (50–80%), stomatostinoma (>70%), growth hormone secreting PNET (> 60%), ACTH secreting PNET (> 95%) [139]. In contrast, insulinomas have a relatively low malignant potential (<10%) [139].

Management of PNETs is complex and requires collaboration within a multidisciplinary team, individualized to patient comorbidities, symptoms, tumor location, grade and malignant potential, and patient goals. Small (< 2 cm) low grade non-functional PNETs are usually indolent and can be routinely surveyed [139]. Management of larger or clinically apparent PNETs should include medical management and curative intent resection when possible. Metastatic disease does not preclude curative intent surgery [139]. Resection of metastatic hepatic metastases is appropriate in select cases [138, 139]. Liver transplantation for unresectable hepatic metastases can be considered in very select patients after resection of primary disease, however, recurrent disease is likely [140].

5.5.4 Pancreas Cystic Neoplasms

Pancreatic cystic neoplasms (PCN) derive from pancreatic exocrine cells and are classified as either epithelial or non-epithelial, and neoplastic or non-neoplastic [141]. Common PCNs without malignant potential include serous cystadenoma (<3% incidence of invasive cancer, SCN), pseudocyst (sequela from pancreatitis), lymphoepithelial cysts, and epidermoid cysts. Common PCNs with malignant potential include mucinous cystic neoplasm (MCN), intraductal mucinous papillary neoplasm (IPMN), solid pseudopapillary tumor [142].

The management of PCNs with malignant potential is complex and despite the publication of many society-based guidelines, a formal consensus on best management practices is still lacking [143]. Management should be approached from a collaborative multidisciplinary team of radiologists, pathologists, surgeons, and gastroenterologists catered to PCN type, the presence or absence of features concerning for invasive cancer, patient symptoms, comorbidities, and goals. Given the complexity of both pathogenesis and management of PCNs, the following is a brief summary of defining features of the most common PCNs whose management may include surgery.

5.5.4.1 Intraductal Papillary Mucinous Neoplasm

IPMNs are mucin producing neoplasms that have the greatest malignant potential (30–68% incidence of progression) and are categorized as intestinal, oncocytic, pancreaticobiliary, or gastric histologic subtypes. The intestinal type is the most common, while the rare pancreaticobiliary subtype has the highest recurrence rate (32–71%) and lowest 5 year survival (36–52%) due to its association with invasive cancer (present in 63% of cases) [142]. IPMNs may be associated with the main pancreatic duct or a side branch duct, and may occur in isolation or involve the entire duct. IPMN features that are concerning for malignant transformation and may serve as indications for surgical resection include jaundice, enhancing mural nodule or associated solid mass, dysplasia or malignant cells on cytology, dilated main pancreatic duct >5–10 mm, however, society-specific guidelines vary and are more nuanced (Fig. 5.5) [141–143]. Invasive IPMN (intraductal papillary mucinous cystadenocarcinoma) has a better prognosis than patients with pancreatic ductal adenocarcinoma (5 year overall survival of 28–68% versus approximately <10% in pancreatic ductal adenocarcinoma) [142].

5.5.4.2 Mucinous Cystic Neoplasm

MCNs derive from ductal epithelial mucin-producing cells and can be distinguished from IPMNs by lack of communication with a pancreatic duct and a predominance in the pancreatic tail. Invasive cancer is found in approximately 17% of MCNs and is associated with larger size (≥ 3 cm) and the presence of mural nodules [142, 144, 145]. Indications for surgery include associated symptoms, mural nodules, or tumor size >3–4 cm but vary by guideline [141–143]. Prognosis for invasive MCN (mucinous cystadenocarcinoma) is similar to that of invasive IPMN and 5 year survival ranges from 26–57% [144, 145].

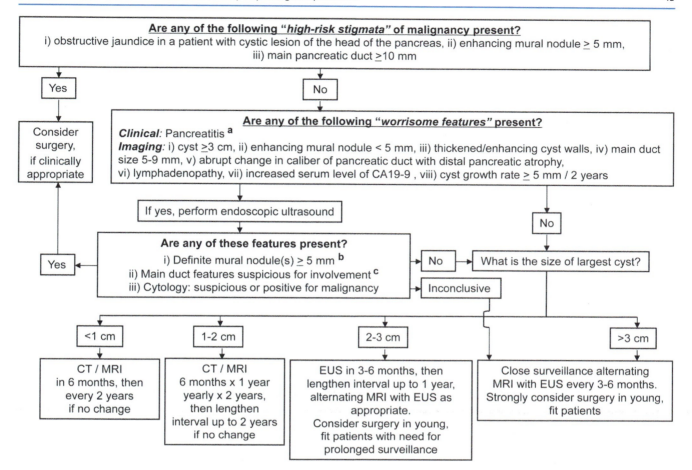

Fig. 5.5 Fukuoko guidelines for the management of IPMN of the pancreas. (**a**) Pancreatitis may be an indication for surgery for relief of symptoms. (**b**) Differential diagnosis includes mucin. Mucin can move with change in patient position, may be dislodged on cyst lavage and does not have Doppler flow. Features of true tumor nodule include lack of mobility, presence of Doppler flow and FNA of nodule showing tumor tissue. (**c**) Presence of any one of thickened walls, intraductal mucin or mural nodules is suggestive of main duct involvement. In their absence main duct involvement is inconclusive. Abbreviations: *BD-IPMN* branch duct intraductal papillary mucinous neoplasm, *FNA* fine needle aspiration

5.5.4.3 Solid Pseudopapillary Neoplasm

Solid pseudopapillary neoplasms lack glandular cells, are defined by degenerative pseudopapillary structures, have a relatively good prognosis with low malignant potential (8–20% incidence of solid pseudopapillary carcinoma at resection and a 5 year overall survival of >95%) [141]. Given the excellent prognosis, surgery is the standard of care and may even be recommended for highly-selected patients with locally advanced, metastatic, or recurrent disease [141, 142].

5.6 Malignant Pancreas Disease: Pathophysiology and Indications for Surgical Treatment

The most common primary pancreas cancer is pancreatic ductal adenocarcinoma, but other types of pancreas cancer can develop from cystic neoplasms (intraductal papillary mucinous cystadenocarcinoma, mucinous cystadenocarcinoma, solid pseudopapillary carcinoma, and even serous cystadenocarcinoma, although this is exceedingly rare), and neuroendocrine neoplasms (discussed previously).

5.6.1 Pancreas Adenocarcinoma

Pancreatic ductal adenocarcinoma (PDAC) arises from malignant transformation of ductal epithelial cells in association with PCN or pancreatic intraepithelial neoplasia (PanIN). Kras mutations are thought to promote dysplastic transformation of ductal epithelial cells to form PanIN-1 lesions which propagate to PanIN-2 and PanIN-3 lesions before progressing to invasive ductal adenocarcinoma. This propagation may be further promoted by other genetic aberrancies (i.e. CDKN2A, TP53, SMAD4, BRCA2, PRSS1) and synergistic environmental exposure (i.e. smoking, alcohol, obesity, chronic pancreatitis) [146]. PDAC is also associated with hereditary breast and ovarian cancer syndrome (BRCA1/2 genes), hereditary breast cancer (PALB2 gene), familial atypical multiple mole melanoma (p16/CDKN2A gene), familial pancreatitis (PRSS1 gene), lynch syndrome/HNPCC (MLH1/MLH2 genes), and Peutz-Jeghers syndrome (STK11 gene). Prognosis is stage dependent: 5 year survival is 37% for localized disease, 12% for regional disease, and 3% for metastatic disease [147]. Unfortunately, most patients present with either regional or distant disease [147].

Management should be approached from a multidisciplinary perspective of radiologists, pathologists, medical and radiation oncologists, and pancreas surgeons. Given the advanced stage at time of diagnosis in majority of patients, in addition to a poor prognosis, it is critical that the care team and patient communicate effectively about patient goals. While resection with a negative margin (R0) remains the only hope for longtime survival, systemic therapy is essential to any surgical approach and should be planned in conjunction [148–152]. Surgery based on the location of the tumor might include pancreaticoduodenectomy or distal pancreatectomy with regional lymphadenectomy. Biliary and enteric reconstruction are required for pancreas head cancers. Vascular resection and reconstruction may be required to achieve negative resection margins [153–155]. Unfortunately, despite aggressive surgery and advances in systemic therapy, the median post-treatment survival remains 15–18 months [149, 150, 153–157].

References

1. Talwani R, Gilliam BL, Howell C. Infectious diseases and the liver. Clin Liver Dis. 2011;15:111–30.
2. Toro A, Mahfouz AE, Ardiri A, et al. What is changing in indications and treatment of hepatic hemangiomas. A Rev Ann Hepatol. 2014;13:327–39.
3. Bajenaru N, Balaban V, Savulescu F, Campeanu I, Patrascu T. Hepatic hemangioma-review. J Med Life. 2015;8 Spec Issue:4–11.
4. Marrero JA, Ahn J, Rajender Reddy K, Americal College of G. ACG clinical guideline: the diagnosis and management of focal liver lesions. Am J Gastroenterol. 2014;109:1328–47; quiz 48.
5. Gemer O, Moscovici O, Ben-Horin CL, Linov L, Peled R, Segal S. Oral contraceptives and liver hemangioma: a case-control study. Acta Obstet Gynecol Scand. 2004;83:1199–201.
6. Lee JH, Yoon CJ, Kim YH, et al. Living-donor liver transplantation for giant hepatic hemangioma with diffuse hemangiomatosis in an adult: a case report. Clin Mol Hepatol. 2018;24:163–8.
7. Okazaki N, Yoshino M, Yoshida T, Ohno T, Kitagawa T. Radiotherapy of hemangioma cavernosum of the liver. Gastroenterology. 1977;73:353–6.
8. Biswal BM, Sandhu M, Lal P, Bal CS. Role of radiotherapy in cavernous hemangioma liver. Indian J Gastroenterol. 1995;14:95–8.
9. Gaspar L, Mascarenhas F, da Costa MS, Dias JS, Afonso JG, Silvestre ME. Radiation therapy in the unresectable cavernous hemangioma of the liver. Radiother Oncol. 1993;29:45–50.
10. Mathieu D, Kobeiter H, Maison P, et al. Oral contraceptive use and focal nodular hyperplasia of the liver. Gastroenterology. 2000;118:560–4.
11. Cole CA, Wirth PH. Health care litigation: recent trends in the law of noneconomic damages – emotional distress. Med Staff Couns. 1990;4:41–9.
12. Lantinga MA, Gevers TJ, Drenth JP. Evaluation of hepatic cystic lesions. World J Gastroenterol. 2013;19:3543–54.
13. Carrim ZI, Murchison JT. The prevalence of simple renal and hepatic cysts detected by spiral computed tomography. Clin Radiol. 2003;58:626–9.
14. Rawla P, Sunkara T, Muralidharan P, Raj JP. An updated review of cystic hepatic lesions. Clin Exp Hepatol. 2019;5:22–9.
15. Macedo FI. Current management of noninfectious hepatic cystic lesions: a review of the literature. World J Hepatol. 2013;5:462–9.
16. Choi HK, Lee JK, Lee KH, et al. Differential diagnosis for intrahepatic biliary cystadenoma and hepatic simple cyst: significance of cystic fluid analysis and radiologic findings. J Clin Gastroenterol. 2010;44:289–93.
17. Moorthy K, Mihssin N, Houghton PW. The management of simple hepatic cysts: sclerotherapy or laparoscopic fenestration. Ann R Coll Surg Engl. 2001;83:409–14.
18. Ardito F, Bianco G, Vellone M, et al. Long-term outcome after laparoscopic fenestration of simple liver cysts. Surg Endosc. 2013;27:4670–4.
19. Zhang JY, Liu Y, Liu HY, Chen L, Su DW, Wang YB. Comparison of the recurrence rates of nonparasitic hepatic cysts treated with laparoscopy or with open fenestration: a meta-analysis. Surg Laparosc Endosc Percutan Tech. 2018;28:67–72.
20. Liau SS, Qureshi MS, Praseedom R, Huguet E. Molecular pathogenesis of hepatic adenomas and its implications for surgical management. J Gastrointest Surg. 2013;17:1869–82.
21. Chang CY, Hernandez-Prera JC, Roayaie S, Schwartz M, Thung SN. Changing epidemiology of hepatocellular adenoma in the United States: review of the literature. Int J Hepatol. 2013;2013:604860.
22. Lee PJ. Glycogen storage disease type I: pathophysiology of liver adenomas. Eur J Pediatr. 2002;161(Suppl 1):S46–9.
23. Bieze M, Phoa SS, Verheij J, van Lienden KP, van Gulik TM. Risk factors for bleeding in hepatocellular adenoma. Br J Surg. 2014;101:847–55.
24. Stoot JH, Coelen RJ, De Jong MC, Dejong CH. Malignant transformation of hepatocellular adenomas into hepatocellular carcinomas: a systematic review including more than 1600 adenoma cases. HPB (Oxford). 2010;12:509–22.
25. Vedie AL, Sutter O, Ziol M, Nault JC. Molecular classification of hepatocellular adenomas: impact on clinical practice. Hepat Oncol. 2018;5:HEP04.
26. Park YS, Lee CH, Kim JW, Shin S, Park CM. Differentiation of hepatocellular carcinoma from its various mimickers in liver magnetic resonance imaging: What are the tips when using hepatocyte-specific agents? World J Gastroenterol. 2016;22:284–99.
27. Bieze M, van den Esschert JW, Nio CY, et al. Diagnostic accuracy of MRI in differentiating hepatocellular adenoma from focal nodular hyperplasia: prospective study of the additional value of gadoxetate disodium. AJR Am J Roentgenol. 2012;199:26–34.
28. Dhingra S, Fiel MI. Update on the new classification of hepatic adenomas: clinical, molecular, and pathologic characteristics. Arch Pathol Lab Med. 2014;138:1090–7.
29. Wang X, Hassan W, Zhao J, et al. The impact of hepatocyte nuclear factor-1alpha on liver malignancies and cell stemness with metabolic consequences. Stem Cell Res Ther. 2019;10:315.
30. Zucman-Rossi J, Jeannot E, Nhieu JT, et al. Genotype-phenotype correlation in hepatocellular adenoma: new classification and relationship with HCC. Hepatology. 2006;43:515–24.

31. Shang S, Hua F, Hu ZW. The regulation of beta-catenin activity and function in cancer: therapeutic opportunities. Oncotarget. 2017;8:33972–89.
32. Farges O, Dokmak S. Malignant transformation of liver adenoma: an analysis of the literature. Dig Surg. 2010;27:32–8.
33. Bossen L, Gronbaek H, Lykke Eriksen P, Jepsen P. Men with biopsy-confirmed hepatocellular adenoma have a high risk of progression to hepatocellular carcinoma: A nationwide population-based study. Liver Int. 2017;37:1042–6.
34. Tsilimigras DI, Rahnemai-Azar AA, Ntanasis-Stathopoulos I, et al. Current approaches in the management of hepatic adenomas. J Gastrointest Surg. 2019;23:199–209.
35. van Aalten SM, Witjes CD, de Man RA, Ijzermans JN, Terkivatan T. Can a decision-making model be justified in the management of hepatocellular adenoma? Liver Int. 2012;32:28–37.
36. Rhim H, Lim HK, Kim YS, Choi D. Percutaneous radiofrequency ablation of hepatocellular adenoma: initial experience in 10 patients. J Gastroenterol Hepatol. 2008;23:e422–7.
37. van Vledder MG, van Aalten SM, Terkivatan T, de Man RA, Leertouwer T, Ijzermans JN. Safety and efficacy of radiofrequency ablation for hepatocellular adenoma. J Vasc Interv Radiol. 2011;22:787–93.
38. van Rosmalen BV, Coelen RJS, Bieze M, et al. Systematic review of transarterial embolization for hepatocellular adenomas. Br J Surg. 2017;104:823–35.
39. Arnaoutakis DJ, Kim Y, Pulitano C, et al. Management of biliary cystic tumors: a multi-institutional analysis of a rare liver tumor. Ann Surg. 2015;261:361–7.
40. Thomas KT, Welch D, Trueblood A, et al. Effective treatment of biliary cystadenoma. Ann Surg. 2005;241:769–73; discussion 73–5.
41. Guglielmi A, Ruzzenente A, Conci S, Valdegamberi A, Iacono C. How much remnant is enough in liver resection? Dig Surg. 2012;29:6–17.
42. Shindoh J, Tzeng CW, Aloia TA, et al. Optimal future liver remnant in patients treated with extensive preoperative chemotherapy for colorectal liver metastases. Ann Surg Oncol. 2013;20:2493–500.
43. Kamath PS, Kim WR, Advanced Liver Disease Study G. The model for end-stage liver disease (MELD). Hepatology. 2007;45:797–805.
44. Kamath PS, Wiesner RH, Malinchoc M, et al. A model to predict survival in patients with end-stage liver disease. Hepatology. 2001;33:464–70.
45. Mittal S, El-Serag HB. Epidemiology of hepatocellular carcinoma: consider the population. J Clin Gastroenterol. 2013;47(Suppl):S2–6.
46. Varbobitis I, Papatheodoridis GV. The assessment of hepatocellular carcinoma risk in patients with chronic hepatitis B under antiviral therapy. Clin Mol Hepatol. 2016;22:319–26.
47. Teufel A, Staib F, Kanzler S, Weinmann A, Schulze-Bergkamen H, Galle PR. Genetics of hepatocellular carcinoma. World J Gastroenterol. 2007;13:2271–82.
48. Llovet JM, Montal R, Sia D, Finn RS. Molecular therapies and precision medicine for hepatocellular carcinoma. Nat Rev Clin Oncol. 2018;15:599–616.
49. Pons F, Varela M, Llovet JM. Staging systems in hepatocellular carcinoma. HPB (Oxford). 2005;7:35–41.
50. Jarnagin W, Chapman WC, Curley S, et al. Surgical treatment of hepatocellular carcinoma: expert consensus statement. HPB (Oxford). 2010;12:302–10.
51. de Ridder J, de Wilt JH, Simmer F, Overbeek L, Lemmens V, Nagtegaal I. Incidence and origin of histologically confirmed liver metastases: an explorative case-study of 23,154 patients. Oncotarget. 2016;7:55368–76.
52. Petrowsky H, Gonen M, Jarnagin W, et al. Second liver resections are safe and effective treatment for recurrent hepatic metastases from colorectal cancer: a bi-institutional analysis. Ann Surg. 2002;235:863–71.
53. Lemke J, Cammerer G, Ganser J, et al. Survival and prognostic factors of colorectal liver metastases after surgical and nonsurgical treatment. Clin Colorectal Cancer. 2016;15:e183–e92.
54. Ueno S, Sakoda M, Kitazono M, et al. Is delayed liver resection appropriate for patients with metachronous colorectal metastases? Ann Surg Oncol. 2011;18:1104–9.
55. Tan MC, Castaldo ET, Gao F, et al. A prognostic system applicable to patients with resectable liver metastasis from colorectal carcinoma staged by positron emission tomography with [18F] fluoro-2-deoxy-D-glucose: role of primary tumor variables. J Am Coll Surg 2008;206:857-68; discussion 68–9.
56. Hallet J, Sa Cunha A, Adam R, et al. Factors influencing recurrence following initial hepatectomy for colorectal liver metastases. Br J Surg. 2016;103:1366–76.
57. House MG, Ito H, Gonen M, et al. Survival after hepatic resection for metastatic colorectal cancer: trends in outcomes for 1,600 patients during two decades at a single institution. J Am Coll Surg. 2010;210(744–52):52–5.
58. Imai K, Allard MA, Benitez CC, et al. Early recurrence after hepatectomy for colorectal liver metastases: what optimal definition and what predictive factors? Oncologist. 2016;21:887–94.
59. Vigano L, Capussotti L, Lapointe R, et al. Early recurrence after liver resection for colorectal metastases: risk factors, prognosis, and treatment. A LiverMetSurvey-based study of 6,025 patients. Ann Surg Oncol. 2014;21:1276–86.
60. Yu X, Gu J, Wu H, Fu D, Li J, Jin C. Resection of liver metastases: a treatment provides a long-term survival benefit for patients with advanced pancreatic neuroendocrine tumors: a systematic review and meta-analysis. J Oncol. 2018;2018:6273947.
61. Fairhurst K, Leopardi L, Satyadas T, Maddern G. The safety and effectiveness of liver resection for breast cancer liver metastases: a systematic review. Breast. 2016;30:175–84.
62. de Groen PC, Gores GJ, LaRusso NF, Gunderson LL, Nagorney DM. Biliary tract cancers. N Engl J Med. 1999;341:1368–78.
63. Khan SA, Toledano MB, Taylor-Robinson SD. Epidemiology, risk factors, and pathogenesis of cholangiocarcinoma. HPB (Oxford). 2008;10:77–82.
64. Patel T. New insights into the molecular pathogenesis of intrahepatic cholangiocarcinoma. J Gastroenterol. 2014;49:165–72.
65. Weber SM, Ribero D, O'Reilly EM, Kokudo N, Miyazaki M, Pawlik TM. Intrahepatic cholangiocarcinoma: expert consensus statement. HPB (Oxford). 2015;17:669–80.
66. Rahnemai-Azar AA, Weisbrod AB, Dillhoff M, Schmidt C, Pawlik TM. Intrahepatic cholangiocarcinoma: current management and emerging therapies. Expert Rev Gastroenterol Hepatol. 2017;11:439–49.
67. Kumar A, Sharma B, Samant H. Cancer, liver angiosarcoma. StatPearls Treasure Island (FL). 2020.
68. Venneman NG, van Erpecum KJ. Pathogenesis of gallstones. Gastroenterol Clin N Am. 2010;39:171–83, vii.
69. Lee SP, LaMont JT, Carey MC. Role of gallbladder mucus hypersecretion in the evolution of cholesterol gallstones. J Clin Invest. 1981;67:1712–23.
70. Ostrow JD. The etiology of pigment gallstones. Hepatology. 1984;4:215S–22S.
71. Sjodahl R, Tagesson C, Wetterfors J. On the pathogenesis of acute cholecystitis. Surg Gynecol Obstet. 1978;146:199–202.
72. den Hoed PT, Boelhouwer RU, Veen HF, Hop WC, Bruining HA. Infections and bacteriological data after laparoscopic and open gallbladder surgery. J Hosp Infect. 1998;39:27–37.
73. Reinders JS, Kortram K, Vlaminckx B, van Ramshorst B, Gouma DJ, Boerma D. Incidence of bactobilia increases over time after endoscopic sphincterotomy. Dig Surg. 2011;28:288–92.

74. Yokoe M, Hata J, Takada T, et al. Tokyo Guidelines 2018: diagnostic criteria and severity grading of acute cholecystitis (with videos). J Hepatobiliary Pancreat Sci. 2018;25:41–54.
75. Strasberg SM. Commentary on: feasibility and value of the critical view of safety in difficult cholecystectomies. Ann Surg. 2019;269:e42.
76. Strasberg SM, Brunt LM. The critical view of safety: why it is not the only method of ductal identification within the standard of care in laparoscopic cholecystectomy. Ann Surg. 2017;265:464–5.
77. Strasberg SM, Brunt LM. Rationale and use of the critical view of safety in laparoscopic cholecystectomy. J Am Coll Surg. 2010;211:132–8.
78. Rosen M, Brody F, Ponsky J. Predictive factors for conversion of laparoscopic cholecystectomy. Am J Surg. 2002;184:254–8.
79. Alponat A, Kum CK, Koh BC, Rajnakova A, Goh PM. Predictive factors for conversion of laparoscopic cholecystectomy. World J Surg. 1997;21:629–33.
80. Kanaan SA, Murayama KM, Merriam LT, et al. Risk factors for conversion of laparoscopic to open cholecystectomy. J Surg Res. 2002;106:20–4.
81. Strasberg SM, Pucci MJ, Brunt LM, Deziel DJ. Subtotal cholecystectomy-"fenestrating" vs "reconstituting" subtypes and the prevention of bile duct injury: definition of the optimal procedure in difficult operative conditions. J Am Coll Surg. 2016;222:89–96.
82. van Dijk AH, Donkervoort SC, Lameris W, et al. Short- and long-term outcomes after a reconstituting and fenestrating subtotal cholecystectomy. J Am Coll Surg. 2017;225:371–9.
83. Byrne MF, Suhocki P, Mitchell RM, et al. Percutaneous cholecystostomy in patients with acute cholecystitis: experience of 45 patients at a US referral center. J Am Coll Surg. 2003;197:206–11.
84. Hatzidakis AA, Prassopoulos P, Petinarakis I, et al. Acute cholecystitis in high-risk patients: percutaneous cholecystostomy vs conservative treatment. Eur Radiol. 2002;12:1778–84.
85. Vauthey JN, Lerut J, Martini M, Becker C, Gertsch P, Blumgart LH. Indications and limitations of percutaneous cholecystostomy for acute cholecystitis. Surg Gynecol Obstet. 1993;176:49–54.
86. Patil R, Ona MA, Papafragkakis C, Anand S, Duddempudi S. Endoscopic ultrasound-guided placement of the lumen-apposing self-expandable metallic stent for gallbladder drainage: a promising technique. Ann Gastroenterol. 2016;29:162–7.
87. St George CM, Shaffer EA. Spontaneous obesity and increased bile saturation in the ground squirrel. J Surg Res. 1993;55:314–6.
88. Agarwal AK, Kalayarasan R, Javed A, Sakhuja P. Mass-forming xanthogranulomatous cholecystitis masquerading as gallbladder cancer. J Gastrointest Surg. 2013;17:1257–64.
89. Hale MD, Roberts KJ, Hodson J, Scott N, Sheridan M, Toogood GJ. Xanthogranulomatous cholecystitis: a European and global perspective. HPB (Oxford). 2014;16:448–58.
90. Parithivel VS, Gerst PH, Banerjee S, Parikh V, Albu E. Acute acalculous cholecystitis in young patients without predisposing factors. Am Surg. 1999;65:366–8.
91. Ryu JK, Ryu KH, Kim KH. Clinical features of acute acalculous cholecystitis. J Clin Gastroenterol. 2003;36:166–9.
92. Savoca PE, Longo WE, Zucker KA, McMillen MM, Modlin IM. The increasing prevalence of acalculous cholecystitis in outpatients. Results of a 7-year study. Ann Surg. 1990;211:433–7.
93. Gu MG, Kim TN, Song J, Nam YJ, Lee JY, Park JS. Risk factors and therapeutic outcomes of acute acalculous cholecystitis. Digestion. 2014;90:75–80.
94. Hakala T, Nuutinen PJ, Ruokonen ET, Alhava E. Microangiopathy in acute acalculous cholecystitis. Br J Surg. 1997;84:1249–52.
95. Warren BL. Small vessel occlusion in acute acalculous cholecystitis. Surgery. 1992;111:163–8.
96. Wang AJ, Wang TE, Lin CC, Lin SC, Shih SC. Clinical predictors of severe gallbladder complications in acute acalculous cholecystitis. World J Gastroenterol. 2003;9:2821–3.
97. Colonna AL, Griffiths TM, Robison DC, et al. Cholecystostomy: Are we using it correctly? Am J Surg. 2019;217:1010–5.
98. Ziessman HA. Hepatobiliary scintigraphy in 2014. J Nucl Med Technol. 2014;42:249–59.
99. Middleton GW, Williams JH. Diagnostic accuracy of 99Tcm-HIDA with cholecystokinin and gallbladder ejection fraction in acalculous gallbladder disease. Nucl Med Commun. 2001;22:657–61.
100. Collins C, Maguire D, Ireland A, Fitzgerald E, O'Sullivan GC. A prospective study of common bile duct calculi in patients undergoing laparoscopic cholecystectomy: natural history of choledocholithiasis revisited. Ann Surg. 2004;239:28–33.
101. European Association for the Study of the Liver. Electronic address eee. EASL Clinical Practice Guidelines on the prevention, diagnosis and treatment of gallstones. J Hepatol. 2016;65:146–181.
102. Dasari BV, Tan CJ, Gurusamy KS, et al. Surgical versus endoscopic treatment of bile duct stones. Cochrane Database Syst Rev. 2013:CD003327.
103. Tranter SE, Thompson MH. Spontaneous passage of bile duct stones: frequency of occurrence and relation to clinical presentation. Ann R Coll Surg Engl. 2003;85:174–7.
104. Kochar B, Akshintala VS, Afghani E, et al. Incidence, severity, and mortality of post-ERCP pancreatitis: a systematic review by using randomized, controlled trials. Gastrointest Endosc. 2015;81(143-9):e9.
105. Cotton PB, Durkalski V, Romagnuolo J, et al. Effect of endoscopic sphincterotomy for suspected sphincter of Oddi dysfunction on pain-related disability following cholecystectomy: the EPISOD randomized clinical trial. JAMA. 2014;311:2101–9.
106. Geenen JE, Hogan WJ, Dodds WJ, Toouli J, Venu RP. The efficacy of endoscopic sphincterotomy after cholecystectomy in patients with sphincter-of-Oddi dysfunction. N Engl J Med. 1989;320:82–7.
107. Neoptolemos JP, Bailey IS, Carr-Locke DL. Sphincter of Oddi dysfunction: results of treatment by endoscopic sphincterotomy. Br J Surg. 1988;75:454–9.
108. Todani T, Watanabe Y, Narusue M, Tabuchi K, Okajima K. Congenital bile duct cysts: Classification, operative procedures, and review of thirty-seven cases including cancer arising from choledochal cyst. Am J Surg. 1977;134:263–9.
109. Soares KC, Arnaoutakis DJ, Kamel I, et al. Choledochal cysts: presentation, clinical differentiation, and management. J Am Coll Surg. 2014;219:1167–80.
110. Singham J, Yoshida EM, Scudamore CH. Choledochal cysts: part 1 of 3: classification and pathogenesis. Can J Surg. 2009;52:434–40.
111. Todani T, Tabuchi K, Watanabe Y, Kobayashi T. Carcinoma arising in the wall of congenital bile duct cysts. Cancer. 1979;44:1134–41.
112. Dyson JK, Beuers U, Jones DEJ, Lohse AW, Hudson M. Primary sclerosing cholangitis. Lancet. 2018;391:2547–59.
113. Lee YM, Kaplan MM. Primary sclerosing cholangitis. N Engl J Med. 1995;332:924–33.
114. Rosen CB, Nagorney DM. Cholangiocarcinoma complicating primary sclerosing cholangitis. Semin Liver Dis. 1991;11:26–30.
115. Razumilava N, Gores GJ, Lindor KD. Cancer surveillance in patients with primary sclerosing cholangitis. Hepatology. 2011;54:1842–52.
116. Marsh JW Jr, Iwatsuki S, Makowka L, et al. Orthotopic liver transplantation for primary sclerosing cholangitis. Ann Surg. 1988;207:21–5.
117. Ponsioen CY, Arnelo U, Bergquist A, et al. No superiority of stents vs balloon dilatation for dominant strictures in patients with primary sclerosing cholangitis. Gastroenterology. 2018;155:752–9 e5.
118. Pawlik TM, Olbrecht VA, Pitt HA, et al. Primary sclerosing cholangitis: role of extrahepatic biliary resection. J Am Coll Surg 2008;206:822–30; discussion 30–2.

119. Bjoro K, Schrumpf E. Liver transplantation for primary sclerosing cholangitis. J Hepatol. 2004;40:570–7.
120. Costamagna G, Boskoski I. Current treatment of benign biliary strictures. Ann Gastroenterol. 2013;26:37–40.
121. Bismuth H, Nakache R, Diamond T. Management strategies in resection for hilar cholangiocarcinoma. Ann Surg. 1992;215:31–8.
122. Sahani D, Prasad SR, Tannabe KK, Hahn PF, Mueller PR, Saini S. Thorotrast-induced cholangiocarcinoma: case report. Abdom Imaging. 2003;28:72–4.
123. Welzel TM, Graubard BI, El-Serag HB, et al. Risk factors for intrahepatic and extrahepatic cholangiocarcinoma in the United States: a population-based case-control study. Clin Gastroenterol Hepatol. 2007;5:1221–8.
124. Soares KC, Kamel I, Cosgrove DP, Herman JM, Pawlik TM. Hilar cholangiocarcinoma: diagnosis, treatment options, and management. Hepatobiliary Surg Nutr. 2014;3:18–34.
125. Valero V 3rd, Cosgrove D, Herman JM, Pawlik TM. Management of perihilar cholangiocarcinoma in the era of multimodal therapy. Expert Rev Gastroenterol Hepatol. 2012;6:481–95.
126. Nagino M, Nimura Y, Nishio H, et al. Hepatectomy with simultaneous resection of the portal vein and hepatic artery for advanced perihilar cholangiocarcinoma: an audit of 50 consecutive cases. Ann Surg. 2010;252:115–23.
127. Ebata T, Ercolani G, Alvaro D, Ribero D, Di Tommaso L, Valle JW. Current status on cholangiocarcinoma and gallbladder cancer. Liver Cancer. 2016;6:59–65.
128. Meyer CG, Penn I, James L. Liver transplantation for cholangiocarcinoma: results in 207 patients. Transplantation. 2000;69:1633–7.
129. Heimbach JK, Gores GJ, Haddock MG, et al. Liver transplantation for unresectable perihilar cholangiocarcinoma. Semin Liver Dis. 2004;24:201–7.
130. D'Angelica M, Dalal KM, DeMatteo RP, Fong Y, Blumgart LH, Jarnagin WR. Analysis of the extent of resection for adenocarcinoma of the gallbladder. Ann Surg Oncol. 2009;16:806–16.
131. Ishihara S, Horiguchi A, Miyakawa S, Endo I, Miyazaki M, Takada T. Biliary tract cancer registry in Japan from 2008 to 2013. J Hepatobiliary Pancreat Sci. 2016;23:149–57.
132. Elfar M, Gaber LW, Sabek O, Fischer CP, Gaber AO. The inflammatory cascade in acute pancreatitis: relevance to clinical disease. Surg Clin North Am. 2007;87:1325–40, vii.
133. Banks PA, Bollen TL, Dervenis C, et al. Classification of acute pancreatitis – 2012: revision of the Atlanta classification and definitions by international consensus. Gut. 2013;62:102–11.
134. van Santvoort HC, Besselink MG, Bakker OJ, et al. A step-up approach or open necrosectomy for necrotizing pancreatitis. N Engl J Med. 2010;362:1491–502.
135. Bakker OJ, van Santvoort HC, van Brunschot S, et al. Endoscopic transgastric vs surgical necrosectomy for infected necrotizing pancreatitis: a randomized trial. JAMA. 2012;307:1053–61.
136. Whitcomb DC, Frulloni L, Garg P, et al. Chronic pancreatitis: an international draft consensus proposal for a new mechanistic definition. Pancreatology. 2016;16:218–24.
137. Andersen DK, Frey CF. The evolution of the surgical treatment of chronic pancreatitis. Ann Surg. 2010;251:18–32.
138. Vinik A, Perry RR, Casellini C, Hughes MS, Feliberti E. Pathophysiology and Treatment of Pancreatic Neuroendocrine Tumors (PNETs): new developments. In: Feingold KR, Anawalt B, Boyce A, et al., eds. Endotext. South Dartmouth (MA) 2000.
139. Falconi M, Eriksson B, Kaltsas G, et al. ENETS consensus guidelines update for the management of patients with functional pancreatic neuroendocrine tumors and non-functional pancreatic neuroendocrine tumors. Neuroendocrinology. 2016;103:153–71.
140. Kim J, Zimmerman MA, Hong JC. Liver transplantation in the treatment of unresectable hepatic metastasis from neuroendocrine tumors. J Gastrointest Oncol. 2020;11:601–8.
141. European Study Group on Cystic Tumours of the P. European evidence-based guidelines on pancreatic cystic neoplasms. Gut. 2018;67:789–804.
142. Pusateri AJ, Krishna SG. Pancreatic cystic lesions: pathogenesis and malignant potential. Diseases. 2018;6.
143. Hasan A, Visrodia K, Farrell JJ, Gonda TA. Overview and comparison of guidelines for management of pancreatic cystic neoplasms. World J Gastroenterol. 2019;25:4405–13.
144. Crippa S, Salvia R, Warshaw AL, et al. Mucinous cystic neoplasm of the pancreas is not an aggressive entity: lessons from 163 resected patients. Ann Surg. 2008;247:571–9.
145. Jang KT, Park SM, Basturk O, et al. Clinicopathologic characteristics of 29 invasive carcinomas arising in 178 pancreatic mucinous cystic neoplasms with ovarian-type stroma: implications for management and prognosis. Am J Surg Pathol. 2015;39:179–87.
146. Maitra A, Hruban RH. Pancreatic cancer. Annu Rev Pathol. 2008;3:157–88.
147. Society AC. Cancer Facts & Figures 2020. Atlanta, GA: American Cancer Society; 2020.
148. Ghaneh P, Kleeff J, Halloran CM, et al. The impact of positive resection margins on survival and recurrence following resection and adjuvant chemotherapy for pancreatic ductal adenocarcinoma. Ann Surg. 2019;269:520–9.
149. Neoptolemos JP, Moore MJ, Cox TF, et al. Effect of adjuvant chemotherapy with fluorouracil plus folinic acid or gemcitabine vs observation on survival in patients with resected periampullary adenocarcinoma: the ESPAC-3 periampullary cancer randomized trial. JAMA. 2012;308:147–56.
150. Neoptolemos JP, Palmer DH, Ghaneh P, et al. Comparison of adjuvant gemcitabine and capecitabine with gemcitabine monotherapy in patients with resected pancreatic cancer (ESPAC-4): a multicentre, open-label, randomised, phase 3 trial. Lancet. 2017;389:1011–24.
151. Neoptolemos JP, Stocken DD, Dunn JA, et al. Influence of resection margins on survival for patients with pancreatic cancer treated by adjuvant chemoradiation and/or chemotherapy in the ESPAC-1 randomized controlled trial. Ann Surg. 2001;234:758–68.
152. Neoptolemos JP, Stocken DD, Tudur Smith C, et al. Adjuvant 5-fluorouracil and folinic acid vs observation for pancreatic cancer: composite data from the ESPAC-1 and -3(v1) trials. Br J Cancer. 2009;100:246–50.
153. Martin RC 2nd, Scoggins CR, Egnatashvili V, Staley CA, McMasters KM, Kooby DA. Arterial and venous resection for pancreatic adenocarcinoma: operative and long-term outcomes. Arch Surg. 2009;144:154–9.
154. Kluger MD, Rashid MF, Rosario VL, et al. Resection of locally advanced pancreatic cancer without regression of arterial encasement after modern-era neoadjuvant therapy. J Gastrointest Surg. 2018;22:235–41.
155. Yekebas EF, Bogoevski D, Cataldegirmen G, et al. En bloc vascular resection for locally advanced pancreatic malignancies infiltrating major blood vessels: perioperative outcome and long-term survival in 136 patients. Ann Surg. 2008;247:300–9.
156. Bockhorn M, Burdelski C, Bogoevski D, Sgourakis G, Yekebas EF, Izbicki JR. Arterial en bloc resection for pancreatic carcinoma. Br J Surg. 2011;98:86–92.
157. Psarelli EE, Jackson R, Neoptolemos JP, et al. Beyond ESPAC-4: better surgery and systemic therapy. Lancet. 2017;389:1517–8.

Biliary Tract Functions and Impairment

6

Hideo Ohtsuka and Michiaki Unno

Abstract

The biliary tract includes the entire biliary excretion route from the liver to the duodenum. Bile is secreted from hepatocytes into the bile canaliculi. It is eventually excreted into the duodenum after passing through the biliary tract. The main components of bile include bile acids, phospholipids, cholesterols, and bilirubin. Some of these substances are reabsorbed in the intestine and returned to the liver via the portal vein, a cycle termed enterohepatic circulation. Enterohepatic circulation involves physiologically active substances and ensures its effective use. The function of the biliary tract is controlled by the autonomic nervous system. Branches from the hepatic plexus, which is formed by the sympathetic nerves and the vagus nerve, are distributed across the biliary tract. The sphincter of Oddi at the papilla and gallbladder play important roles in the control of the bile efflux, and dysfunctions can occur when their motility is inhibited. The gallbladder dysfunction is a motility disorder and causes pain similar to chronic cholecystitis. The sphincter of Oddi regulates the excretion of bile and prevents the regurgitation of duodenal juice. In papillary dysfunction, the sphincter of Oddi is excessively contracted, which inhibits the excretion of bile and pancreatic juice. Pancreaticobiliary maljunction is a congenital malformation in which the pancreatic duct and the bile duct join outside the duodenal wall. In this condition, the sphincter of Oddi does not regulate the confluence of the pancreatic duct and bile duct, resulting in bidirectional regurgitation of bile and pancreatic juice and various complications in the bile duct and the pancreas.

H. Ohtsuka · M. Unno (✉)
Department of Surgery, Tohoku University, Sendai, Miyagi, Japan
e-mail: m_unno@surg.med.tohoku.ac.jp

6.1 The Structure of the Biliary Tract

The biliary tract collectively refers to the bile ducts and the gallbladder. It includes the entire biliary excretion route from the liver to the duodenum. Bile is secreted into the bile canaliculi, which are located between hepatocytes. Bile passes through the terminal cholangioles (canals of Haring ductules, diameter < 15 μm) and interlobular ductules (15–100 μm) before entering the intrahepatic bile ducts and then passes through the left and right hepatic ducts and the common hepatic duct to the duodenum [1, 2] (Fig. 6.1). The intrahepatic bile ducts course parallel to a branch of the portal vein and with one or two branches of the hepatic artery, forming Glisson's triads, which are also referred to as portal triads. The cystic duct joins the gallbladder to the common hepatic duct. The cystic duct is approximately 2–3 cm long and 2–3 mm in diameter. The confluence of the cystic duct and the common hepatic duct forms the common bile duct, which opens into the duodenal cavity through the pancreatic parenchyma after coursing through the posterior side of the first part of the duodenum. The opening of the common bile

Classification of Bile ducts	
Intrahepatic bile ducts	
Small bile ducts (peribiliary grands(-))	
terminal cholangioles (canals of Haring ductules)	15 μm >
Interlobular bile duct	15 – 100 μm
Septal duct	100 – 300 μm
Large bile ducts (peribiliary grands(+))	
Area duct	300 – 400 μm
Segmental duct	400 – 800 μm
Extrahepatic bile ducts	
Left and Right hepatic duct	800 μm <
Common hepatic duct	

Fig. 6.1 Classification of the bile ducts according to the ductal diameter

M. Makuuchi et al. (eds.), *The IASGO Textbook of Multi-Disciplinary Management of Hepato-Pancreato-Biliary Diseases*,
https://doi.org/10.1007/978-981-19-0063-1_6

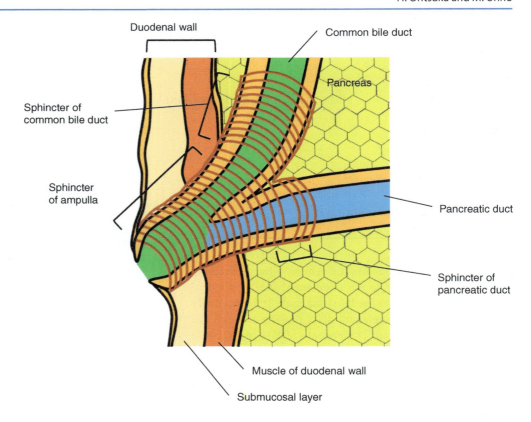

Fig. 6.2 Anatomy of the sphincter of Oddi and ampulla of Vater

duct and the pancreatic duct in the duodenum form the ampulla of Vater. In approximately 80% of individuals, the common bile duct joins the pancreatic duct in the duodenal wall and forms the common channel [3]. The sphincter of Oddi is located in the ampulla of Vater and it serves to prevent regurgitation of both bile and pancreatic juice in the common bile and pancreatic ducts, respectively (Fig. 6.2). The function of the biliary tract is controlled by the autonomic nervous system, specifically the celiac ganglia of the sympathetic nervous system and the vagus nerve of the parasympathetic nervous system. Branches from the hepatic plexus, which is formed by the sympathetic nerves and the vagus nerve, are distributed across the gallbladder, bile ducts, and papilla to control the biliary tract [4].

6.2 The Functions of the Biliary Tract

6.2.1 Gallbladder

The efflux of bile into the duodenum is controlled via the functional integration of the gastrointestinal and neuroendocrine systems. The gallbladder, which is contracted by muscular tissue, and the sphincter of Oddi at the duodenal papilla play important roles in the control of the efflux of bile.

The gallbladder is comprised of a single layer of epithelial cells, a lamina propria layer, a muscularis propria layer, a layer of perimuscular connective tissue, and a serosa layer [5]. The epithelium of the gallbladder absorbs water and electrolytes and concentrates the gallbladder bile, which contains bile acids. The epithelium is also involved in the uptake of bile acid and cholesterol [6]. Bile acid is the main component of bile and is made of several different specific acids. Hydrophobic bile acids are cytotoxic. The epithelium of the gallbladder and bile ducts secrete mucin, which protects the epithelial cells by inactivating free radicals produced by the hydrophobic bile acids.

The contraction and relaxation of the gallbladder are controlled by the vagus nerve, visceral nerves, and cholecystokinin (CCK), a gastrointestinal hormone. Between periods of digestion, the sphincter of Oddi is contracted and the gallbladder is relaxed. This leads to the secretion of bile from the liver into the gallbladder via the hepatic ducts. Approximately 90% of bile flows into the gallbladder and is stored there. The gallbladder maintains a moderate level of tonic contraction between periods of digestion. It repeatedly relaxes and contracts with the cycle of the migrating motor complex (MMC) in the upper gastrointestinal tract [7]. The concentrated bile tends to precipitate in the fundus and the body of the gallbladder. The repeated contraction and relaxation improves the concentration efficiency of the bile by replacing precipitated bile with a relatively lower concentration of bile in the upper gallbladder. The repeated contraction and relaxation also prevents cholesterol deposition, which can lead to the formation of insoluble bile components, including gallstones [8]. When food reaches the duodenum, CCK is secreted from the duodenum and jejunum. CCK induces the contraction of the gallbladder and the relaxation of the sphincter of Oddi, leading to the excretion of the stored bile into the duodenum. As in the other parts of the gastrointestinal tract, the motility of the gallbladder during digestion is affected by the cephalic phase, antral phase, and duodenal phase of digestion [9]. The cephalic phase is initiated by stimulation from the central nervous system, such as olfactory and taste sensations. The gallbladder contracts upon stimulation from the vagus nerve system, and approximately 30–40% of bile is released from the gallbladder at this stage. When food reaches the stomach, a reflex is induced in the area from the pyloric antrum to the gallbladder (the antral phase). During the duodenal phase, when food reaches the duodenum, CCK is released from the duodenum and proximal jejunum and almost all of the remaining content of the gallbladder is excreted [10].

6.2.2 Sphincter of Oddi

The sphincter of Oddi is a smooth muscle structure that is approximately 1 cm long. It regulates the junction of the bile duct and pancreatic duct at the duodenum, preventing regurgitation of bile and pancreatic fluid as well as contents of the duodenum (Fig. 6.2). The functions of the sphincter of Oddi are regulated by the neuroendocrine system [11]. Between periods of digestion, the sphincter of Oddi contracts in a peristaltic manner, which regulates the outflow of bile into the duodenum and helps store the bile in the gallbladder. During digestion, CCK and autonomic nerves relax the sphincter of Oddi and the adjacent segment of the duodenum in a coordinated manner. This helps excrete bile into the duodenum efficiently. The relaxation of the sphincter of Oddi by autonomic nerves involves stimulation mediated by nonadrenergic inhibitory neurons from the vagus nerve and the neurospinal reflex with visceral nerves as afferent and efferent pathways. Morphine and pentazocine contract the sphincter of Oddi and increase the internal pressure of the biliary tract. In contrast, atropine, butylscopolamine bromid, nitroglycerin, and calcium channel blockers relax muscles, leading to reduced tension and inhibited motility [12].

6.3 Impairment of Biliary Tract

6.3.1 Gallbladder Dysfunction

The gallbladder and sphincter of Oddi contain muscle fibers. Dysfunctions of these organs can occur when their motility is inhibited. Gallbladder dysfunction is a motility disorder caused by metabolic abnormalities or a direct motility disturbance of the gallbladder, though this condition has not been clearly defined. Gallbladder dysfunction causes pain similar to chronic cholecystitis [13]. According to the Rome IV criteria, a set of diagnostic criteria used to diagnose functional gastrointestinal disorders, gallbladder motility disorders should be diagnosed when moderate-to-severe pain persists for 30 min or longer in an area from the epigastric region to the right hypochondrium region [14]. Furthermore, gallstones and other organic abnormalities need to be ruled out via imaging examinations (such as an abdominal ultrasonography) before motility disorders can be diagnosed. A reduced gallbladder ejection fraction is observed on provocative cholescintigraphy in patients with gallbladder motility disorders when CCK is administered intravenously. A laparoscopic cholecystectomy relieves the symptoms of gallstones and gallbladder motility disorders.

6.3.2 Dysfunction of the Sphincter of Oddi

The sphincter of Oddi regulates the excretion of bile and pancreatic juice and prevents the regurgitation of duodenal juice into the bile ducts and pancreatic duct. In papillary dysfunction, the sphincter of Oddi is excessively contracted, which inhibits the excretion of bile and pancreatic juice [14, 15]. This leads to increased internal pressure of the bile ducts and the pancreatic duct, causing various symptoms. Dysfunction of the sphincter of Oddi can be broadly classified into pancreatic and biliary types. The pancreatic type is characterized by an increase in the blood pancreatic enzymes, amylase, and lipase, accompanied by symptoms such as abdominal pain. The biliary type is frequently observed in patients who have developed persistent or recurrent abdominal pain after a cholecystectomy and is characterized by elevations of alanine transaminase (ALT) and alkaline phosphatase (ALP), as well as dilation of the bile ducts. Nifedipine and nitroglycerin can be administered to treat dysfunction of the sphincter of Oddi. An endoscopic papillotomy can be performed if the drugs are ineffective, and surgery is performed if the papillotomy is ineffective.

6.3.3 Pancreaticobiliary Maljunction

Pancreaticobiliary maljunction is a congenital malformation in which the pancreatic duct and the bile duct join outside the duodenal wall, forming a long common channel. In patients with pancreaticobiliary maljunction, the sphincter of Oddi does not regulate the confluence of the pancreatic duct and bile duct, resulting in bidirectional regurgitation of bile and pancreatic juice. Due to the reciprocating flow of pancreatic juices and bile, various complications may develop in the bile duct and the pancreas. Reflux of pancreatic juice into the biliary tract is associated with a high incidence of cholangitis and cholangiocarcinoma. Congenital biliary dilatation, which is also known as "congenital choledochal cyst," is a disease in which the extrahepatic bile duct, or both the extra and intrahepatic bile ducts, is dilated in various ways and involves pancreaticobiliary maljunction. In cases with congenital biliary dilatation, because there is an increased incidence of extrahepatic bile duct cancer or gallbladder cancer, prophylactic resection of the dilated extrahepatic biliary duct and gallbladder followed by hepaticojejunostomy is considered as a standard treatment [16].

6.4 The Functions of Bile

6.4.1 The Physiology of Bile

Bile is weakly alkaline (pH: 7.1–7.3) and the total amount of bile produced and secreted per day is 600–1200 mL. The main components of bile include bile acids, phospholipids, cholesterols, and bilirubin. Bile also contains proteins, inorganic salts, and metabolized or detoxified drugs. Hepatic bile is excreted into the bile canaliculi and stored in the gallbladder via the bile ducts. Water and electrolytes are reabsorbed in the gallbladder by the epithelium and concentrated 5- to 10-fold to form gallbladder bile. Bile can be divided into bile in the canaliculi, which is produced by hepatocytes, and bile secreted from the cholangiocytes of the epithelium. The secretion of bile in the canaliculi consists of bile acid-dependent bile flow and bile acid-independent bile flow [17]. These two types of bile flow lead to the excretion of sodium ions and water into the bile ducts. Bile acid-dependent bile flow uses bile acid, which is actively excreted from the hepatocytes; bile acid-independent bile flow uses glutathione, which is also excreted from the hepatocytes. Bile secreted from the cholangiocytes contains a large amount of bicarbonate and is secreted via Cystic fibrosis transmembrane conductance regulator (CFTR), a chloride ion channel [18] (Fig. 6.3). Secretin, a digestive hormone, facilitates the secretion of bile in the bile ducts via cyclic adenosine monophosphate (cAMP); in contrast somatostatin, gastrin, and insulin block secretin receptors and suppress the secretion of bile in the bile ducts [19, 20].

6.4.2 Enterohepatic Circulation

Bile is secreted from hepatocytes into the bile canaliculi. It is eventually excreted into the duodenum after passing through the biliary system. Bile contains biological substances and drugs that are metabolized in the liver. Some of these sub-

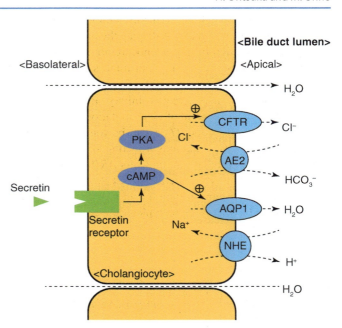

Fig. 6.3 Regulation of cholangiocyte bicarbonate secretion by secretin. *AQP* aquaporin, *AE2* Cl^-/HCO_3^- anion exchanger 2, *NHE* Na^+/H^+ exchanger, *PKA* protein kinase A

stances are reabsorbed in the intestine and returned to the liver via the portal vein to be secreted second time, a cycle termed enterohepatic circulation. Enterohepatic circulation involves bile acid that is synthesized in the liver and physiologically active substances, including vitamin D3, vitamin B12, and folic acid, and ensures the effective use of these substances. Drugs such as morphine, warfarin, and digoxin are metabolized in the liver and enter the enterohepatic circulation. These drugs are excreted into bile after being conjugated with glucuronide in the hepatocytes. Glucuronide conjugates are highly polar and not easily absorbed in the small intestine. However, they are hydrolyzed by β-glucuronidase from the enteric bacteria and metabolized to parent compounds. This increases the lipid solubility and intestinal absorption of the compounds.

6.4.3 Bile Acids

Bile acid consists of primary bile acids (cholic acid and chenodeoxycholic acid) and secondary bile acids (deoxycholic acid and lithocholic acid). Primary bile acids are synthesized from cholesterol in the hepatocytes, and secondary bile acids are produced through the biotransformation of primary bile acid by the enteric bacteria. Bile acid is amphiphilic, containing both hydrophilic and hydrophobic parts within its molecules. Therefore, bile acid acts as a biological surfactant, forming micelles that have an outer hydrophilic part and an inner hydrophobic part. Human bile acid contains a large number of conjugated amino acids, such as glycine and taurine. Compared to free bile acid, conjugated bile acid is highly polar with increased solubility. Bile acid is excreted into the intestine, and the majority of bile acid is reabsorbed in the small intestine through enterohepatic circulation. Uptake in the sinusoidal membrane and the excretory system in the canalicular membranes of hepatocytes play an important role in this mechanism. Sodium-dependent taurocholate co-transporting polypeptide (NTCP), a sodium-dependent transport carrier, and organic anion transporting polypeptide (OATP), a sodium-independent transport carrier, are involved in the uptake of bile acids in the sinusoidal membrane [21]. While NTCP has a high substrate-specificity for bile acid, OATP is also involved in the uptake of hydrophobic organic compounds, such as bilirubin and indocyanine green. The excretion of bile acid from hepatocytes is regulated by drug transporters, such as bile salt export pump (BSEP) and multidrug resistance-associated proteins 2 and 3 (MRP2 and MRP3). BSEP and MRP2 are expressed in the bile canaliculi, and MRP3 is expressed in the sinusoidal membrane of hepatocytes [20]. These efflux transporters are considered to perform ATP-dependent primary active transport.

6.4.4 Cholesterol and Bile Pigments

The cholesterol in the bile is in the hydrophobic free form rather than the hydrophilic ester form. Cholesterol is one of the hydrophobic substances that are dissolved by the mixed micelles formed by bile acids and phospholipids. Cholesterol precipitates as crystals and forms gallstones when the cholesterol content in bile is higher than the number of bile acids and phospholipids.

The color of bile and stool is affected by bile pigments. One of the most important bile pigments is bilirubin. Bilirubin is derived from heme proteins, such as hemoglobin, catalase, and cytochrome. It is taken up by OATPs, which are expressed in the cell membrane on the vascular side of hepatocytes. Bilirubin is secreted into bile by the efflux transporter MRP2 after being conjugated with glucuronide. Conjugated bilirubin is reduced and metabolized to urobilinogen by the enteric bacteria and excreted in the feces. Part of the bilirubin is reabsorbed through enterohepatic circulation.

6.4.5 Nuclear Receptors and Bile Acid Metabolism

The metabolism of cholesterol and bile acid is primarily regulated by the nuclear receptors Liver X Receptor (LXR) and Farnesoid X Receptor (FXR) [22] (Fig. 6.4). LXR is activated by the ligand oxysterol. LXR facilitates the synthesis of bile acid by upregulating the activity of cholesterol-7α-

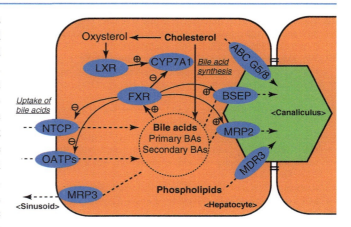

Fig. 6.4 Cholesterol and bile acid metabolism in the hepatocyte

hydroxylase (CYP7A1). FXR is activated by the ligand bile acid. FXR inhibits CYP7A1 and reduces the expression of NTCP and OATP. Together, these regulatory mechanisms lead to increased or decreased hepatic cholesterol levels. The synthesis of bile acid increases when hepatic cholesterol levels are high. In contrast, when bile acid levels are high, bile acid synthesis decreases.

References

1. Saxena R and Theise. Canals of Hering: recent insights and current knowledge. Semin Liver Dis. 2004;24:43–48.
2. Ludwig J. New concepts in biliary cirrhosis. Semin Liver Dis. 1987;7:293–301.
3. RienHoff WF, Pickrell KR. Pancreatitis; an anatomic study of the pancreatic and extrahepatic biliary systems. Arch Surg. 1945;51:205–19.
4. Berthoud HR, Kressel M, Neuhuber WL. An anterograde tracing study of the vagal innervation of rat liver, portal vein and biliary system. Anat Embryol (Berl). 1992;186:431–42.
5. Odze RD, Goldblum JR, editors. Surgical pathology of the GI tract, liver, biliary tract and pancreas, chapter 29, part 2. Philadelphia, PA: Saunders; 2009.
6. Svanvik J, Pellegrini CA, Allen R, et al. Transport of fluid and biliary lipids in the canine gallbladder in experimental cholecystitis. J Surg Res. 1986;41:425–31.
7. Itoh Z, Takahashi I. Periodic contractions of the canine gallbladder during the interdigestive state. Am J Phys. 1981;240:183–9.
8. Behar L, Lee KY, Thompson WR, et al. Gallbladder contraction in patients with pigment and cholesterol stones. Gastroenterology. 1989;97:1479–84.
9. Takahashi I, Kern MK, Dodds WJ, et al. Contraction pattern of opossum gallbladder during fasting and after feeding. Am J Phys. 1986;250:227–35.
10. Burhol PG, Rayford PL, Jorde R, et al. Radioimmunoassay of plasma cholecystokinin (CCK), duodenal release of CCK, diurnal variation of plasma CCK, and immunoreactive plasma CCK components in man. Hepato-Gastroenterology. 1980;27:300–9.
11. Peeters TL, Vantrappen G, Janssens J. Bile acid output and the interdigestive migrating motor complex in normals and in cholecystectomy patients. Gastroenterology. 1980;79:678–81.

12. Toouli J, Baker RA. Innervation of the sphincter of Oddi: physiology and considerations of pharmacological intervention in biliary dyskinesia. Pharmac Ther. 1991;49:269–81.
13. Wu JM, Wu YM, Lee CY. Is early laparoscopic cholecystectomy a safe procedure in patients when the duration of acute cholecystitis is more than three days? Hepato-Gastroenterology. 2012;59:10–2.
14. Cotton PB. Gallbladder and sphincter of Oddi disorders. Gastroenterology. 2016;150:1420–9.
15. Sherman S, Troiano FP, Hawes RH, et al. Frequency of abnormal sphincter of Oddi manometry compared with the clinical suspicion of sphincter of Oddi dysfunction. Am J Gastroenterol. 1991;86:586–90.
16. Kamisawa T, Kaneko K, Itoi T, et al. Pancreaticobiliary maljunction and congenital biliary dilatation. Lancet Gastroenterol Hepatol. 2017;2:610–8.
17. Nathanson MH, Boyer JL. Mechanisms and regulation of bile secretion. Hepatology. 1991;14:551–66.
18. Kanno N, LeSege G, Glaser S, et al. Secretin regulation of Cholangiocyte bicarbonate secretion. Am J Phys. 2001;281:G612–25.
19. Glaser SS, Rodgers RE, Phinizy JL, et al. Gastrin inhibits secretin-induced ductal secretion by interaction with specific receptors on rat cholangiocytes. Am J Phys. 1997;273:G1061–70.
20. Lesage GD, Marucci L, Alvaro D, et al. Insulin inhibits secretin-induced ductal secretion by activation of PKC alpha and inhibition of PKA activity. Hepatology. 2002;36:641–51.
21. Paumgarter G. Biliary physiology and disease: reflactions of a physician-scientist. Hepatology. 2010;51:1095–106.
22. Calkin AC, Tontonoz P. Transcriptional integration of metabolism by the nuclear sterol-activated receptors LXR and FXR. Nat Rev Mol Cell Biol. 2012;13:213–24.

Preinvasive Intraductal Biliary Neoplasm: Biliary Intraepithelial Neoplasm and Intraductal Papillary Neoplasm of Bile Duct

Yasuni Nakanuma, Katsuhiko Uesaka, and Takuro Terada

Abstract

Biliary intraepithelial neoplasm (BilIN) and intraductal papillary neoplasm of the bile duct (IPNB), an intraductal non-invasive neoplasm, are being established pathologically as precursor lesions of invasive cholangiocarcinoma (CCA). These premalignant lesions are found in the extrahepatic and intrahepatic large bile duct but not in the intrahepatic small bile duct. BilINs are a microscopical lesion and can be classified into low-grade and high-grade. High-grade BilIN was previously called "*in situ carcinoma*" of the bile duct. This lesion is presumed to be followed by periductal nodular/sclerosing growth of CCA. The preoperative detection of high-grade BilIN may be an important step in the determination of the risk of CCA. In contrast, IPNB shows grossly exophytic growth in a dilated bile duct lumen, with histologically villous/papillary neoplastic epithelia with tubular components covering fine fibrovascular stalks. Interestingly, approximately half of IPNBs show stromal invasion (IPNB associated with invasive carcinoma) at the time of surgical resection. IPNBs are classified into low-grade and high-grade dysplasia. The recent subclassification of IPNB into types 1 (low-grade dysplasia and high-grade dysplasia with regular architecture) and 2 (high-grade dysplasia with irregular architecture) may be more practically applicable in the clinical field than two-tiered system (low- and high-grade dysplasia). The outcome of postoperative IPNBs is more favorable in IPNBs than in CCA via BilIN processes. The recent recognition of two preinvasive biliary neoplasms may facilitate further clinical and basic studies of CCA.

7.1 Introduction

The concept of epithelial tumors arising from non-invasive intraepithelial dysplasia or neoplasm is well-established in various human cancers [1]. Recent studies have shown that there are at least two types of preinvasive neoplasms of the bile ducts preceding cholangiocarcinoma (CCA): biliary intraepithelial neoplasm (BilIN) and intraductal papillary neoplasm of bile duct (IPNB) [2–5]. BilINs are microscopically identifiable epithelial neoplasm, while IPNBs are grossly visible epithelial neoplasms covering fine fibrovascular stalks (Figs. 7.1, 7.2). BilIN may be the most common precursor in nodular-sclerosing, perihilar and distal CCA (p/dCCA) and large-duct intrahepatic CCA (iCCA). IPNBs present unique pathological features, and about half of IPNBs present stromal invasion at the time of surgical resection. Recently, the World Health Organization (WHO) published the Classification of Digestive System Tumours fifth edition (2019), in which BilIN and IPNB were introduced in separate chapters [3, 4].

We herein review the pathological features of BilIN and IPNB, based on this WHO classification, with reference to the clinical and molecular and genetic features.

Y. Nakanuma (✉)
Department of Diagnostic Pathology, Shizuoka Cancer Center, Shizuoka, Japan

Department of Diagnostic Pathology, Fukui Prefecture Saiseikai Hospital, Fukui, Japan

K. Uesaka
Department of Hepatobiliary Pancreatic Surgery, Shizuoka Cancer Center, Shizuoka, Japan

T. Terada
Department of Gastrointestinal Surgery, Fukui Prefecture Saiseikai Hospital, Fukui, Japan

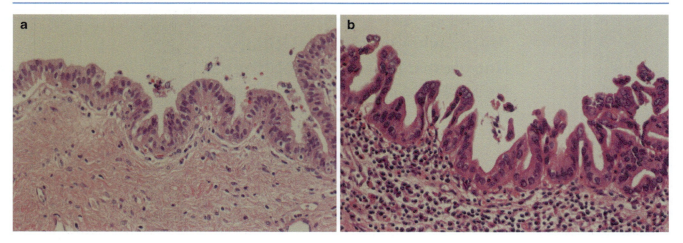

Fig. 7.1 Biliary intraepithelial neoplasm (BilIN) of bile duct. (**a**) Low-grade BilIN showing mild nuclear stratification and hyperchromasia. H&E. (**b**) High grade BilIN showing disordered nuclear polarity and pleomorphism. H&E

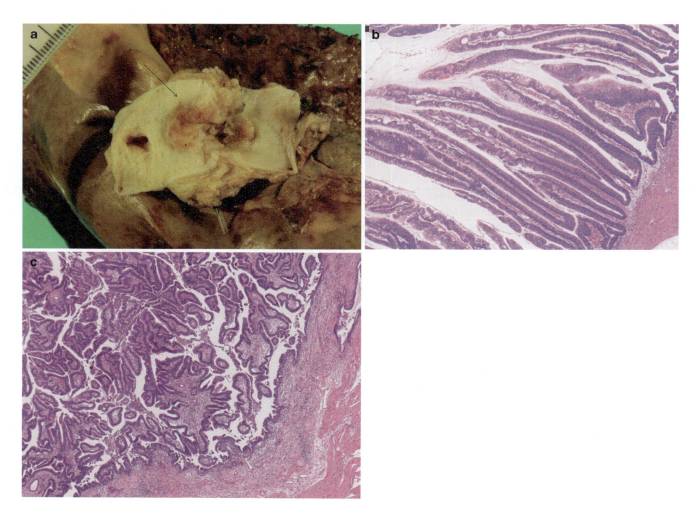

Fig. 7.2 Intraductal papillary neoplasm of bile duct (IPNB). (**a**) Grossly, papillary tumorous lesion (→) is found in the extrahepatic bile duct. (**b**) Type 1 IPNB. Regular papillary neoplasm is found in the bile duct. H&E. (**c**) Type 2 IPNB. Irregular papillary neoplasm with tubular component and widened stroma is found in the bile duct. H&E

7.1.1 Clinical Features, Risks, and Background Lesions and Imaging Findings of BilINs and IPNBs

7.1.1.1 Clinical Features, Risks, and Background Lesions

BilINs

There have been no reports on the clinical or laboratory features characteristic to BilINs. In the background in cases not associated with invasive CCAs, BilINs, particularly high-grade ones, are occasionally found in patients with hepatolithiasis, primary sclerosing cholangitis (PSC), liver fluke infection, and anomalous union of the pancreatic biliary duct and can also be found incidentally in bile duct and gallbladder specimens that are resected for other reasons [5, 6]. In addition, BilIN is often encountered in the mucosa adjacent to nodular/sclerosing CCA. BilINs are generally not associated with excessive mucin secretion.

IPNBs

IPNBs typically affect middle-aged to elderly adults and show a male predominance [7]. Intermittent or recurrent, right-upper-quadrant abdominal pain and acute cholangitis or jaundice are the most common clinical manifestations, but a certain percentage of patients have no symptoms at the diagnosis [7]. Elevated levels of alkaline phosphatase and CEA and CA19-9 have been reported, although they are unlikely to have high sensitivity or specificity for the diagnosis of IPNB [7].

IPNBs account for 10–38% of all bile duct tumors in East Asian populations but only 7–12% of all bile duct tumors in Western populations [8]. Hepatolithiasis and liver fluke infection (*Clonorchiasis sinensis* [CS] or *Opisthorchis viverrini* [OV] infection) are major risk factors of IPNB in Far Eastern countries [8]. IPNBs also reportedly develop in PSC and congenital biliary tract disease. Interestingly, these etiologic factors are also known as major risk factors for nodular-sclerosing p/dCCA and large-duct iCCA [2], suggesting that these factors may be causally related to the development of IPNB and also of CCA via the BilIN process [9].

Recently, an outbreak of IPNB was reported among young adult workers in the offset color proof-printing department at a printing company in Japan [10]. They were chronically exposed to chlorinated organic solvents, including dichloromethane and 1,2-dichloropropane. Interestingly, IPNB or IPNB associated with invasive carcinoma was predominantly observed in the dilated intrahepatic and perihilar bile ducts.

7.1.1.2 Imaging Findings

BilINs

BilIN lesions cannot be accurately identified preoperatively by existing imaging modalities. Occasionally, they are detected as focal bile duct stenosis or dilatation in cases not associated with CCA [11].

IPNB

The most important morphological changes are the presence of (a) bile duct dilatation, (b) intraductal mass(es), (c) cystic lesion(s), and (d) macro-invasion of the liver [12, 13]. The patterns of bile duct dilatation are diffuse duct ectasia, localized duct dilatation, and cystic dilatation. IPNB lesions were found more commonly at the right than left intrahepatic ducts and had more peripheral than central locations in patients with OV [11]. On US, IPNB was more variable with hyperechoic nodules (37.5%), focal bile duct dilatation (37.5%), and diffuse bile duct dilatation with intraductal nodules (25%) [11]. Magnetic resonance imaging (MRI) reveals IPNB as isointense to hypointense masses on T1-weighted images and hyperintense masses on T2-weighted images. On computed tomography (CT), the enhancement pattern of IPNB is isodense or hyperdense during the late arterial phase and not hyperdense during the portal-venous and delayed phase. Other findings obtained by CT are infiltration of the neoplasm along the duct wall and intense rim enhancement at the base of the lesion.

7.1.2 Pathologies of BilINs and IPNBs

7.1.2.1 Gross

BilIN

While BilIN lesions cannot be accurately identified grossly, they may be recognized as subtle and nonspecific granular or rough bile duct mucosa, particularly around invasive CCA [5, 6]. As for the anatomical location, the majority of BilIN cases not associated with CCA arose from the right intrahepatic duct, specifically from a peripheral branch of the inferoposterior and superoposterior segments in cases with OV infection [11].

IPNB

The majority of IPNBs (67%) were located at the intrahepatic bile ducts in Asian countries, while in Western countries, they were more common in the extrahepatic bile ducts or hepatic hilum [12–14]. Some cases simultaneously involved the intrahepatic and extrahepatic bile ducts. When

IPNB exists in the intrahepatic bile ducts, it tends to be found in the left-sided biliary ductal system [7]. However, IPNB in OV-infected patients was found more commonly at the right than left intrahepatic ducts and had more peripheral than central locations [11].

Generally, IPNBs present papillary or villous or polypoid, exophytic growth (range, 1–6 cm) (Fig. 7.2a) [2, 3, 5]; height, at least 5 mm from the adjacent biliary mucosa in the dilated bile ducts is typical; however, some papillary neoplasms with a similar histopathology that are <5 mm but >3 mm in height are occasionally encountered [15]. These exophytic lesions are usually conglomerates of smaller or higher polypoid lesions, but single or isolated polypoid lesions are also encountered. IPNBs located in the intrahepatic bile ducts tend to be larger in both mass and length than those in the extrahepatic bile ducts.

The gross features of IPNBs depend on their anatomical location, state of excessive mucin secretion, and macro-invasion of the liver [3, 12]. Some IPNBs, particularly those arising in the extrahepatic bile ducts, are associated with cylindrical or fusiform morphology with moderate dilatation of the affected bile ducts and appear as cast-like structures, while other IPNBs, particularly those in the intrahepatic bile duct, present with marked macroscopic dilatation or unilocular or multilocular cystic changes. These cystic changes represent cystic dilatation of the bile ducts and usually show luminal communication with the adjacent bile duct. The internal surfaces of the cystic lesions are smooth or finely granular, and papillary mural nodules are commonly observed. IPNBs may present separate multiple lesions of various stages along the biliary tree, both synchronously and dyssynchronously [7]. Some may represent multiple occurrences of IPNB in the bile duct mucosa with a neoplastic predisposition, while others are due to intraluminal implantation or dissemination of neoplastic cells of the main papillary tumor along the biliary tree [16]. Excessive mucin hypersecretion is more frequently observed in intrahepatic IPNBs than in extrahepatic IPNBs. Bile ducts with excessive mucin secretion located upstream and downstream from IPNBs are significantly dilated due to the large amount of mucin in the duct lumen.

A variable proportion of the mucosa around the main papillary conglomerate lesions shows visible granular or small papillary lesions, suggesting neoplastic mucosal changes that are continuous with the main lesion [3].

Controversial Cases: BilIN or IPNB
Some intraductal preinvasive biliary neoplasms present diffuse dilatation of the bile ducts without visible intraductal tumors on imaging and macroscopic observation because of their microscopic size [17]. Indeed, several case reports have described extensive bile duct dilatation filled with mucin and lined by a superficially spreading, microscopically identifiable, non-invasive biliary neoplasm despite no grossly visible identifiable papillary neoplasms [18]. Whether these cases correspond to a variant of BilIN with bile duct dilatation and mucin hypersecretion or should be regarded as a variant of IPNB with microscopic neoplastic size remains unclear.

7.1.2.2 Histologies

BilINs
BilINs show a flat or micropapillary, intraepithelial biliary neoplasm occasionally with glandular formation and are composed of enlarged columnar or cuboidal epithelial cells with stratified hyperchromatic nuclei and a high nucleus/cytoplasm ratio (Fig. 7.1a, b) [2, 4, 5]. Nuclear pleomorphism and nucleoli may be also found. The intramural peribiliary glands may be continuously involved. BilINs usually occur in the extrahepatic and intrahepatic large bile ducts but are also found in the gallbladder. While a majority of BIIINs are of pancreatobiliary phenotype, the gastric and intestinal phenotypes are also encountered.

Grading and Invasion A two-tiered grading system of "low" versus "high" is applied to BilINs in order to delineate the clinically significant examples from the insignificant ones. High-grade BilIN was previously called "*in situ carcinoma*" of the bile duct. The main differential features are shown in Table 7.1 [2, 4]. High-grade BilIN usually forms a field of lesional spread of neoplastic epithelial cells on the biliary mucosa. Immunohistologically, high-grade BilINs are constantly diffusely and strongly positive for S100P, a differential point from low-grade BilIN or reactive changes [5]. High-grade BilINs express CEA and MUC1 [19] and also selectively stain for insulin-like growth factor II mRNA binding protein (IMP3) [19].

High-grade BilINs are frequently found in the bile duct mucosa around nodular-sclerosing CCAs [2, 5, 16], with

Table 7.1 Comparison between low-grade BilIN and high-grade BilIN

Characters	Low-grade BilIN (BilIN-1/2)	High-grade BilIN (BilIN-3)
Histology	Flat/pseudopapillary/micropapillary	Flat/pseudopapillary/micropapillary
	Hyperchromatic nuclei	Hyperchromatic and irregular nuclei
	Increased N/C ratio	Increased N/C ratio, pleomorphic, bizarre nuclei
	Stratified or multi-layered nuclei	Single layered or stratified nuclei
	Reserved nuclear polarity	Disturbed nuclear polarity
Distribution in biliary mucosa	Relatively small foci or area	Relatively extensive area or spread
S-100P expression	Weakly or scattered expression	Strongly and diffusely positive

high-grade BilINs likely being a preceding lesion of these CCAs. Indeed, microscopic stromal invasion of tubular adenocarcinoma is occasionally found beneath high-grade BilINs in patients without grossly visible CCA, suggesting the actual development of invasion from high-grade BilIN resulting in conventional CCA.

IPNB.

IPNBs are a preinvasive, papillary/villous biliary neoplasm with variable tubular components covering fine fibrovascular stalks or with fibrous stroma in dilated bile ducts (Fig. 7.2b, c). Some cases of IPNB, particularly oncocytic subtype, show mildly widened stroma due to edema with inflammatory cell infiltration [3]. The histology of IPNB is heterogeneous, depending on the subtypes and grade of atypia.

Four Subtypes IPNBs are histologically classifiable into four subtypes based on their cell lineages: intestinal IPNB (iIPNB), gastric IPNB (gIPNB), pancreatobiliary IPNB (pbIPNB), and oncocytic IPNB (oIPNB) [2, 3]. While many cases are predominantly composed of an individual subtype, admixtures of foci of other subtypes and cases with controversial subtyping are sometimes observed. This subtyping is facilitated by immunohistochemistry to detect mucus core proteins and cytokeratins. As for the incidence, iIPNB is the most common subtype, followed by gIPNB, pbIPNB, and oIPNB. There are no apparent differences in sex or age among the four subtypes of IPNB.

Grading of Atypia IPNBs are traditionally classified into low-grade and high-grade, mainly based on the cellular atypia and structural alterations, particularly nuclear atypia and alteration [2, 3, 20]. For example, the high-grade IPNBs show hyperchromatic nuclei, nucleoli, nuclear and cellular pleomorphism, and a loss of polarity, while the low-grade IPNBs do not. Some IPNBs are low-grade, while others are high-grade or high-grade with low-grade foci.

IPNBs show structural changes or alterations: some cases show regular papillary, villous or tubular structures, and a relatively homogeneous appearance (type 1), while others show irregular papillary, villous or tubular structures, and a heterogeneous appearance (type 2). Mainly based on these structural alterations, Japan–Korea biliary pathologists propose a new subclassification of IPNB into types 1 and 2 [15]. IPNBs with a low-grade (about 10% of all IPNBs) and those with a high-grade with regular structures (30%) belong to type 1, while the remaining IPNBs with a high grade and irregular structures (60%) belong to type 2. In type 1, papillary fibrovascular stalks are generally thin (depending on the subtype), while fibrovascular stalks are variably widened at the basal side in some cases. In addition, type 2 does not

Table 7.2 Type 1 and 2 subclassification of intraductal papillary neoplasms of bile duct (IPNB)

	Type 1 IPNB	Type 2 IPNB
Structures	* Regular villous, papillary, or tubular structures * Homogeneous appearance	* Irregular and complicated villous, papillary or tubular structures * Heterogeneous appearance
Atypia of intraepithelial neoplasm	* Low-grade dysplasia * High-grade dysplasia with regular histologies	* High-grade dysplasia with irregular histologies
Location at the biliary tree	*Usually intrahepatic bile duct	*Intrahepatic and extrahepatic bile duct
Mucin overproduction	* Frequent	* Infrequent
Stromal invasion	* Rare	* Common
Subtypes		
• Intestinal subtype	* Infrequent	* Frequent
• Gastric subtype	* Equal	* Equal
• PB subtype	* Infrequent	* Frequent
• Oncocytic subtype	* Frequent	* Infrequent
Similarities to prototypic subtypes of IPMN	* Similar (depending on subtypes)	* Different variably (depending on subtype)
Poor differentiation such as solid or cribriform pattern, coagulative necrosis, overt malignant features, cystic changes	* Almost absent	* Frequent
Highly atypical cellular and nuclear changes	* Absent	* Infrequent
Fibrovascular stalks	* Thin (depending on subtype)	* Thin to widened (depending on subtype)

infrequently show foci of complicated lesions, such as cribriform and solid components, and relatively large cystic changes and foci of bizarre cells and nuclear changes. Coagulative necrosis is also experienced in type 2. Neuroendocrine differentiation has been reported in type 2 IPNB. The main differential features between types 1 and 2 are shown in Table 7.2.

As for other characteristics, type 1 tends to arise in the intrahepatic bile ducts, while type 2 develops similarly in the extrahepatic and intrahepatic bile ducts. Furthermore, according to recent studies, types 1 and 2 show other clinicopathological and molecular-genetic differences [21–23]: Type 1 IPNBs were frequently associated with a noninvasive, intestinal and oncocytic subtypes, development in the intrahepatic bile ducts, mucin hypersecretion, a relatively good prognosis and old age, while type 2 IPNBs were associated with an invasive, pancreatobiliary subtype, frequent development within the extrahepatic bile ducts and a worse prognosis than type 1 IPNBs.

Invasion A surgical series demonstrated high rates of invasive cancer arising from IPNB, with rates ranging from 40% to 70% [7]. However, the incidence of invasion differs according to the anatomical location of IPNB, with approximately 30% of cases of intrahepatic IPNBs invasive, while many extrahepatic IPNBs show at least focal stromal invasion at the time of surgical resection [15, 19, 23], implying that intrahepatic IPNBs are less aggressive than extrahepatic IPNBs. The invasive parts of IPNBs usually show tubular adenocarcinoma with a desmoplastic reaction and only occasionally show foci of colloid carcinoma. The oncocytic subtype shows invasion of oncocytic adenocarcinoma.

7.1.3 Pathogenesis: Molecular and Genetic Alterations of BilINs and IPNBs

BilIN and IPNB share key pathogenetic and molecular pathways but show some differences.

7.1.3.1 Progression of BilINs and IPNBs
The growth pattern of BilIN progresses from flat/micropapillary projections to eventually develop the periductal growth pattern of CCA showing tubular adenocarcinoma [2, 4]. IPNB may also sequentially progress from low-grade to high-grade and then to invasive adenocarcinoma (IPNB associated with invasive carcinoma) [3]. Chronic biliary inflammation may induce neoplastic changes of the biliary epithelia including BilINs in chronic biliary diseases.

7.1.3.2 Molecular Alterations in BilINs and IPNBs
BilIN and IPNB have shown the stepwise acquisition of molecular alterations affecting common oncogenic pathways, such as cell-cycle related molecules [3, 14, 24]. For example, p21, cyclin D1, and Dpc4 were shown to be involved in the carcinogenesis of BilIN and IPNB, while the p53 expression was regulated differently between BilIN and IPNB. The loss of SMAD4 is a late molecular change in BilIN lesions. A decreased membranous expression of β-catenin and E-cadherin is an early event in the tumorigenesis of both BilIN and IPNB lineages. Cyclin D1 and c-myc, target molecules of Wnt signaling, were frequently positive in the IPNB lineage, and interestingly, nuclear β-catenin staining was observed only in the IPNB lineage, suggesting the importance of Wnt signaling in the tumorigenesis of the IPNB lineage. The increased expression of autophagy-related proteins in low- and high-grade BilIN, IPNB, and invasive carcinoma suggests the role of dysregulated autophagy at an early stage of BilIN and IPNB in hepatolithiasis [24].

The overexpression of the polycomb group protein enhancer of zeste homolog 2 (EZH2) is also involved in the progression of BilIN and IPNB [19, 25]. The expression of p16 INK4a was decreased in high-grade BilIN and invasive carcinoma, while EZH2 expression showed a stepwise increase from low-grade to high-grade BilIN to invasive carcinoma, suggesting that the overexpression of EZH2 may induce hypermethylation of p16 INK4a promoter followed by decreased expression of p16 INK4a in the progression of BilIN in hepatolithiasis. The overexpression of EZH2 may also be associated with malignant behavior in IPNB in parallel with the upregulated MUC1 expression and downregulated MUC6 expression [24, 25].

7.1.3.3 Genetic Changes in BilIN and IPNB

BilIN
KRAS mutations are already identifiable in low-grade BilIN and slightly increase during progression to high-grade BilIN and invasive adenocarcinoma in hepatolithiasis cases [26]. In contrast to IPNB, BilIN lesions do not seem to harbor GNAS1 mutations. The downregulation of miR-451a and miR-144-3p, a tumor suppressor, was recently reported along with the progression of BilIN supporting the concept of BilIN as a direct precursor of invasive dCCA [1].

IPNB
Yang et al. identified frequent mutations of *KRAS* (49%), *GNAS* (32%), *RNF43* (24%), *APC* (24%), *TP53* (24%), and *CTNNB1* (11%) in IPNBs [21]. *KRAS* and *p16* alterations occur early and in tumors with low-grade IPNB and precede the increased expression of *PT53* [27].

Four Subtypes of IPNB In eastern Asia, *GNAS* mutations were detected in fewer than half of all cases of IPNB, and all cases with *GNAS* mutations had intestinal differentiation [22, 28–30]. Mutations in RNF43, a tumor suppressor gene, were also frequent in the intestinal IPNB [29, 30]. When divided into the intrahepatic and extrahepatic classifications, in intestinal IPNBs arising in the intrahepatic bile ducts, *GNAS* and *KRAS* mutations are frequent, as is observed in intestinal IPMN [28]. As for non-intestinal IPNBs, mutations in *APC* or *CTNNB1*, both of which belong to the Wnt/β-catenin pathway, were observed in one-fourth of IPNBs and were mutually exclusive [31]. Interestingly, *APC* and *CTNNB1* alterations were unique to IPNB [31]. Mutations of genes also seen in colorectal neoplasms, such as *SMAD4*, *PIK3CA*, *APC*, and *CTNNB1*, were frequent in intestinal IPNBs of the extrahepatic bile ducts [28], and the pancreatobiliary subtype arising in the extrahepatic bile ducts also showed a *CTNNB1* mutation [30, 31]. Given these previous findings, the activation of the Wnt/β-catenin signaling pathway may be relevant to the development and progression of non-intestinal-type IPNBs as well as iIPNBs arising in the extrahepatic bile ducts [31].

7.1.4 The Prognosis and Outcomes of BilINs and IPNBs

7.1.4.1 BilIN

Although high-grade BilIN group is a neoplasia with malignant potential, the prognostic significance remains controversial. While the survival and recurrence outcomes of patients with high-grade BilIN at the surgical margin were shown to be similar to those without it in one report [32], high-grade dysplasia of the bile duct margin in patients with surgically resected node-negative perihilar CCA was associated with a poor survival in another study [33]. Yoon et al. reported that the presence of BilIN lesions was not uncommon in CCA patients and was significantly associated with a better disease-free survival and overall survival in extrahepatic CCA patients [34]. A meta-analysis with unified criteria is necessary in order to evaluate the significance of high-grade BilIN at the surgical margin of nodular/sclerosing CCA.

7.1.4.2 IPNB

The median postoperative survival of IPNB patients is favorable compared with conventional CCA via BilIN carcinogenesis [7, 35, 36]. Luvira et al. reported that the median postoperative survival of 102 IPNB patients was 1728 days, with 1-, 3-, and 5-year overall survival rates of 86.3%, 63.7%, and 44.8%, respectively [8]. Factors that have been reported to be associated with adverse outcomes include high serum CA19-9, lymph node metastasis, R0 or R1/2 resection, invasive IPNB, tumor multiplicity, and the high expression of MUC1 in the tumor tissue [2, 7, 20]. The survival of IPNB patients with cystic variant with micropapillary lesions was shown to be favorable, and intrahepatic IPNB shows a favorable prognosis compared with IPNBs arising in the extrahepatic bile ducts. Type 1 is known to be associated with a favorable prognosis, while type 2 is associated with a worse prognosis [15], and recent studies have validated the significance [22, 23]. Recurrence of IPNB or CCA after surgical resection of IPNB may occur due to the implantation or cancerization of neoplastic cells.

7.2 Conclusion

BilIN and IPNB are main precursor lesions of CCA: BilINs are microscopic lesions, while IPNBs are grossly visible lesions. IPNBs are divided into intestinal, gastric, pancreatobiliary, and oncocytic subtypes, with the intestinal subtype the most common followed by the other subtypes; in contrast, a majority of BilINs are of the pancreatobiliary type. Both BilINs and IPNBs are graded by a two-tiered system: low-grade and high-grade. In addition, IPNBs are subclassified into types 1 and 2, with type 1 composed of low-grade IPNB and high-grade IPNB with regular structures and type 2 composed of high-grade IPNB with irregular structures. Type 1 and 2 IPNBs show differing clinicopathological features, including a different mucus overproduction and postoperative survival and unique genetic alterations. Recognition of these two intraductal preinvasive biliary epithelial neoplasms will encourage the better understanding of the clinicopathological features and therapeutic approach to CCA.

References

1. Loeffler MA, Hu J, Kirchner M, et al. miRNA profiling of biliary intraepithelial neoplasia reveals stepwise tumorigenesis in distal cholangiocarcinoma via the miR-451a/ATF2 axis. J Pathol. 2020;252(3):239–51.
2. Nakanuma Y, Sudo Y. Biliary tumors with pancreatic counterparts. Semin Diagn Pathol. 2017;34(2):167–75.
3. Nakanuma Y, Basturk O, Esposito I, et al. Intraductal papillary neoplasm of the bile duct. In: The WHO Classification of Tumours Editoral Board. WHO Classification of Tumors, Digestive System Tumours . 5th ed., Lyon: International Agency for Research on Cancer. 2019. pp. 279–82.
4. Basturk O, Aishima S, Esposito I. Biliary intraepithelial neoplasia. In: The WHO Classification of Tumours Editoral Board. WHO Classification of Tumors, Digestive System Tumours. 5th ed., Lyon: International Agency for Research on Cancer. 2019. pp. 273–5.
5. Hucl T. Precursors to cholangiocarcinoma. Gastroenterol Res Pract. 2019 Nov 13; eCollection 2019.
6. Nakanuma Y, Uchida T, Sato Y, et al. An S100P-positive biliary epithelial field is a preinvasive intraepithelial neoplasm in nodular-sclerosing cholangiocarcinoma. Hum Pathol. 2017;60:46–57.
7. Gordon-Weeks AN, Jones K, Harriss E, et al. Systematic review and meta-analysis of current experience in treating IPNB: Clinical and pathological correlates. Ann Surg. 2016;263(4):656–63.
8. Luvira V, Pugkhem A, Bhudhisawasdi V, et al. Long-term outcome of surgical resection for intraductal papillary neoplasm of the bile duct. J Gastroenterol Hepatol. 2017;32(2):527–33.
9. Nakanuma Y, Kakuda Y. Pathologic classification of cholangiocarcinoma: New concepts. Best Pract Res Clin Gastroenterol. 2015;29(2):277–93.
10. Kubo S, Nakanuma Y, Takemura S, et al. Case series of 17 patients with cholangiocarcinoma among young adult workers of a printing company in Japan. J Hepatobiliary Pancreat Sci. 2014;21(7):479–88.
11. Siripongsakun S, Sapthanakorn W, Mekraksakit P, et al. Premalignant lesions of cholangiocarcinoma: characteristics on ultrasonography and MRI. Abdom Radiol (NY). 2019;44(6):2133–46.
12. Luvira V, Somsap K, Pugkhem A, et al. Morphological classification of intraductal papillary neoplasm of the bile duct with survival correlation. Asian Pac J Cancer Prev. 2017;18(1):207–13.
13. Yoon HJ, Kim YK, Jang KT, et al. Intraductal papillary neoplasm of the bile ducts: description of MRI and added value of diffusion-weighted MRI. Abdom Imaging. 2013;38(5):1082–90.
14. Schlitter AM, Born D, Bettstetter M, et al. Intraductal papillary neoplasms of the bile duct: stepwise progression to carcinoma involves common molecular pathways. Mod Pathol. 2014;27(1):73–86.
15. Nakanuma Y, Jang KT, Fukushima N, et al. A statement by the Japan-Korea expert pathologists for future clinicopathological and molecular analyses toward consensus building of intraductal papillary neoplasm of the bile duct through several opinions at the present stage. J Hepatobiliary Pancreat Sci. 2018;25(3):181–7.

16. Yokode M, Yamashita Y, Zen Y. Biliary intraductal papillary neoplasm with metachronous multiple tumors – true multicentric tumors or intrabiliary dissemination: a case report and review of the literature. Mol Clin Oncol. 2017;6(3):315–20.
17. Tsuyuguchi T, Sakai Y, Sugiyama H, et al. Endoscopic diagnosis of intraductal papillary mucinous neoplasm of the bile duct. J Hepatobiliary Pancreat Sci. 2010;17(3):230–5.
18. Nanashima A, Sumida Y, Tamaru N, et al. Intraductal papillary neoplasm of the bile duct extending superficially from the intrahepatic to extrahepatic bile duct. J Gastroenterol. 2006;41(5):495–9.
19. Sasaki M, Matsubara T, Yoneda N, et al. Overexpression of enhancer of zeste homolog 2 and MUC1 may be related to malignant behaviour in intraductal papillary neoplasm of the bile duct. Histopathology. 2013;62(3):446–57.
20. Nakanuma Y, Kakuda Y, Uesaka K. Characterization of intraductal papillary neoplasm of the bile duct with respect to the histopathologic similarities to pancreatic intraductal papillary mucinous neoplasm. Gut Liver. 2019;13(6):617–27.
21. Yang CY, Huang WJ, Tsai JH, et al. Targeted next-generation sequencing identifies distinct clinicopathologic and molecular entities of intraductal papillary neoplasms of the bile duct. Mod Pathol. 2019;32(11):1637–45.
22. Aoki Y, Mizuma M, Hata T, Aoki T, et al. Intraductal papillary neoplasms of the bile duct are consisted of two distinct types specifically associated with clinicopathological features and molecular phenotypes. J Pathol. 251(1):38–48.
23. Kubota K, Jang JY, Nakanuma Y, et al. Clinicopathological characteristics of intraductal papillary neoplasm of the bile duct: a Japan-Korea collaborative study. J Hepatobiliary Pancreat Sci. 2020;27(9):581–97.
24. Sasaki M, Nitta T, Sato Y, Nakanuma Y. Autophagy may occur at an early stage of cholangiocarcinogenesis via biliary intraepithelial neoplasia. Hum Pathol. 2015;46(2):202–9.
25. Sasaki M, Yamaguchi J, Itatsu K, et al. Over-expression of polycomb group protein EZH2 relates to decreased expression of p16 INK4a in cholangiocarcinogenesis in hepatolithiasis. J Pathol. 2008;215(2):175–83.
26. Hsu M, Sasaki M, Igarashi S, et al. KRAS and GNAS mutations and p53 overexpression in biliary intraepithelial neoplasia and intrahepatic cholangiocarcinomas. Cancer. 2013 May 1;119(9):1669–74.
27. Sasaki M, Matsubara T, Nitta T, et al. GNAS and KRAS mutations are common in intraductal papillary neoplasms of the bile duct. PLoS One. 2013 Dec 2, eCollection.
28. Nakanuma Y, Kakuda Y, Fukumura Y, et al. The pathologic and genetic characteristics of the intestinal subtype of intraductal papillary neoplasms of the bile duct. Am J Surg Pathol. 2019;43(9):1212–20.
29. Tsai JH, Liau JY, Yuan CT, et al. RNF43 mutation frequently occurs with GNAS mutation and mucin hypersecretion in intraductal papillary neoplasms of the bile duct. Histopathology. 2017;70(5):756–65.
30. Tsai JH, Yuan RH, Chen YL, et al. GNAS Is frequently mutated in a specific subgroup of intraductal papillary neoplasms of the bile duct. Am J Surg Pathol. 2013;37(12):1862–70.
31. Fujikura K, Akita M, Ajiki T, et al. Recurrent mutations in APC and CTNNB1 and activated Wnt/β-catenin signaling in intraductal papillary neoplasms of the bile duct: a whole exome sequencing study. Am J Surg Pathol. 2018;42(12):1674–85.
32. Shin D, Lee S, Lee JH, et al. Prognostic implication of high grade biliary intraepithelial neoplasia in bile duct resection margins in patients with resected perihilar cholangiocarcinoma. J Hepatobiliary Pancreat Sci. 2020;27(9):604–13.
33. Higuchi R, Yazawa T, Uemura S, et al. High-grade dysplasia/carcinoma in situ of the bile duct margin in patients with surgically resected node-negative perihilar cholangiocarcinoma is associated with poor survival: a retrospective study. J Hepatobiliary Pancreat Sci. 2017;24(8):456–65.
34. Yoon KC, Yu YD, Kang WH, et al. Prevalence and clinical significance of Biliary Intraepithelial Neoplasia (BilIN) in Cholangiocarcinoma. Am Surg. 2019;85(5):511–7.
35. Kubota K, Nakanuma Y, Kondo F, et al. Clinicopathological features and prognosis of mucin-producing bile duct tumor and mucinous cystic tumor of the liver: a multi-institutional study by the Japan Biliary Association. J Hepatobiliary Pancreat Sci. 2014;21(3):176–85.
36. Paik KY, Heo JS, Choi SH, et al. Intraductal papillary neoplasm of the bile ducts: the clinical features and surgical outcome of 25 cases. J Surg Oncol. 2008;97(6):508–12.

Pathology of Biliary Tract Cancers

Claudio Luchini, Michele Simbolo, and Aldo Scarpa

Abstract

Biliary tract cancers are highly malignant tumors that comprise bile duct cancers (so called cholangiocarcinoma, CCA) and gallbladder carcinomas. Based on their anatomical location, bile duct cancers fall into two main categories: intrahepatic and extrahepatic cholangiocarcinomas. Each type displays peculiar clinic-pathologic and molecular features. Intrahepatic cholangiocarcinoma (iCCA) is further subvided in small duct and large duct iCCA. Small duct iCCA usually involves septal and interlobar bile ducts, produces mass-forming lesions, has a better prognosis than large-duct iCCA and has no known precursor lesions. Large duct iCCA usually involves the first to third branches of hepatic bile ducts, shows a periductal-infiltrating pattern of invasion, has a poorer prognosis than the small duct counterpart and can derive from two types of precursor lesions: biliary intraepithelial neoplasia and intraductal papillary neoplasms. Extrahepatic cholangiocarcinomas (eCCA) includes perihilar eCCA (so-called Klatskin tumors) and distal eCCA. Histologically, eCCA display the morphology of a classic pancreatico-biliary adenocarcinoma. Gallbladder carcinomas (GBC) are malignant tumors mostly involving the gallbladder fundus (70% of cases), with the typical histology of a pancreatico-biliary adenocarcinoma. From the molecular point of view, mutations affecting the driver genes *KRAS* and *TP53* can be found in all CCA subtypes. Of note, mutations affecting *IDH1* and *IDH2* genes and the chromatin-remodelers *ARID1A*, *BAP1* and *PBRM1* are typically enriched in iCCA, whereas *ELF3* and *ARID1B* are more common in eCCA. In GBC, amplification of *ERBB2* is more typical and also represent a therapeutic target.

C. Luchini · M. Simbolo · A. Scarpa (✉)
Department of Pathology, University of Verona, Verona, Italy
e-mail: Aldo.Scarpa@univr.it

8.1 Introduction

Biliary tract cancers are among the most deadly solid malignancies of the gastrointestinal tract [1], and are represented by bile duct cancers and gallbladder carcinomas.

Based on their anatomical location, bile duct cancers fall into two main categories: intrahepatic bile duct cholangiocarcinomas, furtherly subdivided into large duct and small duct subtypes, and extrahepatic bile duct carcinomas [2].

Clinically, intrahepatic bile duct carcinomas are often encountered in the context of differential diagnosis of liver masses; extrahepatic bile duct carcinomas represent, along with pancreatic head carcinomas, the deadliest cause of obstructive jaundice. Gallbladder carcinomas represent the most common biliary tract carcinomas, accounting for 80% of biliary tract cancers, and are characterized by a subtle clinical presentation, which unfortunately leads to late-stage diagnosis [3].

Herein, we will describe the main pathological and molecular features of biliary cancers. A specific focus will regard the distinctive features that guide practicing pathologists in the histopathologic diagnostics of such malignancies.

8.2 Intrahepatic Cholangiocarcinoma

8.2.1 Gross Features

Two main subtypes of intrahepatic cholangiocarcinoma (iCCA) are recognized: small duct iCCA (Fig. 8.1a) and large duct iCCA (Fig. 8.1b).

Small duct iCCAs involve septal and interlobar bile ducts, and are lodged deep inside the hepatic parenchyma; large duct iCCAs involve from the first to third branches of hepatic bile ducts, and are therefore located near the hepatic hilum [1].

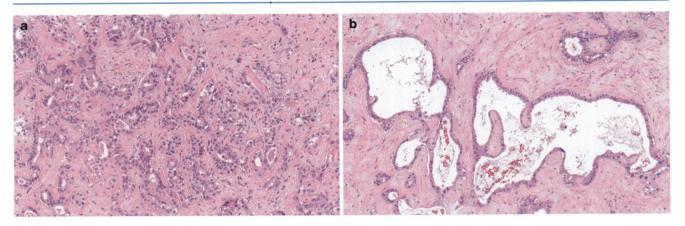

Fig. 8.1 Representative images of the two main subtypes of intrahepatic cholangiocarcinoma are here shown: small duct (**a**) and large duct (**b**). Hematoxylin-Eosin, original magnification 10X

Two macroscopic patterns of growth are described: the periductal infiltrating (PI) type, characterized by whitish sclerosing lesions which encase and obliterate the proximal branches of the left and right hepatic ducts in a longitudinal modality; the mass-forming (MF) type, characterized by white-grayish solid nodular mass lesions involving the hepatic parenchyma.

Large duct carcinomas mostly show a PI pattern, sometimes along with a MF component; small duct carcinomas manifest almost exclusively as MF lesions [3].

ICCAs, particularly the MF types, should be distinguished from other mass-forming malignancies involving the liver: the main differential diagnosis is represented by hepatocellular carcinoma (HCC), followed by metastatic colorectal adenocarcinoma. Cholangiocarcinomas are un-encapsulated white-grayish sclerotic lesions, usually with very scant or absent necrosis, mostly occurring in non-cirrhotic livers. HCCs almost always occur in cirrhotic livers as solitary or multiple nodules with a yellowish to green-brown color, and are often partially or totally encapsulated and/or necrotic. Furthermore, the so-called nodule-in-nodule pattern of growth is characteristic of HCCs and is never seen in iCCAs. Metastatic colonic adenocarcinomas may resemble iCCAs due to their white-yellowish color and lobulated margins; the frequent presence of necrosis and a simple clinical correlation are the most reliable tools for a gross differential diagnosis between these two entities.

8.2.2 Microscopic Features

Regardless of localization, iCCAs share a three-tiered grading system and a common microscopic appearance, which is that of an invasive adenocarcinoma with tubular or ductal pattern, accompanied by abundant fibrous stroma and intense desmoplastic reaction. However, differences are recognized between the main subtypes.

Large duct iCCAs show mucin-secreting glands with columnar to cuboidal epithelium; lymphatic and perineural invasion are frequent, as are lymph node metastasis. Therefore, they have a poorer prognosis compared to the small-duct counterpart [1]. Moreover, large duct iCCAs have two known precursor lesions: biliary intraepithelial neoplasia (BilIN) and intraductal papillary neoplasm of the bile ducts. Similarly to its pancreatic counterpart, BilIN is a microscopic lesion of large bile ducts characterized by flat or micropapillary architecture; here the dysplasia is classified as low-grade or high-grade, but a three-tiered system (BilIN-1,2,3) is also accepted [4]. Intraductal papillary neoplasm of the bile ducts is a grossly visible premalignant papillary lesion, which may progress from low-grade to high-grade dysplasia, and eventually adenocarcinoma [5].

Small duct iCCAs have no known precursor lesions. Two microscopic subtypes are recognized: i) cholangiolocarcinoma, which is characterized by a bland-looking proliferation of small ductular units resembling benign ductular reaction, and ii) ductal plate malformation-like pattern, characterized by ectatic and irregular neoplastic glands, lined with a single layer of cuboidal or low columnar carcinoma cells and irregular protrusions [6, 7].

8.2.3 Molecular Features

The most frequently mutated gene in iCCAs is *TP53* [8]. This gene is also altered with similar frequency in small duct iCCA, extrahepatic cholangiocarcinoma (eCCA) and gallbladder carcinoma (GBC), and cannot be considered a subtype-specific marker. Similarly, *KRAS* mutations can be found in all types of CCAs. On the other hand, *IDH1* and

IDH2 mutations are highly subtype-specific, being altered almost exclusively in iCCA [9–11]. Mutations in these two genes are concentrated in specific hotspots (R132 for *IDH1* and R172 for *IDH2*), with a mutation prevalence ranging between 5% and 40% of iCCA. Another molecular hallmark of iCCAs is represented by alterations of specific chromatin-remodelling genes: *ARID1A*, *BAP1* and *PBRM1* (6–26%) [12]. Interestingly, different studies have clarified that alterations in such genes are mutually exclusive with *IDH1/2* mutations and in most cases with *KRAS* mutations [9, 11–14]. Furthermore, several tyrosine kinase receptors (TKIs) were reported to be amplified in the iCCA subgroup; among them, and in order of frequency: *ERBB2* (4–22%), *EGFR* (2–12%), *ERBB3* (7%) and *MET* (2–7%). In addition, a small proportion of iCCA harbour amplifications of *CCND1* gene (13%) [14]. Among the different subtypes of CCA, fusion genes were mainly observed in iCCA. *FGFR2* gene fusions (14–23%) represent another hallmark of this subcategory, where *BICC1* is the most frequent rearrangement's partner [15]. Other studies pointed out that iCCA can be divided according to its etiologic environment and to the genomic alterations developed during tumorigenesis. Infection by liver flukes such as Opisthorchis viverrini and Clonorchis sinensis concurs to distinguish iCCA into two large genetic subgroups. Specifically, fluke-positive iCCA had a higher rate of single-nucleotide variant, alterations of *TP53* and other genes involved in DNA repair, *ERBB2* amplification and mutations involving *AKT1*, *CTNNB1* and *WNT5B*. In contrast, mutations in *BAP1* and *IDH1/2* genes and *FGFR* rearrangements were observed almost exclusively in fluke-negative samples, which also had a higher rate of gene copy number alterations. These alterations were observed to influence also the methylation type of the genome. It was hypothesized that fluke-positive tumours had a hypermethylation of the CpG islands caused by a longer and multi-step process involving cytosine's deamination and mutation [13].

8.3 Extrahepatic Cholangiocarcinoma

8.3.1 Gross Features

Extrahepatic cholangiocarcinomas (eCCAs) can involve the extrahepatic segment of the hepatic ducts or, less commonly, the common bile duct. Macroscopically, they tend to present as a sclerosing lesion causing an ill-defined stricture of the involved duct; nodular and papillary lesions are also recognized, albeit less common [3].

The main location of eCCAs is the perihilar region (perihilar eCCA), close to the confluence of the left and right hepatic bile ducts [16]. These lesions are also denominated Klatskin tumors, and have been subdivided by Bismuth et al. into four main types, based on the stricture pattern [17]:

Type I: stricture does not interrupt the main hepatic confluence.

Type II: stricture interrupts the main hepatic confluence.

Type III: (a) stricture interrupts the main and the right secondary hepatic confluence; (b) stricture interrupts the main and the left secondary hepatic confluence.

Type IV: primary and both right and left secondary hepatic confluence are interrupted.

Lesions located in the distal portion of the common bile duct (distal eCCA) cause obstructive jaundice, and may be amenable to surgical resection by Whipple's pancreatectomy.

8.3.2 Microscopic Features

In most cases, the histologic picture of eCCAs is that of a classic pancreatico-biliary adenocarcinoma, with irregular angulated glands embedded in a dense desmoplastic stroma with frequent perineural and intravascular invasion (Fig. 8.2a).

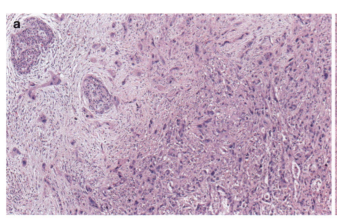 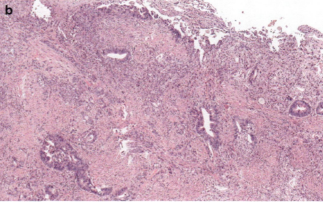

Fig. 8.2 Representative images of an extrahepatic cholangiocarcinoma (**a**), in this case extending from the intra-pancreatic choledochus to the surrounding parenchyma, and of a gallbladder carcinoma (**b**), in which it is usually associated with areas of high-grade dysplasia of the biliary epithelium. Hematoxylin-Eosin, original magnification 10X

Multiple rare histological patterns have also been described, such as intestinal-type, foveolar-type, pyloric gland-type, hepatoid, micropapillary, and signet ring [18–21]. Other rare non-adenocarcinoma tumor types are also on record, albeit exceedingly rare, such as squamous, adenosquamous, sarcomatoid and undifferentiated carcinoma [3, 22].

Extrahepatic CCAs can arise from the same precursor lesions previously described in the context of iCCAs: biliary intraepithelial neoplasia (BilIN) and intraductal papillary neoplasm of the bile ducts.

Due to its striking resemblance to pancreatic ductal adenocarcinoma, eCCA arising in the distal portion of the choledochus may be difficult to distinguish from a pancreatic primary; moreover, both cancers tend to express the same pattern of cytokeratin (CK7, CK19) and mucins (such as MUC1 and MUC4) [23]. The key to the differential diagnosis lies in the identification of precursor lesions in the surgical specimen: the presence of high grade PanIN favors the hypothesis of a pancreatic primary; conversely, the presence of high grade dysplasia in the biliary epithelium of the choledochus supports a biliary primary.

8.3.3 Molecular Features

To date, major molecular studies investigating the eCCAs molecular landscape have combined perihilar and distal eCCAs, without highlighting their differences. This subtypes share genetic alterations in *TP53* (18–45%), *KRAS* (8–47%), *ARID1A/B* (5–16%), *BRCA1/2* (1–4%), *SMAD4* (11–25%) *ELF3* (8%) and *PIK3CA* (7–9%), with *ELF3* and *ARID1B* mutations showing a specifically-higher frequency in distal eCCAs [9]. Recurrent chromosomal amplifications were observed in *YEATS4* (6%), *MDM2* (5%), *CCNE1* (3%), *CDK4* (1%) and *ERBB2* (1%), where *ERBB2* mutations and amplifications were more prevalent in tumors with papillary histology (33%) [24]. Analysis of the fusion genes revealed the presence of rearrangements involving *PRKACA* and *PRKACB* genes, observed, in the biliary tumor spectrum, only in eCCA [9]. Direct comparison between perihilar eCCA and distal eCCA has shown conflicting results and needs to be clarified [24]. The expression profile of these tumors has recently been analyzed. The analysis conducted with an unsupervised approach with respect to the anatomical site, highlighted the presence of 4 molecular groups: (i) metabolic, (ii) proliferative, (iii) mesenchymal and (iv) immune [24]. The Metabolic class presented an overexpression of hepatocyte markers and appears as enriched in gene signatures linked to the deregulated metabolism of bile acids. Conversely, overexpression of *MYC* targets, *ERBB2* aberrations, and enrichment of oncogenic mTOR, DNA repair and cell cycle pathways were observed in the Proliferation class.

In this subgroup a high prevalence of eCCA and papillary histology samples was observed. Furthermore, the Mesenchymal group showed aberrant Hedgehog and TNF-alfa signaling, and was associated with a worse prognosis, whereas the Immune class had several immune-related features, comprising overexpression of PD-1/PD-L1 and a higher lymphocyte infiltration.

8.4 Gallbladder Carcinoma

8.4.1 Gross Features

The most common location of gallbladder carcinomas (GBCs) is the fundus, accounting for 70% of cases; approximately one third arises in the body and the remaining 10% involves the neck.

GBCs are typically accompanied by calculi and tend to grow with an infiltrative pattern. Interestingly, up to 30% of GBCs are grossly unapparent [25]; thus, an extensive sampling is strongly suggested in the case of a cholecystectomy specimen characterized by calculi and by firm, thickened walls with gritty consistency and whitish color. Nodular, papillary and fleshy polypoid lesions are less common; their presence is more often associated with sarcomatoid and undifferentiated variants [3].

8.4.2 Microscopic Features

The vast majority of GBCs are adenocarcinomas.

The most common pattern encountered is pancreatico-biliary adenocarcinoma, which shares the morphology and the dismal clinical behavior with its pancreatic counterpart (Fig. 8.2b).

Pancreatico-biliary GBCs may have a wide range of differentiation: poorly differentiated cases show marked pleomorphism, bizarre nuclei and single-cell or sheet-like pattern of infiltration; well-differentiated cases may resemble benign lesions, sometimes with a foamy gland appearance [26]. However, most cases present a tubular pattern akin to pancreatic adenocarcinoma. The presence of the micropapillary pattern is typically associated with a more aggressive course [3].

Other types of adenocarcinomas encountered in the gallbladder include: (i) intestinal-type adenocarcinoma, a diagnosis which requires the exclusion of a colonic primary; (ii) mucinous adenocarcinoma, composed of >50% extracellular mucin and characterized by a poorer prognosis compared to ordinary GBCs; (iii) clear cell carcinoma, which is virtually always accompanied by foci of conventional GBCs; (iv) poorly cohesive carcinoma with or without signet-ring cells.

Adenosquamous carcinomas (defined by the presence of >25% of squamous elements) and pure squamous cell carcinomas are extremely rare; they tend to show extensive keratinization and have a poorer prognosis compared to ordinary GBCs [27]. Hepatoid carcinomas are very rare and must be distinguished from hepatocellular carcinomas involving the gallbladder; sarcomatoid carcinomas have also been described, and may show cell pleomorphism or heterologous differentiation [3].

The main differential diagnosis in the evaluation of well differentiated GBCs is represented by benign entities mimicking infiltration.

Rokitansky-Aschoff sinuses are the result of hyperplasia and herniation of epithelial cells through the fibromuscular layer of the gallbladder wall, and are usually referred to as adenomyomatosis. They can show glandular hyperplasia and features mimicking a perineural invasion, and therefore must be carefully evaluated and distinguished from foci of adenocarcinoma [28]. Luschka ducts are a development abnormality and can be found in up to 10% of cholecystectomy specimens. They appear as biliary ducts measuring 1–2 mm in diameter, and are typically located within the gallbladder fossa in the lower part of the right hepatic lobe. In the case of a florid proliferation of the epithelium, they may closely resemble a pancreatico-biliary GBC. Therefore, it is important to be aware of histologic aspects and typical anatomic locations of these non-neoplastic entities [29].

8.4.3 Molecular Features

The molecular characterization of GBCs is still evolving. The most recent studies have indicated the *TP53* gene as the most frequently altered (29–50%) [9, 30]. Like all biliary tract cancers, a not-negligible proportion of cases show *KRAS* mutations (up to 20% of cases) [11, 31, 32]. On the other hand, alterations in the genes of the *ERBB* family and of *ELF3* were much more frequent in GBC (up to 11%) than in other biliary cancers [9, 31, 32]. Fusion genes have also been found in GBC. Most of them involve the breakpoint between exon 1 of *TPP* and intron 9 of *BRD9*, observed in up to 19% of cases [30]. A supervised survival outcome-based approach showed the existence of 3 different molecular profiles [30–32]. These three groups were related to a different histo-morphology: (i) biliary-like, (ii) gastric foveolar-like and (iii) intestinal-like. The gastric foveolar-like group showed the best survival and had a high frequency of cases displaying *TPPP-BRD9* fusions. The other two show more frequently alterations affecting the hypoxia pathway. Furthermore, the intestinal-like group was distinguished by a strong association with smoking and with an advanced stage of the neoplasia at the time of diagnosis, indicating a more aggressive behavior.

References

1. Aishima S, Oda Y. Pathogenesis and classification of intrahepatic cholangiocarcinoma: different characters of perihilar large duct type versus peripheral small duct type. J Hepato-Biliary-Pancreat Sci. 2015;22:94–100.
2. Akita M, Fujikura K, Ajiki T, Fukumoto T, Otani K, Azuma T, Itoh T, Ku Y, Zen Y. Dichotomy in intrahepatic cholangiocarcinomas based on histologic similarities to hilar cholangiocarcinomas. Mod Pathol Off J U S Can Acad Pathol Inc. 2017;30:986–97.
3. WHO Classification of Tumours Editorial Board: Digestive System Tumours. International Agency for Research on Cancer; 2019.
4. Nakanuma Y, Sudo Y. Biliary tumors with pancreatic counterparts. Semin Diagn Pathol. 2017;34:167–75.
5. Jung G, Park K-M, Lee SS, Yu E, Hong S-M, Kim J. Long-term clinical outcome of the surgically resected intraductal papillary neoplasm of the bile duct. J Hepatol. 2012;57:787–93.
6. Sempoux C, Fan C, Singh P, Obeidat K, Roayaie S, Schwartz M, Fiel MI, Thung SN. Cholangiolocellular carcinoma: an innocent-looking malignant liver tumor mimicking ductular reaction. Semin Liver Dis. 2011;31:104–10.
7. Nakanuma Y, Sato Y, Ikeda H, Harada K, Kobayashi M, Sano K, Uehara T, Yamamoto M, Ariizumi S, Park YN, Choi JH, Yu E. Intrahepatic cholangiocarcinoma with predominant «ductal plate malformation» pattern: a new subtype. Am J Surg Pathol. 2012;36:1629–35.
8. Banales JM, Marin JJG, Lamarca A, Rodrigues PM, Khan SA, Roberts LR, Cardinale V, Carpino G, Andersen JB, Braconi C, Calvisi DF, Perugorria MJ, Fabris L, Boulter L, Macias RIR, Gaudio E, Alvaro D, Gradilone SA, Strazzabosco M, Marzioni M, Coulouarn C, Fouassier L, Raggi C, Invernizzi P, Mertens JC, Moncsek A, Rizvi S, Heimbach J, Koerkamp BG, Bruix J, Forner A, Bridgewater J, Valle JW, Gores GJ. Cholangiocarcinoma 2020: the next horizon in mechanisms and management. Nat Rev Gastroenterol Hepatol. 2020;17:557–88.
9. Nakamura H, Arai Y, Totoki Y, Shirota T, Elzawahry A, Kato M, Hama N, Hosoda F, Urushidate T, Ohashi S, Hiraoka N, Ojima H, Shimada K, Okusaka T, Kosuge T, Miyagawa S, Shibata T. Genomic spectra of biliary tract cancer. Nat Genet. 2015;47:1003–10.
10. Churi CR, Shroff R, Wang Y, Rashid A, Kang HC, Weatherly J, Zuo M, Zinner R, Hong D, Meric-Bernstam F, Janku F, Crane CH, Mishra L, Vauthey J-N, Wolff RA, Mills G, Javle M. Mutation profiling in cholangiocarcinoma: prognostic and therapeutic implications. PLoS One. 2014;9:e115383.
11. Simbolo M, Fassan M, Ruzzenente A, Mafficini A, Wood LD, Corbo V, Melisi D, Malleo G, Vicentini C, Malpeli G, Antonello D, Sperandio N, Capelli P, Tomezzoli A, Iacono C, Lawlor RT, Bassi C, Hruban RH, Guglielmi A, Tortora G, de Braud F, Scarpa A. Multigene mutational profiling of cholangiocarcinomas identifies actionable molecular subgroups. Oncotarget. 2014;5:2839–52.
12. Jiao Y, Pawlik TM, Anders RA, Selaru FM, Streppel MM, Lucas DJ, Niknafs N, Guthrie VB, Maitra A, Argani P, Offerhaus GJA, Roa JC, Roberts LR, Gores GJ, Popescu I, Alexandrescu ST, Dima S, Fassan M, Simbolo M, Mafficini A, Capelli P, Lawlor RT, Ruzzenente A, Guglielmi A, Tortora G, de Braud F, Scarpa A, Jarnagin W, Klimstra D, Karchin R, Velculescu VE, Hruban RH, Vogelstein B, Kinzler KW, Papadopoulos N, Wood LD. Exome sequencing identifies frequent inactivating mutations in BAP1, ARID1A and PBRM1 in intrahepatic cholangiocarcinomas. Nat Genet. 2013;45:1470–3.
13. Jusakul A, Cutcutache I, Yong CH, Lim JQ, Huang MN, Padmanabhan N, Nellore V, Kongpetch S, Ng AWT, Ng LM, Choo SP, Myint SS, Thanan R, Nagarajan S, Lim WK, Ng CCY, Boot A, Liu M, Ong CK, Rajasegaran V, Lie S, Lim AST, Lim TH, Tan J, Loh JL, McPherson JR, Khuntikeo N, Bhudhisawasdi V, Yongvanit

P, Wongkham S, Totoki Y, Nakamura H, Arai Y, Yamasaki S, Chow PK-H, Chung AYF, Ooi LLPJ, Lim KH, Dima S, Duda DG, Popescu I, Broet P, Hsieh S-Y, Yu M-C, Scarpa A, Lai J, Luo D-X, Carvalho AL, Vettore AL, Rhee H, Park YN, Alexandrov LB, Gordân R, Rozen SG, Shibata T, Pairojkul C, Teh BT, Tan P. Whole-genome and epigenomic landscapes of etiologically distinct subtypes of cholangiocarcinoma. Cancer Discov. 2017;7:1116–35.
14. Farshidfar F, Zheng S, Gingras M-C, Newton Y, Shih J, Robertson AG, Hinoue T, Hoadley KA, Gibb EA, Roszik J, Covington KR, Wu C-C, Shinbrot E, Stransky N, Hegde A, Yang JD, Reznik E, Sadeghi S, Pedamallu CS, Ojesina AI, Hess JM, Auman JT, Rhie SK, Bowlby R, Borad MJ, Cancer Genome Atlas Network, Zhu AX, Stuart JM, Sander C, Akbani R, Cherniack AD, Deshpande V, Mounajjed T, Foo WC, Torbenson MS, Kleiner DE, Laird PW, Wheeler DA, McRee AJ, Bathe OF, Andersen JB, Bardeesy N, Roberts LR, Kwong LN. Integrative genomic analysis of cholangiocarcinoma identifies distinct IDH-mutant molecular profiles. Cell Rep. 2017;19:2878–80.
15. Abou-Alfa GK, Sahai V, Hollebecque A, Vaccaro G, Melisi D, Al-Rajabi R, Paulson AS, Borad MJ, Gallinson D, Murphy AG, Oh D-Y, Dotan E, Catenacci DV, Van Cutsem E, Ji T, Lihou CF, Zhen H, Féliz L, Vogel A. Pemigatinib for previously treated, locally advanced or metastatic cholangiocarcinoma: a multicentre, open-label, phase 2 study. Lancet Oncol. 2020;21:671–84.
16. Kondo S, Takada T, Miyazaki M, Miyakawa S, Tsukada K, Nagino M, Furuse J, Saito H, Tsuyuguchi T, Yamamoto M, Kayahara M, Kimura F, Yoshitomi H, Nozawa S, Yoshida M, Wada K, Hirano S, Amano H, Miura F. Japanese Association of Biliary Surgery, Japanese Society of Hepato-Biliary-Pancreatic Surgery, Japan Society of Clinical Oncology: Guidelines for the management of biliary tract and ampullary carcinomas: surgical treatment. J Hepato-Biliary-Pancreat Surg. 2008;15:41–54.
17. Bismuth H, Nakache R, Diamond T. Management strategies in resection for hilar cholangiocarcinoma. Ann Surg. 1992;215:31–8.
18. Albores-Saavedra J, Chablé-Montero F, Méndez-Sánchez N, Mercado MÁ, Vilatoba-Chapa M, Henson DE. Adenocarcinoma with pyloric gland phenotype of the extrahepatic bile ducts: a previously unrecognized and distinctive morphologic variant of extrahepatic bile duct carcinoma. Hum Pathol. 2012;43:2292–8.
19. Wang Y, Liu Y-Y, Han G-P. Hepatoid adenocarcinoma of the extrahepatic duct. World J Gastroenterol. 2013;19:3524–7.
20. Yoshizawa T, Toyoki Y, Hirai H, Haga T, Toba T, Sakuraba S, Okano K, Wu Y, Seino H, Morohashi S, Hakamada K, Kijima H. Invasive micropapillary carcinoma of the extrahepatic bile duct and its malignant potential. Oncol Rep. 2014;32:1355–61.
21. Ogata S, Kimura A, Hatsuse K, Yamamoto J, Shimazaki H, Nakanishi K, Kawai T. Poorly differentiated adenocarcinoma with signet-ring cell carcinoma of the extrahepatic bile duct in a 42-year-old Japanese female: a case report. Acta Med Okayama. 2010;64:63–5.
22. Goto T, Sasajima J, Koizumi K, Sugiyama Y, Kawamoto T, Fujibayashi S, Moriichi K, Yamada M, Fujiya M, Kohgo Y. Primary poorly differentiated squamous cell carcinoma of the extrahepatic bile duct. Int Med Tokyo Jpn. 2016;55:1581–4.
23. Yonezawa S, Higashi M, Yamada N, Yokoyama S, Goto M. Significance of mucin expression in pancreatobiliary neoplasms. J Hepato-Biliary-Pancreat Sci. 2010;17:108–24.
24. Montal R, Sia D, Montironi C, Leow WQ, Esteban-Fabró R, Pinyol R, Torres-Martin M, Bassaganyas L, Moeini A, Peix J, Cabellos L, Maeda M, Villacorta-Martin C, Tabrizian P, Rodriguez-Carunchio L, Castellano G, Sempoux C, Minguez B, Pawlik TM, Labgaa I, Roberts LR, Sole M, Fiel MI, Thung S, Fuster J, Roayaie S, Villanueva A, Schwartz M, Llovet JM. Molecular classification and therapeutic targets in extrahepatic cholangiocarcinoma. J Hepatol. 2020;73:315–27.
25. Bal MM, Ramadwar M, Deodhar K, Shrikhande S. Pathology of gallbladder carcinoma: current understanding and new perspectives. Pathol Oncol Res POR. 2015;21:509–25.
26. Adsay V, Logani S, Sarkar F, Crissman J, Vaitkevicius V. Foamy gland pattern of pancreatic ductal adenocarcinoma: a deceptively benign-appearing variant. Am J Surg Pathol. 2000;24:493–504.
27. Roa JC, Tapia O, Cakir A, Basturk O, Dursun N, Akdemir D, Saka B, Losada H, Bagci P, Adsay NV. Squamous cell and adenosquamous carcinomas of the gallbladder: clinicopathological analysis of 34 cases identified in 606 carcinomas. Mod Pathol Off J US Can Acad Pathol Inc. 2011;24:1069–78.
28. Albores-Saavedra J, Keenportz B, Bejarano PA, Alexander AAZ, Henson DE. Adenomyomatous hyperplasia of the gallbladder with perineural invasion: revisited. Am J Surg Pathol. 2007;31:1598–604.
29. Singhi AD, Adsay NV, Swierczynski SL, Torbenson M, Anders RA, Hruban RH, Argani P. Hyperplastic Luschka ducts: a mimic of adenocarcinoma in the gallbladder fossa. Am J Surg Pathol. 2011;35:883–90.
30. Nepal C, Zhu B, O'Rourke CJ, Bhatt DK, Lee D, Song L, Wang D, Van Dyke A, Choo-Wosoba H, Liu Z, Hildesheim A, Goldstein AM, Dean M, LaFuente-Barquero J, Lawrence S, Mutreja K, Olanich ME, Bermejo JL, CGR Exome Studies Group(,), Ferreccio C, Roa JC, Rashid A, Hsing AW, Gao Y-T, Chanock SJ, Araya JC, Andersen JB, Koshiol J. Integrative molecular characterization of gallbladder cancer reveals microenvironment-associated subtypes. J Hepatol. 2020.
31. Li M, Zhang Z, Li X, Ye J, Wu X, Tan Z, Liu C, Shen B, Wang X-A, Wu W, Zhou D, Zhang D, Wang T, Liu B, Qu K, Ding Q, Weng H, Ding Q, Mu J, Shu Y, Bao R, Cao Y, Chen P, Liu T, Jiang L, Hu Y, Dong P, Gu J, Lu W, Shi W, Lu J, Gong W, Tang Z, Zhang Y, Wang X, Chin YE, Weng X, Zhang H, Tang W, Zheng Y, He L, Wang H, Liu Y, Liu Y. Whole-exome and targeted gene sequencing of gallbladder carcinoma identifies recurrent mutations in the ErbB pathway. Nat Genet. 2014;46:872–6.
32. Pandey A, Stawiski EW, Durinck S, Gowda H, Goldstein LD, Barbhuiya MA, Schröder MS, Sreenivasamurthy SK, Kim S-W, Phalke S, Suryamohan K, Lee K, Chakraborty P, Kode V, Shi X, Chatterjee A, Datta K, Khan AA, Subbannayya T, Wang J, Chaudhuri S, Gupta S, Shrivastav BR, Jaiswal BS, Poojary SS, Bhunia S, Garcia P, Bizama C, Rosa L, Kwon W, Kim H, Han Y, Yadav TD, Ramprasad VL, Chaudhuri A, Modrusan Z, Roa JC, Tiwari PK, Jang J-Y, Seshagiri S. Integrated genomic analysis reveals mutated ELF3 as a potential gallbladder cancer vaccine candidate. Nat Commun. 2020;11:4225.

Multifocal Hepatocellular Carcinoma: Genomic and Transcriptional Heterogeneity

Ming Kuang, Lixia Xu, Sui Peng, Manling Huang, Xin Liu, and Guanrui Liao

Abstract

Hepatocellular carcinoma (HCC) often presents with multiple nodules within the liver, with limited effective intervention. The high tumor heterogeneity of multifocal HCC might be the major cause of treatment failure. Studies using next-generation sequencing identify genomic and transcriptional heterogeneity among tumor nodules in multifocal HCC patients including mutational profiles, copy number alterations (CNAs), structure variations (SVs), tumor evolutionary trajectory, RNA expression patterns, and tumor immune microenvironment profiles. In addition, recent data indicate that the heterogeneity of druggable targets and immune landscape might help interpret the clinical responsiveness to targeted drugs and immunotherapy for multifocal HCC patients. Thus, a comprehensive and precise understanding of genomic and transcriptional heterogeneity is crucial to improve the treatment of patients with multifocal HCC and is particularly helpful to the development of personalized therapies. This Chapter reviews previous studies of genomic and transcriptional heterogeneity of multifocal HCC and discusses how we can leverage this information to improve the clinical management of patients with multifocal HCC.

9.1 Introduction of Multifocal Hepatocellular Carcinoma

Hepatocellular carcinoma (HCC) is the fourth leading cause of cancer death worldwide [1]. About 50–75% of HCC is reported to be multifocal when diagnosed, of which only 20–30% can undergo surgical resection [2–4]. For advanced multifocal HCC patients who have lost the chance of surgery, targeted therapy is the first-line recommended treatment, offering a median progression free survival of only 3.6–7.3 months [5, 6]. Immunotherapy represents a promising option for HCC. Targeting immune checkpoint programmed cell death protein-1 (PD-1) for advanced HCC patients demonstrated an overall survival of 28.6 months as a first-line treatment and 12.9–15 months as a second-line treatment [7–9]. However, the overall response rate for the anti-PD-1 treatment in advanced HCC patients is less than 20% [8, 9]. Recently, the results of clinical trial IMbrave150 are encouraging as they significantly improve the overall survival in advanced liver cancer through combination of immunotherapy and VEGF inhibitor [10]. This finding further underscores the importance of combination therapy in HCC. Compared to previous single-agent strategy, emerging

M. Kuang (✉)
Center of Hepatopancreatobiliary Surgery, The First Affiliated Hospital, Sun Yat-sen University,
Guangzhou, Guangdong Province, China

Cancer Center, The First Affiliated Hospital, Sun Yat-sen University, Guangzhou, Guangdong Province, China

Institute of Precision Medicine, The First Affiliated Hospital, Sun Yat-sen University, Guangzhou, Guangdong Province, China
e-mail: kuangm@mail.sysu.edu.cn

L. Xu
Cancer Center, The First Affiliated Hospital, Sun Yat-sen University, Guangzhou, Guangdong Province, China

Department of Gastroenterology and Hepatology, The First Affiliated Hospital, Sun Yat-sen University, Guangzhou, Guangdong Province, China

S. Peng
Institute of Precision Medicine, The First Affiliated Hospital, Sun Yat-sen University, Guangzhou, Guangdong Province, China

Department of Gastroenterology and Hepatology, The First Affiliated Hospital, Sun Yat-sen University, Guangzhou, Guangdong Province, China

Clinical Trials Unit, The First Affiliated Hospital, Sun Yat-sen University, Guangzhou, Guangdong Province, China

M. Huang
Cancer Center, The First Affiliated Hospital, Sun Yat-sen University, Guangzhou, Guangdong Province, China

X. Liu · G. Liao
Center of Hepatopancreatobiliary Surgery, The First Affiliated Hospital, Sun Yat-sen University, Guangzhou, Guangdong Province, China

combination therapies can act on more targets, thus could simultaneously treat multiple heterogeneous tumor clones.

Tumor heterogeneity means that different tumor cells can have distinct morphological and phenotypic profiles, including gene expression, metabolism, proliferation, metastatic potential, and so on [11]. Tumor heterogeneity might be more complex in multifocal HCC patients than that in patients with single tumor [12–14]. Some recent studies have evaluated genomic heterogeneity of multifocal HCC based on mutational, copy number alterations (CNAs) profiles, structure variations (SVs), and HBV DNA integrations [15–19]. In addition, transcriptional heterogeneity, especially immune heterogeneity has been reported in multifocal HCC recently and proved to be implicated in different immunotherapies response [18–20].

Here, we review genomic and transcriptional heterogeneity in multifocal HCC to elucidate the internodular heterogeneity of multifocal HCC at the molecular level and discuss how we can leverage this information to improve the treatment and management of patients with multifocal HCC.

9.2 Heterogeneity of Multifocal HCC

9.2.1 Genomic Heterogeneity of Multifocal HCC

Multifocal HCC may result from multicentric occurrence (MO-HCC) or intrahepatic metastases (IM-HCC). Next-generation sequencing (NGS)-based studies have shown substantial genomic heterogeneity in mutational profiles, CNAs, SVs, and tumor clonal evolution among tumors separated by anatomical locations within the same patient. The extent of mutations shared by all tumor nodules in multifocal HCC varied significantly. Recent studies have revealed that the actual shared mutation rates ranged from 8% to 97% in IM-HCC, with nearly no common mutations in MO-HCC [3, 21, 22]. Extensive heterogeneity of copy number aberrations, with highly variable percentages of genomic alteration has also been reported among multifocal lesions. For example, the percentage of ubiquitous CNAs ranged from 22.2% to 100% in IM-HCC and it could reach as high as 46.7% in MO-HCC [23]. In our previous study, we have reported variable extent of heterogeneity in mutations and CNA patterns among tumors of multifocal HCC patients by whole exome sequencing [18]. For patients with HBV infection, HBV-DNA was found to integrate into human host chromosomes in the early stage of natural course of acute hepatitis B infection [13, 14], making the junctional information specific to each tumor clone. As such, tumors with the same HBV DNA integration site are supposed to be intrahepatic metastasis nodules [21]. It has been reported that tumors in IM-HCC exhibited the same HBV DNA integrations, while different patterns of HBV DNA integration were found in tumors of MO-HCC, which is consistent with what we found in our research using whole genome sequencing [23, 24]. In parallel, different genomic structural variations (SVs) were observed among multiple lesions [16]. Moreover, we found that there was a tendency that the tumor with smaller size had increased SV numbers as compared to the large tumor in the same patient in our recent study [19].

Phylogenetic trees which were constructed based on all somatic mutations also indicate great genomic heterogeneity of multifocal HCC [18, 22, 23, 25]. Well-known driver alterations, including druggable targets were further mapped to each phylogenetic tree. The result showed that only 9–85% of the driver alterations were truncal events, indicating multiple tumors follow the scenario of branched tumor evolution [21, 23]. Our recent study also showed that only 30% (18/60) of the driver alterations were truncal events and only 20% (3/15) of druggable alterations were mapped to trunks, refining the great heterogeneity of different tumors among multifocal HCC patient.

9.2.2 Transcriptional Heterogeneity of Multifocal HCC

In recent studies, RNA-sequencing is performed on multiple tumor samples and their adjacent normal liver tissue samples to characterize the transcriptomic profile of multifocal HCC [18, 25]. The differentially expressed genes between all tumors and normal samples are compared and up-regulated genes and down-regulated genes in tumor samples are identified. Gene sets from Gene Ontology (GO) reveal downregulated genes in tumors are mainly concentrated in immune response and protein/metabolic process pathways in our recent study [18]. Consistently, Miao et al. found immune response and metabolism pathways are enriched in multifocal HCC [25], which is supported by the results of a large-scale liver cancer integrative research [26]. We also found that proliferation-related pathways were enriched in the large nodules in multifocal HCC, such as angiogenesis pathway, VEGF signaling pathway, PI3K-AKT signaling pathway, while more immune-related pathways were enriched in small nodules, including TNFα signaling pathway, IFN-α signaling pathway, T cell and B cell receptor signaling pathway [19]. This result partially explains the heterogeneity of clinical responses to targeted therapy or immunotherapy among multiple tumor nodules within the same multifocal HCC patient.

Moreover, RNA expression profile can also predict the proliferation and invasion ability of multifocal HCC, providing new perspectives for postoperative adjuvant therapy [27].

In our recent study, after hierarchical clustering analysis of 34 HCC lesions in 6 patients based on RNA expression, we found that patients with Edmondson–Steiner grade 2 and grade 3 were clearly distinguished, suggesting that RNA expression pattern is associated with tumor differentiation [3]. Moreover, the authors in a retrospective study utilized transcriptome sequencing to associate the sequencing data with clinical outcomes in a cohort of Chinese patients with HBV-related HCC. They found up-regulation of cytoskeletal remodeling and extracellular matrix organization is associated with tumor metastasis, and worse prognosis may be related to up-regulation of cell proliferation, nucleic acid metabolism, protein translation, and macromolecular assembly, suggesting that RNA expression profile helps predict the clinical characteristics of tumor [25].

Immunotherapy is emerging as a promising strategy in HCC, but its relatively low response rate and mixed responses among different tumor nodules remained to be a major challenge. Immune discrepancies among different nodules vary within HCC patients, including cytokines, immunosuppressive cells, stromal cells, growth factors, which together shape the heterogenous immune microenvironment of multifocal HCC. Immune features of multifocal HCC are important for understanding immune-escape mechanisms and developing more effective immunotherapy [3].

A recent study based on immuno-transcriptomic analysis divided multifocal HCC into three subtypes: immunocompetent subtype, immunodeficient subtype, and immunosuppressive subtype. The compositions of immune cells in different subtypes are quite different, which provides a good classification reference for further study. The immunocompetent subtype has normal T cell infiltration, but poor B cell infiltration; the lymphocyte infiltration in immunodeficient subtype is lower, but has higher dendritic cells and natural killing cells; the immunosuppressive subtype had higher frequencies of Treg cells, Breg cells, and M2 macrophages, with up-regulated expressions of PD-1, PD-L1, CTLA-4, and Tim-1 [21]. Besides, it has been reported that there are fewer T cells and more M2 macrophage infiltration, neoantigens, and TCR repertoires in IM-HCC, while more immune checkpoint inhibitory molecules and immune editing are present in MO-HCC [3]. Our study also revealed that there is significant immune heterogeneity in multifocal HCC, with various degrees of immune cell infiltration among different nodules. Interestingly, in $CD8^+$ T cell-rich nodules, the expression of inhibitory immune molecules such as CTLA-4, PD-1, and PD-L1 is also up-regulated, making it difficult for infiltrating $CD8^+$ T cells to exert antitumor function [18]. Therefore, for tumors with high infiltrated $CD8^+$ T cells, PD-1/PD-L1 inhibitor treatment may be able to relieve immunosuppression and enhance the killing effect of infiltrating $CD8^+$ T cells.

9.3 The Influences of Genomic and Transcriptional Heterogeneity on Management of Multifocal HCC

The number of tumors in multifocal HCC is significantly correlated with patients' overall survival [28, 29]. Surgical resection is recommended as the first choice for multifocal HCC patients with less than 3 nodules. For patients with more than 3 tumor nodules, if these tumors are confined to the same segment or ipsilateral liver lobe, or intraoperative radiofrequency ablation can be performed simultaneously to remove lesions outside the resection range, surgical resection may be more effective than other treatment approaches [28, 30]. With the development in surgical techniques and perioperative management, some cancer centers in Asia advocate a relatively more active management of intermediate-stage HCC and have observed better outcomes in patients [31–34]. Anatomical resection of HCC is very important in surgical treatment, which was first proposed by the distinguished Japanese hepatic surgeon, Prof. Makuuchi [35, 36]. This advanced concept has been widely applied in multifocal HCC resection [37, 38], making it possible to analyze the clonal evolution and internodular heterogeneity of multifocal HCC with surgical specimens.

Based on the multi-omics analysis of surgical specimens from multifocal HCC, the understanding of genetic heterogeneity has been deepened, and correspondingly, more insights have been brought to the management of advanced unresectable multifocal HCC. Searching for truncal druggable targets based on NGS sequencing data would help in prevention of postoperative recurrence or treatment selection for multifocal HCC. Our recent study revealed that sorafenib-targeted alterations (including BRAF amplification, PDGFRB amplification, and VEGFA amplification) were identified in the trunk of only one out of six patients, which may explain the relative low treatment response rate to sorafenib in clinical practice [18]. These data indicate that the heterogeneity of druggable targets might help interpret the clinical responsiveness to targeted drugs for multifocal HCC patients.

As the era of immune combination therapy has come in the treatment of HCC, there is an increasing need for a precise analysis to choose the optimal immunotherapy strategy, such as non-invasive imaging test combined with artificial intelligence, circulating tumor DNA, and other signatures to predict therapeutic targets and monitor the treatment efficacy. Our multi-omics study revealed that the small nodules had higher immune cell infiltration and up-regulation of immune pathways as compared to the large nodule of the same multifocal HCC case, which may partially explain the different responses of small and large nodules to anti-PD-1 treatment. We further demonstrated the synergistic effect of combined immunotherapy and anti-proliferation/oncogenic therapy such as tyrosine kinase inhibitors (TKIs) in multifo-

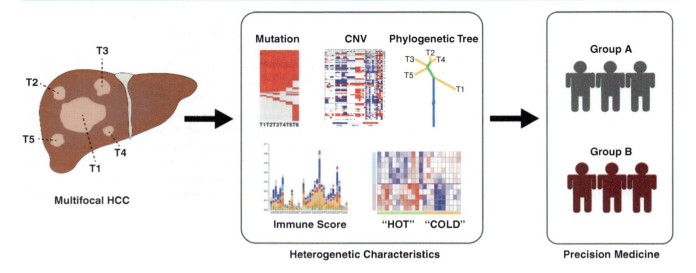

Fig. 9.1 Genomic and transcriptional heterogeneity in multifocal HCC

cal HCC [19]. The heterogenous immune microenvironment of multifocal HCC demands different or combinational immunotherapies for different patients [19, 21]. As immune checkpoint inhibitors can reactivate antitumor immunity in an immunosuppressive microenvironment, it is very crucial to adopt personalized immunotherapy strategies to patients with multifocal HCC for better clinical response.

Moreover, the result of clinical trial IMbrave150 "atezolizumab plus bevacizumab in unresectable hepatocellular carcinoma" brings hope to patients with advanced HCC [10]. This immune combination therapy was recently approved by the National Medical Products Administration in China and Food and Drug Administration in the USA as the first-line treatment of advanced HCC, highlighting the importance of combination immunotherapy in advanced and multifocal unresectable liver cancer. The success of clinical trial IMbrave150 has shed light on future research to improve the prognosis of multifocal HCC, emphasizing the importance of immune combination therapy.

In conclusion, increasing studies have explored the genomic and transcriptional heterogeneity among different nodules in multifocal HCC through multi-omics sequencing. The characteristics of the drug targets distribution and immune microenvironment may help accurately predict the efficacy of targeted drugs and immunotherapy in multifocal HCC patients (Fig. 9.1).

References

1. International Agency For Research On Cancer WHO. Cancer today. https://gco.iarc.fr/today/home
2. Kudo M, Izumi N, Ichida T, Ku Y, Kokudo N, et al. Report of the 19th follow-up survey of primary liver cancer in Japan. Hepatol Res. 2016;46:372–90.
3. Dong LQ, Peng LH, Ma LJ, Liu DB, Zhang S, et al. Heterogeneous immunogenomic features and distinct escape mechanisms in multifocal hepatocellular carcinoma. J Hepatol. 2020;72:896–908.
4. Xie DY, Fan HK, Ren ZG, Fan J, Gao Q. Identifying clonal origin of multifocal hepatocellular carcinoma and its clinical implications. Clin Transl Gastroenterol. 2019;10:e6.
5. Kudo M, Finn RS, Qin S, Han KH, Ikeda K, et al. Lenvatinib versus sorafenib in first-line treatment of patients with unresectable hepatocellular carcinoma: a randomised phase 3 non-inferiority trial. Lancet. 2018;391:1163–73.
6. Llovet JM, Ricci S, Mazzaferro V, Hilgard P, Gane E, et al. Sorafenib in advanced hepatocellular carcinoma. N Engl J Med. 2008;359:378–90.
7. Crocenzi TS, El-Khoueiry AB, Yau TC, Melero I, Sangro B, et al. Nivolumab (nivo) in sorafenib (sor)-naive and -experienced pts with advanced hepatocellular carcinoma (HCC): CheckMate 040 study. J Clin Oncol. 2017;15:4013.
8. El-Khoueiry AB, Sangro B, Yau T, Crocenzi TS, Kudo M, et al. Nivolumab in patients with advanced hepatocellular carcinoma (CheckMate 040): an open-label, non-comparative, phase 1/2 dose escalation and expansion trial. Lancet. 2017;389:2492–502.
9. Zhu AX, Finn RS, Edeline J, Cattan S, Ogasawara S, et al. Pembrolizumab in patients with advanced hepatocellular carcinoma previously treated with sorafenib (KEYNOTE-224): a non-randomised, open-label phase 2 trial. Lancet Oncol. 2018;19:940–52.
10. Finn RS, Qin S, Ikeda M, Galle PR, Ducreux M, et al. Atezolizumab plus bevacizumab in unresectable hepatocellular carcinoma. N Engl J Med. 2020;382:1894–905.
11. Marusyk A, Polyak K. Tumor heterogeneity: causes and consequences. Biochim Biophys Acta. 2010;1805:105–17.
12. Lin DC, Mayakonda A, Dinh HQ, Huang P, Lin L, et al. Genomic and epigenomic heterogeneity of hepatocellular carcinoma. Cancer Res. 2017;77:2255–65.
13. Huang A, Zhao X, Yang XR, Li FQ, Zhou XL, et al. Circumventing intratumoral heterogeneity to identify potential therapeutic targets in hepatocellular carcinoma. J Hepatol. 2017;67:293–301.
14. Torrecilla S, Sia D, Harrington AN, Zhang Z, Cabellos L, et al. Trunk mutational events present minimal intra- and inter-tumoral heterogeneity in hepatocellular carcinoma. J Hepatol. 2017;67:1222–31.
15. Gao Q, Wang ZC, Duan M, Lin YH, Zhou XY, et al. Cell culture system for analysis of genetic heterogeneity within hepatocellular car-

cinomas and response to pharmacologic agents. Gastroenterology. 2017;152:232–42.
16. Furuta M, Ueno M, Fujimoto A, Hayami S, Yasukawa S, et al. Whole genome sequencing discriminates hepatocellular carcinoma with intrahepatic metastasis from multi-centric tumors. J Hepatol. 2017;66:363–73.
17. Zhai W, Lim TK, Zhang T, Phang ST, Tiang Z, et al. The spatial organization of intra-tumour heterogeneity and evolutionary trajectories of metastases in hepatocellular carcinoma. Nat Commun. 2017;8:4565.
18. Xu LX, He MH, Dai ZH, Yu J, Wang JG, et al. Genomic and transcriptional heterogeneity of multifocal hepatocellular carcinoma. Ann Oncol. 2019;30:990–7.
19. Huang ML, He MH, Guo Y, Li HP, Shen SL et al. The influence of immune heterogeneity on the effectiveness of immune checkpoint inhibitors in multifocal hepatocellular carcinomas. Clin Cancer Res. 2020.
20. Sia D, Jiao Y, Martinez-Quetglas I, Kuchuk O, Villacorta-Martin C, et al. Identification of an immune-specific class of hepatocellular carcinoma. Based Mol Features Gastroenterol. 2017;153:812–26.
21. Zhang Q, Lou Y, Yang J, Wang J, Feng J, et al. Integrated multiomic analysis reveals comprehensive tumour heterogeneity and novel immunophenotypic classification in hepatocellular carcinomas. Gut. 2019;68:2019–31.
22. Xue R, Li R, Guo H, Guo L, Su Z, et al. Variable intra-tumor genomic heterogeneity of multiple lesions in patients with hepatocellular carcinoma. Gastroenterology. 2016;150:998–1008.
23. Duan M, Hao J, Cui S, Worthley DL, Zhang S, et al. Diverse modes of clonal evolution in HBV-related hepatocellular carcinoma revealed by single-cell genome sequencing. Cell Res. 2018;28:359–73.
24. Chen XP, Long X, Jia WL, Wu HJ, Zhao J, et al. Viral integration drives multifocal HCC during the occult HBV infection. J Exp Clin Cancer Res. 2019;38:261.
25. Miao R, Luo H, Zhou H, Li G, Bu D, et al. Identification of prognostic biomarkers in hepatitis B virus-related hepatocellular carcinoma and stratification by integrative multi-omics analysis. J Hepatol. 2014;61:840–9.
26. Comprehensive and Integrative Genomic Characterization of Hepatocellular Carcinoma. Cell. 2017;169:1327–41.
27. Feo F, Pascale RM. Multifocal hepatocellular carcinoma: intrahepatic metastasis or multicentric carcinogenesis? Ann Transl Med. 2015;3:4.
28. Yin L, Li H, Li AJ, Lau WY, Pan ZY, et al. Partial hepatectomy vs. transcatheter arterial chemoembolization for resectable multiple hepatocellular carcinoma beyond Milan Criteria: a RCT. J Hepatol. 2014;61:82–8.
29. Zhao WC, Yang N, Zhu N, Zhang HB, Fu Y, et al. Patients with multiple hepatocellular carcinomas within the UCSF criteria have outcomes after curative resection similar to patients within the BCLC early-stage criteria. World J Surg. 2012;36:1811–23.
30. Torzilli G, Belghiti J, Kokudo N, Takayama T, Capussotti L, et al. A snapshot of the effective indications and results of surgery for hepatocellular carcinoma in tertiary referral centers: is it adherent to the EASL/AASLD recommendations?: an observational study of the HCC East-West study group. Ann Surg. 2013;257:929–37.
31. Ohkubo T, Midorikawa Y, Nakayama H, Moriguchi M, Aramaki O, et al. Liver resection of hepatocellular carcinoma in patients with portal hypertension and multiple tumors. Hepatol Res. 2018;48:433–41.
32. Wada H, Eguchi H, Noda T, Ogawa H, Yamada D, et al. Selection criteria for hepatic resection in intermediate-stage (BCLC stage B) multiple hepatocellular carcinoma. Surgery. 2016;160:1227–35.
33. Liu W, Wang K, Bao Q, Sun Y, Xing BC. Hepatic resection provided long-term survival for patients with intermediate and advanced-stage resectable hepatocellular carcinoma. World J Surg Oncol. 2016;14:62.
34. Ho MC, Huang GT, Tsang YM, Lee PH, Chen DS, et al. Liver resection improves the survival of patients with multiple hepatocellular carcinomas. Ann Surg Oncol. 2009;16:848–55.
35. Makuuchi M, Hasegawa H, Yamazaki S. Ultrasonically guided subsegmentectomy. Surg Gynecol Obstet. 1985;161:346–50.
36. Makuuchi M. Surgical treatment for HCC – special reference to anatomical resection. Int J Surg. 2013;11(Suppl 1):S47–9.
37. Makuuchi M, Sano K. The surgical approach to HCC: our progress and results in Japan. Liver Transpl. 2004;10:S46–52.
38. Ishizawa T, Hasegawa K, Aoki T, Takahashi M, Inoue Y, et al. Neither multiple tumors nor portal hypertension are surgical contraindications for hepatocellular carcinoma. Gastroenterology. 2008;134:1908–16.

Intraductal Neoplasms of the Pancreas

Toru Furukawa

Abstract

Here described are definitions, epidemiology, etiology, clinical features, radiology, pathology, and treatment and prognosis of intraductal neoplasms of the pancreas, namely, intraductal papillary mucinous neoplasms (IPMNs), intraductal oncocytic papillary neoplasms (IOPNs), and intraductal tubulopapillary neoplasms (ITPNs). IPMNs are grossly visible intraductal epithelial neoplasms of mucin-producing cells. IPMNs are fairly common without known etiologic factors. Imaging studies show cystically dilated ducts involving branch ducts, the main duct, or the both of ducts. Microscopically, the neoplastic cells grow in papillae with various atypical degree ranging from low-grade to high-grade. The papillae show various morphologic features with expression of characteristic mucin proteins, which are classified into gastric, intestinal, and pancreatobiliary types. Mutations in *KRAS* and *GNAS* are frequently found. IPMNs often become invasive, which show adenocarcinoma with ductal or mucinous elements. Disease-specific survivals of patients with surgically resected IPMNs are fairly good in low-grade IPMNs, modest in high-grade IPMNs, however, poor in invasive IPMNs. IOPNs show cystically dilated mucinous ducts with arborizing papillae consist of eosinophilic cells. IOPN is a rare tumor with an average age of patients <65 years. Imaging studies of IOPNs show the same feature as those of IPMNs. Pathologically, IOPNs show high-grade atypia occasionally with invasive elements. IOPNs often harbor fusion genes of *ATP1B1-PRKACB*, *DNAJB1-PRKACA*, and *ATP1B1-PRKACA*. Disease-specific survival rates of patients with surgically resected IOPNs are reported to be 84% for 5-year and 73% for 10-year. ITPNs are intraductal, grossly visible solid neoplasms arising in the MPD or its branches. ITPN is a rare tumor. Imaging studies show characteristic features called the two-tone duct sign and the cork-in-wine bottle sign. Pathologically, ITPNs show packed tubulopaillary glands consist of cuboidal cells with enlarged atypical nuclei and no visible mucin in cytoplasm. ITPNs often harbor mutations in *PIK3CA*, *KMT2C*, *KMT2D*, and *BAP*. ITPNs are often with invasion, and such cases show poor prognosis.

10.1 Intraductal Papillary Mucinous Neoplasm (IPMN)

10.1.1 Definition

IPMN is a grossly visible, intraductal epithelial neoplasm of mucin-producing cells, found in the main pancreatic duct (MPD), or its branches [1, 2]. The neoplastic epithelium is usually papillary, but may include tubular glands, and the extent of mucin secretion, duct dilatation, and dysplasia can vary [3] (Fig. 10.1). Non-invasive IPMNs are classified into two categories, based on the degree of cyto-architectural atypia: low-grade and high-grade (carcinoma *in situ*) [4]. If there is a component of invasive carcinoma, these are designated as IPMN with associated invasive carcinoma [4].

10.1.2 Epidemiology

IPMNs are fairly common, particularly in the elderly. Incidence was reported to be 1.7–2.8% in consecutive CT scans [5, 6]. The incidence doubled among the patients in their sixties, and tripled in the seventies [6].

T. Furukawa (✉)
Department of Investigative Pathology, Tohoku University Graduate School of Medicine, Sendai, Japan
e-mail: toru.furukawa@med.tohoku.ac.jp

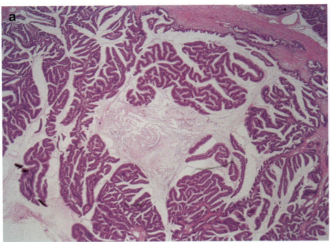 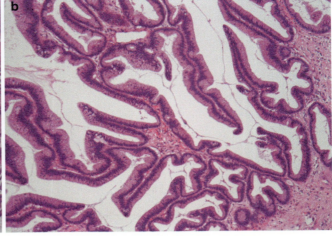

Fig. 10.1 Histological images of IPMN. (**a**) IPMN shows a cystically dilated duct filled with mucin. Well-formed neoplastic papillae are observed inside the dilated duct. (**b**) The neoplastic papillae are consisted of mucin containing tall columnar cells. Grade of atypia may vary from low-grade to high-grade. Hematoxylin and eosin staining. Original magnifications were × 20 (**a**) and ×100 (**b**)

10.1.3 Etiology

No definite etiological environmental factors associated with IPMNs are known. However, patients with Peutz-Jeghers syndrome, familial adenomatous polyposis, and McCune Albright syndrome have a greater risk of IPMNs [7–9]. Individuals with familial predisposition to pancreatic cancer often harbor cystic lesions in their pancreas that are presumably IPMNs [10].

10.1.4 Clinical Features

Clinical manifestations of the dilated main duct include epigastric pain, chronic pancreatitis, weight loss, diabetes mellitus, and jaundice [11–15], whereas the dilated branch ducts are often discovered fortuitously during clinical evaluation of some other conditions [16].

10.1.5 Radiology

Radiological imaging reveals three distinct types of IPMN, including branch duct-type, main duct-type, and mixed type [16–18]. Branch duct IPMNs show dilated secondary pancreatic ducts of >5 mm size, without the dilatation of the main duct, while the main duct IPMNs show segmental or diffused dilation of the MPD, without any other causes of obstruction. Mixed type IPMNs show the characteristics of both these types of IPMNs [16, 18]. Mural nodules and/or irregular ductal wall thickening can be the sign of high-grade or invasive neoplasms [19, 20].

10.1.6 Pathology

10.1.6.1 Macroscopic Appearance

IPMNs show dilated ducts containing mucin. Dilated branch ducts are seen as cysts anywhere in the pancreas. IPMNs involving the main duct can be identified as segmental/fusiform or diffuse/tortuous dilatation of the duct, often accompanied by dilated secondary branch ducts [3], containing mural nodules or polypoid tumors.

10.1.6.2 Microscopic Appearance and Variations

Papillary proliferation of mucin-containing tall columnar cells is a characteristic histopathological feature of IPMNs [1] (Fig. 10.1). Shapes of papillae are diverse, and cellular atypia also vary. According to the shapes of papillae, IPMNs are subdivided into gastric, intestinal, and pancreatobiliary types [21–23]. Gastric-type IPMNs show thick, finger-like papillae, resembling the gastric foveolar cells, or tubular structures of the pyloric glands. Intestinal-type IPMNs show villous papillae mimicking a villous colonic tumor, whereas pancreatobiliary-type show complex, arborizing papillae.

10.1.6.3 Immunohistochemistry

Ductal markers, including cytokeratins 7 and 19, CA19-9, and CEA, are strongly expressed in most of the IPMNs [24, 25]. Mucin glycoproteins MUC1, MUC2, MUC5AC, and MUC6, show subtype-specific expression patterns among IPMNs [21, 26–28]. Gastric-type of IPMNs express MUC5AC and MUC6, while those of the intestinal-type IPMNs contain MUC2 and MUC5AC. Pancretobiliary-type IPMNs express MUC1, MUC5AC, and MUC6 [22, 29].

10.1.6.4 Grading

IPMNs can be low- or high-grade, based on the degree of cytoarchitectural atypia [4]. A high-grade lesion corresponds to carcinoma in situ. Existence of invasive carcinoma with IPMN leads to designation of IPMN with associated invasive carcinoma [4].

10.1.6.5 Differential Diagnosis

Mucinous cystic neoplasm (MCN), oligocystic serous cystic neoplasm (OSC), intraductal tubulopapillary neoplasm (ITPN), lymphoepithelial cyst (LEC), and chronic pancreatitis (CP) with a retention cyst or pseudocyst should be differentially diagnosed from IPMN. MCNs have characteristic ovarian-type stroma in the cyst wall [30]. OSCs are lined by distinct glycogen-rich cuboidal cells [31]. ITPN is a solid intraductal tumor clogging the duct, composed of high-grade cuboidal cells that form tubulopapillae [32]. LECs are lined by keratinized squamous epithelium with lymphoid stroma [33]. When the cysts in CP have flat epithelial lining, they are identified as retention cysts, and when no lining cells are present, they are called pseudocysts [34].

10.1.6.6 Molecular Pathology

Sixty to eighty percent of the IPMNs harbor somatic mutations in *KRAS*, while 50–70% have mutations in *GNAS* [35, 36]. Although *KRAS* mutations are prevalent in the pancreatic ductal adenocarcinomas (PDAC) as well, *GNAS* mutations are rarely found here, which makes them a specific characteristic of IPMN [36–38]. In 14% of the IPMNs, *RNF43* also shows somatic mutations [36, 39, 40]. Overexression of p53, which presumably indicates missense mutations of *TP53*, is found in 10–40% of the high-grade IPMNs and in 40–60% of the associated invasive carcinomas [29, 38, 41, 42]. While loss of SMAD4 is rare [43, 44], nuclear expression of ß-catenin is seen in 18–39% of the IPMNs [38, 45].

10.1.6.7 Treatment and Prognosis

IPMNs with high-grade dysplasia or invasive carcinoma should be surgically resected. According to the international consensus guidelines for management of patients with IPMN [16], surgery is indicated by high-risk stigmata and worrisome features, such as cysts ≥3 cm, enhancing mural nodules <5 mm, thickened enhanced cyst walls, MPD with a size of 5–9 mm, abrupt change in the MPD caliber with distal pancreatic atrophy, lymphadenopathy, elevated serum level of CA19-9, and a rapidly growing cyst at the rate of >5 mm/2 years. High-risk stigmata are usually associated with obstructive jaundice, an enhanced solid component, and MPD with a size ≥10 mm. IPMNs with high-risk stigmata should be resected immediately, while those with worrisome features should be evaluated by endoscopic ultrasound, to further risk-stratify the lesions, whether they have mural nodules or involvement of the MPD. High-grade lesions can be evaluated with cyst fluid or pancreatic juice cytology [16].

Five-year survival rate for patients with surgical resection of the low-grade IPMNs is 100%, and 95–85% with high-grade IPMNs [22, 46, 47]. Survival rate varies between 36–90% when the IPMNs are associated with invasive carcinoma, depending on the stage [22, 46–48]. The morphological subtypes of IPMNs can be a prognostic indicator; 5-year survival rate is 94% for the gastric-type, 90% for the intestinal-type, and 50% for the pancreatobiliary-type [22, 48].

10.2 Intraductal Oncocytic Papillary Neoplasms (IOPN)

10.2.1 Definition

IOPN is an intraductal neoplasm of eosinophilic epithelial cells that form arborizing papillae [49] (Fig. 10.2). It is categorized as a variant of IPMNs, as it shows a grossly visible intraductal neoplasm with mucin production [21], similar to IPMN. However, a number of studies have reported that IOPNs have distinct molecular features that distinguish them from IPMNs in the current fifth edition of the World Health Organization classification of tumors of the digestive system [50].

10.2.2 Epidemiology

IOPNs are fairly infrequent, making up only 4.5–8.4% of the cystic neoplasms of the pancreas [22, 51]. They occur more frequently in men than in women, between 20–80 years of age. With an average age of <65 years, patients with IOPNs are younger than those with IPMNs (> 65 years) [49, 51–53].

10.2.3 Etiology

No etiological factor associated with IOPN is known.

10.2.4 Clinical Features

Clinical manifestations of IOPN are the same as those of IPMNs, including abdominal pain, weight loss, diabetes mellitus, and jaundice [49, 51].

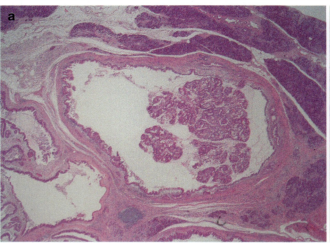

Fig. 10.2 Histological images of IOPN. (**a**) IOPN shows mucinous dilated ducts. Arborising papillae are seen inside them. (**b**) The neoplastic papillae of IOPN consist of eosinophilic cells with enlarged nuclei and prominent nucleoli, which show high-grade atypia. Intraepithelial lumina are often seen in the cells. Hematoxylin and eosin staining. Original magnifications were × 20 (**a**) and ×100 (**b**)

10.2.5 Radiology

Like IPMNs, IOPNs show cystic dilatation of the pancreatic duct, and can be of branch duct type, main duct type, and mixed type. Mural nodules are often seen inside the dilated duct [53].

10.2.6 Pathology

10.2.6.1 Macroscopic Appearance
IOPNs show cystic dilation of ducts filled with mucin [49, 53], which is indistinguishable from IPMNs, and may involve branch ducts or the main duct. Polypoid tortuous tumors are often seen inside them.

10.2.6.2 Microscopic Appearance
In IOPNs, the dilated ducts are lined by arborizing papillae, consisting of eosinophilic cells with enlarged nuclei and prominent nucleoli [21, 49], and show high-grade atypia. Intraepithelial lumina are often seen in the neoplastic papillae (Fig. 10.2). Occasionally, the neoplasm invades the parenchymal stroma, resulting in a diagnosis of IOPN with associated invasive carcinoma. The invading mass usually shows clusters of eosinophilic cells in the mucin pools [54].

10.2.6.3 Immunohistochemistry
Neoplastic cells frequently express HepPar1 and mesothelin [54]. The expression of mucin proteins MUC5AC and MUC6 are consistently positive, while MUC1 and MUC2 are infrequently and focally positive [21, 54].

10.2.6.4 Differential Diagnosis
IOPN should be distinguished from cystic neoplasms, including IPMN, mucinous cystic neoplasm, oligocystic serous cystic neoplasm, lymphoepithelial cyst, and solid pseudopapillary neoplasm.

10.2.6.5 Molecular Pathology
IOPNs infrequently show somatic mutations in *KRAS* and *GNAS* unlike IPMNs [36, 40]. Instead, they carry fusion genes of *ATP1B1-PRKACB*, *DNAJB1-PRKACA*, and *ATP1B1-PRKACA* [55, 56]. Interestingly, these fusion genes upregulate the protein kinase A pathway, which is the main target of *GNAS* that shows frequent gain-of-function mutations in IPMNs, indicating that both IOPNs and IPMNs, are driven by activation of the protein kinase A pathway. Aberrant expression of p53 or SMAD4 is observed in up to 10% of IOPNs [52], and about 30% of these show nuclear accumulation of ß-catenin [48], whereas *RNF43* mutations are not reported [40, 57]. A patient with a germline *SMAD4* mutation was reported to have developed IOPN [58].

10.2.6.6 Treatment and Prognosis
IOPN should be surgically resected. Disease-specific survival rates of patients with surgically resected IOPNs are reported to be 84% for 5-year and 73% for 10-year [22].

10.3 Intraductal Tubulopapillary Neoplasms (ITPN)

10.3.1 Definition

ITPN is an intraductal, grossly visible solid neoplasm arising in the MPD or its branches [32]. Cystic lesions are infrequent and are only focally and peripherally observed. The neoplastic epithelium has the mixture of tubular and papillary configurations, and the neoplastic cells show uniformly high-grade atypia [32] (Fig. 10.3). The neoplasm is often

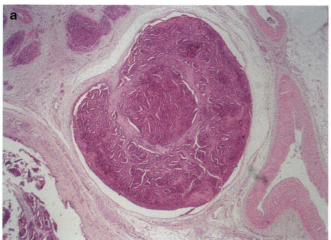 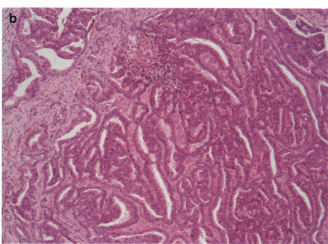

Fig. 10.3 Histological images of ITPN. (a) ITPNs show a solid tumor clogged in dilated pancreatic ducts, without visible mucin. Cystic ducts are occasionally seen in the periphery of a neoplasm-obstructed duct. (b) ITPN consist of cuboidal to columnar cells with enlarged nuclei, with little cytoplasmic mucin, exhibiting solid tubulopapillary growth. Necrotic foci are often seen. Hematoxylin and eosin staining. Original magnifications were ×20 (a) and ×100 (b)

invasive, and is designated as intraductal tubulopapillary neoplasm with associated invasive carcinoma.

10.3.2 Epidemiology

ITPN is rare, barely accounting for 0.9% of the exocrine neoplasms and 3% of the intraductal neoplasms of the pancreas [32].

10.3.3 Etiology

No definite etiological factors of ITPNs are known.

10.3.4 Clinical Features

Clinical manifestations include abdominal pain, nausea, vomiting, jaundice, weight loss, and exacerbation of diabetes mellitus [32, 59]. Some patients have a history of acute pancreatitis [32].

10.3.5 Radiology

In CT scan, patients with ITPN show a solid enhanced mass, packed in a dilated duct. Magnetic resonance cholangiopancreatography indicates a filling defect in a dilated duct or an abrupt disruption of the dilated duct. Images of the dilated duct packed with tumor, are known as the two-tone duct sign and the cork-in-wine bottle sign [60]. ITPNs that involve the MPD show a sausage-like image in magnetic resonance imaging [61].

10.3.6 Pathology

10.3.6.1 Macroscopic Appearance
ITPNs show a solid tumor packed in dilated pancreatic ducts, without visible mucin. Cystic ducts are occasionally seen in the periphery of a neoplasm-obstructed duct [32, 59].

10.3.6.2 Microscopic Appearance and Variations
Cuboidal to columnar cells with enlarged nuclei, with little cytoplasmic mucin, exhibit solid tubulopapillary growth [32, 59]. Some may consist of tubular glands. The neoplastic cells show uniformly high-grade atypia (Fig. 10.3). Intraductal comedo-like necrosis is often present. Stromal invasion can be seen in the periductal parenchyma, which shows clusters of tubulopapillary glands. Tumor emboli are occasionally evident in the veins [32].

10.3.6.3 Immunohistochemistry
Cytokeratin (CK) 7 and CK19 are consistently positive. Mucin glycoproteins, MUC1 and MUC6 are positive, while MUC2 and MUC5AC are negative [32, 59]. Trypsin, an acinar marker, is negative.

10.3.6.4 Differential Diagnosis
A solid intraductal neoplasm can be observed in the intraductal variant of acinar cell carcinoma and intraductal neuroendocrine tumors [62, 63]. Histologically, neuroendocrine

tumors can be easily differentiated; however, the intraductal variant of acinar cell carcinoma may show solid tubular growth with necrosis, mimicking ITPNs. Acinar cell carcinomas usually express trypsin, an immunohistochemical marker of differentiation [32]. IPMNs occasionally show solid nodules inside the dilated duct. IPMN of the pyloric gland variant may particularly show a polypoid tumor in a dilated duct, mainly consisting of tubular glands. However, it can be distinguished from ITPNs by its well-formed tubular glands with low-grade atypia and the expression pattern of mucin which is negative for MUC1 and positive for MUC5AC [64].

10.3.6.5 Molecular Pathology

ITPNs often show somatic mutations in *PIK3CA*, *KMT2C*, *KMT2D*, and *BAP1* [65, 66]. Some tumors also harbor *FGFR2* fusion genes [66]. *KRAS* or *GNAS* mutations that are common in IPMNs, are not seen in ITPNs. Aberrant expression of p16 and p53 is reported in up to 70% of the cases [59], while the atypical expression of SMAD4 is rare [32, 59].

10.3.7 Treatment and Prognosis

Surgery is the treatment of choice for patients with ITPN, but some of them may experience a recurrence in the remnant tissue after pancreatectomy [32, 59]. ITPNs diffusely involving the pancreatic duct, need total pancreatectomy [32, 59, 67]. Efficacy of the adjuvant therapy is not known. About 10% of the patients with ITPN die of the disease [32, 59], and all of them are reported to have invasive tumors.

References

1. Hruban RH, Takaori K, Klimstra DS, Adsay NV, Albores-Saavedra J, Biankin AV, et al. An illustrated consensus on the classification of pancreatic intraepithelial neoplasia and intraductal papillary mucinous neoplasms. Am J Surg Pathol. 2004;28(8):977–87.
2. Tanaka M, Chari S, Adsay V, Fernandez-del Castillo C, Falconi M, Shimizu M, et al. International consensus guidelines for management of intraductal papillary mucinous neoplasms and mucinous cystic neoplasms of the pancreas. Pancreatology. 2006;6(1–2):17–32.
3. Furukawa T, Takahashi T, Kobari M, Matsuno S. The mucus-hypersecreting tumor of the pancreas. Development and extension visualized by three-dimensional computerized mapping. Cancer. 1992;70(6):1505–13.
4. Basturk O, Hong SM, Wood LD, Adsay NV, Albores-Saavedra J, Biankin AV, et al. A revised classification system and recommendations from the baltimore consensus meeting for neoplastic precursor lesions in the pancreas. Am J Surg Pathol. 2015;39(12):1730–41.
5. Laffan TA, Horton KM, Klein AP, Berlanstein B, Siegelman SS, Kawamoto S, et al. Prevalence of unsuspected pancreatic cysts on MDCT. AJR Am J Roentgenol. 2008;191(3):802–7.
6. Chang YR, Park JK, Jang JY, Kwon W, Yoon JH, Kim SW. Incidental pancreatic cystic neoplasms in an asymptomatic healthy population of 21,745 individuals: large-scale, single-center cohort study. Medicine (Baltimore). 2016;95(51):e5535.
7. Su GH, Hruban RH, Bansal RK, Bova GS, Tang DJ, Shekher MC, et al. Germline and somatic mutations of the STK11/LKB1 Peutz-Jeghers gene in pancreatic and biliary cancers. Am J Pathol. 1999;154(6):1835–40.
8. Maire F, Hammel P, Terris B, Olschwang S, O'Toole D, Sauvanet A, et al. Intraductal papillary and mucinous pancreatic tumour: a new extracolonic tumour in familial adenomatous polyposis. Gut. 2002;51(3):446–9.
9. Wood LD, Noe M, Hackeng W, Brosens LA, Bhaijee F, Debeljak M, et al. Patients with McCune-Albright syndrome have a broad spectrum of abnormalities in the gastrointestinal tract and pancreas. Virchows Arch. 2017;470(4):391–400.
10. Canto MI, Hruban RH, Fishman EK, Kamel IR, Schulick R, Zhang Z, et al. Frequent detection of pancreatic lesions in asymptomatic high-risk individuals. Gastroenterology. 2012;142(4):796–804; quiz e14–5.
11. Kloppel G. Clinicopathologic view of intraductal papillary-mucinous tumor of the pancreas. Hepato-Gastroenterology. 1998;45(24):1981–5.
12. Traverso LW, Peralta EA, Ryan JA Jr, Kozarek RA. Intraductal neoplasms of the pancreas. Am J Surg. 1998;175(5):426–32.
13. Yasuda H, Takada T, Amano H, Yoshida M. Surgery for mucin-producing pancreatic tumor. Hepato-Gastroenterology. 1998;45(24):2009–15.
14. Salvia R, Fernandez-del Castillo C, Bassi C, Thayer SP, Falconi M, Mantovani W, et al. Main-duct intraductal papillary mucinous neoplasms of the pancreas: clinical predictors of malignancy and long-term survival following resection. Ann Surg. 2004;239(5):678–685; discussion 85–7.
15. Sohn TA, Yeo CJ, Cameron JL, Hruban RH, Fukushima N, Campbell KA, et al. Intraductal papillary mucinous neoplasms of the pancreas: an updated experience. Ann Surg. 2004;239(6):788–97; discussion 97–9.
16. Tanaka M, Fernandez-Del Castillo C, Kamisawa T, Jang JY, Levy P, Ohtsuka T, et al. Revisions of international consensus Fukuoka guidelines for the management of IPMN of the pancreas. Pancreatology. 2017;17(5):738–53.
17. Kobari M, Egawa S, Shibuya K, Shimamura H, Sunamura M, Takeda K, et al. Intraductal papillary mucinous tumors of the pancreas comprise 2 clinical subtypes: differences in clinical characteristics and surgical management. Arch Surg. 1999;134(10):1131–6.
18. Tanaka M, Fernandez-del Castillo C, Adsay V, Chari S, Falconi M, Jang JY, et al. International consensus guidelines 2012 for the management of IPMN and MCN of the pancreas. Pancreatology. 2012;12(3):183–97.
19. Furukawa T, Oohashi K, Yamao K, Naitoh Y, Hirooka Y, Taki T, et al. Intraductal ultrasonography of the pancreas: development and clinical potential. Endoscopy. 1997;29(6):561–9.
20. Koito K, Namieno T, Nagakawa T, Hirokawa N, Ichimura T, Syonai T, et al. Pancreas: imaging diagnosis with color/power Doppler ultrasonography, endoscopic ultrasonography, and intraductal ultrasonography. Eur J Radiol. 2001;38(2):94–104.
21. Furukawa T, Kloppel G, Adsay NV, Albores-Saavedra J, Fukushima N, Horii A, et al. Classification of types of intraductal papillary-mucinous neoplasm of the pancreas: a consensus study. Virchows Arch. 2005;447(5):794–9.
22. Furukawa T, Hatori T, Fujita I, Yamamoto M, Kobayashi M, Ohike N, et al. Prognostic relevance of morphological types of intraductal papillary mucinous neoplasms of the pancreas. Gut. 2011;60(4):509–16.
23. Basturk O, Tan M, Bhanot U, Allen P, Adsay V, Scott SN, et al. The oncocytic subtype is genetically distinct from other pancreatic

intraductal papillary mucinous neoplasm subtypes. Mod Pathol. 2016;29(9):1058–69.
24. Terada T, Ohta T, Nakanuma Y. Expression of oncogene products, anti-oncogene products and oncofetal antigens in intraductal papillary-mucinous neoplasm of the pancreas. Histopathology. 1996;29(4):355–61.
25. Terada T, Ohta T, Kitamura Y, Ashida K, Matsunaga Y. Cell proliferative activity in intraductal papillary-mucinous neoplasms and invasive ductal adenocarcinomas of the pancreas: an immunohistochemical study. Arch Pathol Lab Med. 1998;122(1):42–6.
26. Adsay NV, Merati K, Basturk O, Iacobuzio-Donahue C, Levi E, Cheng JD, et al. Pathologically and biologically distinct types of epithelium in intraductal papillary mucinous neoplasms: delineation of an "intestinal" pathway of carcinogenesis in the pancreas. Am J Surg Pathol. 2004;28(7):839–48.
27. Nakamura A, Horinouchi M, Goto M, Nagata K, Sakoda K, Takao S, et al. New classification of pancreatic intraductal papillary-mucinous tumour by mucin expression: its relationship with potential for malignancy. J Pathol. 2002;197(2):201–10.
28. Adsay NV, Merati K, Andea A, Sarkar F, Hruban RH, Wilentz RE, et al. The dichotomy in the preinvasive neoplasia to invasive carcinoma sequence in the pancreas: differential expression of MUC1 and MUC2 supports the existence of two separate pathways of carcinogenesis. Mod Pathol. 2002;15(10):1087–95.
29. Furukawa T, Fujisaki R, Yoshida Y, Kanai N, Sunamura M, Abe T, et al. Distinct progression pathways involving the dysfunction of DUSP6/MKP-3 in pancreatic intraepithelial neoplasia and intraductal papillary-mucinous neoplasms of the pancreas. Mod Pathol. 2005;18(8):1034–42.
30. Compagno J, Oertel JE. Mucinous cystic neoplasms of the pancreas with overt and latent malignancy (cystadenocarcinoma and cystadenoma). A clinicopathologic study of 41 cases. Am J Clin Pathol. 1978;69(6):573–80.
31. Lewandrowski K, Warshaw A, Compton C. Macrocystic serous cystadenoma of the pancreas: a morphologic variant differing from microcystic adenoma. Hum Pathol. 1992;23(8):871–5.
32. Yamaguchi H, Shimizu M, Ban S, Koyama I, Hatori T, Fujita I, et al. Intraductal tubulopapillary neoplasms of the pancreas distinct from pancreatic intraepithelial neoplasia and intraductal papillary mucinous neoplasms. Am J Surg Pathol. 2009;33(8):1164–72.
33. Truong LD, Rangdaeng S, Jordan PH Jr. Lymphoepithelial cyst of the pancreas. Am J Surg Pathol. 1987;11(11):899–903.
34. Kloppel G. Pseudocysts and other non-neoplastic cysts of the pancreas. Semin Diagn Pathol. 2000;17(1):7–15.
35. Wu J, Matthaei H, Maitra A, Dal Molin M, Wood LD, Eshleman JR, et al. Recurrent *GNAS* mutations define an unexpected pathway for pancreatic cyst development. Sci Tansl Med. 2011;3(92):92ra66.
36. Furukawa T, Kuboki Y, Tanji E, Yoshida S, Hatori T, Yamamoto M, et al. Whole-exome sequencing uncovers frequent *GNAS* mutations in intraductal papillary mucinous neoplasms of the pancreas. Sci Rep. 2011;1:161.
37. Wu J, Jiao Y, Dal Molin M, Maitra A, de Wilde RF, Wood LD, et al. Whole-exome sequencing of neoplastic cysts of the pancreas reveals recurrent mutations in components of ubiquitin-dependent pathways. Proc Natl Acad Sci USA. 2011;108(52):21188–93.
38. Kuboki Y, Shimizu K, Hatori T, Yamamoto M, Shibata N, Shiratori K, et al. Molecular biomarkers for progression of intraductal papillary mucinous neoplasm of the pancreas. Pancreas. 2015;44(2):227–35.
39. Amato E, Molin MD, Mafficini A, Yu J, Malleo G, Rusev B, et al. Targeted next-generation sequencing of cancer genes dissects the molecular profiles of intraductal papillary neoplasms of the pancreas. J Pathol. 2014;233(3):217–27.
40. Sakamoto H, Kuboki Y, Hatori T, Yamamoto M, Sugiyama M, Shibata N, et al. Clinicopathological significance of somatic RNF43 mutation and aberrant expression of ring finger protein 43 in intraductal papillary mucinous neoplasms of the pancreas. Mod Pathol. 2015;28(2):261–7.
41. Biankin AV, Biankin SA, Kench JG, Morey AL, Lee CS, Head DR, et al. Aberrant p16(INK4A) and DPC4/Smad4 expression in intraductal papillary mucinous tumours of the pancreas is associated with invasive ductal adenocarcinoma. Gut. 2002;50(6):861–8.
42. Abe K, Suda K, Arakawa A, Yamasaki S, Sonoue H, Mitani K, et al. Different patterns of p16INK4A and p53 protein expressions in intraductal papillary-mucinous neoplasms and pancreatic intraepithelial neoplasia. Pancreas. 2007;34(1):85–91.
43. Iacobuzio-Donahue CA, Klimstra DS, Adsay NV, Wilentz RE, Argani P, Sohn TA, et al. Dpc-4 protein is expressed in virtually all human intraductal papillary mucinous neoplasms of the pancreas: comparison with conventional ductal adenocarcinomas. Am J Pathol. 2000;157(3):755–61.
44. Inoue H, Furukawa T, Sunamura M, Takeda K, Matsuno S, Horii A. Exclusion of SMAD4 mutation as an early genetic change in human pancreatic ductal tumorigenesis. Genes Chromosomes Cancer. 2001;31(3):295–9.
45. Chetty R, Serra S, Salahshor S, Alsaad K, Shih W, Blaszyk H, et al. Expression of Wnt-signaling pathway proteins in intraductal papillary mucinous neoplasms of the pancreas: a tissue microarray analysis. Hum Pathol. 2006;37(2):212–7.
46. Chari ST, Yadav D, Smyrk TC, DiMagno EP, Miller LJ, Raimondo M, et al. Study of recurrence after surgical resection of intraductal papillary mucinous neoplasm of the pancreas. Gastroenterology. 2002;123(5):1500–7.
47. Maire F, Hammel P, Terris B, Paye F, Scoazec JY, Cellier C, et al. Prognosis of malignant intraductal papillary mucinous tumours of the pancreas after surgical resection. Comparison with pancreatic ductal adenocarcinoma. Gut. 2002;51(5):717–22.
48. Mino-Kenudson M, Fernandez-del Castillo C, Baba Y, Valsangkar NP, Liss AS, Hsu M, et al. Prognosis of invasive intraductal papillary mucinous neoplasm depends on histological and precursor epithelial subtypes. Gut. 2011;60(12):1712–20.
49. Adsay NV, Adair CF, Heffess CS, Klimstra DS. Intraductal oncocytic papillary neoplasms of the pancreas. Am J Surg Pathol. 1996;20(8):980–94.
50. Basturk O, Esposito I, Fukushima N, Furukawa T, Hong SM, Klöppel G, et al. Pancreatic intraductal oncocytic papillary neoplasm. In: Gill AJ, Klimstra DS, Lam AK, Washington MK, editors. WHO Classification of Digestive System Tumours. WHO Classification of Tumours 1. Lyon: International Agency for Research on Cancer; 2019. p. 315–6.
51. Marchegiani G, Mino-Kenudson M, Ferrone CR, Warshaw AL, Lillemoe KD, Fernandez-del CC. Oncocytic-type intraductal papillary mucinous neoplasms: a unique malignant pancreatic tumor with good long-term prognosis. J Am Coll Surg. 2015;220(5):839–44.
52. Xiao HD, Yamaguchi H, Dias-Santagata D, Kuboki Y, Akhavanfard S, Hatori T, et al. Molecular characteristics and biological behaviours of the oncocytic and pancreatobiliary subtypes of intraductal papillary mucinous neoplasms. J Pathol. 2011;224(4):508–16.
53. D'Onofrio M, De Robertis R, Tinazzi Martini P, Capelli P, Gobbo S, Morana G, et al. Oncocytic intraductal papillary mucinous neoplasms of the pancreas: imaging and histopathological findings. Pancreas. 2016;45(9):1233–42.
54. Basturk O, Chung SM, Hruban RH, Adsay NV, Askan G, Iacobuzio-Donahue C, et al. Distinct pathways of pathogenesis of intraductal oncocytic papillary neoplasms and intraductal papillary mucinous neoplasms of the pancreas. Virchows Arch. 2016;469(5):523–32.
55. Singhi AD, Wood LD, Parks E, Torbenson MS, Felsenstein M, Hruban RH, et al. Recurrent rearrangements in *PRKACA* and *PRKACB* in intraductal oncocytic papillary neoplasms of the pancreas and bile duct. Gastroenterology. 2020;158(3):573–82 e2.
56. Vyas M, Hechtman JF, Zhang Y, Benayed R, Yavas A, Askan G, et al. *DNAJB1-PRKACA* fusions occur in oncocytic pancreatic and

57. Chang XY, Wu Y, Jiang Y, Wang PY, Chen J. RNF43 mutations in IPMN cases: a potential prognostic factor. Gastroenterol Res Pract. 2020;2020:1457452.
58. Takai E, Nakamura H, Chiku S, Kubo E, Ohmoto A, Totoki Y, et al. Whole-exome sequencing reveals new potential susceptibility genes for japanese familial pancreatic cancer. Ann Surg. 2020.
59. Basturk O, Adsay V, Askan G, Dhall D, Zamboni G, Shimizu M, et al. Intraductal tubulopapillary neoplasm of the pancreas: a clinicopathologic and immunohistochemical analysis of 33 cases. Am J Surg Pathol. 2017;41(3):313–25.
60. Motosugi U, Yamaguchi H, Furukawa T, Ichikawa T, Hatori T, Fujita I, et al. Imaging studies of intraductal tubulopapillary neoplasms of the pancreas: 2-tone duct sign and cork-of-wine-bottle sign as indicators of intraductal tumor growth. J Comput Assist Tomogr. 2012;36(6):710–7.
61. Lu ZF, Kang B, Li JM, Sun C. Intraductal tubulopapillary neoplasm of the pancreas presenting as sausage. Am J Gastroenterol. 2020.
62. Basturk O, Zamboni G, Klimstra DS, Capelli P, Andea A, Kamel NS, et al. Intraductal and papillary variants of acinar cell carcinomas: a new addition to the challenging differential diagnosis of intraductal neoplasms. Am J Surg Pathol. 2007;31(3):363–70.
63. Fabre A, Sauvanet A, Flejou JF, Belghiti J, Palazzo L, Ruzniewski P, et al. Intraductal acinar cell carcinoma of the pancreas. Virchows Arch. 2001;438(3):312–5.
64. Yamaguchi H, Kuboki Y, Hatori T, Yamamoto M, Shimizu K, Shiratori K, et al. The discrete nature and distinguishing molecular features of pancreatic intraductal tubulopapillary neoplasms and intraductal papillary mucinous neoplasms of the gastric type, pyloric gland variant. J Pathol. 2013;231(3):335–41.
65. Yamaguchi H, Kuboki Y, Hatori T, Yamamoto M, Shiratori K, Kawamura S, et al. Somatic mutations in PIK3CA and activation of AKT in intraductal tubulopapillary neoplasms of the pancreas. Am J Surg Pathol. 2011;35(12):1812–7.
66. Basturk O, Berger MF, Yamaguchi H, Adsay V, Askan G, Bhanot UK, et al. Pancreatic intraductal tubulopapillary neoplasm is genetically distinct from intraductal papillary mucinous neoplasm and ductal adenocarcinoma. Mod Pathol. 2017;30(12):1760–72.
67. Kosmidis C, Varsamis N, Atmatzidis S, Koimtzis G, Mantalovas S, Anthimidis G, et al. Total pancreatectomy with splenectomy for multifocal Intraductal Tubulopapillary Neoplasm (ITPN) of the pancreas associated with invasive component: report of a rare case. Am J Case Rep. 2020;21:e924760.

Mucinous Cystic Neoplasms

Noriyoshi Fukushima

Abstract

Mucinous cystic neoplasm (MCN) of the pancreas is one of the three most common primary cyst-forming epithelial neoplasms of the pancreas including intraductal papillary mucinous neoplasm (IPMN), serous cystic neoplasm (SCN) and MCN. From another point of view, MCN is one of the three precursors of invasive adenocarcinoma of the pancreas including pancreatic intraepithelial neoplasia (PanIN), IPMN and MCN. MCNs occur almost exclusively in the distal pancreas of middle-aged women. Grossly, MCNs typically show a "cyst-in-cyst" pattern of growth, and are well encapsulated by a thick fibrous wall. In histology, MCNs are composed of mucinous neoplastic epithelial cells and subepithelial cellular stroma called as "ovarian-type" stroma. The epithelium is dysplastic and the grade can be divided into low- and high-grade, and some MCNs have an associated invasive carcinoma. MCNs harbor several characteristic genetic and epigenetic alterations, some of which are shared with conventional invasive pancreatic ductal adenocarcinoma. Several studies suggest steroidogenesis in the "ovarian-type" stroma. A 5-year survival rate of non-invasive MCN is 100%, and MCN with T1a and T1b carcinoma also had an excellent prognosis. However, in one study, MCN with invasive carcinoma show aggressive clinical course; a 3-year and 5-year survival rate are 44% and 26%, respectively. In European guidelines, MCNs <40 mm are treated conservatively when other risk factors are absent. In international and American guidelines, on the other hand, an MCN of any size is an absolute indication for resection. Better knowledge of the pathology and molecular alterations could help in the management of patients with MCN.

11.1 Introduction

Most cystic lesions of the pancreas, increasingly being recognized with improvements in diagnostic imaging, are non-neoplastic benign cysts such as retention cysts and pseudocysts [1]. Cystic neoplastic lesions are a minority of the cystic lesions of the pancreas. Mucinous cystic neoplasms (MCNs) is one of the three most common primary cyst-forming epithelial neoplasms of the pancreas including intraductal papillary mucinous neoplasm (IPMN), serous cystic neoplasm (SCN) and MCN [1, 2]. Compagno and Oertel clarified the distinction between serous and mucin-producing cystic neoplasms in 1978 [3]. In 1982 Ohashi et al. first described "mucous secreting pancreatic cancer" that is now classified into IPMN [4]. Through most of the 1990s, the distinction between MCNs and branch-duct type IPMNs was unclear and controversial, because stromal component of MCN had not been noticed well. Then now we recognize, as current WHO guideline describes, "MCN is a grossly visible, multilocular cystic lesion, with no communication to the ductal system; a cystic lesion with cuboidal and columnar neoplastic epithelia, staining at least partly positive for mucin, with variable atypia; ovarian-like, mesenchymal stroma, at least focally positive for ER and/or PR [2]."

From another point of view, MCN is one of the three precursors of invasive adenocarcinoma of the pancreas including pancreatic intraepithelial neoplasia (PanIN), IPMN and MCN. Namely, MCN can develop and have invasive carcinoma as PanIN and IPMN. So clinical decision making, surgical resection or follow up, is very important.

In this article, clinicopathologic characteristics of MCNs are reviewed.

N. Fukushima (✉)
Department of Pathology, Jichi Medical University, Shimotsuke, Tochigi, Japan
e-mail: nfukushima@jichi.ac.jp

11.2 Clinical Aspects

MCNs are noticed most frequently in young or middle-aged (mean about 48 years old) women [2, 5, 6]. Patients with invasive carcinoma are 5–10 years older than patients with a non-invasive MCN. Most MCN are located in the body and tail of the pancreas [1, 2]. Small MCNs are usually found incidentally, and larger tumors may produce symptoms including a palpable mass and discomfort due to compression of adjacent structures. General fatigue and weight loss are rarely seen.

In imaging studies, the classic appearance of MCN is a thickened wall, which enhances on contrast-enhanced CT and MR imaging. Calcification is occasionally seen at the edge of the cyst. Cysts are unilocular or multilocular and show so-called "cyst-in -cyst" appearance as described in macroscopical features.

The incidence of associated invasive carcinoma in resected MCN was various up to about 30%, which is considered to be depending on the criteria for surgical resection because there are relatively many early lesions may have been detected by diagnostic imaging in recent years. Findings associated with malignancy are reported that 56 years or older, high serum carcinoembryonic antigen level, high carbohydrate antigen 19–9 level, tumor size of 51 mm or greater, and the presence of mural nodules [7].

11.3 Pathological Findings

11.3.1 Macroscopical Features

MCNs are well-encapsulated round cystic mass and usually large-ranging up to 35 cm, although there is a tendency to be detected smaller size recently [8–11]. The cut surface shows uni- or multilocular cysts, so-called "cyst-in-cyst appearance", with fibrous cyst wall and/or septum with variable thickness and frequent calcifications (Fig. 11.1a and b). Cysts typically contain mucus, but watery fluid, or hemorrhagic and/or necrotic material are often seen. The internal surface can show smooth or be with papillary growing soft tumors or solid nodules. The presence of larger papillary projections correlates with higher grade of neoplasm and possible invasive components. Usually no communicate with the pancreatic ductal system is seen.

11.3.2 Histological Features

MCN is composed of mucinous neoplastic epithelium and subepithelial ovarian-type stroma (OS). Especially this OS is the most characteristic histologic feature of MCN distinct from IPMN or other cystic neoplasms [1, 2].

The internal surface of the cysts is lined by columnar mucinous epithelium, which may occur in a single layer with some areas showing papillary growth (Fig. 11.2a and b). The neoplastic epithelium shows gastric foveolar, pyloric-type glandular, intestinal or pancreatobiliary type epithelium, similar to IPMN, in each case and sometimes mixed with several components within the same tumor. Each neoplasm is graded as low-grade or high-grade on the basis of the highest degree of dysplasia of the neoplastic epithelium (Fig. 11.2a and b). According to the current WHO classification, carcinoma in situ (non-invasive carcinoma) of MCN is acceptable as a synonym high-grade MCN [2].

The OS that underlines the mucinous epithelium is a typically cellular stroma [5, 12, 13] (Figs. 11.2a, b, 11.3a). It is occasionally hard to identify this "ovarian-type" stroma because the stroma can be changed into hyalinous fibrous bandles over time and/or by intracystic pressure. In those

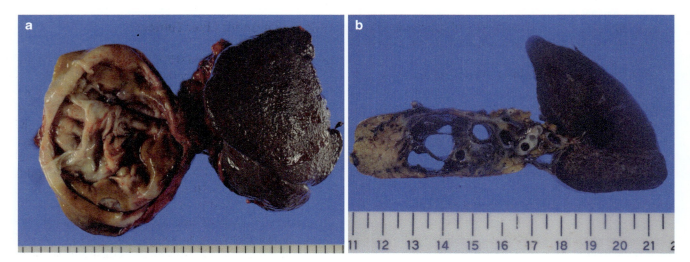

Fig. 11.1 Macroscopic feature of mucinous cystic neoplasm (MCN). (**a**) A case of large unilocular MCN. (**b**) The cut surface shows multilocular cysts, so-called "cyst-in-cyst appearance" in this case

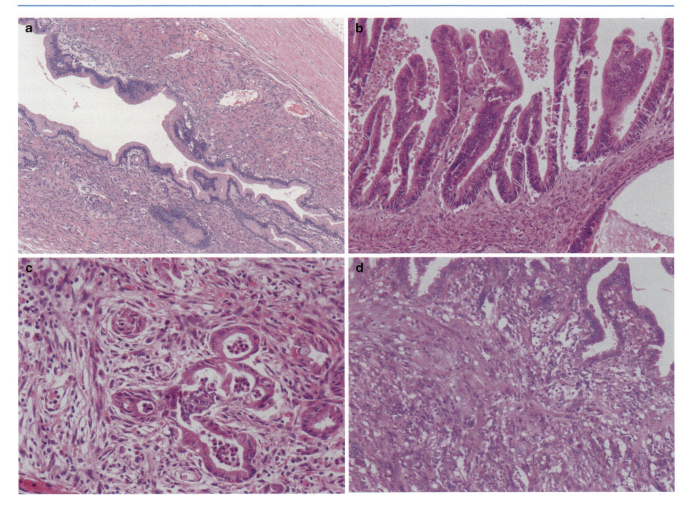

Fig. 11.2 Histology of mucinous cystic neoplasm (MCN). (**a**) Columnar mucinous epithelium with low-grade dysplasia and subepithelial "ovarian type" stroma are seen. (**b**) MCN with high-grade dysplasia. The epithelial component has an irregular papillary growth with severe cellular atypia. (**c**) Invasive component shows tubular adenocarcinoma. (**d**) This case has an associated invasive component of spindle carcinomatous cells with irregularity enlarged nuclei (undifferentiated carcinoma)

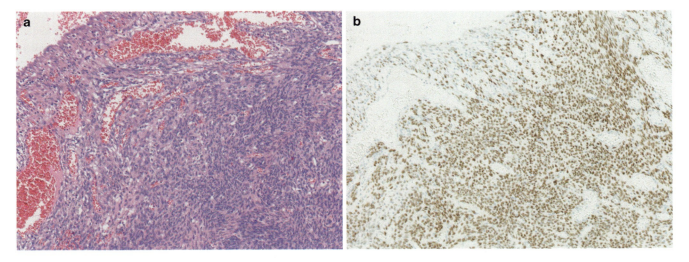

Fig. 11.3 (**a**) Cellular stroma is present but surface epithelial component is denuded. (**b**) Nuclear expression of progesterone receptor (PR) in the cells of the cellular stroma is seen. This finding allows us to determine that this is an MCN

cases, the features described as follows are useful to identify "ovarian-type" stroma: a layered structure (OS is usually located immediately beneath the epithelial layer), the presence of small round, eosinophilic cells resembling luteinized cells, overlapping cell nuclei in some areas, being intermingled with capillaries, and the waviness of the spindle cells [5].

Spindle cells of OS show immunoreactivity for vimentin, smooth-muscle actin [12], progesterone receptors (PR) (Fig. 11.2b), and estrogen receptors (ER) [1, 2, 5]. Occasional "luteinized cells" are expressing alpha-inhibin and/or steroidogenic acute regulatory protein (STAR) [13].

Invasive features usually resemble the common ductal adenocarcinoma (Fig. 11.2c), and colloid/mucinous carcinomas are rare, though focal expression of CDX2 in neoplastic epithelium is found in half of MCN [14]. MCNs with malignant "sarcomatous stroma" have been reported, but are likely spindle cell carcinomas rather than mesenchymal neoplasms (Fig. 11.2d) [15].

The staging of the MCNs with an associated invasive carcinoma should be determined by the UICC/AJCC. The overall size of the invasive carcinoma should be recorded and categorized into pT1a (< 0.5 cm), pT1b (0.5 to 1 cm) and pT1c (> 1 cm), and pT2 (>2 cm) and beyond [16].

11.4 Molecular Abnormalities

During the last three decades, significant advances have been made in our understanding of the molecular biology of pancreatic neoplasms including MCN. For pancreatic ductal adenocarcinomas arising through the conventional PanIN pathway, the most frequent recurring alterations occur in the following 4 genes: *KRAS, TP53, CDKN2A,* and *SMAD4* [17]. According to the studies using next-generation sequencing analysis, the recurring molecular alterations in high-risk MCN were similar to those described in PanINs and in PDAC [17, 18]. Jimenez et al. reported KRAS alterations in 20% of tumors considered benign and 89% considered malignant [19]. The low frequency of KRAS mutations in low-grade MCN suggests a low risk for malignant progression. KRAS gene has an important role in the pathogenesis of pancreatic adenocarcinomas arising from MCN. TP53 was mutated in more than 50% of high-grade MCNs and may also be a useful marker of high-grade and/or MCN with an invasive carcinoma [19]. RNF43, a gene coding for a protein with intrinsic E3 ubiquitin ligase activity, alterations are largely in non-invasive lesions of MCN [18, 20]. Several studies have reported somatic mutations in the PIK3CA gene in several neoplasms including MCN [21], but not in PDAC. Furthermore, there is a tendency for PIK3CA gene mutations to occur in higher grade lesions. Guanine nucleotide binding protein, alpha stimulating (GNAS) gene mutations are common and early genetic changes in IPMNs, and especially in most intestinal type of IPMN [22, 23]. On the other hand, MCNs do not harbor GNAS gene mutations.

We previously reported several gene expression in OS, which included estrogen receptor 1 (ESR1) and STAR [12, 13]. The STAR protein has a key role in steroid hormone synthesis. Furthermore, 3 beta-hydroxysteroid dehydrogenase (3 beta-HSD), 17 alpha-hydroxylase (17 alpha-H) and 5α-reductase-1 (5αRED-1) were also reported to be overexpressed in OS of MCNs [24, 25].

Although the origin of the OS remains unknown, one possibility is that MCN may arise from ectopic ovarian stroma in the pancreas, and the other is that MCNs may arise from periductal immature stroma stimulated by female hormones in the pancreas during embryogenesis. Ectopic ovarian stroma may release kinds of hormones and growth factors, and proliferate epithelium and form cystic tumors. The expression of ER and other steroidogenesis-associated proteins in OS, and several cases of MCNs associated with pregnancy showing rapid growth have been reported [26], and it is suggest an association with effect of female hormones in pathogenesis.

11.5 Treatment and Prognosis

The majority of MCNs show an indolent clinical course. Almost all of MCNs without invasive carcinoma are cured by surgical resection [10]. MCNs are more often low-grade and less common having associated invasive component comparing to IPMNs. Furthermore, MCN with T1a and T1b carcinoma (<1 cm in size) were reported as showing an excellent prognosis similar to MCNs without invasive carcinoma [10, 11]. This suggests that close follow up rather than aggressive systemic therapy may be a better approach to manage the patients with a MCN with small invasive carcinoma arising in MCN. In relatively young age of most patients, considering the risk of progression to invasive MCN, surgical resection is recommended. MCNs are usually located in the pancreatic body and tail, and thus require distal pancreatectomy that can be performed safely.

On the other hand, patients with MCN showing aggressive clinical course have been reported. Jang et al. reported that 3- and 5-year survival rates of the patient with MCN with an invasive carcinoma are 44% and 26%, respectively. This study cases, however, included 12 cases having advanced invasion (>2 cm), and furthermore 5 out 29 case with undifferentiated carcinoma [27]. And all reports described above were examined in surgically resected cases and may be significantly affected by the criteria for surgical indication.

There are several guidelines for management of pancreatic cystic lesions especially in IPMN and MCN [28–30]. Based on the recent studies, these guidelines suggest a possibility of nonoperative management for small MCNs without high-risk features and especially in elderly patients. However there are several differences among those proposal. European guidelines and American Gastroenterological Association (AGA) guidelines have been designed for pancreatic cystic lesions in general, on the other hand, the International Association of Pancreatology (IAP) guidelines mainly focuses on the management of branch-duct type IPMN. In European guidelines say that MCN ≥40 mm (size of the cyst) should undergo surgical resection. Resection is also recommended for MCN irrespective of their size which are symptomatic or have risk factors such as mural nodule [29]. MCN measuring <40 mm without a mural nodule or symptoms may undergo imaging studies with MRI and/or EUS. Surveillance is recommended every 6 months for the first year, then annually if no changes are observed. In AGA guidelines only recommend surgery if two concerning features, such as increase size (>3 cm) or main-duct dilatation and solid component, are present and cytologic analysis of the fluid or cyst wall is either malignant or suspicious for high-grade dysplasia [30]. In IAP guidelines, observation may be considered in elderly patients. However, given the relatively young age of most patients surgical resection is recommended for all surgically appropriate patients, and it would require years of follow-up based on high-resolution imaging [28].

Better knowledge of the pathology and molecular alterations could help in the management of patients with MCN.

References

1. Hruban RH, Pitman MB, Klimstra DS. Tumors of the Pancreas (AFIP Atlas of Tumor Pathology; 4th Series Fascicle 6) American Registry of Pathology; 2007.
2. Gill AJ, Klimstra DS, Lam AK, Washington MK (eds). Tumours of the pancreas. In WHO classification of tumours – 5th edition – Digestive System, 294–373, IARC Press, Lyons, 2019.
3. Compagno J, Oertel JE. Microcystic adenomas of the pancreas (glycogen-rich cystadenomas): a clinicopathologic study of 34 cases. Am J Clin Pathol. 1978;69:289–98.
4. Ohashi K, Murakami Y, Maruyama M. Four cases of a mucous secreting pancreatic cancer [in Japanese]. Prog Dig Endosc. 1982;20:348–51.
5. Zamboni G, Scarpa A, Bogina G, et al. Mucinous cystic tumors of the pancreas: clinicopathological features, prognosis, and relationship to other mucinous cystic tumors. Am J Surg Pathol. 1999;23:410–22.
6. Thompson LD, Becker RC, Przygodzki RM, Adair CF, Heffess CS. Mucinous cystic neoplasm (mucinous cystadenocarcinoma of low-grade malignant potential) of the pancreas: a clinicopathologic study of 130 cases. Am J Surg Pathol. 1999;23:1–16.
7. Ohtsuka T, Nakamura M, Hijioka S, et al. Prediction of the probability of malignancy in mucinous cystic neoplasm of the pancreas with ovarian-type stroma: a nationwide multicenter study in Japan. Pancreas. 2020;49(2):181–6.
8. Crippa S, Salvia R, Warshaw AL, et al. Mucinous cystic neoplasm of the pancreas is not an aggressive entity: lessons from 163 resected patients. Ann Surg. 2008;247(4):571–9.
9. Yamao K, Yanagisawa A, Takahashi K, et al. Clinicopathological features and prognosis of mucinous cystic neoplasm with ovarian-type stroma: a multi-institutional study of the Japan pancreas society. Pancreas. 2011;40:67–71.
10. Griffin JF, Page AJ, Samaha GJ, et al. Patients with a resected pancreatic mucinous cystic neoplasm have a better prognosis than patients with an intraductal papillary mucinous neoplasm: a large single institution series. Pancreatology. 2017;17(3):490–6.
11. Hui L, Rashid A, Foo WC, et al. Significance of T1a and T1b carcinoma arising in mucinous cystic neoplasm of pancreas. Am J Surg Pathol. 2018;42(5):578–86.
12. Fukushima N, Mukai K, Kanai Y, et al. Intraductal papillary tumors and mucinous cystic tumors of the pancreas. Clinicopathologic study of 38 cases. Hum Pathol. 1997;28:1010–7.
13. Fukushima N, Sato N, Yeo CJ, Cameron JL, Hruban RH, Goggins M. Characterization of mucinous cystic neoplasms (MCNs) of the pancreas using oligonucleotide-microarrays. Oncogene. 2004;23:9042–51.
14. Baker ML, Seeley ES, Pai R, et al. Invasive mucinous cystic neoplasms of the pancreas. Exp Mol Pathol. 2012;93:345–9.
15. Albores-Saavedra J, Manivel C, Dorantes-Heredia R, et al. Nonmucinouscystadenomas of the pancreas with pancreatobiliary phenotype and ovarian-like stroma. Am J Clin Pathol. 2013;139:599–604.
16. Brierley J, Gospodarowicz MK, Wittekind C. TNM classification of malignant tumours. 8th ed. Hoboken, New Jersey: Wiley-Blackwell; 2017. p. 93–5.
17. Hruban RH, Adsay NV, Esposito I, et al. Pancreatic ductal adenocarcinoma. In WHO classification of tumours – 5th edition – Digestive System (Eds: the WHO classification of tumours editorial board), 322–332, IARC Press, Lyons, 2019.
18. Wu J, Jiao Y, Dal Molin M, et al. Whole-exome sequencing of neoplastic cysts of the pancreas reveals recurrent mutations in components of ubiquitin-dependent pathways. Proc Natl Acad Sci USA. 2011;108(52):21188–93.
19. Conner JR, Mariño-Enríquez A, Mino-Kenudson M, et al. Characterization of low- and high-grade pancreatic mucinous cystic neoplasms reveals recurrent KRAS alterations in "high-risk" lesions. Pancreas. 2017;46(5):665–71.
20. Noë M, Niknafs N, Fischer CG, et al. Genomic characterization of malignant progression in neoplastic pancreatic cysts. Nat Commun. 2020;14;11(1):4085.
21. Garcia-Carracedo D, Chen ZM, Qiu W, et al. PIK3CA mutations in mucinous cystic neoplasms of the pancreas. Pancreas. 2014;43(2):245–9.
22. Furukawa T, Kuboki Y, Tanji E, et al. Whole-exome sequencing uncovers frequent GNAS mutations in intraductal papillary mucinous neoplasms of the pancreas. Sci Rep. 2011;1:161.
23. Dal Molin M, Matthaei H, Wu J, et al. Clinicopathological correlates of activating GNAS mutations in intraductal papillary mucinous neoplasm (IPMN) of the pancreas. Ann Surg Oncol. 2013;20(12):3802–8.
24. Ishiguro H, Kato K, Kishimoto T, et al. Expression of steroidogenic enzymes by luteinizing cells in the ovarian-type stroma of a mucin-producing cystic tumour of the pancreas. Histopathology. 2003;43:94–100.
25. Kumata H, Murakami K, Ishida K, et al. Steroidogenesis in ovarian-like mesenchymal stroma of hepatic and pancreatic mucinous cystic neoplasms. Hepatol Res. 2018;48(12):989–99.
26. Revoredo F, de Vinatea J, Reaño G, et al. Mucinous cystic neoplasms of the pancreas associated with pregnancy: two case reports. Medicine (Baltimore). 2020;31;99(31):e21471.
27. Jang KT, Park SM, Basturk O, et al. Clinicopathologic characteristics of 29 invasive carcinomas arising in 178 pancreatic mucinous cystic neoplasms with ovarian-type stroma: implications for management and prognosis. Am J Surg Pathol. 2015;39(2):179–87.

28. Tanaka M, Fernández-del Castillo C, Adsay V, et al. International consensus guidelines 2012 for the management of IPMN and MCN of the pancreas. Pancreatology. 2012;12(3):183–97.
29. European evidence-based guidelines on pancreatic cystic neoplasms. European Study Group on Cystic Tumours of the Pancreas. Gut. 2018;67:789–804.
30. Scheiman JM, Hwang JH, Moayyedi P. American gastroenterological association technical review on the diagnosis and management of asymptomatic neoplastic pancreatic cysts. Gastroenterology. 2015;148(4):824–48.e22.

Pathology of Pancreatic Cancer

Ralph H. Hruban and Elizabeth Thompson

Abstract

Pathology provides remarkable insight into the biology of ductal adenocarcinomas of the pancreas, and pathology is the basis for the clinical management of patients with the disease. An understanding of the pathology of pancreatic cancer is therefore critical to those studying the disease, as well as those treating pancreatic cancer patients. This chapter will review the pathology of pancreatic cancer with an emphasis on clinical implications. We will also delve more deeply into several unique features of the disease, including the intense desmoplastic stroma these cancers elicit as they invade into tissues, and the propensity of the neoplastic cells to invade the venous system. These two features may provide insight into the poor sensitivity of pancreatic cancer to chemotherapy, and help explain why these cancers so frequently metastasize to the liver.

12.1 Introduction

Pancreatic cancer is one of the deadliest of all of the solid malignancies, and yet histologically many pancreatic cancers appear deceptively bland and can be hard to diagnose [1, 2]. This is one of the great mysteries in pathology—how can such a deadly cancer look so harmless under the microscope? In this chapter we will provide an overview of the pathology of ductal adenocarcinoma of the pancreas, referred to here as "pancreatic cancer."

We will first describe the gross and microscopic appearance of pancreatic cancer, as well as the features that are used by practicing pathologists to diagnose ductal adenocarcinomas of the pancreas. We will then highlight pathologic features that can help guide patient care. Finally, looking forward, we will discuss several of the distinctive features that characterize pancreatic cancer, but are rare in other tumor types, as these may provide avenues for future advances. The first of these features is the intense desmoplastic reaction that almost universally accompanies pancreatic cancer [3]. The second is the propensity for pancreatic cancer to invade veins [4, 5]. While lymphatic invasion is unfortunately all too common in most cancer types, venous invasion, the invasion of the neoplastic cells into veins with muscular walls, in particularly common in pancreatic cancer and may explain why it is so deadly [4].

Finally, it is important to recognize that among pancreatic cancers there can be significant variation. It used to be said that, "if you have seen one pancreatic cancer you have seen them all." In fact, although pancreatic cancers superficially often have a uniform appearance of tubules embedded in dense stroma, a number of clinically important variants have been recognized. Some of these variants have been associated with specific genetic alterations, helping to establish them as separate entities [6–14].

12.1.1 General Features

Grossly, most pancreatic cancers form firm, white and ill-defined infiltrative masses [2, 15]. When they involve the main pancreatic duct they can cause upstream ductal dilatation (Fig. 12.1a). Central necrosis may occur in larger lesions, and the infiltrative edges of the cancers often encase blood vessels (Fig. 12.1b).

Microscopically, by definition, these are infiltrative gland-forming neoplasms [2, 15]. The neoplastic glands are haphazardly arranged, infiltrative and they induce an intense desmoplastic stroma (Fig. 12.2a and b). They can even grow from the stroma back into the ductal system, a process designated "cancerization of the ducts" [16]. Of interest, it appears

R. H. Hruban (✉) · E. Thompson
Department of Pathology, The Sol Goldman Pancreatic Cancer Research Center, Baltimore, MD, USA

Department of Oncology, The Johns Hopkins University School of Medicine, Baltimore, MD, USA
e-mail: rhruban@jhmi.edu

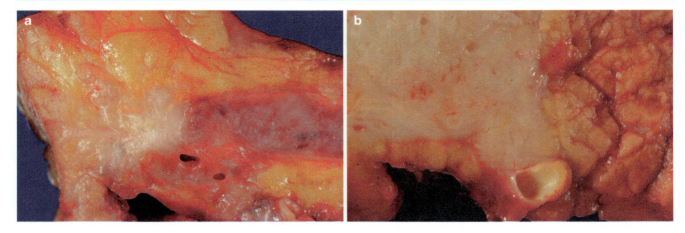

Fig. 12.1 Gross photographs of infiltrating ductal adenocarcinoma. Note the ductal dilitation secondary to the carcinoma stenosing the pancreatic duct in panel **a**, and the involvement of large vessels in panel **b**

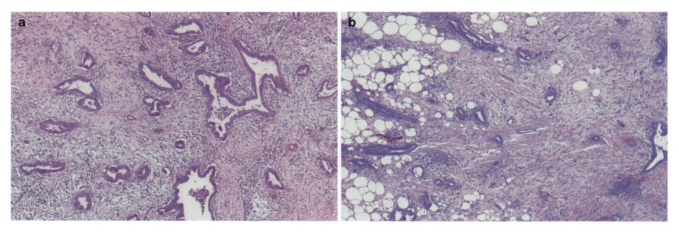

Fig. 12.2 Histologic sections of infiltrating ductal adenocarcinoma. Note the haphazard arrangement of the glands (panel **a**), and the intense desmoplastic stroma (panel **b**). Both are hemotoxylin and eosin stained

that these cancer cells in ducts appear to be less responsive to therapy [17].

In well-differentiated carcinomas, the glands are lined by well-oriented uniform mucin-producing cells with relatively uniform nuclei. In moderately differentiated examples, the gland formation is less well-developed, the neoplastic cells have visible pleomorphism, and mitotic figures can be seen. The pleomorphism is more pronounced in poorly-differentiated carcinomas, with numerous mitoses, poorly formed glands and areas showing single cell infiltration.

Immunolabeling can demonstrate a typical phenotype in pancreatic cancer. Pancreatic cancers typically label with antibodies to cytokeratins 7, 8, 18 and 19 (CK7, CK8, CK18 and CK19), with antibodies to the mucins MUC1, MUC3, MUC4 and MUC5AC, with antibodies to the glycoproteins carcinoembryonic antigen (CEA), carcinoma antigen 19–9 (CA19–9), B72.3 and CA125, and with antibodies to mesothelin and claudin 4 [2, 15, 18, 19]. In addition, immunolabeling can also be used as a surrogate marker for gene status, as labeling for the smad4 protein correlates with *SMAD4* gene status, and labeling for the p53 protein correlates with *TP53* gene status [20, 21].

12.1.2 Diagnostic Features

The diagnosis of pancreatic cancer carries such a grim prognosis and therapies are so debilitating, making it critically important that clear and precise criteria are used when establishing the diagnosis [2, 15]. As highlighted in Table 12.1, seven histologic features can be used to distinguish ductal adenocarcinoma from reactive glands.

First, the haphazard growth of pancreatic cancer, as appreciated at low magnification, contrasts with the lobular arrangement of normal pancreatic parenchyma and the orderly branching growth of non-neoplastic glands. Benign glands retain an organized lobular pattern even when there is severe atrophy, as seen in chronic pancreatitis. We like to think of benign glands as similar to orderly grapes on vine. Even when the grapes have dried up (atrophied), the vine retains a lobular arrangement of bunches of grapes. By contrast, there is no rhyme or reason to the organization of neoplastic glands (Fig. 12.2a).

A second helpful feature is a gland located immediately adjacent to a muscular vessel (Fig. 12.3a). The ducts of normal pancreas are surrounded by lobules of acinar cells and are thus separated from blood vessels with smooth muscle media. By contrast, it is common in pancreatic cancer to see a gland immediately adjacent to a vessel [2, 15, 22, 23]. Three-dimensional analyses of cleared human pancreatic cancers has reveals that this finding occurs because the invasive glands of pancreatic cancer preferentially grow parallel to blood vessels [5, 22].

Perineural invasion is the third feature that can be used to distinguish benign from malignant glands. With extremely rare exceptions, benign glands do not grow into nerves in the pancreas [2, 15, 24–26]. In addition to diagnostic utility, perineural invasion in the pancreas has further clinical relevance as it has been associated with pain, and extension of the cancer out of the pancreas and into the retroperitoneum [27–29]

Vascular invasion is the fourth feature that can be used to distinguish benign from malignant glands [2, 15]. What is remarkable is that the neoplastic glands growing within vessels often grow along the inner lining of the vessels, replacing the endothelial cells, and forming well oriented duct-like structures within the channel of the invaded vessel (Fig. 12.3b) [5, 30]. The foci are easy to pass over because this pattern of vascular invasion mimics a benign duct until one realizes that the cells are in a vessel!

Significant pleomorphism, the variation of nuclear size and shape from cell to cell, is the fifth feature [2, 15]. Known as the "four-to-one rule," a four-fold variation in nuclear area supports the diagnosis of cancer [31]. This feature is very helpful, but unfortunately is not seen when it is needed most: differentiating well-differentiated cancers from benign glands.

The sixth feature is the presence of necrotic debris in the lumen of glands ("luminal necrosis") and the seventh the incomplete epithelial lining of a lumen ("incomplete lumina") [2, 15].

When rigorously applied these seven features produce very sensitive and specific diagnosis of pancreatic cancer [2, 15, 31].

12.1.3 Clinical Implications

Pathologic findings provide significant prognostic information that can be used to guide therapy. As recognized in the American Joint Commission on Cancer (AJCC) staging

Table 12.1 Histologic features supporting the diagnosis of infiltrating ductal adenocarcinoma over reactive glands

Feature	Infiltrating ductal adenocarcinoma	Reactive glands
Organization	Haphazard	Lobular
Relation to muscular vessel	Immediately adjacent	Separated by parenchyma or stroma
Relation to nerves	Perineural invasion	Separated from nerves
Relation to vessels	Vascular invasion	No vascular invasion
Variation in nuclear size	Can be greater than 4 to 1	Less than 4 to 1
Completeness of glands	Can be incomplete with lumen touching stroma	Complete. Always epithelial cells between lumen and stroma.
Luminal necrosis	Necrotic cellular debris can be found in lumen	No necrosis

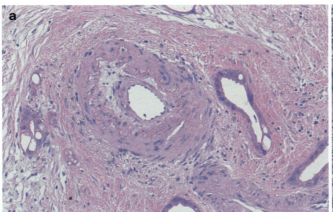 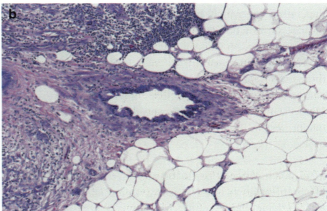

Fig. 12.3 Histologic sections of infiltrating ductal adenocarcinoma. Note the neoplastic gland immediately adjacent to a muscular vessel (panel **a**), and the venous invasion (panel **b**). Both are hemotoxylin and eosin stained

system, tumor size, lymph node status, and presence or absence of distant metastases are the most important prognostic features [32]. The degree of histologic differentiation, margin status, and the presence or absence of venous invasion are also important prognosticators [30]. Several somatic genetic alterations also provide prognostic information, including loss of *SMAD4*, associated with poor survival, and mutations in one of the chromatin-regulating genes (*MLL*, *MLL2*, *MLL3* and *ARID1A*), associated with improved survival [33, 34]. High *GATA6* expression is associated with the "classical" RNA subtype and with better responses to chemotherapy [35, 36]. As useful as these features are, the reality is that the vast majority of patients succumb to their disease [1]. We need to do more than just prognosticate, we need to improve prognosis.

We believe that insights gained from the unique pathologic features of pancreatic cancer, as described in the next sections, will provide clues into how to improve outcomes for patients with pancreatic cancer.

12.1.4 Desmoplastic Stroma

The dramatic desmoplastic stroma that characterizes pancreatic cancer (Fig. 12.2b) has a number of important implications that deserve additional discussion [2, 3, 15]. First, the non-neoplastic stroma is usually so abundant that bulk pancreatic cancer tumors, in fact, contain relatively few neoplastic cells [2, 15, 37]. This has implications in the interpretation of small biopsies, as rare cancer cells scattered in abundant stroma may be inadequately sampled, and it has profound implications for the study of pancreatic cancer as studies of bulk tumors actually end up studying the stroma not cancer. This problem is nicely illustrated in recent studies of RNA expression patterns in pancreatic cancer [35, 36, 38–40]. As shown in The Cancer Genome Atlas (TCGA) study of pancreatic cancer, non-neoplastic stromal contamination can lead to the incorrect subtyping of pancreatic cancers as, depending on which part of the cancer the sample was harvested from, it will have varying amounts of stromal contamination [35, 36, 38–40].

The desmoplastic stroma also has significant clinical implications as it may hinder the access of systemically administered drugs to the cancer cells [3, 37]. For example, Hingorani and colleagues have shown that high levels of hyaluronan in the stroma can reduce the perfusion of small molecule therapeutics in pancreatic cancer [41]. They, and others, have even suggested that therapies to deplete stroma may increase tumor perfusion and increase the efficacy of chemotherapies [41–43]. Clearly, future studies of stromal biology have the potential to unlock new approaches to the treatment of pancreatic cancer.

12.1.5 Venous Invasion

A second dramatic feature that is present in virtually all pancreatic cancers is venous invasion (Fig. 12.3). Almost all, even early stage, pancreatic cancers invade into the small veins in the pancreas [4, 5, 22, 30, 44]. In routine hematoxylin and eosin stained sections, venous invasion is identified in ~65% of surgically resectable pancreatic cancers [30, 44]. When one examines pancreatic cancers in three-dimensions, using techniques such as tissue clearing, the percentage of positive cases goes up to >90% [4, 5, 22].

The high prevalence of venous invasion in pancreatic cancer has profound implications. First, it may explain the poor blood flow to pancreatic cancer [45]. If the veins are occluded by neoplastic cells, blood cannot get into the cancers as it cannot get out. Second, since the veins in the pancreas drain directly into the liver, it may also explain the extremely high prevalence of liver metastases present in patients with pancreatic cancer [4]. Future studies of the biology of venous invasion have the potential to unlock new approaches to the treatment of pancreatic cancer that address this deadly propensity for early metastatic spread to the liver.

12.1.6 Variants

Several variants of pancreatic cancer deserve special note as they have clinical implications.

Adenosquamous carcinomas are, as the name suggests, characterized by a significant component of the carcinoma (at least 30%) having squamous differentiation (Fig. 12.4a) [6]. These carcinomas label with p63, p40 and CK5/6 in the areas of squamous differentiation and have low levels of GATA6 expression. Although they tend to be extremely aggressive with a poor prognosis, some respond to platinum-containing chemotherapies [7, 35, 36, 38–40].

Colloid carcinomas are characterized by the production of copious amounts of extracellular mucin (Fig. 12.4b). These carcinomas often arise in association with an intestinal-type intraductal papillary mucinous neoplasm (IPMN), and they tend to have a better prognosis than usual ductal adenocarcinomas of the pancreas [8, 9]. Since colloid carcinomas arise in association with IPMNs, they often harbor mutations in the IPMN-related genes *GNAS* and *RNF43* [46].

Medullary carcinomas are a third variant of note. These carcinomas are characterized by a syncytial pattern of growth (the cells seem to blend into each other), pushing boarders, and a brisk inflammatory infiltrate (Fig. 12.4c) [47, 48]. They are important to recognize because these cancers often, but not always, have microsatellite instability (MSI high), and

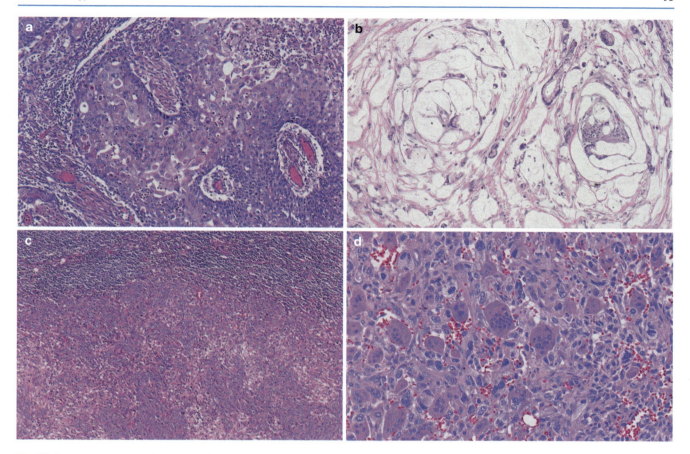

Fig. 12.4 Variants of pancreatic cancer include adenosquamous carcinoma (panel **a**), colloid carcinoma (panel **b**), medullary carcinoma (panel **c**), and undifferentiated carcinoma with osteoclast-like giant cells (panel **d**). All are hemotoxylin and eosin stained

they have a relatively good prognosis [47, 48]. Critically, MSI high cancers appear to be exquisitely sensitive to immunotherapy [49].

Undifferentiated carcinomas, as the name indicates, lack a definitive direction of differentiation. Of note, undifferentiated carcinomas with rhabdoid features often have a distinctive genetic change with loss of at least one member of the SWI/SNF complex [12–14]. This includes loss of SMARCB1 (INI1), SMARCA2 (BRM), SMARCA4 (BRG1) or ARID1A [12–14]. Looking forward, these alterations may make these cancers susceptible to targeted therapy.

Undifferentiated carcinomas with osteoclast-like giant cells have a dramatic microscopic appearance with giant osteoclast-like cells scattered amongst highly atypical mononuclear cells (Fig. 12.4d) [11]. Molecular studies have shown that the atypical mononuclear cells are the neoplastic cells, and that the osteoclast-like cells are reactive, non-neoplastic cells [11]. These distinctive cancers likely have a worse prognosis than usual ductal adenocarcinomas, but recent literature suggests that the prognosis may not be as dire as initially thought [11, 50].

12.1.7 Pathology in Familial Syndromes

Before we close, we should note that pancreatic pathology has been studied in individuals with a family history of pancreatic cancer and in patients with germline mutations, such as germline variants in *BRCA2* and *CDKN2A*, known to predispose to the disease [51–53]. Both of these groups appear to have increased numbers of precursor lesions (IPMNs and pancreatic intraepithelial neoplasia), suggesting that screening efforts may detect early, curable, lesions in these patients and save lives [51–55]. The association of medullary histology with MSI high status was noted above, and some MSI high cancers arise in patients with Lynch syndrome [56].

12.2 Conclusions

Pancreatic cancer pathology forms the basis for patient prognostication and it provides unique insights into why this cancer is so deadly [4]. Looking forward, we believe that the integration of germline and somatic changes with tumor morphology will lead to more precise treatment of patients, and further studies into the desmoplastic stroma and into venous invasion will lead to both better understanding of the aggressive biology of pancreatic cancer as well as identify new therapeutic approaches. In the end, we believe that a better understanding of pancreatic pathology will reduce patient mortality.

References

1. Siegel RL, Miller KD, Jemal A. Cancer statistics, 2020. CA Cancer J Clin. 2020;70:7–30.
2. Hruban RH, Pitman MB, Klimstra DS. Tumors of the pancreas. American Registry of Pathology: Washington, DC, 2007. 422 pp.
3. Whittle MC, Hingorani SR. Fibroblasts in pancreatic ductal adenocarcinoma: biological mechanisms and therapeutic targets. Gastroenterology. 2019;156:2085–96.
4. Hruban RH, Gaida MM, Thompson E, et al. Why is pancreatic cancer so deadly? The pathologist's view. J Pathol. 2019;248:131–41.
5. Hong SM, Jung D, Kiemen A, et al. Three-dimensional visualization of cleared human pancreas cancer reveals that sustained epithelial-to-mesenchymal transition is not required for venous invasion. Mod Pathol. 2020;33:639–47.
6. Brody JR, Costantino CL, Potoczek M, et al. Adenosquamous carcinoma of the pancreas harbors KRAS2, DPC4 and TP53 molecular alterations similar to pancreatic ductal adenocarcinoma. Mod Pathol. 2009;22:651–9.
7. Voong KR, Davison J, Pawlik TM, et al. Resected pancreatic adenosquamous carcinoma: clinicopathologic review and evaluation of adjuvant chemotherapy and radiation in 38 patients. Hum Pathol. 2010;41:113–22.
8. Seidel G, Zahurak M, Iacobuzio-Donahue C, et al. Almost all infiltrating colloid carcinomas of the pancreas and periampullary region arise from in situ papillary neoplasms: a study of 39 cases. Am J Surg Pathol. 2002;26:56–63.
9. Adsay NV, Merati K, Nassar H, et al. Pathogenesis of colloid (pure mucinous) carcinoma of exocrine organs: Coupling of gel-forming mucin (MUC2) production with altered cell polarity and abnormal cell-stroma interaction may be the key factor in the morphogenesis and indolent behavior of colloid carcinoma in the breast and pancreas. Am J Surg Pathol. 2003;27:571–8.
10. Hruban RH, Molina JM, Reddy MN, Boitnott JK. A neoplasm with pancreatic and hepatocellular differentiation presenting with subcutaneous fat necrosis. Am J Clin Pathol. 1987;88:639–45.
11. Westra WH, Sturm P, Drillenburg P, et al. K-ras oncogene mutations in osteoclast-like giant cell tumors of the pancreas and liver: genetic evidence to support origin from the duct epithelium. Am J Surg Pathol. 1998;22:1247–54.
12. Agaimy A, Daum O, Markl B, et al. SWI/SNF complex-deficient undifferentiated/rhabdoid carcinomas of the gastrointestinal tract: a series of 13 cases highlighting mutually exclusive loss of SMARCA4 and SMARCA2 and frequent co-inactivation of SMARCB1 and SMARCA2. Am J Surg Pathol. 2016;40:544–53.
13. Agaimy A, Haller F, Frohnauer J, et al. Pancreatic undifferentiated rhabdoid carcinoma: KRAS alterations and SMARCB1 expression status define two subtypes. Mod Pathol. 2015;28:248–60.
14. Sano M, Homma T, Hayashi E, et al. Clinicopathological characteristics of anaplastic carcinoma of the pancreas with rhabdoid features. Virchows Arch. 2014;465:531–8.
15. Bosman FT, Carneiro F, Hruban RH, Theise ND. WHO classification of tumours of the digestive system. 4th ed. Lyon: International Agency for Research on Cancer; 2010.
16. Hutchings D, Waters KM, Weiss MJ, et al. Cancerization of the pancreatic ducts: demonstration of a common and under-recognized process using immunolabeling of paired duct lesions and invasive pancreatic ductal adenocarcinoma for p53 and Smad4 expression. Am J Surg Pathol. 2018;42:1556–61.
17. Fujikura K, Hutchings D, Braxton AM, et al. Intraductal pancreatic cancer is less responsive than cancer in the stroma to neoadjuvant chemotherapy. Mod Pathol. 2020;
18. Swartz MJ, Batra SK, Varshney GC, et al. MUC4 expression increases progressively in pancreatic intraepithelial neoplasia. Am J Clin Pathol. 2002;117:791–6.
19. Argani P, Iacobuzio-Donahue C, Ryu B, et al. Mesothelin is overexpressed in the vast majority of ductal adenocarcinomas of the pancreas: identification of a new pancreatic cancer marker by serial analysis of gene expression (SAGE). Clin Cancer Res. 2001;7:3862–8.
20. Wilentz RE, Su GH, Dai JL, et al. Immunohistochemical labeling for dpc4 mirrors genetic status in pancreatic adenocarcinomas: a new marker of DPC4 inactivation. Am J Pathol. 2000;156:37–43.
21. Baas IO, Hruban RH, Offerhaus GJ. Clinical applications of detecting dysfunctional p53 tumor suppressor protein. Histol Histopathol. 1999;14:279–84.
22. Noë M, Rezaee N, Asrani K, et al. Immunolabeling of cleared human pancreata provides insights into three-dimensional pancreatic anatomy and pathology. Am J Pathol. 2018;188:1530–5.
23. Sharma S, Green KB. The pancreatic duct and its arteriovenous relationship: an underutilized aid in the diagnosis and distinction of pancreatic adenocarcinoma from pancreatic intraepithelial neoplasia. A study of 126 pancreatectomy specimens. Am J Surg Pathol. 2004;28:613–20.
24. Liebig C, Ayala G, Wilks JA, Berger DH, Albo D. Perineural invasion in cancer: a review of the literature. Cancer. 2009;115:3379–91.
25. Jurcak NR, Rucki AA, Muth S, et al. Axon guidance molecules promote perineural invasion and metastasis of orthotopic pancreatic tumors in mice. Gastroenterology. 2019;157:838–50 e6.
26. Nagakawa T, Mori K, Nakano T, et al. Perineural invasion of carcinoma of the pancreas and biliary tract. Br J Surg. 1993;80:619–21.
27. Liang D, Shi S, Xu J, et al. New insights into perineural invasion of pancreatic cancer: More than pain. Biochim Biophys Acta. 2016;1865:111–22.
28. Tanaka M, Mihaljevic AL, Probst P, et al. Meta-analysis of recurrence pattern after resection for pancreatic cancer. Br J Surg. 2019;106:1590–601.
29. Demir IE, Friess H, Ceyhan GO. Neural plasticity in pancreatitis and pancreatic cancer. Nat Rev Gastroenterol Hepatol. 2015;12:649–59.
30. Hong SM, Goggins M, Wolfgang CL, et al. Vascular invasion in infiltrating ductal adenocarcinoma of the pancreas can mimic pancreatic intraepithelial neoplasia: a histopathologic study of 209 cases. Am J Surg Pathol. 2012;36:235–41.
31. Cioc AM, Ellison EC, Proca DM, Lucas JG, Frankel WL. Frozen section diagnosis of pancreatic lesions. Arch Pathol Lab Med. 2002;126:1169–73.
32. Allen PJ, Kuk D, Castillo CF, et al. Multi-institutional validation study of the American Joint Commission on Cancer (8th edition) changes for T and N staging in patients with pancreatic adenocarcinoma. Ann Surg. 2017;265:185–91.
33. Blackford A, Serrano OK, Wolfgang CL, et al. SMAD4 gene mutations are associated with poor prognosis in pancreatic cancer. Clin Cancer Res. 2009;15:4674–9.
34. Sausen M, Phallen J, Adleff V, et al. Clinical implications of genomic alterations in the tumour and circulation of pancreatic cancer patients. Nat Commun. 2015;6:7686.
35. Collisson EA, Sadanandam A, Olson P, et al. Subtypes of pancreatic ductal adenocarcinoma and their differing responses to therapy. Nat Med. 2011;17:500–3.

36. Collisson EA, Bailey P, Chang DK, Biankin AV. Molecular subtypes of pancreatic cancer. Nat Rev Gastroenterol Hepatol. 2019;16:207–20.
37. Seymour AB, Hruban RH, Redston M, et al. Allelotype of pancreatic adenocarcinoma. Cancer Res. 1994;54:2761–4.
38. Moffitt RA, Marayati R, Flate EL, et al. Virtual microdissection identifies distinct tumor- and stroma-specific subtypes of pancreatic ductal adenocarcinoma. Nat Genet. 2015;47:1168–78.
39. Rashid NU, Peng XL, Jin C, et al. Purity Independent Subtyping of Tumors (PurIST), a clinically robust, single-sample classifier for tumor subtyping in pancreatic cancer. Clin Cancer Res. 2020;26:82–92.
40. Cancer Genome Atlas Research Network. Electronic address aadhe, Cancer Genome Atlas Research N. Integrated Genomic Characterization of Pancreatic Ductal Adenocarcinoma. Cancer Cell. 2017;32:185–203 e13.
41. Maloney E, DuFort CC, Provenzano PP, et al. Non-invasive monitoring of stromal biophysics with targeted depletion of hyaluronan in pancreatic ductal adenocarcinoma. Cancers (Basel) 2019;11.
42. Ireland L, Santos A, Ahmed MS, et al. Chemoresistance in pancreatic cancer is driven by stroma-derived insulin-like growth factors. Cancer Res. 2016;76:6851–63.
43. Neesse A, Algul H, Tuveson DA, Gress TM. Stromal biology and therapy in pancreatic cancer: a changing paradigm. Gut. 2015;64:1476–84.
44. Yamada M, Sugiura T, Okamura Y, et al. Microscopic venous invasion in pancreatic cancer. Ann Surg Oncol. 2018;25:1043–51.
45. Olive KP, Jacobetz MA, Davidson CJ, et al. Inhibition of Hedgehog signaling enhances delivery of chemotherapy in a mouse model of pancreatic cancer. Science. 2009;324:1457–61.
46. Amato E, Molin MD, Mafficini A, et al. Targeted next-generation sequencing of cancer genes dissects the molecular profiles of intraductal papillary neoplasms of the pancreas. J Pathol. 2014;233:217–27.
47. Goggins M, Offerhaus GJ, Hilgers W, et al. Pancreatic adenocarcinomas with DNA replication errors (RER+) are associated with wild-type K-ras and characteristic histopathology. Poor differentiation, a syncytial growth pattern, and pushing borders suggest RER+. Am J Pathol. 1998;152:1501–7.
48. Wilentz RE, Goggins M, Redston M, et al. Genetic, immunohistochemical, and clinical features of medullary carcinoma of the pancreas: a newly described and characterized entity. Am J Pathol. 2000;156:1641–51.
49. Le DT, Uram JN, Wang H, et al. PD-1 blockade in tumors with mismatch-repair deficiency. N Engl J Med. 2015;372:2509–20.
50. Reid MD, Muraki T, HooKim K, et al. Cytologic features and clinical implications of undifferentiated carcinoma with osteoclastic giant cells of the pancreas: an analysis of 15 cases. Cancer Cytopathol. 2017;125:563–75.
51. Brune K, Abe T, Canto M, et al. Multifocal neoplastic precursor lesions associated with lobular atrophy of the pancreas in patients having a strong family history of pancreatic cancer. Am J Surg Pathol. 2006;30:1067–76.
52. Singhi AD, Ishida H, Ali SZ, et al. A histomorphologic comparison of familial and sporadic pancreatic cancers. Pancreatology. 2015;15:387–91.
53. Hutchings D, Jiang Z, Skaro M, et al. Histomorphology of pancreatic cancer in patients with inherited ATM serine/threonine kinase pathogenic variants. Mod Pathol. 2019;32:1806–13.
54. Canto MI, Almario JA, Schulick RD, et al. Risk of neoplastic progression in individuals at high risk for pancreatic cancer undergoing long-term surveillance. Gastroenterology. 2018;155:740–51 e2.
55. Goggins M, Overbeek KA, Brand R, et al. Management of patients with increased risk for familial pancreatic cancer: updated recommendations from the International Cancer of the Pancreas Screening (CAPS) Consortium. Gut. 2020;69:7–17.
56. Kastrinos F, Mukherjee B, Tayob N, et al. Risk of pancreatic cancer in families with Lynch syndrome. JAMA. 2009;302:1790–5.

CT in Hepato-Bilio-Pancreatic Surgical Pathology

Ioana G. Lupescu and Mugur C. Grasu

Abstract

Computed tomography (CT) represents the most current modality used to evaluate hepato-biliary tree and pancreatic (HBP) surgical pathology. Multidetector CT (MDCT) is a very quick, robust, reproducible and reliable method for the pretherapeutic and postsurgical hepato-biliary tree and pancreatic diagnostic. Using a correct and a specific CT protocol for the HBP region in correlation with multiplanar reconstructions, maximum intensity and 3D reconstructions, CT provides detailed and consistent information's regarding the type of mass, its characteristics, volumetry and local extension, allowing to appreciate the vascular involvement and tumor resectability but also in malignant tumoral pathology the presence of distant metastasis.

13.1 Technical CT Considerations in Hepato-Bilio-Pancreatic Evaluation

Computed tomography (CT) is the fastest and most accessible imaging method of hepato-biliary-pancreatic (HBP) evaluation, currently used in medical and surgical emergencies, and in the therapeutic treatment of expansive lesion(s) [1–4]. Multidetector CT (MDCT) exam of the HBP region involves, after the nonenhanced CT (NECT), a multiphase dynamic acquisition, with non-ionic iodinated contrast material (CM) injected i.v. in late arterial phase (AP) at 30–35 seconds (s) after the start of the CM injection, portal venous phase (PVP) at 50–70 s and late phase (LP) at 3–5 min post-contrast injection, using a dose of 1.5 ml/kgc CM, in bolus, with a flow rate of 2.5–3 ml/s (Fig. 13.1).

Multiplanar reconstructions (MPR), three-dimensional (3D), Maximum Intensity Projection (MIP), VRT (Volume Rendering Transparency) reconstructions together with post-contrast source CT images analysis allow a complete lesion (s) characterization, vascular and biliary mapping, hepatic segmentation, specification of vascular and biliary tree anatomical variants, volumetry of the liver parenchyma or of a tumor, with the elaboration of a virtual surgical plan, and appreciation of the remaining hepatic volume, being particularly important in liver surgery and indispensable in liver transplantation with living donor [1–10]. In pre-therapy, in patients who are suspected with a tumoral mass of the HBP region, the role of CT is to make a complete assessment of the mass, by assessing: tumor location, size, number, involvement of adjacent vascular and biliary structures, the presence of lymphadenopathies or extrahepatic metastases [4, 10–14].

In cirrhotic patients with hepatocellular carcinoma (HCC) who meet the criteria for liver transplantation (LT), the optimal treatment is LT [9]. MPR, especially the coronal and sagittal plane, are very useful in assessing vascular invasion [4, 10–18]. Thrombosis and invasion of the portal vein (PV) trunk, portal carrefour, hepatic veins (HV) or inferior vena cava (IVC) are associated with an unfavorable prognosis compared to cases in which only the secondary portal branches are involved. CT evaluation allows the detection of steatosis, fibrosis and liver cirrhosis, in association with the detection of all the anatomical variants [8, 19]. For example, the origin of the right hepatic artery (HA) in the superior mesenteric artery (SMA) involves additional steps of surgical technique for the donor and recipient. According to the Michel classification, the HA variants with increased surgical risk are type 2, 3, 5 and 9. For the PV it is important to specify in the CT report the presents of variants such as trifurcation, abnormal right configuration or accessory veins [3, 8, 19, 20]. Accessory HA and HV should be reported. It is also necessary to specify the existing variants at the level of the intra-/extrahepatic bile ducts (BD), aspect of biliary trifurcation, accessory BD (risk of biliary fistula) or low implantation of the cystic duct [3, 20]. The identification of ascites, hydrotho-

I. G. Lupescu (✉) · M. C. Grasu
Radiology, Medical Imaging and Interventional Imaging Department of Fundeni Clinical Institute, University of Medicine and Pharmacy "Carol Davila", Bucharest, Romania

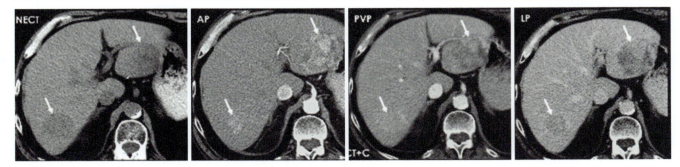

Fig. 13.1 CT technique for liver focal lesions evaluation: nonenhanced CT and CT with non-ionic iodinated contrast material in late arterial phase, (AP) portal venous phase (PVP) and late phase (LP) in a patient with hepatocellular carcinoma-macronodular type, located in the right and left liver lobe (white arrows)

rax, portal hypertension (splenomegaly, gastro-esophageal varices, porto-systemic anastomoses) are suggestive for severe hepatic dysfunction [8]. It is also important, in the CT report to specify the liver lesion (s) type knowing that there are 5 categories of LI-RADS lesions: LR-1: definitely benign lesion; LR-2: probably benign; LR-3: intermediate probability for HCC; LR-4: probably HCC; LR-5: definitely HCC. A definite tumor into a vein correspond to LR-TIV. LR-M represent a malignant lesion, not suggestive for HCC. A liver tumor which has been treated by a loco-regional procedure correspond to a LR-treated lesion (treatment). The lesional description must contain the following elements: nodule size (smaller or larger than 2 cm), postcontrast behaviour: early enhancement (hypervascularity) or iso/hypovascularity of the nodule, with washout in PVP or in LP, the presence or absence of a capsule, the dimensional increase of the lesion equal to/ or greater than 50% of the diameter at the re-evaluation imaging exam compared to the previous evaluation after an interval less than 6 months; more or equal 100% dimensional increasement of the nodule at the follow up imaging examination performed at an interval larger than 6 months, or newly appeared lesion, with dimensions equal to or larger than 10 mm discovered after less than 24 months in relation to the last imaging evaluation [9].

For pancreatic tumors, the location of the tumor (head, isthmus, body, tail), the dimensions of the tumoral process (cm), the post-contrast aspect must be specified: hypo/iso/hyperenhancing, involvement of the BD (yes/no), appearance of the Wirsung duct (WD), presence of lymphadenopathies (yes/no), presence of metastases (yes/no), presence of ascites/peripancreatic fluid (yes/no); involvement of vascular structures (90°, 180°, 360°)—yes/no: celiac trunk (CT), SMA, superior mesenteric vein (SMV), other vascular invasions (yes/no), existence of vascular thrombosis (yes/no), anatomical variants, presence of venous collaterals, atherosclerosis of the CT and SMA, distance measurement between the tumor and the SMV (mm) [1–3, 5–8].

In cases of malignant tumoral pathology of the biliary tree (cholangiocarcinoma), the CT report must specify the type of tumor: intrahepatic mass forming, periductal, intraductal type, the cranio-caudal extension of the tumoral process, the invasion of adjacent structures, native and postcontrast aspect of the tumor (hypodense, moderate peripheral enhancement, central enhancement in the LP and peripheral washout ring), associating capsular retraction, vascular embedding without thrombosis at the level of the PV or HV, the presence of satellite nodules [1–3, 5–8].

13.2 CT in Focal Liver Mass

13.2.1 Benign Liver Tumors

Hepatic cyst (HC) represents the second liver benign tumor after haemangioma (incidence: 2–5%). HC can be congenital, associated with tuberous sclerosis, polycystic kidney disease, polycystic liver (over 10 cysts) or acquired in a post-traumatic, post-inflammatory, parasitic context [1–3, 5–8]. *CT aspects:* circumscribed round or oval shape lesion with homogeneous structure and fluid density (0–10 HU); the cyst wall is often invisible. The simple cyst doesn't enhance; dimensions varies from a few mm to 20 cm [1–3, 5–8, 12]. *CT report* must contain localization, semiology of the cyst, single/multiple, complications (hemorrhage, infection) exclusion of a cystic tumoral lesion (metastases, cystadenoma), other associated lesions.

Hemangioma represents the most common benign liver tumor (incidence: 5–7% of the population). *CT aspects*. On NECT, small hemangioma is homogeneous, hypodense (density close to that of the circulating blood); large hemangiomas are heterogeneous; postcontrast, small hemangiomas (<1 cm) show complete and rapid filling; hemangiomas over 2 cm have an intense contrast enhancement in the periphery which progresses towards the center; in the late phase there is a total filling of the lesion, with intralesional persistence of the CM. Cavernous hemangioma present a heterogeneous structure (central fibrosis area, calcifications) and is not fully enhanced with CM in the LP. *CT report*: must contain semiological appearance, number, exclusion of hypervascularized primary or secondary liver malignancies; other associated lesions (Fig. 13.2).

Focal nodular hyperplasia (FNH) represents 8% of primary liver tumors in adults and the second cause of benign solid hepatic tumor, mainly affecting decades 3 and 4. FNHs are generally solitary and <5 cm; may be associated with hemangiomas. The central stellar scar is present in 20–30% of cases [1–3, 5–8, 12]. *CT aspects*: spontaneous hypodense to isodense liver mass; intense enhancement in the AP, with discreetly washout in the PVP, and isodense aspect in the LP; the central scar appear spontaneously hypodense and enhance in the LP. *CT report*: must contain location and semiology of the lesion, single/multiple, exclusion of hypervascularized malignant tumors or liver perfusion disorders.

Hepatocellular adenoma (HA) is the most common tumor in young women (20–40 years) who use oral contraceptive treatment; presents a risk of malignant degeneration. HA are generally unique and voluminous (up to 30 cm), with heterogeneous structure through areas of lipomatous infiltration, necrosis and hemorrhage [1–3, 5–8]. Hepatic adenomatosis is a rare disorder characterized by the presence of more than 10 liver adenomas. *CT aspects*: frequent bulky tumor (over 5 cm), hypodense (may contain fat or areas of necrosis) or hyperdense in case of intratumoral haemorrhage; heterogeneous enhancement in AP with wash out in LP; peripheral capsule. *CT report*: in some cases, there are difficulties to delineate between liver HA, FNH or HCC [1–3, 5–8, 12].

Angiomyolipoma (AML) is a rare, benign mesenchymal tumor with a myoid, angioid and lipomatous component; associated with Bourneville tuberous sclerosis [1, 5, 6]. *CT aspects*: lipomatous intratumoral islands have negative densities: −40/−80 UH, the angio component enhance very early with CM. *CT report*-semiological analysis of the tumor (lipomatous and angio components), exclusion of aggressive tumors that may have lipomatous inclusions [4, 11].

13.2.2 Malignant Liver Tumors

Hepatocellular carcinoma (HCC) is the most common primary liver tumor malignancy (80–90%). 60–90% of HCC is developed on a cirrhotic liver, in a context of B or C virus hepatitis, following the evolution and conversion of regeneration nodules into small/high-grade dysplastic nodules and then into small HCC [3, 9, 14, 18]. Simultaneously, there is a decrease in portal flow and an increase of arterial intratumoral vascularisation. HCC may be single, multiple, or diffuse in shape. 24% of the HCC are encapsulated; calcifications are present in 10–20% of cases; vascular invasion is encountered in ~48% of cases. HCC metastasizes into the lungs, adrenal glands, bone and lymph nodes [1–12]. *CT aspects*: hypodense/rarely isodense/hyperdense mass (hemorrhage, lipomatous areas); AP hyperenhancement (80%) with PVP washing and hypoattenuation appearance in LP (Fig. 13.3); heterogeneous appearance in large HCC (see Fig. 13.1); spontaneous hypodense peritumoral capsule which enhance in LP [13, 17, 21, 22]. *CT report*: positive diagnosis (Li-RADS criteria: hypervascularized mass in AP with wash out in PVP and LP [23]; may associate tumoral invasion of the adjacent PV, HV or IVC; staging; exclusion of pseudotumors or benign liver tumors [3, 7–9, 12].

Fibrolamellar hepatocellular carcinoma (FLC) is a rare primary liver malignancy (incidence: 1–9% of all HCC) which affects young people. General characteristics: encapsulated, hypervascularized mass; central scar (45–60%); nodular, stellate, dotted calcifications (35–55%); dimensions between 5–20 cm; capsular retraction (10%); satellite nodules are present in 10–20% of cases; vascular invasion is rare (less than 5%). Lymph node (50–70%), pulmonary and peritoneal metastases [1–3, 5–7]. *CT aspects*: spontaneous hypodense mass; heterogeneous postcontrast aspect in AP and PVP; the absence of scar enhancement. *CT report*: exclusion of other tumors or hypervascular liver lesions [23]; associated injuries.

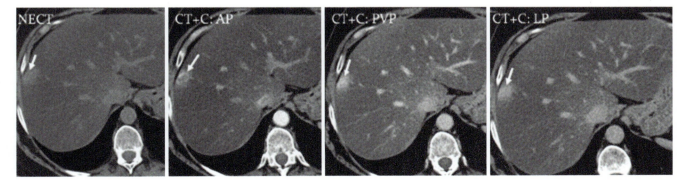

Fig. 13.2 Liver hemangioma (white arrow) and liver steatosis: intense contrast enhancement in the periphery of the nodule, progressing towards the center, with total filling in the LP and persistence of the CM into the nodule

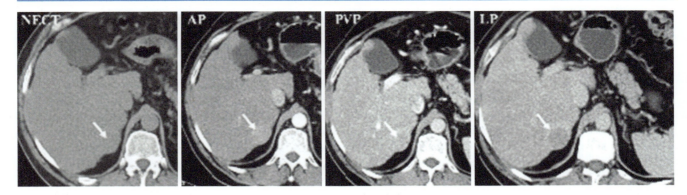

Fig. 13.3 Hepatocellular carcinoma: nodular type: isodense nodule with enhancement in arterial phase and wash-out in the late phase (white arrow)

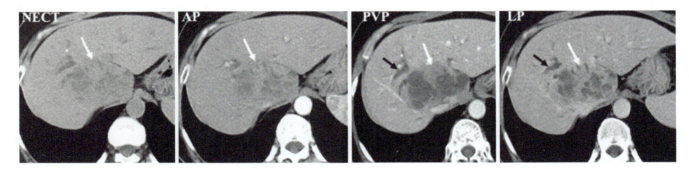

Fig. 13.4 Intrahepatic cholangiocarcinoma. Large heterogeneous and hypovascular mass, with solid portion and cystic component, involving the caudate lobe (white arrow) which associate dilatation of adjacent BD (black arrow)

Hepatoblastoma (HB) is the most common primary liver tumor of the child, usually voluminous, unique, with a well-defined, lobulated contour; in 20% of cases the HB is multifocal [3, 6]. Amorphous calcifications are present in 50% of cases. *CT aspects*: hypodense, heterogeneous mass with multiple amorphous calcifications and septa, and peripheral enhancement. *CT report* must contain tumoral location, postcontrast behaviour, signs of vascular invasion; exclusion of other heterogeneous liver tumors; associated injuries.

Intrahepatic cholangiocarcinoma (IHCC). IHCC represents 15% of malignant tumors of the liver; 20–30% of biliary ducts (BD) carcinomas originate into the small IHBD epithelium; occurs more frequently in patients with primary sclerosing cholangitis (PSC) and intrahepatic gallstones. IHCC forms: nodular (Fig. 13.4); infiltrative with periductal extension; intraductal, polypoid [1–3, 5–7, 12]. *CT aspects*: round homogeneous mass, hypodense, with irregular edges; hypovascular; fugitive early enhancement in the periphery of the mass, with progressive filling enhancement and washout in the periphery (the sign of peripheral wash out). Late homogeneous enhancement (74% of cases). *CT report*: location of the tumor, semiological aspect, resectability criteria, elimination of a hepatocellular carcinoma.

Liver metastasis (LM) are the most common malignant tumors of the liver, being 20 times more common than primitive malignant liver tumors; dissemination may be by systemic or portal vascular system. The most common primary tumors that metastasize into the liver are lung, breast, gastrointestinal, pancreatic, melanoma, or sarcoma neoplasms. *Types of metastases. Cystic LM*: mucinous ovarian carcinoma; colon carcinoma; sarcoma; melanoma; lung carcinoma; carcinoid. *Hemorrhagic LM*: colon carcinoma; thyroid carcinoma; breast carcinoma; choriocarcinoma; melanoma; renal carcinoma. *Hypervascularized LM*: renal cell carcinoma; carcinoid; pancreatic endocrine tumors; melanoma; thyroid cancer; choriocarcinoma; cystadenocarcinoma; sarcoma; pheochromocytoma. *Hypovascularized LM*: stomach; colon; pancreas; lung; breast [1–3, 5–7]. *CT aspects*: iso-/spontaneous hypodense, most of LM are hypovascular; hypervascular metastases: intense enhancement in AP and hypovascular appearance in PVP and LP [4]. *CT report* must contain: number of nodules, location, size, other associated lesions (Fig. 13.5).

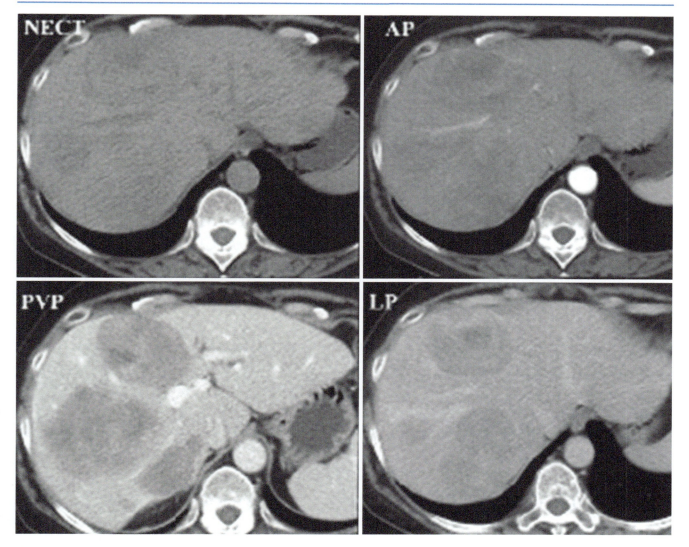

Fig. 13.5 Liver metastasis: multiple large and heterogeneous liver tumors involving the right hepatic lobe and the IV segment, in a patient with colon cancer

13.2.3 Infectious and Parasitic Hepatic Pathology

13.2.3.1 Liver Abscess

Pyogenic abscesses (Fig. 13.6): may occur after biliary, digestive surgery, in a context of cholangitis, secondary to choledochal lithiasis or intrahepatic BD stones, in patients with inflammatory bowel disease or diverticulitis [1–3, 5–7, 12].

Fungal abscesses (*candidiasis, cryptococcosis, aspergillosis*) occur in immunocompromised patients [3]. *CT aspects*: nonenhanced central hypodense area (density: 20–40 UH), surrounded by a capsule, with a uniform thickness (2–4 mm), spontaneously hypodense which enhance moderately after CM i.v. injection. In fungal abscesses: multiple circumscribed hypodense lesions, small, without enhancement distributed throughout the liver parenchyma but also in the splenic one. *Amoebic abscess*: low-density mass with peripheral enhancing rim; unilocular/multilocular; debris, wall irregularities. *CT report* must contain the findings in favour of an abscess and highlighting of the underlying cause/pathology.

Hepatic hydatic cyst (HHC) is an endemic parasitic infection caused by *Echinococcus granulosus*. The hepatic and pulmonary parenchyma are the location of choice. *CT aspects:* Fluid density, with frequent peripheral focal calcifications, daughter cysts may be visualized. The water-lily sign indicates a cyst with a floating, undulating membrane, caused by a detached endocyst. Rupture of the cyst in the BD is a major complication (10–15% c). The direct sign: biliary-cystic communication. Indirect signs: flattening of the cyst wall and dilation of IHBD. Infection of the cyst materializes by increasing the intracystic density and appearance of a horizontal level between air and cystic fluid. *CT report*: pointing the CT diagnostic criteria and the exclusion of a simple liver cyst.

13.2.4 CT in Pre-/and Post Liver Transplantation

Liver transplantation (LT) is the only curative treatment for acute fulminant and chronic liver disease as well and in patients with HCC who do not have enough liver function reserve [5]. Medical imaging plays a major role in performing the pretransplant balance as well as in monitoring of posttransplant patients [2, 7, 19, 22–25].

CT evaluation of the liver in pretransplant At *the donor*, MDCT angiography (MDCTA) provides a complete mapping of liver parenchyma, vascular anatomy (HA, PV, HV), allowing accuracy measurements of the liver volume, very important elements for virtual surgical planning. Knowing these anatomical variants, the surgeon can elaborate an adequate arterial, venous and biliary reconstruction plan [2, 7, 19, 20, 24]. At *the receiver*, CT imaging allow exclusion of absolute contraindications in LT: extrahepatic malignancy, infiltrating or diffuse hepatic tumor, extensive venous thrombosis of the PV axis and of the SMV [2, 7, 20, 25].

CT evaluation of the liver in post-transplant Aspects encountered early in LT are represented by periportal oedema (21%), fluid collections at the level of the liver hilum; peri-/subhepatic hematoma; small left pleural fluid [25–30].

Vascular complications (VC). MDCTA is the method of choice; VC are represented by: HA stenosis; HA thrombosis (Fig. 13.7); HA pseudoaneurysm; stenosis of the inferior vena cava (IVC), PV stenosis at anastomosis level; thrombosis of PV or IVC [25–31].

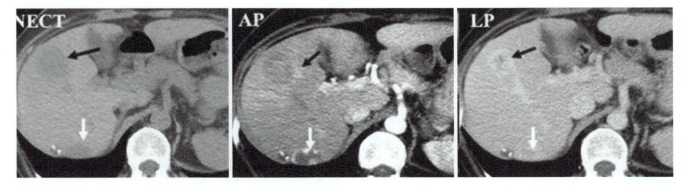

Fig. 13.6 Liver abscess: nonenhanced central hypodense area surrounded by a capsule, with a uniform thickness that enhance after CM injection (black arrow). Note also the perfusion abnormalities adjacent to the abscess and the hemangioma (white arrow).

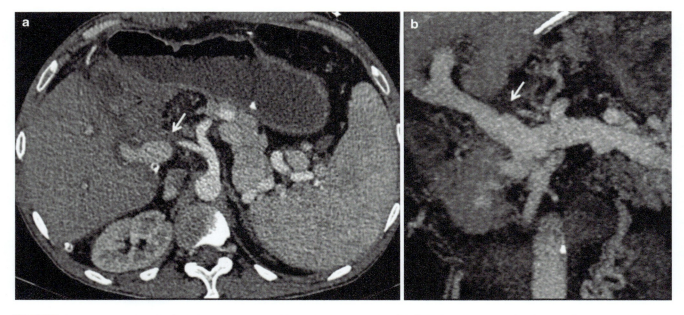

Fig. 13.7 Hepatic artery thrombosis (white arrow) in a patient with liver transplant-MDCTA in axial plane (**a**) and coronal reconstruction (**b**)

Biliary complications after LT are evaluated using ultrasound and MRI and are represented by biliary obstruction, biliary fistula, biliary tree lithiasis [3, 31].

Intraparenchymal complications (IPC). The main IPCs are: liver graft infection, liver infarction, acute and chronic rejection. *Malignancies*. The most common neoplasms are HCC recurrence and lymphoproliferative syndromes [32, 33].

13.3 CT in Liver, Biliary Tree and Pancreatic Traumatic Injuries

Liver trauma MDCT is the best imaging modality to evaluate liver trauma. *CT aspects*. Lacerations appear as irregular linear/branching areas of hypoattenuation; different grade of parenchymal disruption; vascular liver injury (arterial, venous) or active bleeding. Acute hematomas appear as a hyperdense accumulation compared to normal liver parenchyma located between the liver and its capsule or can be intraparenchymal [3, 12]. *CT report* must contain the complete list of parenchymal and vascular liver injuries and of others associates intrabdominal posttraumatic or nontraumatic lesions.

CT in pancreatic trauma (PT) *CT aspects*. Direct signs of PT are represented by: enlargement of the pancreas with hypodense laceration of the pancreatic parenchyma; heterogeneous parenchymal enhancement; fluid collections (pseudocyst, abscess or hematoma); pancreatic duct disruption. Secondary signs: peripancreatic fat stranding, fluid or hematoma between the pancreas and splenic vein, peripancreatic fluid, thickening of perirenal fascia's [3, 6].

CT in biliary trauma *Gallbladder (GB) injury*. *CT aspects*. Presence of pericholecystic free fluid, intraluminal or pericholecystic high-density hematoma, or GB wall thickening. Poor definition of GB, GB wall contour abnormal, or collapsed GB, particularly with surrounding pericholecystic fluid, raises suspicion for GB perforation. Unusual position of the GB or separation of GB from the normal location in cases of avulsion. **Bile duct injuries**. *CT aspects*. Free fluid or loculated collection (bilioma) in right upper quadrant adjacent to biliary tree [3, 7].

13.4 CT in Acquired Biliary Tract Pathology

Primitive sclerosing cholangitis (PSC) is an autoimmune disease in which the IHBD and EHBD become inflamed, scarred, narrowed or blocked. *CT aspects and report*: alternation of dilatations and areas of stenosis, appearance of "winter tree"; lobar atrophy in the affected area; abscesses, development of liver cirrhosis and portal HT, development of BD carcinoma [3, 5, 34]. *Secondary sclerosing cholangitis*. Occur as a result of chronic bacterial cholangitis secondary to biliary strictures/choledocholithiasis; by postischemic BD changes; infectious cholangitis from AIDS; secondary to congenital bile duct abnormalities; in BD neoplasms; secondary to postoperative changes of the BD [3, 31].

CT aspects and report: BD dilation with inequalities of calibre, contrast enhancement of the BD walls; hyperdense biliary lithiasis [3, 5, 31].

Biliary tree lithiasis Composition of gallstones: cholesterol (70%): transparent (93%), calcified (7%); discreetly hypodense compare to the biliary fluid; pure cholesterol stones (transparencies); small stones (cholesterol + bilirubin + calcium)—spontaneous hyperdense in CT. Location: intrahepatic lithiasis, extrahepatic BD, in the gallbladder, in the cystic duct [3, 5]. *CT aspects*: gallstones are visible in 60–70% of cases. CT report: location, appearance, size of the stone(s), signs of obstruction, complications (Fig. 13.8), associated lesions [3, 5, 7, 8].

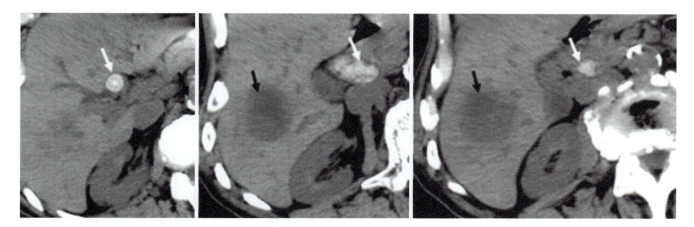

Fig. 13.8 Calcified biliary lithiasis involving the CHD and the choledoc (white arrow) and liver abscess (black arrow)

Acute cholecystitis (AC). *CT aspects*: GB distention; GB wall over 3 mm thick, hyperdense; mucosal hyperenhancement; densified gallbladder (GB) content; pericolecistic fat stranding or fluid; changes in hepatic perfusion in the early AP, with transient enhancement in the pericolecistic liver parenchyma.

Complications: emphysematous cholecystitis (hypertransparent air accumulations in the GB projection area); pericolecistic abscess; Mirizzi syndrome; gangrene; Bouveret's syndrome (calculus that eroded the GB wall, migrated into the duodenal lumen with obstruction); biliary ileus: migration of the GB stone in the gastrointestinal tract secondary to bilio-digestive fistula and inclusion in the narrowing areas of the digestive tract: Treitz angle, ileocecal valve, sigmoid colon, characterised by diagnostic triad: occlusive syndrome, aerobilia and hyperdense lithiasis [3, 6–8]. *Gangrenous cholecystitis*: occurs in immunocompromised patients; evolves into parietal necrosis and perforation; vesicular perforation can be done intraperitoneally, in the digestive tract (duodenum, colon) or can be collected in the GB bed in the form of a perivesicular abscess [3, 6]. *CT report*: calculus embedded in the cystic duct, pericholecystic inflammatory changes, complications, exclusion of acute pancreatitis or of a perforated duodenal ulcer.

Chronic cholecystitis is a chronic inflammation of the GB walls. The causes of chronic cholecystitis are GB stones and cystic duct obstruction; the GB wall is increased in thickness (average 5 mm), with regular or irregular contour. *Particular forms. Xanthogranulomatous cholecystitis* is part of the chronic inflammations of the GB, simulating both clinically and imagistically a GB carcinoma [3, 7, 8]. The *porcelain bladder* represents the deposition of calcium carbonate in the GB wall; associated with GB stones in 90% of cases [3].

CT aspects and report: parietal GB changes associated with density content changes (hyperdense content in porcelain GB), exclusion of a GB carcinoma [3, 7, 8].

13.4.1 Biliary Tree Tumors

Cholangiocarcinoma (CC). CC are malignant tumors originating in the BD epithelium with peripheral (intrahepatic), centrohilar topography (Klatskin tumor) or located at the extrahepatic BD (EHBD) level: common hepatic duct (CHD) or choledochus. Intrahepatic CC represents approximately 20% of all CC, being the second most common liver tumor after HCC. In the Klatskin tumors or in tumors of EHBD level, there are the following forms: obstructive with amputation in U or V (70–85%); stenotic (10–25%) with irregular edges appearance; polypoid (5–6%), with upstream BD dilation. The incidence of Klatskin's tumor represents 70% of CC cases. Lymphatic extension (48%), infiltration in the liver parenchyma (23%); peritoneal determinations (9%); hematogenous disseminations are rare (liver, lung, peritoneum).

CT aspects. Intrahepatic CC: focal or segmental dilation of IHBD (see Fig. 13.4); segmental BD stenosis or presence of endoluminal polypoid mass [35]; spontaneous hypodense mass; after CM i.v. injection the tumor demonstrate heterogeneous peripheral enhancement with gradual centripetal enhancement. The rate and extent of enhancement depend on the degree of central fibrosis; segmental atrophy may be associated; portal invasion is rare [2, 3, 5–8, 36, 37]. *Central CC*: IHBD dilation, without distal EHBD dilation. Staging of the central CC (Bismuth and Corlette classification). Type I: tumor at CHD level with respect of the bifurcation. Type II: the tumor infiltrates CHD extending to the bifurcation. Type III a: infiltration of the CHD, bifurcation with right BD extension and right second-order branches involvements. Type III b: infiltration of the CHD, bifurcation, left hepatic duct, and left second-order BD branches. Type IV: tumor at the level of CHD, R and LCHD and of the second order BD branches [2, 3, 5–8, 36, 37]. *CC at CHD level*: mass circumscribing the CHD, infiltrative or polypoid type (Fig. 13.9),

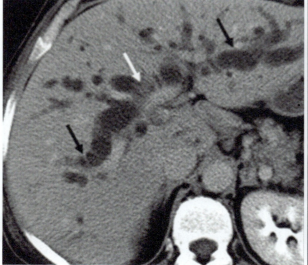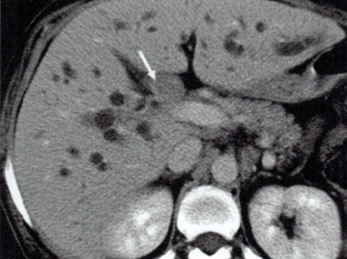

Fig. 13.9 Central cholangiocarcinoma-polypoid type (white arrow) involving the CHD and the bifurcation with symmetrical IHBD dilatation (black arrow)

with upstream BD dilatation. *Choledochal CC*: more frequently infiltrative lesion, rarely polypoid lesion. Dilation of the GB, CHD and IHBD are associated [2, 3, 5–8, 36, 37].

CT report: correct and complete evaluation of the tumor, resectability criteria, exclusion of benign BT pathologies, associated lesions [12].

Gallbladder carcinoma Represents the fifth tumor, in frequency, from malignant tumors of the gastrointestinal tract [5, 6]. There are two forms of GB neoplasm: nodular and infiltrative with localized or diffuse thickening of the wall, difficult to differentiate from a scleroatrophic GB. The extension is made quickly towards the hilum, the hepatic pedicle and into the hepatic parenchyma (in the V, VI or IV liver segments). Regional lymphadenopathies may be present in the hepatic and peripancreatic pedicles. The mechanisms of EHBD involvement are represented by direct contiguous invasion or compression on CHD or choledocus, given by lymphadenopathies or by the tumor mass itself [2, 3, 5–8, 36, 37].

13.5 CT in Pancreatic Pathology

Acute pancreatitis (AP) represents the acute inflammation of the pancreatic tissue that causes changes in structure and function [1, 5, 6].

CT aspects and report. The Balthazar classification groups 5 stages: A and B correspond to the oedematous form of AP; stage C corresponds to AC that associates peripancreatic inflammation; stages D and E correspond to extensive complicated AC with poorly defined-phlegmon-type collections. CT visualizes the pancreas in 98% of cases. CT scan highlight: diffuse increasement with convex edges of the pancreas; hypodense/or absence of enhancement of the pancreatic tissue in necrotic areas; peripancreatic fat infiltration; thickening of the perirenal fascia's; hyperdense areas (50–70UH) in hemorrhagic AP; intra-/peripancreatic fluid collections (Fig. 13.10); identification of fluid collection, pseudocyst (s) or of abscesses; assess the opportunity and the optimal approaches in the post AC encysted collections [1, 3, 5–8].

Chronic pancreatitis (CP) is a persistent and progressive inflammation of the pancreatic tissue that leads to irreversible alterations in anatomical architecture and pancreatic function. There are several types of CP: calcified, obstructive, autoimmune, pseudotumoral, groove pancreatitis [1, 3, 5, 6]. *CT aspects and report*: moniliform dilatation of Wirsung duct (WD); intrapancreatic, intraductal calcifications (CT +++); atrophic appearance of pancreatic tissue; intra-/peripancreatic pseudocyst, focal/diffuse enlargement of the pancreas; moderate dilation of choledoc; others lesions: splenomegaly; splenic vein thrombosis; formation of arterial pseudoaneurysms; thickening of the peripancreatic fascia [1, 3, 5, 6, 12, 38, 39].

Pancreatic pseudocyst is an encapsulated fluid collection delimited by fibrous tissue with dimensions generally between 2–10 cm. Location: 2/3 are located in the pancreas; atypical topography: intraperitoneal, retroperitoneal, subcapsular (hepatic, splenic, renal), mediastinal, in the cervical region. It can communicate with the stomach, duodenum, spleen [1, 3, 5–8, 12].

CT aspects and report: fluid/parafluid density (0–30 UH) collection with well delineated wall, extremely rare parietal calcifications; changes in peripancreatic fat. Complications: rupture, hemorrhage, infection, intestinal obstruction [1, 3, 5–8, 12].

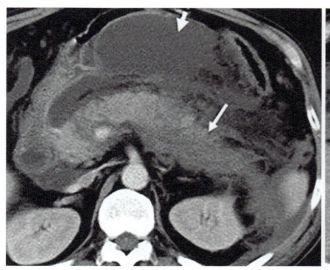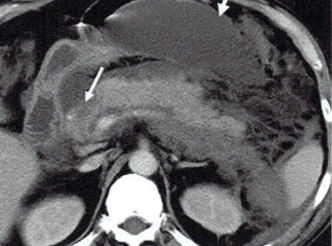

Fig. 13.10 Acute pancreatitis with necrotic areas (white arrow) and multiple peripancreatic fluid collections (dotted arrow)

13.5.1 Pancreatic Tumors

Serous cystadenoma represents 50% of all pancreatic cystic tumors and 1–2% of exocrine tumors of the pancreas; may be associated with von Hippel Lindau syndrome [1, 5, 6].

CT aspect: honeycomb cystic areas; after contrast, the septa and the periphery enhance; characteristic: central fibrous scar sometimes calcified.

Mucinous cystadenoma/cystadenocarcinoma corresponds to a single cystic or multiloculated mass, delimited by a thick wall, sometimes with dense nodules on the internal contour, containing mucin in the cystic areas [1, 3, 5–8, 12]. *CT aspect*: intratumoral septa; fluid densities into the cysts; the tumor is generally hypovascular; positive enhancement of the walls and septa of the cysts; calcifications. Liver metastases are cystic, round with a regular thick wall.

Intraductal papillary mucinous neoplasm (IPMN) represent a mucinous ductal ectasia, with malignant potential. The location is in the WD causing global or focal dilation, or in the afferent branches [3, 6, 12]. *CT aspects and report*. Cystic dilatation of WD and related branches; presence of mural nodules and thick septa in malignant lesions; pancreatic tissue atrophy [3, 6, 12, 40].

Pseudopapillary solid tumor is a cystic and solid tumor with a low degree of malignancy [3, 7, 8, 12]. *CT aspect*: heterogeneous mass with important contrast uptake in the venous phase (Fig. 13.11); presence of calcifications in 30% of cases.

Pancreatic ductal adenocarcinoma (PDAC) is the most common malignancy of the pancreas. 65% of cases are invasive tumors which presents at the time of diagnosis distant metastases. 21% of cases have lymph node invasion. Only 14% have a tumor located strictly into the pancreas. *CT aspects*: pancreatic mass (95%), diffuse enlargement (4%), normal appearance (1%); hypodense, hypovascularized; dilation of choledoc and WD without noticeable tumor mass (4%); dilatation of EBD and IHBD (38%), dilatation of WD (67%); pancreatic body and tail atrophy of (20%); pseudocyst (11%); calcifications (2%); arterial and venous invasion (Fig. 13.12); invasion of lymphatics; venous collateral circulation; thickening of the Gerota fascia; posterior tumor extension; extension to the splenic hilum and hepatic hilum; contiguous invasion of adjacent organs (duodenum, stomach, root of the mesentery).

CT report: 1. establishing *resectability criteria*: no contact with the celiac axis (CA), SMA, or common hepatic artery. Vein: no contact or abutment to the SMV or PV. 2. *unresectable locally advanced*-see Fig. 13.12). Artery: encasement (tumor–vascular contact>180°) of the SMA, HA or CA, abutment or encasement of the first jejunal SMA branch, or abutment of the CA and aortic involvement. Vein: occlusion or tumor thrombosis of SMV or PV or abutment or encasement of the first jejunal SMV branch; *unresectable metastatic*-distant metastasis including nonregional lymph node metastasis. 3. *borderline resectable*: abutment (tumor–vascular contact<180°) or short encasement of the common HA without extension to the CA or HA bifurcation or abutment of the SMA or variant artery; abutment or encasement of the CA without involvement of the aorta, GDA, and SMA. Vein: abutment, impingement, short encasement of the SMV or PV, or short segment venous occlusion [1, 3, 5–8, 12, 41–47].

Pancreatic endocrine tumors Pancreatic neuroendocrine tumors are rare tumors that produce hormonal secretion with specific symptoms; the most common are insulinomas and gastrinomas. Associated with MEN I syndrome; von Hippel Lindau disease, neurofibromatosis and tuberous sclerosis. The degree of malignancy is variable [1, 3, 5–8, 12]. *CT aspects*. Frequently are tumors with a diameter of less than 3 cm, hypervascularized; bulky tumors have necrotic and hemorrhagic areas; In most cases there are no signs of WD obstruction. *CT aspect*: location, number, semiological appearance of the tumor/tumors, signs of malignant degeneration, distant metastases.

Pancreatic non-secreting endocrine tumors are often larger than secretory neuroendocrine tumors; 80% of tumors are hypervascularized; 20% are hypovascularized; cystic/

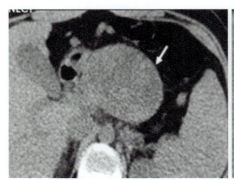 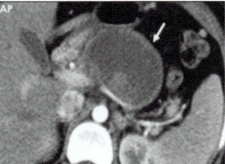 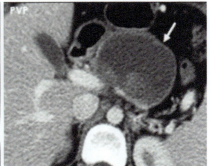

Fig. 13.11 Pseudopapillary solid tumor-large heterogenous pancreatic mass with cystic and solid areas (white arrow)

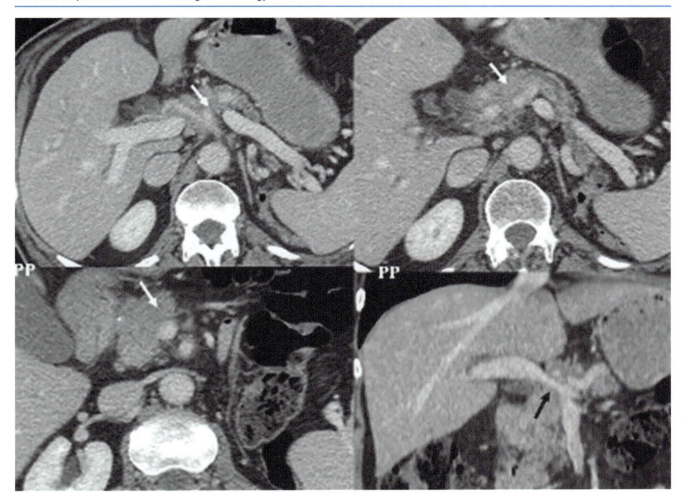

Fig. 13.12 Invasive pancreatic adenocarcinoma: cephalo-isthmic pancreatic mass (white arrow) with invasion of celiac axis, HA, SMV and PV

necrotic components are common; bulky tumors may have calcifications; tumors over 5 cm are frequently malignant and can cause WD obstruction and dilation [1, 5, 6].

CT aspects: intense enhancement in 80% of cases; bulky tumors are heterogeneous with necrotic areas and calcifications. *CT report:* location, number, semiological appearance of the tumor/tumors, signs of malignant degeneration, distant metastases.

Pancreatic metastases occur in the terminal stages of a primary tumor, more commonly in renal cell carcinoma. Primary tumors: renal, lung, breast, colon carcinoma, melanoma, soft tissue sarcoma [1, 3, 5–8, 12]. *CT aspects:* nodules with heterogeneous appearance (60%), homogeneous (17%), iso-/hypodense; hypo-/hypervascularised [1, 3, 5–8, 12].

13.6 CT of Postoperative Complications in HBP Surgery

Postoperative complications in HBP surgery are not uncommon, due to high complexity of surgical procedures. MDCT is the most effective postoperative imaging procedure used in early postoperative period in case of fever, leukocytosis, abdominal pain, jaundice or suspicion of bleeding or peritonitis. Early complications include collections, vascular thromboses, biliary, pancreatic or vascular injuries. Late complications are related mainly to the initial disease relapse. MDCT protocol include a nonenhanced phase (to detect hyperdense collection like hematoma), an AP to assess active bleedings and a PVP to detect and characterize complications like liver abscesses or venous thromboses (portal, mesenteric).

Liver injuries Pneumobilia, periportal edema and soft-tissue stranding can be normal findings during the early postoperative period in patients with HBP surgery. Transient fluid collections are often seen after HBP surgery and drainage is not required, unless clinically indicated. *CT aspects. Fluid collections* are commonly represented by seromas, hematomas, bilioma, pancreatic fistula or abscesses (Fig. 13.13). MDCT is more accurate than ultrasound for diagnosis and characterization of complex collection and is used to perform invasive procedure if necessary. CT allows assessment of the size, location and content of the collection.

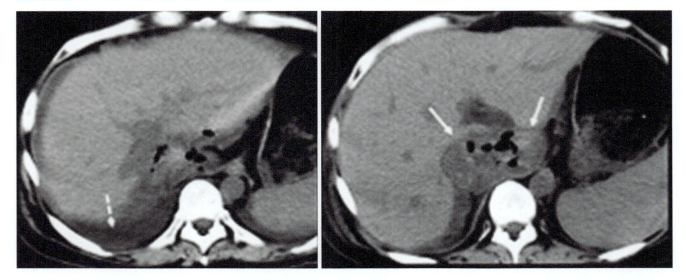

Fig. 13.13 Heterogenous encapsulated collection with multiple aeric bubbles, suggestive for abscess (white arrow). Small right pleural fluid (dotted arrow)

The diagnostic should be correlated with clinical status, laboratory values and surgical procedure. CT-guided procedures (puncture with aspiration, percutaneous drainage) are often required for diagnostic confirmation. *Hematomas* are hyperdense (attenuation between 50–70 HU) on NECT and may show extravasations of CM when active bleeding is present. Fluid collections related with leakages from biliary or pancreatic fistula have lower attenuation (10–20 HU) and located near biliary or pancreatic anastomosis. *Biliomas* are commonly located in the upper right quadrant and appears on MDCT as a well-defined fluid collection, rounded or oval shaped. Complicated bilioma with hemorrhage or infection may have attenuation higher than 20 HU. Collections with gas bubbles and wall enhancement are highly suggestive for *abscesses* (see Fig. 13.13). Typical aspect on MDCT of an abscess is a well-defined, rounded hypodense mass, with gas bubbles inside (in <20% of cases) and wall enhancement after administration of intravenous contrast.

Vascular injuries and thromboses Postoperative vascular thromboses may include PV, SV, HV, HA, SMA. Vascular thrombosis following HBP surgery are rare. MDCTA is used for a precise evaluation of the vascular tree. *CT aspects.* A thrombus typically appears as a nonenhancing filling defect within the lumen of the vessel, an acute thrombus is hyperdense on NECT. MDCT may document associated signs like ischemia of the small bowel or perfusion abnormalities of the liver.

Biliary injuries The post-cholecystectomy BD injuries may be caused by mistakenly placed clips generating stenosis of the CHD or erroneous section of BD. *CT aspects.* MDCT with contrast visualizes the fluid collections and dilatation of the biliary tract and may detect the level of lesion and the associate vascular damage (arterio-venous fistula, vasculo-biliary fistula) if exists.

Pancreatic injuries The most common complications of pancreatic surgery are pancreatic fistula (related to the WD damage), abdominal abscesses, intraabdominal bleeding and anastomotic leakage producing peritonitis and pancreatitis of the remanent gland. *CT aspect.* Pancreatic fistula is the most common complication after the partial pancreatectomy. The most important CT finding is the presence of persistent perianastomotic collection, sometimes with gas bubbles included.

References

1. Catalano OA, Singh AH, Uppot RN, et al. Vascular and biliary variants in the liver: implications for liver surgery. Radiographics. 2008;28:359–78.
2. Lupescu IG, Boros M, Georgescu SA. Imagistica Ficatului, în Tratat de Chirurgie sub redacția Popescu I, vol IX, Chirurgie generala (partea a II-a). Editura Academiei Romane. 2009;51:580–634.
3. Federle MP, Jeffrey RB, Tublin ME, Borhani AA. Hepatobiliary and pancreas. Amyrsis. 2013;I-54-74, I240-329, II-2-172:3-2-63.
4. Murakami T, Kim T, Takamura M, et al. Hypervascular hepatocellular carcinoma: detection with double arterial phase multi-detector row helical CT. Radiology. 2001;218(763–76):18.
5. Brambs H-J. Foie, Vesicule et voies biliaire, pancreas în Appareil Digestif. Lavoisier. 2010:1–137.
6. Choi BI (editor). Radiology illustrated: hepatobiliary and pancreatic radiology. Springer 2014, 3–719.
7. Lupescu IG, Stoica ZS. Radiologia gastrointestinală și abdominală, în Radiologie Imagistică Medicală sub redacția Dudea SM. Editura Medicală. 2015;I(7):672–704.
8. Ioana G Lupescu. Imagistica in patologia chirurgicala hepato-bilio-pancreatica., in Tratat de chirurgie hepato-biliopancreatica si

transplant heptic, coordonator Irinel Popescu. Editura Academiei Romane, 2016;cap 3:38 pag.
9. CT/MRI LI-RADS® v2018. https://www.acr.org/Clinical-Resources/Reporting-and-Data-Systems/LI-RADS/CT-MRI-LI-RADS-v2018
10. Iannaccone R, Laghi A, Catalano C, et al. Hepatocellular carcinoma: role of unenhanced and delayed phase multidetector row helical CT in patients with cirrhosis. Radiology. 2005;234:460–7.
11. Hayashi M, Matsui O, Ueda K, Kawamori Y, Gabata T, Kadoya M. Progression to hypervascular hepatocellular carcinoma: correlation with intranodular blood supply evaluated with CT during intra-arterial injection of contrast material. Radiology. 2002;225:143–9.
12. Erturk SM, Ichikawa T. Teaching Atlas of hepatobiliary and pancreatic Imaging, Springer 2016, 1–221.
13. Matsui O, Kobayashi S, Sanada J, et al. Hepatocelluar nodules in liver cirrhosis: hemodynamic evaluation (angiography-assisted CT) with special reference to multi-step hepatocarcinogenesis. Abdom Imaging 2011; 36(3): 264–272. 27.
14. Taouli B, Goh JS, Lu Y, et al. Growth rate of hepatocellular carcinoma: evaluation with serial computed tomography or magnetic resonance imaging. J Comput Assist Tomogr. 2005;29:425–9.
15. Jha RC, et al. LI-RADS categorization of benign and likely benign findings in patients at risk of hepatocellular carcinoma: a pictorial Atlas. AJR. 2014;203:W48–69.
16. Brancatelli G, Baron RL, Peterson MS, Marsh W. Helical CT screening for hepatocellular carcinoma in patients with cirrhosis: frequency and causes of false-positive interpretation. AJR. 2003;180:1007–14.
17. Hwang GJ, Kim MJ, Yoo HS, Lee JT. Nodular hepatocellular carcinomas: detection with arterial-, portal-, and delayed-phase images at spiral CT. Radiology. 1997;202:383.
18. Lim JH, Kim MJ, Park CK, Kang SS, Lee WJ, Lim HK. Dysplastic nodules in liver cirrhosis: detection with triple phase helical dynamic CT. Br J Radiol. 2004;77(911–916):47.
19. Erbay N, Raptopoulos V, Pomfret EA, et al. Liver donor-liver transplantation in adults: vascular variants important in surgical planning for donors and recipients. AJR. 2003;16(181):109–14.
20. Singh AK, Cronin CG, Verma HA, et al. Imaging of preoperative liver transplantation in adults: What radiologists should know. Radiographics. 2011;31:1017–30.
21. Iannaccone R, Laghi A, Catalano C, et al. Hepatocellular carcinoma: role of unenhanced and delayed phase multidetector row helical CT in patients with cirrhosis. Radiology. 2005;234:460–7.
22. Vitale A, Cucchetti A, et al. Is resectable hepatocellular carcinoma a contraindication to liver transplantation? A novel decision model based on "number of patients needed to transplant" as measure of transplant benefit. J Hepatol. 2014;60:1165–71.
23. Li JP, Zhao DL, et al. Assessment of tumor vascularization with functional computed tomography perfusion imaging in patients with cirrhotic liver disease. Hepatobiliary Pancreat Dis Int. 2011;10(1):43–9.
24. Araújo CCV, Balbi E, Pacheco-Moreira LF, et al. Evaluation of living donor liver transplantation: causes for exclusion. Transpl Proc. 2010;42(2):424–5.
25. Zamboni GA, Pedrosa I, Kruskal JB, et al. Liver transplantation in imaging in transplantation, Editor Bankier A Springer, 2008, 99–134.
26. Caiado AH, et al. Complications of liver transplantation: multimodality imaging approach. Radiographics. 2007;27(5):1401–17.
27. Dani G, Sun RMM, Bennett AE. Imaging of liver transplant and its complications. Semin Ultrasound CT MRI. 2013;4:365–77.
28. Quiroga S, Sebastia MC, Margarit C, et al. Complications of orthotopic liver transplantation: spectrum of findings with helical CT. Radiographics. 2001;21(1085–2201):72.
29. Itri JN, Heller TM, Tublin ME. Hepatic transplantation: postoperative complications. Abdom Imaging. 2013;38:1300–33.
30. Camacho JC, et al. Nonvascular PostLiver transplantation complications: from US screening to crosssectional and interventional imaging. Radiographics. 2015;35:87–104.
31. Catalano OA, et al. Biliary infections: spectrum of imaging findings and management. Radiographics. 2009;29(7):2059–80.
32. Aberg F, Pukkala E, Höckerstedt K, Sankila R, Isoniemi H. Risk of malignant neoplasms after liver transplantation: a population-based study. Liver Transpl. 2008;14(10):1428–36.
33. McCaughan GW, Vajdic CM. De novo malignant disease after liver transplantation? Risk and surveillance strategies. Liver Transpl. 2013;19(suppl 2):S62–7.
34. Nakazawa T, Ohara H, Sano H, Ando T, Joh T. Schematic classification of sclerosing cholangitis with autoimmune pancreatitis by cholangiography. Pancreas. 2006;32(2):229.
35. Lim JH, Yoon KH, Kim SH, et al. Intraductal papillary mucinous tumor of the bile ducts. Radiographics. 2004; 24(1):53–67. 3.
36. Kim JH, Kim TK, Eun HW, et al. CT findings of cholangiocarcinoma associated with recurrent pyogenic cholangitis. AJR Am J Roentgenol. 2006;187(6):1571–7.
37. Chung YE, Kim M-J, Park YN. Varying appearances of cholangiocarcinoma: radiologic pathologic correlation. Radiographics. 2009;29:683–700.
38. Shanbhogue AKS, Najla Fasih N, Surabhi VR, et al. A clinical and radiologic review of uncommon types and causes of pancreatitis. Radiographics. 2009;29:1003–26.
39. Kim JK, Altun E, Elias J, et al. Focal pancreatic mass: distinction of pancreatic cancer from chronic pancreatitis using gadolinium-enhanced 3D-gradient-echo MRI. J Magn Reson Imaging. 2007;26:313–22.
40. Ichikawa T, Sou H, Araki T, et al. Duct-penetrating sign at MRCP: usefulness for differentiating inflammatory pancreatic mass from pancreatic carcinomas. Radiology. 2001;221:107–16.
41. Park HS, Lee JM, Choi JY, et al. Preoperative evaluation of bile duct cancer: MRI combined with MR cholangiopancreatography versus MDCT with direct cholangiography. AJR. 2008;190(2):396–405.
42. Tajima Y, Kuroki T, Tsutsumi R, Kim T, et al. Pancreatic carcinoma coexisting with chronic pancreatitis versus tumor forming pancreatitis: diagnostic utility of the timesignal intensity curve from dynamic contrast-enhanced MR imaging. World J Gastroenterol. 2007;13:858–65.
43. Leung TK, Lee CM, Wang FC, et al. Difficulty with diagnosis of malignant pancreatic neoplasms coexisting with chronic pancreatitis. World J Gastroenterol. 2005;11:5075–8.
44. Chun YS, Milestone BN, Watson JC, et al. Defining venous involvement in borderline resectable pancreatic cancer. Ann Surg Oncol. 2010;17(11):2832–8.
45. Morgan DE, Waggoner CN, Canon CL, et al. Resectability of pancreatic adenocarcinoma in patients with locally advanced disease downstaged by preoperative therapy: a challenge for MDCT. AJR. 2010;194(3):615–22.
46. Cassinotto C, Cortade J, Belleannée G, et al. An evaluation of the accuracy of CT when determining resectability of pancreatic head adenocarcinoma after neoadjuvant treatment. Eur J Radiol. 2013;82(4):589–93.
47. Hong SB, Lee SS, Kim JH, et al. Pancreatic cancer CT: prediction of resectability according to NCCN criteria. Radiology. 2018;289(3):710–8.

Magnetic Resonance Elastography (MRE) to Assess Hepatic Fibrosis

Aliya Qayyum

Abstract

Chronic liver disease and cirrhosis are a major worldwide health problem and represent the 11th leading cause of death in the USA based on data from 1999 to 2018 [1]. There are many etiologies of chronic liver disease including hepatotoxic factors such as viral hepatitis B and C, alcohol, nonalcoholic fatty liver disease, hemochromatosis, and autoimmune hepatitis, as well as biliary factors (toxicities) such as primary sclerosing cholangitis and primary biliary cirrhosis. While liver biopsy is the standard of reference for diagnosis and monitoring of liver fibrosis, it is an invasive procedure associated with a non-negligible complication risk [2]. Bleeding occurs in ~1 of 500 liver biopsies, which may be severe in 1 of 2500 to 10,000 liver biopsies [3]. Additional important complications include sepsis, pneumothorax, and hemothorax. The reported mortality risk from liver biopsy is up to 0.3% [4]. Aside from complications, liver biopsy is not an accurate reference standard. Important limitations of liver biopsy include small sample size (~1/50,000 part of liver) resulting in sampling errors due to the heterogeneity of diffuse liver disease, and high intra- and inter-observer variability in interpretation [5–12].

Cross-sectional imaging with ultrasound, CT, and MRI can depict morphologic changes that can be present in some but not all patients with cirrhosis but liver morphology usually is normal with earlier stages of fibrosis. MR elastography (MRE) is an non-invasive technique for quantitatively assessing the stiffness of tissue and is now deployed on more than 1500 MRI systems around the world. MRE is often included as part of a standard liver MRI for evaluation of chronic liver disease. The normal liver is a soft organ with structural support mainly from the extracellular matrix of the parenchyma, which is comprised largely of collagen and a thin connective tissue capsule. In chronic liver injury, activation of the hepatic stellate cells to myofibroblasts results in fibrosis. The fibrosis is associated with alteration of liver blood flow. Both of these factors contribute to an increase in liver stiffness. Additional pathological processes that can contribute to liver stiffness include venous congestion, biliary obstruction, and inflammation within the liver [13]. The premise for clinical MRE is based on the altered mechanical properties of diseased tissues. The most successful application of MRE to date is in the detection and staging of liver fibrosis, which has driven the use of MRE over the last decade. A normal liver typically has a stiffness of approximately 2 kPa (similar to subcutaneous fat), whereas a cirrhotic liver may have a stiffness value of >5 kPa. Shear waves propagating in tissues with higher stiffness will have a greater wavelength and a faster speed. The basis of MRE exploits the faster propagation of shear waves in stiffer tissue and slower propagation in softer tissue. During MRE, applied vibration to the organ of interest is synchronized with a modified phase-contrast MRI pulse sequence used to image the propagating shear waves. MRE measures the speed of the propagating shear waves. The MRE data is used to generate an "elastogram" which is a grayscale or color "stiffness" map (i.e., magnitude of the tissue shear modulus in kilopascals/kPa, commonly known as "shear stiffness" or simply "stiffness"). Liver stiffness is independent of magnetic field strength and MRE can be performed on either 1.5T or 3T clinical scanners. However, it is necessary to perform liver MRE at the same frequency of vibration to achieve comparable measurements (stiffness

A. Qayyum (✉)
MD Anderson Cancer Center, Houston, TX, USA
e-mail: AQayyum@mdanderson.org

depends on frequency). Reportedly, a well-performed liver MRE study should "achieve a 95% confidence interval for a true change in stiffness when there is a measured change in hepatic stiffness of 19% or larger" [13–16]. The diagnostic accuracy of MRE (0.994 for fibrosis stage >2, 0.985 for fibrosis stage >3, and 0.998 for fibrosis stage >4) is reported to be greater than that of other tests such as transient elastography (TE), serum aspartate aminotransferase to platelets ratio index (APRI), and the combination of TE with APRI [16].

14.1 MRE Technique

There are three key components to MRE: (1) transducers, (2) pulse sequences for data acquisition, and (3) postprocessing for converting raw images into an elastogram or stiffness map. The transducer generates and transmits mechanical waves into an organ of interest in the body (e.g., liver). All current commercially available MRE systems use an "active driver" located outside the magnet room to generate the low frequency pressure waves. These waves are transmitted by a coupling tube to a small drum-like device ("passive driver") placed on the chest wall overlying the liver (Fig. 14.1). The passive driver converts the pressure waves into vibrations in the chest wall which generate shear waves in the liver.

MRE is based on a phase-contrast pulse sequence, with superimposed cyclic motion encoding gradients synchronized with the mechanical waves from the transducer. An MRE pulse sequence can be either 2-dimensional (2D) or 3-dimensional (3D). A typical MRE sequence involves a modified 2D echo-planar (EPI) imaging (TR/TE 600 ms/min full (~554.4); slice/gap 8/2 mm; flip angle default (90); field of view 42 cm; matrix 64×64; bandwidth 250 kHz; number of excitations (NEX) 2; 4–6 slices acquired through largest portion of the liver) (Fig. 14.1). The acquisition time is 16–19 seconds (1 breath-hold).

MRE postprocessing involves the following steps: (1) converting the raw phase data into displacement; (2) generating shear-wave images by removing the compressive wave component; (3) generating wave speed from the shear waves at the different phase offsets, and (4) generating the elastogram from the wave speed with an inversion algorithm (measurement units in kilopascals, kPa). The standard MRE

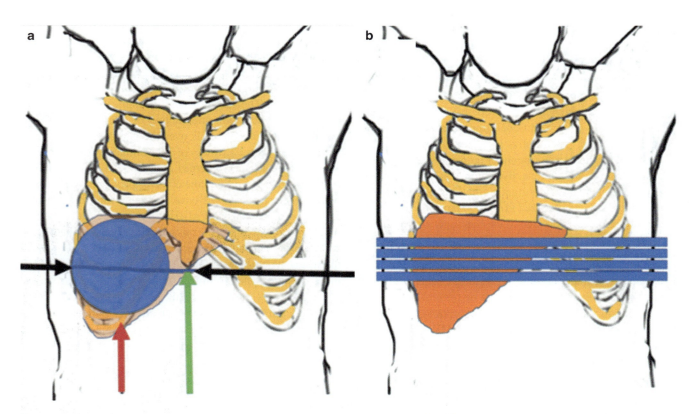

Fig. 14.1 (a) The passive driver (blue circle) is placed on the right lower chest wall overlying the liver. The vertical center of the driver is in line with the right mid-clavicle (red arrow). The horizontal level of the driver (black arrows) is in line with the tip of the xiphisternum (green arrow). (b) MRE images are acquired as 4–6 slices (8 mm slices with 2 mm gap) at the level of the widest extent of the liver (blue lines), while avoiding the liver dome and inferior liver tip

postprocessing employs a multimodel direct inversion (MMDI) algorithm [17]. A confidence map, indicating where the inversion algorithm is unreliable (noisy data), is displayed as a checkerboard overlay on the stiffness map to highlight regions of low confidence. Liver stiffness is calculated as an average of measurements from ROIs placed at multiple liver slice levels while avoiding the checkered regions [14].

14.2 MRE Performance

Technical failure rates with MRE are small, reportedly occurring in 2–5% of scans [14, 18]. Liver MRE is repeatable and reproducible with high inter- and intra-observer agreement [19–22]. Liver stiffness measurements with MRE have also shown to be comparable across vendors [23, 24], and the reported accuracy is superior to routine serum liver function tests for detection of significant and advanced fibrosis [25–27]. The major advantage of MRE over ultrasound-based techniques is the large field of view enabling assessment over a much larger liver volume. This is particularly important given the heterogeneous distribution of diffuse liver disease. Patient factors are also less likely to affect MRE compared to ultrasound-based quantitative elastography. In a review of 153 studies, MRE was the only non-invasive technique with reasonable accuracy for diagnosis of mild fibrosis [27]. Furthermore, it has been suggested that MRE may be useful for predicting inflammatory change in patients with nonalcoholic steatohepatitis before development of fibrosis [28].

Fibrosis detection and staging: The normal liver is soft and has a mean stiffness value of 2.05–2.44 kPa with reported ranges from 1.54 to 2.87 [23, 29–31]. Liver stiffness increases with the development of fibrosis. MRE detects liver fibrosis before the development of morphological changes seen on cross-sectional imaging. MRE has a reported accuracy of 89–99%, sensitivity of 80–98%, and specificity of 90–100% [13, 25, 26, 28–32]. The threshold for detecting liver fibrosis ranges from 2.4 to 2.93 kPa [13, 16, 25, 28–33]. The variation in threshold for detection may be related to population variation with different liver disease etiologies. MRE stiffness thresholds used for staging liver fibrosis are shown in Fig. 14.2 [14]. The overlap between threshold values for fibrosis stage indicates the importance of interpreting liver stiffness measurements within clinical context and test results.

Liver stiffness is calculated as an average using regions-of-interest placed at four to six axial levels through the liver. A liver stiffness of less than 2.5 kPa is generally considered normal. Images from a patient with an average liver stiffness of 1.6 kPa consistent with normal liver (no fibrosis) are shown in Fig. 14.3.

The severity of liver fibrosis can be readily identified with application of a color scale to the stiffness values of the elastogram. For example, the images of two patients with a different fibrosis stage due to chronic liver disease are shown in Fig. 14.4.

Typically, diffuse liver disease is heterogeneous as shown in Fig. 14.5. The variation in liver fibrosis can be readily

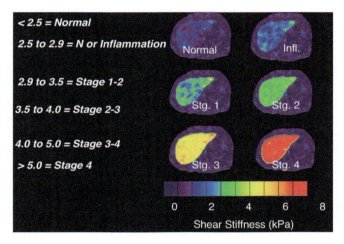

Fig. 14.2 Range of MRE stiffness values (kPa) used to stage liver fibrosis and color representation of liver stiffness range on elastograms associated with fibrosis stage

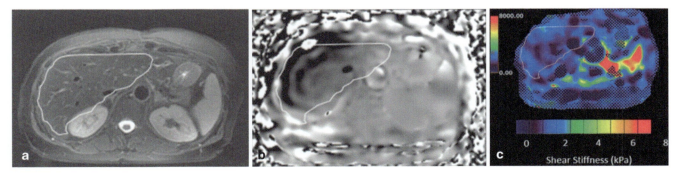

Fig. 14.3 MRI images from a patient with a normal liver. (**a**) Axial T2-weighted image showing liver outlined by a white line. (**b**) MRE phase/wave image through the liver. (**c**) Color elastogram with checkerboard overlay to highlight regions of low confidence; the liver is purple/blue based on the color scale. The average liver stiffness was 1.6 kPa indicating normal stiffness

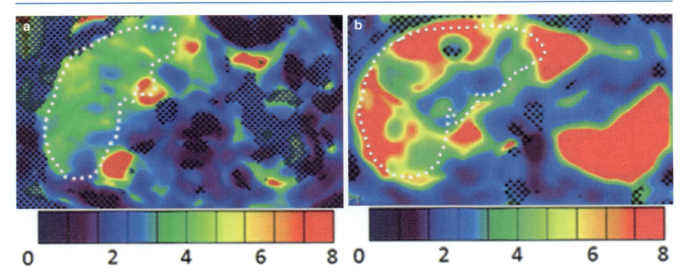

Fig. 14.4 Color elastograms from two patients with chronic liver disease. (**a**) In the first patient, the average stiffness of the liver (outlined by broken line) was 3.5 kPa (mainly green) corresponding to a fibrosis stage of 2–3. (**b**) In the second patient, the average liver stiffness was 8 kPa (mainly red) corresponding to fibrosis stage 4

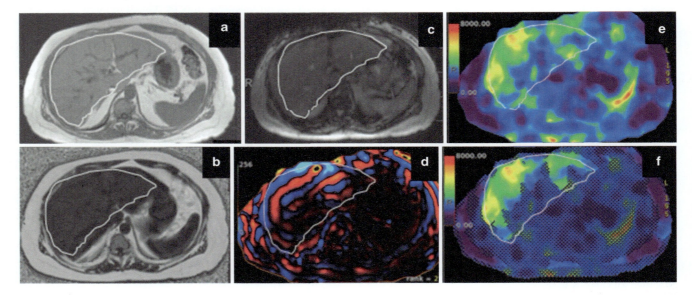

Fig. 14.5 Patient with nonalcoholic steatohepatitis. (**a**) T1-weighted image of the liver (outlined by a white line). (**b**) Fat fraction map; the estimated liver fat fraction was seven (mild steatosis). (**c**) MRE magnitude image. (**d**) MRE wave image. (**e**) Color MR elastogram demonstrating heterogeneous liver color/stiffness. (**f**) MR elastogram with checkerboard overlay to highlight regions of low confidence. The liver biopsy of this patient demonstrated stage 1 portal fibrosis. However, the average liver stiffness derived from measurements obtained at multiple levels in the liver was 3.9 kPa corresponding to a higher overall fibrosis stage of 2–3

identified on the color MRE elastogram and highlights how a liver biopsy can result in incorrect estimation of fibrosis stage depending on the region sampled.

As mentioned above, shear waves propagate faster in stiffer tissue and are associated with a longer wavelength. The longer wavelength is represented by the width of propagating waves on the MRE wave as shown in Fig. 14.6. The longer wavelength is reflected in the arbitrary color scale assigned to the shear stiffness values.

Liver fibrosis that is detected on MRE may not be apparent on conventional MR images as shown in Fig. 14.7. The greater sensitivity of MRE for detection of liver fibrosis has

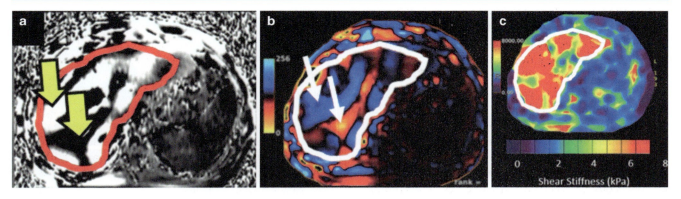

Fig. 14.6 Patient with stage 4 fibrosis. (**a**) Gray scale and (**b**) Color MRE wave images demonstrate wide shear waves (arrows) in the liver due to long wavelength. (**c**) Color elastogram with large regions of red arbitrarily selected to indicate higher stiffness within the liver (outlined by white line). The liver stiffness was 6.8 kPa consistent with stage 4 fibrosis

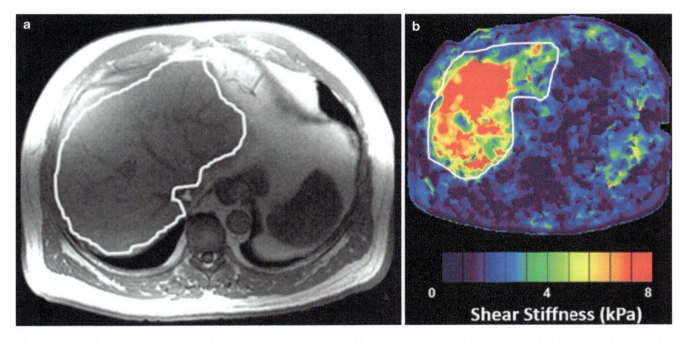

Fig. 14.7 Liver images from a patient with nonalcoholic fatty liver disease, which affects one in three Americans. The conventional liver MRI exam showed no evidence of fibrosis. (**a**) T1-weighted image of the liver (outlined in white). (**b**) MRE color elastogram demonstrating extensive red color within the liver consistent with increased liver stiffness and advanced fibrosis

resulted in an increased incorporation of MRE to routine liver MRI for assessment of liver disease.

14.3 Pitfalls in Stiffness Measurement

Liver stiffness measurements require manual segmentation of the liver on the MR images while avoiding regions of low confidence in the liver. It is also important to avoid nonhepatocyte tissues such as major blood vessels, and areas susceptible to artifact such as the left liver (cardiac pulsation artifact), diaphragm and liver edges (partial volume averaging effect causing an artificial increased stiffness). Tumors within the liver should not be included when assessing background liver stiffness since tumors and tumor thrombus are associated with higher stiffness levels compared to nontumor liver parenchyma. For example, Fig. 14.8 shows images from a patient with extensive infiltrating hepatocellular carcinoma (HCC) and portal vein tumor thrombus resulting in marked increased stiffness of the liver. However, the

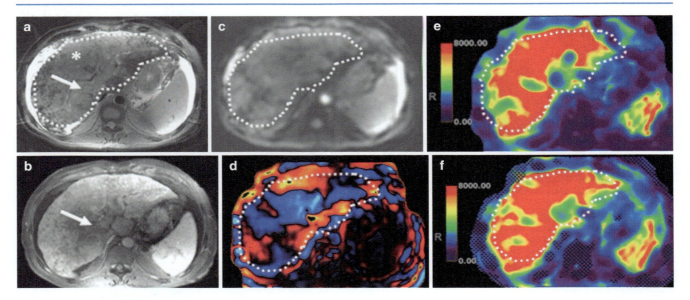

Fig. 14.8 A 44-year-old man with infiltrating HCC and tumor thrombus. (**a**) T2-weighted image. The liver (outlined by white broken line) has extensive high T2-signal intensity due to infiltrating HCC (asterisk). Expansile tumor thrombus (arrow) is seen in the right and left portal vein. (**b**) Contrast-enhanced image. (**c**) MRE magnitude image. (**d**) MRE wave image with color. The wide bands of color indicate longer wavelength and faster wave speed. (**e**) Color elastogram showing predominantly red color within the liver consistent with increased stiffness. (**f**) Color elastogram with checkerboard overlay to highlight regions of low confidence. Although the liver stiffness is measured at >6 kPa, this cannot be interpreted as fibrosis since the tumor and portal vein tumor thrombus will contribute to the high liver stiffness

increased stiffness is likely due to tumor and tumor thrombus in the portal vein rather than reflecting liver fibrosis. When measuring liver stiffness, it is helpful to use the magnitude image for anatomical guidance in order to correctly match locations to the elastogram (use table position/slice location parameters). Matching anatomy facilitates identification of focal lesions on the elastogram. Follow-up imaging should use similar liver locations to the baseline scan [34].

14.4 Technical Limitations

There are several technical and biological factors that can affect the success of an MRE exam including:

1. Transducer failure and incorrect settings (e.g., incorrect wave frequency and amplitude) and incorrect placement of the passive driver (driver does not overlie the liver). Additional factors that result in MRE failure are poor contact between the passive driver and patient, loose connection between the plastic tube and passive driver and failure to synchronize the active driver with the MRE sequence (Fig. 14.9).
2. Patient motion, as shown in Fig. 14.10, can degrade the MRE image, and intrinsic confounders, e.g. increased liver iron (reduces MRI signal), and post-prandial increased portal blood flow to the liver (increases liver stiffness). In the past, failure rates were more common at higher field strengths (3T) but these have been addressed by the improvement in pulse sequences. For example, ascites and high BMI are not significant causes of technical failure with up-to-date MRE techniques. Based on a recent meta-analyses, the overall technical failure rate of MRE is approximately 2%, and most commonly due to iron overload in the liver.

Several tactics can enhance the diagnostic quality of MRE exams. MRE data should be obtained at end expiration since this enables a more repeatable diaphragm position than end-inspiration and reduces respiratory motion artifact. Performing MRE with sequences that have a shorter echo time, such as spin-echo echo-planar imaging (EPI), reduces signal loss from increased liver iron. Imaging patients in a fasting state (4–6 h) reduces the likelihood of post-prandial portal blood flow related artificial increase in liver stiffness [35, 36]. The time-to-echo (TE) for MRE should be near or at the TE of in-phase imaging to maximize signal intensity of the liver parenchyma and avoid loss of signal from liver fat. Updated postprocessing techniques should be used as they continue to evolve. For example, the newer multimodel direct inversion (MMDI) algorithm has better image quality and slightly lower stiffness values compared to the previously used multiscale direct inversion algorithm (MSDI) at 3T magnet strengths [17]. An average liver stiffness should be obtained using multiple regions-of-interest carefully placed in the liver to reduce the effects of heterogeneous disease distribution.

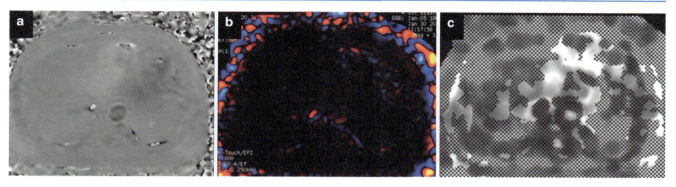

Fig. 14.9 Driver failure due to improper connection of coupling tube. (**a**) Phase image which appears "flat" without wave visualization. (**b**) Color map of waves on phase image showing signal loss (dark region). (**c**) Elastogram with checkerboard overlay showing regions of low confidence throughout the image. Stiffness measurements are not possible

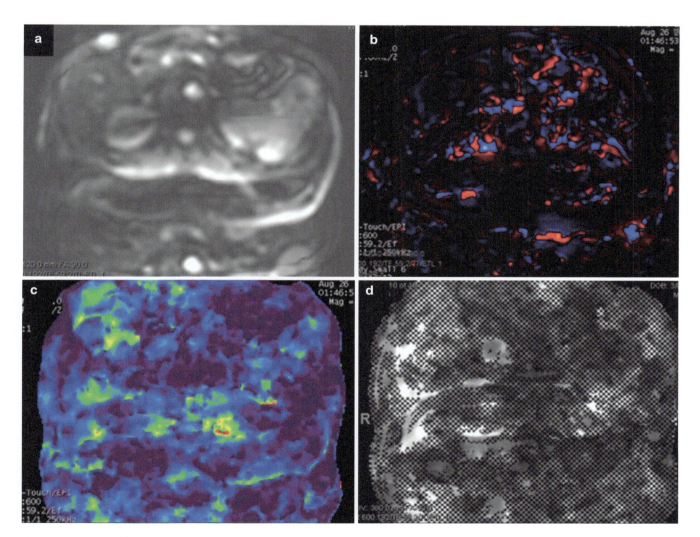

Fig. 14.10 MRE failure due to severe respiratory motion artifact. (**a**) Magnitude image demonstrating phase encoding artifact causing an overlap/ghosting in the image. (**b**) Color map of waves on phase image showing signal loss (dark region). (**c**) Color map of elastogram (stiffness map) with motion artifact. (**d**) Elastogram with checkerboard overlay highlights regions of low confidence throughout the image. Stiffness measurements are not possible

Advances in MRE: Current commercially available MRE packages employ a two-dimensional wave propagation model (2D MRE), which assumes that shear waves propagate in the plane of acquisition while ignoring waves traveling in an oblique direction. This assumption may result in an overestimation of liver stiffness. More recently, 3D MRE has been introduced, employing imaging the wave motion and processing the wave images in three dimensions to calculate tissue stiffness. The 3D MRE offers more reliable and repeatable measures of liver stiffness with larger liver coverage, as well more accurate assessment of focal liver lesions. In addition, 3D MRE allows measurement of the subcomponents of the complex shear modulus, i.e. the real and imaginary components, which represent the elastic (storage modulus, G') and viscous (loss modulus, G") properties of tissue, respectively. Such quantitative biomarkers are promising for the non-invasive assessment of histopathologic processes such as inflammation UCSF [14, 37, 38].

14.5 Summary

Liver MRE is a robust technique for liver stiffness quantification. Currently MRE is the most accurate non-invasive method for detection and staging of liver fibrosis. Advances in MRE technology may further our understanding of diffuse and focal liver disease and improve patient management in the future.

Acknowledgments Richard L. Ehman, M.D. Mayo Clinic, Rochester, MN.

References

1. Centers for Disease Control and Prevention, National Center for Health Statistics. Underlying Cause of Death 1999-2018 on CDC WONDER Online Database, released in 2020. Data are from the Multiple Cause of Death Files, 1999-2018, as compiled from data provided by the 57 vital statistics jurisdictions through the Vital Statistics Cooperative Program. http://wonder.cdc.gov/ucd-icd10.html. Accessed 7 Nov 2020.
2. Chi H, Hansen BE, Tang WY, Schouten JN, Sprengers D, Taimr P, et al. Multiple biopsy passes and the risk of complications of percutaneous liver biopsy. Eur J Gastroenterol Hepatol. 2017;29(1):36–41.
3. Rockey DC, Caldwell SH, Goodman ZD, Nelson RC, Smith AD. American Association for the Study of Liver Diseases position paper: liver biopsy. Hepatology. 2009;49(3):1017–44.
4. West J, Card TR. Reduced mortality rates following elective percutaneous liver biopsies. Gastroenterology. 2010;139:1230–7.
5. Cadranel JF, Rufat P, Degos F. Practices of liver biopsy in France: results of a prospective nationwide survey. For the Group of Epidemiology of the French Association for the Study of the Liver (AFEF). Hepatology (Baltimore, MD). 2000;32(3):477–81.
6. Bedossa P, Dargere D, Paradis V. Sampling variability of liver fibrosis in chronic hepatitis C. Hepatology (Baltimore, MD). 2003;38(6):1449–57.
7. Castera L, Negre I, Samii K, Buffet C. Pain experienced during percutaneous liver biopsy. Hepatology (Baltimore, MD). 1999;30(6):1529–30.
8. Poynard T, Ratziu V, Bedossa P. Appropriateness of liver biopsy. Can J Gastroenterol. 2000;14(6):543–8.
9. Regev A, Berho M, Jeffers LJ, Milikowski C, Molina EG, Pyrsopoulos NT, et al. Sampling error and intraobserver variation in liver biopsy in patients with chronic HCV infection. Am J Gastroenterol. 2002;97(10):2614–8.
10. Maharaj B, Maharaj RJ, Leary WP, Cooppan RM, Naran AD, Pirie D, et al. Sampling variability and its influence on the diagnostic yield of percutaneous needle biopsy of the liver. Lancet (London, England). 1986;1(8480):523–5.
11. Rousselet MC, Michalak S, Dupre F, Croue A, Bedossa P, Saint-Andre JP, et al. Sources of variability in histological scoring of chronic viral hepatitis. Hepatology (Baltimore, MD). 2005;41(2):257–64.
12. Puche JE, Saiman Y, Friedman SL. Hepatic stellate cells and liver fibrosis. Compr Physiol. 2013;3(4):1473–92.
13. Yin M, Talwalkar JA, Glaser KJ, Manduca A, Grimm RC, Rossman PJ, et al. Assessment of hepatic fibrosis with magnetic resonance elastography. Clin Gastroenterol Hepatol. 2007;5(10):1207–13.e2.
14. Hoodeshenas S, Meng Y, Venkatesh SK. Magnetic resonance elastography of liver- current update. Top Magn Reson Imaging. 2018;27(5):319–33. https://doi.org/10.1097/RMR.0000000000000177.
15. Rouviere O, Yin M, Dresner MA, Rossman PJ, Burgart LJ, Fidler JL, et al. MR elastography of the liver: preliminary results. Radiology. 2006;240(2):440–8.
16. Huwart L, Sempoux C, Vicaut E, Salameh N, Annet L, Danse E, et al. Magnetic resonance elastography for the noninvasive staging of liver fibrosis. Gastroenterology. 2008;135:32–40. https://doi.org/10.1053/j.gastro.2008.03.076.
17. Yoshimitsu K, Shinagawa Y, Mitsufuji T, Mutoh E, Urakawa H, Sakamoto K, et al. Preliminary comparison of multi-scale and multi-model direct inversion algorithms for 3T MR elastography. Magn Reson Med Sci. 2017;16(1):73–7.
18. Kim DW, Kim SY, Yoon HM, Kim KW, Byun JH. Comparison of technical failure of MR elastography for measuring liver stiffness between gradient-recalled echo and spin-echo echo-planar imaging: a systematic review and meta-analysis. J Magn Reson Imaging. 2020;51(4):1086–102. https://doi.org/10.1002/jmri.26918.
19. Hines CD, Bley TA, Lindstrom MJ, Reeder SB. Repeatability of magnetic resonance elastography for quantification of hepatic stiffness. J Magn Reson Imaging. 2010;31(3):725–31.
20. Shire NJ, Yin M, Chen J, Railkar RA, Fox-Bosetti S, Johnson SM, et al. Test-retest repeatability of MR elastography for noninvasive liver fibrosis assessment in hepatitis C. J Magn Reson Imaging. 2011;34(4):947–55.
21. Venkatesh SK, Wang G, Teo LL, Ang BW. Magnetic resonance elastography of liver in healthy Asians: normal liver stiffness quantification and reproducibility assessment. J Magn Reson Imaging. 2014;39(1):1–8.
22. Lee Y, Lee JM, Lee JE, Lee KB, Lee ES, Yoon JH, et al. MR elastography for noninvasive assessment of hepatic fibrosis: reproducibility of the examination and reproducibility and repeatability of the liver stiffness value measurement. J Magn Reson Imaging. 2014;39(2):326–31.
23. Yasar TK, Wagner M, Bane O, Besa C, Babb JS, Kannengiesser S, et al. Interplatform reproducibility of liver and spleen stiffness measured with MR elastography. J Magn Reson Imaging. 2016;43(5):1064–72.
24. Trout AT, Serai S, Mahley AD, Wang H, Zhang Y, Zhang B, et al. Liver stiffness measurements with MR elastography: agreement and repeatability across imaging systems, field strengths, and pulse sequences. Radiology. 2016;281(3):793–804.

25. Venkatesh SK, Wang G, Lim SG, Wee A. Magnetic resonance elastography for the detection and staging of liver fibrosis in chronic hepatitis B. Eur Radiol. 2014;24:70–8.
26. Huwart L, Sempoux C, Salameh N, Jamart J, Annet L, Sinkus R, et al. Liver fibrosis: noninvasive assessment with MR elastography versus aspartate aminotransferase-to-platelet ratio index. Radiology. 2007;245:458–66.
27. Bonekamp S, Kamel I, Solga S, Clark J. Can imaging modalities diagnose and stage hepatic fibrosis and cirrhosis accurately? J Hepatol. 2009;50:17–35.
28. Chen J, Talwalkar JA, Yin M, Glaser KJ, Sanderson SO, Ehman RL. Early detection of nonalcoholic steatohepatitis in patients with nonalcoholic fatty liver disease by using MR elastography. Radiology. 2011;259:749–56.
29. Lee DH, Lee JM, Han JK, Choi BI. MR elastography of healthy liver parenchyma: normal value and reliability of the liver stiffness value measurement. J Magn Reson Imaging. 2013;38(5):1215–23.
30. Kim BH, Lee JM, Lee YJ, Lee KB, Suh KS, Han JK, et al. MR elastography for noninvasive assessment of hepatic fibrosis: experience from a tertiary center in Asia. J Magn Reson Imaging. 2011;34(5):1110–6.
31. Herzka DA, Kotys MS, Sinkus R, Pettigrew RI, Gharib AM. Magnetic resonance elastography in the liver at 3 tesla using a second harmonic approach. Magn Reson Med. 2009;62(2):284–91.
32. Asbach P, Klatt D, Schlosser B, Biermer M, Muche M, Rieger A, et al. Viscoelasticity-based staging of hepatic fibrosis with multifrequency MR elastography. Radiology. 2010;257(1):80–6.
33. Huwart L, Peeters F, Sinkus R, Annet L, Salameh N, ter Beek LC, et al. Liver fibrosis: non-invasive assessment with MR elastography. NMR Biomed. 2006;19(2):173–9.
34. Tan CH, Venkatesh SK. Magnetic resonance elastography and other magnetic resonance imaging techniques in chronic liver disease: current status and future directions. Gut Liver. 2016;10(5):672–86.
35. Yin M, Talwalkar JA, Glaser KJ, Venkatesh SK, Chen J, Manduca A, Ehman RL. Dynamic postprandial hepatic stiffness augmentation assessed with MR elastography in patients with chronic liver disease. AJR Am J Roentgenol. 2011;197(1):64–70.
36. Mederacke I, Wursthorn K, Kirschner J, Rifai K, Manns MP, Wedemeyer H, et al. Food intake increases liver stiffness in patients with chronic or resolved hepatitis C virus infection. Liver Int. 2009;29:1500–6.
37. Fovargue D, Nordsletten D, Sinkus R. Stiffness reconstruction methods for MR elastography. NMR Biomed. 2018;31(10):e395. https://doi.org/10.1002/nbm.3935.
38. Morisaka H, Motosugi U, Glaser KJ. Comparison of diagnostic accuracies of 2D and 3D MR elastography of the liver. J Magn Reson Imaging. 2017;45(4):1163–70.

FDG-PET for Management on Hepato-Pancreato-Biliary Disease

15

Koji Murakami

Abstract

PET (Positron Emission Tomography) has a unique feature that is visualized "metabolic activities" of cell, or tissue. Malignant tumors including hepato-pancreato-biliary cancer (HPBC) usually shows hypermetabolism of glucose to be depicted clearly by using FDG-PET. PET has the advantage of being able to survey the entire body because it covers a wide area, but on the other hand, because of its low spatial resolution, it is not suitable for detecting small lesions. From such features on FDG-PET, the major roles for HPBC are staging (detecting lymph node, distant metastases), response assessment for chemo(radiation) therapy, and early detection of recurrence (surveillance). But recent advancement of PET/CT camera enables us to detect small lesions which were missed by other imaging modalities. We should have a good understanding of the characteristics of FDG-PET and use it successfully in the management on HPBC patients.

15.1 Introduction

FDG-PET is said to be one of the most rapidly popular diagnostic imaging modalities in this century not only in Japan but in major advanced countries. However, since PET examination requires a large amount of capital investment, facilities at which PET is available are still limited. PET equipment has been introduced mainly in major institutions or diagnostic imaging centers in big cities. Although numerous middle-sized and small hospitals cannot economically afford to introduce PET, physicians can refer their patients to facilities where PET is available. Therefore, it is essential for general physicians to gain accurate knowledge about PET, including the appropriate indications for PET in order to select patients for referral to PET facilities.

General speaking, PET is not always a useful tool especially for detecting small lesions because of its low spatial resolutions. Main purpose of performing PET in malignant tumor are to detect lymph node and distant metastases for staging, response assessment for chemo (and/or radiation) therapy, and early detection of recurrence (surveillance). But these indications of PET are a little bit different according to the organs and disease. In this article, we review the indications for PET (or PET/computed tomography [CT]) using FDG of the liver, biliary tract, and pancreas.

15.2 FDG-PET Examination for Liver Cancer

15.2.1 PET for Hepatocellular Carcinoma (HCC)

HCC is known to show low FDG accumulation. This can be explained based on the mechanism of FDG uptake in tumors. FDG is an analogue of glucose, and when injected into the body, it is taken up by the cells and phosphorylated in the same pathway as glucose. The metabolic process of FDG is the same as that of glucose up to this point, but the reactions of FDG do not proceed further (Fig. 15.1). In other words, the FDG remains in the cells as phosphorylated FDG. On the other hand, because dephosphorylating enzyme activity is higher in hepatocytes than in other tissues, it is likely that the glucose accumulated in normal hepatocyte is dephosphorylated again and excreted out of the cells. As activity of dephosphorylating enzyme is retained in well-differentiated HCC, the tumor shows relatively low FDG accumulation (Fig. 15.2). Another reason of low FDG uptake in well-differentiated HCC is that the expression of the glucose transporter at the surface of cell is fewer compared to other types of malignant tumors. On the other hand, poorly-differentiated HCC has

K. Murakami (✉)
Department of Radiology, Graduate School of Medicine, Juntendo University, Tokyo, Japan
e-mail: k-murakami@juntendo.ac.jp

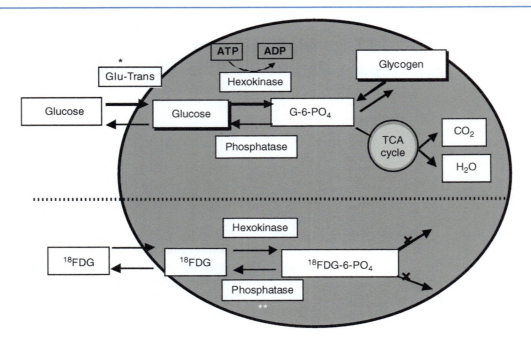

Fig. 15.1 Schema of metabolic pathway in cells of glucose and 18-F-FDG. FDG take same pathway as glucose till phosphorylation, though it does not progress further. Most malignant cell is known to have overexpression of glucose transporter (asterisk) and low activity of phosphatase (double asterisk)

weak enzyme activity to show strong FDG uptake [1, 2]. As the FDG uptake vary with the degree of differentiation of HCC, we may be able to predict, to some extent the degree of differentiation of HCC by the degree of FDG uptake, even though FDG-PET is not useful for the detection. Furthermore, because poorly differentiated HCC is frequently associated with metastasis and recurrence, FDG/PET is useful for detecting such metastasis/recurrence to be able to survey whole body (Fig. 15.3) [3]. The degree of histological differentiation is thought to be correlated with the prognosis, and the poorer the degree of differentiation of the HCC, the poorer the prognosis is. Thus, FDG-PET offers the promising tool for predicting the prognosis of HCC [4, 5].

15.2.2 PET for Cholangiocellular Carcinoma (CCC)

CCC is histologically classified as adenocarcinoma, and usually shows increased FDG uptake (Fig. 15.4) [6, 7]. However, since both poorly differentiated HCC and metastatic hepatic carcinoma usually shows marked FDG uptake, it is difficult to differentiate these malignant liver tumors based on the uptake of FDG alone. Other morphological diagnostic imaging such as dynamic CT or magnetic resonance imaging (MRI) are indispensable for reference.

Moreover, diagnostic "high-resolution" imaging tools, such as direct contrast radiography, endoscopic ultrasound (EUS), intraductal ultrasound (IDUS), contrast-enhanced CT and MRI, are sufficient for diagnosing the stage of primary lesions, so that clinical significance of PET is of little value for the diagnosis of the T factor in CCC. On the other hand, PET may be used as a complementary diagnostic tool for the diagnosis of lymph node metastases when diameter of which are below 10 mm. FDG positive lymph nodes less than 10 mm in diameter suggests a high probability of metastatic lymph node that is difficult to estimate as metastasis only by CT criteria.

PET is also expected to be useful for detecting the presence/absence of distant metastases and diagnosing recurrent disease in CCC. In particular, PET is useful for the diagnosis of distant metastasis, as demonstrated by a study which showed that the treatment policy was determined by PET in 17% of the cases [8], or changing the treatment policy in 30% of the cases [9]. PET also has an excellent ability to diagnose recurrent disease, which is difficult to detect after hepatic resection or bile duct resection, in view of its excellent contrast resolution.

There are two major pitfalls to be known. One is FDG uptake in inflammatory tissue, such as cholangitis which causes false positive. Another is weak FDG uptake in slow growing or fibrosis abundant tumor which cause false negative.

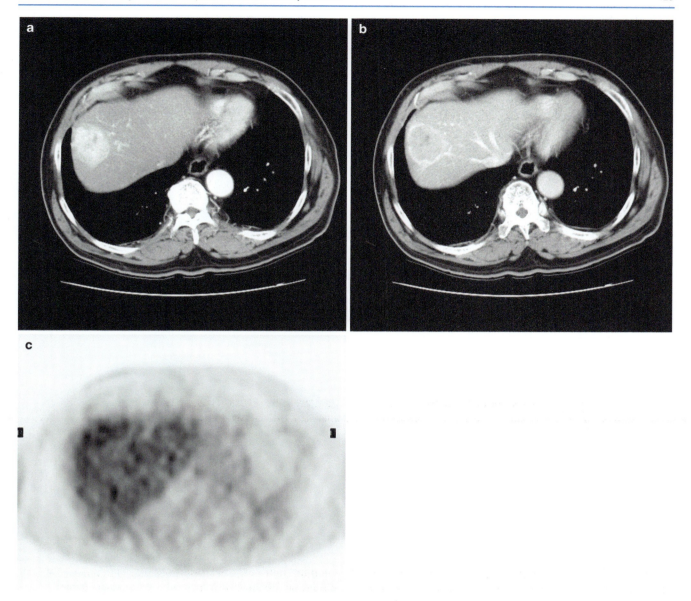

Fig. 15.2 A case of well-differentiated HCC. (**a**, **b**) Arterial and portal phase of dynamic CT. Typical enhancement pattern of HCC was shown; (**c**) FDG-PET. There was no FDG uptake

15.2.3 PET Examination for Metastatic Liver Cancer

The visualization of liver metastases may depend on the histological characters of the primary lesion. In general, when the primary lesion shows marked FDG uptake, the metastases also shows increased FDG uptake. However, the visualization of metastases on PET is also influenced by other factors, e.g., such as the tumor size, cell density, presence of bleeding/necrosis as tumor-related factors, and the blood glucose level, respiratory movements during data acquisition as external factors, so and so. Thus, the FDG uptake may differ between the primary and metastatic lesions depending on the aforementioned factors.

As compared with other imaging modalities, PET is not the most suitable for the detection of small lesions because of its poor spatial resolution. Even if liver tumors show FDG avidity, tumor uptake of FDG must be stronger than the physiological liver uptake to be clearly recognized. Even considering these factors, it is sure that both the contrast

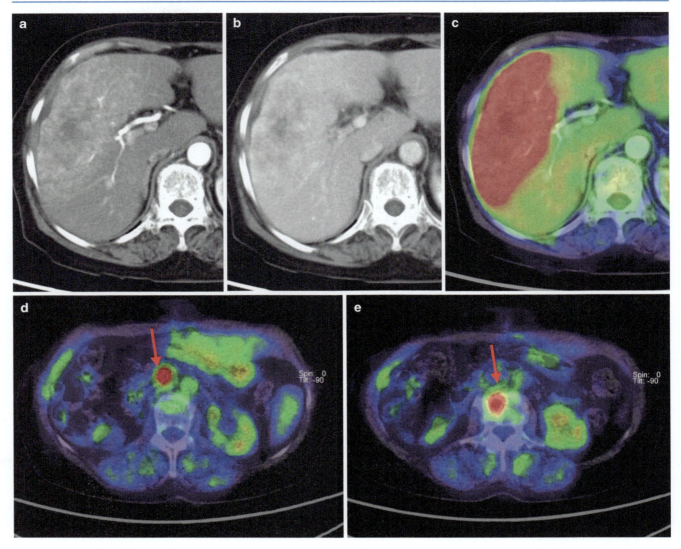

Fig. 15.3 A case of mixed type HCC with extrahepatic metastases. (**a**) Arterial phase of dynamic CT; (**b**) Portal phase of dynamic CT. A tumor showed early enhancement which is a feature of HCC, though it also had lobular border and delayed enhancement that are the features of CCC (cholangiocellular carcinoma). Pathological diagnosis was mixed type HCC; (**c**) This type of HCC showed strong FDG accumulation; (**d, e**) This case also had lymph node and bone matastases (arrow)

resolution and specificity of PET is superior to that offered by plain or contrast-enhanced CT (Fig. 15.5). In addition, recent technological advances in PET cameras have significantly improved spatial resolution, and the detection rate of small lesions is improving year by year.

CT alone is sometimes inadequate for differentiating small liver tumors, such as cysts from hemangiomas or hepatic metastases even if dynamic contrast imaging is performed, because small tumors do not always show characteristic hemodynamics. MRI (especially contrast MRI and diffusion weighted MRI) may be currently the best imaging method for detecting small liver metastases, but it is also difficult to make differential diagnosis of small liver tumor by means of MR signal. In such cases, FDG-PET is highly useful for deciding diagnosis due to its high specificity, though it should be noted that it is effective for tumors with strong FDG accumulation such as colon cancer and pancreatic cancer, but weak accumulation such as renal cell cancer.

PET has another advantage of being able to screen the whole body. Ruers et al. [10] focusing on the usefulness of PET for the detection of metastatic lesions in addition to primary hepatic tumors. There is a literature also emphasis of the merit of FDG-PET to find restaging disease and it has additional clinical value in management of solitary liver metastases [11].

PET is expected to play an important role in the future for assessment of the therapeutic response of molecular-targeted drugs. Molecular-targeted drugs have been reported to show

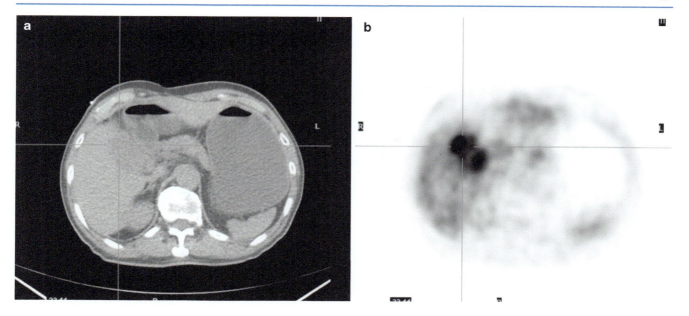

Fig. 15.4 A case of cholangiocellular carcinoma (CCC). (**a**) Non-contrast CT obtained by PET/CT (low-dose CT); (**b**) FDG-PET. CCC is usually depicted as FDG-avid tumor unlike HCC

less effective for decreasing tumor size compared to conventional cytotoxic anticancer drugs because of its cytostatic feature. Consequently, the findings of PET have attracted attention as surrogate markers for evaluating the effects of the molecular-targeted drugs. At present, molecular-targeted drugs are widely used in the treatment of lung cancer, breast cancer and gastrointestinal stromal tumors, which are frequently happens liver metastases. Since PET allows detection of not only liver metastases but also metastases elsewhere in the body, it is expected to play a more important role in the future as surrogate markers [12].

15.3 FDG-PET Examination for Biliary Cancer

According to the report of Petrowsky et al. [8], the diagnostic accuracy of FDG-PET was 53% for extrahepatic bile duct cancer that is indicative of a poor diagnostic performance. The flat "infiltrating" type, which is the most common histological type of extrahepatic bile duct cancer, is characterized with abundant fibrosis and endoluminal extension not to form "mass". Such histological and morphological features are major reasons for the poor diagnostic value in FDG-PET of this tumors.

On the other hand, the papillary type (one of minor subtype of bile duct cancer) that are characterized by a massive form and protruding growth into the lumen sometimes shows increased uptake of FDG. PET has been shown to have a high sensitivity for the detection of this histological type of bile duct cancer [9, 13].

PET examination for bile duct cancer is desirable to be performed prior to the insertion of PTCD tube, because stimulation to the tip of the inserted tube causes cholangitis. It may cause pseudo-positive result.

Although FDG also accumulate to the lymph node metastases of extrahepatic bile duct cancer, it is incapable of revealing microscopic metastases. In other words, FDG-PET is not useful for the detection of lymph node metastases from extrahepatic bile duct cancer because of its low sensitivity [13]. Thus, FDG-PET appears to be limited usefulness for the diagnosis of bile duct cancer for staging before therapy.

Most valuable occasion to perform PET in biliary cancer is to find distant metastases or early detection of recurrence. Though morphological or anatomical change caused by surgical procedure sometimes makes difficult to find tumor recurrence, PET can play a great role to find missed tumors [14].

15.4 FDG-PET Examination for Gallbladder Cancer

FDG-PET has a sensitivity of 75–100% and specificity of 80–89% for the detection of primary gallbladder cancer in the literature (Fig. 15.6). However, ultrasound, MRI, and contrast-enhanced CT would be better for the detection of this cancer because of its high spatial resolutions. FDG-PET is reported to be useful for differentiating benign from malignant gallbladder tumors [15] though acute cholecystitis and mass-forming xanthogranulomatous cholecystitis may also show marked FDG uptake (Fig. 15.7). Thus, the ability of this modality to allow differentiation among these tumors

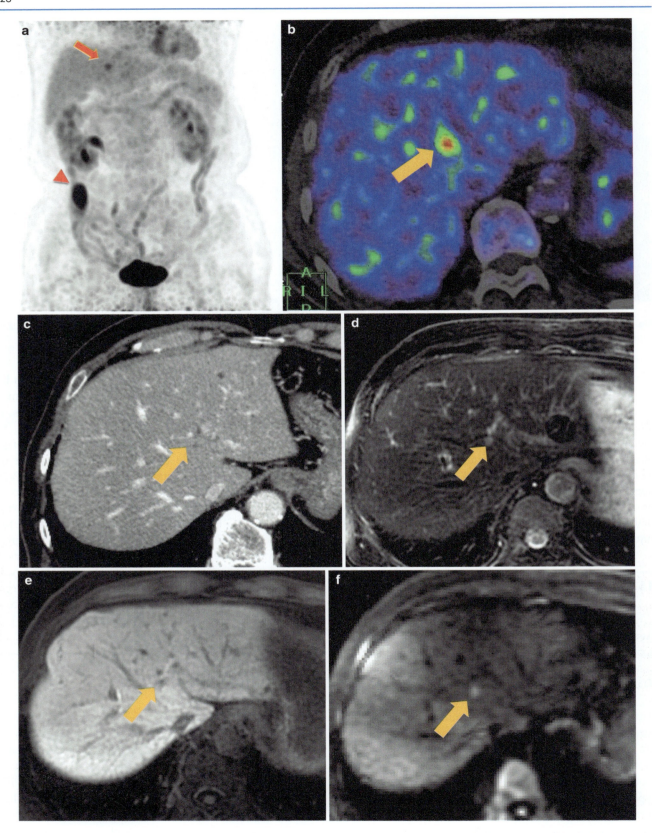

Fig. 15.5 A case of cecum cancer with small liver metastases; (**a**) MIP (Maximum Intensity Projection) image (**b**) fusion image of PET/CT. Both of PET images clearly shows liver metastases (arrow) besides primary cecum cancer (arrow head). (**c**) contrast CT; (**d**) T2WI; (**e**) contrast MRI using EOB-DTPA; (**f**) Diffusion weighted MRI. The small liver lesion is hard to pointed out both by CT and MRI except DWI

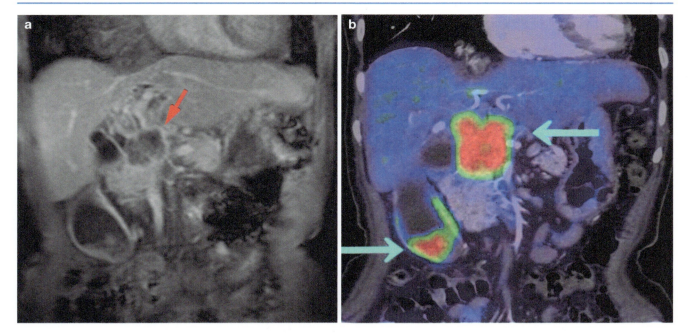

Fig. 15.6 Gall bladder cancer with hilar lymph node metastases. (**a**) CE-MRI (coronal section) showed poorly enhanced tumor near pancreatic head (arrow). The tumor was thought to be primary lesion at first; (**b**) PET/CT (with CE) demonstrated two FDG-avid lesions (arrow). Gall bladder cancer and its metastases usually shows strong FDG deposit

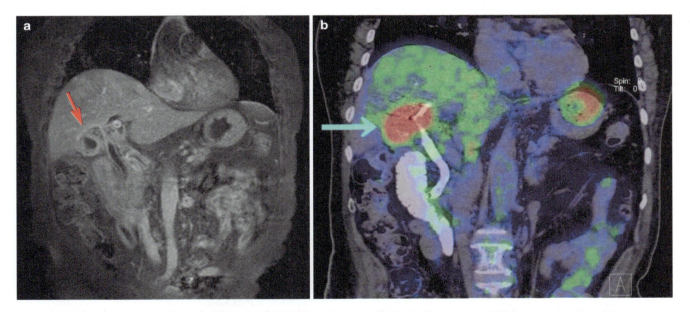

Fig. 15.7 A case of acute cholecystitis. (**a**) CE-MRI (coronal section) showed irregular wall thickening of gall bladder (arrow) with hilar bile duct stenosis; (**b**) PET/CT performed after PTC. Gall bladder showed strong FDG accumulations (arrow) though pathological diagnosis was acute cholecystitis. Discrimination between active inflammation and tumor is difficult by accumulation of FDG

remains controversial. For gallbladder cancer, the primary aim of performing FDG-PET would be to find distant metastases and recurrence same as that of biliary cancer mentioned before.

15.5 FDG-PET Examination for Pancreatic Cancer

The 2019 edition of the Clinical Practice Guidelines for Pancreatic Cancer in Japan [16] recommends contrast-enhanced (dynamic) CT as the first-line diagnostic imaging method in pancreatic cancer practice, followed by MRI and US for detection and qualitative diagnosis. According to this guideline, FDG-PET is "weakly recommended not to be performed" the reason of which is that FDG accumulates in inflammation, so the specificity is insufficient. Other reason includes PET to be economically expensive and having radiation exposure. In other words, if contrast-enhanced dynamic CT is performed and additional examinations such as US, MRI, ERCP, and EUS are performed, it can be said that the information that can be added by FDG-PET is limited.

On the other hand, when the pancreas is not the target organ, plain CT or CT with only one phase contrast-enhancement is often performed. In such cases, small pancreatic cancers are sometimes missed especially in the case of uncinate pancreatic cancer without dilation of the main pancreatic duct. In the past, small pancreatic cancer which is overlooked by CT was also difficult to detect by PET because of its low spatial resolution, but recent advances in PET/CT detectors and image reconstruction algorithm have dramatically improved spatial resolution. Therefore, the number of cases of small pancreatic cancer that is missed by CT but is detected by FDG-PET is increasing (Fig. 15.8).

Regarding to qualitative diagnosis, it is sure that chronic pancreatitis can be differentiated from cancer because of its lower FDG uptake compared to those of cancer. However, the inflammatory cells also show increased FDG uptake because of the accelerated glucose metabolism, differentiation between acute pancreatitis and cancer is difficult. Accordingly, positive findings obtained in patients who have clinical symptoms of pancreatitis or biochemical evidence of inflammation should be interpreted with caution. Imdahl et al. [17] reported that delayed PET imaging is useful for the differentiation of cancer from acute pancreatitis as cancer shows increasing deposit in delayed phase. However, a controversial study has reported that FDG uptake is enhanced in the delayed phase even in cases of inflammation. Thus, FDG-PET cannot be regarded as a reliable imaging tool for differentiation between acute pancreatitis and cancer even though obtaining delayed images.

FDG-PET has been reported to play significant roles in the differentiation of IgG4-related pancreatitis among cases of pancreatitis. This disease has been defined to be a systemic disease complicated by inflammation in various organs other than pancreas. FDG-PET is reported as effective tools for evaluating the lesions [18] because various organs, such as the salivary glands, hilar lymph nodes, lungs (interstitial pneumonia), kidney (nephritis) and retroperitoneum are sometimes suffered simultaneously. In other words, abnormal FDG uptake other than the pancreas may raise a suspicion of IgG4-related pancreatitis rather than pancreatic cancer (Fig. 15.9).

In cases of pancreatic cancer, PET is the most powerful tool for finding distant metastasis (Fig. 15.10) and recurrence (Fig. 15.11). Local recurrence is sometimes difficult to evaluate by conventional morphological imaging alone because it is associated with treatment-related morphological changes,

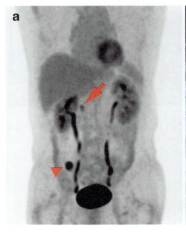
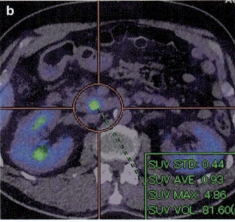
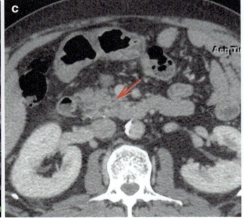

Fig. 15.8 A case of pancreatic uncinate cancer incidentally found by FDG-PET performed for staging of ascending colon cancer. (**a**) MIP (**b**) fusion of PET/CT. Both of FDG-PET image revealed abnormal accumulation at the pancreatic head (arrow) besides ascending colon (arrow head). (**c**) contrast CT performed for staging of colon cancer. It was difficult to detect pancreatic tumor by this image

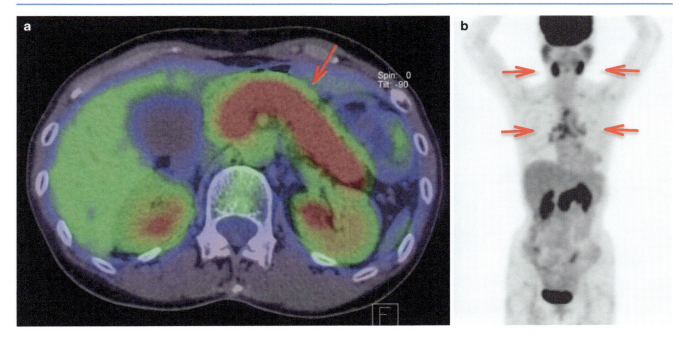

Fig. 15.9 IgG4 related pancreatitis. (**a**) PET/CT showed strong FDG accumulation to whole pancreas with swelling (arrow). (**b**) MIP image of PET. Besides diffuse uptake to pancreas, symmetrical FDG deposit was noted at bilateral salivary glands and hilar, mediastinal lymph nodes (arrow). Distribution of suffered organ is characteristic of this disease

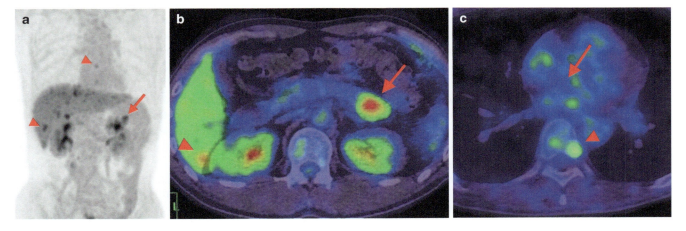

Fig. 15.10 A case of pancreatic tail cancer with multiple metastases. (**a**) MIP image clearly shows all lesions at pancreatic tail (arrow), liver and spine (arrow heads). (**b, c**) fusion image of PET/CT. PET only could be able to point out the bone metastases at the spine

such as fibrosis, hemorrhage, etc. Moreover, as pancreatic cancer has character of poor vascularity, it is difficult to evaluate the tumor based on the dynamic contrast study. Under this circumstance, PET may be of great value for visualizing the lesion because of its high contrast resolution.

Another reason of difficulty to detect distant metastasis based on conventional imaging is difficulty to predict the site of metastasis. The merit of whole body imaging on PET is of great value particularly when recurrence is suspected by clinical symptoms such as the development of pain or increased serum levels of tumor markers, etc. Ruf et al. [19] performed PET, CT and MRI in 23 patients with clinically suspected recurrence of pancreatic cancer based on the development of postoperative pain, decreased body weight and increased serum levels of tumor markers, and confirmed recurrence by PET in 22 of the patients (96%) on PET, but in only nine patients (39%) by CT/MRI.

Besides FDG-PET, Somatostatin Receptor Scintigraphy (SRS) are very beneficial for clinical practice in pancreatic neuroendocrine tumor (PNET). Some advanced countries have already applied SRS as clinical PET imaging using ^{68}Ga-DOTA-TOC or ^{68}Ga-DOTA-TATE.

As FDG accumulation represents the proliferative capacity of tumor cells, low-grade G1 accumulation is low, high-

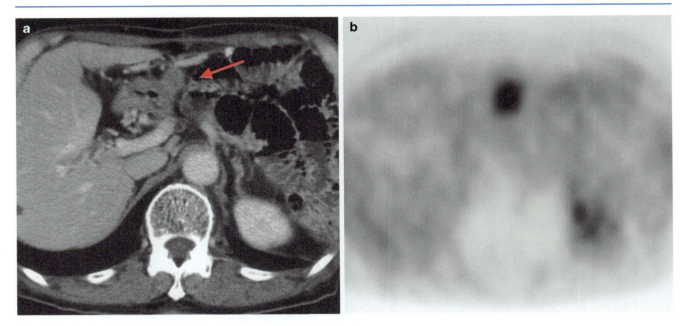

Fig. 15.11 A case of elevating tumor marker after resection of pancreatic cancer. (**a**) Small nodule (arrow) was missed by initial survey by CECT. (**b**) PET could detect the recurrent nodule much more clearly

grade G3 and NEC (Neuroendocrine Cancer) have strong accumulation [20]. Therefore, FDG-PET is effective for searching metastasis of high-grade PNET, and is recommended as Grade A in "Pancreatic and gastrointestinal neuroendocrine tumor (NEN) clinical guidelines 2nd edition" in Japan [21].

On the other hand, SRS has strong accumulation in G1 with high somatostatin receptor expression and low accumulation in poorly differentiated G3/NEC, which is inversely related to FDG accumulation. Therefore, it is important to use FDG-PET and SRS properly according to the degree of differentiation and malignancy of the tumor, and they play complementary roles.

Since this chapter focuses on FDG, details are omitted, though SRS using PET is very promising modality in the future because it is directly linked to internal radiation therapy if the labeled radioisotope is replaced from positron emitter to α-ray or β-ray emitting nuclides, the therapy of which is called peptide receptor radionuclide therapy (PRRT) [22].

15.6 Conclusion

In this review, the usefulness and limitations of PET/CT for the evaluation of lesions in the liver, gallbladder, and pancreas were outlined. Ultrasound and dynamic CT are the simplest and most economical imaging modalities for the diagnosis of lesions in these organs. In addition, many other imaging tools, such as MRI, EUS and IDUS, are also available for detailed evaluation of these organs. All of these methods are used as "high-resolution" diagnostic imaging for visualizing "locoregional areas," and PET is unlikely to play an important role in the local diagnosis of the lesion. On the contrary, PET (PET/CT) involves whole-body imaging and is quite useful for visualizing distant metastases and unexpected recurrences. Therefore, PET/CT appears to be of significance in the evaluation of the whole body in cases with somewhat advanced or atypical tumors. On the other hands, recent advancement in PET/CT dramatically improved spatial resolution and enable us to find unexpected pancreatic lesions. SRS using PET/CT also is very promising modality in the future because it is directly linked to PRRT for PNET.

References

1. Trojan J, Schroeder O, Raedle J, et al. Fluorine-18 FDG positron emission tomography for imaging of hepatocellular carcinoma. Am J Gastroenterol. 1999;94(11):3314–9.
2. Torizuka T, Tamaki N, Inokuma T, et al. In vivo assessment of glucose metabolism in hepatocellular carcinoma with FDG-PET. J Nucl Med. 1995;36(10):1811–7.
3. Iwata Y, Shiomi S, Sasaki N, et al. Clinnical usefulness of posiron emission tomograohy with fluorine-18-fluorodeoxiglucose in the diagnosis of liver tumors. Ann Nucl Med. 2000;14(2):121–6.
4. Hatano E, Ikai I, Higashi T, et al. Preoperative positron emission tomography with fluorine-18-fluorodeoxyglucose is predictive of prognosis in patients with hepatocellular carcinoma after resection. World J Surg. 2006;30(9):1736–41.

5. Sugiyama M, Sakahara H, Torizuka T, et al. 18F-FDG PET in the detection of extrahepatic metastases from hepatocellular carcinoma. J Gastroenterol. 2004;39(10):961–8.
6. Keiding S, Hansen SB, Rasmussen HH, et al. Detection of cholangiocarcinoma in primary sclerosing cholangitis by positron emission tomography. Hepatology. 1998;28:700–6.
7. Kim YJ, Yun M, Lee WJ, et al. Usefulness of 18F-FDG PET in intrahepatic cholangiocarcinoma. Eur J Nucl Med Mol Imaging. 2003;30(11):1467–72.
8. Petrowsky H, Wildbertt P, Husrik DB, et al. Impact of integrated positron emission tomography and computed tomography on staging and management of gall bladder cancer and cholangiocarcinoma. J Hepatol. 2006;45:43–50.
9. Anderson CD, Rice MH, Pinson CW, et al. Fluorodeoxyglucose PET imaging in the evaluation of gall bladder carcinoma and cholangiocarcinoma. J Gastrointestinal Surg. 2004;8:90–7.
10. Ruers TJ, Langenhoff BS, Neeleman N, et al. Value of positron emission tomography with [F-18]fluorodeoxyglucose in patients with colorectal liver metastases: a prospective study. J Clin Oncol. 2002;20(2):388–95.
11. Grassetto G, Fornasiero A, Bonciarelli G, et al. Additional value of FDG-PET/CT in management of "solitary" liver metastases: preliminary results of a prospective multicenter study. Mol Imaging Biol. 2010;12(2):139–44.
12. Heinicke T, Wardelmann E, Sauerbruch T, et al. Very early detection of response to imatinib mesylate therapy of gastrointestinal stromal tumours using 18fluoro-deoxyglucose-positron emission tomography. Anticancer Res. 2005;25(6C):4591–4.
13. Kato T, Tsukamoto E, Kuge Y, et al. Clinical role of 18F-FDG PET for initial staging of extrahepatic bile duct cancer. Eur J Nucl Med. 2002;29:1047–54.
14. Kitajima K, Murakami K, Kanegae K, et al. Clinical impact of whole body FDG-PET for recurrent biliary cancer: a multicenter study. Ann Nucl Med. 2009;23(8):709–15.
15. Koh T, Taniguchi H, Yamaguchi A, et al. Differential diagnosis of gall bladder cancer using positron emission tomography with fluorine-18-labeled fluoro- deoxyglucose (FDG-PET). J Surg Oncol. 2003;84:74–81.
16. Japan Pancreatic Society. Clinical practice guidelines for pancreatic cancer. Tokyo: Kanehara & Co. Ltd; 2019.
17. Imdahl A, Nitzsche E, Krautmann F, et al. Evaluation of positron emission tomography with 2-[18F]fluoro-2-deoxy-D-glucose for the differentiation of chronic pancreatitis and pancreatic cancer. Br J Surg. 1999;86(2):194–9.
18. Nakajo M, Jinnouchi S, Noguchi M, et al. FDG PET and PET/CT monitoring of autoimmune pancreatitis associated with extrapancreatic autoimmune disease. Clin Nucl Med. 2007;32(4):282–5.
19. Ruf J, Lopez Hänninen E, Oettle H, et al. Detection of recurrent pancreatic cancer: comparison of FDG-PET with CT/MRI. Pancreatology. 2005;5:266–72.
20. Tomimaru Y, Eguchi H, Tatsumi M, et al. Clinical utility of 2-[(18)F] fluoro-2-deoxy-D- glucose positron emission tomography in predicting World Health Organization grade in pancreatic neuroendocrine tumors. Surgery. 2016;157(2):269–76.
21. Japan Neuroendocrine Tumor Society. Clinical practice guideline for gastroenteropancreatic neuroendocrine neoplasms. Tokyo: Kanehara & Co. Ltd; 2019.
22. Strosberg J, El-Haddad G, Wolin E, et al. Phase 3 trial of (177)Lu-Dotatate for midgut neuroendocrine tumors. N Engl J Med. 2017;376(2):125–35.

Endoscopic Ultrasound for Hepato-Pancreato-Biliary Diseases

Yasunobu Yamashita and Masayuki Kitano

Abstract

Endoscopic ultrasound (EUS) equipped with an ultrasound transducer at the tip of gastrointestinal endoscopy plays crucial roles for diagnosis of hepato-pancreato-biliary diseases because of high spatial resolution. In particular, EUS has advantages over the other imaging methods in detection of small lesions. In addition, recent advances in ultrasound technology such as contrast enhancement and tissue elastography allowed characterization of the undetermined lesions. EUS-guided fine-needle aspiration has a high sensitivity and specificity in pathological diagnosis of pancreatic tumors with <1% of complications. This technique has been extensively applied to treatment of hepato-pancreato-biliary diseases with puncture of a needle, through which we can perform injection with liquid materials and ablation of the tumors as well as drainage of pancreato-biliary ducts and abdominal abscess.

16.1 Introduction

Owing to its high spatial resolution, endoscopic ultrasound (EUS) equipped with an ultrasound transducer at the tip of a gastrointestinal endoscope plays a crucial role in the diagnosis of hepato-pancreato-biliary diseases. In particular, EUS has advantages over other imaging methods with respect to the detection of small lesions. Furthermore, recent advances in ultrasound technology such as contrast enhancement and tissue elastography has enabled the characterization of undetermined lesions.

EUS-guided fine-needle aspiration (EUS-FNA) for the pathological diagnosis of lesions with a complication rate of <1% has a high sensitivity and specificity (Fig. 16.3). EUS-FNA with needle puncture, through which liquid material injection, tumor ablation, and pancreatobiliary duct and abdominal abscess drainage can all be performed, has been extensively applied to the treatment of hepato-pancreato-biliary diseases.

16.2 Diagnosis

16.2.1 Pancreatic Cancers

16.2.1.1 Imaging

EUS images of pancreatic cancer show heterogeneous hypoechoic lesions with irregular margins. The sensitivity of EUS has been reported to be superior to that of computed tomography (CT) (98% vs. 74%) in 19 studies and abdominal ultrasound (94% vs. 67%) in four studies [1]. EUS is a particularly valuable tool for diagnosing early pancreatic cancers. Kanno et al. reported stage 0 pancreatic tumor detection rates of 8.8%, 10%, 10.9%, and 24.4% as well as stage I pancreatic tumor detection rates of 67.3%, 65.8%, 57.5%, and 92.4% for abdominal ultrasound, CT, magnetic resonance imaging (MRI), and EUS, respectively [2]. A meta-analysis focusing on the diagnostic performance of EUS in detecting pancreatic cancers missed on CT reported a pooled sensitivity of 85%, pooled specificity of 58%, and area under the curve (AUC) of 0.8 [3].

Considering the usefulness of EUS in diagnosing pancreatic cancers that are not detectable on CT, EUS is strongly recommended to be performed in patients with indirect findings (e.g., dilated main pancreatic duct with no visible lesion on other imaging modalities) in order to diagnose pancreatic cancer (Fig. 16.1). Nonetheless, characterization of pancreatic lesions is difficult with conventional EUS because most solid pancreatic lesions are detected as hypoechoic lesions on EUS. In this regard, contrast-enhanced harmonic EUS

Y. Yamashita · M. Kitano (✉)
Second Department of Internal Medicine, Wakayama Medical University, Wakayama, Japan
e-mail: kitano@wakayama-med.ac.jp

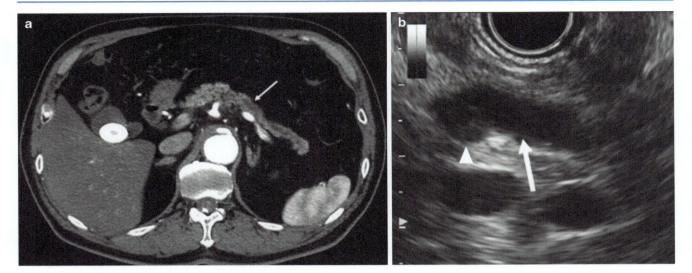

Fig. 16.1 Representative endoscopic images of a small pancreatic carcinoma which contrast-enhanced multidetector-row computed tomography (MDCT) detected only main pancreatic duct dilation (indirect findings) without depiction of the lesion. (**a**) MDCT: Although the main pancreatic duct dilation (arrow) was detected by contrast-enhanced MDCT, it failed to depict the pancreatic lesion. (**b**) Endoscopic ultrasonography (EUS): EUS shows a hypoechoic lesion of 8 mm in size (arrowhead) with main pancreatic duct dilation (arrow)

(CH-EUS) and EUS elastography can improve the ability to characterize pancreatic lesions.

Signals from microbubbles produced by intravenously administered contrast agents are detected and selectively filtered in CH-EUS. Pancreatic cancer, inflammatory masses, and neuroendocrine tumors generally exhibit hypo-enhancement, iso-enhancement, and hyper-enhancement patterns, respectively (Fig. 16.2), on CH-EUS. A meta-analysis involving 887 patients from nine articles investigating the differential diagnosis of pancreatic lesions reported a pooled sensitivity of 93%, pooled specificity of 80%, and area under the summary receiver operating characteristic (SROC) curve of 0.97 [4]. Moreover, CH-EUS is superior to contrast-enhanced CT and MRI in patients with contraindications, such as renal failure and contrast allergy, given that adverse reactions to contrast agents for CH-EUS are rare in humans [5]. Hence, CH-EUS is both useful and effective in the differential diagnosis of pancreatic carcinomas.

As malignant tumors are generally harder than benign tumors, EUS elastography can enhance the ability to characterize elastic pancreatic lesions. With respect to the underlying principle, the strain created by the compression of target tissues with the EUS probe or cardiovascular pulsation through the aorta is expressed on ultrasound images [6], with a higher strain indicating softer tissues and a lower strain reflecting harder tissues [7]. A meta-analysis of 19 studies enrolling 1687 patients reported a pooled sensitivity of 98%, pooled specificity of 63%, and area under the SROC curve of 0.91 for the differential diagnosis of pancreatic lesions using EUS elastography [8]. Thus, EUS elastography is also effective for the differential diagnosis of pancreatic cancers.

16.2.1.2 EUS-FNA

EUS-FNA is employed for the acquisition of tissue samples from pancreatic lesions using 19–25 G needles and is currently regarded as the most effective method for obtaining pancreatic samples with a complication rate of <1% [9]. A meta-analysis involving 31 studies reported a pooled sensitivity of 89%, specificity of 96%, and AUC of 0.97 for the ability of EUS-FNA to diagnose pancreatic cancers [10]. Therefore, EUS-FNA is useful for the pathological diagnosis of pancreatic lesions (Fig. 16.3).

A previous study investigating needle tract seeding after preoperative EUS-FNA in patients who underwent surgery for pancreatic body and tail cancers reported a five-year cumulative needle tract seeding rate of 3.8% (95% confidence interval [CI], 1.6–7.8%), which was estimated using the Fine and Gray method, and showed no significant difference in the median recurrence-free survival or overall survival between the EUS-FNA and non-EUS-FNA groups [11]. Preoperative EUS-FNA for pancreatic body and tail cancers has no negative effect on recurrence-free survival or overall survival; nevertheless, needle tract seeding after EUS-FNA was observed to have a non-negligible rate. Hence, we should always consider the possibility of needle tract seeding when performing EUS-FNA for pancreatic cancers.

16.2.1.3 Staging

Pooled summary estimates from a meta-analysis indicated a sensitivity of 85%, specificity of 91%, and AUC of 0.94 for the assessment of vascular invasion with EUS and a sensitivity of 69%, specificity of 81%, and AUC of 0.83 for nodal

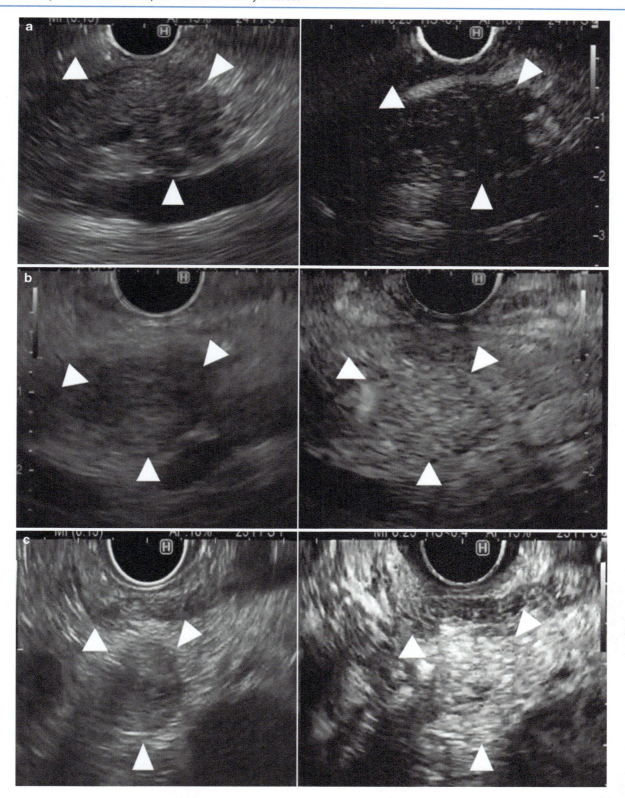

Fig. 16.2 Typical patterns for contrast-enhanced endoscopic ultrasonography (CH-EUS) findings of pancreatic solid lesions. (**a**) Typical case of hypo-enhancement (a pancreatic cancer). CH-EUS image: CH-EUS (right) shows that the lesion (arrowhead) has a lower intensity echo signal than that of the surrounding pancreatic tissue. (**b**) Typical case of iso-enhancement (an inflammatory mass). CH-EUS image: CH-EUS (right) shows that the lesion (arrowhead) has signals of iso-intensity compared to that of the surrounding pancreatic tissue. (**c**) Typical case of hyper-enhancement (a neuroendocrine tumor). CH-EUS image: CH-EUS (right) shows that the lesion (arrowhead) has a higher intensity echo signal than that of the surrounding pancreatic tissue

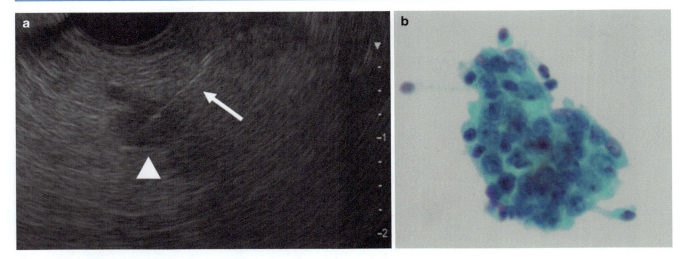

Fig. 16.3 Endoscopic ultrasonography-guided fine-needle aspiration (EUS-FNA) for a small pancreatic lesion. (**a**) Image during EUS-FNA: EUS-FNA was performed for the diagnosis of small pancreatic lesion of 6 mm in size (arrowhead). The arrow indicates the EUS-FNA needle. (**b**) Cytology of EUS-FNA sample: Papanicolaou staining revealed adenocarcinoma with high nuclear-to-cytoplasmic ratio and irregular nuclear contours

staging with EUS in patients with pancreatic cancers [12]. Minaga et al. reported that the diagnostic accuracy of CT, conventional EUS, and CH-EUS for staging metastasis in the left hepatic lobe was 90.6%, 93.4%, and 98.4%, respectively, and showed that the sensitivity and accuracy of CH-EUS for diagnosing metastasis in the left hepatic lobe were significantly higher than those of conventional EUS or CT. In particular, the sensitivity of CH-EUS for the detection of small liver metastasis (<10 mm) was considerably higher than that of CT or conventional EUS ($P < 0.001$). In 2.1% of patients, only CH-EUS could detect a single distant metastasis in the left hepatic lobe, thereby upgrading tumor staging and altering clinical management [13]. With respect to resectability, a meta-analysis of eight studies enrolling 4903 patients indicated that EUS alone identified unresectable diseases in 19% of patients after they were diagnosed with resectable pancreatic cancer by CT [14]. Hence, EUS is an important tool for the determination of pancreatic cancer stage.

16.2.2 Intraductal Papillary Mucinous Neoplasms (IPMNs)

16.2.2.1 Imaging

Mural nodules (MNs) in IPMNs are important factors for the determination of surgical indications and have a positive predictive value of 62.2% for malignancy according to a meta-analysis of 70 studies involving 2297 resected IPMNs. The MN size also has a considerable effect on the prediction of IPMNs with both invasive cancer and high-grade dysplasia, with a standardized mean difference of 0.79. However, no reliable cut-off value for the MN size was identified owing to the heterogeneity of proposed thresholds. Multivariate analysis revealed that MN was the only independent predictor of invasive cancer and high-grade dysplasia for all IPMN types [15]. Additionally, all studies included in the meta-analysis used CH-EUS for MN assessment. Therefore, CH-EUS is the best tool for characterizing size and has the best accuracy for predicting malignancy in IPMNs.

Kamata et al. followed up 102 patients with branch-duct IPMNs for a median of 42 months and concluded that EUS was useful for the early detection of newly developed concomitant pancreatic carcinomas, reporting 3- and 5-year rates of 4% and 8.8%, respectively. In their study, the sensitivity and specificity for pancreatic cancer detection in patients with IPMNs were 100%, 100% on EUS and 39%, 99% on abdominal ultrasound and 56%, 100% on CT and 50%, 100% on MRI, respectively. EUS was significantly superior to other modalities [16].

16.2.2.2 EUS-FNA

EUS-FNA is also performed to diagnose cystic lesions. A meta-analysis of eight studies including a total of 1438 patients evaluated the diagnostic accuracy of EUS-FNA for distinguishing mucinous from non-mucinous cystic lesions with cyst-fluid analysis for cytology and carcinoembryonic antigen (CEA). The most promising cystic fluid biomarker was CEA level, which was increased in mucinous cysts but was low in serous cystadenomas and benign lesions. The optimum threshold for cyst-fluid CEA level was 192 ng/mL in this study, indicating high discriminatory accuracy. Furthermore, the pooled sensitivity and specificity were 54% and 93% for cytology and 63% and 88%, for CEA level, respectively [17]. EUS-FNA, when used in conjunction with cross-sectional imaging, is a useful diagnostic tool for the correct identification of mucinous cysts.

16.2.3 Ampullary Cancers

Ampullary cancers without submucosal or ductal infiltration that are confined to the ampulla are considered amenable to endoscopic resection [18–22] because neither vascular invasion, lymphatic permeation, nor lymph node metastasis is observed in patients when the lesions are restricted to the duodenal mucosa [22, 23]. A meta-analysis of 14 studies investigating ampullary cancer staging by EUS in 422 patients reported a pooled sensitivity and specificity of 77% and 78% for T1 staging, 73% and 76% for T2 staging, 79% and 76% for T3 staging, 84% and 74% for T4 staging, and 70% and 74% for N staging, respectively [24]. Therefore, EUS is important for prognostic prediction and determination of the most appropriate therapeutic approach for ampullary cancers.

16.2.4 Bile Duct Cancers

A comparison of different diagnostic tools for the detection of cholangiocellular carcinomas indicated the following accuracy rates: 92% for endoscopic retrograde cholangiopancreatography (ERCP)/intraductal ultrasound (IDUS), 74% for endoscopic transpapillary forceps biopsy (ETP), 92% for IDUS + ETP, 70% for EUS, and 79% for CT. An analysis of accuracy rates with respect to localization of bile duct stenosis revealed that the accuracy rate of EUS for proximal versus distal stenosis was significantly higher than that for distal stenosis (79% vs. 57%; $P < 0.0001$) [25]. ERCP/IDUS is superior to EUS and CT in establishing accurate diagnoses of bile duct strictures of uncertain etiology. Hence, multimodal diagnostic imaging is recommended for bile duct cancers.

16.2.5 Gallbladder Cancers

Diagnosis using imaging modalities is important because preoperative pathological diagnosis is difficult in gallbladder cancers. Malignancy diagnosis with conventional EUS and CH-EUS for 36 gallbladder wall thickening lesions had been reported to have an overall sensitivity of 61–87% and 90–97%, specificity of 65–83% and 56–98% ($P < 0.001$), and accuracy of 73–86% and 94–96%, respectively [26–28]. An inhomogeneous enhanced pattern on CH-EUS was a strong predictive factor for malignant gallbladder wall thickening. CH-EUS has the potential to improve preoperative diagnostic accuracy in the differential diagnosis of gallbladder wall thickening.

16.3 Therapy

16.3.1 Drainage

16.3.1.1 EUS-Guided Biliary Drainage (EUS-BD)

Transpapillary drainage with ERCP is generally performed for malignant biliary obstruction. Nonetheless, some previous studies have reported difficulty in biliary cannulation in 15–22% of patients [29, 30], occurrence of post-ERCP pancreatitis (PEP) in 3–15% of patients [31], and an inaccessible biliary orifice due to duodenal stenosis in 7–13% of patients with pancreatic head cancers [32].

Percutaneous transhepatic biliary drainage is conventionally performed when ERCP fails; however, this procedure has several disadvantages, including tube dislocation, external drainage, and cosmetic problems. The recently developed EUS-BD is carried out when endoscopic transpapillary drainage fails in patients with distal malignant biliary obstruction. Important advantages of this method over other procedures include internal drainage and prevention of PEP (Fig. 16.4). A meta-analysis of four studies enrolling 302 patients revealed no difference in technical success (risk ratio [RR], 1.00; 95% CI, 0.93–1.08), clinical success (RR, 1.00; 95% CI, 0.94–1.06), and total adverse events (RR, 0.68; 95% CI, 0.31–1.48) between EUS-BD and ERCP drainage as primary treatment for distal malignant biliary obstruction. EUS-BD was associated with lower rates of PEP (RR, 0.12; 95% CI, 0.02–0.62), stent dysfunction (RR, 0.54; 95% CI, 0.32–0.91), and tumor ingrowth and overgrowth (RR, 0.22; 95% CI, 0.07–0.76). No differences in reinterventions (RR, 0.59; 95% CI, 0.21–1.69), procedural duration (weighted mean difference, −2.11; 95% CI, −9.51–5.29), stent patency (hazard ratio, 0.61; 95% CI, 0.34–1.11), and overall survival (hazard ratio, 1.00; 95% CI, 0.66–1.51) were observed [33]. With adequate expertise in endoscopy, EUS-BD can show the same efficacy and safety as ERCP for the primary palliation of distal malignant biliary obstruction and exhibits several clinical advantages with respect to complications.

16.3.1.2 EUS-Guided Pancreatic Duct Drainage (EUS-PD)

EUS-PD is considered a feasible alternative to percutaneous drainage (PCD) or surgical drainage when endoscopic retrograde pancreatography is unsuccessful in patients with pancreatic ductal obstruction (Fig. 16.5). The overall technical and clinical success rates of EUS-PD had been reported to be 85% (339/401; range, 63–100%) and 88% (328/372; range, 76–100%), respectively. Additionally, 25% (102/401) of cases experienced short-term adverse events, including abdominal pain ($n = 45$), acute pancreatitis ($n = 17$), bleeding ($n = 10$), and problems associated with pancreatic juice leakage such as perigastric or peripancreatic fluid collection

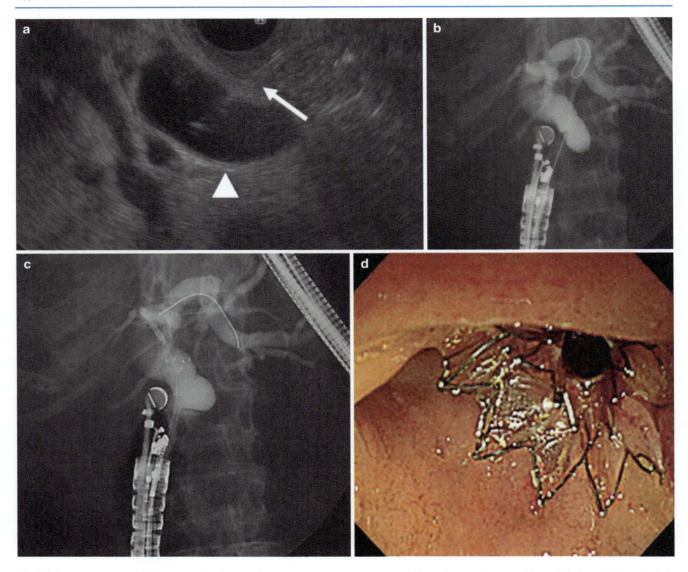

Fig. 16.4 Endoscopic ultrasonography (EUS)-guided choledochoduodenostomy. (**a**) EUS showing a 19-gauge needle (arrows) inserted into the dilating extrahepatic bile duct (arrowhead). (**b**) Fluoroscopic image showing a guidewire inserted into the dilating bile duct. (**c**) Fluoroscopic image showing stent placement. (**d**) Endoscopic image showing the fully opened stent in duodenum

(PFC; n = 9) [34]. EUS-PD continues to be a challenging procedure associated with a high risk of adverse events; nonetheless, it is an alternative tool for pancreatic duct drainage in patients with altered anatomy or selected patients for whom ERCP conducted by experts at high-volume centers is unsuccessful.

16.3.1.3 EUS-Guided PFC Drainage

EUS-guided drainage has become a widely accepted treatment option for PFC. In the early days, EUS-guided PFC drainage was performed using double-pigtail plastic stents (DPPSs) to minimize migration risk. However, endoscopists eventually recognized the limitations of DPPSs. Consequently, fully covered self-expanding metal stents (FCSEMSs) and lumen-apposing metal stents (LAMSs) were developed to overcome these limitations (Fig. 16.6). A meta-analysis that included 15 studies (1746 patients) identified no significant difference in clinical success between LAMSs and DPPSs (RR, 1.04; 95% CI, 0.99–1.11) or between LAMSs and FCSEMSs (RR, 0.96; 95% CI, 0.91–1.03). FCSEMSs were superior to DPPSs with respect to clinical success (RR, 1.09; 95% CI, 1.02–1.15). Furthermore, no significant difference in PFC recurrence was observed among the groups. As for adverse events, LAMSs exhibited a higher bleeding risk than FCSEMSs (RR, 6.70; 95% CI, 1.77–36.27) and tended to have a higher bleeding risk than DPPSs (RR, 2.67; 95% CI, 0.71–9.28) [35]. LAMSs were considered a breakthrough in the endoscopic management of walled-off necrosis (WON), as their larger drainage diameter was expected to result in effective necrotic material drainage.

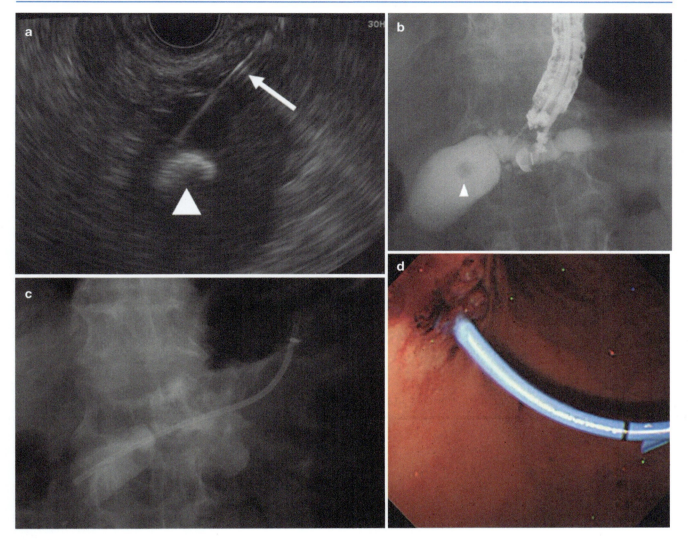

Fig. 16.5 Endoscopic ultrasonography (EUS)-guided pancreatic duct drainage. (**a**) EUS showing a 19-gauge needle inserted into the dilating main pancreatic duct (arrows). EUS showing pancreatic stone (arrow head) in main pancreatic duct. (**b**) Fluoroscopic image showing dilating main pancreatic duct and stone (arrowhead). (**c**) Fluoroscopic image showing stent placement. (**d**) Endoscopic image showing the plastic stent in stomach

Rana et al. reported that LAMSs were associated with a significantly shorter time to resolution; however, with respect to technical success, the WON resolution and complication rates were similar between patients treated with multiple plastic stents and LAMSs [36]. Moreover, large WON or WON with a high proportion of solid debris may be a good indication for direct endoscopic necrosectomy through LAMS with large inner diameter [37] (Fig. 16.7).

16.3.1.4 EUS-Guided Postoperative Pancreatic Fluid Collection (POPFC) Drainage

POPFC is an important complication following abdominal surgery. While PCD is the traditional mainstay of treatment, EUS-guided drainage for POPFC has recently been performed. EUS and PCD were used in the management of POPFC in 10 (239 patients) and 6 (267 patients) out of 13 studies included in a meta-analysis. The pooled clinical success rate was significantly higher with EUS than with PCD (93.2% vs. 79.8%; $P = 0.002$). Furthermore, the recurrence rate was significantly lower with EUS than with PCD (9.4% vs. 25.7%) [38]. The pooled technical success and adverse event rates were similar between EUS and PCD. EUS has significantly better clinical outcomes in terms of clinical success and disease recurrence than PCD in the management of POPFC. Therefore, EUS-guided drainage plays a role in the management of POPFC.

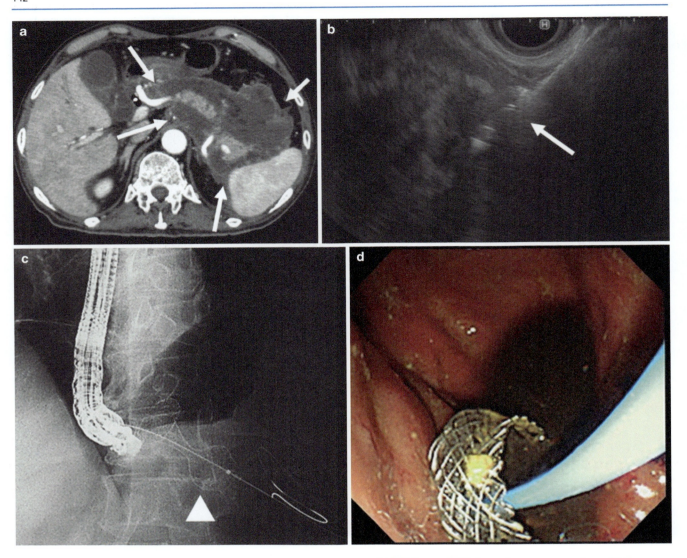

Fig. 16.6 Peripancreatic fluid collection (PFC) drainage and endoscopic necrosectomy through lumen-apposing metal stent (LAMS) for walled-off necrosis. (**a**) MDCT showing large walled-off necrosis (WON) with a high proportion of solid debris (arrow) in peripancreatic area. (**b**) EUS image: EUS shows electrocautery-enhanced delivery system (arrow) was inserted into WON with a high proportion of solid debris. (**c**) Fluoroscopic image showing stent placement (arrowhead). (**d**) Endoscopic image showing the fully opened stent in stomach

16.3.1.5 EUS-Guided Celiac Plexus Neurolysis (EUS-CPN)

EUS-CPN is widely employed to reduce pain originating from upper abdominal organs. In particular, EUS-CPN using the central or bilateral approach is accepted as a common pain control measure for patients with pancreatic cancer and chronic pancreatitis. Some of its advantages include real-time guidance; short puncture distance; use of anterior pathway, thereby avoiding puncture through the posterior diaphragm space; and color Doppler, thus preventing vascular damage. Absolute ethanol is injected through the FNA needle at the base of the celiac artery in the central approach and on both sides of the celiac artery in the bilateral approach. A meta-analysis extracted data from eight studies (238 patients) evaluating EUS-CPN for the relief of pain due to pancreatic cancer and from nine studies (376 patients) investigating EUS-CPN for the relief of pain due to chronic pancreatitis. Overall, 80.12% of patients with pancreatic cancer (95% CI, 74.47–85.22) and 59.45% of patients with chronic pancreatitis (95% CI, 54.51–64.30) showed pain relief [39]. Wyse et al. reported that the relief of pain due to pancreatic cancer was significantly greater at three months in the EUS-CPN group than in the morphine group [40]. Hence, EUS-CPN offers a safe alternative technique for pain relief in patients with chronic pancreatitis or pancreatic cancer.

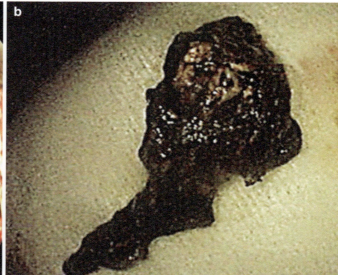

Fig. 16.7 Endoscopic necrosectomy via lumen-apposing metal stent (LAMS) for walled-off necrosis (WON). (**a**) Endoscopic image: Endoscopy is inserted into WON via LAMS and shows a large amount of necrotic tissue. (**b**) Necrotic tissues are removed from inside of WON by endoscopic necrosectomy

16.3.1.6 EUS-Guided Ablation Therapy

EUS-guided ablation therapy is considered a safe alternative treatment for patients deemed unsuitable to undergo surgery. According to a meta-analysis of 14 studies that included 158 patients, the major types of solid pancreatic tumors were nonfunctional pancreatic neuroendocrine tumors ($n = 78$, 49.4%), pancreatic cancers ($n = 48$, 30.4%), and insulinomas ($n = 26$, 16.5%). Overall, the pooled clinical success and complication rates were 85.9% (95% CI, 75.4–92.4%) and 29.1% (95% CI, 18.6–42.3%), respectively. A subgroup analysis of ablation methods indicated clinical success rates of 83.5% (95% CI, 67.9–92.4%) and 87.9% (95% CI, 66.2–96.4%) and complication rates of 32.2% (95% CI, 19.4–48.4%) and 21.2% (95% CI, 6.8–49.9%) for radiofrequency ablation and ethanol ablation, respectively [41]. EUS-guided ablation therapy may be an alternative treatment for solid pancreatic tumors, particularly neuroendocrine tumors and insulinomas <2 cm with rarely severe complications. Further prospective studies with long-term follow-up are warranted in the future owing to the small number of studies.

16.4 Conclusions

EUS plays an important role in the diagnosis and staging of pancreaticobiliary lesions, offers advantages over other imaging methods in the detection of small lesions, and is superior to any other modality with respect to spatial resolution. With a high accuracy rate and a low complication rate, EUS-FNA can be regarded as the final tool for decision-making regarding the therapeutic strategy and is extensively applied as treatment for hepato-pancreato-biliary diseases. EUS-guided drainage for PFC is a widely accepted treatment option, and EUS-guided pancreatobiliary duct drainage has become an alternative to conventional drainage in difficult cases. Further studies investigating the role of EUS ablation in solid pancreatic lesions are required in the future.

References

1. Kitano M, Yoshida T, Itonaga M, Tamura T, Hatamaru K, Yamashita Y. Impact of endoscopic ultrasonography on diagnosis of pancreatic cancer. J Gastroenterol. 2019;54:19–32.
2. Kanno A, Masamune A, Hanada K, et al. Multicenter study of early pancreatic cancer in Japan. Pancreatology. 2018;18:61–7.
3. Krishna SG, Rao BB, Ugbarugba E, et al. Diagnostic performance of endoscopic ultrasound for detection of pancreatic malignancy following an indeterminate multidetector CT scan: a systemic review and meta-analysis. Surg Endosc. 2017;31:4558–67.
4. Yamashita Y, Shimokawa T, Napoléon B, et al. Value of contrast-enhanced harmonic endoscopic ultrasonography with enhancement pattern for diagnosis of pancreatic cancer: a meta-analysis. Dig Endosc. 2019;31:125–33.
5. Reddy NK, Ioncica AM, Saftoiu A, et al. Contrast-enhanced endoscopic ultrasonography. World J Gastroenterol. 2011;17:42–8.
6. Shiina T, Nitta N, Ueno E, Bamber JC. Real time tissue elasticity imaging using the combined autocorrelation method. J Med Ultrason (2001). 2002;29:119–28.
7. Hirooka Y, Kuwahara T, Irisawa A, et al. JSUM ultrasound elastography practice guidelines: pancreas. J Med Ultrason (2001). 2015;42:151–74.

8. Zhang B, Zhu F, Li P, Yu S, Zhao Y, Li M. Endoscopic ultrasound elastography in the diagnosis of pancreatic masses: a meta-analysis. Pancreatology. 2018;18:833–40.
9. Wang KX, Ben QW, Jin ZD, et al. Assessment of morbidity and mortality associated with EUS-guided FNA: a systematic review. Gastrointest Endosc. 2011;73:283–90.
10. Chen G, Liu S, Zhao Y, Dai M, Zhang T. Diagnostic accuracy of endoscopic ultrasound-guided fine-needle aspiration for pancreatic cancer: a meta-analysis. Pancreatology. 2013;13:298–304.
11. Yane K, Kuwatani M, Yoshida M, et al. Non-negligible rate of needle tract seeding after endoscopic ultrasound-guided fine-needle aspiration for patients undergoing distal pancreatectomy for pancreatic cancer. Dig Endosc. 2020;32:801–11.
12. Nawaz H, Fan CY, Kloke J, et al. Performance characteristics of endoscopic ultrasound in the staging of pancreatic cancer: a meta-analysis. JOP. 2013;14:484–97.
13. Minaga K, Kitano M, Nakai A, et al. Improved detection of liver metastasis using Kupffer-phase imaging in contrast-enhanced harmonic EUS in patients with pancreatic cancer (with video). Gastrointest Endosc. 2021;93(2):433–41.
14. James PD, Meng ZW, Zhang M, et al. The incremental benefit of EUS for identifying unresectable disease among adults with pancreatic adenocarcinoma: a meta-analysis. PLoS One. 2017;12:e0173687.
15. Marchegiani G, Andrianello S, Borin A, et al. Systematic review, meta-analysis, and a high-volume center experience supporting the new role of mural nodules proposed by the updated 2017 international guidelines on IPMN of the pancreas. Surgery. 2018;163:1272–9.
16. Kamata K, Kitano M, Kudo M, et al. Value of EUS in early detection of pancreatic ductal adenocarcinomas in patients with intraductal papillary mucinous neoplasms. Endoscopy. 2014;46:22–9.
17. Thornton GD, McPhail MJ, Nayagam S, Hewitt MJ, Vlavianos P, Monahan KJ. Endoscopic ultrasound guided fine needle aspiration for the diagnosis of pancreatic cystic neoplasms: a meta-analysis. Pancreatology. 2013;13:48–57.
18. Norton ID, Gostout CJ, Baron TH, Geller A, Petersen BT, Wiersema MJ. Safety and outcome of endoscopic snare excision of the major duodenal papilla. Gastrointest Endosc. 2002;56:239–43.
19. Catalano MF, Linder JD, Chak A, et al. Endoscopic management of adenoma of the major duodenal papilla. Gastrointest Endosc. 2004;59:225–32.
20. Jung S, Kim MH, Seo DW, Lee SK. Endoscopic snare papillectomy of adenocarcinoma of the major duodenal papilla. Gastrointest Endosc. 2001;54:622.
21. Binmoeller KF, Boaventura S, Ramsperger K, Soehendra N. Endoscopic snare excision of benign adenomas of the papilla of Vater. Gastrointest Endosc. 1993;39:127–31.
22. Wee E, Lakhtakia S, Gupta R, et al. The diagnostic accuracy and strength of agreement between endoscopic ultrasound and histopathology in the staging of ampullary tumors. Indian J Gastroenterol. 2012;31:324–32.
23. Ito K, Fujita N, Noda Y, et al. Preoperative evaluation of ampullary neoplasm with EUS and transpapillary intraductal US: a prospective and histopathologically controlled study. Gastrointest Endosc. 2007;66:740–7.
24. Trikudanathan G, Njei B, Attam R, Arain M, Shaukat A. Staging accuracy of ampullary tumors by endoscopic ultrasound: meta-analysis and systematic review. Dig Endosc. 2014;26:617–26.
25. Heinzow HS, Kammerer S, Rammes C, Wessling J, Domagk D, Meister T. Comparative analysis of ERCP, IDUS, EUS and CT in predicting malignant bile duct strictures. World J Gastroenterol. 2014;20:10495–503.
26. Imazu H, Mori N, Kanazawa K, et al. Contrast-enhanced harmonic endoscopic ultrasonography in the differential diagnosis of gallbladder wall thickening. Dig Dis Sci. 2014;59:1909–16.
27. Kamata K, Takenaka M, Kitano M, et al. Contrast-enhanced harmonic endoscopic ultrasonography for differential diagnosis of localized gallbladder lesions. Dig Endosc. 2018;30:98–106.
28. Leem G, Chung MJ, Park JY, et al. Clinical value of contrast-enhanced harmonic endoscopic ultrasonography in the differential diagnosis of pancreatic and gallbladder masses. Clin Endosc. 2018;51:80–8.
29. Halttunen J, Meisner S, Aabakken L, et al. Difficult cannulation as defined by a prospective study of the Scandinavian Association for Digestive Endoscopy (SADE) in 907 ERCPs. Scand J Gastroenterol. 2014;49:752–8.
30. Bailey AA, Bourke MJ, Williams SJ, et al. A prospective randomized trial of cannulation technique in ERCP: effects on technical success and post-ERCP pancreatitis. Endoscopy. 2008;40:296–301.
31. Morales SJ, Sampath K, Gardner TB. A review of prevention of post-ERCP pancreatitis. Gastroenterol Hepatol. 2018;14:286–92.
32. Tuca A, Guell E, Martinez-Losada E, Codorniu N. Malignant bowel obstruction in advanced cancer patients: epidemiology, management, and factors influencing spontaneous resolution. Cancer Manag Res. 2012;4:159–69.
33. Jin Z, Wei Y, Lin H, et al. Endoscopic ultrasound-guided versus endoscopic retrograde cholangiopancreatography-guided biliary drainage for primary treatment of distal malignant biliary obstruction: a systematic review and meta-analysis. Dig Endosc. 2020;32:16–26.
34. Imoto A, Ogura T, Higuchi K. Endoscopic ultrasound-guided pancreatic duct drainage: techniques and literature review of transmural stenting. Clin Endosc. 2020;53:525–34.
35. Park CH, Park SW, Nam E, Jung JH, Jo JH. Comparative efficacy of stents in endoscopic ultrasonography-guided peripancreatic fluid collection drainage: a systematic review and network meta-analysis. J Gastroenterol Hepatol. 2020;35:941–52.
36. Rana SS, Sharma R, Dhalaria L, Gupta R. Efficacy and safety of plastic versus lumen-apposing metal stents for transmural drainage of walled-off necrosis: a retrospective single-center study. Ann Gastroenterol. 2020;33:426–32.
37. Rerknimitr R. Endoscopic transmural necrosectomy: timing, indications, and methods. Clin Endosc. 2020;53:49–53.
38. Mohan BP, Shakhatreh M, Dugyala S, et al. EUS versus percutaneous management of postoperative pancreatic fluid collection: a systematic review and meta-analysis. Endosc Ultrasound. 2019;8:298–309.
39. Puli SR, Reddy JB, Bechtold ML, Antillon MR, Brugge WR. EUS-guided celiac plexus neurolysis for pain due to chronic pancreatitis or pancreatic cancer pain: a meta-analysis and systematic review. Dig Dis Sci. 2009;54:2330–7.
40. Wyse JM, Carone M, Paquin SC, Usatii M, Sahai AV. Randomized, double-blind, controlled trial of early endoscopic ultrasound-guided celiac plexus neurolysis to prevent pain progression in patients with newly diagnosed, painful, inoperable pancreatic cancer. J Clin Oncol. 2011;29:3541–6.
41. Zhang L, Tan S, Huang S, et al. The safety and efficacy of endoscopic ultrasound-guided ablation therapy for solid pancreatic tumors: a systematic review. Scand J Gastroenterol. 2020;55:1121–31.

Intraoperative Imaging Techniques in Liver Surgery

Florin Botea, Alexandru Barcu, and Irinel Popescu

Abstract

Despite tremendous development of preoperative imaging techniques in liver tumors, the high complexity liver surgery, including techniques to increase resectability and the minimal invasive approach, as well as the significant intraoperative risk, demand the development and implementation of intraoperative imaging techniques, such as intraoperative cholangiography, intraoperative ultrasound, intraoperative fluorescence, and intraoperative navigation.

Despite tremendous development of preoperative imaging techniques in liver tumors, the high complexity liver surgery, including techniques to increase resectability and the minimal invasive approach, as well as the significant intraoperative risk, demand the development and implementation of intraoperative imaging techniques, such as intraoperative cholangiography, intraoperative ultrasound, intraoperative fluorescence, and intraoperative navigation.

17.1 Intraoperative Cholangiography

The first report on depiction of the biliary ducts was published in 1918 by Reich [1], who used bismuth and petrolatum to define a biliary fistula. Mirizzi advanced the field by reporting in 1932 the first series of routine intraoperative cholangiography (IOC) is using lipiodol during cholecystectomy [2]. Berci, Shore, Hamlin, and Morgenstern [3] reported in 1978 a series of patients in whom a C-arm mobile image intensifier was used for IOC, obtaining high-definition X-rays.

Intraoperative cholangiography (IOC) is currently the most frequently used technique for intraoperative assessment of the biliary anatomy. Being safe, effective, and helpful in evaluating the biliary anatomy and guiding the surgical procedures that involves the bile ducts.

The diagnostic accuracy of a static X-ray method is 50–70%, but the digitized image intensifier fluoroscopic method increases the accuracy to 95–100%. The time decreased from 20–30 min for a static cholangiogram to 3–5 min with fluoroscopic IOC. Dynamic fluoroscopy speeds up the IOC and provides high-resolution images that more accurately depict the biliary anatomy [4].

The advantages of IOC are [4]:

- identification of the anatomy and aberrant anatomy of the extrahepatic bile ducts,
- identification of pathology and injuries of the common bile duct or Oddi's sphincter,
- data storage for documentation and review,
- landmarks for further surgical dissection.

However, IOC has several drawbacks, preventing the routine use of IOC:

- does not allow 3-dimensional (3D) anatomical viewing;
- the spatial relationships between the bile ducts and liver parenchyma, as well as the location of the bile ducts passing through the liver, are difficult to understand because only the bile duct can be imaged [5].
- the caudate bile ducts, that may cause biliary leakage after bile duct division, are not always clearly delineated;
- poor detection of variants of intrahepatic biliary anatomy [6],
- risk of false positive results,
- risk of iatrogenic bile duct injuries.
- time consuming procedure;
- a large C-arm fluoroscopy device and additional human resources are required,
- the patient and medical staff are exposed to radiation.

F. Botea (✉) · A. Barcu · I. Popescu
"Dan Setlacec" Center of General Surgery and Liver Transplantation, Fundeni Clinical Institute, Bucharest, Romania

However, in the era of laparoscopy and of no tolerance for complications in living donor, IOC is extremely important in case of unclear or aberrant biliary anatomy [4].

17.2 Intraoperative Ultrasound

Intraoperative ultrasonography (IOUS) was introduced in liver surgery in 1980′ by Makuuchi [7] and had proven to be fundamental for making a complete diagnosis during liver surgery, but also for guiding the liver resection (LR), with a low rate of intraoperative incidents and postoperative complications, while increasing the resectability [8].

IOUS usually uses high-frequency probes (7.5–10 MHz), due to the high resolution and, therefore, the highest detection rate, especially in case of small relatively superficial lesions. The low-frequencies probes (3.5–5 MHz) may be used for initial exploration, allowing a panoramic view of the liver and the detection of deep located structures and lesion (such as segment 1). They also are used for contrast-enhance IOUS.

It is worth mentioning that IOUS has difficulties in detecting small subcapsular lesions; however, these are usually easily detected at inspection and palpation. If IOUS is intended to be used for detecting such lesions, especially in case of a fibrotic liver that impedes lesion palpation, a surgical glove filled with sterile saline solution can be used as an interface between the probe and the liver surface, making the lesion visible.

IOUS is performed using specific devices, either in open approach or in laparoscopy (Fig. 17.1), after partial mobilization of the liver by sectioning the round and falciform ligaments, and the triangular and coronary ligaments. It involves four main steps:

1. evaluation of liver anatomy: exploration of vessels and bile ducts at hilum and intrahepatic levels, establishing the liver segmentation;
2. diagnosis: detection, diagnosis and mapping (according to liver segmentation and relation to major intrahepatic structures) of all liver lesions; Contrast-enhanced IOUS may detect additional lesions and/or ensure a positive diagnosis of the detected lesions [9]. Additionally, IOUS evaluates the background liver, assessing its impairments, such as cirrhosis and steatosis,
3. guidance of liver resection: resection planning, and real-time guidance of the transection plane using specific techniques, such as the hooking technique for vessel identification during transection [10],
4. control of post-resection results in terms of tumor clearance, including the control of the specimen for very small

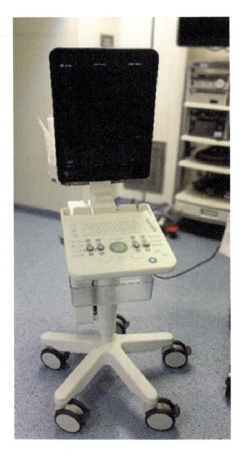
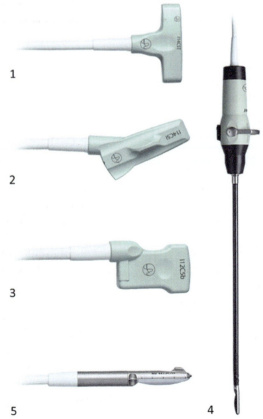

Fig. 17.1 BK 5000 ultrasound machine designed for intraoperative ultrasound. of the liver, with various probes: T-shaped convex intraoperative probe (1); I-shaped convex intraoperative probe (2); biplane convex intraoperative probe (3); laparoscopic 4-way convex probe (4); convex probe for (5)

lesions using the "water-bath" technique [11] and vessel and bile duct integrity of the remnant liver.

17.2.1 Anatomy

IOUS examination is started by placing the ultrasound probe on the diaphragmatic face of the liver in the central portion (at the level of segment 4) to obtain an ultrasound section of the main portal bifurcation. From here, the examination continues following the left portal vein and its branches for segments 2, 3 and 4 (upper and lower) and then the left and middle hepatic veins, thus achieving the precise delimitation of the segments of the left hemiliver. After repositioning the ultrasound probe at the portal bifurcation, the examination follows the right portal vein with its branches for the right anterior section (with the portal branches for segments 8 and 5), and then, after returning to the right portal bifurcation, for the right posterior section (with the corresponding branches for segments 6 and 7). Then, the right and middle hepatic veins are followed to the confluence with the inferior vena cava, achieving the delimitation of the segments of the right hemiliver. The examination is completed with segment 1 exploration.

Intraoperative ultrasound can be performed before any dissection and repeated at will to guide the surgeon especially when hilar mapping is difficult due to fibrosis, inflammation or tumor infiltration. IOUS may be repeated as many times as needed during surgery, prior, during and after the resection, assisting in mapping the biliary, arterial, portal and hepatic veins system, in detecting all their aberrant anatomy [12], guiding the resection plane in order to prevent biliary and vascular injuries, controlling the results after resection, and, as discussed in this paper, identifying the corresponding drainage territories of the bile duct stumps on the liver cut surface for a proper biliary reconstruction.

17.2.2 Diagnosis

IOUS is superior to preoperative imaging methods, detecting 10–50% more focal liver lesions (FLL) [13, 14]. While percutaneous ultrasound, computed tomography (CT) and magnetic resonance imaging (MRI) are limited in identifying FLL <2 cm, IOUS easily detects FLL of 3–5 mm [15, 16] (Fig. 17.2). The sensitivity of CT in the FLL detection is 72%, while for IOUS is 98%. CT sensitivity decreases with tumor size, reaching 35% for tumor of 1 cm, while IOUS sensitivity is maintained in this scenario [17]. Moreover, thrombosis of any vascular and/or biliary structure is easily identified at IOUS, and helps in establishing its tumoral feature. IOUS also effectively assesses the background liver,

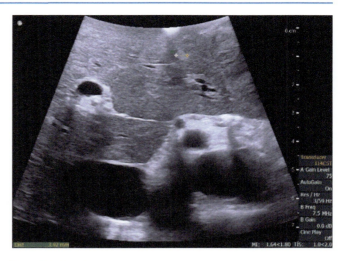

Fig. 17.2 IOUS detection of a 4 mm colorectal liver metastasis

diagnosing impairments such as cirrhosis, cholestasis, and steatosis. The use of contrast agent further increases the sensitivity and specificity of IOUS [18]. New generation liver-specific contrast agents, such as perfluorobutane (Sonazoid, Daiichi Sankyo, Tokyo) further improves the detection and differential diagnosis of focal liver lesions [19, 20].

Additionally, IOUS precisely defines the 3D relationships between the FLLs and the surrounding main vessels, helping in establishing the proper strategy and resection planning, while maximizing the volume of the future liver remnant (FLR). IOUS can change the resection planning in up to 72% of cases [21].

17.2.3 Resection Guidance

This step involves IOUS techniques that guide the liver resection planned based on information gathered by IOUS, IOUS-guided techniques that are integrated in the surgical technique as follows:

1. Demarcation of the resection area.
2. Resection guidance.
3. Identification of intrahepatic vessels.
4. Evaluation of post-resection results.

17.2.3.1 Demarcation of the Resection Area
IOUS-guided demarcation of the resection area is achieved by using:

- IOUS-guided placement of the tip of the electrocautery: the tip is placed between the ultrasound probe and the liver surface, generating a specific artefact at ultrasound exploration that helps the precise positioning of the tip at

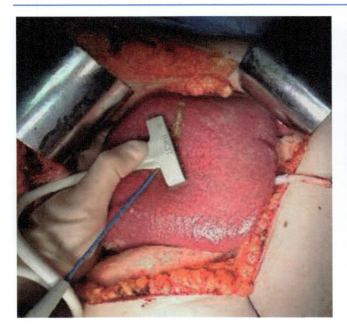

Fig. 17.3 Electrocautery tip placement between the ultrasound probe and the liver surface, generating a specific artefact at ultrasound exploration that helps the precise positioning of the tips at the level of the planned resection plane, in a patient with HCC on HBV-related cirrhosis

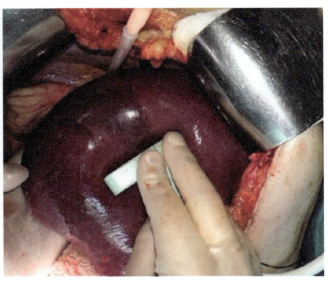

Fig. 17.4 Demarcation for S7 subsegmentectomy based on the ischemia induced by ultrasound-guided portal pedicle compression, in a patient with HCC on HBV chronic hepatitis

the level of the planned resection plane (Fig. 17.3). In this way, multiple key points are marked onto the liver surface, that are afterwards united by a closed-shaped line (demarcating the resection area) in a such manner that this area includes the lesion/lesions to be resected with safety margins, while excluding key structures of the future liver remnant (FLR), thus insuring its viability and function. The resection volume is virtually delimited, based on the demarcated resection area and intrahepatic landmarks identified at IOUS; these landmarks are few key points located in vicinity of the deepest part of the lesion to be resected, and/or of a key vascular element that is to be preserved for the FLR and exposed on the resection plane. This technique is used commonly used for non-anatomical LR;

- tattooing technique [22]—consists in puncturing the portal branch(es) that vascularize(s) the (sub)segments that encompasses the tumor, and injecting a dye (carmine blue) that colors the anatomical territory to be resected both on the liver surface and in depth (intraparenchymal delimitation is not as clear), thus guiding the resection plane. When this technique is not feasible, the counterstaining may be used, consisting in puncturing and injecting the portal branches that serve the segments/subsegments adjacent to the resection territory. This technique was designed for anatomical liver resection, particularly recommended in hepatocellular carcinoma [23, 24];

- IOUS-guided digital compression of intrahepatic vessels:
  - of intrahepatic portal pedicles—alternative to the tattooing technique: IOUS locates the portal branch(es) for the (sub)segment to be resected, and clamped between the ultrasound probe and the surgeon's finger placed opposite to the probe onto the liver surface; the induced transient ischemia of the corresponding parenchyma allows the demarcation of the resection area (Fig. 17.4). When not feasible, the counter-compression may be used as an alternative (the concept is analogous to the counterstaining) [25];
  - of the hepatic veins (HV)—while the HV planned to be resected is finger clamped under IOUS-guidance, the identification at eco-Doppler of hepato-hepatic shunts (between the branches of the clamped HV and those of the neighboring HV) and certification of a normal flow in the portal branch(es) related to the drained parenchyma of the finger-occluded HV allows to preserve the drained territory of the HV to be resected [26].

17.2.3.2 Resection Guidance

Using IOUS-guidance, the resection plane is established between the border of the resection area marked by electrocautery (and easily visualized in IOUS, similarly to the tip of the electrocautery), the deepest point of the future specimen, and the key intrahepatic vessels in relation to the resection plane which are to be preserved for the FRL, that are usually exposed on the cut surface. The transection plane is visualized at IOUS as a hyperechoic irregular line, due to the presence of air and coagulated blood between the two hepatic tranches [27]. Thus, under ultrasound control, the transection plane is guided and changed in real-time if necessary, adapting it in real time in such way to correspond to the planned resection.

17.2.3.3 Identification of Intrahepatic Vessels

During transection, any significant vessel exposed on the transection plane can be identified by the hooking technique [10]: a reference surgical thread placed around the key vessel is visualized at IOUS as a hyperechoic point with a posterior shadow cone; by gently pulling the thread during IOUS, the traction point on the vessel is identified [10].

17.2.3.4 Evaluation of Post-Resection Results

The IOUS evaluation of immediate postresection results consists of:

- control of tumor clearance: IOUS exploration of the remnant liver identifies potentially missed lesions. In case of very small lesion, IOUS certifies its presence in the specimen immersed in saline solution (the "water-bath" technique) (Fig. 17.5), and guides the sectioning the specimen, allowing the marking of the lesion, so the pathologist wouldn't miss it.
- control of the vascularization and biliary drainage of the remnant liver: control of vascularization is performed by intraoperative Doppler echo, any significant alteration of vascularization found at Doppler IOUS is sanctioned by repositioning the remaining liver (in case of torsion, angulation or traction of vessels), thrombectomy (in the case of portal thrombosis), or resection of the ischemic/congested territory. Detection of any significant biliary dilatation usually involves the resection of the corresponding territory.

IOUS ensures optimal tumor clearance. In case of non-assisted IOUS LR, positive oncological safety margins were registered in 16–18% of cases, while no such case was recorded after IOUS-guided LR [28]. Postoperative morbidity also appears to be lower with IOUS-guided LR [29]. The main advantage of such LR is the maximization of functional residual liver volume, preventing the risk of liver failure [29], while allowing extensive multiple resections to be performed in a single operation [30, 31]. Another important benefit is the possibility of repeated liver resections in the case recurrences, with a significant impact on the oncological outcome [32, 33]. The disadvantages of such procedure are represented by the cost of the equipment, and the slow learning curve. We emphasize that, unlike the diagnostic IOUS that can be performed by the radiologist, the IOUS guidance of LR can be done only by the liver surgeon.

Literature analysis proved ultrasound as a safe, quick, non-irradiating, cost-effective technique, which is well known but largely under-utilized, probably due to the perception of a difficult learning curve.

IOUS is a precise real-time method of diagnosis and guidance of LR, that must be part of the arsenal of liver surgery, being optimally exploited when performed by the liver surgeon.

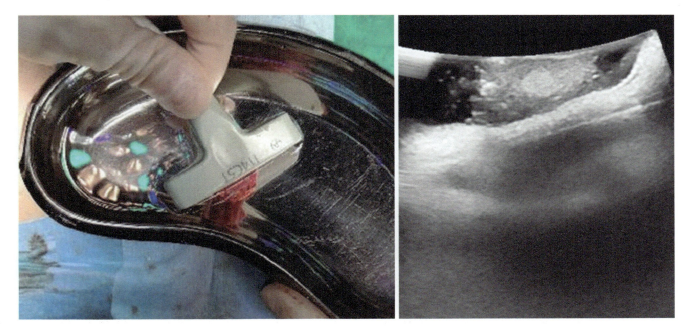

Fig. 17.5 "Water-bath" technique for detecting a 5-mm colorectal liver metastasis in the specimen

17.3 Intraoperative Fluorescence Imaging

The use of intraoperative fluorescence imaging (IFI) in liver surgery has significantly increased and improved, offering new perspectives. In selected patients, especially during minimally invasive surgery, IFI adds useful data to visual inspection, palpation, and intraoperative ultrasound, limited to a depth of 5–10 mm [34]. IFI is based on the visualization at a special infrared camera of certain areas where indocyanine green (ICG) injected intravenously accumulates or not.

The main use of IFI is the visualization of the biliary anatomy, due to ICG biliary excretion starting approximately 30 min after intravenous injection (Fig. 17.6). This is useful especially resections of centrally located liver tumors and hilar cholangiocarcinoma [35, 36]. IFI cholangiography can detect bile duct leakages during hepatectomies, that are missed by other routine tests [37].

IFI may also be used as an alternative to the tattooing technique, by injecting ICG into the portal branch (instead of the colored dye) [38]. However, one of the disadvantages of this procedure is difficult tracking of the stained plane during transection. The ICG within the targeted segment gradually disappears and repeated ICG injection or temporally clamping the hepatic artery (for reducing washout of the dye) is necessary to continuously track the transection plane. Additionally, a small amount of ICG recirculates the liver after the initial passage through the portal vein branch, that lead eventually to the staining of the entire liver. To avoid this, intermittent Pringle maneuver is recommended [39] in order to obtains continuous fluorescence tracking during transection, allowing a persistent visualization of the segmental boundaries [40].

Moreover, IFI enables identification of subcapsular liver tumors through accumulation of ICG administered preoperatively in malignant tissues, as in case of hepatocellular carcinoma (HCC), or in the surrounding parenchyma in case of intrahepatic cholangiocarcinoma and liver metastases (Fig. 17.7). However, only tumors located 5 mm or closer to the liver surface are usually detected at IFI, while tumors located ≥ 8 mm from the liver surface cannot be identified [41]. Nevertheless, in this thin superficial zone of the liver, IFI may detect up to 29% more liver metastasis with diameter ≤ 3 mm [42].

Fluorescens patterns are related to the type of cancer and its grade of differentiation [43]. Impaired bile excretion in HCC cells retains the ICG within the tumor, therefore well-differentiated HCCs appears at IFI as strong, homogenous fluorescence emissions. In contrast, in poorly-differentiated

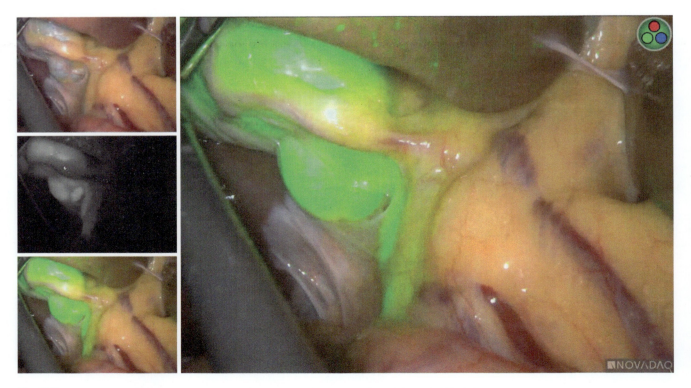

Fig. 17.6 Intraoperative fluorescence imaging depicting the gallbladder, cystic and the main bile ducts

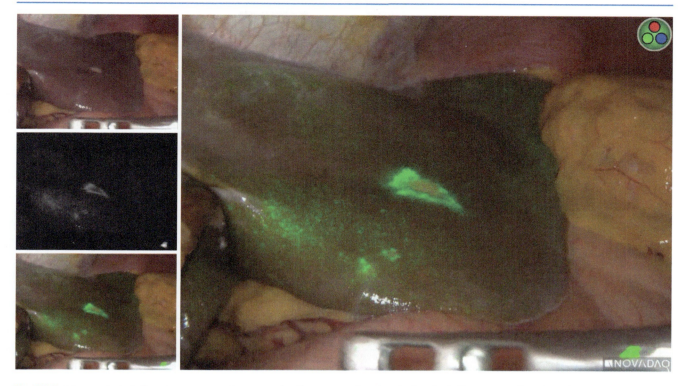

Fig. 17.7 Liver metastasis from breast cancer: intraoperative fluorescence imaging depicts the hallow surrounding the lesion

HCCs and liver metastases, ICG is retained in the cytoplasm of the surrounding parenchyma, inducing a rim type fluorescence pattern.

Recent experimental study showed that IFI may be used as a drug delivery system in combination with photodynamic therapy may not only detect cancer tissue but also treat it [44].

17.4 Navigation Assisted Liver Resection

Some attempts were made on computer-aided navigation-assisted LR, using preoperative imaging superimposed intraoperatively onto the anatomical structures of the liver [45–47]. However, the implementation of this procedure in liver surgery is impeded by intraoperative organ shift and deformation, and differences of total liver volume and vascular anatomy (when compared to the preoperative imaging), the respiratory movements during surgery, along with the lack of intraoperative external liver landmarks. Efforts are made to overcome these obstacles, but still remains only a future perspective [48, 49].

References

1. Reich A. Accidental injection of bile ducts with petrolatum and bismuth paste. JAMA. 1918;71:1555.
2. Mirizzi PL. La Cholangiografia Durante las Operaciones de las Vias Biliares. Bol Soc Cir Buenos Aires. 1932;16:1133.
3. Berci G, Shore JM, Hamlin JA, Morgenstern J. Operative fluoroscopy and cholangiography. Am Surg. 1978;135:32.
4. MacFadyen BV. Intraoperative cholangiography: past, present, and future. Surg Endosc. 2006;20(Suppl 2):S436–40.
5. Urade T, Fukumoto T, Kido M, Takebe A, Tanaka M, Kuramitsu K, Kinoshita H, Toyama H, Ajiki T, Iwasaki T, Tominaga M, Ku Y. Contrast-enhanced intraoperative ultrasonic cholangiography in living donor hepatectomy. Liver Transpl. 2016;22(10):1437–42.
6. Sanjay P, Tagolao S, Dirkzwager I, Bartlett A. A survey of the accuracy of interpretation of intraoperative cholangiograms. HPB (Oxford). 2012;14:673–6.
7. Makuuchi M, Torzilli G, Machi J. History of intraoperative ultrasound. Ultrasound Med Biol. 1998;24(9):1229–42. https://doi.org/10.1016/s0301-5629(98)00112-4.
8. Torzilli G, Makuuchi M, Inoue K, et al. No-mortality liver resection for hepatocellular carcinoma in cirrhotic and noncirrhotic patientsis there a way? A prospective analysis of our approach. Arch Surg. 1999;134:984–92.
9. Torzilli G, Botea F, Donadon M, et al. Criteria for the selective use of contrast-enhanced intra-operative ultrasound during surgery for colorectal liver metastases. HPB (Oxford). 2014;16(11):994–1001.
10. Torzilli G, Takayama T, Hui AM, et al. A new technical aspect of ultrasound-guided liver surgery. Am J Surg. 1999;178:341–3.
11. Makuuchi M. Abdominal intraoperative ultrasonography. New York: Igaku-Shoin; 1987.
12. Pfluke JM, Bowers SP Jr. Laparoscopic intraoperative biliary ultrasonography: findings during laparoscopic cholecystectomy for acute disease. J Laparoendosc Adv Surg Tech A. 2011;21(6):505–9.
13. Gozzetti G, Mazziotti A, Bolondi L, et al. Intraoperative ultrasonography in surgery for liver tumors. Surgery. 1986;99:523–30.
14. Ravikumar TS, Buenaventura S, Salem RR, et al. Intraoperative ultrasonography of liver, detection of occult liver tumors and treatment by cryosurgery. Cancer Detect Prev. 1994;18:131.
15. Clarke MP, Kane RA, Steele G, et al. Prospective comparison of preoperative imaging and intraoperative ultrasonography in the detection of liver tumors. Surgery. 1989;106:849–55.

16. Wernecke K, Rummeny E, Bongartz G, et al. Detection of hepatic masses in patients 48 with carcinoma: comparative sensitivities of sonography, CT, and MR imaging. AJR Am J Roentgenol. 1991;157:731.
17. Hata S, Imamura H, Aoki T, et al. Value of visual inspection, bimanual palpation, and intraoperative ultrasonography during hepatic resection for liver metastases of colorectal carcinoma. World J Surg. 2011;35:2779–87.
18. Torzilli G. Contrast-enhanced intraoperative ultrasonography in surgery for liver tumors. Eur J Radiol. 2004;51(Suppl):S25–9.
19. Hatanaka K, Kudo M, Minami Y, Maekawa K. Sonazoid-enhanced ultrasonography for diagnosis of hepatic malignancies: comparison with contrast-enhanced CT. Oncology. 2008;75(Suppl 1):42–7. https://doi.org/10.1159/000173423.
20. Nakano H, Ishida Y, Hatakeyama T, et al. Contrast-enhanced intraoperative ultrasonography equipped with late Kupffer-phase image obtained by sonazoid in patients with colorectal liver metastases. World J Gastroenterol. 2008;14(20):3207–11. https://doi.org/10.3748/wjg.14.3207.
21. Cervone A, Sardi A, Conaway GL. Intraoperative ultrasound (IOUS) is essential in the management of metastatic colorectal liver lesions. Am Surg. 2000;66:611–5.
22. Makuuchi M, Hasegawa H, Yamazaki S. Ultrasonically guided subsegmentectomy. Surg Gynecol Obstet. 1985;161(4):346–50.
23. Makuuchi M. Remodeling the surgical approach to hepatocellular carcinoma. Hepatogastroenterology. 2002;49(43):36–40.
24. Makuuchi M, Imamura H, Sugawara Y, Takayama T. Progress in surgical treatment of hepatocellular carcinoma. Oncology. 2002;62(Suppl 1):74–81. https://doi.org/10.1159/000048280.
25. Torzilli G, Donadon M, Cimino M, Del Fabbro D, Procopio F, Botea F. Systematic subsegmentectomy by ultrasound-guided finger compression for hepatocellular carcinoma in cirrhosis. Ann Surg Oncol. 2009;16(7):1843.
26. Torzilli G, Montorsi M, Del Fabbro D, et al. Ultrasonographically guided surgical approach to liver tumours involving the hepatic veins closet o the caval confluence. Br J Surg. 2006;93:1238–46.
27. Vauthey JN, Pawlik TM, Abdalla EK, et al. Is extended hepatectomy for hepatobiliary malignancy justified? Ann Surg. 2004;239(5):722–39.
28. Lau WY, Leung KL, Lee TW, et al. Ultrasonography during liver resection for hepatocellular carcinoma. Br J Surg. 1993;80:493–4.
29. Torzilli G, Montorsi M, Donadon M, et al. "Radical but conservative" is the main goal for ultrasonography guided liver resection: prospective validation of this approach. Am Coll Surg. 2005;201(4):517–28.
30. Jaeck D, Oussoultzoglou E, Rosso E, et al. A two-stage hepatectomy procedure combined with portal vein embolization to achieve curative resection for initially unresectable multiple and bilobar colorectal liver metastases. Ann Surg. 2004;240:1037–49.
31. Adam R, Laurent A, Azoulay D, et al. Two-stage hepatectomy: a planned strategy to treat irresectable liver tumors. Ann Surg. 2000;232:777–85.
32. Suzuki S, Sakaguchi T, Yokoi Y, et al. Impact of repeat hepatectomy on recurrent colorectal liver metastases. Surgery. 2001;129:421–8.
33. Nakajima Y, Ko S, Kanamura T, et al. Repeat liver resection for hepatocellular carcinoma. J Am Coll Surg. 2001;192:339–44.
34. Mitsuhashi N, Kimura F, Shimizu H, et al. Usefulness of intraoperative fluorescence imaging to evaluate local anatomy in hepatobiliary surgery. J Hepatobiliary Pancreat Surg. 2008;15:508–14.
35. Ashitate Y, Stockdale A, Choi HS, et al. Real-time simultaneous near-infrared fluorescence imaging of bile duct and arterial anatomy. J Surg Res. 2012;176:7–13.
36. Ishizawa T, Bandai Y, Ijichi M, Kaneko J, Hasegawa K, Kokudo N. Fluorescent cholangiography illuminating the biliary tree during laparoscopic cholecystectomy. Br J Surg. 2010;97:1369–77.
37. Kaibori M, Ishizaki M, Matsui K, Kwon AH. Intraoperative indocyanine green fluorescent imaging for prevention of bile leakage after hepatic resection. Surgery. 2011;150:91–8.
38. Aoki T, Murakami M, Yasuda D, et al. Intraoperative fluorescent imaging using indocyanine green for liver mapping and cholangiography. J Hepatobiliary Pancreat Sci. 2010;17:590–4.
39. Miyata A, Ishizawa T, Tani K, et al. Reappraisal of a dye-staining technique for anatomic hepatectomy by the concomitant use of indocyanine green fluorescence imaging. J Am Coll Surg. 2015;221:e27–36.
40. Aoki T, Yasuda D, Shimizu Y, et al. Image-guided liver mapping using fluorescence navigation system with indocyanine green for anatomical hepatic resection. World J Surg. 2008;32:1763–7.
41. Kudo H, Ishizawa T, Tani K, et al. Visualization of subcapsular hepatic malignancy by indocyanine-green fluorescence imaging during laparoscopic hepatectomy. Surg Endosc. 2014;28:2504–8.
42. Peloso A, Franchi E, Canepa MC, et al. Combined use of intraoperative ultrasound and indocyanine green fluorescence imaging to detect liver metastases from colorectal cancer. HPB (Oxford). 2013;15(12):928–34. https://doi.org/10.1111/hpb.12057.
43. Lim C, Vibert E, Azoulay D, et al. Indocyanine green fluorescence imaging in the surgical management of liver cancers: current facts and future implications. J Visc Surg. 2014;151:117–24.
44. Kaibori M, Kosaka H, Matsui K, et al. Near-infrared fluorescence imaging and photodynamic therapy for liver tumors. Front Oncol. 2021;11:638327. https://doi.org/10.3389/fonc.2021.638327.
45. Kleemann M, Deichmann S, Esnaashari H, et al. Laparoscopic navigated liver resection: technical aspects and clinical practice in benign liver tumors. Case Rep Surg. 2012;2012:8. https://doi.org/10.1155/2012/265918
46. Kingham TP, Scherer MA, Neese BW, et al. Image-guided liver surgery: intraoperative projection of computed tomography images utilizing tracked ultrasound. HPB (Oxford). 2012;14(9):594–603. https://doi.org/10.1111/j.1477-2574.2012.0048.
47. Peterhans M, vom Berg A, Dagon B, et al. A navigation system for open liver surgery: design, workflow and first clinical applications. Int J Med Robot. 2011;7:7–16.
48. Heizmann O, Zidowitz S, Bourquain H, et al. Assessment of intraoperative liver deformation during hepatic resection: prospective clinical study. World J Surg. 2010;34(8):1887–93. https://doi.org/10.1007/s00268-010-0561-x.
49. Mise Y, Tani K, Aoki T, et al. Virtual liver resection: computer-assisted operation planning using a three-dimensional liver representation. J Hepatobiliary Pancreat Sci. 2013;20(2):157–64. https://doi.org/10.1007/s00534-012-0574-y.

Use of Radiotherapy Alone and in Combination with Other Therapies for Hepatocellular Carcinoma: Rationale and Future Directions

Dan G. Duda and Franziska D. Hauth

Abstract

The continuous rise in incidence of hepatocellular carcinoma (HCC) worldwide has led to renewed efforts to improve therapeutic strategies. The gold standard of curative therapy for patients with HCC is surgery. However, in HCC patients with tumors with specific anatomical locations, such as near gastrointestinal structures or vessels, or with vascular occlusions, surgery may be particularly challenging. Poor baseline liver function is often an additional limiting factor for many established treatment modalities, especially for liver resection. Therefore, available treatment options have been very limited in efficacy, which led to dismal survival rates. In recent years, radiotherapy has emerged as a new and promising local treatment option for certain patients with HCC. Advances in technology and delivery techniques have aided in establishing radiotherapy as a safe and effective treatment modality. As a painless, non-invasive, outpatient treatment procedure, radiotherapy may have many advantages over other treatment modalities. This chapter will discuss recent developments and advances in establishing radiotherapy as a new pillar of treatment for patients with HCC, review available data from retrospective and prospective trials, and give an overview of potential future combinational treatment approaches with systemic therapies to further expand the benefits.

D. G. Duda (✉)
Department of Radiation Oncology, Massachusetts General Hospital Research Institute, Boston, MA, USA

Edwin L. Steele Laboratories for Tumor Biology, Massachusetts General Hospital, Boston, MA, USA
e-mail: duda@steele.mgh.harvard.edu

F. D. Hauth
Department of Radiation Oncology, Massachusetts General Hospital Research Institute, Boston, MA, USA

Edwin L. Steele Laboratories for Tumor Biology, Massachusetts General Hospital, Boston, MA, USA

Department of Radiation Oncology, University Clinic Tuebingen, Tuebingen, Germany

18.1 Introduction

Hepatocellular carcinoma (HCC) is a primary cancer of the liver and is often associated with chronic liver injury. The etiology of chronic liver injury is different in various regions of the world. While in Eastern areas the development of HCC is often based on viral infections of the liver (Hepatitis B and C), the rising incidence of liver tumors (~42,800 cases/year) in the US is linked to increased rates of non-alcoholic fatty liver disease (NAFLD) [1]. Although, therapeutic options have evolved in the last decade, mortality from liver cancer is still high (6% of all cancer related deaths in men in the USA) [1], and five-year survival ranges between 20% (after ablation) and 67% (after liver transplantation) [2].

The gold standard for curative therapy remain total resection of the tumor or liver transplantation for patients within Milan criteria (single tumor <5 cm or up to three lesions <3 cm, no angioinvasion, no extrahepatic disease) [3, 4]. However, less than one-third of patients are eligible for these treatments, mainly due to limited overall health status or underlying liver disfunction [2, 5]. Moreover, HCC tumors are often multifocal, including pre-cancerous and cancerous areas, further limiting surgical options [2]. Other local treatment options include radiofrequency ablation (RFA), percutaneous ethanol injection (PEI), microwave ablation and trans-arterial chemoembolization (TACE) [6]. Especially for RFA and TACE, treatment efficacy is limited in patients with portal vein thrombosis or vascular invasion due to delivery technique via the vascular system. Another limitation of these treatment approaches is tumor size, as they are less effective against larger tumors [7, 8].

In recent years, technological advances in radiation oncology have led to the establishment of radiotherapy as a locoregional treatment option for patients with HCC. In particular, hypofractionated image-guided radiotherapy (HIGRT), better known as stereotactic body radiotherapy (SBRT), has been shown to be a safe and effective way to deliver ablative doses of radiation to liver tumors. In general, hypofractionated (stereotactic) radiotherapy refers to delivery of high radiation doses in few, usually in less than 10 fractions. These fractions may be delivered daily or spaced apart by several days, generally between two to seven days. Precision and accuracy are at the heart of this new therapy. Improvements in treatment planning and delivery techniques as well as the establishment of new imaging solutions during radiotherapy have accelerated its implementation for liver cancer treatment. This holds especially true for tumors in challenging locations including tumors near blood vessels or GI organs. As a non-invasive, painless, outpatient treatment procedure with short treatment periods the benefits for patients are indisputable. While efficacy of RFA greatly diminishes with tumor diameters above 3 cm, radiotherapy has been shown to achieve high local control rates also in locally advanced patients [9–11].

In this chapter, we provide an overview of the advances in liver cancer radiotherapies, including photon and charged particle therapy, review the available data from retrospective and prospective studies, and point to potential future combination with novel systemic therapies.

18.2 Photon Therapy

Photon radiotherapy is the most readily available form of radiotherapy. Historically, patients have been treated with conventionally fractionated radiotherapy, resulting in generally low local control (LC) rates. This was mainly due to the inability to deliver tumor ablative radiation doses within the constraints of normal tissue tolerance. Technological advancements in recent years have made it possible to precisely deliver higher radiation doses and to improve normal tissue preservation, therefore reducing risk of liver-associated side effects.

Efficacy of SBRT has been shown both for patients with single site HCC as well as for patients with large or locally advanced tumors. Currently available data is summarized in Table 18.1. Overall survival (OS) rates after irradiation in these studies shows very promising results with local control rates between 65% and 100%. In a Phase II trial, Takeda and his group reported high LC as well as OS rates in patients with solitary HCC with a maximal dimension of 4 cm. Good treatment outcomes were independent of pretreatment or residual tumor burden or treatment in recurrent settings [33]. Similarly, Kang et al. and Bujold et al. reported high local control rates for patients with large or multiple HCC lesions [34, 35]. As with many other treatment modalities, local control rates largely depend on tumor size. In a retrospective analysis Yoon and colleagues reported 76.3%, 93.3% and 100% local recurrence-free survival rates for patients with HCC > 3 cm, between 2.1–3 cm, and ≤ 2 cm, respectively [17].

Possible side effects after liver irradiation include elevation of liver enzymes, increase of Child-Pugh (CP) score and worsening of liver function and hematologic toxicities as well as fatigue and erythema. In general, side effects could be separated into early (within 90 days after treatment) and late toxicities (>90 days after treatment). Whereas early side effects have the potential to resolve without treatment, late onset toxicities are more likely to persist. A summary of side effects Grade 3 or more is provided in Table 18.1.

The optimal radiation dose as well as the timing of radiation in relation to other treatments remains unclear to date [39]. However, studies have indicated a distinct dose-dependence of tumor response for HCC. In this context, Park and colleagues observed increasing response rates correlating to radiation dose (<40 Gy: 29%; 40–50 Gy: 69%; >50 Gy: 77%) [40]. In line with this observation, Kang and his group reported a dose-dependence of two-year LC rates for patients treated with SBRT: Patients receiving >54 Gy showed a LC of 100% whereas patients treated with doses <54 Gy had a LC rate of 81.7% [34]. However, in this study patients were treated in a primary tumor setting and results are unlikely relevant for adjuvant treatment settings. Similar results from other studies led to the assumption that a radiation dose >50 Gy is required to achieve effective LC for HCC patients [24, 41, 42]. A retrospective analysis by Su and colleagues indicated that a biologically effective dose (BED_{10}) ≥100 Gy and an equivalent dose in 2 Gy fractions (EQD_2) ≥ 74 Gy are correlated with longer OS [20]. Similarly, Kim et al. reported significant higher two-year PFS and OS for patients treated with BED_{10} > 105 Gy [15]. In this study, a gross tumor volume < 214 cm^3 was also correlated with OS. Of note, a review of the national cancer database for patients treated with SBRT revealed no association between a BED > 100 and overall survival. Further studies are needed to clarify the relationship between dose, fractionation and patient survival and to answer the outstanding questions.

In addition, the majority of previous studies have focused on the treatment of patients with low grade liver cirrhosis (mainly CP class A patients) due to the increased risk of development of side effects after radiotherapy. A small study by Culleton et al. in 29 patients with CP class B and C tested SBRT with a median dose of 30 Gy in six fractions. They reported favorable survival data with a median OS of 7.9 month in this patient cohort with very limited treatment options. However, 63% of treated patients showed a worsening of CP sore of at least two points after treatment. Whether these changes were correlated with treatment toxicity or due to natural decline of liver function in these patients with underlying liver diseases remained uncertain. The authors argued for the application of the lowest effective radiation dose in this very vulnerable patient population, and postulated that use of combinational treatment approaches may allow further dose reduction [22]. In line with this conclu-

Table 18.1 Overview over current data on photon therapy

	n	Dose (fractionation) [Gy]	Tumor size median (range) [cm]	Baseline liver function (CPA/CPB/CPC) [%]	LC [%]	OS [%]	Toxicities
Retrospective analysis							
Lou et al. 2019 [12]	75	30–48 (3–4 Gy/fx)	NA	88/12/0	NA	10 months (median)	• No ≥ grade 3
Hara et al. 2019 [11]	374	34/40 (5 fx)	1.7 (1.0–3.0)	96/4/0	NA	63.6 (3 y)	• 8.2% worsening of CP score • 4 deaths (liver failure)
Park et al. 2018 [13]	77	35–50 (10 fx)	2.4 (0.8–5.6)	56/21/0	72.6 (5 y)	52.3 (3 y) 40.9 (5 y)	• 1.3% grade 3
Bae et al. 2012 [14]	20	50 (10 fx)	80% <3 cm	90/10/0	85	100 (1 y) 87.9 (2 y)	• No ≥ grade 3
Kim et al. 2017 [15]	72	33–60 (3–10 fx)	7 (5.0–10.0)	87.5/12.5/0	NA	70.1 (1 y) 45.2 (2 y)	• 29.1% worsening of CPC score ≥ 2 pt • 1 patient grade 4 GI toxicity
Andolino et al. 2011 [16]	66	CPA: 44 (3 fx) CPB: 40 (5 fx)	3.2	54.5/36.4/0	90 (2 y)	67 (2 y)	• 20% progression CTP class • 13% increase hepatic dysfunction
Yoon et al. 2013 [17]	93	30–60 Gy (3–4 fx)	2 (1.0–6.0)	74.2/25.8/0	92.1 (3 y)	86 (1 y) 53.8 (3 y)	• 6.5% ≥ grade 3
Sanuki et al. 2014 [18]	185	CPA: 40 CPB: 35 (5 fx)	35 Gy: 2.7 (1.0–5.0) 40 Gy: 2.4 (0.8–5.0)	35 Gy: 48/52/0 40 Gy: 99/1/0	91 (3 y)	70 (3 y)	• 13% ≥ grade 3 • 10.3% worsening of CP score by 2 • Grade 5 liver failure 2 patients
Huertas et al. 2015 [19]	77	45 (3 fx)	2.4	85.7/14.3/0	99 (1/2 y)	81.8 (1 y) 56.6% (2 y)	• Acute: 2.6% ≥ grade 3 • Long-term: 2.6% ≥ grade 3
Su et al. 2016 [20]	50	30–50 (3–5 fx)	8.5 (5.1–21.0)	82/18/0	NA	62.4% (1 y) 32.9% (3 y) 32.9% (5 y)	• 1/50 death (RILD) • 5/50 grade ≥ 3
Jacob et al. 2015 [21]	37	36/45/60 (3 fx)	7.8 ± 3.3 (mean + SD)	NA	89.2	33 months (median)	• 1/37 ≥ grade 3
Culleton et al. 2014 [22]	29	30 (6 fx)	8.6 (4.1–26.6)	0/28/1	NA	32.3 (1 y)	• 63% worsening of CP score ≥ 2 • Grade 3 thrombocytopenia 14/17% (1/3 months) • Grade 3/4 elevated transaminases 10.3% • Grade 3 and 4 hyperbilirubinemia 17/28% and 14/3.5% (1/3 months)
Park et al. 2013 [23]	26	40–50 (10 fx)	2.8 (1.1–5.7)	73.1/26.9/0	87.6 (2 y)	88.5 (1 y) 67.2 (2 y)	• 3.8% grade 3 hepatic toxicity • 3.8% worsening of CP score ≥ 2
Huang et al. 2013 [24]	40	40–66 (14–23 fx)	<5: 62.5% 5–10: 35% >10: 2.5%	62.5/37.5/0	73 (1 y) 62 (2 y) 56 (5 y)	60 (1 y) 40 (2 y) 21 (5 y)	• 20% worsening of CP score ≥ 2 • 2.5% duodenal ulcer
Yao et al. 2018 [25]	33	39–45 (3–5 fx)	NA	100/0/0	84.8 (6 m)	75.8 (1 y) 45.5 (2 y)	• 24.2% fatigue grade 1–2 • 33.3% grade 1–2 GI toxicity
Katz et al. 2012 [26]	18	50 (10 fx)	4 (1.2–6.5)	16.7/44.4/22.2	NA	NA	• 5.5% grade 3 increase of hepatic enzymes

(continued)

Table 18.1 (continued)

	n	Dose (fractionation) [Gy]	Tumor size median (range) [cm]	Baseline liver function (CPA/CPB/CPC) [%]	LC [%]	OS [%]	Toxicities
Prospective studies							
Mendez-Romero et al. 2006 [27]	25 (8 HCC, 17 metastasis)	12.5/10 (3 fx), 5 (5 fx)	3.2 (0.5–7.2)	5(8)/2(8)/0	94% (1 y) 82% (2 y)	82%(1 y) 54% (2 y)	• 1 grade 5 (death) • 16% ≥ grade 3
Tse et al. 2008 [28]	41	36 (24–54) (6 fx)	173 ml (9–1913 ml)	41/0/0	65% (1 y)	51% (1 y)	• 7% increase CP class • 12% grade 3 increase liver enzymes.
Scorsetti et al. 2015 [29]	48	48–75 (3 fx), 36–60 (6 fx)	4.8 (1–12.5)	53/47/0	85.8 (1 y) 64.4 (2 y)	77.9 (1 y) 45.3 (2 y)	• 16% ≥ grade 3 • 4.2% worsening of CP score
Lee et al. 2020 [30]	23	40 (5 fx)	3.1 (1–10)	0/78.3/21.7	92.3 (1 y)	56.5 (1 y)	• 43% CP score progression • 17% worsening of CP score ≥ 2 • 7 liver related deaths
Seo et al. 2008 [31]	65	61 (34 fx)	10.8 (6.1–15.5)	66.2/33.8/0	NA	34.7(1 y)	• 15.4% did not complete RT (HCC/liver function detoriation) • 6.2% ≥ grade 3 Hepatic events • 9.2% ≥ grade 3 Hematologic events
Cardenes et al. 2010 [32]	17	40/48 (3–5 fx)	4 (2–6)	35.3/64.7/0	100 (2 y)	75 (1 y) 60 (2 y)	• 17.6% RILD • 47% grade 3 • 11.8% grade 4
Takeda et al. 2016 [33]	101	35–40 (5 fx)	2.3 (1–4)	91/9/0	96.3 (3 y)	66.7 (3 y)	• 8.9% worsening of CP score ≥ 2 • 6.6% grade 3
Kang et al. 2012 [34]	50	42–60 (3 fx)	2.9 (1.3–7.8)	87.2/12.8/0	94.6 (2 y)	68.7 (2 y)	• 6.4% grade 3 GI toxicity • 4.3% grade 4 gastric ulcer perforation.
Bujold et al. 2013 [35]	102	24–54 (6 fx)	9.9 (1.8–43.3)	100/0/0	87% (1 y)	17 months (median)	• 30% > grade 3 • 6.9% grade 5 • 7 patient's death possibly related to SBRT
Lasely et al. 2015 [36]	59	40 (5 fx), 48 Gy (3 fx)	NA	64.4/35.6/0	CPA: 92 (6 m) CPB: 93 (6 m)	CPA: 94/72/61.3 (1/2/3 y) CPB: 57.1/32.7/26.1 (1/2/3 y)	• 50%/33.3% worsening of CP score (CPA/CPB) • 10.5/38% ≥ grade 3 hepatic toxicity (CPA/CPB) • 5.1% RILD
Weiner et al. 2016 [37]	26	55 (5 fx)	5 (1.6–12.3)	88/12/0	91 (1 y)	45 (1 y)	• 23/19.2% ≥ grade 3 GI toxicity (acute/late) • 65.4/69.2% ≥ grade 3 (acute/late) • 34.6% worsening of CP score ≥ 2
Takeda et al. 2008 [38]	16	35–50 (5–7 fx)	(1.9–7)	87.5/12.5/0	NA	NA	• 37.5% transient elevation of CP score

sion, a recent study by Lee and colleagues reported slightly longer OS rate at one year of 56.5% and worsening of CP sore by at least two points in only 17% of patients with CP score B and C after treatment with SBRT. Of note, patients in this cohort had less advanced disease compared to the cohort reported by Culleton et al. (tumor diameter: 3.1 vs. 8.6 cm; portal vein thrombosis: 4.3% vs. 76%) [30].

18.3 Charged Particles Therapy

In recent years, charged particle therapy in form of Proton Beam Therapy (PBT) and Carbon Ion Radiotherapy (CIRT) has been developed into an exciting new treatment modality to overcome the limitations of photon-based radiotherapy in HCC.

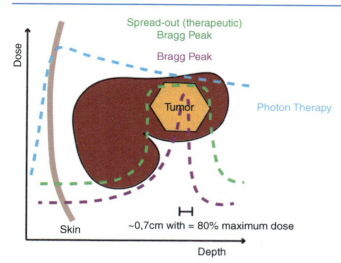

Fig. 18.1 Figure showing overview over depth dose distribution of photon and proton therapy

PBT is a form of radiotherapy that utilizes protons instead of photon beams to deliver therapeutic doses of radiation. The advantage to this modality is the characteristic depth-dose curve with a pronounced dose peak, also known as Bragg peak, and a very fast dose demarcation in the periphery, which provides significant normal tissue dose sparing [43, 44] (Fig. 18.1). In the clinic, multiple proton beams with differences in energies are applied together to create a spread-out Bragg peak and therefore a "treating field". Due to the low radiation tolerance of normal liver tissue, PBT has unique beneficial capabilities for HCC patients [45, 46]. This technique seems to be especially beneficial for patients with large tumors or multiple lesions, as a decrease of the tumor target dose often has to be accepted in photon-based therapies in order to comply with dose constraints in the surrounding normal liver tissue [47, 48].

Several studies have reported promising efficacy of PBT with high local control rates (61.9–100%) (Table 18.2). The high efficacy of local PBT was histologically proven in a phase II study, where explants after liver transplantation following PBT showed a pathological complete response in 33% and only microscopic residual disease in an additional 39% of patients [56]. Of note, Chadha and colleagues reported that BED>90 GyE led to significantly higher OS and showed a trend towards higher LC after two years compared to patients treated with lower doses of radiation [54]. Based on this data, authors hypothesized that further dose escalation beyond 90 GyE might be beneficial to improve outcomes.

Conversely, the frequency and severity of adverse effects are comparatively lower. In a prospective phase II study reported by Bush and colleagues, which included patients with CP-C liver cirrhosis, only 5 out of 76 patients experienced Grade 2 GI adverse reactions after PBT, and no Grade 3 or higher toxicities were reported in the treatment cohort [56]. Similarly, a retrospective, propensity matched analysis showed significantly higher biological equivalent doses for patients treated with protons in combination with lower risk of RILD compared to the photon group, again highlighting the potentially better protection properties of normal tissue [63]. In another retrospective analysis, authors reported higher OS in combination with lower risk of RILD after irradiation with protons compared to photons. Of note, LC rates did not differ between the groups [64]. However, a meta-analysis by Qi et al. reported similar OS rates between PBT and SBRT patients [65]. Currently, a clinical study directly comparing photon vs. proton SBRT for patients with HCC is underway, led by our institution (clinicaltrials.gov identifier NCT03186898). This study will prospectively evaluate which treatment modality has higher efficacy with lower risk of severe side effects and has integrated biomarker evaluations such as plasma hepatocyte growth factor (HGF) [66], discussed below.

Another study directly compared PBT with TACE, one of the most common treatment modalities for irresectable HCC patients, found a trend towards higher two-year LC rate (88% vs. 45%) while OS rates did not significantly differ between the two groups in an interim analysis. Of note, the number of days patients had to be hospitalized was significantly lower in the PBT group (24 vs 166 days) [58].

However, there are also limitations and disadvantages of PBT compared to photon-based therapies. These primarily include significantly higher costs and comparatively lower availability of PBT. Furthermore, PBT is more susceptible to range uncertainties due to daily changes in abdominal anatomy causing changes in tissue density (e.g., bowel movement). The relative added benefit of PBT vs. photon therapy remains to be yet determined.

Similar to PBT, CIRT also creates a Bragg peak and dose falls of rapidly after reaching it. The main advantage of CIRT over PBT lies however in its increased relative biological effectiveness (RBE), through induction of higher cellular damage [67, 68]. Generally, a RBE of three is assumed for CIRT [44]. Clinical data from patients treated with CIRT for HCC is relatively spare and studies have been mainly conducted in Asia resulting in potential differences to Western patients due to different etiologies of disease. Applied radiation doses for CIRT range from 40–79.5 GyE with acceptable side effects in patients (Table 18.3). Of note, several studies excluded patients with known risk factors for acute and long-term toxicities including close proximity to GI organs (<1 cm), portal vein invasion and/or thrombosis as well as patients with poor baseline liver function. Furthermore, especially for CIRT, radiation dose is largely based on retrospective analysis of Japanese patient data and further, prospective larger clinical trials are needed to define dose-constraints as well as optimal treatment dose. In this

Table 18.2 Overview over current studies on proton irradiation of HCC patients

	n	Dose (fractionation)	tumor size median (range) [cm]	Baseline liver function (CPA/CPB/CPC) [%]	LC [%]	OS [%]	Toxicities	Ref
Retrospective analysis								
Fukuda et al. 2017	129	66–77 GyE (10–35 fx)	3.9 (1.0–13.5)	78.3/21.7/0	94/87/75 (5 y) (CPA/CPB/CPC)	69/66/25 (5 y) (CPA/CPB/CPC)	• No grade 3	[49]
Lee et al. 2014	27	55 GyE (20–22 fx)	7 (3–16)	66.7/33.3/0	70.7 (1 y) 61.9 (2 y)	55.6 (1 y) 33.3 (2 y)	• No grade 3	[50]
Sekino et al. 2020	21	72.6 Gy (RBE)	8 (3.9–20)	57.1/42.9/0	NA	62 (1 y) 33 (2 y) 19 (3 y)	• No grade 3	[51]
Hata et al. 2006	21	73 Gy (18 fx)	4 (2.5–10)	28.6/28.6/42.8	93 (5 y)	62 (2 y) 33 (5 y)	• No grade 3	[52]
Chiba et al. 2005	162	72 Gy (16 fx)	<3.0:26.6% 3–5: 56.3% >5: 17.2%	50.6/38.3/6.2	86.9 (5 y)	23.5 (5 y)	• 1.1% infection Biloma • 1.1% GI Bleeding • 0.5% common bile Duct stenosis	[53]
Chadha et al. 2019	46	97.7 GyE (15 fx)	6 (1.5–21)	83/17/0	81 (2 y)	62 (2 y)	• 13% worsening CP score • 13% acute grade 3	[54]
Mizuhata et al 2018	40	60–80 CGE (20–38 fx)	3.7 (1.1–12.4)	70/30/0	94% (2 y)	76% (2 y)	• 2.5% grade 3 GI toxicity and aszites	[55]
Sugahara et al. 2009	22	72.6 GyE (22 fx)	11 (10–14)	50/50/0	87% (2 y)	36% (2 y)	• No grade 3	[48]
Prospective studies								
Bush et al. 2011	76	63 Gy (15 fx)	5.5 (mean)	29/47.4/23.7	NA	34/13/12 mo (CPA/CPB/CPC)	• No grade 3	[56]
Hong et al. 2016	83	67.5 GyE (15 fx)	5 (1.9–12)	79.5/15.7/0	94.8 (2 y)	63.2 (2 y)	• 4.8% grade 3	[47]
Kim et al. 2020	45	70 GyE (10 fx)	1.6 (1.0–6.8)	100/0/0	95.2 (3 y)	86.4 (3 y)	• No grade 3 • 4.4% worsening CP score	[57]
Kim et al. 2015	27	60 GyE (20 fx) 66 GyE (22 fx) 72 GyE (24 fx)	(1.3–7)	88.9/11.1/0	79.9 (3 y) 63.9 (5 y)	56.4 (3 y) 42.3 (5 y)	• No grade 3 • 3.7% worsening CP score	[46]
Bush et al. 2016	69	70.2 Gy (15 fx)	3.2 (1.8–6.5)	NA	88 (2 y)	59 (2 y)	• 2 pt. hospitalized within 30 days	[58]
Mizumoto et al. 2011	266	66 GyE (10 fx) 72.6 GyE (22 fx) 77 GyE (35 fx)	3.4 (0.6–13)	76/23/1	98 (1 y) 87 (3 y) 81 (5 y)	87 (1 y) 61 (3 y) 48 (5 y)	• 0.8% grade 3 erythema • 1.1% rib fractures • 1.1% grade 3 GI toxicity	[59]
Kawashima et al. 2005	30	76 CGE (20 fx)	4.5 (2.5–8.2)	66.7/33.3/0	96% (2 y)	66% (2 y)	• 4 deaths • 40% grade 3 acute toxicity	[60]
Fukumitsu et al. 2009	51	66 GyE (10 fx)	<5: 88.2% >5: 11.8%	80.4/19.6/0	94.5 (3 y) 87.8 (5 y)	49.2 (3 y) 38.7 (5 y)	• 15.7% worsening of CP class	[61]
Hata et al. 2007	21	60 Gy (10 fx) 66 Gy (22 fx) 70 Gy (35 fx)	4 (1–13.5)	71.4/23.8/4.8	100% (3 y)	62% (3 y)	• 9.5% grade 3 thrombopenia	[62]

context Shibuya and colleagues reported feasibility of a 60 Gy (RBE) in four fractions schedule, equivalent to 125 Gy in EQD2 ($\alpha/\beta = 10$), which is the highest dose-escalation protocol to date. Promising results were also reported recently in patients with large HCC tumors (median tumor diameter 5.3 cm) treated with doses between 52.8 and 60 GyE [77]. Of note, a matched-pair analysis revealed that for stage IIIB patients with inferior vena cava thrombus

Table 18.3 Overview over current data on carbon ion therapy

	n	Dose (fractionation)	Tumor size median (range) [cm]	Baseline liver function (CPA/CPB/CPC) [%]	LC [%]	OS [%]	Toxicities	Ref.
Retrospective analysis								
Shiba et al. 2017	31	52.8/60 Gy (RBE) (4 fx); 50 Gy (12 fx)	4.5 (1.5–9.3)	87.1/12.9/0	89.2 (2 y)	82.3 (2 y)	• 9.7% grade 3 encephalopathia • 3.2% progressed from CPA to CPB	[69]
Shibuya et al. 2018	174	48 Gy (RBE) (2 fx) 52.8/60 Gy (RBE) (4 fx)	3 (0.8–10.3)	88/12/0	94.6/87.7/81 (1/2/3 y)	94.5/82.5/73.3 (1/2/3 y)	• 5.7% grade ¾ • 1.7% RILD	[70]
Shiba et al. 2020	11	52.8/60 Gy (RBE) (4 fx); 50 Gy (RBE) (12 fx)	5.3 (2.7–11.9)	90.9/9.1/0	78 (3 y)	64 (3 y)	• No grade 3	[67]
Prospective studies								
Kato et al. 2004	24	49.5–79.5 GyE (15 fx)	5 (2.1–8.5)	66.7/33.3/0	92/81/81 (1/3/5 y)	92/50/25 (1/3/5 y)	• 22%/25% worsening of CP score ≥ 2 (acute/late) • 4% grade 3 early skin reaction • 20.8% grade 3 hematologic	[71]
Habermehl et al. 2013	6	40 Gy (RBE) (4 fx)	3.5 (0.9–4.5)	66.7/16.7/0	100 (11 mo)	11 mo (mean OS)	• 83% mild fatigue • No grade 3	[72]
Shibuya et al. 2019	21	60 Gy (RBE) (4 fx)	4.8 mean (3–7.8)	100/0/0	92.3 (2 y)	80 (2 y)	• No grade 3	[73]
Kasuya et al. 2017	124	52.8 Gy (RBE) (4 fx)	4 (1–12)	77/23/0	94.7/91.4/90.0 (1/3/5 y)	90.3/50/25 (1/3/5)	• 4 deaths of liver failure • 2% grade 3: Skin • 1.6% rib fracture • 29/22% change in CP score + 1 (3/6 mo) • 3/5% change in CP score + 2 (3/6 mo)	[74]
Imada et al. 2010	64	52.8 GyE (4 fx)	4 (1.2–12)	92.2/7.8/0	87.8/95.7 (5 y) (porta hepatis group/non-porta hepatis group)	44.4/22.2; 60.9/34.8 (3/5 y) (porta hepatis group/non-porta hepatis group)	• No grade 3 • 84.4% change in CP score + 1 • 15.6% change in CP score + 2	[75]
Komatsu et al. 2011	16	52.8 GyE (4 fx); 52.8 GyE (8 fx)	NA	75/18.75/6.25	NA	61.1/36.7 (1/3 y)	• No grade 3	[76]

median OS was higher in patients treated with either PBT or CIRT compared to surgery, and resulted in significantly lower treatment-related side effects (0% vs. 26%) [78].

18.4 MRI Guided Therapy

One of the main challenges for radiotherapy in liver cancer is the inter- and intra-fractional variability as well as poor resolution of tumors in x-ray images. The simplest method to overcome this issue is to increase therapeutic margins—resulting in increased non-targeted liver irradiation and thus risk of developing radiation-induced liver damage (RILD) and liver failure. In recent years, a new system combining a linear accelerator with an MRI system—called MR linear accelerator (MR Linac)—has been developed by industry to address this gap. First promising results of studies utilizing this hybrid system on treatment of liver cancers, including HCC, have been published [79, 80]. Another advantage of this system is the option to adapt the radiation plan to the daily anatomy of the patient [81]. In this context, Henke and colleagues reported a phase 1 study showing improved sparing of organs at risk as well as good feasibility of their online-adapted radiation system in 20 patients [82].

18.5 Combination Strategies Using Cytotoxics

Combination of trans-arterial chemoembolization (TACE) with irradiation—either conventionally fractionated radiotherapy and SBRT [34]—has shown improved outcomes in patients with HCC compared to TACE alone [83]. This advantage is most likely due to tumor-shrinkage after TACE, resulting in smaller target volumes for radiotherapy. Of note, a direct comparison between conventional fractionated and hypofractionated radiotherapy in combination with TACE revealed higher OS for patients treated with SBRT in advanced HCC [84]. Another important factor influencing efficacy of combination treatment may be tumor size. For tumors >3 cm, Jacob and colleagues showed a significant increase of OS in the combination group compared to TACE alone (33 vs. 20 months) [21]. Similarly, in a retrospective analysis, Su et al. observed significant differences in OS between combination therapies (SBRT + TAE/TACE or TAE/TACE+SBRT) and SBRT alone (p = 0.047), indicating that a combinational approach might be beneficial for patients with large tumors (>5 cm longest tumor diameter).

Radiotherapy has also been successfully used as a bridging strategy for patients who were not eligible for other types of treatments [85, 86]. In this context, a BEDs between 15.7 and 124.8 Gy have been used showing good local control rates for medium sized HCC tumors [26, 87].

18.6 Radioimmunotherapy

Over the last decade, systemic treatment options for advanced HCC have rapidly evolved starting with the approval of the multi-tyrosine kinase inhibitor (mTKI) sorafenib. Since then, several more agents have been successfully tested in phase III trials including the mTKIs lenvatinib, regorafenib and cabozantinib and the anti-VEGFR2 antibody ramucirumab [88]. Furthermore, several phase I/II studies with immune checkpoint blockers (ICB), such as the anti- Programmed cell Death protein 1 (PD-1) antibodies pembrolizumab and nivolumab as well as ipilimumab, an anti-cytotoxic T lymphocyte antigen 4 (CTLA-4) antibody, have shown promising results with durable responses in patients with advanced HCC [89, 90]. However, the randomized phase 3 trials on nivolumab and pembrolizumab monotherapy missed their predefined primary endpoints despite significant activity in a minority of the advanced HCC patients [91, 92]. These results suggested that the efficacy of ICB therapy needs to be enhanced by combinational treatment approaches. In this context, a promising approach is combining different ICBs, for example ipilimumab and nivolumab [93]. In addition, ICB with atezolizumab (an anti-PD ligand 1 antibody) combined with an anti-VEGF antibody (bevacizumab) showed substantial and significant improvement in OS and PFS in a randomized phase III trial in advanced HCC [94].

The availability of these systemic drugs has raised the feasibility of combinations with radiotherapy. In particular, over recent years, increasing evidence has supported the rationale of combining radiotherapy with immunotherapy for earlier stages of the disease. The unique characteristics of radiotherapy offer the great potential to boost immunotherapeutic responses in patients. These include induction of immunogenic cell death, supporting a pro-inflammatory tumor microenvironment and increased availability of tumor antigen [95]. In brief, radiotherapy has the potential to support the conversion of an immunologically "cold" tumor into an immunologically "hot" tumor [96]. Radiotherapy has also been shown to upregulate PD-L1 expression in vivo and combination of radiation with anti-PD-L1 treatment led to significantly increased survival in a murine HCC mouse model [97]. In a first clinical case study of five patients treated with SBRT followed by anti-PD1 antibody treatment, two patients showed complete response, while three patients had partial responses according to modified RECIST criteria. The one-year LC and OS rates were both 100% [98]. These results are in line with a report by Yu and colleagues, who observed significantly longer PFS and OS in patients with previous or concurrent radiotherapy during application of nivolumab for advanced HCC [99]. To further enhance synergy of radiotherapy and ICB approaches with triple-combinational treatments are also under evaluation. In a preclinical study by Sheng and colleagues, authors reported further improvement of survival of tumor bearing mice after adding an ATR inhibitor (AZD6738) to radioimmunotherapy (radiation + αPD-L1) [100].

Clearly, further preclinical and clinical studies are needed to elucidate the potential synergy of radiation and ICB and to clarify optimal treatment schedules, dosing and fractionation.

18.7 Challenges and Opportunities

Radiotherapy for liver malignancies, including HCC, is limited by various factors including radiation field size and underlying liver damage. One of the most severe side effects of liver irradiation is the induction of RILD. While the etiology remains largely unclear up to date, the clinical presentation in patients ranges from pain in the right upper quadrant to subacute onset of liver failure and death. Retrospective analysis of patient data presumes a threshold for onset of

RILD at a total liver irradiation dose above 30 Gy and probability of developing RILD increases with radiation dose and irradiated volume. Bujold and colleagues reported worsening of Child-Pugh Score in 29% of patients three months after SBRT and seven patient deaths were possibly related to radiotherapy [35]. Similar side effect profiles were reported by other groups [16, 37]. Of note, several groups reported a correlation between either treated or spared liver volume with worsening of CP scores [101–103]. This "volume-response" relationship seemed to be independent of treatment modality (photons vs. protons) and was also shown for patients treated with PBT [104]. However, treatment doses and regimes differed greatly diminishing comparability of studies and transferability to other patient groups. Other risk factors for development of RILD seem to be underlying viral hepatitis [24, 105], portal vein thrombosis and tumor morphology (singular vs. multi-site HCC).

Many groups have attempted to establish biomarkers to predict occurrence and severity of RILD. Sanuki and his group for example proposed Grade 3 elevated transaminases and thrombocytopenia as well as a CP score above eight to be predictive for severe liver damage after irradiation [106]. Another promising biomarker is circulating HGF level as a direct measure for hepatic function. HGF is a ligand mainly produced by activated stromal cells in the liver. It has been shown previously to be associated with high CP scores and liver fibrosis [107, 108]. In our recent study of PBT, we found that high plasma HGF level was associated with lower two-year OS compared to patients with low plasma level (14% to 69%) [66, 109]. Currently, a phase III trial is underway trying to validate these results in a larger patient cohort (clinicaltrials.gov identifier NCT03186898).

Underlying liver damage, e.g., cirrhosis, further increases the risk of (fatal) liver failure after radiotherapy. In a phase I study by Cárdenes and his group, the treatment protocol for patients with CP-B disease had to be amended to lower doses after two patients developed Grade 3 hepatic toxicity at 42 Gy, whereas dose could be escalated to 48 Gy in patients with CP-A disease without dose-limiting toxicity [32]. A worsening of CP scores after radiotherapy has also been shown to be associated with decreased OS in patients [22]. Taken together, these findings resulted in a recommendation to treat CP-B patients with lower doses and fractionation sizes, in acceptance of resulting lower LC rates.

Another possibly severe side effect of liver radiotherapy is gastrointestinal toxicity. Patients with underlying portal hypertension due to liver cirrhosis seem to be susceptible to developing gastroduodenal complications including ulcers, bleeding and perforation. This is likely related to impaired function and defense mechanisms of the gastrointestinal mucosa. As a result, it has been recommended that patients with impaired liver function should undergo esophagogastroduodenoscopy prior to SBRT to determine underlying health concerns and subsequently adopting fractionated radiotherapy and normal tissue constraints if warranted [34]. Indeed, the study of Weiner and colleagues showed that only 81% of patients could receive the prescribed dose of 55 Gy due to dose constraints [37]. Park and colleagues specifically addressed this question in a study and showed that radiotherapy could be safely administered also for tumors within 2 cm of radiosensitive organs, including the stomach, duodenum, large bowel and esophagus, with an adapted fractionation regime (35/40/50 Gy in 10 fraction over a two-week period) [23]. Of note, long-term local control rates were slightly lower compared to studies delivering higher doses/fraction [13].

18.8 Summary

In conclusion, radiotherapy has shown promise as a therapeutic option for liver cancers, including in patients with less favorable disease and underlying liver cirrhosis. Further studies are needed to clarify the optimal treatment option for these patients, including the type of radiation technique and specific combination with other treatment modalities. Currently, evidence indicates that for patients with small tumors photon radiotherapy may be effective, particularly as MR-guided radiotherapy. For patients with advanced and large tumors, charged particle therapies can result in very promising survival data in combination with a favorable side effect profile.

References

1. Siegel RL, Miller KD, Jemal A. Cancer statistics, 2020. CA Cancer J Clin. 2020;70:7–30.
2. Schwarz RE, Smith DD. Trends in local therapy for hepatocellular carcinoma and survival outcomes in the US population. Am J Surg. 2008;195:829–36.
3. Mazzaferro V, Bhoori S, Sposito C, et al. Milan criteria in liver transplantation for hepatocellular carcinoma: an evidence-based analysis of 15 years of experience. Liver Transpl. 2011;17(Suppl 2):S44–57.
4. Mazzaferro V, Regalia E, Doci R, et al. Liver transplantation for the treatment of small hepatocellular carcinomas in patients with cirrhosis. N Engl J Med. 1996;334:693–9.
5. El-Serag HB, Siegel AB, Davila JA, et al. Treatment and outcomes of treating of hepatocellular carcinoma among medicare recipients in the United States: a population-based study. J Hepatol. 2006;44:158–66.
6. Vogel A, Cervantes A, Chau I, et al. Hepatocellular carcinoma: ESMO clinical practice guidelines for diagnosis, treatment and follow-up. Ann Oncol. 2019;30:871–3.
7. Rou WS, Lee BS, Moon HS, Lee ES, Kim SH, Lee HY. Risk factors and therapeutic results of early local recurrence after transcatheter arterial chemoembolization. World J Gastroenterol. 2014;20:6995–7004.

8. Ayav A, Germain A, Marchal F, et al. Radiofrequency ablation of unresectable liver tumors: factors associated with incomplete ablation or local recurrence. Am J Surg. 2010;200:435–9.
9. Lu DS, Yu NC, Raman SS, et al. Radiofrequency ablation of hepatocellular carcinoma: treatment success as defined by histologic examination of the explanted liver. Radiology. 2005;234:954–60.
10. Wahl DR, Stenmark MH, Tao Y, et al. Outcomes after stereotactic body radiotherapy or radiofrequency ablation for hepatocellular carcinoma. J Clin Oncol. 2016;34:452–9.
11. Hara K, Takeda A, Tsurugai Y, et al. Radiotherapy for hepatocellular carcinoma results in comparable survival to radiofrequency ablation: a propensity score analysis. Hepatology (Baltimore, Md). 2019;69:2533–45.
12. Lou J, Li Y, Liang K, et al. Hypofractionated radiotherapy as a salvage treatment for recurrent hepatocellular carcinoma with inferior vena cava/right atrium tumor thrombus: a multi-center analysis. BMC Cancer. 2019;19:668.
13. Park J, Jung J, Kim D, et al. Long-term outcomes of the 2-week schedule of hypofractionated radiotherapy for recurrent hepatocellular carcinoma. BMC Cancer. 2018;18:1040.
14. Bae SH, Park HC, Lim DH, et al. Salvage treatment with hypofractionated radiotherapy in patients with recurrent small hepatocellular carcinoma. Int J Radiat Oncol Biol Phys. 2012;82:e603–7.
15. Kim M, Kay CS, Jang WI, Kim MS, Lee DS, Jang HS. Prognostic value of tumor volume and radiation dose in moderate-sized hepatocellular carcinoma: a multicenter analysis in Korea (KROG 14-17). Medicine. 2017;96:e7202.
16. Andolino DL, Johnson CS, Maluccio M, et al. Stereotactic body radiotherapy for primary hepatocellular carcinoma. Int J Radiat Oncol Biol Phys. 2011;81:e447–53.
17. Yoon SM, Lim YS, Park MJ, et al. Stereotactic body radiation therapy as an alternative treatment for small hepatocellular carcinoma. PLoS One. 2013;8:e79854.
18. Sanuki N, Takeda A, Oku Y, et al. Stereotactic body radiotherapy for small hepatocellular carcinoma: a retrospective outcome analysis in 185 patients. Acta Oncol. 2014;53:399–404.
19. Huertas A, Baumann AS, Saunier-Kubs F, et al. Stereotactic body radiation therapy as an ablative treatment for inoperable hepatocellular carcinoma. Radiother Oncol. 2015;115:211–6.
20. Su TS, Lu HZ, Cheng T, et al. Long-term survival analysis in combined transarterial embolization and stereotactic body radiation therapy versus stereotactic body radiation monotherapy for unresectable hepatocellular carcinoma >5 cm. BMC Cancer. 2016;16:834.
21. Jacob R, Turley F, Redden DT, et al. Adjuvant stereotactic body radiotherapy following transarterial chemoembolization in patients with non-resectable hepatocellular carcinoma tumours of ≥ 3 cm. HPB. 2015;17:140–9.
22. Culleton S, Jiang H, Haddad CR, et al. Outcomes following definitive stereotactic body radiotherapy for patients with child-Pugh B or C hepatocellular carcinoma. Radiother Oncol. 2014;111:412–7.
23. Park JH, Yoon SM, Lim YS, et al. Two-week schedule of hypofractionated radiotherapy as a local salvage treatment for small hepatocellular carcinoma. J Gastroenterol Hepatol. 2013;28:1638–42.
24. Huang BS, Tsang NM, Lin SM, et al. High-dose hypofractionated X-ray radiotherapy for hepatocellular carcinoma: tumor responses and toxicities. Oncol Lett. 2013;6:1514–20.
25. Yao E, Chen J, Zhao X, et al. Efficacy of stereotactic body radiotherapy for recurrent or residual hepatocellular carcinoma after transcatheter arterial chemoembolization. Biomed Res Int. 2018;2018:5481909.
26. Katz AW, Chawla S, Qu Z, Kashyap R, Milano MT, Hezel AF. Stereotactic hypofractionated radiation therapy as a bridge to transplantation for hepatocellular carcinoma: clinical outcome and pathologic correlation. Int J Radiat Oncol Biol Phys. 2012;83:895–900.
27. Méndez Romero A, Wunderink W, Hussain SM, et al. Stereotactic body radiation therapy for primary and metastatic liver tumors: a single institution phase i-ii study. Acta Oncol. 2006;45:831–7.
28. Tse RV, Hawkins M, Lockwood G, et al. Phase I study of individualized stereotactic body radiotherapy for hepatocellular carcinoma and intrahepatic cholangiocarcinoma. J Clin Oncol. 2008;26:657–64.
29. Scorsetti M, Comito T, Cozzi L, et al. The challenge of inoperable hepatocellular carcinoma (HCC): results of a single-institutional experience on stereotactic body radiation therapy (SBRT). J Cancer Res Clin Oncol. 2015;141:1301–9.
30. Lee P, Ma Y, Zacharias I, et al. Stereotactic body radiation therapy for hepatocellular carcinoma in patients with child-Pugh B or C cirrhosis Adv Radiat Oncol. 2020;5:889–96.
31. Seo YS, Kim JN, Keum B, et al. Radiotherapy for 65 patients with advanced unresectable hepatocellular carcinoma. World J Gastroenterol. 2008;14:2394–400.
32. Cárdenes HR, Price TR, Perkins SM, et al. Phase I feasibility trial of stereotactic body radiation therapy for primary hepatocellular carcinoma. Clin Transl Oncol. 2010;12:218–25.
33. Takeda A, Sanuki N, Tsurugai Y, et al. Phase 2 study of stereotactic body radiotherapy and optional transarterial chemoembolization for solitary hepatocellular carcinoma not amenable to resection and radiofrequency ablation. Cancer. 2016;122:2041–9.
34. Kang JK, Kim MS, Cho CK, et al. Stereotactic body radiation therapy for inoperable hepatocellular carcinoma as a local salvage treatment after incomplete transarterial chemoembolization. Cancer. 2012;118:5424–31.
35. Bujold A, Massey CA, Kim JJ, et al. Sequential phase I and II trials of stereotactic body radiotherapy for locally advanced hepatocellular carcinoma. J Clin Oncol. 2013;31:1631–9.
36. Lasley FD, Mannina EM, Johnson CS, et al. Treatment variables related to liver toxicity in patients with hepatocellular carcinoma, child-Pugh class a and B enrolled in a phase 1-2 trial of stereotactic body radiation therapy. Pract Radiat Oncol. 2015;5:e443–9.
37. Weiner AA, Olsen J, Ma D, et al. Stereotactic body radiotherapy for primary hepatic malignancies - report of a phase I/II institutional study. Radiother Oncol. 2016;121:79–85.
38. Takeda A, Takahashi M, Kunieda E, et al. Hypofractionated stereotactic radiotherapy with and without transarterial chemoembolization for small hepatocellular carcinoma not eligible for other ablation therapies: preliminary results for efficacy and toxicity. Hepatol Res. 2008;38:60–9.
39. Sheth N, Osborn V, Lee A, Schreiber D. Stereotactic ablative radiotherapy fractionation for hepatocellular carcinoma in the United States. Cureus. 2020;12:e8675.
40. Park HC, Seong J, Han KH, Chon CY, Moon YM, Suh CO. Dose-response relationship in local radiotherapy for hepatocellular carcinoma. Int J Radiat Oncol Biol Phys. 2002;54:150–5.
41. Park W, Lim DH, Paik SW, et al. Local radiotherapy for patients with unresectable hepatocellular carcinoma. Int J Radiat Oncol Biol Phys. 2005;61:1143–50.
42. Liu MT, Li SH, Chu TC, et al. Three-dimensional conformal radiation therapy for unresectable hepatocellular carcinoma patients who had failed with or were unsuited for transcatheter arterial chemoembolization. Jpn J Clin Oncol. 2004;34:532–9.
43. Hu M, Jiang L, Cui X, Zhang J, Yu J. Proton beam therapy for cancer in the era of precision medicine. J Hematol Oncol. 2018;11:136.
44. Skinner HD, Hong TS, Krishnan S. Charged-particle therapy for hepatocellular carcinoma. Semin Radiat Oncol. 2011;21:278–86.
45. Wang X, Krishnan S, Zhang X, et al. Proton radiotherapy for liver tumors: dosimetric advantages over photon plans. Med Dosim. 2008;33:259–67.
46. Kim JY, Lim YK, Kim TH, et al. Normal liver sparing by proton beam therapy for hepatocellular carcinoma: comparison with heli-

cal intensity modulated radiotherapy and volumetric modulated arc therapy. Acta Oncol. 2015;54:1827–32.
47. Hong TS, Wo JY, Yeap BY, et al. Multi-institutional phase II study of high-dose hypofractionated proton beam therapy in patients with localized, unresectable hepatocellular carcinoma and intrahepatic cholangiocarcinoma. J Clin Oncol. 2016;34:460–8.
48. Sugahara S, Oshiro Y, Nakayama H, et al. Proton beam therapy for large hepatocellular carcinoma. Int J Radiat Oncol Biol Phys. 2010;76:460–6.
49. Fukuda K, Okumura T, Abei M, et al. Long-term outcomes of proton beam therapy in patients with previously untreated hepatocellular carcinoma. Cancer Sci. 2017;108:497–503.
50. Lee SU, Park JW, Kim TH, et al. Effectiveness and safety of proton beam therapy for advanced hepatocellular carcinoma with portal vein tumor thrombosis. Strahlenther Onkol. 2014;190:806–14.
51. Sekino Y, Okumura T, Fukumitsu N, et al. Proton beam therapy for hepatocellular carcinoma associated with inferior vena cava tumor thrombus. J Cancer Res Clin Oncol. 2020;146:711–20.
52. Hata M, Tokuuye K, Sugahara S, et al. Proton beam therapy for hepatocellular carcinoma with limited treatment options. Cancer. 2006;107:591–8.
53. Chiba T, Tokuuye K, Matsuzaki Y, et al. Proton beam therapy for hepatocellular carcinoma: a retrospective review of 162 patients. Clin Cancer Res. 2005;11:3799–805.
54. Chadha AS, Gunther JR, Hsieh CE, et al. Proton beam therapy outcomes for localized unresectable hepatocellular carcinoma. Radiother Oncol. 2019;133:54–61.
55. Mizuhata M, Takamatsu S, Shibata S, et al. Respiratory-gated proton beam therapy for hepatocellular carcinoma adjacent to the gastrointestinal tract without fiducial markers. Cancers. 2018;10:58.
56. Bush DA, Kayali Z, Grove R, Slater JD. The safety and efficacy of high-dose proton beam radiotherapy for hepatocellular carcinoma: a phase 2 prospective trial. Cancer. 2011;117:3053–9.
57. Kim TH, Park JW, Kim BH, et al. Phase II study of hypofractionated proton beam therapy for hepatocellular carcinoma. Front Oncol. 2020;10:542.
58. Bush DA, Smith JC, Slater JD, et al. Randomized clinical trial comparing proton beam radiation therapy with transarterial chemoembolization for hepatocellular carcinoma: results of an interim analysis. Int J Radiat Oncol Biol Phys. 2016;95:477–82.
59. Mizumoto M, Okumura T, Hashimoto T, et al. Proton beam therapy for hepatocellular carcinoma: a comparison of three treatment protocols. Int J Radiat Oncol Biol Phys. 2011;81:1039–45.
60. Kawashima M, Furuse J, Nishio T, et al. Phase II study of radiotherapy employing proton beam for hepatocellular carcinoma. J Clin Oncol. 2005;23:1839–46.
61. Fukumitsu N, Sugahara S, Nakayama H, et al. A prospective study of hypofractionated proton beam therapy for patients with hepatocellular carcinoma. Int J Radiat Oncol Biol Phys. 2009;74:831–6.
62. Hata M, Tokuuye K, Sugahara S, et al. Proton beam therapy for aged patients with hepatocellular carcinoma. Int J Radiat Oncol Biol Phys. 2007;69:805–12.
63. Cheng JY, Liu CM, Wang YM, et al. Proton versus photon radiotherapy for primary hepatocellular carcinoma: a propensity-matched analysis. Radiat Oncol (London, England). 2020;15:159.
64. Sanford NN, Pursley J, Noe B, et al. Protons versus photons for unresectable hepatocellular carcinoma: liver decompensation and overall survival. Int J Radiat Oncol Biol Phys. 2019;105:64–72.
65. Qi WX, Fu S, Zhang Q, Guo XM. Charged particle therapy versus photon therapy for patients with hepatocellular carcinoma: a systematic review and meta-analysis. Radiother Oncol. 2015;114:289–95.
66. Hong TS, Grassberger C, Yeap BY, et al. Pretreatment plasma HGF as potential biomarker for susceptibility to radiation-induced liver dysfunction after radiotherapy. NPJ Precis Oncol. 2018;2:22.
67. Shiba S, Shibuya K, Kawashima M, et al. Comparison of dose distributions when using carbon ion radiotherapy versus intensity-modulated radiotherapy for hepatocellular carcinoma with macroscopic vascular invasion: a retrospective analysis. Anticancer Res. 2020;40:459–64.
68. Abe T, Saitoh J, Kobayashi D, et al. Dosimetric comparison of carbon ion radiotherapy and stereotactic body radiotherapy with photon beams for the treatment of hepatocellular carcinoma. Radiat Oncol (London, England). 2015;10:187.
69. Shiba S, Abe T, Shibuya K, et al. Carbon ion radiotherapy for 80 years or older patients with hepatocellular carcinoma. BMC Cancer. 2017;17:721.
70. Shibuya K, Ohno T, Terashima K, et al. Short-course carbon-ion radiotherapy for hepatocellular carcinoma: a multi-institutional retrospective study. Liver Int. 2018;38:2239–47.
71. Kato H, Tsujii H, Miyamoto T, et al. Results of the first prospective study of carbon ion radiotherapy for hepatocellular carcinoma with liver cirrhosis. Int J Radiat Oncol Biol Phys. 2004;59:1468–76.
72. Habermehl D, Debus J, Ganten T, et al. Hypofractionated carbon ion therapy delivered with scanned ion beams for patients with hepatocellular carcinoma - feasibility and clinical response. Radiat Oncol (London, England). 2013;8:59.
73. Shibuya K, Ohno T, Katoh H, et al. A feasibility study of high-dose hypofractionated carbon ion radiation therapy using four fractions for localized hepatocellular carcinoma measuring 3 cm or larger. Radiother Oncol. 2019;132:230–5.
74. Kasuya G, Kato H, Yasuda S, et al. Progressive hypofractionated carbon-ion radiotherapy for hepatocellular carcinoma: combined analyses of 2 prospective trials. Cancer. 2017;123:3955–65.
75. Imada H, Kato H, Yasuda S, et al. Comparison of efficacy and toxicity of short-course carbon ion radiotherapy for hepatocellular carcinoma depending on their proximity to the porta hepatis. Radiother Oncol. 2010;96:231–5.
76. Komatsu S, Fukumoto T, Demizu Y, et al. The effectiveness of particle radiotherapy for hepatocellular carcinoma associated with inferior vena cava tumor thrombus. J Gastroenterol. 2011;46:913–20.
77. Shiba S, Shibuya K, Okamoto M, et al. Clinical impact of Hypofractionated carbon ion radiotherapy on locally advanced hepatocellular carcinoma. Radiat Oncol (London, England). 2020;15:195.
78. Komatsu S, Kido M, Asari S, et al. Particle radiotherapy, a novel external radiation therapy, versus liver resection for hepatocellular carcinoma accompanied with inferior vena cava tumor thrombus: a matched-pair analysis. Surgery. 2017;162:1241–9.
79. Feldman AM, Modh A, Glide-Hurst C, Chetty IJ, Movsas B. Real-time magnetic resonance-guided liver stereotactic body radiation therapy: an institutional report using a magnetic resonance-Linac system. Cureus. 2019;11:e5774.
80. Hal WA, Straza MW, Chen X, et al. Initial clinical experience of Stereotactic Body Radiation Therapy (SBRT) for liver metastases, primary liver malignancy, and pancreatic cancer with 4D-MRI based online adaptation and real-time MRI monitoring using a 1.5 Tesla MR-Linac. PLoS One. 2020;15:e0236570.
81. Mittauer K, Paliwal B, Hill P, et al. A new era of image guidance with magnetic resonance-guided radiation therapy for abdominal and thoracic malignancies. Cureus. 2018;10:e2422.
82. Henke L, Kashani R, Robinson C, et al. Phase I trial of stereotactic MR-guided online adaptive radiation therapy (SMART) for the treatment of oligometastatic or unresectable primary malignancies of the abdomen. Radiother Oncol. 2018;126:519–26.
83. Guo WJ, Yu EX, Liu LM, et al. Comparison between chemoembolization combined with radiotherapy and chemoembolization alone for large hepatocellular carcinoma. World J Gastroenterol. 2003;9:1697–701.

84. Wang C, Li S, Sun A, et al. The comparison of outcomes between hypofractionated and conventional 3D-CRT regimens used in combination with TACE as first-line treatment of advanced hepatocellular carcinoma. Tumour Biol. 2015;36:4967–72.
85. Guarneri A, Franco P, Romagnoli R, et al. Stereotactic ablative radiation therapy prior to liver transplantation in hepatocellular carcinoma. Radiol Med. 2016;121:873–81.
86. Gresswell S, Tobillo R, Hasan S, et al. Stereotactic body radiotherapy used as a bridge to liver transplant in patients with hepatocellular carcinoma and child-Pugh score ≥8 cirrhosis. J Radiosurg SBRT. 2018;5:261–7.
87. O'Connor JK, Trotter J, Davis GL, Dempster J, Klintmalm GB, Goldstein RM. Long-term outcomes of stereotactic body radiation therapy in the treatment of hepatocellular cancer as a bridge to transplantation. Liver Transpl. 2012;18:949–54.
88. Yang JD, Hainaut P, Gores GJ, Amadou A, Plymoth A, Roberts LR. A global view of hepatocellular carcinoma: trends, risk, prevention and management. Nat Rev Gastroenterol Hepatol. 2019;16:589–604.
89. El-Khoueiry AB, Sangro B, Yau T, et al. Nivolumab in patients with advanced hepatocellular carcinoma (CheckMate 040): an open-label, non-comparative, phase 1/2 dose escalation and expansion trial. Lancet. 2017;389:2492–502.
90. Zhu AX, Finn RS, Edeline J, et al. Pembrolizumab in patients with advanced hepatocellular carcinoma previously treated with sorafenib (KEYNOTE-224): a non-randomised, open-label phase 2 trial. Lancet Oncol. 2018;19:940–52.
91. Finn RS, Ryoo BY, Merle P, et al. Pembrolizumab as second-line therapy in patients with advanced hepatocellular carcinoma in KEYNOTE-240: a randomized, double-blind, phase III trial. J Clin Oncol. 2020;38:193–202.
92. Yau T, Park JW, Finn RS, et al. LBA38_PR - CheckMate 459: a randomized, multi-center phase III study of nivolumab (NIVO) vs sorafenib (SOR) as first-line (1L) treatment in patients (pts) with advanced hepatocellular carcinoma (aHCC). Ann Oncol. 2019;30:v874–5.
93. Yau T, Kang YK, Kim TY, et al. Efficacy and safety of nivolumab plus ipilimumab in patients with advanced hepatocellular carcinoma previously treated with sorafenib: the CheckMate 040 randomized clinical trial. JAMA Oncol. 2020;6(11):e204564.
94. Finn RS, Qin S, Ikeda M, et al. Atezolizumab plus bevacizumab in unresectable hepatocellular carcinoma. N Engl J Med. 2020;382:1894–905.
95. Chajon E, Castelli J, Marsiglia H, De Crevoisier R. The synergistic effect of radiotherapy and immunotherapy: a promising but not simple partnership. Crit Rev Oncol Hematol. 2017;111:124–32.
96. Demaria S, Coleman CN, Formenti SC. Radiotherapy: changing the game in immunotherapy. Trends Cancer. 2016;2:286–94.
97. Kim KJ, Kim JH, Lee SJ, Lee EJ, Shin EC, Seong J. Radiation improves antitumor effect of immune checkpoint inhibitor in murine hepatocellular carcinoma model. Oncotarget. 2017;8:41242–55.
98. Chiang CL, Chan ACY, Chiu KWH, Kong FS. Combined stereotactic body radiotherapy and checkpoint inhibition in unresectable hepatocellular carcinoma: a potential synergistic treatment strategy. Front Oncol. 2019;9:1157.
99. Yu JI, Lee SJ, Lee J, et al. Clinical significance of radiotherapy before and/or during nivolumab treatment in hepatocellular carcinoma. Cancer Med. 2019;8:6986–94.
100. Sheng H. Huang Y, Xiao Y, et al. ATR inhibitor AZD6738 enhances the antitumor activity of radiotherapy and immune checkpoint inhibitors by potentiating the tumor immune microenvironment in hepatocellular carcinoma. J Immunother Cancer. 2020;8:e000340.
101. Son SH, Choi BO, Ryu MR, et al. Stereotactic body radiotherapy for patients with unresectable primary hepatocellular carcinoma: dose-volumetric parameters predicting the hepatic complication. Int J Radiat Oncol Biol Phys. 2010;78:1073–80.
102. Dyk P, Weiner A, Badiyan S, Myerson R, Parikh P, Olsen J. Effect of high-dose stereotactic body radiation therapy on liver function in the treatment of primary and metastatic liver malignancies using the Child-Pugh score classification system. Pract Radiat Oncol. 2015;5:176–82.
103. Velec M, Haddad CR, Craig T, et al. Predictors of liver toxicity following stereotactic body radiation therapy for hepatocellular carcinoma. Int J Radiat Oncol Biol Phys. 2017;97:939–46.
104. Hsieh CE, Venkatesulu BP, Lee CH, et al. Predictors of radiation-induced liver disease in Eastern and Western patients with hepatocellular carcinoma undergoing proton beam therapy. Int J Radiat Oncol Biol Phys. 2019;105:73–86.
105. Cheng JC, Wu JK, Lee PC, et al. Biologic susceptibility of hepatocellular carcinoma patients treated with radiotherapy to radiation-induced liver disease. Int J Radiat Oncol Biol Phys. 2004;60:1502–9.
106. Sanuki N, Takeda A, Oku Y, et al. Influence of liver toxicities on prognosis after stereotactic body radiation therapy for hepatocellular carcinoma. Hepatol Res. 2015;45:540–7.
107. Krawczyk M, Zimmermann S, Hess G, et al. Panel of three novel serum markers predicts liver stiffness and fibrosis stages in patients with chronic liver disease. PLoS One. 2017;12:e0173506.
108. Prystupa A, Kiciński P, Sak J, Boguszewska-Czubara A, Toruń-Jurkowska A, Załuska W. Proinflammatory cytokines (IL-1α, IL-6) and hepatocyte growth factor in patients with alcoholic liver cirrhosis. Gastroenterol Res Pract. 2015;2015:532615.
109. Hong TS, Grassberger C, Yeap BY, et al. Hepatocyte growth factor is associated with liver dysfunction and survival: biomarker results of a phase 2 study of proton beam therapy in patients with hepatocellular carcinoma and intrahepatic cholangiocarcinoma. Int J Radiati Oncol Biol Phys. 2017;99:S89.

Recent Update in Chemotherapy of Cholangiocarcinoma

Jung Hyun Jo, Seungmin Bang, and Si Young Song

Abstract

Cholangiocarcinoma (CCA) is a relatively rare form of cancer arising from epithelial cells lining the biliary tree that connects the liver and gallbladder to the small intestine and can be categorized into intrahepatic CCA (iCCA), perihilar CCA (pCCA), and distal CCA (dCCA). While only surgical resection can provide a cure, most CCAs are detected at inoperable stages and are associated with poor prognosis with median survival of less than two years in patients with advanced stages. Moreover, CCA has a high recurrence rate, even after radical surgery. Therefore, chemotherapy has an important role in the treatment but presently the available systemic medical therapies for advanced and metastatic CCA have very limited efficacy. Even though scientists and physicians have made tremendous efforts to reveal genetic factors of tumor progression and identify CCA specific biomarkers and novel therapeutic targets to develop novel drugs, we are still in the dark when it comes to this cancer. In this chapter, we summarize the latest updates on chemotherapy-based strategies for CCA, and discuss therapeutic targets that may be relevant for the future development of personalized treatments.

19.1 Introduction

Approximately 10,000 new cases of cholangiocarcinoma (CCA) are diagnosed annually in the USA, and a five-year survival rate is below 20% [1, 2]. In Korea, there are 11.2 new cases per 100,000 people annually, and a five-year survival rate is 29.2% according to cancer statistics in 2014 [3]. CCA usually presents at an advanced stage, with less than 20% of patients considered resectable at presentation. Additionally, in applicable cases, adjuvant chemotherapy indicated improved rates of relapse-free survival and overall survival (OS). In inoperable patients, stent placement can be offered to treat obstructive jaundice, control symptoms such as pruritus, cholangitis, and decrease related secondary morbidity. Endobiliary techniques have made notable progress, improving stent median patency with self-expanding metal stents.

The standard therapy using gemcitabine and platinum-based chemotherapy showed a median OS of 12 months for inoperable CCA. Namely, there are only few therapeutic options that establish an effective chemotherapy for advanced CCA failed to standard therapy.

In recent years, some studies have focused on CCA behavior and their prognosis by anatomical site, their responsivity to chemotherapeutic agents and their molecular pathophysiology, finding new treatment options, the carcinogenic role of some genes, and genes affected by copy number alterations which can benefit from targeted therapy. Common gene alterations beyond Kras and TP53 have been identified. These include potentially actionable mutations in the HER and FGFR families, MAPK, PI3K/AKT/mTOR pathway, and epigenetic alterations (e.g., IDH). Interestingly, the molecular changes are dependent on the anatomical location of the tumor with iCCA shown to have IDH1/2 and FGFR2 alterations, whereas eCCA and gallbladder cancers are more likely to have ERBB2 or catenin beta 1 alterations. We herein discuss these latest therapeutic strategies and their possible future applications.

J. H. Jo · S. Bang · S. Y. Song (✉)
Division of Gastroenterology, Department of Internal Medicine, Yonsei University College of Medicine, Seoul, South Korea
e-mail: sysong@yuhs.ac

19.2 Systemic Chemotherapy

19.2.1 Adjuvant Therapy

Necessity of adjuvant chemotherapy for CCA is based on prognosis after surgical treatments. Surgery is only a curative therapy; however, two-year survival after radical resection was reported to be very poor [4]. A meta-analysis data from retrospective studies presented a survival benefit in high-risk patients with node-positive disease and R1 resection status after surgery [5].

Several randomized clinical trials were reported, but could provide only limited evidence of adjuvant chemotherapy for CCA. In ESPAC-3 trial [6], of the 428 patients included in the primary analysis, 144 patients were assigned to the observation group, and 143 patients received 5-FU chemotherapy and the other 141 patients received gemcitabine chemotherapy. Median survival for the observation group was 35.2 months; for patients treated with 5-FU plus folinic acid, 38.9 months; and for patients treated with gemcitabine, 45.7 months, without significant differences by log-rank analysis across the three groups (p = 0.23). In secondary analyses adjusting for prognostic variables using multiple regression analysis, the HR for chemotherapy compared with observation was 0.75 (p = 0.03) and for gemcitabine, 0.70 (p = 0.03). In the BCAT trial [7], 226 patients with eCCA were randomly selected to either receive gemcitabine or were assigned to the observation group, only after surgery. There were no significant differences between groups in median OS (62.3 vs. 63.8 months, p = 0.964) and median disease-free survival (DFS) (36.0 vs 39.9 months, p = 0.693). The PRODIGE-12/ACCORD-18 trial [8] reported no significant differences between gemcitabine and oxaliplatin (GEM/OX) versus observation only after surgical resection of CCA in 196 patients (DFS, 30.4 vs. 18.5, p = 0.48). The BILCAP study [9], which enrolled 447 patients, also could not show survival benefits of the capecitabine arm compared to the observational arm in terms of OS by the intention-to-treat (ITT) analysis. However, the per-protocol analysis presented an increased median OS in the capecitabine arm (53 vs. 36 months, p = 0.028). Despite the native difficulties in research about CCA which has anatomical heterogeneity, adjuvant chemotherapy for CCA is considered effective with limited evidences, and the nodal involvements and histologic margin status after surgery are suggested as the most important conditions for indication of adjuvant therapy. Further large randomized trials are required for confirmative prospection, and one of the largest ongoing RCT, the ACTICCA study (gemcitabine/cisplatin versus capecitabine, NCT02170090) is expected to report further evidences for adjuvant chemotherapy in CCA.

19.2.2 First-Line Therapy

Currently recommended standard treatment for patients with advanced CCA is gemcitabine and cisplatin combination therapy. The phase III ABC-02 trial [10] revealed that the combination of gemcitabine with cisplatin improved the OS by 3.6 months compared to gemcitabine alone. The median OS was 11.7 months in the cisplatin–gemcitabine group and 8.1 months among the gemcitabine group (p < 0.001). The median progression survival (8.0 versus 5.0 months, p < 0.001) and tumor control rate (81.4 versus 71.8%, p = 0.049) were improved in the cisplatin–gemcitabine group.

Further studies are ongoing to develop more effective chemotherapy. The phase III FUGA-BT trial [11] presented non-inferiority of gemcitabine/S1 chemotherapy compared to gemcitabine/cisplatin chemotherapy. Of a total 354 patients, there was no difference between gemcitabine/S1 and gemcitabine/cisplatin in median OS (15.1 vs. 13.4 months, p = 0.046 for non-inferiority). In the phase II trial of gemcitabine/cisplatin plus nanoparticle albumin-bound (nab)-paclitaxcel [12], sixty CCA patients showed prolonged median progression-free survival (PFS) and median OS (11.8 months and 19.2 months) compared to historical controls. Phase III randomized clinical trial is ongoing to compare this regimen to gemcitabine/cisplatin (S1815 clinical trial, NCT03768414). In the ongoing Phase II/III AMEBICA trial, modified FOLFIRINOX (5-FU, irinotecan, and oxaliplatin) is currently tested as a first-line treatment for patients with CCA (NCT02591030).

19.2.3 Second-Line Therapy

Still, there is no effective second-line anti-cancer drugs that could be used for patients who have failed to respond to the gemcitabine-based first-line chemotherapy. Moreover, cisplatin is associated with severe toxicity, including dose-dependent nephrotoxicity and neurotoxicity, which may limit the opportunities for second-line treatment after disease progression. In a systematic review of second-line chemotherapy in advanced CCA including 25 studies comprising of 14 phase II clinical trials [13], nine retrospective analyses, and two case reports evaluate the level of evidence for the use of second-line chemotherapy. A total of 761 patients were evaluated and the mean OS was 7.2 months while the mean PFS, response rate, and disease control rate were 3.2 months, 7.7%, and 49.5%, respectively.

Several novel anti-cancer strategies are being tried. The phase III ABC-06 trial [14] reported mFOLFOX (5-FU and oxaliplatin) showed a benefit in terms of OS compared to active supportive care (HR 0.69, 95% CI [0.50–0.97], p = 0.031) in 162 CCA patients following progression after first-line gemcitabine/cisplatin therapy. Median OS (months), 6 m and 12 m OS-rate (%) were 6.2 m, 50.6%, and 25.9% for the mFOLFOX and 5.3 m, 35.5%, and 11.4% for the active supportive care, respectively. Other novel regimens, such as FOLFIRINOX (5-FU, irinotecan, and oxaliplatin) [15], and nal-irinotecan based regimens (the NALIRICC trial; NCT03043547, the NAPOLI-2 trial; NCT04005339) are currently under investigation as second-line chemotherapy for CCA.

19.3 Targeted Therapy

Recently the advent of next-generation sequencing has substantially improved the ability of scientists to understand the complex molecular events occurring in CCA, including interactions between gene mutations and disease risk factors. Among the discoveries regarding the important mutations associated with the pathogenesis of CCA are mutations in isocitrate dehydrogenase (IDH) 1/2, as well as mutations in the genes involved in chromatin remodeling, such as ARID1A, PBRM1, and BAP1. The deregulation of several growth factor tyrosine kinases, noted in various malignancies including CCA, also plays a critical role in tumor initiation and progression. These include the FGFR pathway and EGFR and HGFR pathways. The most promising target for CCA identified in recent years is within the FGF signaling pathway.

Molecular profiles of CCA have been recently investigated. In addition to the combination of cytotoxic chemotherapeutic agents, combination regimen with target agents was studied in several trials. A couple of studies evaluated possibility of growth factor inhibitors as combination agent with conventional chemotherapeutic agents, such as EGFR [16–18] and VEGF receptor inhibiting agents [19, 20]. However, there was not enough evidence yet to use these target agents in advanced CCA.

Recent updates about fusion genes as therapeutic target of CCA are notable. Research has shown that fibroblast growth factor receptor (FGFR) or neurotropic tyrosine kinase receptor (NTRK) fusions and IDH-1/2 or BRAF mutations may be potential therapeutic targets in CCA [21–23]. A phase II study of BGJ398 [24], an pan-FGFR kinase inhibitor, has shown clinical activity against CCA with FGFR alterations. Sixty-one patients with FGFR2 fusion, mutation, or amplification were enrolled and the overall response rate was 14.8%, disease control rate was 75.4%, and median PFS was 5.8 months (95% CI, 4.3 to 7.6 months). Another phase II trial with Derazantinib (ARQ 087) [25], a pan-FGFR kinase inhibitor, presented encouraging anti-tumor activity with 29 iCCA patients with FGFR2 fusion. Overall response rate was 20.7%, disease control rate was 82.8%, median PFS was 5.7 months (95% CI: 4.04–9.2 months). Currently, there are several ongoing trials of FGFR inhibitors; Infigratinib, pemigatinib, and futibatinib have been studied in the Phase III trials as first-line therapy (NCT03773302, NCT03656536, and NCT04093362). In the Phase III ClarIDHy trial [26], ivosidenib (AG-120), a targeted inhibitor of mutated IDH1, was evaluated in 230 patients with IDH1-mutant, chemotherapy-refractory CCA. Median PFS was significantly improved with ivosidenib compared with placebo (2.7 vs. 1.4 months; hazard ratio 0.37; one-sided p < 0.0001). Other ongoing clinical trials targeting the IDH1 mutation in CCA are also being investigated (NCT03212274 and NCT03878095) and results are expected. However, FGFR and IHD inhibitors have only proven to be effective in about 20% of iCCA patients with FGFR fusion and IHD mutations. Other druggable targets need to be developed to oppose CCA for the future.

19.4 Immunotherapy

Advances in the field of cancer immunology has made it possible to apply immunotherapy as a new therapeutic option for CCA. Immunotherapy strengthens the immune system of patients to struggle against cancer through personalized vaccination, adoptive immunotherapy, or immune checkpoint inhibitor therapy. Pembrolizumab, an immune checkpoint inhibitor that blocks programmed cell death 1 (PD-1) pathway and its ligands (PD-L1 and PD-L2), has been reported as a possible promising anti-tumor agent in patients with advanced CCA in the interim results of the clinical trial, KEYNOTE-028. In the study, objective response rate was 17% (four partial response and four had stable disease) [27]. Recently, final result from the KEYNOTE-158 (NCT02628067; phase II) and KEYNOTE-028 (NCT02054806; phase Ib) studies [28] reported the efficacy and safety of pembrolizumab for the treatment of advanced CCA. Total 104 patients from KEYNOTE-158 and 24 patients from KENOTE-028 presented ORR; 5.8%, median OS/PFS; 7.5/2.0 months and ORR; 13%, median OS/PFS; 5.7/1.8 months, respectively. The response of pembrolizumab was not related to PD-L1 expression of the tumor.

The therapeutic efficacy of immunotherapy as monotherapy is a disappointment so far. Consequently, combinations of immunotherapy and other therapies are under evaluation. Nivolumab alone or in combination with cisplatin plus gemcitabine was tested in phase I trial with 30 advanced CCA patients [29]. The median OS and PFS were much longer in combined therapy cohort than nivolumab monotherapy (OS; 15.4 vs. 5.2 months, PFS; 4.2 vs. 1.4 months). In the phase I JVDF study [30], ramucirumab, a VEFG inhibitor, in combination with pembrolizumab was used to treat advanced CCA. Of the total 26 patients, objective response rate was

4%. Median PFS and OS were 1.6 months and 6.4 months, respectively. Immunotherapy and chemotherapy combinations are currently ongoing in phase III studies, TOPAZ-1 (Durvalumab with Gemcitabine/Cisplatin, NCT03875235) and KEYNOTE-966 (Pembrolizumab with Gemcitabine/Cisplatin, NCT04003636). In addition to the immune checkpoint inhibitor, NK cell, T-cell, and dendritic cell based therapies have been tested to treat CCA. Depending on the findings of ongoing research, immunotherapy may be a new treatment option for CCA.

19.5 Precision Medicine

Personalized therapy has come into focus with the recent advances in targeted therapy and immunotherapy, in conjunction to systemic chemotherapy or chemoradiation for the treatment of CCA. Understanding the molecular pathways associated with the development and progression of CCA may help identify novel biomarkers and develop potential therapeutic targets. With further development of gene sequencing technic, it is expected that precision therapy will be possible by judging the presence or absence of a specific gene and selecting an optimized therapeutic drug accordingly. So far, most previous studies have viewed cholangiocarcinoma and gallbladder cancer as a group of biliary tract cancers. However, recent studies revealed that molecular profiling of CCA is different from gallbladder cancer. Furthermore, several studies reported that iCCA and eCCA have different molecular features. Jusakul et al. reported their research combining whole-genome sequencing and epigenomic analysis of CCA with 489 patients from 10 countries [31]. In the study, CCA was subgrouped into four clusters according to their molecular features. Cluster 1 comprised mostly fluke positive tumors with enrichment of ARID1A and BRCA1/2 mutations. Cluster 2 was characterized by a mix of fluke positive and negative tumors with upregulated CTNNB1, WNT5B, and NKT1. Clusters 1 and 2 were enriched in TP53 mutation and ERBB2 gene expression. Clusters 3 and 4 were mostly fluke negative tumors, and cluster 3 exhibited specific upregulation of immune checkpoint genes; PD-1, PD-L2, and BTLA. Cluster 4 had BAP1, IDH1/2 mutations, and FGFR alterations. Anatomical classification of CCA was associated with clusters. Clusters 1 and 2 were enriched in eCCA, whereas clusters 3 and 4 consisted almost of iCCA. Moreover, iCCA was more frequently mutated in BAP1 and KRAS. Clinically, each clusters had different OS; clusters 3 and 4 had significantly better OS than clusters 1 and 2. These findings suggest heterogenic clinical features of CCA were also based on genetic and epigenetic variance of tumors, and further studies have to focus on classifying subgroups according to treatment strategy and identifying novel therapeutic targets for personalized therapy.

19.6 Summary and Conclusion

Adjuvant chemotherapy is effective in patients with CCA after curative surgery, especially with lymph node-positive and resection margin-positive disease. Although there are limited clinical trial data to establish a standard chemotherapy regimen for CCA after surgery, current recommended regimens are 5-FU-based or gemcitabine-based chemotherapies.

Palliative chemotherapy has an important role in the treatment of advanced and recurrent CCA. According to the results of randomized controlled phase III trial, gemcitabine plus cisplatin combination became the standard treatment option for first-line chemotherapy of advanced and metastatic CCA. The efficacy of second-line chemotherapy was not definite until now. Novel targeted therapies reported promising results especially with fusion gene targets in iCCA but immunotherapies demonstrated disappointing results so far.

Precision medicine is recently on the rise in addition to cytotoxic systemic chemotherapy or chemoradiation. The identification of novel therapeutic targets based on next-generation sequencing technology and immunologic assessment is actively being researched. In the future, anti-cancer therapy for CCA will develop to identify specific genes expressed in individual patients and provide personalized therapies accordingly.

However, the therapeutic landscape for CCA has expanded considerably in recent years after being nearly forgotten for a few decades. Combined therapy with chemotherapy, locoregional treatment, and immunotherapy are promising strategies. The knowledge of the biology of CCA is still limited compared to that of other solid cancers, but the available data on target therapies have added hopes for the future management of CCA and will likely continue to improve patient outcomes. Results from ongoing clinical trials are eagerly awaited to further elucidate the optimal management of this aggressive malignancy.

References

1. Jo JH, Song SY. Chemotherapy of cholangiocarcinoma: current management and future directions. Topics in the surgery of the biliary tree. IntechOpen. 2018;2:35–52.
2. Siegel RL, Miller KD, Jemal A. Cancer statistics, 2017. CA Cancer J Clin. 2017;67:7–30.

3. Korea Central Cancer Registry NCC. Annual report of cancer statistics in Korea in 2014. Ministry of Health and Welfare; 2016.
4. Jarnagin WR, Fong Y, DeMatteo RP, Gonen M, Burke EC, Bodniewicz BJ, et al. Staging, resectability, and outcome in 225 patients with hilar cholangiocarcinoma. Ann Surg. 2001;234:507–17. discussion 517–509
5. Horgan AM, Amir E, Walter T, Knox JJ. Adjuvant therapy in the treatment of biliary tract cancer: a systematic review and meta-analysis. J Clin Oncol. 2012;30:1934–40.
6. Neoptolemos JP, Moore MJ, Cox TF, Valle JW, Palmer DH, McDonald AC, et al. Effect of adjuvant chemotherapy with fluorouracil plus folinic acid or gemcitabine vs observation on survival in patients with resected periampullary adenocarcinoma: the espac-3 periampullary cancer randomized trial. JAMA. 2012;308:147–56.
7. Ebata T, Hirano S, Konishi M, Uesaka K, Tsuchiya Y, Ohtsuka M, et al. Randomized clinical trial of adjuvant gemcitabine chemotherapy versus observation in resected bile duct cancer. Br J Surg. 2018;105:192–202.
8. Edeline J, Benabdelghani M, Bertaut A, Watelet J, Hammel P, Joly JP, et al. Gemcitabine and oxaliplatin chemotherapy or surveillance in resected biliary tract cancer (PRODIGE 12-ACCORD 18-UNICANCER GI): a randomized phase III study. J Clin Oncol. 2019;37:658–67.
9. Primrose JN, Fox RP, Palmer DH, Malik HZ, Prasad R, Mirza D, et al. Capecitabine compared with observation in resected biliary tract cancer (BILCAP): a randomised, controlled, multicentre, phase 3 study. Lancet Oncol. 2019;20:663–73.
10. Valle J, Wasan H, Palmer DH, Cunningham D, Anthoney A, Maraveyas A, et al. Cisplatin plus gemcitabine versus gemcitabine for biliary tract cancer. N Engl J Med. 2010;362:1273–81.
11. Morizane C, Okusaka T, Mizusawa J, Katayama H, Ueno M, Ikeda M, et al. Combination gemcitabine plus s-1 versus gemcitabine plus cisplatin for advanced/recurrent biliary tract cancer: the FUGA-BT (JCOG1113) randomized phase III clinical trial. Ann Oncol. 2019;30:1950–8.
12. Shroff RT, Javle MM, Xiao L, Kaseb AO, Varadhachary GR, Wolff RA, et al. Gemcitabine, cisplatin, and nab-paclitaxel for the treatment of advanced biliary tract cancers: a phase 2 clinical trial. JAMA Oncol. 2019;5:824–30.
13. Lamarca A, Hubner RA, David Ryder W, Valle JW. Second-line chemotherapy in advanced biliary cancer: a systematic review. Ann Oncol. 2014;25:2328–38.
14. Lamarca A, Palmer DH, Wasan HS, Ross PJ, Ma YT, Arora A, et al. ABC-06 | a randomised phase III, multi-centre, open-label study of active symptom control (ASC) alone or asc with oxaliplatin / 5-FU chemotherapy (ASC+mFOLFOX) for patients (pts) with locally advanced / metastatic biliary tract cancers (ABC) previously-treated with cisplatin/gemcitabine (CisGem) chemotherapy. J Clin Oncol. 2019;37:4003.
15. Belkouz A, Vos-Geelen J, Eskens F, Mathot RAA, van Gulik T, van Oijen MGH, et al. Efficacy and safety of FOLFIRINOX in advanced biliary tract cancer after failure of gemcitabine plus cisplatin: a phase II trial. J Clin Oncol. 2019;37:4086.
16. Sohal DP, Mykulowycz K, Uehara T, Teitelbaum UR, Damjanov N, Giantonio BJ, et al. A phase II trial of gemcitabine, irinotecan and panitumumab in advanced cholangiocarcinoma. Ann Oncol. 2013;24:3061–5.
17. Gruenberger B, Schueller J, Heubrandtner U, Wrba F, Tamandl D, Kaczirek K, et al. Cetuximab, gemcitabine, and oxaliplatin in patients with unresectable advanced or metastatic biliary tract cancer: a phase 2 study. Lancet Oncol. 2010;11:1142–8.
18. Malka D, Cervera P, Foulon S, Trarbach T, de la Fouchardiere C, Boucher E, et al. Gemcitabine and oxaliplatin with or without cetuximab in advanced biliary-tract cancer (bingo): a randomised, open-label, non-comparative phase 2 trial. Lancet Oncol. 2014;15:819–28.
19. Valle JW, Wasan H, Lopes A, Backen AC, Palmer DH, Morris K, et al. Cediranib or placebo in combination with cisplatin and gemcitabine chemotherapy for patients with advanced biliary tract cancer (abc-03): a randomised phase 2 trial. Lancet Oncol. 2015;16:967–78.
20. Moehler M, Maderer A, Schimanski C, Kanzler S, Denzer U, Kolligs FT, et al. Gemcitabine plus sorafenib versus gemcitabine alone in advanced biliary tract cancer: a double-blind placebo-controlled multicentre phase II AIO study with biomarker and serum programme. Eur J Cancer. 2014;50:3125–35.
21. Lamarca A, Barriuso J, McNamara MG, Valle JW. Molecular targeted therapies: ready for "prime time" in biliary tract cancer. J Hepatol. 2020;73:170–85.
22. Sia D, Losic B, Moeini A, Cabellos L, Hao K, Revill K, et al. Massive parallel sequencing uncovers actionable FGFR2-PPHLN1 fusion and ARAF mutations in intrahepatic cholangiocarcinoma. Nat Commun. 2015;6:6087.
23. Wang Y, Ding X, Wang S, Moser CD, Shaleh HM, Mohamed EA, et al. Antitumor effect of FGFR inhibitors on a novel cholangiocarcinoma patient derived xenograft mouse model endogenously expressing an FGFR2-CCDC6 fusion protein. Cancer Lett. 2016;380:163–73.
24. Javle M, Lowery M, Shroff RT, Weiss KH, Springfeld C, Borad MJ, et al. Phase II study of BGJ398 in patients with fgfr-altered advanced cholangiocarcinoma. J Clin Oncol. 2018;36:276–82.
25. Mazzaferro V, El-Rayes BF, Droz Dit Busset M, Cotsoglou C, Harris WP, Damjanov N, et al. Derazantinib (ARQ 087) in advanced or inoperable fgfr2 gene fusion-positive intrahepatic cholangiocarcinoma. Br J Cancer. 2019;120:165–71.
26. Abou-Alfa GK, Macarulla T, Javle MM, Kelley RK, Lubner SJ, Adeva J, et al. Ivosidenib in idh1-mutant, chemotherapy-refractory cholangiocarcinoma (ClarIDHy): a multicentre, randomised, double-blind, placebo-controlled, phase 3 study. Lancet Oncol. 2020;21:796–807.
27. Bang YJ, Doi T, De Braud F, Piha-Paul S, Hollebecque A, Razak ARA, et al. Safety and efficacy of pembrolizumab (mk-3475) in patients (pts) with advanced biliary tract cancer: interim results of keynote-028. Eur J Cancer. 2015;51:S112.
28. Piha-Paul SA, Oh DY, Ueno M, Malka D, Chung HC, Nagrial A, et al. Efficacy and safety of pembrolizumab for the treatment of advanced biliary cancer: results from the keynote-158 and keynote-028 studies. Int J Cancer. 2020;147:2190–8.
29. Ueno M, Ikeda M, Morizane C, Kobayashi S, Ohno I, Kondo S, et al. Nivolumab alone or in combination with cisplatin plus gemcitabine in Japanese patients with unresectable or recurrent biliary tract cancer: a non-randomised, multicentre, open-label, phase 1 study. Lancet Gastroenterol Hepatol. 2019;4:611–21.
30. Arkenau HT, Martin-Liberal J, Calvo E, Penel N, Krebs MG, Herbst RS, et al. Ramucirumab plus pembrolizumab in patients with previously treated advanced or metastatic biliary tract cancer: nonrandomized, open-label, phase I trial (JVDF). Oncologist. 2018;23:1407–e1136.
31. Jusakul A, Cutcutache I, Yong CH, Lim JQ, Huang MN, Padmanabhan N, et al. Whole-genome and epigenomic landscapes of etiologically distinct subtypes of cholangiocarcinoma. Cancer Discov. 2017;7:1116–35.

Chemotherapy in Pancreatic Ductal Adenocarcinoma

Hee Seung Lee, Seung Woo Park, and Si Young Song

Abstract

Pancreatic ductal adenocarcinoma (PDAC) can be divided into four groups: (1) resectable, (2) borderline, (3) locally advanced, and (4) disseminated. Resection followed by adjuvant chemotherapy remains the standard of care for resectable PDAC. All patients with resected PDAC should be offered six months of adjuvant chemotherapy in the absence of contraindications. The modified FOLFIRINOX (mFOLFIRINOX) is preferred in the absence of concerns for toxicity or tolerance. Alternatively, combination therapy with gemcitabine and capecitabine, monotherapy with gemcitabine alone or (Fluorouracil) plus folinic acid can be offered as adjuvant chemotherapy. Recently, there has been increasing interest in neoadjuvant treatment due to the inability of some patients from adjuvant chemotherapy and the possibility of early micrometastasis even in resectable and borderline resectable PDAC. Patients at high risk for positive surgical margins are not considered to be good candidates for an upfront resection but may be potentially downstaged and safely resected following neoadjuvant therapy. Recent clinical trials suggested that neoadjuvant chemotherapy with FOLFIRINOX, gemcitabine plus nanoparticle albumin-bound paclitaxel (nab-paclitaxel), and S-1 might be useful. However, future confirmative prospective studies are required. Unfortunately, most PDAC patients are metastatic at their diagnosis. FOLFIRINOX and gemcitabine plus nab-paclitaxel are the first recommended chemotherapeutic drugs. FOLFIRINOX and gemcitabine plus nab-paclitaxel combination therapy has shown remarkable effects in patients with advanced PDAC with relatively good systemic conditions, bringing new hope in the treatment of advanced PDAC. In addition, new targeted treatments and immune treatments using cancer cell-specific targets, and new treatments for desmoplastic characteristics of PDAC tissues are being attempted.

20.1 Introduction

PDAC is a highly lethal malignancy originating from the exocrine pancreas [1]. Radical resection is the only hope to expect long-term survival; however, at the time of diagnosis, resectable PDAC accounts for only about 20% of all patients, and most patients were diagnosed as advanced stages [2–4]. Even, cancer recurrence occurs in 70–80% of patients with PDAC discovered in the early stages after radical surgery [5]. Including surgery, chemotherapy, radiation therapy, chemo-combined radiotherapy, and palliative care are treatment options depending on the stage of PDAC [6, 7]. For decades, various types of anti-cancer treatment have been tried. However, PDAC shows a remarkable resistance to established therapeutic options due to various innate mechanisms of resistance like genetic and epigenetic alterations and a complex and dense tumor microenvironment. Here, we aimed to discuss briefly the present and future of anticancer therapy in PDAC.

20.2 Chemotherapy in PDAC

20.2.1 Neoadjuvant Chemotherapy

The benefits of neoadjuvant therapy include the potential to downsize tumors in order to increase the possibility of a margin-free resection, select PDAC patients with more stable disease, and to treat micrometastases at an earlier stage [8]. Preoperative chemotherapy in borderline resectable PDAC can be effective and well-tolerated [8, 9]. Patients with borderline resectable PDAC demonstrated a higher possibility for an R0 resection after neoadjuvant therapies, and

H. S. Lee · S. W. Park · S. Y. Song (✉)
Division of Gastroenterology, Department of Internal Medicine, Yonsei University College of Medicine, Seoul, South Korea
e-mail: sysong@yuhs.ac

survival of patients who underwent surgical resection was better than that of those who did not [10]. However, further research is necessary to discover the best regimens to use in a neoadjuvant setting.

Recently, neoadjuvant chemotherapy was also used in patients with resectable cases, especially in those with high-risk features. The phase III study (Prep-02/JSAP-05) of neoadjuvant gemcitabine plus S-1 conducted in Japan [11] demonstrated a significant survival benefit of neoadjuvant chemotherapy, with a median overall survival (OS) of 36.7 months vs. 26.6 months for upfront surgery (Hazard ratio (HR) 0.72, p = 0.015). Approximately 80% of patients enrolled in this study had resectable PDAC at diagnosis. On the other hand, perioperative mFOLFIRINOX and gemcitabine/nab-paclitaxel showed similar efficacy, with acceptable safety and resectability rates. The 2-year OS was 41.6% with mFOLFIRINOX (p = 0.42) and 48.8% with gemcitabine/nab-paclitaxel (p = 0.12) [12]. Median OS was 22.4 months and 23.6 months, respectively. Median disease-free survival (DFS) after resection was 10.9 months with mFOLFIRINOX and 14.2 months with gemcitabine/nab-paclitaxel. Neither arm's two-year OS estimate was statistically significantly higher than the prior historical threshold of 40%. The National Comprehensive Cancer Network (NCCN) guideline of the USA recommends neoadjuvant therapy for selected patients who appear technically resectable but have poor prognostic features (i.e., markedly elevated CA 19–9, large primary tumors, large regional lymph nodes, excessive weight loss, and extreme pain) [13].

20.2.2 Adjuvant Chemotherapy

Postoperative adjuvant chemotherapy is routinely performed in all resectable PDAC. It was proven effective by improving recurrence free survival and OS after curative resection. The ESPAC-1 trial demonstrated a benefit of adjuvant chemotherapy with 5-FU and folinic acid (leucovorin) in patients following resection. The CONKO-001 trial showed increased DFS and OS with the use of adjuvant gemcitabine for six cycles compared with no adjuvant treatment [14].

The Japan Adjuvant Study Group of Pancreatic Center (JASPAC) conducted a phase III comparative study of postoperative adjuvant chemotherapy with gemcitabine alone versus S-1 alone in patients who had undergone resection for PDAC [15, 16]. A total of 385 patients were enrolled, and the five-year survival rate and median survival time were 44.1% vs. 24.4% and 46.5 vs. 25.5 months in both groups. It has been reported that S-1 is superior to gemcitabine (HR 0.56, p < 0.0001). The ESPAC-4 trial demonstrated that the combined gemcitabine plus capecitabine regimen yielded a significantly prolonged OS after PDAC resection as compared to gemcitabine monotherapy (25.5 vs. 28.0 months, HR 0.82, p = 0.032) [17, 18].

In the phase III PRODIGE 24/Canadian Cancer Trials Group (CCTG) PA.6 trial, patients aged 18–79 years with resected (R0 or R1) PDAC, who had not received prior chemotherapy or radiation therapy were randomly assigned to receive six months of adjuvant therapy with either gemcitabine or mFOLFIRINOX [19]. Median DFS, the primary end point of the study, was significantly prolonged for patients receiving mFOLFIRINOX compared with gemcitabine monotherapy (21.6 vs. 12.8 months, HR 0.58, p < 0.001). Furthermore, median OS, a secondary end point of the study, was 54.4 months and 35.0 months for those receiving mFOLFIRINOX and gemcitabine, respectively (HR 0.64, p = 0.003). However, grade 3/4 adverse events were more frequent in the mFOLFIRINOX compared with the gemcitabine (75.9% vs. 52.9%), including fatigue, diarrhea, nausea, vomiting, abdominal pain, sensory peripheral neuropathy, paresthesia, mucositis, and increased γ-glutamyl transferase level.

The global phase III APACT trial evaluated adjuvant chemotherapy with gemcitabine plus nab-paclitaxel versus gemcitabine alone in patients with resectable PDAC [20]. The primary endpoint, DFS by independent assessment, was not met. The median DFS was 19.4 months with gemcitabine plus nab-paclitaxel compared to 18.8 months with gemcitabine monotherapy (HR = 0.88, p = 0.1824). However, in the prespecified sensitivity analysis of investigator-assessed DFS, a benefit was shown for the combination, with a median DFS of 16.6 months vs. 13.7 months for gemcitabine monotherapy (HR = 0.82, p = 0.0168). OS data are immature, yet. The interim median OS was 40.5 vs. 36.2 months, respectively (HR = 0.82, p = 0.045).

20.2.3 Palliative Chemotherapy

In the majority of patients with PDAC, the cancer is already at an advanced unresectable stage at the time of diagnosis. Therefore, chemotherapy is the mainstay of treatment for metastatic PDAC [21, 22]. After a landmark clinical trial to compare gemcitabine and 5-FU in 1997, gemcitabine has been a standard of chemotherapy, and numerous clinical trials have compared novel regimens against gemcitabine monotherapy [23]. In a phase III trial, the addition of erlotinib to gemcitabine improved progression-free survival (PFS) and OS compared with gemcitabine alone, although this benefit was marginal.

In the phase III ACCORD-11 trial, the FOLFIRINOX regimen (oxaliplatin 85 mg/m^2, folinic acid 400 mg/m^2, irinotecan 180 mg/m^2, bolus fluorouracil 400 mg/m^2, infusional 5-FU 2400 mg/m^2 over 46 hr., every 14 days) had a median OS of 11.1 months when compared to the existing standard therapy, gemcitabine alone, which was significantly improved compared to 6.8 months in the gemcitabine alone group (HR 0.57, p < 0.001) [24]. Median PFS was 6.4 months, showing a prolonged effect compared to 3.3 months of the gemcitabine alone group (HR 0.47, p < 0.001). However, treatment-related toxicity was also significantly worse with FOLFIRINOX, including grade 3/4 neutropenia (45.7%), thrombocytopenia (9.1%), and diarrhea (12.7%). Therefore, this regimen is recommended for relatively younger patients with good performance status. Another phase III trial, the MPACT trial, showed that gemcitabine plus nab-paclitaxel was superior to gemcitabine alone in terms of response, PFS, and OS in patients with metastatic PDAC [25, 26]. The median OS was significantly improved at 8.5 vs. 6.7 months (HR 0.72, p < 0.001), and the median PFS was also at 5.5 vs. 3.7 months (HR 0.69, p < 0.001). Some studies investigated the biological effects of gemcitabine plus nab-paclitaxel and suggested that this regimen decreases cancer associated fibroblast (CAF) content inducing a marked alteration in cancer stroma that results in tumor softening. Since the two drugs showed an improvement in survival time compared to the gemcitabine alone group, FOLFIRINOX and gemcitabine plus nab-paclitaxel could be considered as first-line chemotherapeutic agents.

Recently, efficacy of maintenance Olaparib (PARP inhibitor) in patients with a germline BRCA mutation and metastatic PDAC that had not progressed after at least 16 weeks of first-line platinum-based chemotherapy was reported (POLO trial) [27]. This was an international, double-blind, placebo-controlled, phase III trial that randomized a total of 154 patients to either Olaparib (n = 92) or placebo (n = 62). If there is a germline BRCA1 or BRCA2 mutation, Olaparib (300 mg twice a day) was used as maintenance therapy. The median PFS was 7.4 months, which was significantly longer than the placebo group, 3.8 months (HR 0.53, p = 0.004). POLO is the first randomized trial to study the efficacy of PARP inhibitors in germline BRCA-mutated patients. The study is the first proof of concept of the feasibility of an individualized strategy in the choice of therapy based on a genomic marker in PDAC.

For patients who are refractory to first-line chemotherapeutic regimen, it is reasonable to consider further second-line chemotherapy in patients who maintain a good performance status. For patients with advanced disease who have received prior gemcitabine-based therapy, 5-FU-based chemotherapy regimens are acceptable second-line options. Alternatively, gemcitabine-based therapy can be given to those previously treated with 5-FU-based therapy. However, there are no widely accepted optimal regimens for second-line therapy yet. In the recent NAPOLI-1 phase III randomized trial, the effects of nanoliposomal irinotecan were examined in patients with metastatic PDAC who previously received gemcitabine-based therapy [28]. Median PFS (3.1 vs. 1.5 months, HR 0.56, p < 0.001) and OS (6.2 vs. 4.2 months, HR 0.75, p = 0.042) were significantly greater for patients who received nanoliposomal irinotecan with 5-FU/leucovorin, compared to patients who did not receive irinotecan. When the above treatments are not suitable, gemcitabine alone therapy, TS-1 therapy, gemcitabine combined with other drugs (erlotinib, cisplatin, or capecitabine) are also possible [29–32].

Second-line treatment options for patients with good performance status and previously treated with gemcitabine-based therapy include: 5-FU/leucovorin/liposomal irinotecan, FOLFIRI, FOLFIRINOX, 5-FU/leucovorin/oxaliplatin (OFF), FOLFOX, CapeOx, capecitabine, and continuous infusion 5-FU [7, 33, 34]. Options for patients with good performance status and previously treated with 5-FU-based therapy include: gemcitabine/albumin-bound paclitaxel, gemcitabine/cisplatin, gemcitabine/erlotinib, and gemcitabine monotherapy [13].

20.3 Immunotherapy

Immunotherapy is one of the emerging therapeutic options. However, previous clinical trials of immunotherapy did not show benefit in OS in PDAC. Immunotherapy stimulates a host immune response that results in long-term tumor destruction [35, 36]. The stroma of PDAC is particularly rich in inflammatory cells that are proposed to mediate drug resistance and tumor progression. Therefore, immune cells—such as T-cells and macrophages—infiltrating the peritumoral stroma represent a promising target for immunotherapeutic approaches. T-cell mediated immunity includes multiple sequential steps that are regulated by counterbalancing stimulatory and inhibitory signals that fine-tune the response [37, 38]. These inhibitory pathways are referred to as immune checkpoints and these are crucial for maintaining self-tolerance and modulating the duration and amplitude of physiological immune responses.

A new treatment option uses human immune-check point-inhibitor antibodies that inhibit the interactions between immune cells and antigen-presenting cells, including tumor cells. There is evidence that PD-1 blockade with pembrolizumab may be effective in tumors with mismatch repair deficiency (dMMR) [39, 40]. Pembrolizumab is an anti-PD-1 receptor antibody which blocks its interaction with PD-L1 and PD-L2, releasing the PD-1-mediated inhibition of the immune response, which improves antitumor immunity. The results of a phase II study in patients with 12 different dMMR advanced cancers, including pancreas, found that treatment with pembrolizumab resulted in durable responses (ORR in 53% of patients, with 21% complete response). There were six patients with PDAC with an ORR in 62% of patients (two had complete response and three had progressive disease).

Cytotoxic T-lymphocyte-associated antigen 4 (CTLA-4) is an immune checkpoint that plays a critical role in regulating and limiting immune responses, and it can be blocked by specific antibodies such as ipilimumab, a fully human antibody [41, 42]. The binding of ipilimumab to CTLA-4 blocks the immune limiting activity of CTLA-4, thereby sustaining an active immune response against the cancer cells. Early phase trials are currently underway in PDAC for ipilimumab (NCT01473940). Another promising immune-modulatory target is CD40, which is a co-stimulatory molecule for antigen presenting cells [43, 44]. Gemcitabine treatment combined with CD40 agonist-activated T-cells reduced the tumor burden in advanced PDAC patients in a phase I study by decreasing tumor stroma and increasing the tumor infiltration of activated macrophages [45]. In addition to enhancing the systemic immune response, attracting selected antitumor cytokines is also a promising concept that is currently under intense preclinical and clinical investigation. One of the most tumor selective antigens that can be used to guide cytokines to the site of a tumor is the extradomain B (ED-B) of fibronectin. The fusion product consisting of the ED-B antibody fragment L19 and interleukin-2 is currently being tested in a phase I/II trial in PDAC (NCT01198522).

20.4 Tumor Microenvironment

Other promising novel approaches to PDAC treatment include therapies targeting the desmoplastic stroma [46]. PDAC is characterized by the presence of a dense fibrous stromal tissue that represents up to 90% of the tumor volume [38]. This pancreatic extracellular matrix, produced by CAF, is predominantly made of collagen, hyaluronic acid, and fibronectin [47]. The full implications of this extracellular matrix and associated cells are still under investigation, but this dense stroma has been shown to limit efficacy of standard cytotoxic, immune, and targeted agents [48, 49]. Inefficient drug deliveries due to the intense stromal reaction may be an important contributor to chemo-resistance in PDAC [50]. The inhibition of stroma-related signaling pathways is considered to be a promising tool to decrease stromal density and to facilitate the access of cytotoxic drugs to the tumor cells. A cellular matrix component is currently being evaluated as targets for therapeutic intervention. Human recombinant PH20 hyaluronidase (PEGPH20) enzymatically depletes hyaluronan (highly abundant in the extracellular matrix of both human and murine PDAC tissues), thereby inducing the re-expansion of tumor blood vessels and increasing the concentration of gemcitabine within the tumor [51]. PEGPH20 resulted in significantly diminished tumor growth and prolonged survival in mice. Increased hyaluronic acid is associated with decreased survival in patients with PDAC, probably through increased interstitial pressure that impedes diffusion of therapeutic agents and nutrients into the tumor microenvironment. Hyaluronidase was investigated to break down hyaluronic acid. A phase 1b study of PEGPH20 in combination with gemcitabine showed an OS of 6.6 months in all-comers, but an OS of 13 months in the six patients with elevated hyaluronic acid concentrations [52]. This study was followed by a randomized phase II trial of gemcitabine and nab-paclitaxel with or without PEGPH20 [53]. The PEGPH20 group of this trial had an improvement in PFS (6.0 vs. 5.3 m), which was amplified in patients with tumors with high hyaluronic acid expression (9.2 vs. 5.2 m). But phase III trial evaluating PEGPH20 in combination with gemcitabine and nab-paclitaxel in patients who have tumors with high hyaluronic acid concentrations reported no improvement in OS compared with gemcitabine alone, leading to a suspension of further exploration of PEGPH20.

20.5 Summary

As the landscape of cancer treatment continues to evolve, understanding and targeting driver mutations will become the cornerstone of anticancer chemotherapy. In cancers such as PDAC that have an extremely poor prognosis and limited treatment options, molecular targeted therapy is even more important. Multiple clinical trials are currently under way, and more promising data will soon be available.

References

1. Ryan DP, Hong TS, Bardeesy N. Pancreatic adenocarcinoma. N Engl J Med. 2014;371:1039–49.
2. Rahib L, Smith BD, Aizenberg R, Rosenzweig AB, Fleshman JM, Matrisian LM. Projecting cancer incidence and deaths to 2030: the unexpected burden of thyroid, liver, and pancreas cancers in the United States. Cancer Res. 2014;74:2913–21.
3. Kamisawa T, Wood LD, Itoi T, Takaori K. Pancreatic cancer. Lancet. 2016;388:73–85.
4. Ferlay J, Soerjomataram I, Dikshit R, et al. Cancer incidence and mortality worldwide: sources, methods and major patterns in GLOBOCAN 2012. Int J Cancer. 2015;136:E359–86.
5. Siegel RL, Miller KD, Jemal A. Cancer statistics, 2020. CA Cancer J Clin. 2020;70:7–30.
6. Hartwig W, Werner J, Jager D, Debus J, Buchler MW. Improvement of surgical results for pancreatic cancer. Lancet Oncol. 2013;14:e476–85.
7. Kalser MH, Ellenberg SS. Pancreatic cancer. Adjuvant combined radiation and chemotherapy following curative resection. Arch Surg. 1985;120:899–903.
8. Muller PC, Frey MC, Ruzza CM, et al. Neoadjuvant chemotherapy in pancreatic cancer: an appraisal of the current high-level evidence. Pharmacology. 2020;106(3–4):143–53.

9. Christians KK, Tsai S, Mahmoud A, et al. Neoadjuvant FOLFIRINOX for borderline resectable pancreas cancer: a new treatment paradigm? Oncologist. 2014;19:266–74.
10. Tinchon C, Hubmann E, Pichler A, et al. Safety and efficacy of neoadjuvant FOLFIRINOX treatment in a series of patients with borderline resectable pancreatic ductal adenocarcinoma. Acta Oncol. 2013;52:1231–3.
11. Motoi F, Kosuge T, Ueno H, et al. Randomized phase II/III trial of neoadjuvant chemotherapy with gemcitabine and S-1 versus upfront surgery for resectable pancreatic cancer (Prep-02/JSAP05). Jpn J Clin Oncol. 2019;49:190–4.
12. Ahmad SA, Duong M, Sohal DPS, et al. Surgical outcome results from SWOG S1505: a randomized clinical trial of mFOLFIRINOX versus gemcitabine/nab-paclitaxel for perioperative treatment of resectable pancreatic ductal adenocarcinoma. Ann Surg. 2020;272(3):481–6.
13. Tempero MA, Malafa MP, Chiorean EG, et al. Pancreatic adenocarcinoma, version 1.2019. J Natl Compr Cancer Netw. 2019;17:202–10.
14. Neoptolemos JP, Stocken DD, Friess H, et al. A randomized trial of chemoradiotherapy and chemotherapy after resection of pancreatic cancer. N Engl J Med. 2004;350:1200–10.
15. Oettle H, Post S, Neuhaus P, et al. Adjuvant chemotherapy with gemcitabine vs observation in patients undergoing curative-intent resection of pancreatic cancer: a randomized controlled trial. JAMA. 2007;297:267–77.
16. Uesaka K, Boku N, Fukutomi A, et al. Adjuvant chemotherapy of S-1 versus gemcitabine for resected pancreatic cancer: a phase 3, open-label, randomised, non-inferiority trial (JASPAC 01). Lancet. 2016;388:248–57.
17. Neoptolemos JP, Palmer DH, Ghaneh P, et al. Comparison of adjuvant gemcitabine and capecitabine with gemcitabine monotherapy in patients with resected pancreatic cancer (ESPAC-4): a multicentre, open-label, randomised, phase 3 trial. Lancet. 2017;389:1011–24.
18. Valle JW, Palmer D, Jackson R, et al. Optimal duration and timing of adjuvant chemotherapy after definitive surgery for ductal adenocarcinoma of the pancreas: ongoing lessons from the ESPAC-3 study. J Clin Oncol. 2014;32:504–12.
19. Vivaldi C, Fornaro L, Vasile E. FOLFIRINOX adjuvant therapy for pancreatic cancer. N Engl J Med. 2019;380:1187–8.
20. Tempero MA, Reni M, Riess H, et al. APACT: phase III, multicenter, international, open-label, randomized trial of adjuvant nab-paclitaxel plus gemcitabine (nab-P/G) vs gemcitabine (G) for surgically resected pancreatic adenocarcinoma. J Clin Oncol. 2019;37:4000.
21. Sohal DP, Mangu PB, Khorana AA, et al. Metastatic pancreatic cancer: American Society of Clinical Oncology Clinical Practice Guideline. J Clin Oncol. 2016;34(23):2784–96.
22. Ko AH. Progress in the treatment of metastatic pancreatic cancer and the search for next opportunities. J Clin Oncol. 2015;33:1779–86.
23. Burris HA 3rd, Moore MJ, Andersen J, et al. Improvements in survival and clinical benefit with gemcitabine as first-line therapy for patients with advanced pancreas cancer: a randomized trial. J Clin Oncol. 1997;15:2403–13.
24. Conroy T, Desseigne F, Ychou M, et al. FOLFIRINOX versus gemcitabine for metastatic pancreatic cancer. N Engl J Med. 2011;364:1817–25.
25. Von Hoff DD, Ervin T, Arena FP, et al. Increased survival in pancreatic cancer with nab-paclitaxel plus gemcitabine. N Engl J Med. 2013;369:1691–703.
26. Von Hoff DD, Ramanathan RK, Borad MJ, et al. Gemcitabine plus nab-paclitaxel is an active regimen in patients with advanced pancreatic cancer: a phase I/II trial. J Clin Oncol. 2011;29:4548–54.
27. Golan T, Hammel P, Reni M, et al. Maintenance olaparib for germline BRCA-mutated metastatic pancreatic cancer. N Engl J Med. 2019;381:317–27.
28. Wang-Gillam A, Hubner RA, Siveke JT, et al. NAPOLI-1 phase 3 study of liposomal irinotecan in metastatic pancreatic cancer: final overall survival analysis and characteristics of long-term survivors. Eur J Cancer. 2019;108:78–87.
29. Cunningham D, Chau I, Stocken DD, et al. Phase III randomized comparison of gemcitabine versus gemcitabine plus capecitabine in patients with advanced pancreatic cancer. J Clin Oncol. 2009;27:5513–8.
30. Herrmann R, Bodoky G, Ruhstaller T, et al. Gemcitabine plus capecitabine compared with gemcitabine alone in advanced pancreatic cancer: a randomized, multicenter, phase III trial of the Swiss Group for Clinical Cancer Research and the Central European Cooperative Oncology Group. J Clin Oncol. 2007;25:2212–7.
31. Moore MJ, Goldstein D, Hamm J, et al. Erlotinib plus gemcitabine compared with gemcitabine alone in patients with advanced pancreatic cancer: a phase III trial of the National Cancer Institute of Canada Clinical Trials Group. J Clin Oncol. 2007;25:1960–6.
32. Ueno H, Ioka T, Ikeda M, et al. Randomized phase III study of gemcitabine plus S-1, S-1 alone, or gemcitabine alone in patients with locally advanced and metastatic pancreatic cancer in Japan and Taiwan: GEST study. J Clin Oncol. 2013;31:1640–8.
33. Louvet C, Labianca R, Hammel P, et al. Gemcitabine in combination with oxaliplatin compared with gemcitabine alone in locally advanced or metastatic pancreatic cancer: results of a GERCOR and GISCAD phase III trial. J Clin Oncol. 2005;23:3509–16.
34. Oettle H, Riess H, Stieler JM, et al. Second-line oxaliplatin, folinic acid, and fluorouracil versus folinic acid and fluorouracil alone for gemcitabine-refractory pancreatic cancer: outcomes from the CONKO-003 trial. J Clin Oncol. 2014;32:2423–9.
35. Ribas A. Releasing the brakes on cancer immunotherapy. N Engl J Med. 2015;373:1490–2.
36. Wu J, Cai J. Dilemma and challenge of immunotherapy for pancreatic cancer. Dig Dis Sci. 2021;66(2):359–68.
37. Balachandran VP, Beatty GL, Dougan SK. Broadening the impact of immunotherapy to pancreatic cancer: challenges and opportunities. Gastroenterology. 2019;156:2056–72.
38. Immunotherapy shows promise in pancreatic cancer. Cancer Discov. 2019;9:1330.
39. Le DT, Durham JN, Smith KN, et al. Mismatch repair deficiency predicts response of solid tumors to PD-1 blockade. Science. 2017;357:409–13.
40. Asaoka Y, Ijichi H, Koike K. PD-1 blockade in tumors with mismatch-repair deficiency. N Engl J Med. 2015;373:1979.
41. Bengsch F, Knoblock DM, Liu A, McAllister F, Beatty GL. CTLA-4/CD80 pathway regulates T cell infiltration into pancreatic cancer. Cancer Immunol Immunother. 2017;66:1609–17.
42. Bajor DL, Vonderheide RH. Cracking the stone: combination vaccination and CTLA-4 blockade in pancreatic cancer. J Immunother. 2013;36:362–4.
43. Beatty GL, Chiorean EG, Fishman MP, et al. CD40 agonists alter tumor stroma and show efficacy against pancreatic carcinoma in mice and humans. Science. 2011;331:1612–6.
44. Van Audenaerde JR, Marcq E, von Scheidt B, et al. Novel combination immunotherapy for pancreatic cancer: potent anti-tumor effects with CD40 agonist and interleukin-15 treatment. Clin Transl Immunology. 2020;9:e1165.
45. Vonderheide RH, Bajor DL, Winograd R, Evans RA, Bayne LJ, Beatty GL. CD40 immunotherapy for pancreatic cancer. Cancer Immunol Immunother. 2013;62:949–54.
46. Karamitopoulou E. The tumor microenvironment of pancreatic cancer. Cancers (Basel). 2020;12:3076.

47. Karamitopoulou E. Tumour microenvironment of pancreatic cancer: immune landscape is dictated by molecular and histopathological features. Br J Cancer. 2019;121:5–14.
48. Christenson ES, Jaffee E, Azad NS. Current and emerging therapies for patients with advanced pancreatic ductal adenocarcinoma: a bright future. Lancet Oncol. 2020;21:e135–45.
49. DuFort CC, DelGiorno KE, Hingorani SR. Mounting pressure in the microenvironment: fluids, solids, and cells in pancreatic ductal adenocarcinoma. Gastroenterology. 2016;150:1545–57.e2.
50. Ligorio M, Sil S, Malagon-Lopez J, et al. Stromal microenvironment shapes the intratumoral architecture of pancreatic cancer. Cell. 2019;178:160–75.e27.
51. PEGPH20 may improve standard-of-care therapy in pancreatic cancer. Cancer Discov. 2018;8:136.
52. Hingorani SR, Harris WP, Beck JT, et al. Phase Ib study of PEGylated recombinant human hyaluronidase and gemcitabine in patients with advanced pancreatic cancer. Clin Cancer Res. 2016;22:2848–54.
53. Hingorani SR, Zheng L, Bullock AJ, et al. HALO 202: randomized phase II study of PEGPH20 plus nab-paclitaxel/gemcitabine versus nab-paclitaxel/gemcitabine in patients with untreated, metastatic pancreatic ductal adenocarcinoma. J Clin Oncol. 2018;36:359–66.

21

Immune-Checkpoint Inhibitors in Hepatocellular Carcinoma

Rubens Copia Sperandio, Roberto Carmagnani Pestana, and Ahmed O. Kaseb

Abstract

Hepatocellular carcinoma (HCC) is a major cause of cancer-related death worldwide. Prognosis is grim, with 5-year overall survival <10% for patients with advanced disease, and the management is complex, demanding a multidisciplinary approach. Recently, a better understanding of the pathophysiology and immune microenvironment of HCC has led to advances in systemic treatment with the incorporation of immunotherapeutic strategies. The rationale behind immunotherapy as a treatment modality for HCC include the immunosuppressive effects of chronic inflammatory conditions associated with cirrhosis and hepatitis. Initially, anti-PD-1 immune-checkpoint inhibitors (ICIs)—nivolumab and pembrolizumab—were evaluated in single-arm early-phase trials, with promising efficacy. However, larger confirmatory studies of anti-PD1 ICI alone have yielded disappointing results. This insufficient activity of single-agent ICI led to interest in combination strategies, and the association of atezolizumab (an anti-PD-L1 ICI) and bevacizumab (an anti-VEGF antibody) has been established as the new standard of care for first-line systemic therapy in advanced HCC. Furthermore, there is increasing interest in assessing the usefulness of ICIs as an option to earlier stages—either in the neoadjuvant or adjuvant settings or combined with locoregional approaches. In this chapter, we aim to review the rationale, efficacy data and future perspectives regarding the use of ICI for HCC.

R. C. Sperandio · R. C. Pestana
Centro de Oncologia e Hematologia Einstein Familia Dayan-Daycoval, Hospital Israelita Albert Einstein, São Paulo, Brazil

A. O. Kaseb (✉)
Department of Gastrointestinal Medical Oncology, The University of Texas MD Anderson Cancer Center, Houston, TX, USA
e-mail: akaseb@mdanderson.org

21.1 Background

Hepatocellular carcinoma (HCC) is the fourth leading cause of cancer-related mortality worldwide, accountable for over 780,000 deaths in 2018 [1]. The major risk factor is cirrhosis from any etiology, most notably viral hepatitis, environmental toxins, alcohol abuse, and metabolic factors leading to non-alcoholic fatty liver disease (NAFLD) [2]. As a heterogeneous disease that most commonly arises in this background of chronic inflammatory liver conditions, the management of HCC is complex and demands a multidisciplinary approach. Regrettably, less than 20% of patients are diagnosed at early stages, when a curative treatment with surgical resection, ablation or liver transplantation is feasible [3]; the majority get the diagnosis when disease is already locally advanced or metastatic and prognosis is grim, with 5-year overall survival of less than 10% [4]. Additionally, over 70% of patients will experience recurrence following curative-intent therapy [5].

Historically, effective systemic therapies for advanced HCC have been scarce. HCC is a chemotherapy-refractory tumor and no cytotoxic agent has been shown to meaningfully improve survival [6, 7]. A more refined understanding of the pathophysiology of HCC lead to the discovery that hypervascularity and vascular abnormalities such as arterialization and sinusoidal capillarization, mediated by the action of proangiogenic factors such as vascular endothelial growth factor (VEGF), are common findings in HCC and shed light on angiogenesis as a potential therapeutic target [8]. In fact, the treatment landscape of advanced, unresectable HCC substantially evolved with clinical development of tyrosine-kinase inhibitors (TKI) that target the VEGF pathway. Initially, in 2008, sorafenib, an orally-available TKI, was approved based on data from the phase III SHARP trial, demonstrating a modest but significant overall survival benefit versus best supportive care alone (10.7 versus 7.9 months, HR 0.69; $p < 0.001$) [9]. This targeted-therapy became the standard of care and was the only first-line approved systemic approach until 2018, when the therapeutic arsenal against HCC was broadened with the approval of lenvatinib as first-line, after demonstrating non-inferiority versus sorafenib in the phase III REFLECT study [10]. Moreover, since 2017, a plethora of anti-angiogenic agents were approved in second-line settings, with overall survival improvements ranging from 1.6 to 2.8 months versus placebo; subsequent options include regorafenib [11], ramucirumab [12] and cabozantinib [13]. Nevertheless, the impact of these agents is modest, and no reliable biomarker for selection of patients has been identified. Therefore, progress is needed and effective therapy against HCC remains an unmet need.

With the recognition of cancer as an immunogenic disease, the role of immune modulation as a part of oncologic management was explored. In the early 2000s, local and systemic immunotherapy with interferon [14] and cytokines such as IL-12 [15] were studied, with poor results. More recently, cancer treatment was revolutionized by the introduction of immune checkpoint inhibitors (ICI) [16]. This group of agents is composed by immunomodulatory antibodies with the primary function of blocking immune inhibitory pathways and therefore unleashing the body's response against malignancies, with particular success in melanoma [17], renal cell carcinoma [18], and non-small cell lung cancer [19]. Strikingly, ICI has demonstrated potential for long-term disease control and even cure in metastatic chemotherapy-refractory solid tumors [20]. In light of the limited treatment options and an improved understanding of liver immune biology, ICI's use soon expanded to HCC. In this chapter, we will review the rationale, efficacy data and future perspectives regarding the use of ICI for HCC.

21.2 Rationale and the Evolving Role of Immunotherapy in Cancer Treatment

A better understanding of how innate and adaptive immune surveillance interplay with cancer development has led to major therapeutic advances across many cancer types [21]. The intricated mechanisms underlying this process initiate with the immune system's ability to recognize self and non-self antigens. The interface between the immune and tumor cells is mediated by antigen-presenting cells (APC) and components of major histocompatibility complex (MHC) classes I and II, responsible for recognition and consequent activation/inhibition of the immune response, comprising the "immune synapse". The primary connection between T cells and APC is through the MHC and the T cell receptor (TCR) complexes [22]. To ensure meticulous regulation of this process, the initial signal depends on additional costimulatory and co-inhibitory molecules, collectively known as "immune checkpoints". These bindings may produce, respectively, two opposing effects as a final result: immune activation through effector T cells; or immune evasion through increased participation of regulatory and suppressing cells [23]. These pathways create a dynamic balance between carcinogenesis and immune destruction, exemplifying a phenomenon called "cancer immunoediting"—a relationship described in three phases: elimination, equilibrium, and escape. The latter is characterized by tumor growth that is no longer blocked by adaptive immunity and is able to cause clinical manifestations of disease [24]. The most representative and studied negative immune checkpoints to date are cytotoxic T-lymphocyte associated protein 4 (CTLA-4), programmed cell-death receptor (PD-1) and its ligand programmed cell-death ligand 1 (PD-L1) (Table 21.1).

CTLA-4 blockade is a hallmark to immunotherapy as it represents the first-ever approved drug of ICI class—ipilimumab [25]. CTLA-4 is constitutively expressed in regulatory T cells, and by activated CD4+ and CD8+ lymphocytes. CTLA-4 competitively binds to CD80 (also known as B7-1) and CD86 (B7-2), thus decreasing the costimulatory signal of CD28 on APCs [26]. Upregulation of CTLA-4 occurs mediated by pro-effector cytokines IL-12, IFN-gamma and the degree of TCR activation, which leads to a feedback inhibition loop on effector T cells and, consequently, impairment of the immune response [27].

PD-1 is expressed in lymphocytes (T cells, B cells and NK cells) and is paramount for immunomodulation in tumor microenvironment. PD-1 is a co-inhibitory receptor that binds to the PDL-1 (also known as B7-H1 or CD274) and PDL-2 (B7-H2 or CD273), promoting peripheral T effector cell exhaustion [28]. While PDL-2 is mostly found in hematopoietic cells, PDL-1 is expressed across many tissues, including tumor cells. PDL-1 expression in the tumor microenvironment is also enhanced by IL-12 and IFN-gamma, highlighting its role as a physiological brake to effector T cells and as a mechanism for immune evasion [29, 30]. Chronic presented antigens as seen in chronic viral infections or neoplastic clones may induce feedback inhibition of effector T cells, in a process called "immune exhaustion" [23].

Table 21.1 Immune checkpoint inhibitors

Anti-PD1	Anti-PDL-1	Anti-CTLA-4
Pembrolizumab	Atezolizumab	Ipilimumab
Nivolumab	Avelumab	Tremelimumab
Cemiplimab	Durvalumab	

21.3 The Unique Microenvironment and Immune System of the Liver

ICI have yielded better responses when used in solid tumors with high mutational burden cancers, such as melanoma and non-small cell lung cancer. In such tumors, there is a predicted higher burden of neoantigens to be recognized by immune effector cells. Most cases of HCC arise in the background of a chronically inflamed liver, with underlying cirrhosis. A correlation between an inflamed tumor microenvironment and more neoantigens leading to higher IFN-gamma and PD-L1 expression has suggested—in a broad analysis of over 100,000 cancer genomes, the tumor mutational burden for HCC was found to be moderate [31].

Due to unique features of the hepatic tissue, such as self-tolerance, the immunological landscape of HCC is a key feature to the effectiveness of this class of agents. There is a myriad of cells found in HCCs, which include malignant hepatocytes, endothelial cells and infiltrating immune cells such as dendritic cells, lymphocytes, macrophages and monocytes (Fig. 21.1). The immune microenvironment in HCC is also characterized by upregulation and overexpression of PD-1 in intrahepatic lymphocytes, PD-L1 and PD-L2 in Kupffer cells, liver sinusoidal endothelium and leucocytes [32].

Recent advances in gene profiling and identification of gene signatures and other molecular features allow a phenotype classification that intend to better select subsets of patients which are more likely to respond. There has been evidence for classifying microenvironment-based immune subtypes in distinct phenotype groups. A study found that 25% of HCC samples show features of inflammatory response with overexpression of PD-1 and PD-L1. This so-called "Immune Class" is subdivided in two groups accordingly to immune status: (1) active (~65%, with overexpression of adaptive immune response genes) or (2) exhaustion of immunological activity (~35%, with predominance of immunosuppressive features such as TGF-ß expression and M2 macrophages infiltration) [33].

21.4 Single-Agent Immune Checkpoint Inhibitors Trials

Efficacy and safety of ICI in treating HCC were initially assessed in single-arm trials. Published in 2017, the CheckMate-040 [34] was a phase I/II study that evaluated nivolumab (an anti-PD1 ICI) after sorafenib failure in 262 patients. Results were promising, with an overall response rate of 20%, and disease control rate of 64%. The median

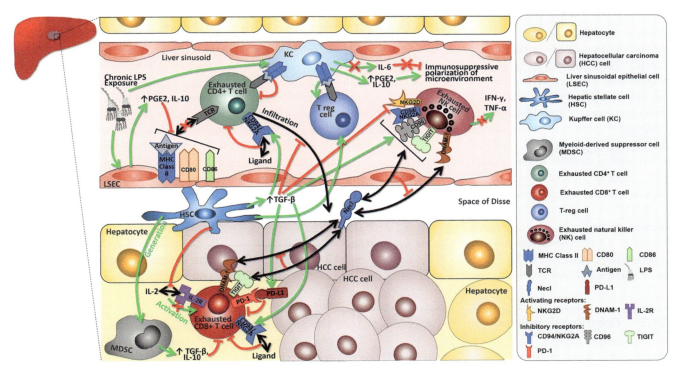

Fig. 21.1 The complex and multi-faceted functional interactions guiding cancer immune tolerogenesis in hepatocellular carcinoma. Cellular and functional heterogeneity of the HCC tumour microenvironment. Reused with permission from: Pinato DJ, Guerra N, Fessas P, et al. Immune-based therapies for hepatocellular carcinoma. *Oncogene*. 2020;39(18):3620–3637. https://doi.org/10.1038/s41388-020-1249-9. License at: http://creativecommons.org/licenses/by/4.0/

progression-free survival was 4.0 months, and the median duration of response was 9.9 months, highlighting the ICI's potential for long-term responses. Overall survival at 6 months and at 9 months were 83% and 74%, respectively, which compared favorably to published trials in the later line setting. Moreover, treatment was well tolerated, and only 3% of subjects had to discontinue treatment due to drug-related adverse events. A particular safety concern was the risk of immune-related hepatitis, but this event was rare and mostly low grade [35].

In 2018, the results of the single-arm phase II KEYNOTE-224 trial [36] were reported. In this study, 104 patients that had progressed on sorafenib were treated with pembrolizumab (an anti-PD-1 ICI). Overall response rate was 17%, and disease control rate 62%. Median time to response was 2.1 months and median duration of response was not reached, with 77% of patients continuing to respond for ≥9 months. Median overall survival was 12.9 months. Similarly to nivolumab, only 3% of patients showed increased alanine aminotransferase concentration attributable to immune-mediated hepatitis, with no viral flares or further complications.

Unfortunately, larger confirmatory trials of single-agent anti-PD-1 ICI yielded disappointing results, both in first- and second-line settings. KEYNOTE-240 [37] was a multicenter, randomized phase III study that assigned 413 patients to pembrolizumab or placebo as second-line therapy, after progression to sorafenib. The trial was negative for the co-primary endpoints of overall survival and progression-free survival. Notwithstanding, secondary efficacy data was consistent with prior reports—response rate was 16.9, with median duration of response of 13.8 months. Regarding frontline therapy, CheckMate-459 [38] was a phase III trial comparing nivolumab versus sorafenib for 743 systemic-therapy naive patients with advanced HCC. This study has also failed to meet its primary endpoint of overall survival, with median overall survival of 16.4 months versus 14.8 months for the nivolumab and sorafenib groups, respectively (HR 0.85; p = 0.0522 not significant). At 33 months, overall survival rates were 29% for nivolumab and 21% for sorafenib. Grade 3–4 treatment-related adverse events were reported in 82 patients (22.3%) of the nivolumab group and in 180 patients (49.6%) of the sorafenib group.

21.5 Combination Strategies

Despite the initial high expectations and relatively good response rates, ICI as single agents so far failed to demonstrate improvement in survival endpoints. Consequently, there has been a growing interest towards diversifying strategies and combining agents in order to improve efficacy (Fig. 21.2).

There is a strong scientific rationale suggesting that combined VEGF/PD-L1 blockade may be beneficial in a number of solid cancers, including HCC. It is recognized that HCC is a highly vascularized tumor [39], and the VEGF pathway plays a crucial role in exerting and maintaining an immunosuppressive tumor microenvironment through several mechanisms [40]. In May 2020, a combination therapy has become the new standard of care for advanced and unresectable HCC as the FDA approved atezolizumab (an anti-PD-L1 ICI) and bevacizumab (an anti-VEGF monoclonal antibody) as first-line therapy. This approval followed results of the phase III IMbrave150 trial [41], which assessed the aforementioned combination versus sorafenib as a first-line treatment in 501 previously untreated patients. Median overall survival was significantly better for the combined therapy (NR vs 13 months; HR 0.58, p < 0.001), translating into an overall survival benefit of 12% at 1 year (67% vs 55%). Combination therapy also yielded longer progression-free survival (6.8 vs 4.3 months, HR 0.59; p < 0.001). Moreover, the combined therapy doubled the objective response rate (27% vs 12%). Importantly, authors also reported a benefit in quality of life and physical/role functioning [42].

Further, a novel ICI combination has been approved in the later-line setting. In March 2020, the FDA granted accelerated approval to the combination of nivolumab plus ipilimumab (an anti-CTLA-4 ICI) for previously treated advanced HCC patients, based on a cohort of the CheckMate-040 study [43]. Overall response rate was 33%, including four complete responses and 12 partial responses. More than 30% of responses persist for at least 24 months, with median response duration of 17 months. This combination was associated with higher occurrence of immune-related adverse events, requiring the use of steroids, including grade 3–4 increased levels of aspartate aminotransferase and lipase [44].

Currently, in 2020, there are multiple ongoing clinical trials assessing different combinatory schemes incorporating ICI—either in combination with other ICIs or with targeted-therapies—, and more approvals are anticipated in the near future.

21.6 ICIs Use in the Neoadjuvant and Adjuvant Settings in Resectable HCC

The approval of ICIs for most malignancies initially took place in the context of advanced disease. More recently, ICI have been assessed in the management of earlier stages of cancer, and are approved for the (neo)adjuvant treatment of melanoma [45, 46] and non-small cell lung cancer [47]. Incorporating ICI earlier in HCC is of special interest as tumor recurrence is common and 5-year recurrence rates for resected HCC have been reported to be >70% [5].

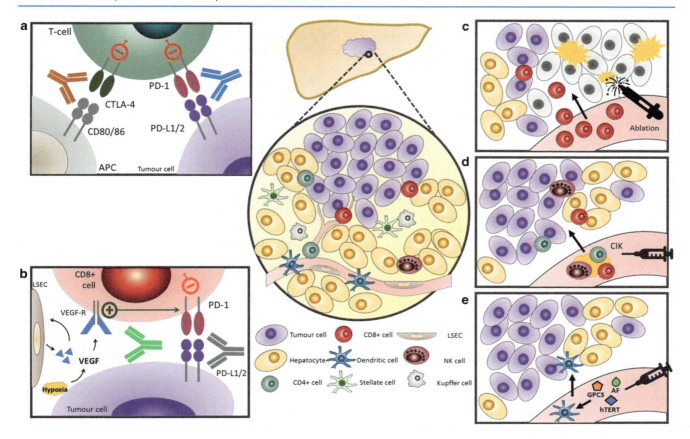

Fig. 21.2 General overview of immune-based therapies for HCC. (**a**) Simultaneous inhibition of CTLA-4 and the PD-1 axis by monoclonal antibodies (brown and blue respectively). The effect of dual checkpoint blockade on T-cell immune reconstitution is demonstrated, with CTLA-4 acting mainly on T-reg cells and antigen-presenting cells, and PD-1 acting on effector CD8+ CTLs. (**b**) Schematic representation of synergy between anti-angiogenic therapy (green antibody) and PD-1/PD-L1-targeted therapy. (**c**) Locoregional therapies, such as ablation and trans-arterial chemoembolisation are loco-regional inducers of immunogenic cell death and drive CD8+ cell infiltration into the tumour microenvironment, providing a rationale for combined anti-PD-1 therapy. (**d**) Autologous T cell transfer involves ex vivo activation of mixed T cell/NK cell populations by cytokines (i.e., CIK cells) and reinfusion into the patient with the intent of bypassing immune-evasion and eliciting an anti-tumour responses. (**e**) Anti-tumour vaccines against immunodominant peptides of oncofoetal proteins, such as AFP, GPC3 and hTERT, have been combined with ex vivo activation of dendritic cells to promote effective antigen presentation. Reused with permission from: Pinato DJ, Guerra N, Fessas P, et al. Immune-based therapies for hepatocellular carcinoma. *Oncogene.* 2020;39(18):3620–3637. https://doi.org/10.1038/s41388-020-1249-9. License at: http://creativecommons.org/licenses/by/4.0/

In the neoadjuvant setting, it is hypothesized that blocking immune checkpoints preoperatively increases systemic T cell response by enhancing neoantigen presentation and T cell priming both at the primary tumor site and draining lymph nodes [48]. The resulting effect would be the elimination of micrometastatic niches that are deposited far from the resectable lesion, which is thought to be the cause of relapse.

An interim analysis of an ongoing phase II pilot trial of preoperative ipilimumab with or without nivolumab has demonstrated a pathological complete response of 29% (4 out of evaluable 14 patients), highlighting the promise of early ICI use. As expected, grade 3 or higher toxicities prior to surgery were more present at the combination arm [49]. Larger confirmatory trials are ongoing. Currently, adjuvant immunotherapy studies in HCC include ICI alone randomized to placebo, including nivolumab (CheckMate-9DX, NCT03383458) and pembrolizumab (KEYNOTE-937, NCT03867084), in addition to atezolizumab plus bevacizumab randomized to placebo (Imbrave-050, NCT04102098).

21.7 Future Perspectives

Based on the new standard of care approved in 2020—atezolizumab plus bevacizumab—, the trend for the near future is towards evaluating diverse combination strategies, such as ICI with other ICI, or in conjunction with molecular targeted therapies such as multi-kinase inhibitors, or locoregional therapies, among others. Despite great excitement regarding the introduction of a novel modality of treatment with immunotherapy after a long time with few and modest options of systemic therapy, there is still a significant cohort of patients who do not respond to ICIs or combinations. Additionally, mechanisms of resistance—tumor intrinsic and extrinsic factors—are relevant and may play an important role in long-term follow-up of HCC patients. Moreover, inducing higher response rate is essential to improving outcome in unresectable HCC since it could downsize tumors to a resectable or transplantable stages and offer cure.

Notably, reliable predictive biomarkers that allow identification and better selection of patients more likely of responding to therapy are currently lacking. There is a number of candidates under investigation—both intratumoral and extratumoral biomarkers; such as PD-L1 expression, Tumor Mutational Burden (TMB), gene signatures, signaling pathways, tumor microenvironment features such as infiltrating lymphocytes. Circulating soluble factors such as cytokines, and immune cells, are other possible biomarkers which are currently under investigation [50]. Imaging predictors are also being assessed—recently, a significant correlation between HCC stiffness at magnetic resonance elastography, presence of intratumoral T lymphocytes, overall survival and time to disease progression has been recently reported and warrants further validation [51].

In summary, the study of immunotherapy for HCC is an active area of interest and has led to the establishment of a new frontline standard of care for unresectable disease. However, survival for patients with advanced HCC is still suboptimal, and there remains a need for novel treatment strategies, highlighting that progress is particularly strenuous due to the challenges of treating patients with underlying cirrhosis.

References

1. Bray F, Ferlay J, Soerjomataram I, Siegel RL, Torre LA, Jemal A. Global cancer statistics 2018: GLOBOCAN estimates of incidence and mortality worldwide for 36 cancers in 185 countries. CA Cancer J Clin. 2018;68(6):394–424.
2. Singal AG, El-Serag HB. Hepatocellular carcinoma from epidemiology to prevention: translating knowledge into practice. Clin Gastroenterol Hepatol. 2015;13(12):2140–51.
3. Bruix J, Sherman M, American Association for the Study of Liver Diseases. Management of hepatocellular carcinoma: an update. Hepatology. 2011;53(3):1020–2.
4. Llovet JM, Bustamante J, Castells A, Vilana R, Ayuso Mdel C, Sala M, et al. Natural history of untreated nonsurgical hepatocellular carcinoma: rationale for the design and evaluation of therapeutic trials. Hepatology. 1999;29(1):62–7.
5. Kumada T, Nakano S, Takeda I, Sugiyama K, Osada T, Kiriyama S, et al. Patterns of recurrence after initial treatment in patients with small hepatocellular carcinoma. Hepatology. 1997;25(1):87–92.
6. Lohitesh K, Chowdhury R, Mukherjee S. Resistance a major hindrance to chemotherapy in hepatocellular carcinoma: an insight. Cancer Cell Int. 2018;18:44.
7. Miyahara K, Nouso K, Yamamoto K. Chemotherapy for advanced hepatocellular carcinoma in the sorafenib age. World J Gastroenterol. 2014;20(15):4151–9.
8. Morse MA, Sun W, Kim R, He AR, Abada PB, Mynderse M, et al. The role of angiogenesis in hepatocellular carcinoma. Clin Cancer Res. 2019;25(3):912–20.
9. Llovet JM, Ricci S, Mazzaferro V, Hilgard P, Gane E, Blanc JF, et al. Sorafenib in advanced hepatocellular carcinoma. N Engl J Med. 2008;359(4):378–90.
10. Kudo M, Finn RS, Qin S, Han KH, Ikeda K, Piscaglia F, et al. Lenvatinib versus sorafenib in first-line treatment of patients with unresectable hepatocellular carcinoma: a randomised phase 3 non-inferiority trial. Lancet. 2018;391(10126):1163–73.
11. Bruix J, Qin S, Merle P, Granito A, Huang YH, Bodoky G, et al. Regorafenib for patients with hepatocellular carcinoma who progressed on sorafenib treatment (RESORCE): a randomised, double-blind, placebo-controlled, phase 3 trial. Lancet. 2017;389(10064):56–66.
12. Zhu AX, Park JO, Ryoo BY, Yen CJ, Poon R, Pastorelli D, et al. Ramucirumab versus placebo as second-line treatment in patients with advanced hepatocellular carcinoma following first-line therapy with sorafenib (REACH): a randomised, double-blind, multicentre, phase 3 trial. Lancet Oncol. 2015;16(7):859–70.
13. Abou-Alfa GK, Meyer T, Cheng AL, El-Khoueiry AB, Rimassa L, Ryoo BY, et al. Cabozantinib in patients with advanced and progressing hepatocellular carcinoma. N Engl J Med. 2018;379(1):54–63.
14. Llovet JM, Sala M, Castells L, Suarez Y, Vilana R, Bianchi L, et al. Randomized controlled trial of interferon treatment for advanced hepatocellular carcinoma. Hepatology. 2000;31(1):54–8.
15. Sangro B, Mazzolini G, Ruiz J, Herraiz M, Quiroga J, Herrero I, et al. Phase I trial of intratumoral injection of an adenovirus encoding interleukin-12 for advanced digestive tumors. J Clin Oncol. 2004;22(8):1389–97.
16. Thallinger C, Fureder T, Preusser M, Heller G, Mullauer L, Holler C, et al. Review of cancer treatment with immune checkpoint inhibitors: current concepts, expectations, limitations and pitfalls. Wien Klin Wochenschr. 2018;130(3-4):85–91.
17. Chang CY, Park H, Malone DC, Wang CY, Wilson DL, Yeh YM, et al. Immune checkpoint inhibitors and immune-related adverse events in patients with advanced melanoma: a systematic review and network meta-analysis. JAMA Netw Open. 2020;3(3):e201611.
18. Wang J, Li X, Wu X, Wang Z, Zhang C, Cao G, et al. Role of immune checkpoint inhibitor-based therapies for metastatic renal cell carcinoma in the first-line setting: a Bayesian network analysis. EBioMedicine. 2019;47:78–88.
19. Dafni U, Tsourti Z, Vervita K, Peters S. Immune checkpoint inhibitors, alone or in combination with chemotherapy, as first-line treatment for advanced non-small cell lung cancer. A systematic review and network meta-analysis. Lung Cancer. 2019;134:127–40.
20. Borcoman E, Kanjanapan Y, Champiat S, Kato S, Servois V, Kurzrock R, et al. Novel patterns of response under immunotherapy. Ann Oncol. 2019;30(3):385–96.
21. Pennock GK, Chow LQ. The evolving role of immune checkpoint inhibitors in cancer treatment. Oncologist. 2015;20(7):812–22.
22. Garcia KC, Adams EJ. How the T cell receptor sees antigen--a structural view. Cell. 2005;122(3):333–6.
23. Wherry EJ. T cell exhaustion. Nat Immunol. 2011;12(6):492–9.
24. Schreiber RD, Old LJ, Smyth MJ. Cancer immunoediting: integrating immunity's roles in cancer suppression and promotion. Science. 2011;331(6024):1565–70.
25. Schadendorf D, Hodi FS, Robert C, Weber JS, Margolin K, Hamid O, et al. Pooled analysis of long-term survival data from phase II and phase III trials of ipilimumab in unresectable or metastatic melanoma. J Clin Oncol. 2015;33(17):1889–94.
26. Walker LS, Sansom DM. The emerging role of CTLA4 as a cell-extrinsic regulator of T cell responses. Nat Rev Immunol. 2011;11(12):852–63.
27. Berkson JD, Slichter CK, DeBerg HA, Delaney MA, Woodward-Davis AS, Maurice NJ, et al. Inflammatory cytokines induce sus-

tained CTLA-4 cell surface expression on human MAIT cells. Immunohorizons. 2020;4(1):14–22.
28. Buchbinder EI, Desai A. CTLA-4 and PD-1 pathways: similarities, differences, and implications of their inhibition. Am J Clin Oncol. 2016;39(1):98–106.
29. Spranger S, Spaapen RM, Zha Y, Williams J, Meng Y, Ha TT, et al. Up-regulation of PD-L1, IDO, and T(regs) in the melanoma tumor microenvironment is driven by CD8(+) T cells. Sci Transl Med. 2013;5(200):200ra116.
30. Kinter AL, Godbout EJ, McNally JP, Sereti I, Roby GA, O'Shea MA, et al. The common gamma-chain cytokines IL-2, IL-7, IL-15, and IL-21 induce the expression of programmed death-1 and its ligands. J Immunol. 2008;181(10):6738–46.
31. Chalmers ZR, Connelly CF, Fabrizio D, Gay L, Ali SM, Ennis R, et al. Analysis of 100,000 human cancer genomes reveals the landscape of tumor mutational burden. Genome Med. 2017;9(1):34.
32. Kassel R, Cruise MW, Iezzoni JC, Taylor NA, Pruett TL, Hahn YS. Chronically inflamed livers up-regulate expression of inhibitory B7 family members. Hepatology. 2009;50(5):1625–37.
33. Sia D, Jiao Y, Martinez-Quetglas I, Kuchuk O, Villacorta-Martin C, Castro de Moura M, et al. Identification of an immune-specific class of hepatocellular carcinoma, based on molecular features. Gastroenterology. 2017;153(3):812–26.
34. El-Khoueiry AB, Sangro B, Yau T, Crocenzi TS, Kudo M, Hsu C, et al. Nivolumab in patients with advanced hepatocellular carcinoma (CheckMate 040): an open-label, non-comparative, phase 1/2 dose escalation and expansion trial. Lancet. 2017;389(10088):2492–502.
35. Colombo M, Lleo A. Is liver injury an affordable risk of immune checkpoint inhibitor therapy for cancer? Gastroenterology. 2018;155(6):2021–3.
36. Zhu AX, Finn RS, Edeline J, Cattan S, Ogasawara S, Palmer D, et al. Pembrolizumab in patients with advanced hepatocellular carcinoma previously treated with sorafenib (KEYNOTE-224): a non-randomised, open-label phase 2 trial. Lancet Oncol. 2018;19(7):940–52.
37. Finn RS, Ryoo BY, Merle P, Kudo M, Bouattour M, Lim HY, et al. Pembrolizumab as second-line therapy in patients with advanced hepatocellular carcinoma in KEYNOTE-240: a randomized, double-blind, phase III trial. J Clin Oncol. 2020;38(3):193–202.
38. Sangro B, Park J, Finn R, Cheng A, Mathurin P, Edeline J, et al. CheckMate 459: Long-term (minimum follow-up 33.6 months) survival outcomes with nivolumab versus sorafenib as first-line treatment in patients with advanced hepatocellular carcinoma. ESMO World Congress on Gastrointestinal Cancer 2020; Virtual (1–4 July) 2020.
39. Asayama Y, Yoshimitsu K, Nishihara Y, Irie H, Aishima S, Taketomi A, et al. Arterial blood supply of hepatocellular carcinoma and histologic grading: radiologic-pathologic correlation. AJR Am J Roentgenol. 2008;190(1):W28–34.
40. Yang J, Yan J, Liu B. Targeting VEGF/VEGFR to modulate antitumor immunity. Front Immunol. 2018;9:978.
41. Finn RS, Qin S, Ikeda M, Galle PR, Ducreux M, Kim TY, et al. Atezolizumab plus bevacizumab in unresectable hepatocellular carcinoma. N Engl J Med. 2020;382(20):1894–905.
42. Galle PR, Finn RS, Qin S, Ikeda M, Zhu AX, Kim TY, et al. Patient-reported outcomes from the phase III IMbrave150 trial of atezolizumab plus bevacizumab vs sorafenib as first-line treatment for patients with unresectable hepatocellular carcinoma. 2020 Gastrointestinal Cancers Symposium; January 24, 2020.
43. FDA grants accelerated approval to nivolumab and ipilimumab combination for hepatocellular carcinoma. U.S. FDA website: https://www.fda.gov/drugs/resources-information-approved-drugs/fda-grants-accelerated-approval-nivolumab-and-ipilimumab-combination-hepatocellular-carcinoma.
44. He AR, Yau T, Hsu C, Kang Y-K, Kim T-Y, Santoro A, et al. Nivolumab (NIVO) + ipilimumab (IPI) combination therapy in patients (pts) with advanced hepatocellular carcinoma (aHCC): subgroup analyses from CheckMate 040. J Clin Oncol. 2020;38(4_suppl):512.
45. Rozeman EA, Menzies AM, van Akkooi ACJ, Adhikari C, Bierman C, van de Wiel BA, et al. Identification of the optimal combination dosing schedule of neoadjuvant ipilimumab plus nivolumab in macroscopic stage III melanoma (OpACIN-neo): a multicentre, phase 2, randomised, controlled trial. Lancet Oncol. 2019;20(7):948–60.
46. Blank CU, Reijers ILM, Pennington T, Versluis JM, Saw RP, Rozeman EA, et al. First safety and efficacy results of PRADO: a phase II study of personalized response-driven surgery and adjuvant therapy after neoadjuvant ipilimumab (IPI) and nivolumab (NIVO) in resectable stage III melanoma. J Clin Oncol. 2020;38(15_suppl):10002.
47. Forde PM, Chaft JE, Smith KN, Anagnostou V, Cottrell TR, Hellmann MD, et al. Neoadjuvant PD-1 blockade in resectable lung cancer. N Engl J Med. 2018;378(21):1976–86.
48. Topalian SL, Taube JM, Pardoll DM. Neoadjuvant checkpoint blockade for cancer immunotherapy. Science. 2020;367(6477):eaax0182.
49. Kaseb AO, Pestana RC, Vence LM, Blando JM, Singh S, Ikoma N, et al. Randomized, open-label, perioperative phase II study evaluating nivolumab alone versus nivolumab plus ipilimumab in patients with resectable HCC. J Clin Oncol. 2019;37(4_suppl):185.
50. Onuma AE, Zhang H, Huang H, Williams TM, Noonan A, Tsung A. Immune checkpoint inhibitors in hepatocellular cancer: current understanding on mechanisms of resistance and biomarkers of response to treatment. Gene Expr. 2020;20(1):53–65.
51. Qayyum A, Hwang KP, Stafford J, Verma A, Maru DM, Sandesh S, et al. Immunotherapy response evaluation with magnetic resonance elastography (MRE) in advanced HCC. J Immunother Cancer. 2019;7(1):329.

Molecularly Targeted Therapy in Cholangiocarcinoma

22

Aakash Desai and Mitesh J. Borad

Abstract

Biliary tract cancers (BTCs) are a heterogeneous group of aggressive malignancies of the liver and biliary tract. While traditional approaches for advanced disease patients have comprised cytotoxic therapies such as gemcitabine and cisplatin, next generation sequencing has revolutionized the field and has cast growing appreciation of the molecular underpinnings of the disease. Towards this end, inhibitors of fibroblast growth factor receptor 2 (FGFR2) and isocitrate dehydrogenase 1 (IDH1) have yielded compelling data in pivotal clinical studies and subsequently garnered regulatory approval across a number of geographies. Enhancing this paradigm are studies that have yielded promising early data for targets such as BRAF and HER2 and microsatellite instability. These trends are expected to continue and the role of precision medicine deepens in the treatment of BTCs and these therapies are studies in relevant combinations, earlier disease settings and as next generation therapies towards these targets are developed.

Biliary tract cancers (BTCs) are a heterogeneous group of malignancies arising from the epithelial cells of the distinct anatomical locations of the biliary tree (intrahepatic, perihilar, distal bile ducts or the gallbladder). BTCs are generally categorized into intrahepatic cholangiocarcinoma (ICCA), extrahepatic cholangiocarcinoma (ECCA), and gallbladder carcinoma (GBC). In 2019, in there was an estimated total of 54,390 new cases (liver cancer and BTC), with approximately 35,740 deaths in the United States [1].

The definition of an ICCA is a cholangiocarcinoma (CCA) detected inside the hepatic parenchyma, whereas ECCA is a type of tumor located outside the liver parenchyma. These tumors can arise in any portion of the extrahepatic bile duct and can be additionally classified as hilar or distal CCA [2].

For localized disease, surgery remains the only curative option. Meanwhile, for advanced inoperable disease, chemotherapy with gemcitabine and cisplatin has emerged as the standard of care [3]. In recent years, a growing number of genomic studies have begun to uncover the molecular underpinnings of BTCs and suggest many potential treatments (Table 22.1). Targeted testing of advanced cholangiocarcinoma for deficient mismatch repair (dMMR)/microsatellite instability (MSI) and for specific molecular alterations (FGFR, IDH and others), for which a targeted treatment might be available (Table 22.2), is indicated for those who might be eligible for molecularly targeted therapy or immunotherapy, preferably within the context of a clinical trial.

In the Molecular Screening for Cancer Treatment Optimization (MOSCATO)-01 trial, 43 of 1035 adults with advanced cancer had a biliary tract malignancy, 34 of whom successfully underwent high-throughput molecular screening. Potentially actionable molecular aberrations were identified in 23 patients (68 percent), 18 of whom received targeted treatment. Median progression-free survival was 5.2 months, and there were six objective responses (33 percent, one complete) [4]. This trial informed on the potential impact of a molecularly targeted approach in patients with advanced biliary tract cancers. Thus, genomic studies of BTCs are ushering in a new era of precision therapy, already playing an emerging role in the treatment and prognostication of BTCs.

A. Desai
Department of Oncology, Mayo Clinic, Rochester, MN, USA

M. J. Borad (✉)
Mayo Clinic Cancer Center, Phoenix, AZ, USA

Center for Individualized Medicine, Mayo Clinic, Rochester, MN, USA

Department of Molecular Medicine, Mayo Clinic, Rochester, MN, USA

Division of Hematology/Oncology, Mayo Clinic, Phoenix, AZ, USA
e-mail: Borad.Mitesh@mayo.edu

Table 22.1 Therapeutic targets and approach to molecular profiling in biliary tract cancers

Molecular target	Frequency	Targeted agents	Molecular test
FGFR pathway	~10–20% of intrahepatic cholangiocarcinoma	Erdafitinib [9] Infigratinib [10] Pemigatinib [11] Futibatinib [13]	Tumor next generation DNA sequencing including FGFR2 intronic region, targeted RNAseq, or FISH testing for FGFR2 translocation
IDH1	~15% of intrahepatic cholangiocarcinoma	Ivosedinib [16]	Tumor next-generation DNA sequencing or targeted sequencing for hotspot mutations in coding region of IDH1
BRAF	~5% of intrahepatic cholangiocarcinoma	Dabrafenib plus Trametinib [18], Vemurafenib [33]	Tumor next-generation DNA sequencing or targeted sequencing for hotspot mutations in coding region of BRAF
MSI-high or MMR deficiency or high TMB	~2% of biliary tract cancers	Pembrolizumab [34]	PCR, immunohistochemistry, or tumor next generation DNA sequencing
ERRB2 (HER2)	~15–20% gallbladder cancer and extrahepatic cholangiocarcinoma cases	Trastuzumab/Pertuzumab	Multiple testing modalities available including immunohistochemistry and FISH for expression and amplification, tumor next generation DNA sequencing for mutations
NTRK	Rare	Entrectinib [31], Larotrectinib [32]	Tumor next-generation DNA sequencing including NTRK intronic region or targeted RNAseq, or FISH testing for NTRK translocation

Table 22.2 Clinical studies for molecularly targeted therapies in cholangiocarcinoma

Drug	Type of trial (n = sample size)	Primary endpoints (95% CI)	Secondary endpoints (95% CI)
FGFR2 fusions or gene rearrangements			
Erdafinitib [9]	Phase 1 (n = 11)	ORR: 27%	–
Infigratinib [8, 10]	Phase 2- cohort 1 (n = 108)	ORR: 23.1% (15.6%–32.2%); DoR: 5.0 months (0.9–19.1)	mPFS: 7.3 months mOS: 12.2 months
Pemigatinib [11]	Phase 2 (n = 146)	ORR: 35.5% (26.5%–45.5%)	mPFS: 6.9 months OS: 21.1 months
IDH1 mutations			
Ivosedinib [16]	Phase 3 (n = 187)	mPFS: 2.7 months vs. 1.4 months; HR: 0.37 (0.25–0.54)	mOS: 10.3 months (vs. 7.5 months), HR: 0.79; (95% CI, 0.56–1.12)
BRAF V600E mutations			
Dabrafenib/Trametinib [18]	Phase 2 (n = 43)	ORR: 51% (36%–67%)	mPFS: 9 months mOS: 14 months
MSI or dMMR/TMB			
Pembrolizumab [20]	Phase 2 (n = 41)	irORR: 40%	mPFS, mOS: NR
Pembrolizumab [23]	Phase 2 (n = 105)	ORR: 29%	3-yr PFS: 32%
ERRB2 (HER2) mutations			
Neratinib [30]	Phase 2 (n = 9)	PR: 2/9 patients (22.2%)	–

ORR overall response rate, irORR immune related ORR, DoR duration of response, mPFS median progression free survival, mOS median overall survival, NR not reached

The NCI-MATCH trial data confirmed the richness of molecular targets in cases of cholangiocarcinoma including: IDH1 mutations (17%), CDKN2A mutations (10%), BRAF mutations (7%), ERBB2 alterations (6%), NRAS mutations (6%), IDH2 mutations (5%), and FGFR2 alterations (3%). Intrahepatic cholangiocarcinoma had an assignment rate of 29.1% to 12 different NCI-MATCH subprotocols [5].

The genes most frequently associated with genomic alterations are TP53, KRAS, ARID1A, SMAD4, CCND1, MET, MDM2, CDKN2A, and CDKN2B, and the most common actionable gene targets are FGFR2 fusions, IDH1 mutations, and ERBB2 (HER-2) and MET amplifications; actionable targets are commonly observed in ICCA (Fig. 22.1) [6].

In this chapter, we discuss evidence for the management of CCA and molecular insights of personalized approaches, including fibroblast growth factor receptor (FGFR) inhibitors, checkpoint inhibitors, and other targets.

22.1 FGFR Alterations

About 13–17% of ICCAs harbor genomic alterations in the FGFR2 gene, with most being fusions, which predict tumor sensitivity to anti-FGFR2 tyrosine kinase inhibitors [7]. Translocations that relieve the FGFR2 gene of its upstream transcriptional regulation result in constitutively active

22 Molecularly Targeted Therapy in Cholangiocarcinoma

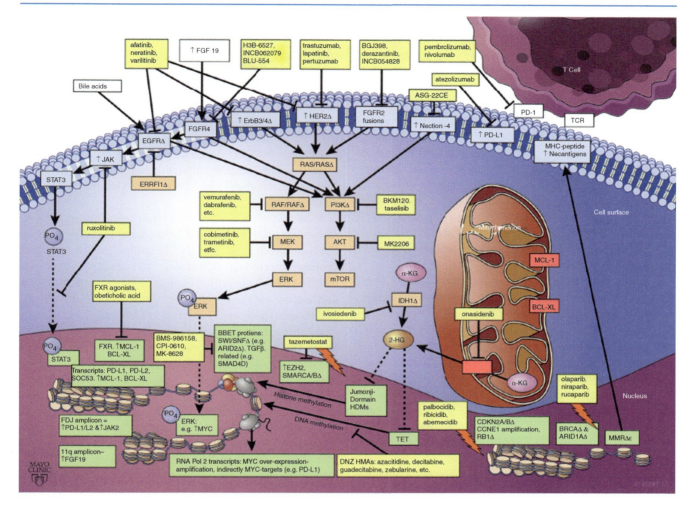

Fig. 22.1 Emerging role of precision medicine in biliary tract cancers. Yellow boxes highlight US FDA-approved drugs and drugs undergoing clinical investigation as reviewed, with arrows indicating pathway/target activation and blocked lines indicating pathway/target inhibition. BTC targets/pathways discussed are shown in color-coded boxes according to subcellular localization, blue = cell surface, orange = cytsolic, red = mitochondrial, and green = nuclear. "Upwards arrow" denotes over-expression, "Delta" denotes copy number aberrations and/or point mutation, a lighting bolt symbol denotes a synthetic lethal interaction between drug(s) and target(s) listed

growth factor pathway signaling, promoting cell proliferation, angiogenesis, and metastasis. Patients with FGFR aberrations may have superior overall survival (OS) with FGFR-targeted therapy as compared to standard non targeted regimens [8]. Multiple inhibitors of FGFR isoforms 1–3 have shown activity in advanced cholangiocarcinoma harboring FGFR2 translocations, including several ATP-competitive, reversible inhibitors (erdafitinib, infigratinib, pemigatinib, and derazantinib) as well as a non-ATP competitive, covalent inhibitor, futibatinib.

Erdafitinib was studied in a phase I trial including 187 patients with advanced solid tumors for which standard antineoplastic therapy was no longer effective. All patients with urothelial carcinoma and cholangiocarcinoma who responded to erdafitinib carried FGFR mutations or fusions. Median duration of response (DoR) was 5.6 months for urothelial carcinoma and 11.4 months for cholangiocarcinoma, clearly demonstrating response in cholangiocarcinoma patients [9].

BJG 398 (infigratinib), an ATP-competitive FGFR1–3-selective oral tyrosine kinase inhibitor has showed good response in the second line setting for patients resistant to frontline gemcitabine-based therapies. This was based on the an open-label, phase 2 trial enrolled 140 patients with unresectable locally advanced or metastatic cholangiocarcinoma who had either progressed on or were intolerant to gemcitabine-based chemotherapy. For eligibility, all participants had to have either FGFR gene fusions or rearrangements. Patients were grouped into three different cohorts: patients with FGFR2 gene fusions or rearrangements comprised cohort 1 (n = 120), those with FGFR1 and FGFR3 gene fusions or rearrangements and/or FGFR mutations comprised cohort 2 (n = 20), and those with FGFR2 gene fusions who had progressed after previous treatment with a selective FGFR inhibitor beyond infigratinib were included in cohort 3 (n = 20). Patients received infigratinib 125 mg orally for 21 days of each 28-day cycle until unacceptable toxicity or disease progression.

Among 61 patients (n = 48 FGFR2 fusions, n = 8 FGFR2 mutations, n = 3 FGFR2 amplifications) with >1 type of FGFR2 aberration detected in three patients the ORR, all partial responses (PRs), was 15%, with 75% of patients experiencing some disease control and a median progression-free survival (PFS) of 5.8 months. Four patients who carried FGFR3 amplifications did not respond. Dose modifications were required for many patients, although AEs were mostly reversible. The most common adverse events (AE) were hyperphosphatemia (72%), with 25% of patients experiencing grade 3 or 4 hyperphosphatemia [10].

The updated results of the largest cohort of FGFR2 gene fusions or rearrangements (cohort 1) were reported recently with median follow up of 10.6 months (range 1.1–55.9 months). Centrally reviewed ORR was 23.1% (95% CI 15.6–32.2) with a median DoR of 5.0 months (range 0.9–19.1 months). Among responders, 8 (32.0%) patients had a DoR of 6 months. Median PFS was 7.3 months (95% CI 5.6–7.6 months). Most common adverse events (AEs, any grade) were hyperphosphatemia (76.9%), eye disorders (67.6%, excluding central serous retinopathy/retinal pigment epithelium detachment [CSR/RPED]), stomatitis (54.6%), and fatigue (39.8%).

Pemigatinib is a selective, potent, oral competitive inhibitor of FGFR1, FGFR2, and FGFR3, which was studied in the multicenter, open-label phase 2 fibroblast Growth factor receptor inhibitor in oncology and Hematology Trial (FIGHT-202) [11]. This trial evaluated the safety and antitumor activity of pemigatinib in previously treated patients with locally advanced or metastatic cholangiocarcinoma, with or without FGF/FGFR alterations. 38 (35.5% [95% CI 26.5–45.4]) patients with FGFR2 fusions or rearrangements achieved an ORR. Overall, hyperphosphatemia was the most common all-grade adverse event irrespective of cause (88 [60%] of 146 patients). Overall, 71 (49%) patients died during the study, most frequently because of disease progression (61 [42%]); no deaths were deemed to be treatment related.

Lastly, activation of FGFR2 kinase domain point mutations occurs as a mechanism of resistance to ATP-competitive FGFR inhibition; these mutations can be polyclonal and heterogeneous [12]. Futibatinib (non-ATP-competitive) shows inhibitory activity against most secondary acquired resistance mutations, suggesting a role in FGFR2-translocated cholangiocarcinoma after progression on ATP-competitive FGFR inhibitors [13], although it is not active against the V565F gatekeeper mutation. Selective FGFR2 kinase inhibitors are in development with more potent FGFR2 inhibition and reduced off-target adverse events.

22.2 IDH Mutations

Gain-of-function mutations in the coding region of IDH1 are present in about 13% of cases of intrahepatic cholangiocarcinoma (almost never in extrahepatic cholangiocarcinoma) based upon a systematic review including 5393 cases of cholangiocarcinoma [14]. The mutant-IDH1 protein catalyzes production of an oncometabolite, D-2-hydroxyglutarate (2-HG), via NADPH-dependent reduction. Accumulation of 2-HG impairs cellular differentiation through effects on chromatin structure and DNA methylation, leading to tumorigenesis.

Ivosidenib is a first-in-class, oral, selective, and reversible mutant-IDH1 inhibitor. In a phase 1 basket study of IDH1-mutated solid tumors, 73 patients with advanced cholangiocarcinoma refractory to standard therapies received ivosidenib [15]. Although objective responses were uncommon (5%), the median progression-free survival (3.8 months) and overall survival (13.8 months) were longer than expected for standard chemotherapy in similar populations. The subsequent phase 3 ivosidenib in IDH1-mutant, chemotherapy-refractory cholangiocarcinoma (ClarIDHy) trial enrolled 185 patients with advanced IDH1-mutant cholangiocarcinoma after 1–2 lines of previous, unsuccessful systemic therapy [16]. Patient were randomized 2:1 to ivosidenib versus placebo and allowance of crossover at progression for patients in the placebo group Ivosidenib improved progression-free survival (the primary endpoint): median 2.7 months for ivosidenib versus 1.4 months for placebo (HR 0.37, 95% CI 0.25–0.54, p < 0.001), and 32% treated with ivosidenib were progression-free at six months (vs none in the placebo group). The updated OS results presented at ASCO GI 2021 showed median OS was 10.3 months in patients who received ivosidenib compared with 7.5 months for those who received placebo (HR, 0.79; 95% CI, 0.56–1.12; 1-sided p = 0.093). Overall, ivosidenib was well tolerated with low rates of grade 3 or higher adverse events and only 8.5% (vs. 6.6%) requiring discontinuation for toxicity attributed to ivosidenib. The most common grade 3 or higher TEAEs reported in the ivosidenib and placebo groups, respectively, were ascites (9.0% vs 6.8%, respectively), blood bilirubin increase (5.4% vs 1.7%), and anemia (7.2% vs 0%). Based on these results, a regulatory approval is anticipated for patients with advanced, IDH1-mutant cholangiocarcinoma after ineffective standard therapy.

22.3 BRAF Alterations

Activating serine/threonine-protein kinase B-raf kinase (BRAF) mutations at the V600E locus are well-known drivers in oncology and an established therapeutic target in

BRAF-V600E-mutant melanoma, colorectal cancer, anaplastic thyroid cancer, and non-small cell lung cancer. 5% of intrahepatic cholangiocarcinoma cases may harbor BRAF-V600E mutations. [8] Reports have shown potential for robust activity of dual BRAF plus MEK inhibition in biliary tract cancer harboring BRAF-V600E mutations [17]. The phase 2 ROAR basket trial of the BRAF inhibitor, dabrafenib, in combination with the MEK inhibitor, trametinib, in multiple tumor type cohorts, included advanced biliary tract cancer refractory to standard therapy [18]. ORR occurred in 51% of cases, with median PFS of 9.2 months and OS of 11.7 months. Common treatment-related adverse events included fever, rash, and nausea.

Similarly, another multicohort "basket" study of the BRAF inhibitor vemurafenib in non-melanoma BRAFV600 mutation–positive solid tumors enrolled 9 (5%) patients with cholangiocarcinoma. Although subgroup analysis is not available at this time, an objective response rate of 32.6% (25.6%–40.1%) was observed across all tumor types with DoR 13.1 months, mPFS 5.8 months and mOS of 17.6 months. These early results warrant further investigation of exploring this molecular target in larger trials for cholangiocarcinoma.

22.4 Microsatellite Instability (MSI) and Tumor Mutation Burden (TMB)

Patients with high microsatellite instability (MSI) or mismatch repair (MMR) deficiency form a special subset with robust response to immunotherapies. Pembrolizumab is FDA-approved for the treatment of patients with metastatic or inoperable solid tumors with these abnormalities. A genetic risk factor for biliary tract cancer includes Lynch syndrome, characterized by MSI and MMR deficiency [19]. The pivotal phase 2 study of pembrolizumab which included four patients with cholangiocarcinoma or ampullary cancer, showed a longer survival in MMR-deficient patients compared with MMR-proficient patients (median OS not reached versus 5.0 months); moreover, radiological responses were exclusively seen in MMR-deficient patients [20]. Another phase 2 basket study of anti-PD1 antibody in advanced MMR-deficient tumors (including n = 8 with biliary tract cancer) showed an ORR of 53% (complete RR, 21%). Responding patients harbored a vast amount of mutation-associated neoantigens making them susceptible to immune checkpoint-blockade [21]. Given this treatment option, determining if patients with biliary tract cancer have high MSI or MMR is important, although this applies to a small minority of only about 2% of patients.

Tumor Mutation Burden (TMB) has been of increasing interest as a potential biomarker of benefit from immune checkpoint inhibitor immunotherapy, and several reports now support a link between high levels of TMB and response to anti-PD-1 therapy [22]. The most compelling data on the predictive capacity of TMB in the response to immune checkpoint inhibitor immunotherapy come from the multicenter open-label phase II KEYNOTE-158 study, which established a link between TMB-high status (as determined by the FoundationOne CDx assay) and overall response rate with pembrolizumab [23]. The trial accrued patients with anal, biliary, cervical, endometrial, salivary, thyroid, or vulvar carcinoma, mesothelioma, a neuroendocrine tumor (NET), or small cell lung cancer (SCLC), who had an Eastern Cooperative Oncology Group performance status (ECOG PS) of 0 or 1, and had progressed or were intolerant of at least one prior line of standard therapy. Pembrolizumab was administered at 200 mg IV every three weeks. For TMB-high patients, the ORR (the primary endpoint) was 29 percent, while the ORR for TMB-low patients was only six percent. Within the context of biliary tract cancers, none of the 63 enrolled patients with biliary tract cancer had TMB-high disease. However, given the recent FDA approval for pembrolizumab for the treatment of adult and pediatric patients with unresectable or metastatic solid tumors that are tissue TMB-high (≥ 10 mut/Mb) by an FDA-approved assay (although the FoundationOne CDx assay was used in the supporting KEYNOTE-158 clinical trial), who have progressed following prior therapy, and who have no satisfactory alternative treatment options, patients with cholangiocarcinoma with this biomarker should be considered for treatment with pembrolizumab.

Currently, many immunotherapeutic agents are under investigation for biliary tract cancers. For example, bintrafusp alfa (M7824) is a first-in-class bifunctional fusion protein composed of the extracellular domain of the tumor growth factor (TGF)βRII receptor (a TGF-β trap) fused to a human IgG1 monoclonal antibody blocking PD-L1. In an expansion cohort from a phase 1 study (NCT02699515), 30 patients with refracted biliary tract cancer were treated with bintrafusp alfa monotherapy [24]. RR was 20% by central assessment (23.3% by investigator assessment), the median PFS was 2.6 months (95% CI 1.3–5.6), and OS was 12.7 months (95% CI 6.7–not reached). There is an ongoing phase 2 study of bintrafusp alfa monotherapy being investigated as a second-line treatment option in patients with advanced biliary tract cancer (NCT03833661).

Additionally, first-line, placebo-controlled phase 3 studies of immunotherapy in combination with cisplatin and gemcitabine chemotherapy include durvalumab (NCT03875235) and pembrolizumab (NCT04003636), and there is a phase 2–3 study of bintrafusp alfa in combination with cisplatin and gemcitabine chemotherapy (NCT04066491) underway.

22.5 HER2 Amplifications and Mutations

The epidermal growth factor receptor (EGFR) pathway is upregulated in preclinical models of biliary tract cancer, however currently no randomized controlled trial data has shown an improvement in OS with the addition of EGFR to standard gemcitabine and platinum chemotherapy [25–27]. The EGFR family member receptor tyrosine-protein kinase erbB-2 (ERBB2; HER2) can be activated by overexpression, amplification, or mutation in subsets of patients with biliary tract cancer. In gallbladder cancer and extrahepatic cholangiocarcinoma, ERBB2 overexpression or gene amplification can occur in ~15–20% of cases, while rates of activation are much lower in intrahepatic cholangiocarcinoma [28]. A small biliary tract cancer cohort (n = 7) treated with trastuzumab plus pertuzumab had an ORR in two patients along with three additional patients experiencing prolonged (>6 months) disease stability [29]. In a basket trial of patients with ERBB2 or ERBB3 mutations treated with neratinib, two of nine patients with biliary tract cancer experienced confirmed PR [30]. Additional studies are needed to determine the efficacy of ERBB2- targeted therapies as monotherapy or in combination for patients with ERBB2-activated biliary tract cancer.

22.6 NTRK and Other Targets

The neurotrophic receptor tyrosine kinase (NTRK) 1–3 genes can undergo fusion events of the NTRK kinase domain to various upstream partners, leading to overexpression of chimeric protein and constitutively active, ligand-independent downstream signaling. NTRK fusions are implicated in many tumor types and occasionally (in <5% cases) in biliary tract cancer [8]. The TRK inhibitors, entrectinib and larotrectinib, achieved high RRs (57% for entrectinib and 75% for larotrectinib) with long DoR (10 months for entrectinib and not reached for larotrectinib), in patients with advanced solid tumors harboring NTRK gene fusions [31, 32]. The robust and durable responses, coupled with overall mild and manageable safety profiles, led to both larotrectinib and entrectinib receiving accelerated approval from the US FDA in 2018 and 2019, for patients with histology-agnostic solid tumors harboring NTRK fusions. Several patients with cholangiocarcinoma were included in the data leading to regulatory approval for both entrectinib and larotrectinib, supporting the role for NTRK fusion testing in cholangiocarcinoma, and treatment, if present.

22.7 Conclusions

In conclusion, cholangiocarcinoma represents a substantial area of unmet need globally. The various entities that constitute cholangiocarcinoma have distinct differences in molecular characteristics. Surgery remains the cornerstone of cure in early-stage disease, however evaluation of advanced disease with the identification of molecular subgroups and associated targeted therapies is rapidly emerging. It is incumbent on clinicians to look for these aberrations. The role of immunotherapy continues to evolve with a focus on better patient selection and the value of its addition to a chemotherapy backbone is under investigation. It is important to realize that many of the mutations/aberrations observed in cholangiocarcinoma's are often indolent drivers alone (e.g., IDH or FGFR2), and even where such drivers may be significantly beneficial to target as monotherapy, combination therapy targeting two or more drivers is likely to yield deeper and more durable responses. Well-designed preclinical models, that recapitulate in vivo properties and thus can accurately interrogate precise genomic contexts to derive and test such combination therapies, will be paramount in moving beyond empirical therapy into a new era of precision therapy for cholangiocarcinoma.

Acknowledgments Illustrations reproduced from Bogenberger et al., *NPJ Precision Oncology* (Springer journal); https://www.nature.com/articles/s41698-018-0064-z

References

1. Siegel RL, Miller KD, Jemal A. Cancer statistics, 2019. CA Cancer J Clin. 2019;69(1):7–34.
2. Benson AB, D'Angelica MI, Abbott DE, Abrams TA, Alberts SR, Anaya DA, Anders R, Are C, Brown D, Chang DT, Cloyd J, Covey AM, Hawkins W, Iyer R, Jacob R, Karachristos A, Kelley RK, Kim R, Palta M, Park JO, Sahai V, Schefter T, Sicklick JK, Singh G, Sohal D, Stein S, Tian GG, Vauthey JN, Venook AP, Hammond LJ, Darlow SD. Guidelines insights: hepatobiliary cancers, version 2.2019. J Natl Compr Cancer Netw. 2019;17(4):302–10. https://doi.org/10.6004/jnccn.2019.0019.
3. Valle J, Wasan H, Palmer DH, Cunningham D, Anthoney A, Maraveyas A, Madhusudan S, Iveson T, Hughes S, Pereira SP, Roughton M, Bridgewater J, Investigators ABCT. Cisplatin plus gemcitabine versus gemcitabine for biliary tract cancer. N Engl J Med. 2010;362(14):1273–81. https://doi.org/10.1056/NEJMoa0908721.
4. Verlingue L, Malka D, Allorant A, Massard C, Ferté C, Lacroix L, Rouleau E, Auger N, Ngo M, Nicotra C. Precision medicine for patients with advanced biliary tract cancers: an effective strategy within the prospective MOSCATO-01 trial. Eur J Cancer. 2017;87 122–30.
5. Flaherty KT, Gray RJ, Chen AP, Li S, LM MS, Patton D, Hamilton SR, Williams PM, Iafrate AJ, Sklar J, editors. Molecular landscape

and actionable alterations in a genomically guided cancer clinical trial: National Cancer Institute Molecular Analysis for Therapy Choice (NCI-MATCH). Alexandria, VA: American Society of Clinical Oncology; 2020.
6. Bogenberger JM, DeLeon TT, Arora M, Ahn DH, Borad MJ. Emerging role of precision medicine in biliary tract cancers. NPJ Precis Oncol. 2018;2(1):1–9.
7. Kennedy L, Hargrove L, Demieville J, Francis N, Seils R, Villamaria S, Francis H. Recent advances in understanding cholangiocarcinoma. F1000Res. 2017;6:1818.
8. Javle M, Bekaii-Saab T, Jain A, Wang Y, Kelley RK, Wang K, Kang HC, Catenacci D, Ali S, Krishnan S, Ahn D, Bocobo AG, Zuo M, Kaseb A, Miller V, Stephens PJ, Meric-Bernstam F, Shroff R, Ross J. Biliary cancer: utility of next-generation sequencing for clinical management. Cancer. 2016;122(24):3838–47. https://doi.org/10.1002/cncr.30254.
9. Bahleda R, Italiano A, Hierro C, Mita A, Cervantes A, Chan N, Awad M, Calvo E, Moreno V, Govindan R. Multicenter phase I study of erdafitinib (JNJ-42756493), oral pan-fibroblast growth factor receptor inhibitor, in patients with advanced or refractory solid tumors. Clin Cancer Res. 2019;25(16):4888–97.
10. Javle M, Lowery M, Shroff RT, Weiss KH, Springfeld C, Borad MJ, Ramanathan RK, Goyal L, Sadeghi S, Macarulla T. Phase II study of BGJ398 in patients with FGFR-altered advanced cholangiocarcinoma. J Clin Oncol. 2018;36(3):276.
11. Abou-Alfa GK, Sahai V, Hollebecque A, Vaccaro G, Melisi D, Al-Rajabi R, Paulson AS, Borad MJ, Gallinson D, Murphy AG. Pemigatinib for previously treated, locally advanced or metastatic cholangiocarcinoma: a multicentre, open-label, phase 2 study. Lancet Oncol. 2020;21(5):671–84.
12. Goyal L, Saha SK, Liu LY, Siravegna G, Leshchiner I, Ahronian LG, Lennerz JK, Vu P, Deshpande V, Kambadakone A. Polyclonal secondary FGFR2 mutations drive acquired resistance to FGFR inhibition in patients with FGFR2 fusion–positive cholangiocarcinoma. Cancer Discov. 2017;7(3):252–63.
13. Goyal L, Shi L, Liu LY, de la Cruz FF, Lennerz JK, Raghavan S, Leschiner I, Elagina L, Siravegna G, Ng RW. TAS-120 overcomes resistance to ATP-competitive FGFR inhibitors in patients with FGFR2 fusion–positive intrahepatic cholangiocarcinoma. Cancer Discov. 2019;9(8):1064–79.
14. Boscoe AN, Rolland C, Kelley RK. Frequency and prognostic significance of isocitrate dehydrogenase 1 mutations in cholangiocarcinoma: a systematic literature review. J Gastrointest Oncol. 2019;10(4):751.
15. Lowery MA, Burris HA III, Janku F, Shroff RT, Cleary JM, Azad NS, Goyal L, Maher EA, Gore L, Hollebecque A. Safety and activity of ivosidenib in patients with IDH1-mutant advanced cholangiocarcinoma: a phase 1 study. Lancet Gastroenterol Hepatol. 2019;4(9):711–20.
16. Abou-Alfa GK, Macarulla T, Javle MM, Kelley RK, Lubner SJ, Adeva J, Cleary JM, Catenacci DV, Borad MJ, Bridgewater J. Ivosidenib in IDH1-mutant, chemotherapy-refractory cholangiocarcinoma (ClarIDHy): a multicentre, randomised, double-blind, placebo-controlled, phase 3 study. Lancet Oncol. 2020;21(6):796–807.
17. Kocsis J, Arokszallasi A, Andras C, Balogh I, Beres E, Deri J, Petak I, Janvary L, Horvath Z. Combined dabrafenib and trametinib treatment in a case of chemotherapy-refractory extrahepatic BRAF V600E mutant cholangiocarcinoma: dramatic clinical and radiological response with a confusing synchronic new liver lesion. J Gastrointest Oncol. 2017;8(2):E32–8. https://doi.org/10.21037/jgo.2017.01.06.
18. Subbiah V, Lassen U, Élez E, Italiano A, Curigliano G, Javle M, de Braud F, Prager GW, Greil R, Stein A. Dabrafenib plus trametinib in patients with BRAFV600E-mutated biliary tract cancer (ROAR): a phase 2, open-label, single-arm, multicentre basket trial. Lancet Oncol. 2020;21(9):1234–43.
19. Shigeyasu K, Tanakaya K, Nagasaka T, Aoki H, Fujiwara T, Sugano K, Ishikawa H, Yoshida T, Moriya Y, Furukawa Y. Early detection of metachronous bile duct cancer in lynch syndrome: report of a case. Surg Today. 2014;44(10):1975–81.
20. Le DT UJN, Wang H, Bartlett BR, Kemberling H, Eyring AD, Skora AD, Luber BS, Azad NS, Laheru D, Biedrzycki B, Donehower RC, Zaheer A, Fisher GA, Crocenzi TS, Lee JJ, Duffy SM, Goldberg RM, de la Chapelle A, Koshiji M, Bhaijee F, Huebner T, Hruban RH, Wood LD, Cuka N, Pardoll DM, Papadopoulos N, Kinzler KW, Zhou S, Cornish TC, Taube JM, Anders RA, Eshleman JR, Vogelstein B, Diaz LA Jr. PD-1 blockade in tumors with mismatch-repair deficiency. N Engl J Med. 2015;372(26):2509–20. https://doi.org/10.1056/NEJMoa1500596.
21. Le DT DJN, Smith KN, Wang H, Bartlett BR, Aulakh LK, Lu S, Kemberling H, Wilt C, Luber BS, Wong F, Azad NS, Rucki AA, Laheru D, Donehower R, Zaheer A, Fisher GA, Crocenzi TS, Lee JJ, Greten TF, Duffy AG, Ciombor KK, Eyring AD, Lam BH, Joe A, Kang SP, Holdhoff M, Danilova L, Cope L, Meyer C, Zhou S, Goldberg RM, Armstrong DK, Bever KM, Fader AN, Taube J, Housseau F, Spetzler D, Xiao N, Pardoll DM, Papadopoulos N, Kinzler KW, Eshleman JR, Vogelstein B, Anders RA, Diaz LA Jr. Mismatch repair deficiency predicts response of solid tumors to PD-1 blockade. Science. 2017;357(6349):409–13. https://doi.org/10.1126/science.aan6733.
22. Goodman AM, Kato S, Bazhenova L, Patel SP, Frampton GM, Miller V, Stephens PJ, Daniels GA, Kurzrock R. Tumor mutational burden as an independent predictor of response to immunotherapy in diverse cancers. Mol Cancer Ther. 2017;16(11):2598–608.
23. Marabelle A, Fakih M, Lopez J, Shah M, Shapira-Frommer R, Nakagawa K, Chung HC, Kindler HL, Lopez-Martin JA, Miller WH Jr, Italiano A, Kao S, Piha-Paul SA, Delord JP, RR MW, Fabrizio DA, Aurora-Garg D, Xu L, Jin F, Norwood K, Bang YJ. Association of tumour mutational burden with outcomes in patients with advanced solid tumours treated with pembrolizumab: prospective biomarker analysis of the multicohort, open-label, phase 2 KEYNOTE-158 study. Lancet Oncol. 2020;21(10):1353–65. https://doi.org/10.1016/s1470-2045(20)30445-9.
24. Yoo C, Oh D-Y, Choi H, Kudo M, Ueno M, Kondo S, Chen L-T, Osada M, Helwig C, Dussault I. M7824 (MSB0011359C), a bifunctional fusion protein targeting PD-L1 and TGF-β, in Asian patients with pretreated biliary tract cancer: preliminary results from a phase I trial. Ann Oncol. 2018;29:viii258–9.
25. Lee J, Park SH, Chang HM, Kim JS, Choi HJ, Lee MA, Jang JS, Jeung HC, Kang JH, Lee HW, Shin DB, Kang HJ, Sun JM, Park JO, Park YS, Kang WK, Lim HY. Gemcitabine and oxaliplatin with or without erlotinib in advanced biliary-tract cancer: a multicentre, open-label, randomised, phase 3 study. Lancet Oncol. 2012;13(2):181–8. https://doi.org/10.1016/s1470-2045(11)70301-1.
26. Malka D, Cervera P, Foulon S, Trarbach T, de la Fouchardière C, Boucher E, Fartoux L, Faivre S, Blanc JF, Viret F, Assenat E, Seufferlein T, Herrmann T, Grenier J, Hammel P, Dollinger M, André T, Hahn P, Heinemann V, Rousseau V, Ducreux M, Pignon JP, Wendum D, Rosmorduc O, Greten TF. Gemcitabine and oxaliplatin with or without cetuximab in advanced biliary-tract cancer (BINGO): a randomised, open-label, non-comparative phase 2 trial. Lancet Oncol. 2014;15(8):819–28. https://doi.org/10.1016/s1470-2045(14)70212-8.

27. Chen JS, Hsu C, Chiang NJ, Tsai CS, Tsou HH, Huang SF, Bai LY, Chang IC, Shiah HS, Ho CL, Yen CJ, Lee KD, Chiu CF, Rau KM, Yu MS, Yang Y, Hsieh RK, Chang JY, Shan YS, Chao Y, Chen LT. A KRAS mutation status-stratified randomized phase II trial of gemcitabine and oxaliplatin alone or in combination with cetuximab in advanced biliary tract cancer. Ann Oncol. 2015;26(5):943–9. https://doi.org/10.1093/annonc/mdv035.

28. Valle JW, Lamarca A, Goyal L, Barriuso J, Zhu AX. New horizons for precision medicine in biliary tract cancers. Cancer Discov. 2017;7(9):943–62. https://doi.org/10.1158/2159-8290.CD-17-0245.

29. Hainsworth JD, Meric-Bernstam F, Swanton C, Hurwitz H, Spigel DR, Sweeney C, Burris H, Bose R, Yoo B, Stein A, Beattie M, Kurzrock R. Targeted therapy for advanced solid tumors on the basis of molecular profiles: results from MyPathway, an open-label, phase IIa multiple basket study. J Clin Oncol. 2018;36(6):536–42. https://doi.org/10.1200/jco.2017.75.3780.

30. Hyman DM, Piha-Paul SA, Won H, Rodon J, Saura C, Shapiro GI, Juric D, Quinn DI, Moreno V, Doger B, Mayer IA, Boni V, Calvo E, Loi S, Lockhart AC, Erinjeri JP, Scaltriti M, Ulaner GA, Patel J, Tang J, Beer H, Selcuklu SD, Hanrahan AJ, Bouvier N, Melcer M, Murali R, Schram AM, Smyth LM, Jhaveri K, Li BT, Drilon A, Harding JJ, Iyer G, Taylor BS, Berger MF, Cutler RE Jr, Xu F, Butturini A, Eli LD, Mann G, Farrell C, Lalani AS, Bryce RP, Arteaga CL, Meric-Bernstam F, Baselga J, Solit DB. HER kinase inhibition in patients with HER2- and HER3-mutant cancers. Nature. 2018;554(7691):189–94. https://doi.org/10.1038/nature25475.

31. Doebele RC, Drilon A, Paz-Ares L, Siena S, Shaw AT, Farago AF, Blakely CM, Seto T, Cho BC, Tosi D. Entrectinib in patients with advanced or metastatic NTRK fusion-positive solid tumours: integrated analysis of three phase 1–2 trials. Lancet Oncol. 2020;21(2):271–82.

32. Drilon A, Laetsch TW, Kummar S, DuBois SG, Lassen UN, Demetri GD, Nathenson M, Doebele RC, Farago AF, Pappo AS. Efficacy of larotrectinib in TRK fusion–positive cancers in adults and children. N Engl J Med. 2018;378(8):731–9.

33. Subbiah V, Puzanov I, Blay J-Y, Chau I, Lockhart AC, Raje NS, Wolf J, Baselga J, Meric-Bernstam F, Roszik J. Pan-cancer efficacy of vemurafenib in BRAFV600-mutant non-melanoma cancers. Cancer Discov. 2020;10(5):657–63.

34. Le DT, Durham JN, Smith KN, Wang H, Bartlett BR, Aulakh LK, Lu S, Kemberling H, Wilt C, Luber BS. Mismatch repair deficiency predicts response of solid tumors to PD-1 blockade. Science. 2017;357(6349):409–13.

Systemic Therapies for Pancreatic Cancer

Faysal Dane and Nazim Can Demircan

Abstract

Pancreatic cancer is a highly deadly cancer with a 5-year survival rate of only about 10%. Most of the patients are diagnosed with advanced disease at the time of admission. Even in resectable cancers, the disease recurs in most patients. Almost all patients with good performance status, whether in the early or advanced stages, need systemic treatments. Advances in systemic treatments have improved median overall survival. Here we review systemic treatment options for both early and advanced pancreatic cancer.

23.1 Introduction

Pancreatic cancer (PC) is the 11th most common cancer worldwide and the seventh leading cause of cancer deaths in developed countries according to GLOBOCAN 2018 statistics [1]. In recent years, its incidence and mortality rates show a trend towards increasing regardless of gender [1]. More than half of patients are diagnosed with metastatic disease and for those with initially localized disease, progression is often inevitable despite multimodal approach. Pancreatic ductal adenocarcinoma (PDA) is the most frequent histologic subtype of PC and carries a dismal prognosis, with a 5-year survival remaining below 10% [2].

Systemic therapy is the mainstay of PC management and largely based on cytotoxic agents. Survival benefit of chemotherapy (CT) for PC was demonstrated in several studies in the last two decades. CT can be administered postoperatively to prevent or delay recurrence (adjuvant setting), preoperatively to downstage tumors and achieve negative surgical margins (neoadjuvant setting) and in a palliative manner for advanced, unresectable disease. This chapter will cover systemic treatment strategies in different settings of PC and review clinical trial data regarding these approaches.

23.2 Adjuvant Systemic Therapy

Surgical resection is the primary treatment for patients with localized PDA whose tumors do not involve mesenteric vessels and who have suitable performance status (PS) and comorbid conditions. Adjuvant CT is recommended for all patients who underwent resection for PDA and did not receive neoadjuvant CT [3, 4]. Although optimal timing and duration of adjuvant CT for PDA has not been established yet, an updated guideline by the American Society of Clinical Oncology (ASCO) recommends six months of postoperative CT preferentially starting within eight weeks of surgery [3].

Early trials which compared adjuvant single-agent CT with observation in resected PDA demonstrated survival benefit of CT. First of those was the ESPAC-1 trial from Europe, which enrolled 541 patients with resected PDA and consisted of three parallel studies: chemoradiotherapy (CRT) vs. no CRT (n = 68), adjuvant CT vs. no CT (n = 188), and a four-arm trial including CRT (n = 73), CT (n = 75), both (n = 72), and observation (n = 69) [5]. Pooled analysis of these trials was published in 2001 and highlighted a median survival of 19.7 months in patients who received adjuvant CT consisting of 5-fluorouracil (5-FU) and folinic acid (FA) and 14 months in patients who did not (p = 0.0005). A subsequent report of ESPAC-1 in 2004 including 289 patients from the four-arm study also showed improved survival with adjuvant CT (20.1 vs. 15.5 months, hazard ratio (HR) = 0.71, p = 0.009) [6]. Another European trial, CONKO-001, included PC patients who had microscopically or macroscopically complete (R0 or R1) resection and were randomized to gemcitabine or observation [7]. First report of

F. Dane (✉)
Division of Medical Oncology, Department of Internal Medicine, Altunizade Acibadem Hospital, Istanbul, Turkey

N. C. Demircan
Division of Medical Oncology, Department of Internal Medicine, Marmara University School of Medicine, Istanbul, Turkey

this study from 2007 showed superior disease-free survival (DFS) in gemcitabine arm (13.4 vs. 6.9 months, p < 0.001) and this translated into improved long-term survival as suggested by the update published in 2013 (22.8 vs. 20.2 months, p = 0.01) [7, 8]. Head-to-head comparison of adjuvant 5-FU plus FA and gemcitabine in the ESPAC-3 trial demonstrated similar efficacy, making both regimens established options in resected PC [9].

Subsequent trials focused on multiagent combination strategies in adjuvant CT for PC. The ESPAC-4 study assigned 730 patients with R0 or R1 resected PC to gemcitabine alone or gemcitabine plus capecitabine [10]. In this trial, the majority of patients had R1 resection and positive lymph nodes and median overall survival (OS) was significantly longer in combination arm (28.0 vs. 25.5 months, p = 0.032), with no remarkable difference in serious toxicities between treatment arms. Updated analysis of ESPAC-4, which was published in 2019, revealed median OS of 30.2 vs. 27.9 months in two-drug and gemcitabine arms, respectively (HR = 0.81, p = 0.03) [11]. On the other hand, the multicenter PRODIGE-24 trial investigated efficacy of modified FOLFIRINOX (mFOLFIRINOX = infusional 5-fluorouracil, leucovorin, irinotecan, and oxaliplatin) compared to gemcitabine [12]. This study enrolled 493 patients with PDA who had R0 or R1 resection along with an ECOG PS of 0 or 1 and its results confirmed superiority of mFOLFIRINOX in both DFS and OS (21.6 and 54.4 months, respectively). Based on the recently published results that indicate improved long-term survival, mFOLFIRINOX and gemcitabine plus capecitabine are both recommended by the National Comprehensive Cancer Network (NCCN) as preferred adjuvant CT regimens for PC, with mFOLFIRINOX requiring an ECOG-PS of 0 or 1 [13]. Clinical trial data regarding adjuvant CT in PC are summarized in Table 23.1.

There are other adjuvant regimens which were evaluated in phase III trials but are not among recommended treatment protocols currently due to limited evidence. One of them is S-1, a fluoropyrimidine approved for gastric cancer treatment in Europe and Japan, which was compared to gemcitabine in 385 Japanese patients with stage I-III resected PC [14]. Although 5-year survival was higher in S-1 arm (44.1% vs. 24.4%, p < 0.0001), these outcomes have not been assessed yet in non-Asian populations. Gemcitabine plus nab-paclitaxel is an active regimen in metastatic PC and it was investigated in adjuvant setting in 866 patients with R0 or R1 resected PC [14]. Here, addition of nab-paclitaxel to six-month gemcitabine did not improve DFS significantly (19.4 vs. 18.8 months, p = 0.18) and although interim analysis of this study suggests improved OS with nab-paclitaxel (40.5 vs. 36.2 months, p = 0.045), additional follow-up is needed [15].

23.3 Neoadjuvant Systemic Therapy

The role of neoadjuvant therapy (NAT) in PC management is growing and it is increasingly used in resectable or borderline resectable disease. The term "borderline resectable," although often variable in definition, generally refers to a tumor that abuts the superior mesenteric artery, encases the gastroduodenal artery up to the hepatic artery, or involves the superior mesenteric/portal vein which is suitable for resection and reconstruction. Borderline resectable disease differs from potentially resectable tumors in that it is more likely to result in positive surgical margins due to abutment of arteries which is associated with poor prognosis; however, it encompasses the majority of tumors initially deemed to be potentially resectable, especially considering the inaccuracy of imaging and high rates of margin positivity with upfront sur-

Table 23.1 Clinical trials evaluating adjuvant systemic therapy in pancreatic cancer

Trial [Reference]	Treatment arms	mDFS/mPFS (Months)	mOS (Months)
ESPAC-1 [5]	5-FU 425 mg/m^2 + FA 20 mg/m^2; d1–5 q4w x6 (n = 238) No CT (n = 235)	NR	19.7 vs. 14 HR = 0.66 p = 0.0005
CONKO-001 [8]	Gemcitabine 1000 mg/m^2; d1,8,15 q4w x6 (n = 179) Observation (n = 175)	13.4 vs. 6.7 HR = 0.55 p < 0.001	22.8 vs. 20.2 HR = 0.76 p = 0.01
ESPAC-3 [9]	5-FU 425 mg/m^2 + FA 20 mg/m^2; d1–5 q4w x6 (n = 551) Gemcitabine 1000 mg/m^2; d1,8,15 q4w x6 (n = 538)	14.1 vs. 14.3 HR = 0.96 p = 0.53	23.0 vs. 23.6 HR = 0.94 p = 0.39
ESPAC-4 [10]	Gemcitabine 1000 mg/m^2; d1,8,15 q4w x6 (n = 366) Gemcitabine 1000 mg/m^2; d1,8,15 + capecitabine 1660 mg/m^2; d1–21 q4w x6 (n = 364)	13.1 vs. 13.9 HR = 0.86 p = 0.082	25.5 vs. 28.0 HR = 0.82 p = 0.032
PRODIGE-24 [12]	mFOLFIRINOX^a q2w x 12 (n = 247) Gemcitabine 1000 mg/m^2; d1,8,15 q4w x6 (n = 246)	21.6 vs. 12.8 HR = 0.58 p < 0.001	54.4 vs. 35.0 HR = 0.64 p = 0.003

5-FU 5-fluorouracil, *FA* folinic acid, *HR* hazard ratio, *mDFS* median disease-free survival, *mPFS* median progression-free survival, *mOS* median overall survival, *NR* not reported
^{a}Modified FOLFIRINOX = 5-fluorouracil 2400 mg/m^2 (46-hour infusion) + leucovorin 400 mg/m^2 + irinotecan 180 mg/m^2 + oxaliplatin 85 mg/m^2

gery. Rationale of NAT is based on that it helps selecting patients for whom surgery would not be beneficial (i.e., disease progression during treatment), increases R0 resection rates, and enables early treatment of micrometastatic disease. However, guidelines have been conflicting in the use of NAT for PC so far: The ASCO recommends it in potentially resectable tumors which have an interface with mesenteric vessels, the European Society of Medical Oncology (ESMO) suggests not to administer it in potentially resectable disease, whereas the NCCN suggests that it could be considered in high-risk potentially resectable tumors, i.e. those with concerning radiological findings, very high CA 19–9 levels, large size, large regional lymph nodes, or accompanying severe symptoms (excessive weight loss, severe pain) [4, 13, 16]. Some of the recent studies demonstrated higher R0 resection rates and longer survival with neoadjuvant approach than upfront surgery, as discussed below, and preoperative therapy is therefore a reasonable option in potentially or borderline resectable PC.

One of the first reports showing benefit of NAT in PC was from 2015 and included 127 patients with locally advanced or borderline resectable disease, 87 of them had upfront resection and 40 had received neoadjuvant FOLFIRINOX, of whom 24 had also received neoadjuvant radiotherapy (RT) with 5-FU [17]. In the FOLFIRINOX arm, 25 patients were locally advanced and 15 were borderline resectable initially, and post-treatment imaging revealed objective response in 36 patients (90%) while there was no progressive disease. Surgical morbidity was lower, rates of aggressive pathological features (lymphovascular invasion, perineural invasion, greater tumor size, and positive lymph nodes) were lower, and overall survival was significantly improved in patients who received FOLFIRINOX ($p = 0.008$); a non-significant increase in R0 resection rate was also observed (92% vs. 86%). An analysis including the largest sample size was derived from the National Cancer Database (NCDB), which was issued in 2017 and matched 2005 patients who received NAT with 6015 patients who underwent surgery first for clinical stage I or II PC [18]. Approximately half of the NAT arm had received multiagent CT and 58% of the arm had completed multimodal therapy (vs. 30% in the surgery-first arm). Patients in the upfront surgery arm had significantly higher pathologic T3 and T4 stage (86% vs. 73%), higher positive lymph nodes (73% vs. 48%), and higher positive margins (24% vs. 17%). Besides, OS was superior in the NAT arm (26 vs. 21 months, HR = 0.72, $p < 0.01$) and this significance persisted when NAT was compared to the group with upfront resection and adjuvant therapy (26 vs. 23 months, HR = 0.83, $p < 0.01$). A second retrospective analysis from NCDB including 593 patients who had clinical stage III PC supported the benefit of NAT, with higher rates of pathologic downstaging (78% vs. 36%), lymph node negativity (63% vs. 25%), and operative margin negativity (79% vs. 54%) along with improved OS (20.7 vs. 13.7 months, HR = 0.68, $p = 0.001$) [19].

Following the above-mentioned studies, the preoperative CT plus CRT strategy in PC continued to be investigated in prospective studies. A phase II trial including 48 patients with borderline resectable PC was designed to administer eight cycles of FOLFIRINOX followed by short-course CRT with capecitabine in cases with resolution of vascular involvement and long-course CRT with 5-FU or capecitabine in cases with persistent vascular involvement upon restaging [20]. Radiographic response to induction CT was partial in 44% of patients and two patients (5%) experienced progression with liver metastasis. R0 resection was accomplished in 65% of patients, median progression-free survival (PFS) and OS were 14.7 and 37.7 months, respectively. Despite the absence of a control group, R0 resection rate in this trial is higher than previously reported rates with upfront surgery for borderline resectable disease [21]. In the Dutch phase III PREOPANC trial, which is the only prospective randomized study to compare NAT with immediate surgery plus adjuvant therapy, 246 patients with resectable or borderline resectable PC were randomized in a 1:1 design to three courses of neoadjuvant (concurrent RT in the second course) and four courses of adjuvant gemcitabine or upfront resection followed by six months of gemcitabine [22]. In this study, radiographic progressive disease was identified in 10 patients who received neoadjuvant CT. Recently published results of this trial demonstrated significantly higher R0 resection rate (71% vs. 40%), longer DFS (8.1 vs. 7.7 months, $p = 0.03$), and longer locoregional failure-free interval (not reached vs. 13.4 months, $p = 0.003$) in the preoperative therapy arm.

Efficacy of neoadjuvant CT without CRT was addressed by two randomized studies. A phase II/III trial from Italy allocated 93 patients with clinical stage I-II PC to surgery followed by six cycles of gemcitabine (arm A), surgery followed by six cycles of PEXG consisting of cisplatin, epirubicin, gemcitabine, and capecitabine (arm B) or three cycles of preoperative and three cycles of postoperative PEXG (arm C) [23]. In arm C, one patient had local progressive disease during preoperative CT and three were unresectable intraoperatively. Highest R0 resection rate, longest median event-free survival, and median OS were in arm C (63%, 16.9 and 38.2 months, respectively). Nevertheless, the authors did not continue with phase III of this trial because the standard of care for adjuvant therapy of PC had changed after the trial had begun. Another phase II/III trial from Japan allocated 364 patients with potentially resectable PC to two courses of neoadjuvant gemcitabine plus S-1 or upfront surgery, with patients undergoing curative resection receiving six months of S-1 in both arms [24]. A preliminary report of his study, presented in 2019, showed an improvement only in OS with preoperative therapy (36.7 vs. 26.6 months, HR = 0.72, $p = 0.015$).

The FOLFIRINOX and gemcitabine plus nabpaclitaxel (Gem-NabP) regimens were compared as perioperative regimens (three months before and three months after surgery) in the phase II SWOG S1505 study which included 102 patients with potentially resectable PC and was presented in 2020 [25]. The study revealed high resectability rates (73% vs. 70%), similar median DFS (10.9 and 14.2 months, p = 0.87) and OS (22.4 vs. 23.6 months, p = 0.42) between two arms. These results emphasized FOLFIRINOX and Gem-NabP as active regimens for preoperative approach and both are preferred NAT protocols as stated by the NCCN guidelines [13].

23.4 Systemic Therapy for Locally Advanced and Metastatic Disease

23.4.1 First-Line Therapy for Locally Advanced and Unresectable Disease

Initial CT is commonly recommended by the ASCO, ESMO, and NCCN guidelines for non-metastatic, locally advanced, and unresectable disease [4, 13, 16]. Preferred first-line regimens for patients with good PS are FOLFIRINOX (ECOG 0–1) and Gem-NabP (ECOG 0–2); however, these recommendations were extrapolated from randomized trials on metastatic PC [26, 27]. A meta-analysis including 315 patients with locally advanced PC (LAPC) who received FOLFIRINOX reported a pooled median PFS of 15 months and median OS of 24.2 months, proportion of surgery was 26% and 74% of these cases had R0 resection [28]. Data regarding gemcitabine combinations in LAPC are scarce and some can be acquired from the German phase II NEOLAP study, final results of which were presented in 2019 [29]. In this trial 130 patients with LAPC were administered two cycles of induction Gem-NabP, cases without disease progression and unacceptable adverse events were then randomly allocated to two additional cycles of Gem-NabP or four cycles of FOLFIRINOX. No significant difference in rates of R0/R1 resection (30.6% vs. 45%, p = 0.13) and OS (17.2 vs. 22.5 months, p = 0.26) was observed between treatment arms.

In patients with LAPC and poor PS, standard or fixed dose rate (FDR) gemcitabine, capecitabine, and continuous 5-FU infusion are among frontline treatment alternatives [13]. Of these agents, gemcitabine was shown to improve clinical benefit and median survival over bolus 5-FU in an early trial including patients with locally advanced or metastatic PC [30]. The rationale of FDR gemcitabine is that it can maximize intracellular concentrations of the active drug and at a dose of 10 mg/m^2/min, it provided a modest survival advantage versus standard gemcitabine infusion over 30 minutes (6.2 vs. 4.9 months, p = 0.04) in advanced PC according to the ECOG-6201 study [31].

23.4.2 First-Line Therapy for Metastatic Disease

Systemic CT is only palliative in metastatic PC (MPC) but can improve symptoms and survival. Similar to LAPC, preferred first-line protocols for patients with good PS are FOLFIRINOX (ECOG 0–1) and Gem-NabP (ECOG 0–2) [13]. These regimens also require a total bilirubin level of ≤1.5 times the upper limit of normal, according to the updated guidelines of the ASCO [32]. In contrast to LAPC, both approaches are supported by phase III trials for MPC. In the phase III PRODIGE trial, 342 patients with MPC were randomized 1:1 to FOLFIRINOX or gemcitabine [26]. FOLFIRINOX was superior in terms of median OS (11.1 vs. 6.8 months, p < 0.001), median PFS (6.4 vs. 3.3 months, p < 0.001), and objective response rate (ORR) (31.6% vs. 9.4%, p < 0.001). The phase III MPACT study, which enrolled 861 patients with MPC, demonstrated significant improvements in OS (8.5 vs. 6.7 months, p < 0.001), PFS (5.5 vs. 3.7 months, p < 0.001), and ORR (23% vs. 7%, p < 0.001) with addition of nab-paclitaxel to gemcitabine [27].

The BRCA1/2 and PALB2 genes are important elements of homologous recombinant repair (HRR) pathway and mutations in them are found in approximately 5–9% of PDA, leading to defective DNA repair [33]. One clinical implication of this is susceptibility to DNA cross-linking agents, especially platinum compounds. In fact, cisplatin plus gemcitabine was tested in a phase II trial including 50 patients with treatment-naive stage III or IV PDA and germline BRCA/PALB2 mutations, where ORR was 74%, median PFS 10.1 months, and median OS 15.5 months [34]. Although a randomized comparison with non-platinum CT has to be performed yet in the specific population, cisplatin plus gemcitabine, along with FOLFIRINOX, is one of the frontline options for MPC as well as LAPC patients with BRCA1/2 or PALB2 mutations and good PS [13].

Other recommended first-line regimens for MPC patients with good PS include gemcitabine, gemcitabine plus capecitabine, FDR gemcitabine plus docetaxel plus capecitabine (GTX), 5-FU plus leucovorin plus oxaliplatin (OFF), capecitabine plus oxaliplatin (CapeOx), and gemcitabine plus erlotinib [13]. A randomized phase III trial assessed addition of capecitabine to gemcitabine in 533 patients with previously untreated LAPC or MPC [35]. In this study, a significant increase in ORR (19.1% vs. 12.4%, p = 0.03) and PFS (5.3 vs. 3.8 months, p = 0.004) was observed in the combination arm; a trend toward better OS was also reported with capecitabine plus gemcitabine (7.1 vs. 6.2 months, p = 0.08). Data regarding the activity of GTX regimen is available from a phase II trial which included 43 patients with previously untreated MPC; ORR was 21.9%, median time to treatment failure 6.9 months, and median OS of 14.5 months [36]. Overexpression human epidermal

Table 23.2 Clinical trials evaluating first-line systemic therapy in metastatic pancreatic cancer

Reference	Treatment arm(s)	ORR (%)	mPFS (months)	mOS (months)
Conroy et al. (PRODIGE) [26]	FOLFIRINOX[b] (n = 171) Gemcitabine 1000 mg/m^2; d1,8,15,22,29,36,43 q8w, then d1,8,15 q4w (n = 171)	31.6 vs 9.4 p < 0.001	6.4 vs. 3.3 HR = 0.47 p < 0.001	11.1 vs. 6.8 HR = 0.57 p < 0.001
Von Hoff et al. (MPACT) [27]	Nab-paclitaxel 125 mg/m^2 + gemcitabine 1000 mg/m^2; d1,8,15 q4w (n = 431) Gemcitabine 1000 mg/m^2; d1,8,15,22,29,36,43 q8w, then d1,8,15 q4w (n = 430)	23 vs. 7 p < 0.001	5.5 vs. 3.7 HR = 0.69 p < 0.001	8.5 vs. 6.7 HR = 0.72 p < 0.001
O'Reilly et al. [34][a]	Cisplatin 60 mg/m^2 + gemcitabine 600 mg/m^2; d3,10 q3w (n = 27, germline BRCA/PALB2+)	74.1	10.1	15.5
Cunningham et al. [35][a]	Capecitabine 1660 mg/m^2/d; d1–21 + gemcitabine 1000 mg/m^2; d1,8,15 q4w (n = 267) Gemcitabine 1000 mg/m^2; d1,8,15,22,29,36,43 q8w, then d1,8,15 q4w (n = 266)	19.1 vs. 12.4 p = 0.03	5.3 vs. 3.8 HR = 0.78 p = 0.004	7.1 vs. 6.2 HR = 0.86 p = 0.08
Fine et al. [36]	Capecitabine 1500 mg/m^2/d; d1–14 + gemcitabine 750 mg/m^2; d4,11 + docetaxel 30 mg/m^2; d4,11 q21	21.9	6.9	14.5
Moore et al. [38][a]	Erlotinib 100 or 150 mg/day (n = 285) or placebo (n = 284) + Gemcitabine 1000 mg/m^2; d1,8,15,22,29,36,43 q8w, then d1,8,15 q4w	8.6 vs. 8.0 p = NR	3.7 vs. 3.5 HR = 0.77 p = 0.004	6.2 vs. 5.9 HR = 0.82 p = 0.038

HR hazard ratio, mPFS median progression-free survival, mOS median overall survival, NR not reported, ORR objective response rate
[a]Also include patients with locally advanced disease
[b]FOLFIRINOX = 5-fluorouracil 2400 mg/m^2 (46-hour infusion) + 5-fluorouracil 400 mg/m^2 (bolus) + leucovorin 400 mg/m^2 + irinotecan 180 mg/m^2 + oxaliplatin 85 mg/m^2

growth factor receptor type 1 (HER1/EGFR) can be found in many pancreatic tumors and it is associated with progressive disease [37]. Based on this perspective, the oral EGFR tyrosine kinase inhibitor erlotinib was added to gemcitabine in a phase III trial including 569 with LAPC or MPC, who were only allowed prior concurrent RT and radiosensitizing agents [38]. The gemcitabine plus erlotinib combination provided a small but significant benefit in terms of OS (6.2 vs. 5.9 months, p = 0.038) and PFS (3.7 vs. 3.5 months, p = 0.004) compared to gemcitabine only, ORRs were similar (8.6% vs 8.0%). Recommendations regarding the OFF and CapeOx regimens are based on trials assessing them in second-line setting, these will be mentioned in the "Second-line Therapy" subsection below.

For MPC cases with poor PS, preferred initial regimens are the same as in LAPC; namely standard or FDR gemcitabine, capecitabine, and continuous 5-FU infusion [13]. Table 23.2 recaps efficacy data of first-line combination regimens in MPC.

23.4.3 Second-Line Therapy

Patients with LAPC or MPC who progress during or after first-line CT and have suitable PS should be offered second-line therapy. Aside from PS, regimens in this setting depend on first-line treatment.

After first-line gemcitabine-based CT, recommended combination regimens for patients with good PS include 5-FU plus leucovorin plus liposomal irinotecan, 5-FU plus leucovorin plus unencapsulated irinotecan (FOLFIRI), FOLFIRINOX, OFF, and CapeOx [13]. The phase III NAPOLI-1 trial was a three-arm study randomizing 417 PDA patients, who progressed with gemcitabine-based therapy, to liposomal irinotecan, 5-FU plus FA, or combination of these agents [39]. The combination arm was superior to 5-FU plus FA arm in terms of OS (6.1 vs. 4.2 months, p = 0.01), PFS (3.1 vs. 1.5 months, p = 0.0001), and ORR (16% vs. 1%, p < 0.0001) whereas efficacy of liposomal irinotecan monotherapy was not better than 5-FU plus FA. In two phase II trials from Italy including a total of 90 patients with gemcitabine-refractory stage III-IV PC, FOLFIRI produced a partial response of 8% and 15%, median PFS of 3.2 and 3.7 months, and median OS of five and six months [40, 41]. Oxaliplatin-based protocols are also active in advanced PC after progression on gemcitabine. OFF did significantly improve OS over best supportive care (4.8 vs. 2.3 months, p = 0.008) in the phase III CONKO-003 trial whereas median PFS and OS were 9.9 and 23 weeks in a phase II study investigating second-line CapeOx [42, 43]. Although no prospective trials assessing FOLFIRINOX after gemcitabine-based therapy in advanced PC exist, it can be active as suggested by a retrospective analysis reporting an ORR of 19% and median PFS of 5.4 months but should be limited to patients with good PS (ECOG 0–1) [13, 44].

For patients who have progressed on first-line fluoropyrimidine-based therapy and have a good PS, recommended regimens are gemcitabine, Gem-NabP, gemcitabine plus erlotinib, gemcitabine plus cisplatin (for known BRCA1/2 or PALB2 mutations), and 5-FU plus leucovorin plus liposomal irinotecan (if irinotecan was not received previously) [13]. Trials evaluating gemcitabine after

Table 23.3 Efficacy data from clinical trials regarding second-line CT in locally advanced or metastatic pancreatic cancer

Reference	Treatment arm(s)	ORR (%)	mPFS	mOS
Wang-Gillam et al. (NAPOLI-1) [39][a]	Liposomal irinotecan 80 mg/m^2 + FA 400 mg/m^2 + 5-FU 2400 mg/m^2 in 46 h; q2w (n = 117) Liposomal irinotecan 120 mg/m^2; q3w (n = 151) FA 200 mg/m^2 + 5-FU 2000 mg/m^2 in 24 h; d1,8,15,22 q6w (n = 149)	16 vs 1[c] p < 0.0001	3.1 vs. 1.5[c] months HR = 0.56 p = 0.0001	6.1 vs. 4.2[c] months HR = 0.67 p = 0.012
Zaniboni et al. [41][a]	Irinotecan 180 mg/m^2; d1 + FA 200 mg/m^2; d1,2 + 5-FU 400 mg/m^2 bolus; d1,2 + 5-FU 600 mg/m^2 in 22 h; d1,2 q2w (n = 50)	8	3.2 months	5 months
Pelzer et al. (CONKO-003) [42][a]	FA 200 mg/m^2 + 5-FU 2000 mg/m^2 in 24 h; d1,8,15,22 + oxaliplatin 85 mg/m^2; d8,22 q6w (n = 23) BSC (n = 23)	NR	NR	4.8 vs. 2.3 months HR = 0.45 p = 0.008
Xiong et al. [43][a]	Capecitabine 2000 mg/m^2/d; d1–14 + oxaliplatin 130 mg/m^2; d1 q3w (n = 39)	3	9.9 weeks	23 weeks
Portal et al. [49][b]	Nab-paclitaxel 125 mg/m^2 + gemcitabine 1000 mg/m^2; d1,8,15 q4w (n = 57)	18	5.1 months	8.8 months
Mita et al. [50][b]	Nab-paclitaxel 125 mg/m^2 + gemcitabine 1000 mg/m^2; d1,8,15 q4w (n = 30)	13	3.8 months	7.6 months

5-FU 5-fluorouracil, *BSC* best supportive care, *FA* folinic acid, *HR* hazard ratio, *mPFS* median progression-free survival, *mOS* median overall survival, *NR* not reported, *ORR* objective response rate
[a]Includes patients who progressed on prior gemcitabine-based therapy
[b]Includes patients who progressed on prior FOLFIRINOX
[c]Combination arm vs. 5-FU + FA arm

FOLFIRINOX failure in PC reported median PFS of 2–2.5 months, median OS of 3.6–5.7 months, and ORR of 11% [45–48]. On the other hand, two trials assessing Gem-NabP after progression on FOLFIRINOX highlighted a median PFS of 3.8 and 5.1 months, median OS of 7.6 and 8.8 months, and ORR of 13% and 18% [49, 50]. Although these outcomes favor Gem-NabP in second-line setting after FOLFIRINOX, it should be noted that these regimens have not been compared in a randomized trial yet.

Patients with LAPC or MPC and a poor PS can be offered single-agent gemcitabine (standard or FDR), capecitabine, or continuous 5-FU as second-line treatment [13]. Efficacy data of second-line CT in advanced PC is summarized in Table 23.3.

23.4.4 Targeted Therapy

Poly (ADP-ribose) polymerase (PARP) as an enzyme is the main repair pathway for DNA single-strand breaks in cells with defective HRR, its inhibition leads to unrepaired DNA breaks and ultimately death of cancer cells harboring BRCA mutations [51, 52]. The multicenter phase III POLO trial investigated efficacy of olaparib, an oral PARP inhibitor, versus placebo in 154 patients with MPC and germline BRCA1/2 mutations whose disease did not progress during at least 16 weeks of first-line platinum-based CT [53]. Olaparib significantly improved PFS (7.4 vs. 3.8 months, p = 0.004) but OS was similar between the two arms (18.9 vs. 18.1 months, p = 0.68), response rate was also higher with olaparib (20% vs. 10%). Subsequently, olaparib was approved by the Food and Drug Administration (FDA) for maintenance treatment after first-line platinum-based CT in patients with MPC and germline BRCA1/2 mutations, it is also among recommendations in the NCCN guidelines [13].

Enhancing anti-tumor immunity is a potential therapeutic strategy and targeting programmed death receptor 1 (PD-1) or its ligand PD-L1, which limit immune response, is a common method to restore immunologic activity against cancer cells. Predictive value of mismatch repair deficiency (dMMR) for immunotherapy in solid tumors was demonstrated; however, only 2% or less of PCs have dMMR [54, 55]. Nevertheless, activity of the anti PD-1 monoclonal antibody pembrolizumab was observed in 22 PC patients with dMMR or high microsatellite instability (MSI-H) enrolled in the phase II KEYNOTE-158 trial [56]. Four of these subjects (18%) experienced objective response and median duration of response was 13.4 months. Thus, pembrolizumab is an alternative for patients with advanced PC whose tumors are dMMR or MSI-H and who progressed on first-line therapy, regardless of PS [13].

The neurotrophic tropomyosin receptor kinase (NTRK) gene fusion is found in <1% of PC but responses can be achieved with NTRK inhibitors entrectinib and larotrectinib [57–59]. As recommended by the NCCN, entrectinib and larotrectinib are second-line options in patients with LAPC or MPC and NTRK gene fusion [1].

In conclusion, pancreatic cancer is fatal for the majority of patients. Systemic chemotherapies are currently used as standard therapy in adjuvant, neoadjuvant, and palliative treatments. Clinical studies investigating the benefit of targeted therapies and immunotherapy strategies have resulted in significant benefits in a small percentage of patients. Ongoing studies on tumor biology and tumor microenvironment are promising for treatment options that will yield clinical benefit in this cancer.

References

1. Bray F, Ferlay J, Soerjomataram I, et al. Global cancer statistics 2018: GLOBOCAN estimates of incidence and mortality worldwide for 36 cancers in 185 countries. CA Cancer J Clin. 2018;68:394–424.
2. Ilic M, Ilic I. Epidemiology of pancreatic cancer. World J Gastroenterol. 2016;22:9694–705.
3. Khorana AA, Mangu PB, Berlin J, et al. Potentially curable pancreatic cancer: American society of clinical oncology clinical practice guideline update. J Clin Oncol. 2017;35:2324.
4. Ducreux M, Cuhna AS, Caramella C, et al. Cancer of the pancreas: ESMO clinical practice guidelines for diagnosis, treatment and follow-up. Ann Oncol. 2015;26 Suppl 5:v56.
5. Neoptolemos JP, Dunn JA, Stocken DD, et al. Adjuvant chemoradiotherapy and chemotherapy in resectable pancreatic cancer: a randomised controlled trial. Lancet. 2001;358:1576.
6. Neoptolemos JP, Stocken DD, Friess H, et al. A randomized trial of chemoradiotherapy and chemotherapy after resection of pancreatic cancer. N Engl J Med. 2004;350:1200.
7. Oettle H, Post S, Neuhaus P, et al. Adjuvant chemotherapy with gemcitabine vs observation in patients undergoing curative-intent resection of pancreatic cancer: a randomized controlled trial. JAMA. 2007;297:267.
8. Oettle H, Neuhaus P, Hochhaus A, et al. Adjuvant chemotherapy with gemcitabine and long-term outcomes among patients with resected pancreatic cancer: the CONKO-001 randomized trial. JAMA. 2013;310:1473.
9. Neoptolemos JP, Stocken DD, Bassi C, et al. Adjuvant chemotherapy with fluorouracil plus folinic acid vs gemcitabine following pancreatic cancer resection: a randomized controlled trial. JAMA. 2010;304:1073.
10. Neoptolemos JP, Palmer DH, Ghaneh P, et al. Comparison of adjuvant gemcitabine and capecitabine with gemcitabine monotherapy in patients with resected pancreatic cancer (ESPAC-4): a multicentre, open-label, randomised, phase 3 trial. Lancet. 2017;389:1011.
11. Jones RP, Psarelli EE, Jackson R, et al. Patterns of recurrence after resection of pancreatic ductal adenocarcinoma: a secondary analysis of the ESPAC-4 randomized adjuvant chemotherapy trial. JAMA Surg. 2019;154:1038.
12. Conroy T, Hammel P, Hebbar M, et al. FOLFIRINOX or gemcitabine as adjuvant therapy for pancreatic cancer. N Engl J Med. 2018;379:2395.
13. National Comprehensive Cancer Network (NCCN). NCCN clinical practice guidelines in oncology. https://www.nccn.org/professionals/physician_gls. Accessed 12 Aug 2020.
14. Uesaka K, Boku N, Fukutomi A, et al. Adjuvant chemotherapy of S-1 versus gemcitabine for resected pancreatic cancer: a phase 3, open-label, randomised, non-inferiority trial (JASPAC 01). Lancet. 2016;388:248–57.
15. Tempero MA, Reni M, Riess H, et al. APACT: phase III, multicenter, international, open-label, randomized trial of adjuvant nab-paclitaxel plus gemcitabine (nab-P/G) vs gemcitabine (G) for surgically resected pancreatic adenocarcinoma. J Clin Oncol. 2019;37(15_suppl):4000.
16. Khorana AA, Mangu PB, Berlin J, et al. Potentially curable pancreatic cancer: American society of clinical oncology clinical practice guideline. J Clin Oncol. 2016;34:2541.
17. Ferrone CR, Marchegiani G, Hong TS, et al. Radiological and surgical implications of neoadjuvant treatment with FOLFIRINOX for locally advanced and borderline resectable pancreatic cancer. Ann Surg. 2015;261:12–7.
18. Mokkad AA, Minter RM, Zhu H, et al. Neoadjuvant therapy followed by resection versus upfront resection for resectable pancreatic cancer: a propensity score matched analysis. J Clin Oncol. 2017;35:515–22.
19. Shubert CR, Bergquist JR, Groeschl RT, et al. Overall survival is increased among stage III pancreatic adenocarcinoma patients receiving neoadjuvant chemotherapy compared to surgery first and adjuvant chemotherapy: an intention to treat analysis of the National Cancer Database. Surgery. 2016;160:1080–96.
20. Murphy JE, Wo JY, Ryan DP, et al. Total Neoadjuvant therapy with FOLFIRINOX followed by individualized chemoradiotherapy for borderline resectable pancreatic adenocarcinoma: a phase 2 clinical trial [published correction appears in JAMA Oncol. 2018;4:1439]. JAMA Oncol. 2018;4:963–9.
21. Yamada S, Fujii T, Sugimoto H, et al. Aggressive surgery for borderline resectable pancreatic cancer: evaluation of National Comprehensive Cancer Network guidelines. Pancreas. 2013;42:1004–10.
22. Versteijne E, Suker M, Groothuis K, et al. Preoperative chemoradiotherapy versus immediate surgery for resectable and borderline resectable pancreatic cancer: results of the Dutch randomized phase III PREOPANC trial. J Clin Oncol. 2020;38:1763–73.
23. Reni M, Balzano G, Zanon S, et al. Safety and efficacy of preoperative or postoperative chemotherapy for resectable pancreatic adenocarcinoma (PACT-15): a randomised, open-label, phase 2-3 trial. Lancet Gastroenterol Hepatol. 2018;3:413–23.
24. Unno M, Motoi F, Matsuyama Y, et al. Randomized phase II/III trial of neoadjuvant chemotherapy with gemcitabine and S-1 versus upfront surgery for resectable pancreatic cancer (Prep-02/JSAP-05). J Clin Oncol. 2019;37S:ASCO #189.
25. Sohal D, Duong MT, Ahmad SA, et al. SWOG S1505: results of perioperative chemotherapy (peri-op CTx) with mFOLFIRINOX versus gemcitabine/nab-paclitaxel (Gem/nabP) for resectable pancreatic ductal adenocarcinoma (PDA). J Clin Oncol. 2020;38S:ASCO #4504.
26. Conroy T, Desseigne F, Ychou M, et al. FOLFIRINOX versus gemcitabine for metastatic pancreatic cancer. N Engl J Med. 2011;364:1817–25.
27. Von Hoff DD, Ervin T, Arena FP, et al. Increased survival in pancreatic cancer with nab-paclitaxel plus gemcitabine. N Engl J Med. 2013;369:1691–703.
28. Suker M, Beumer BR, Sadot E, et al. FOLFIRINOX for locally advanced pancreatic cancer: a systematic review and patient-level meta-analysis. Lancet Oncol. 2016;17:801–10.
29. Kunzmann V, Algül H, Goekkurt E, et al. Conversion rate in locally advanced pancreatic cancer (LAPC) after nab-paclitaxel/gemcitabine- or FOLFIRINOX-based induction chemotherapy (NEOLAP): final results of a multicenter randomised phase II AIO trial (abstract 671O). Data presented at the 2019 European Society for Medical Oncology (ESMO) Congress, Barcelona, Spain; September 27 through October 1, 2019. Abstract available online at https://academic.oup.com/annonc/article/30/Supplement_5/mdz247/5577841. Accessed 19 Aug 2020.
30. Burris HA 3rd, Moore MJ, Andersen J, et al. Improvements in survival and clinical benefit with gemcitabine as first-line therapy for patients with advanced pancreas cancer: a randomized trial. J Clin Oncol. 1997;15:2403–13.
31. Poplin E, Feng Y, Berlin J, et al. Phase III, randomized study of gemcitabine and oxaliplatin versus gemcitabine (fixed-dose rate infu-

sion) compared with gemcitabine (30-minute infusion) in patients with pancreatic carcinoma E6201: a trial of the Eastern Cooperative Oncology Group [published correction appears in J Clin Oncol. 2009 Dec 1;27(34):5859]. J Clin Oncol. 2009;27:3778–85.
32. Sohal DPS, Kennedy EB, Khorana A, et al. Metastatic pancreatic cancer: ASCO clinical practice guideline update. J Clin Oncol. 2018;36:2545–56.
33. Wong W, Raufi AG, Safyan RA, et al. BRCA mutations in pancreas cancer: spectrum, current management, challenges and future prospects. Cancer Manag Res. 2020;12:2731–42.
34. O'Reilly EM, Lee JW, Zalupski M, et al. Randomized, multicenter, phase II trial of gemcitabine and cisplatin with or without veliparib in patients with pancreas adenocarcinoma and a germline BRCA/PALB2 mutation. J Clin Oncol. 2020;38:1378–88.
35. Cunningham D, Chau I, Stocken DD, et al. Phase III randomized comparison of gemcitabine versus gemcitabine plus capecitabine in patients with advanced pancreatic cancer. J Clin Oncol. 2009;27:5513–8.
36. Fine RL, Moorer G, Sherman W, et al. Phase II trial of GTX chemotherapy in metastatic pancreatic cancer. J Clin Oncol. 2009;27(15_suppl):4623.
37. Fjällskog ML, Lejonklou MH, Oberg KE, et al. Expression of molecular targets for tyrosine kinase receptor antagonists in malignant endocrine pancreatic tumors. Clin Cancer Res. 2003;9:1469–73.
38. Moore MJ, Goldstein D, Hamm J, et al. Erlotinib plus gemcitabine compared with gemcitabine alone in patients with advanced pancreatic cancer: a phase III trial of the National Cancer Institute of Canada clinical trials group. J Clin Oncol. 2007;25:1960–6.
39. Wang-Gillam A, Li CP, Bodoky G, et al. Nanoliposomal irinotecan with fluorouracil and folinic acid in metastatic pancreatic cancer after previous gemcitabine-based therapy (NAPOLI-1): a global, randomised, open-label, phase 3 trial [published correction appears in lancet. 2016;387:536]. Lancet. 2016;387:545–57.
40. Gebbia V, Maiello E, Giuliani F, et al. Irinotecan plus bolus/infusional 5-fluorouracil and leucovorin in patients with pretreated advanced pancreatic carcinoma: a multicenter experience of the Gruppo Oncologico Italia Meridionale. Am J Clin Oncol. 2010;33:461–4.
41. Zaniboni A, Aitini E, Barni S, et al. FOLFIRI as second-line chemotherapy for advanced pancreatic cancer: a GISCAD multicenter phase II study. Cancer Chemother Pharmacol. 2012;69:1641–5.
42. Pelzer U, Schwaner I, Stieler J, et al. Best supportive care (BSC) versus oxaliplatin, folinic acid and 5-fluorouracil (OFF) plus BSC in patients for second-line advanced pancreatic cancer: a phase III-study from the German CONKO-study group. Eur J Cancer. 2011;47:1676–81.
43. Xiong HQ, Varadhachary GR, Blais JC, et al. Phase 2 trial of oxaliplatin plus capecitabine (XELOX) as second-line therapy for patients with advanced pancreatic cancer. Cancer. 2008;113:2046–52.
44. Assaf E, Verlinde-Carvalho M, Delbaldo C, et al. 5-fluorouracil/leucovorin combined with irinotecan and oxaliplatin (FOLFIRINOX) as second-line chemotherapy in patients with metastatic pancreatic adenocarcinoma. Oncology. 2011;80:301–6.
45. Da Rocha LA, Abrahão CM, Brandão RM, et al. Role of gemcitabine as second-line therapy after progression on FOLFIRINOX in advanced pancreatic cancer: a retrospective analysis. J Gastrointest Oncol. 2015;6:511–5.
46. Viaud J, Brac C, Artru P, et al. Gemcitabine as second-line chemotherapy after folfirinox failure in advanced pancreatic adenocarcinoma: a retrospective study. Dig Liver Dis. 2017;49:692–6.
47. Gilabert M, Chanez B, Rho YS, et al. Evaluation of gemcitabine efficacy after the FOLFIRINOX regimen in patients with advanced pancreatic adenocarcinoma. Medicine (Baltimore). 2017;96:e6544.
48. Sarabi M, Mais L, Oussaid N, et al. Use of gemcitabine as a second-line treatment following chemotherapy with folfirinox for metastatic pancreatic adenocarcinoma. Oncol Lett. 2017;13:4917–24.
49. Portal A, Pernot S, Tougeron D, et al. Nab-paclitaxel plus gemcitabine for metastatic pancreatic adenocarcinoma after Folfirinox failure: an AGEO prospective multicentre cohort. Br J Cancer. 2015;113:989–95.
50. Mita N, Iwashita T, Uemura S, et al. Second-line gemcitabine plus nab-paclitaxel for patients with Unresectable advanced pancreatic cancer after first-line FOLFIRINOX failure. J Clin Med. 2019;8:761.
51. Fisher AE, Hochegger H, Takeda S, et al. Poly(ADP-ribose) polymerase 1 accelerates single-strand break repair in concert with poly(ADP-ribose) glycohydrolase. Mol Cell Biol. 2007;27:5597–605.
52. Farmer H, McCabe N, Lord CJ, et al. Targeting the DNA repair defect in BRCA mutant cells as a therapeutic strategy. Nature. 2005;434:917–21.
53. Golan T, Hammel P, Reni M, et al. Maintenance olaparib for germline BRCA-mutated metastatic pancreatic cancer. N Engl J Med. 2019;381:317–27.
54. Hu ZI, Shia J, Stadler ZK, et al. Evaluating mismatch repair deficiency in pancreatic adenocarcinoma: challenges and recommendations. Clin Cancer Res. 2018;24:1326–36.
55. Le DT, Durham JN, Smith KN, et al. Mismatch repair deficiency predicts response of solid tumors to PD-1 blockade. Science. 2017;357:409–13.
56. Marabelle A, Le DT, Ascierto PA, et al. Efficacy of pembrolizumab in patients with noncolorectal high microsatellite instability/mismatch repair-deficient cancer: results from the phase II KEYNOTE-158 study. J Clin Oncol. 2020;38:1–10.
57. Solomon JP, Linkov I, Rosado A, et al. NTRK fusion detection across multiple assays and 33,997 cases: diagnostic implications and pitfalls. Mod Pathol. 2020;33:38–46.
58. O'Reilly EM, Hechtman JF. Tumour response to TRK inhibition in a patient with pancreatic adenocarcinoma harbouring an NTRK gene fusion. Ann Oncol. 2019;30:viii36–40.
59. Doebele RC, Drilon A, Paz-Ares L, et al. Entrectinib in patients with advanced or metastatic NTRK fusion-positive solid tumours: integrated analysis of three phase 1-2 trials [published correction appears in lancet Oncol. 2020;21:e70] [published correction appears in lancet Oncol. 2020;21:e341] [published correction appears in lancet Oncol. 2020;21:e372]. Lancet Oncol. 2020;21:271–82.

Endoscopic Biliary Drainage and Associated Procedures Required for Patients with Malignant Biliary Strictures

Hiroyuki Isayama, Toshio Fujisawa, Shigeto Ishii, Ko Tomishima, Muneo Ikemura, Hiroto Ota, Daishi Kabemura, Mako Ushio, Sho Takahashi, Yusuke Takasaki, Akinori Suzuki, Koichi Ito, Kazushige Ochiai, and Hiroaki Saito

Abstract

Endoscopic biliary drainage of a malignant biliary obstruction (MBO) is a common procedure, but a recognized standard of evaluation is lacking. To this end, the Tokyo criteria have been newly proposed and include certain definitions. Recurrent biliary obstruction (RBO) is defined as stent occlusion and migration, and the time to RBO is employed rather than the duration of stent patency. For patients with distal MBO, the preoperative management has changed to incorporate new developments in neoadjuvant chemotherapies for pancreatic cancer. Self-expandable metallic stents (SEMSs) serve as the current standard. Palliative management requires long-term stent patency, and SEMS use is thus indicated. A covered SEMS serves as the standard for palliative cases with distal MBO because such stents afford a time to RBO that is similar or superior to those of other stents, with a similar rate of adverse events. Furthermore, SEMSs are removable. However, the optimal covered SEMS is not yet available, and covered large-bore SEMSs with anti-migration and anti-reflux properties remain under evaluation. There is currently no standard management for hilar MBO (in either the preoperative or palliative context). Recently, an inside stent placed above the papilla was reported to afford better results than those of conventional stents, but strong evidence is lacking. Endoscopic ultrasound-guided biliary drainage (EUS-BD) serves as a salvage technique when routine endoscopic retrograde cholangiopancreatography fails or is difficult. Recent clinical practice guidelines for EUS-BD are becoming accepted gradually. However, dedicated devices and strong evidence of efficacy and safety are required.

24.1 Introduction

Endoscopic biliary drainage (EBD) of a malignant biliary obstruction (MBO) is a common procedure. However, the surgical strategy is affected by patient anatomy, disease characteristics, and overall health status. Various types of stents are available. Here, we review the various strategies and stents used for EBD of MBO in an effort to increase the effectiveness, efficiency, and safety of our procedures.

24.2 The Tokyo Criteria: A Standard Reporting System

Evaluation of the various available biliary stents is crucial. No standard criteria have been defined until recently. The first authors (H.I) proposed the use of the Tokyo criteria for evaluating biliary stents in terms of both efficacy and safety (Table 24.1) [1]. Although many different evaluations have been published, a meta-analysis is difficult given the large variations in the stents examined and the study methods. The Tokyo criteria propose the use of the phrase "recurrent biliary obstruction (RBO)" to define stent occlusion and migration, replacing terms such as "stent occlusion" and "stent dysfunction". Complications are classified as RBO or other (pancreatitis, cholecystitis, and cholangitis). We propose using the time to RBO (TRBO) when evaluating stent patency. Technical and clinical successes and other items are

H. Isayama (✉) · T. Fujisawa · S. Ishii · K. Tomishima · M. Ikemura · H. Ota · D. Kabemura · M. Ushio · S. Takahashi · Y. Takasaki · A. Suzuki · K. Ito · K. Ochiai · H. Saito
Department of Gastroenterology, Graduate School of Medicine, Juntendo University, Tokyo, Japan
e-mail: h-isayama@juntendo.ac.jp

Table 24.1 Factors affect the endoscopic biliary drainage

Causative disease
    Papillary cancer (distal stricture)
    Pancreatic cancer (distal stricture)
    Cholangiocarcinoma (distal and hilar stricture)
    Gallbladder cancer (distal and hilar stricture)
    Metastatic lymph node (distal and hilar stricture)
    Direct invasion of another malignant tumor (distal and hilar stricture)
    Hepatocellular carcinoma (hilar stricture)
    Metastatic liver cancer (hilar stricture)
Tumor status
    Resectable
    Borderline resectable (only pancreatic cancer)
    Palliation
Stricture location
    Distal
    Hilar (bismuth type 1–4)
Anatomy affected endoscopic procedure
    Normal
    Surgically altered (B-1, B-2, Leu-en-Y)
    Duodenal invasion
Patients' condition
    Performance status (1–4)
    High age
    Frail

Table 24.2 Kinds of self-expandable metallic stent

Structure
    Braided type
        Cross wire design
        Hook wire design
        Zigzag & Spiral-Zigzag wire design
    Laser cut type
        Zigzag wire design
Covering membrane
    Covered type (partially-, fully-covered)
    Uncovered type
Anchoring system
    Flare & Square flare
    Flare and bank
    Flap
Other function
    Drug eluting
    Anti-reflux

also defined in the Tokyo criteria. We hope that many future reports on biliary stents will employ the Tokyo criteria, as this would greatly aid meta-analyses.

24.3 Biliary Drainage in Patients with Malignant Biliary Strictures

Many factors affect selection of the procedure and stent in patients requiring EBD (Table 24.2). It is essential to consider the tumor type, patient's condition, stricture location, and surgical skills available. Distal strictures are most commonly caused by pancreatic cancer but also by distal cholangiocarcinoma, gallbladder and papillary cancers, and metastatic lymph nodes. Hilar strictures are caused by various malignant tumors including hilar cholangiocarcinoma, gallbladder cancer, metastatic lymph nodes, and liver metastases. The resectability status must be considered when developing a drainage strategy. Resectable cancers, borderline resectable cancers (requiring neoadjuvant chemotherapy/chemoradiotherapy [NAC]), and unresectable cancers require different drainage strategies and stents.

Individual patient anatomies must also be considered. It is difficult to attain the papilla if a patient presents with a surgically altered anatomy and/or duodenal tumor obstruction. Device-assisted enteroscopy is required if the anatomy is surgically altered, and percutaneous trans-hepatic biliary drainage (PTBD) is indicated for duodenal tumor obstruction. If the papilla can be accessed via the duodenal obstruction, double stenting is required (for both the duodenal and biliary strictures). Recently, endosonography/endoscopic ultrasound (EUS)-guided biliary drainage (EUS-BD) has become possible [2]. Finally, the performance status of the patient is used to guide the selection of one of several possible anti-cancer treatments; the performance status also affects biliary drainage, as do older age and frailty status.

24.4 The Various Stents Available

The stent is selected by reference to the stricture location, stage of the causative disease, patients' condition, etc. Table 24.3 lists the various stents available. Basically, two stent types are used for EBD: plastic stents (PSs) and self-expandable metallic stents (SEMSs). Both straight and double-pigtail PSs are commonly employed. SEMSs may be either braided or laser-cut. Braiding varies by the wire pattern, which may be a cross, hook, combined cross and hook, zigzag, or spiral zigzag (Fig. 24.1). Laser-cut stents feature zigzag wires. The differences described above affect the mechanical properties of SEMSs, particularly their ability to withstand radial force (RF) and axial force [3]. Some SEMSs feature a covering membrane to prevent tumor ingrowth via the stent mesh and to facilitate stent removal [4].

The Achilles' heel of a covered SEMS is stent migration. Tumor and hyperplastic tissues invade uncovered SEMSs via the mesh, rendering the stents difficult to remove. However, the membrane prevents tumor and tissue ingrowth; therefore, covered SEMSs do not become occluded by ingrowing tissue and may be easily removed. Some covered SEMSs feature anti-migration systems [5, 6]. However, the optimal covered SEMS is not yet available.

Table 24.3 Evaluating items of biliary metallic stents (Modified citation from Tokyo Criteria [1]

Technical and functional success rates	
Recurrent biliary obstruction (RBO)	The incidence of RBO during the observed period. (required the description of observational time)
	Median time to RBO (TRBO) estimated using the Kaplan-Meier method
	Non-obstruction rates at the time of 3, 6 and 12 months estimated using the Kaplan-Meier method
	Comparison using the log-rank test
Causes of RBO ✓ Rate of each cause ✓ Median time from the placement ✓ Early (within 30 days) or late (31 days or later)	Occlusion ✓ Tumor ingrowth/mucosal hyperplasia ✓ Tumor overgrowth ✓ Sludge with/without stone ✓ Food impaction ✓ Hemobilia ✓ Kinking of bile duct ✓ Others Symptomatic migration (required any intervention) ✓ Proximal ✓ Distal
Complications other than RBO ✓ Rate of each cause ✓ Median time from the placement ✓ Early (within 30 days) or late (31 days or later) ✓ Severity (Table 24.2) Survival time	✓ Pancreatitis ✓ Cholecystitis ✓ Non-occlusion cholangitis ✓ Others (bleeding, ulceration, penetration, perforation, etc.) ✓ Complications associated with stent placement procedure (peroration, bleeding with scope, desaturation of oxygen, aspiration pneumonia, etc.)

24.5 Preoperative Management of a Distal Stricture

Previously, the basic management of a preoperative distal MBO featured the use of PSs [7, 8], which can be easily placed and removed/exchanged. However, the TRBO of a PS is shorter than that of a SEMS, and thus PS placement should be performed soon after surgery. A SEMS may be indicated by pathological evaluation of the resected specimen. However, NAC has recently become indicated for patients with resectable or borderline resectable pancreatic cancers [9]. The duration of stent placement prior to surgery is thus prolonged, and the stenting strategy must be reconsidered if the patient becomes unfit for surgery. Initially, a SEMS should be chosen for patients with pancreatic cancers that are resectable or borderline resectable [10, 11]. Both covered and uncovered SEMSs have been used, but very few comparative studies have been published. A randomized controlled trial (RCT) of covered and uncovered SEMSs placed in patients receiving NAC revealed no significant difference in the cumulative stent patency [12]. However, the complication profiles of the two groups differed. Stent migration and cholecystitis were the principal causes of complications in the covered SEMS group versus tumor ingrowth in the uncovered SEMS group. Both types of SEMSs were used, but for patients receiving NAC, over 40% of the tumors were never resected [12]. In such cases, covered SEMSs are optimal.

Critically, stent selection must be based on patient and disease status. However, NAC is not a standard therapy for patients with distal cholangiocarcinoma; PSs remain the standard.

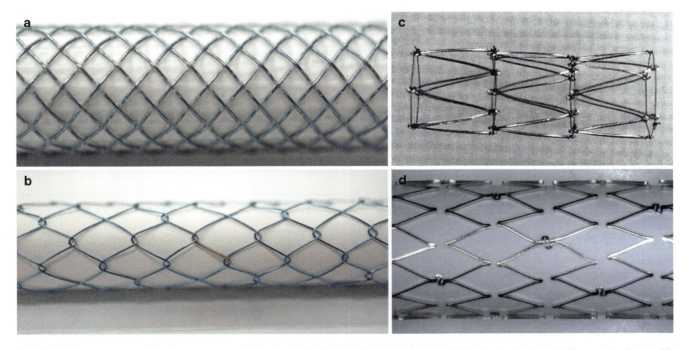

Fig. 24.1 Basic structures of self-expandable metallic stent (SEMS). (**a**) Cross wire design; (**b**) Hook wire design; (**c**) Zigzag wire design; (**d**) Zigzag wire design (Laser-cut type SEMS)

24.6 Palliative Management of Distal Strictures

A few RCTs and meta-analyses have compared PSs with SEMSs for patients with unresectable distal MBOs [13–16]. The SEMSs were clearly superior, but the choice of covered versus uncovered SEMS remains controversial. Although covered SEMSs prevent tumor ingrowth via the stent mesh [4] and thus are easily removable, this renders them prone to migration. RCTs that found no superiority of covered SEMSs over uncovered SEMSs reported a high incidence of migration. However, RCTs showed significantly longer cumulative TRBOs when using covered SEMSs with anti-migration systems compared with SEMSs lacking the anti-migration modification [6, 17].

24.7 Efforts to Prolong the TRBOs of Covered SEMSs

Despite the introduction of anti-migration systems, the TRBOs of covered SEMSs remain inadequate. Recently, effective chemotherapies have been used to manage unresectable pancreatobiliary malignancies; the incidence of stent migration is thus expected to increase [18, 19]. Prevention of migration is crucial to maintain patient quality of life and to allow patients to maintain their chemotherapy schedules. We previously showed that a weak RF and chemotherapy were the principal predictors of stent migration [19, 20]. Anti-migration systems effectively prolonged the TRBO. Figure 24.2 shows the various types of covered SEMSs with anti-migration systems, which include flaps, external uncovered regions, flares, and methods of enhancing the RF. No system is yet ideal, and the safety of each system requires further evaluation.

Recently, a larger-diameter fully covered SEMS (FCSEMS) developed by the first author (H.I) has become commercially available in Japan. Mukai et al. evaluated the large-bore covered SEMS (12 mm in diameter); in a pilot study, the TRBO was prolonged (compared with that of a control stent); sludge accumulation in and food impaction of the new stent were slower [21]. The complications associated with stent placement were acceptable. Recently, a 12-mm-diameter FCSEMS with a large flare (16 mm) has become commercially available in Japan, and is considered promising.

FCSEMSs with anti-reflux functions (ARSEMSs) are also promising. Bacterial infection in the FCSEMS cavity attributable to refluxed duodenal contents creates biliary sludge and stones. Food impaction of the stent body and orifice is a prime cause of stent occlusion. In a pilot study, an ARSEMS effectively prevented food impaction soon after placement [22]. RCTs comparing a conventional FCSEMS with an ARSEMS yielded controversial results. Lee and Moon et al. reported that the ARSEMS exhibited a longer cumulative TRBO than that of a conventional FCSEMS, but Hamada et al. found no superiority of the ARSEMS [23, 24]. Efforts to reduce the incidence of RBO and prolong the TRBO are continuing.

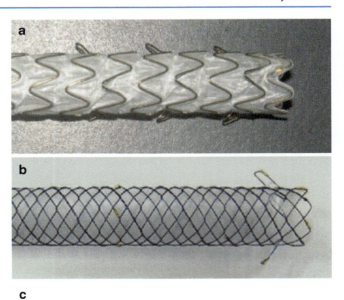
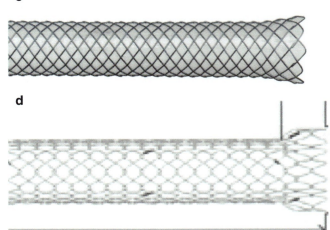

Fig. 24.2 Anti-migration systems of self-expandable metallic stent. (**a**) Flaps; (**b**) Flap; (**c**) Flare design; (**d**) Square flare design

24.8 Hilar Strictures (Resectable Cases)

Prior to hepatectomy, biliary drainage and portal vein embolization are standard to prevent liver dysfunction after surgery. Pre-surgical preparation includes biliary drainage of the future remnant lobe and portal vein embolization of the future resected lobe. Hypertrophy of the future remnant lobe and atrophy of the future resected lobe may reduce liver dysfunction after surgery. Previously,

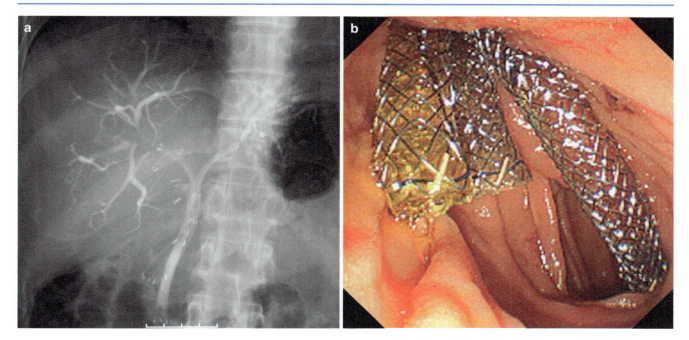

Fig. 24.3 Side-by-side stenting for hilar cholangiocarcinoma with three slim-covered self-expandable metallic stents (6 mm in a diameter). (**a**) X-ray image of side-by-side stenting. (**b**) Endoscopic image of side-by-side stenting

PTBD was employed to thoroughly drain the target biliary branch; however, the incidence of recurrent tract cancer was relatively high [25, 26]. The EBD procedure has gradually improved and is currently the standard treatment. However, stent selection during preoperative EBD remains controversial. Most Japanese institutions employ endonasobiliary drainage to reduce cholangitis before surgery, but this is uncomfortable for patients [27]. In addition, many high-volume cholangiocarcinoma surgery centers in Japan require patients to drink bile juice. Conventional PSs are standard for preoperative cases, but an inside stent placed above the papilla exhibited a longer cumulative TRBO [28]. This type of stent is promising, but more evidence is required.

24.9 Hilar Stricture: Palliative Cases

Drainage of 50% of the liver volume is required to preserve liver function and prevent ineffective stenting [29]. However, stent selection and placement are not standardized. Uncovered SEMSs exhibited longer TRBOs than those of PSs in some RCTs, but re-interventions were required when the uncovered SEMS became occluded. The Japanese clinical practice guidelines for bile duct cancer recommend the use of both PSs and metallic stents because many endoscopists favor PSs.

Two endoscopic stenting methods are used when placing SEMSs in patients with unresectable hilar biliary malignancies: the stent-in-stent (SIS) and side-by-side (SBS) methods. During the SIS method, it is sometimes difficult to place the second stent through the mesh. Certain SEMSs with loose or moveable portions have been developed to facilitate through-the-mesh placement. SBS is easier than SIS, and in some clinical trials, the initial placement success rate was similar to or slightly better than that of the SIS method. A problem with SBS placement is that a second/third SEMS delivery system passes beside the prior SEMS. When uncovered SEMSs are used, the techniques are different, but the clinical results have been similar [30].

Recent advances include slim-covered SEMSs and inside stents. Slim-covered SEMSs of thin diameter (6 mm) are placed in patients with hilar MBOs using the SBS method. Segmental cholangitis caused by obstruction of the biliary branch after covered SEMS placement has been of concern. However, the incidence thereof is not high [31]. Slim-covered SEMSs can be easily removed and exchanged. Inside stents are sutured above the papilla and have been reported to be easily removable (Fig. 24.3). The inside stent also exhibits a longer cumulative TRBO than that of conventional PSs [32] (Fig. 24.4). However, many endoscopists remain concerned about removability, and large-scale studies are warranted. No ideal stent for management of hilar MBO is yet available, thus requiring continued efforts.

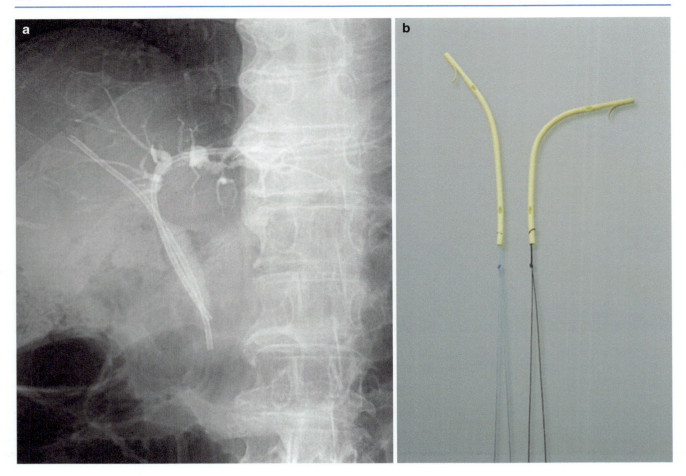

Fig. 24.4 Inside stent placement for the malignant hilar stricture case. (**a**) X-ray image of inside stent placement above the papilla. (**b**) Inside stents. Suture for removal was attached to the distal site. *Right side stent* with deep angle indicates for the left and right-posterior branch. *Left side stent* indicates for right-anterior branch

24.10 Radiofrequency Ablation of the Bile Duct

Radiofrequency ablation of the bile duct was developed to improve stent TRBO [33]. Uncovered SEMSs exhibit tumor ingrowth via the stent mesh, and tumor ablation prior to SEMS placement delayed such ingrowth. Radiofrequency ablation prior to PS placement effectively prolonged the TRBO [34]. More studies and more evidence are needed.

24.11 Endoscopic Ultrasound-Guided Biliary Drainage

EUS-BD was developed as a salvage technique after difficulty or failure of conventional endoscopic drainage. Initially, EUS-BD was indicated only for patients with unresectable MBOs, but currently, the indications are increasing. There are two principal types of EUS-BD: hepaticogastrostomy (EUS-HGS) and choledochogastrostomy (EUS-CDS) [2]. In EUS-HGS, a fistula is created between the liver (the intrahepatic bile duct) and the stomach. The EUS-CDS fistula runs from the common hepatic duct/common bile duct to the duodenum. This procedure is easier than EUS-HGS because the liver parenchyma is not penetrated. Recent Japanese clinical practice guidelines to ensure that EUS-BD is safe were proposed [35]. The procedure should be preferred to PTBD in various situations; however, very few reports on preoperative EUS-BD have appeared. Given recent developments in dedicated devices, two clinical trials have suggested that EUS-BD might serve as a primary drainage method [36, 37], being both effective and promising. The technique and devices must be developed further and standardized by referencing strong clinical and safety evidence.

24.12 Conclusions

EBD remains the standard treatment for patients with biliary obstruction/stricture. As many procedures and stents are available, it is essential to choose them carefully. No standard procedure or stent has yet emerged. EUS-BD is a relatively new biliary drainage modality that should become the drainage method of choice.

The English in this document has been checked by at least two professional editors, both native speakers of English. For a certificate, please see: http://www.textcheck.com/certificate/QZ6lR6

References

1. Isayama H, Hamada T, Yasuda I, Itoi T, Ryozawa S, Nakai Y, Kogure H, Koike K. TOKYO criteria 2014 for transpapillary biliary stenting. Dig Endosc. 2015;27(2):259–64.
2. Kawakubo K, Isayama H, Kato H, Itoi T, Kawakami H, Hanada K, Ishiwatari H, Yasuda I, Kawamoto H, Itokawa F, Kuwatani M, Iiboshi T, Hayashi T, Doi S, Nakai Y. Multicenter retrospective study of endoscopic ultrasound-guided biliary drainage for malignant biliary obstruction in Japan. J Hepatobiliary Pancreat Sci. 2014;21(5):328–34.
3. Isayama H, Nakai Y, Toyokawa Y, Togawa O, Gon C, Ito Y, Yashima Y, Yagioka H, Kogure H, Sasaki T, Arizumi T, Matsubara S, Yamamoto N, Sasahira N, Hirano K, Tsujino T, Toda N, Tada M, Kawabe T, Omata M. Measurement of radial and axial forces of biliary self-expandable metallic stents. Gastrointest Endosc. 2009;70(1):37–44.
4. Isayama H, Komatsu Y, Tsujino T, Sasahira N, Hirano K, Toda N, Nakai Y, Yamamoto N, Tada M, Yoshida H, Shiratori Y, Kawabe T, Omata M. A prospective randomized study of "covered" vs "uncovered" diamond stents for the management of distal malignant biliary obstruction. Gut. 2004;53:729–34.
5. Isayama H, Kawakubo K, Nakai Y, Inoue K, Gon C, Matsubara S, Kogure H, Ito Y, Tsujino T, Mizuno S, Hamada T, Uchino R, Miyabayashi K, Yamamoto K, Sasaki T, Yamamoto N, Hirano K, Sasahira N, Tada M, Koike K. A novel, fully covered laser-cut nitinol stent with antimigration properties for nonresectable distal malignant biliary obstruction: a multicenter feasibility study. Gut Liver. 2013;7(6):725–30.
6. Park DH, Lee SS, Lee TH, Ryu CH, Kim HJ, Seo DW, Park SH, Lee SK, Kim MH, Kim SJ. Anchoring flap versus flared end, fully covered self-expandable metal stents to prevent migration in patients with benign biliary strictures: a multicenter, prospective, comparative pilot study (with videos). Gastrointest Endosc. 2011;73(1):64–70.
7. Sasahira N, Hamada T, Togawa O, Yamamoto R, Iwai T, Tamada K, Kawaguchi Y, Shimura K, Koike T, Yoshida Y, Sugimori K, Ryozawa S, Kakimoto T, Nishikawa K, Kitamura K, Imamura T, Mizuide M, Toda N, Maetani I, Sakai Y, Itoi T, Nagahama M, Nakai Y, Isayama H. Multicenter study of endoscopic preoperative biliary drainage for malignant distal biliary obstruction. World J Gastroenterol. 2016;22(14):3793–802.
8. Kawakami H, Kuwatani M, Onodera M, Haba S, Eto K, Ehira N, Yamato H, Kudo T, Tanaka E, Hirano S, Kondo S, Asaka M. Endoscopic nasobiliary drainage is the most suitable preoperative biliary drainage method in the management of patients with hilar cholangiocarcinoma. J Gastroenterol. 2011;46(2):242–8.
9. Motoi F, Kosuge T, Ueno H, Yamaue H, Satoi S, Sho M, Honda G, Matsumoto I, Wada K, Furuse J, Matsuyama Y, Unno M, Study Group of Preoperative Therapy for Pancreatic Cancer (Prep) and Japanese Study Group of Adjuvant Therapy for Pancreatic Cancer (JSAP). Randomized phase II/III trial of neoadjuvant chemotherapy with gemcitabine and S-1 versus upfront surgery for resectable pancreatic cancer (Prep-02/JSAP05). Jpn J Clin Oncol. 2019;49(2):190–4.
10. Togawa O, Isayama H, Kawakami H, Nakai Y, Mohri D, Hamada T, Kogure H, Kawakubo K, Sakamoto N, Koike K, Kita H. Preoperative biliary drainage using a fully covered self-expandable metallic stent for pancreatic head cancer: a prospective feasibility study. Saudi J Gastroenterol. 2018;24(3):151–6.
11. Saito K, Nakai Y, Isayama H, Yamamoto R, Kawakubo K, Kodama Y, Katanuma A, Kanno A, Itonaga M, Koike K. A prospective multicenter study of partially covered metal stents in patients receiving neoadjuvant chemotherapy for resectable and borderline resectable pancreatic cancer: BTS-NAC study. Gut Liver. 2021;15(1):135–41. https://doi.org/10.5009/gnl19302.
12. Seo DW, Sherman S, Dua KS, Slivka A, Roy A, Costamagna G, Deviere J, Peetermans J, Rousseau M, Nakai Y, Isayama H, Kozarek R, Biliary SEMS During Neoadjuvant Therapy Study Group. Covered and uncovered biliary metal stents provide similar relief of biliary obstruction during neoadjuvant therapy in pancreatic cancer: a randomized trial. Gastrointest Endosc. 2019;90(4):602–12.
13. Almadi MA, Barkun A, Martel M. Plastic vs. self-expandable metal stents for palliation in malignant biliary obstruction: a series of meta-analyses. Am J Gastroenterol. 2017;112(2):260–73.
14. Nakai Y, Isayama H, Wang HP, Rerknimitr R, Khor C, Yasuda I, Kogure H, Moon JH, Lau J, Lakhtakia S, Ratanachu-Ek T, Seo DW, Lee DK, Makmun D, Dy F, Liao WC, Draganov PV, Almadi M, Irisawa A, Katanuma A, Kitano M, Ryozawa S, Fujisawa T, Wallace MB, Itoi T, Devereaux B. International consensus statements for endoscopic management of distal biliary stricture. J Gastroenterol Hepatol. 2020;35(6):967–79.
15. Davids PH, Groen AK, Rauws EA, Tytgat GN, Huibregtse K. Randomised trial of self-expanding metal stents versus polyethylene stents for distal malignant biliary obstruction. Lancet. 1992;340(8834–8835):1488–92.
16. Isayama H, Yasuda I, Ryozawa S, Maguchi H, Igarashi Y, Matsuyama Y, Katanuma A, Hasebe O, Irisawa A, Itoi T, Mukai H, Arisaka Y, Okushima K, Uno K, Kida M, Tamada K. Results of a Japanese multicenter, randomized trial of endoscopic stenting for non-resectable pancreatic head cancer (JM-test): covered Wallstent versus DoubleLayer stent. Dig Endosc. 2011;23(4):310–5.
17. Krokidis M, Fanelli F, Orgera G, Bezzi M, Passariello R, Hatzidakis A. Percutaneous treatment of malignant jaundice due to extrahepatic cholangiocarcinoma: covered Viabil stent versus uncovered Wallstents. Cardiovasc Intervent Radiol. 2010;33(1):97–106.
18. Nakai Y, Isayama H, Mukai T, Itoi T, Maetani I, Kawakami H, Yasuda I, Maguchi H, Ryozawa S, Hanada K, Hasebe O, Ito K, Kawamoto H, Mochizuki H, Igarashi Y, Irisawa A, Sasaki T, Togawa O, Hara T, Kamada H, Toda N, Hamada T, Kogure H. Impact of anticancer treatment on recurrent obstruction in covered metallic stents for malignant biliary obstruction. J Gastroenterol. 2013;48(11):1293–9.
19. Nakai Y, Isayama H, Kogure H, Hamada T, Togawa O, Ito Y, Matsubara S, Arizumi T, Yagioka H, Mizuno S, Sasaki T, Yamamoto N, Hirano K, Tada M, Koike K. Risk factors for covered metallic stent migration in patients with distal malignant biliary obstruction due to pancreatic cancer. J Gastroenterol Hepatol. 2014;29(9):1744–9.
20. Isayama H, Nakai Y, Hamada T, Matsubara S, Kogure H, Koike K. Understanding the mechanical forces of self-expandable metal stents in the biliary ducts. Curr Gastroenterol Rep. 2016;18(12):64.

21. Mukai T, Yasuda I, Isayama H, Iwashita T, Itoi T, Kawakami H, Kogure H, Nakai Y. Pilot study of a novel, large-bore, fully covered self-expandable metallic stent for unresectable distal biliary malignancies. Dig Endosc. 2016;28(6):671–9.
22. Hamada T, Isayama H, Nakai Y, Kogure H, Togawa O, Kawakubo K, Yamamoto N, Ito Y, Sasaki T, Tsujino T, Sasahira N, Hirano K, Tada M, Koike K. Novel antireflux covered metal stent for recurrent occlusion of biliary metal stents: a pilot study. Dig Endosc. 2014;26(2):264–9.
23. Lee YN, Moon JH, Choi HJ, Choi MH, Lee TH, Cha SW, Cho YD, Choi SY, Lee HK, Park SH. Effectiveness of a newly designed antireflux valve metal stent to reduce duodenobiliary reflux in patients with unresectable distal malignant biliary obstruction: a randomized, controlled pilot study (with videos). Gastrointest Endosc. 2016;83(2):404–12.
24. Hamada T, Isayama H, Nakai Y, Iwashita T, Ito Y, Mukai T, Yagioka H, Saito T, Togawa O, Ryozawa S, Hirano K, Mizuno S, Yamamoto N, Kogure H, Yasuda I, Koike K. Antireflux covered metal stent for nonresectable distal malignant biliary obstruction: Multicenter randomized controlled trial. Dig Endosc. 2019;31(5):566–74.
25. Takahashi Y, Nagino M, Nishio H, Ebata T, Igami T, Nimura Y. Percutaneous transhepatic biliary drainage catheter tract recurrence in cholangiocarcinoma. Br J Surg. 2010;97(12):1860–6.
26. Kawakami H, Kondo S, Kuwatani M, Yamato H, Ehira N, Kudo T, Eto K, Haba S, Matsumoto J, Kato K, Tsuchikawa T, Tanaka E, Hirano S, Asaka M. Preoperative biliary drainage for hilar cholangiocarcinoma: which stent should be selected? J Hepatobiliary Pancreat Sci. 2011;18(5):630–5.
27. Nakai Y, Yamamoto R, Matsuyama M, Sakai Y, Takayama Y, Ushio J, Ito Y, Kitamura K, Ryozawa S, Imamura T, Tsuchida K, Hayama J, Itoi T, Kawaguchi Y, Yoshida Y, Sugimori K, Shimura K, Mizuide M, Iwai T, Nishikawa K, Yagioka H, Nagahama M, Toda N, Saito T, Yasuda I, Hirano K, Togawa O, Nakamura K, Maetani I, Sasahira N, Isayama H. Multicenter study of endoscopic preoperative biliary drainage for malignant hilar biliary obstruction: E-POD hilar study. J Gastroenterol Hepatol. 2018;33(5):1146–53.
28. Kobayashi N, Watanabe S, Hosono K, Kubota K, Nakajima A, Kaneko T, Sugimori K, Tokuhisa M, Goto A, Mori R, Taniguchi K, Matsuyama R, Endo I, Maeda S, Ichikawa Y. Endoscopic inside stent placement is suitable as a bridging treatment for preoperative biliary tract cancer. BMC Gastroenterol. 2015;15:8.
29. Vienne A, Hobeika E, Gouya H, Lapidus N, Fritsch J, Choury AD, Chryssostalis A, Gaudric M, Pelletier G, Buffet C, Chaussade S, Prat F. Prediction of drainage effectiveness during endoscopic stenting of malignant hilar strictures: the role of liver volume assessment. Gastrointest Endosc. 2010;72(4):728–35.
30. Lee TH, Moon JH, Choi JH, Lee SH, Lee YN, Paik WH, Jang DK, Cho BW, Yang JK, Hwangbo Y, Park SH. Prospective comparison of endoscopic bilateral stent-in-stent versus stent-by-stent deployment for inoperable advanced malignant hilar biliary stricture. Gastrointest Endosc. 2019;90(2):222–30.
31. Kitamura K, Yamamiya A, Ishii Y, Mitsui Y, Nomoto T, Yoshida H. Side-by-side partially covered self-expandable metal stent placement for malignant hilar biliary obstruction. Endosc Int Open. 2017;5(12):E1211–7.
32. Kaneko T, Sugimori K, Shimizu Y, Miwa H, Kameta E, Koh R, Numata K, Tanaka K, Maeda S. Efficacy of plastic stent placement inside bile ducts for the treatment of unresectable malignant hilar obstruction (with videos). J Hepatobiliary Pancreat Sci. 2014;21(5):349–55.
33. Steel AW, Postgate AJ, Khorsandi S, Nicholls J, Jiao L, Vlavianos P, Habib N, Westaby D. Endoscopically applied radiofrequency ablation appears to be safe in the treatment of malignant biliary obstruction. Gastrointest Endosc. 2011;73(1):149–53.
34. Sofi AA, Khan MA, Das A, Sachdev M, Khuder S, Nawras A, Lee W. Radiofrequency ablation combined with biliary stent placement versus stent placement alone for malignant biliary strictures: a systematic review and meta-analysis. Gastrointest Endosc. 2018;87(4):944–51.
35. Isayama H, Nakai Y, Itoi T, Yasuda I, Kawakami H, Ryozawa S, Kitano M, Irisawa A, Katanuma A, Hara K, Iwashita T, Fujita N, Yamao K, Yoshida M, Inui K. Clinical practice guidelines for safe performance of endoscopic ultrasound/ultrasonography-guided biliary drainage: 2018. J Hepatobiliary Pancreat Sci. 2019;26(7):249–69.
36. Nakai Y, Isayama H, Kawakami H, Ishiwatari H, Kitano M, Ito Y, Yasuda I, Kato H, Matsubara S, Irisawa A, Itoi T. Prospective multicenter study of primary EUS-guided choledochoduodenostomy using a covered metal stent. Endosc Ultrasound. 2019;8(2):111–7.
37. Paik WH, Lee TH, Park DH, Choi JH, Kim SO, Jang S, Kim DU, Shim JH, Song TJ, Lee SS, Seo DW, Lee SK, Kim MH. EUS-guided biliary drainage versus ERCP for the primary palliation of malignant biliary obstruction: a multicenter randomized clinical trial. Am J Gastroenterol. 2018;113(7):987–97.

Endoscopic Management of Peripancreatic Fluid Collection

Yukitoshi Matsunami, Shuntaro Mukai, and Takao Itoi

Abstract

Patients with acute necrotic pancreatitis occasionally develop walled-off necrosis (WON). Traditionally, surgical necrosectomy has been the standard treatment for symptomatic WON. However, open surgical necrosectomy has been associated with high morbidity and mortality rates. In recent years, the endoscopic step-up approach has been developed as an alternative to open surgical necrosectomy, and studies have demonstrated that this method is associated with a high clinical success rate. In the endoscopic step-up approach, endoscopic ultrasonography-guided transmural drainage (EUS-TD) is presently the standard first step. In the absence of improvement by EUS-TD alone, endoscopic necrosectomy is performed. More recently, the electrocautery-enhanced lumen-apposing metal stent was invented for use in EUS-TD. Although there have been advancements in the devices, techniques, and methodology of EUS-TD, the mortality rate of WON still appears to be high owing to the serious complications, including bleeding and perforation. Therefore, multidisciplinary management by endoscopists, surgeons, and interventional radiologists is required.

25.1 Introduction

Peripancreatic fluid collection (PFC) is a well-known clinical consequence of acute necrotizing pancreatitis. In the revised Atlanta classification, PFC is classified into the following four categories [1]. Acute peripancreatic fluid collection, which is the collection of peripancreatic fluid associated with interstitial edematous pancreatitis that is seen within the first four weeks after the onset of pancreatitis, pancreatic pseudocyst (PP), which is a late complication of interstitial edematous pancreatitis that is seen usually more than four weeks after onset, acute necrotic collection, which is the formation of variable amounts of both fluid and necrosis that is associated with necrotizing pancreatitis, and walled-off necrosis (WON), which is a mature encapsulated necrotic collection usually occurring more than four weeks after the onset of pancreatitis. PFC, including WON, has been traditionally managed by open necrosectomy [2]. However, the procedure is associated with high morbidity and mortality [3]. Management of PFC has changed significantly in the previous decade, and endoscopic techniques are increasingly utilized in the management of PFC. Recently, the endoscopic step-up approach has been developed as an alternative to surgical necrosectomy [4]. This method aims to control the PFC by a less invasive approach in the first step of treatment, and then moving to more invasive approaches step by step. This endoscopic step-up approach has been reported to achieve high technical and clinical success rates [5, 6]. Endoscopic ultrasonography-guided transmural drainage (EUS-TD) and endoscopic necrosectomy (EN) play an important role in the endoscopic step-up approach. The lumen-apposing metal stent (LAMS) has been increasingly used for EUS-TD [7, 8]. This stent anchor is designed to distribute pressure evenly over the luminal wall and to securely anchor the stent to prevent migration. The large bore enables the evacuation of debris, and direct scope insertion when performing EN. More recently, the novel electrocautery-enhanced lumen-apposing metal stent (EC-LAMS) was invented and has contributed to enabling simpler and quicker endoscopic procedure [9]. However, determining the indications and timing of drainage, as well the timing of step-up is occasionally difficult. Herein, we describe the present status of the management of PFC, including the indications of drainage and the endoscopic techniques that are used.

Y. Matsunami · S. Mukai · T. Itoi (✉)
Department of Gastroenterology and Hepatology, Tokyo Medical University, Tokyo, Japan
e-mail: itoi@tokyo-med.ac.jp

25.2 Indications of Drainage

In general, drainage of PFC is not recommended in the early phase, owing to the lack of formation of a matured capsule. Well-encapsulated PFCs, i.e., PP and WON, are safely drained and are good indications of intervention. Drainage is recommended for patients with confirmed or clinically suspected infected WON, in whom control by conservative therapy, such as by antibiotics, was unsuccessful. Furthermore, symptomatic WON, such as organ compression, including gastric outlet obstruction, intestinal and biliary obstruction, and pain owing to a large mass is also an indication for drainage. However, the appropriate timing to perform the drainage is controversial. If the patient is tolerating the WON, the intervention is recommended to be delayed for four weeks; however, if the patient's condition is severe and associated with organ failure, it should be drained, as long as it is encapsulated. Contrast-enhanced computed tomography (CT) is often the initial imaging modality used to evaluate the size of the cavity and the presence of a pseudoaneurysm. Magnetic resonance imaging (MRI) is also considered before the intervention, as the contents of PFC, whether liquid or solid, are more accurately characterized by MRI. Pseudoaneurysms are occasionally associated with infected PFC and surrounding artery disruption. If an aneurysm is present, preceding interventional radiology (IVR) and embolization is required to avoid bleeding, which is a common adverse event of drainage. Understanding the differences between PP and WON is also important, as the endoscopic drainage of WON has been demonstrated to have a significantly lower success rate and higher adverse events rate, as well as requires more frequent reinterventions and a longer hospital stay than that of PP. Some contraindications to endoscopic drainage include splenic or portal vein occlusion, gastric varices, and the presence of pseudoaneurysm [10].

25.3 EUS-TD Technique

A linear array echoendoscope is first inserted into the stomach or duodenum, and the diameter of the PFC and the distance between the GI tract and cavity are measured. The distance between the GI tract and cavity wall longer than 1 cm should be avoided. The conventional method is to use a 19-gauge needle to puncture the PFC cavity under EUS guidance. After the needle puncture, a 0.035-inch or 0.025-inch guidewire is advanced within the cavity under fluoroscopic guidance. The tract is dilated using an electrocautery dilator and/or balloon dilator. After tract dilation, plastic stents or fully covered self-expandable metal stents (SEMS) are placed. Plastic stents are usually double-pigtail stents in order to avoid migration. The metal stents used are either fully covered biliary stents, esophageal SEMS, or LAMS [11, 12]. The recently developed EC-LAMS, which has an electrocautery wire at the distal tip of the delivery system, enables one-step stent deployment without needle puncture, guidewire advancement, or tract dilation [9]. EC-LAMS, such as the Hot-AXIOS system (Boston Scientific, Natick, MA, USA), has enabled simplification of the endoscopic drainage procedure (Fig. 25.1).

25.4 EN Technique

In patients in whom there is a poor clinical response to the drainage, EN is performed through the previously placed stent (Fig. 25.2). EN involves direct insertion of the endoscope into the cavity with a combination of suction and removal of the debris using a polypectomy snare, basket catheter, and retrieval forceps. The use of CO_2 instead of air for insufflation during necrosectomy is mandatory to reduce the risk of gas embolism. EN is usually performed once or twice a week, until clinical improvement is achieved. A balance between efficacy and safety is required to avoid injury to the intracavity vessels and retroperitoneal tissue, which leads to bleeding and perforation. In the case of bleeding during the procedure, clip hemostasis, epinephrine injection, and argon plasma coagulation are useful [13]. However, if endoscopic hemostasis is unsuccessful, emergent IVR or surgical hemostasis is required (Fig. 25.3). Contrast-enhanced CT is performed during the interval period of necrosectomy to evaluate the appearance of pseudoaneurysms.

25.5 Treatment Algorithm and Outcomes

The treatment algorithm for symptomatic PFC has evolved from invasive open surgical necrosectomy to a less invasive endoscopic step-up approach. The step-up approach was first introduced by a Dutch group in 2010, in which they reported a randomized controlled trial (RCT) comparing open necrosectomy with minimally invasive endoscopic or percutaneous drainage, and patients in the step-up approach group were found to experience significantly fewer major complications [14]. A recent retrospective study demonstrated that the endoscopic step-up approach is associated with a technical success rate of 99% and a clinical success rate of 96.5% [5]. The European Society of Gastrointestinal Endoscopy guidelines, which are recently released multidisciplinary guidelines for the endoscopic management of acute necrotizing pancreatitis, also recommend the use of the step-up approach [15]. In the step-up approach, the first step is the drainage of the infected fluid endoscopically or percutaneously. Endoscopic transmural drainage appears to be advantageous in patients in whom the PFC is located adjacent to the stomach or duodenum. At present, EUS-TD

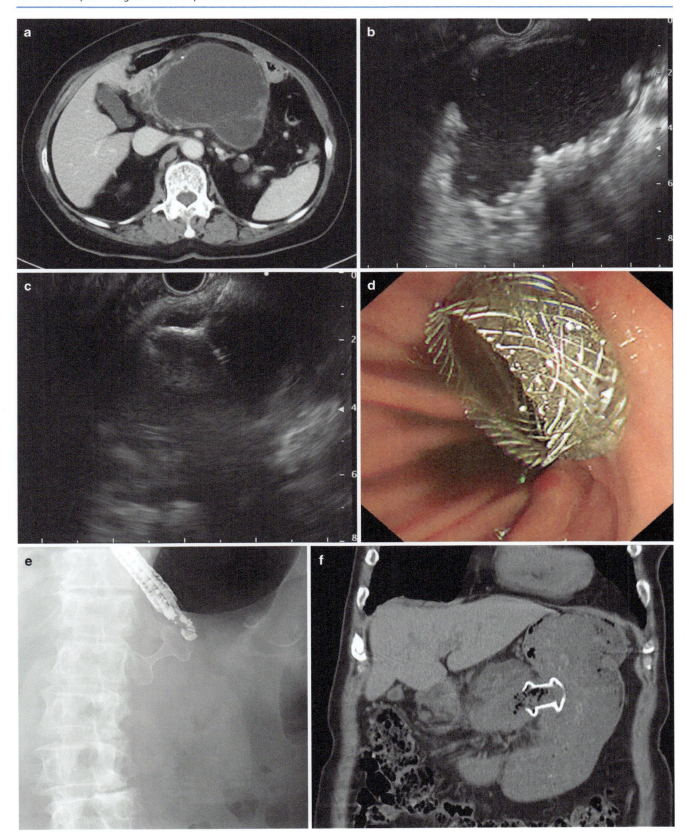

Fig. 25.1 Images of the EUS-TD. (**a**) CT scan axial view of WON. (**b**) EUS image of the encapsulated WON. (**c**) The opened distal stent anchor is visible on EUS. (**d**) Endoscopic image of Hot-AXIOS. (**e**) Fluoroscopic image of Hot-AXIOS. (**f**) CT scan coronal view of Hot-AXIOS

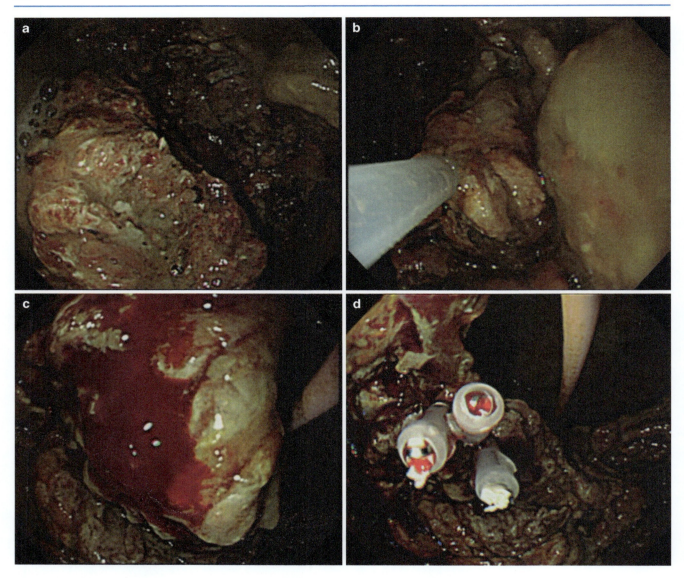

Fig. 25.2 Images of the EN. (**a**) Necrotic debris within the WON cavity. (**b**) Necrosectomy through the stent. Polypectomy snare was used for the debris removal. (**c**) Bleeding from intracavity vessel was seen during the necrosectomy. (**d**) Clip hemostasis was performed

is the optimal transmural drainage approach, replacing the conventional transmural drainage method using a gastroscope, owing to the higher success rate of drainage. Regarding the type of stent, some retrospective studies demonstrated no differences in the treatment success rate of drainage between plastic stents and metal stents, although procedure time was shorter in the metal stents group [16, 17]. However, a recently published systematic review demonstrated that resolution of WON was more likely with the use of metal stents than with plastic stents, with a trend of lower perforation and stent occlusion with metal stents, although there is more migration [18]. Another systematic review demonstrated that the clinical success rate of drainage using metal stents was 93.8% and the adverse events rate was 10.2%, which included bleeding, perforation, stent migration, and infection [19]. At present, most clinical institutions use metal stents, particularly LAMS for the initial drainage. The technical success rate of EUS-TD using EC-LAMS has been demonstrated to be 100% with no procedure-associated complications, and a 96% clinical success rate regarding resolution of the PFC [20]. If the PFC is located far from the stomach or duodenum, percutaneous drainage can be considered as an appropriate first step. The percutaneous procedure is performed under CT or ultrasound guidance. In the case of extended WON to the pelvic area, a combination of EUS-TD with additional percutaneous drainage is considered. In patients with multiple cavities or a large WON showing insufficient response to drainage alone, the multiple transluminal gateway technique (MTGT) and/or single transluminal gateway transcystic multiple

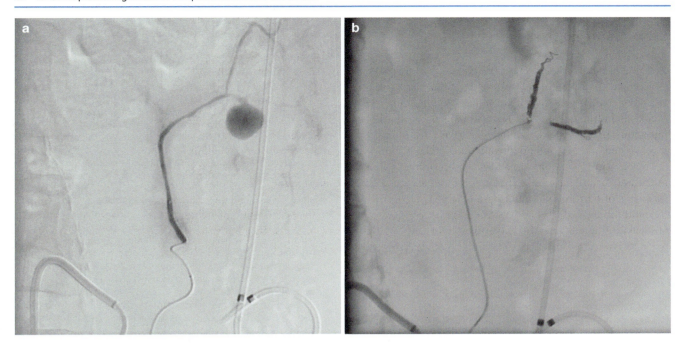

Fig. 25.3 Images of the IVR. (**a**) Rupture of pseudoaneurysm was seen from the marginal artery. (**b**) IVR with hemostatic coiling was conducted

drainage (SGTMD) should be considered [21, 22]. MTGT involves creation of some transmural gateways, and SGTMD involves drainage via one gateway by placing multiple plastic stents for the multiple cavities. Both methods were established from the idea that multiple sites of access to the cavities would achieve more efficient drainage. In the absence of improvement by drainage, EN is the next step of therapy. Patients who require EN tend to have a larger collection with more solid and necrotic debris [6]. Although EN is less invasive than surgical necrosectomy, the rate of adverse events is not low. One study demonstrated that the clinical success rate of endoscopic necrosectomy was 75%, with an adverse events rate of 33% and mortality rate of 11% [23]. The potential serious adverse events, such as bleeding, perforation, and air embolism can be life-threatening. Therefore, the procedures should be performed in a multidisciplinary setting, in which emergency rescue surgery or IVR can be performed. The LAMS should be retrieved within four weeks of placement, to avoid stent-associated complications [24]. If treatment is incomplete after four weeks, the plastic stent should be replaced. If clinical improvement is not achieved by these procedures, the next step is minimally invasive surgery, such as video-assisted retroperitoneal debridement (VARD), which minimizes the surgical incision, usually along the previously placed percutaneous catheter, or open surgical necrosectomy [14]. Indications of surgery have become limited, although surgery plays an important salvage role, such as decompressive laparotomy in cases of abdominal compartment syndrome, which is a less common but lethal complication of acute necrotizing pancreatitis [25]. These studies indicate that the endoscopic step-up approach is a reasonable treatment algorithm. However, a recently reported RCT comparing the endoscopic step-up approach and the surgical step-up approach, which consists of percutaneous catheter drainage followed by VARD if necessary, demonstrated that the endoscopic step-up approach is not superior to the surgical step-up approach in reducing major complications or death, although the rate of pancreatic fistulas and length of hospital stay were lower in the endoscopy group [4]. Regarding the role of endoscopic retrograde cholangiopancreatography (ERCP) for the management of WON, if the patient has disconnected pancreatic duct syndrome (DPDS), which is disruption of the main pancreatic duct (MPD) owing to WON, combining EUS-TD with transpapillary stenting by ERCP for bridging the disruption is considered. ERCP enables management of the underlying source of persistent leakage. A recent retrospective study demonstrated that DPDS occurs more frequently in patients with WON than those with other PFCs [26]. However, routine ERCP with transpapillary drainage is not necessary in patients that do not have DPDS. If transpapillary stenting for the MPD disruption is unsuccessful or if there is complete disruption, EUS-guided pancreatic duct drainage can be considered [27]. Although most of the previous data were from small retrospective studies, and the procedure is technically challenging, the placement of a stent as pancreatico-gastrotomy is feasible for patients with a dilated MPD.

25.6 Conclusion

The step-up approach is useful for the treatment of patients with WON. However, despite advancements in the devices, techniques, and methodology, the mortality of patients with WON is still high owing to its serious complications. Therefore, multidisciplinary management by endoscopists, surgeons, and interventional radiologists is required for successful treatment of WON.

References

1. Banks P, Bollen T, Dervenis C, et al. Classification of acute pancreatitis - 2012: revision of the Atlanta classification and definitions by international consensus. Gut. 2013;62:101–11.
2. Banks PA, Freeman ML. Practice guidelines in acute pancreatitis. Am J Gastroenterol. 2006;101:2379–400.
3. Harrison S, Kakade M, Varadarajulu S, et al. Characteristics and outcomes of patients undergoing debridement of pancreatic necrosis. J Gastrointest Surg. 2010;14:245–51.
4. van Brunschot S, van Grinsven J, van Santvoort HC, et al. Endoscopic or surgical step-up approach for infected necrotising pancreatitis: a multicentre randomised trial. Lancet. 2018;391(10115):51–8.
5. Lakhtakia S, Basha J, Talukdar R, et al. Endoscopic "step-up approach" using a dedicated biflanged metal stent reduces the need for direct necrosectomy in walled-off necrosis (with videos). Gastrointest Endosc. 2017;85:1243–52.
6. Rana SS, Sharma V, Sharma R, et al. Endoscopic ultrasound guided transmural drainage of walled off pancreatic necrosis using a "step - up" approach: a single centre experience. Pancreatology. 2017;17(2):203–8.
7. Itoi T, Binmoeller KF, Shah J, et al. Clinical evaluation of a novel lumen-apposing metal stent for endosonography-guided pancreatic pseudocyst and gallbladder drainage (with videos). Gastrointest Endosc. 2012;75(4):870–6.
8. Sharaiha RZ, Tyberg A, Khashab MA, et al. Endoscopic therapy with lumen-apposing metal stents is safe and effective for patients with pancreatic walled-off necrosis. Clin Gastroenterol Hepatol. 2016;14(12):1797–803.
9. Rinninella E, Kunda R, Dollhopf M, et al. EUS-guided drainage of pancreatic fluid collections using a novel lumen-apposing metal stent on an electrocautery-enhanced delivery system: a large retrospective study (with video). Gastrointest Endosc. 2015;82(6):1039–46.
10. Marino KA, Hendrick LE, Behrman SW. Surgical management of complicated pancreatic pseudocysts after acute pancreatitis. Am J Surg. 2016;211(1):109–14.
11. Itoi T, Reddy DN, Yasuda I, et al. New fully-covered self-expandable metal stent for endoscopic ultrasonography-guided intervention in infectious walled-off pancreatic necrosis (with video). J Hepatobiliary Pancreat Sci. 2013;20(3):403–6.
12. Siddiqui AA, Kowalski TE, Loren DE, et al. Fully covered self-expanding metal stents versus lumen-apposing fully covered self-expanding metal stent versus plastic stents for endoscopic drainage of pancreatic walled-off necrosis: clinical outcomes and success. Gastrointest Endosc. 2017;85(4):758–65.
13. Rana S, Shah J, Kang M, et al. Complication of endoscopic ultrasound-guided transmural drainage of pancreatic fluid collections and their management. Ann Gastroenterol. 2019;32:441–50.
14. van Santvoort HC, Besselink MG, Bakker OJ, et al. A step-up approach or open necrosectomy for necrotizing pancreatitis. N Engl J Med. 2010;362:1491–502.
15. Arvanitakis M, Dumonceau JM, Albert J, et al. Endoscopic management of acute necrotizing pancreatitis: European Society of Gastrointestinal Endoscopy (ESGE) evidence-based multidisciplinary guidelines. Endoscopy. 2018;50:524–46.
16. Bang JY, Hawes R, Bartolucci A, et al. Efficacy of metal and plastic stents for transmural drainage of pancreatic fluid collections: a systematic review. Dig Endosc. 2015;27:486–98.
17. Mukai S, Itoi T, Baron TH, et al. EUS-guided placement of plastic vs biflanged metal stent for therapy of walled-off necrosis: a retrospective single center study. Endoscopy. 2015;47:47–55.
18. Bazerbach F, Sawas T, Vargas E, et al. Metal stents versus plastic stents for the management of pancreatic walled-off necrosis: a systematic review and meta-analysis. Gastrointest Endosc. 2018;87(1):30–42.
19. Saunders R, Ramesh J, Cicconi S, et al. A systematic review and meta-analysis of metal versus plastic stents for drainage of pancreatic fluid collections: metal stents are advantageous. Surg Endosc. 2019;33(5):1412–25.
20. Anderloni A, Leo MD, Carrara S, et al. Endoscopic ultrasound-guided transmural drainage by cautery-tipped lumen-apposing metal stent: exploring the possible indications. Ann Gastroenterol. 2018;31(6):735–41.
21. Varadarajulu S, Phadnis MA, Christein JD, et al. Multiple transluminal gateway technique for EUS-guided drainage of symptomatic walled- off pancreatic necrosis. Gastrointest Endosc. 2011;74:74–80.
22. Mukai S, Itoi T, Sofuni A, et al. Expanding endoscopic interventions for pancreatic pseudocyst and walled-off necrosis. J Gastroenterol. 2015;50:211–20.
23. Yasuda I, Nakashima M, Iwai T, et al. Japanese multicenter experience of endoscopic necrosectomy for infected walled-off pancreatic necrosis: the JENIPaN study. Endoscopy. 2013;45(8):627–34.
24. Bang JY, Hasan M, Navaneethan U, et al. Lumen-apposing metal stents (LAMS) for pancreatic fluid collection (PFC) drainage: may not be business as usual. Gut. 2017;66:2054–6.
25. Van Brunschot S, Schut AJ, Bouwense SA, et al. Abdominal compartment syndrome in acute pancreatitis: a systematic review. Pancreas. 2014;43:665–74.
26. Bang JY, Wilcox CM, Navaneethan U, et al. Impact of disconnected pancreatic duct syndrome on the endoscopic management of pancreatic fluid collections. Ann Surg. 2018;267(3):561–8.
27. Lawrence C, Howell DA, Stefan AM, et al. Disconnected pancreatic tail syndrome: potential for endoscopic therapy and results of long- term follow-up. Gastrointest Endosc. 2008;67:673–9.

26. Endoscopic Ultrasound and Fine Needle Tissue Acquisition for Pancreatic Tumors

Razvan Iacob and Cristian Gheorghe

Abstract

Endoscopic ultrasound (EUS) has emerged as one of the most valuable tools in current clinical practice to assess pancreatic tumors, allowing accurate early diagnosis, tumor staging as well as tissue acquisition for histological and immunohistochemical characterization. The present chapter is focused on EUS in pancreatic solid tumors, reviewing indications of EUS examination, technical recommendations, and available equipment and accessories. Fine needle aspiration or biopsy (FNA/FNB) procedures have dramatically changed the management of patients with pancreatic tumors. Clinical benefit, relevant technical aspects, possible limitations of pancreatic tissue acquisition by the means of EUS-guided FNA/FNB are further detailed. EUS guided tissue sampling methods open the prospect of molecular characterization of pancreatic tumors, even in the absence of a surgical specimen, facilitating the novel personalized treatment approach.

26.1 Background

Pancreatic tumors include multiple solid or cystic primary pancreatic lesions. Solid pancreatic lesions comprise up to 85% of pancreatic tumors, whereas cystic lesions represent 10–15% of cases [1]. Pancreatic adenocarcinoma, neuroendocrine tumors, pancreatic cystic neoplasms, lymphomas, and other rare miscellaneous neoplasms are the main categories of pancreatic tumors. Pancreatic ductal adenocarcinoma represents 85–95% off all malignant pancreatic tumors. Pancreatic neuroendocrine tumors (PanNET) account for approximately 1% of pancreatic cancers by incidence and 10% of pancreatic cancers by prevalence. PanNET are insulinomas, gastrinomas, glucagonomas, somatostatinomas, VIPomas, PPomas (one third) or non-functioning tumors (two thirds) and represent the second cause of malignant pancreatic neoplasms (1–2% of all neoplasms of the pancreas) [2, 3]. Pancreas is also the site of metastasis from other primary tumors, more frequently renal cell carcinomas, or other tumor-like lesions (Table 26.1).

Appropriate management of pancreatic lesions requires adequate imaging techniques performed by experienced radiologists, as well as adequate tissue sampling capabilities. Multidetector-row computed tomography is the most frequently used imaging technique for the assessment of pancreatic tumors [5, 6]. It has a sensitivity of 72–92% for pancreatic cancer, an accuracy of up to 95% for tumor detection, with a negative predictive value in evaluating unresectability of up to 79% [6, 7].

Due to its high soft tissue contrast resolution, magnetic resonance imaging (MRI) including morphologic and functional image acquisitions, is currently preferred for the diagnosis of pancreatic lesions, having a very high accuracy for detection and staging of pancreatic adenocarcinoma (90–100%) [8]. The anatomy of pancreatic ductal system is accurately imaged by the means of magnetic resonance cholangiopancreatography (MRCP), allowing the assessment of relationships between cystic lesions and pancreatic duct as well as the follow-up of pancreatic cystic neoplasms [9, 10].

Positron Emission Tomography (PET) with 2-deoxy-[18F] fluoro-D-glucose (18FDG-PET) was found, in a recent meta-analysis, to have a 95% sensitivity and 100% specificity for pancreatic cancer diagnosis [11]. F-DOPA (3,4-dihydroxy-L-phenylalanine labelled with ^{18}F) or Ga-DOTA peptides (somatostatin analogues) are better suited for PanNET diagnosis, the latter also allowing the evaluation of somatostatin receptors expression to guide treatment [12].

R. Iacob (✉) · C. Gheorghe
University of Medicine and Pharmacy "Carol Davila", Bucharest, Romania

Fundeni Clinical Institute, Digestive Diseases and Liver Transplantation Center, Bucharest, Romania

Table 26.1 Pancreatic tumors and tumor-like lesions (after Scialpi M et al. Reference [4])

Tumor lesions	Primitive	Secondary
	Solid exocrine tumors	• Renal cell carcinoma
	• Ductal adenocarcinoma	• Lung carcinoma
	• Acinar cell carcinoma	• Breast carcinoma
	• Pancreatoblastoma	• Colorectal carcinoma
	• Solid pseudpapillary neoplasm	• Melanoma
	• Pancreatic lymphoma	• Ovarian cancer
	• Miscalaneous carcinoma	• Sarcoma
	Solid endocrine tumors	
	• Insulinoma	
	• Gastrinoma	
	• Glucagonoma	
	• Vipoma	
	• Pancreatic polypeptide secreting tumors (PPoma)	
	• Somatostatinoma	
	• Non-functioning tumors	
	Cystic lesions	
	• Intraductal papillary mucinous neoplasm (IPMN)	
	• Serous cystadenoma	
	• True cyst	
	• Cystic variants of solid tumors (cystic teratoma, cystic ductal adenocarcinoma, cystic NET)	
Tumor-like lesions	• Focal pancreatitis	
	• Fatty infiltration replacement	
	– Pseudocysts	
	– Intrapancreatic accessory spleen	
	– Hydatic cysts	
	– Fibrocystic disease	
	– Duplication cysts and retention cysts	
	– Sarcoidosis	
	– Castelman disease	

The most sensitive technique that allows detection of small pancreatic tumors (less than 2 cm) especially located in the head of the pancreas is endoscopic ultrasound (EUS) [13]. Contrast-enhanced US (CEUS) has emerged as a cost-effective method that allows a real time evaluation and differential diagnosis of pancreatic lesions, being exceptionally accurate to demonstrate PanNET vascularization [14]. A major advantage of EUS over other techniques is that EUS allows tissues sampling during the same diagnostic session, by the means of fine need aspiration or core biopsy [15].

26.2 Short History

EUS was initially developed in 1970 and emerged as an essential diagnostic tool for pancreatic parenchyma in 1980s, when the groups of DiMagno and Hisanaga first described the ability to examine the gastrointestinal wall and the extraluminal space by the means of and US transducer mounted on the tip of a rigid endoscope [16, 17]. The first radial echoendoscope was developed by Olympus (Tokyo, Japan) in 1982, whereas Tytgat and Tio first proposed to use the biopsy channel of the endoscope for cytology [18]. First linear-array echoendoscopes were constructed by the collaboration of Hitachi with Pentax Medical in the 1990s and developed rapidly due to the novel ability to track the biopsy needle in real time across the image plane to target the lesion. Vilmann et al. introduced the first EUS biopsy tool, in collaboration with Medi-Globe GmbH opening an entirely new field for diagnostic EUS [19]. Subsequently Wiersema et al. have published the first EUS-FNA in the United States in 1992 [20]. The importance of on-site cytopathology was assessed also by the Wiersema group in 1994 [21], whereas Giovaninni et al. have documented EUS-FNA as a safe procedure for routine clinical practice [22]. In 1997 Binmoeller et al. have described the first automated biopsy device for pancreatic lesions [23] while the first clinical experience with EUS-guided biopsies in perigastric tissues were reported in 2002 [24]. The initial True-cut biopsy needle with limited flexibility was replaced by the ProCore fine needle biopsy (FNB) needles, available in a wide variety of sizes from 25 to 19G [25].

26.3 EUS Equipment and Accessories

Current echoendoscopes have been designed to overcome technical challenges of older equipment having improved maneuverability, better endoscopic views, and detailed ultrasound images for all investigating frequencies. Different needle designs, including core biopsy needles together with the new optical biopsy concept have revolutionized the field of cytological and histological endoscopic ultrasound tissue sampling.

All three major endoscope manufacturers (Olympus, Pentax and Fujifilm) provide forward viewing endoscopes having electronic 360° radial-array transducers for high resolution EUS images. There are subtle differences in scope designs between the available scopes, concerning mainly the positioning of the suction channel and the optical sensor. Clinical applications for radial EUS scopes remain for primary staging of esophageal, gastric or rectal cancers or for characterization of gastrointestinal submucosal lesions.

The same endoscope manufacturers provide linear echoendoscopes with subtle differences between devices: the tip of the Olympus transducer is more rounded and contoured, allowing for increased imaging of tissue anterior to the echoendoscope. The Hi-Compound feature of Pentax linear echoendoscopes allows the image scanning from multiple angles by combining frequency and spatial compounding. Fijifilm echoendoscopes are characterized by easier maneuverability having similar therapeutic capabilities.

Each EUS platform requires unique ultrasound processors for imaging having defined features and enhancements. Olympus has two distinct ultrasound platforms (Hitachi Aloka ProSound F75 and EU-ME2 and Premier Plus, allowing frequencies up to 12 MHz and many enhanced ultrasound physics capabilities, as well as contrast echo features, to visualize microvascularisation to the capillary level. Pentax uses the Hitachi HI VISION Preirus Ultrasound platform that combines Hi-Compound imaging with Hi-Resolution for enhanced organ boundary visualization and reduced angle-dependent artifacts. Fijifilm promotes scopes using the new generation small Super CCD chip technology for bright, high-resolution endoscopic images, integrating the ZONE Sonography and Sound Speed Correction technologies for ultrasound imaging. The new Sonart Su-1 processor is used for both radial and linear echoendoscopes, having specific features for compound harmonic imaging, sound speed imaging and elastography [26].

The fine needle aspiration needles have been substantially enhanced having different characteristics in term of needle tip, configuration, stylet composition, different sheath materials, different length and attachment to the FNA channel. There are numerous single-use needle devices available in 25-, 22- and 19-G. Some of the features of available FNA needles are presented in Table 26.2. 19G needles may offer advantages over 22G needles in terms of the size and quality of the tissue sample. However, these needles are stiffer and more difficult to use, and as a result, often fail, especially when biopsy is performed with the scope in a bent position, for example in the duodenum.

Fine needle biopsy needles have been developed to overcome the frequent drawback of failure to obtain an adequate sample for analysis, despite advancement in needle designs

Table 26.2 Fine needle aspiration, available needles, main design features and benefits (after Mishra G et al. Reference [26])

Company	Product name	Sizes	Needle design	Main design features and benefits
Cook Medical	EchoTip Ultra	19-, 22-, 25-G	Lancet	Better target and visibility; contoured handle; compatibility with multiple echoendoscopes by sheath adjuster; greater needle flexibility by coiled sheath
Boston Scientific	Expect; Expect Slimline	19-, 19-G Flexible (Nitinol), 22-, 25-G	Lancet	Precise targeting and sampling with echogenic tip and sharp needle grind; better tissue penetration capability by cobalt-chromium construction providing greater hardness and tensile properties; needle resistant to damage; stylet cap with integrated tip
Medronic	Beacon EUS Delivery System	19-G (nitinol), 22-, 25-G (stainless steel)	Lancet	Allows the passage of multiple needles through a single delivery system for improved workflow; only FDA-cleared EUS safety needle with automated safety shield; improved tissue yield for cytology by four cutting edges design
Con-Med	Clearview	19-, 22-, 25-G	Lancet	Laser-etched needle for clear visibility with ultrasound; Nitinol stylet with locking cap; enhanced Luer-Lok design
Olympus	EZ Shot 3 Plus	19-G+, 19-G (side hole), 22G + (side hole), 25-G	Menghini	Less force to pass into torqued endoscope; smooth puncture even from oblique angles; needle remains straight during fanning after multiple passes; greater force transmission by multilayered metal coil sheath
Medi-Globe GmbH	SonoTip Pro Control	19-, 22-, 25-G	Standard cut with back cut without special facet	TLT (Twist-Lock Technology) for needle length and sheath length adjustment; large needle opening for atraumatic puncture and optimal clean yield of cytology specimen; faster stylet insertion time and easier coiling by optimized lighter stylet; specially treated needle for needle visibility

and multiple passage procedures. Fine needle biopsy procedure is now standard for centers that lack on-site cytology capabilities or when molecular characterization of the sample is required for personalized targeted therapy, as it provides adequate amount of tumor cells and desmoplastic stroma suitable for molecular analysis. In suspected autoimmune pancreatitis or in cases requiring molecular staining for metastasis diagnosis (kidney, lung, melanomas) FNB is indicated. Needles have been designed also to allow injection of content rather than only for tissue acquisition, cone shaped tip needles with side-holes being specifically designed to deliver neurolysis agents radially by spray into the celiac plexus. Currently available fine needle biopsy needles with respective design features and intended benefits are depicted in Table 26.3.

Table 26.3 Fine needle biopsy, available needles, available needles, main design features and benefits (after Mishra G et al. Reference [26])

Company	Product name	Sizes and design	Design and benefits
Cook Medical	Echotip ProCore	19-C (Lancet), 20-C (Menghini), 22-C (Lancet), 25-C (Lancet)	Receives sample into the needle using the core trap technology; secure management and minimizing contamination risk using Nitinoil Recoil stylet; coiled sheath which facilitates steel needle flexibility
Boston Scientific	Acquire	19-G, 22-G (All Franseen), 25-G	Maximize tissue capture and minimize fragmentation by the means of the three symmetrical cutting surfaces with fully formed heels; better needle penetration, less kinking and deformation after multiple passes due to the cobalt-chromium needle; optimized control during actuation by Controlzone and Lubricomp polymer ergonomically defined areas
US Endoscopy	Moray	Micro Forceps	Effective tissue grabs by serrated jaws; 0.8 mm stainless steel spring sheath compatible with most 19-G FNA needles; designed to take tissue samples from wall of pancreatic cysts
Medtronic	SharkCore	19-G, 22-G, 25-G	Designed to acquire cohesive units with intact cell architecture having six distal cutting edges; minimizes tissue stacking and fracturing to provide better core samples

26.4 EUS for Pancreatic Solid Tumors

EUS with tissue acquisition is currently considered the diagnostic test of choice for pancreatic masses. A significant minority of these patients do not have PDAC and those who do, are increasingly requiring precision therapy. Pancreatic solid tumors may be malignant, benign, or inflammatory. In prospective EUS-FNA trials 55–70% of pancreatic tumors are adenocarcinomas, 15 to 25% are inflammatory masses, 6 to 15% are PanNET, whereas 5 to 15% are metastasis or rare tumors. It has been shown that neoadjuvant therapy may improve outcomes, so that approximately 46% of borderline resectable tumors are converted to resectable lesions after treatment [27]. EUS is also the best diagnostic modality for PanNETs superior to both CT and MRI.

EUS-guided FNA diagnostic yield can be optimized by specific technical recommendations, like performing FNA by the "fanning technique", by the availability of onsite pathologist for immediate sample processing and analysis or by the means of core biopsy needles use to maximize tissue acquisition. Initially there has been concern that EUS-FNA might led to potential spread of malignant cells but subsequent studies in pancreatic masses have shown that EUS-FNA procedure is not associated with decreased survival due to malignant cells dissemination in patients with resected pancreatic cancer [28]. The recent innovations in core needles allows better tissue sampling especially for tissue acquisition for molecular characterization of tumors and personalized therapy.

26.4.1 Indications for Evaluation of a Suspected Pancreatic Tumor

The ultrasound examination should always investigate key characteristics off visualized masses like maximal diameter of the lesion, lesion border characteristics (irregular or well-defined borders), echogenicity, associated cystic lesions, the presence of ductal dilatation. The relationship with surrounding vessels should be investigated, describing the tumor vessel interface, the vascular tumor invasion or occlusion. Lymph nodes (LN) stations should be examined to establish possible metastatic disease: celiac axis, peripancreatic region, porta hepatis, gastrohepatic ligament, aortocaval, posterior mediastinal stations. Liver examination during EUS could indicate the presence of hypoechoic, well defined metastatic lesions, however only limited transgastric or transduodenal examination is possible.

The presence of an anechoic triangular or irregularly shaped region outside the duodenal or gastric wall, as well as omental nodules could be an indication of peritoneal carcinomatosis, and fluid aspiration or biopsy could be performed for diagnosis.

When performing tissue sampling, the most distant metastatic station should be sampled first, prioritizing sampling for ascites, distant metastatic lymph node, omental nodule or liver nodule followed by sampling of regional lymph node or suspected tumor in case of initial negative result.

For all suspected pancreatic malignant lesions, tumor staging according to the most recent tumor-node-metastasis (TMN) staging classification should be conducted.

26.4.2 Technical Aspects of Endoscopic Ultrasound (EUS)-Guided Sampling

Technical aspects of endoscopic ultrasound (EUS)-guided sampling have been recently reviewed by the European Society of Gastrointestinal Endoscopy (ESGE) in its technical guideline published in March 2017 [29]. For routine EUS-guided sampling of solid masses and lymph nodes ESGE recommends 25G or 22G needles with equal recommendation of fine needle aspiration (FNA) and fine needle biopsy (FNB). Analyzing the results of randomized controlled trials comparing the diagnostic yield and accuracy of EUS-FNA and EUS-FNB there have not been significant differences that could strongly and routinely recommend one or the other technique in term of diagnostic yield [30]. With the aim of obtaining a core tissue specimen 19G FNA or FNB needles or 22G FNB needles are recommended. EUS- FNB needles (Pro-core, Acquire, Shark core) have advantages over FNA needles in improving diagnostic yield in cases with prior negative diagnosis (salvage approach), improving the assessment of tissue architecture and allowing for immunohistochemical stains for autoimmune pancreatitis, lymphoma, metastasis, neuroendocrine tumors, if there is no rapid on site cytological evaluation capability or whenever evaluation of molecular markers and genomic profiling for targeted therapies is desired.

The use of a 10-mL syringe suction for EUS-guided sampling of solid masses and LNs with 25G or 22G FNA needles as well as with other types of needles is suggested. The neutralization of residual negative pressure in the needle before withdrawing the needle from the target lesion should be performed. There is no recommendation in favour or against using the needle stylet for EUS-guided sampling of solid masses and LNs with FNA needles but there is benefit for using the needle stylet for EUS-guided sampling with FNB needles. When sampling solid masses or LNs the "fanning technique" should be used. When the is no on-site cytologic evaluation available, ESGE suggests conducting three to four needle passes with an FNA needle or two to three passes with an FNB needle [29].

The is no ESGE recommendation for routine antibiotic prophylaxis for EUS-guided sampling of solid masses or LNs, but fluoroquinolones or beta-lactam antibiotics should be used as antibiotic prophylaxis when sampling cystic lesions. ESGE recommends not to use smear cytology only for evaluation of tissue obtained by EUS-guided sampling, but instead to include histologic preparations (e. g., cell blocks and/or formalin-fixed and paraffin-embedded tissue fragments) whenever possible [29].

26.4.3 EUS for Pancreatic Ductal Adenocarcinoma

Pancreatic ductal adenocarcinoma has a dismal five-year survival rate of 8%, thus early diagnosis and adequate management planning are of paramount importance for better outcomes. Although usually diagnosed in the seventh decade of life, cases diagnosed in younger patients are associated with a greater disease burden, through the potential years of life lost, emphasizing the importance of an accurate early diagnosis for optimal management [31]. The use in clinical practice of EUS-FNA is currently the most accurate diagnostic modality of pancreatic cancer and had led to a changing paradigm in the management of PDAC patients [32]. EUS - FNA is indicated in PDAC in case of locally irresectable of metastatic lesions prior to chemotherapy, for borderline-resectable tumors before chemotherapy and in case of resectable lesions, only in selected cases, when histology is required for differential diagnosis. Several factors could impact the yield of EUS FNA procedure: the experience of the operator, the technique of the biopsy, the type of needle used and the availability of on-site pathology for rapid sample processing and examination. There is a learning curve in performing adequate EUS-FNA. ASGE guidelines recommend 25 supervised EUS-FNA for the diagnosis of pancreatic adenocarcinoma whereas ESGE guidelines recommend 20–30 supervised procedures. Most experts recommend a 6–24 months "hands-on" training in EUS before achieving competency.

For detection of pancreatic cancer, EUS has a sensitivity of 89–100%, a specificity of 50–100%, an accuracy of 94–96% and a negative predictive value of 100% [33]. EUS suggests pancreatic cancer in case of a hypoechoic tumor with irregular margins (Fig. 26.1) and contrast administration could further enhance the diagnostic accuracy by visualizing a hypoenhancing lesion, allowing differential diagnosis with chronic pancreatitis (isoenhancing or hyperenhancing) [34]. Elastography uses different colors to indicate the degree of stiffness of the tissue, that could be evaluated qualitatively or quantitatively, in comparison to adjacent tissue in the form of a strain ratio [35].

EUS has a well-defined role in the staging algorithm of PDAC as an accurate modality to determine tumor size, to provide a tissue acquisition modality, to assess vascular invasion especially portal vein invasion and to evaluate locore-

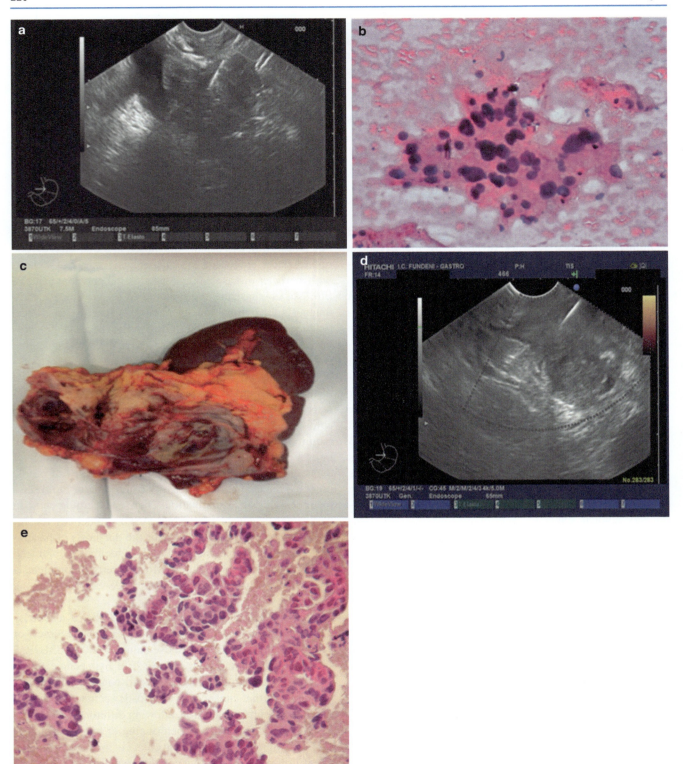

Fig. 26.1 Pancreatic ductal adenocarcinoma, EUS appearance, FNA cytology and surgical specimen. (**a**) EUS appearance of resectable pancreatic ductal adenocarcinoma (PDAC), the FNA needle could be visualized as a hyperechoic tract in the upper right corner of the image. (**b**) Atypical cells at cytologic examination with pleomorphic nuclei suggesting malignancy (HE stain 400×). (**c**) Surgical specimen of resected PDAC. (**d**) EUS appearance of an unresectable PDAC. (**e**) Cell-block cytology—sheets of ductal atypical cells with pleomorphic nuclei and focal acinar structures suggesting PDAC (HE stain, 200×) (*Becheanu G. and Dumbrava M. Collection, Digestive Diseases and Liver Transplantation Center, Fundeni Clinical Institute, Bucharest, Romania*)

gional lymph node stations. The following lymph node stations should be assessed by EUS in case of patients with suspected PDAC: celiac axis, peripancreatic station, porta hepatis, gastro-hepatic ligament and aortocaval stations. The metastatic lymph node EUS appearance is that of round hypoechoic lymph nodes, with well-defined margins and over 1 cm size. EUS has also an important role in establishing the diagnosis of peritoneal carcinomatosis by visualizing the peritoneal fluid even in small volumes and allowing fluid aspiration for cytologic diagnosis [36].

Fine needle aspiration is currently the standard diagnostic procedure for PDAC, using needles of different sizes (19G, 22G or 25G). Although initial meta-analyses have shown that 25G needle systems are more sensitive than 22G needles for diagnosing pancreatic malignancy, more recent RCTs have indicated that FNA yield is comparable between 22G and 25G needles [37]. Pancreatic masses located in the body and tail of the pancreas should be sampled via the transgastric route, whereas lesions located in the head or the uncinate process could be accessed via the trans-duodenal route. Trans-duodenal route poses supplementary problems when using 22G needles due to the torque of the endoscope and the angulation of the echoendoscope's tip. When performing FNA one should take into account that the center of a malignant mass is usually necrotic, while the periphery is often fibrotic (desmoplastic). Repeated sampling along the same trajectory increase bloodiness. The currently recommended sampling technique is the "fanning technique" that consists in the moving of the FNA needle in multiple planes and areas of the tumor, rather than sampling of a single area, thus increasing diagnostic accuracy.

The use of a stylet in EUS FNA of a pancreatic tumor was not associate with a significant improvement of the diagnostic yield, the present recommended approach is to let the stylet in situ for the first pass and to remove it for subsequent passes [38]. The availability of a cytopathologist on site when performing EUS-FNA is increasing the diagnostic accuracy of the procedure. In case he is not available, the FNA aspirate should be placed in a preservative for specimen processing and off-site assessment, however with a reduction in diagnostic yield of up to 20% according to some studies. The use of FNB instead of FNA needles is currently recommended in this setting [39].

Lesions located in the uncinate process could be difficult to sample thus the adoption of an algorithmic approach is recommended, using 25G needles for trans-duodenal sampling and 22G needles for the trans-gastric approach. The presence of chronic pancreatitis is also challenging when assessing suspected pancreatic tumors, due to the high negative FNA samples in case of fibrous modifications or the abundant inflammatory infiltrate that mimics malignant cells. In this setting it is recommended to repeat the FNA to document the diagnosis of malignancy.

FNA is considered a safe procedure as adverse events are cited in up to 1% of cases comprising in acute pancreatitis, abdominal pain, bleeding, fever and infection [40]. Most adverse events are mild in severity and self-limiting, and severe complications are rare [41].

26.4.4 EUS for Pancreatic Neuroendocrine Tumors

PanNET is the second most common pancreatic malignancy, comprising approximately 2% of pancreatic neoplasms, and most lesions arise de novo or as part of multiple endocrine neoplasia type I (MEN-1). The diagnostic workup requires immunohistochemical staining for neuroendocrine markers such as chromogranin, synaptophysin and the assessment of Ki-67 index for tumor grading. PanNETs are a very heterogeneous group of neoplasms, often slow growing, but sometimes may present at advanced, incurable stage. Therapeutic management is mainly guided by symptoms, tumor grade (G1-G3) (EUS-FNA/FNB) and tumor stage (TNM). Surgery is the only curative treatment, whereas systemic therapy can only control disease progression. Observation may represent a reasonable approach for patients with small, low-grade non-functional PanNETs (evaluated by EUS-FNA/FNB). In the presence of unresectable progressive disease, somatostatin analogs, targeted therapies such as everolimus, peptide receptor radionuclide therapy (PRRT) and systemic chemotherapy are useful.

On EUS PanNETs appear as homogenous, vascular, hypoechoic lesions with smooth margins, with peripheric rim enhancement (Fig. 26.2). Some lesions might have a cystic component and, in most cases, do not obstruct the main pancreatic duct, in contrast to PDAC. The sensitivity of EUS for the diagnosis of PanNET is 86–97% and the specificity of 95–98% [42].

As PanNETs are vascular lesions, the FNA samples could be bloody, so that it is recommended not to use 19G needles or suction for tissue sampling. For immunohistochemical diagnosis is required to have at least two dedicated passes and cell block cytology or paraffin embedded tissue samples. In PanNETs EUS has a role in assisting surgical planning, allowing a more limited resection (after excluding PDAC by FNA), accurately assessing the distance to pancreatic capsule and to main pancreatic duct or even allowing endoscopic tattooing.

26.4.5 EUS for Other Pancreatic Tumors

In up to 15% of cases the pancreas could be the site of metastasis for other cancers like renal cell carcinoma, non-small cell lung carcinoma or urogenital cancers, malignant mela-

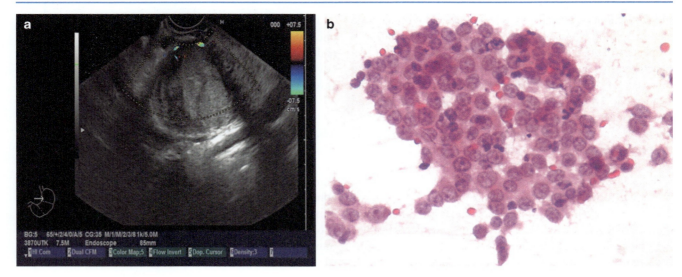

Fig. 26.2 Pancreatic neuroendocrine tumor, EUS appearance and cytology. (**a**) EUS appearance of PanNET as a well-defined lesion with hyperechoic rim. (**b**) Cytology sample with cellular uniformity, "salt and pepper" nuclei (HE stain, 400×) (*Becheanu G. and Dumbrava M. Collection, Digestive Diseases and Liver Transplantation Center, Fundeni Clinical Institute, Bucharest, Romania*)

noma, gastrointestinal cancers, breast cancer, sarcomas and lymphomas, which could occur up to 29 years after the initial tumor was diagnosed [43]. EUS can identify in these cases single or multiple hypoechoic pancreatic lesions, with a round shape and usually without ductal dilation, with well-defined margins. EUS-FNA/FNB has a sensitivity of 88–94% and specificity of 60–100% for diagnosis of pancreatic metastatic lesions and diagnosis is established based on immunohistochemistry staining of cell block specimens or pancreatic biopsy [44].

Pancreatic lymphoma is a rare entity with a uniformly hypoechoic EUS appearance, usually located in the pancreatic head with ill-defined margins. The lesions are usually less than 4 cm in size, could present vascular invasion in up to 40% of cases and peripancreatic lymphadenopathy is encountered in >50% of cases. Atypical lymphocytes could be identified by FNA and diagnosis is established by immunohistochemical staining [45].

26.4.6 Personalized Cancer Treatment

Molecular profiling using EUS-guided tissue acquisition could be used to improve diagnostic accuracy, to establish prognosis and to guide therapy in PDAC. Targeted therapies have shown significant survival benefit in many different cancer types, and there is urgent need to develop and validate personalized therapies also for pancreatic cancer, to improve therapeutic outcome. Initial clinical trials of targeted therapy have failed to establish a survival benefit in PDAC probably due to suboptimal patient selection. Several recent molecular profiling studies, however, have indicated that up to 25% of PDAC patients harbor actionable tumoral alterations, the largest actionable altered gene pathway involving the DNA Damage Response Genes (DDR). Other gene targets could be the Mismatch repair genes (MMR), targeting tumors that carry these mutations by immune checkpoints inhibitors. TRK inhibitors could be prescribed to patients that are diagnosed with tumors harboring ROS1 or NTRK1-3 mutations whereas the new poly(ADP-ribose) polymerase (PARP) inhibitors could represent promising therapeutic alternatives for tumors carrying BRCA1/2 mutations. Other genetic alterations have been linked to prognostic and response to current therapies and could be further used to better tailor individual treatments: KRAS, NRAS, TP53, DYPD [46].

As surgery is possible at diagnosis only in a minority of PDAC patients, EUS-guided tissue acquisition remains the main tool that allows molecular profiling of individual cases, with liquid biopsy showing promising perspectives. The new generation of core-biopsy needles, with the ability to provide a histologic sample, are recommended for tissue acquisition for molecular profiling, although the latest next generation sequencing platforms have been shown to provide robust data, also when FNA samples are used.

References

1. Cho HW, Choi JY, Kim MJ, Park MS, Lim JS, Chung YE, Kim KW. Pancreatic tumors: emphasis on CT findings and pathologic classification. Korean J Radiol. 2011;12(6):731–9.
2. Reddy S, Wolfgang CL. Benign pancreatic tumors. Surg Clin North Am. 2007;87(6):1359–78.
3. Larsson LI. Endocrine pancreatic tumors. Hum Pathol. 1978;9(4):401–16.
4. Scialpi M, Reginelli A, D'Andrea A, Gravante S, Falcone G, Baccari P, Manganaro L, Palumbo B, Cappabianca S. Pancreatic tumors imaging: an update. Int J Surg. 2016;28(Suppl 1):S142–55.

5. Tummala P, Junaidi O, Agarwal B. Imaging of pancreatic cancer: an overview. J Gastrointest Oncol. 2011;2(3):168–74.
6. Fletcher JG, Wiersema MJ, Farrell MA, Fidler JL, Burgart LJ, Koyama T, Johnson CD, Stephens DH, Ward EM, Harmsen WS. Pancreatic malignancy: value of arterial, pancreatic, and hepatic phase imaging with multidetector row CT. Radiology. 2003;229:81–90.
7. Brennan DD, Zamboni GA, Raptopoulos VD, Kruskal JB. Comprehensive preoperative assessment of pancreatic adenocarcinoma with 64-section volumetric CT. Radiographics. 2007;27(6):1653–66.
8. Wang Y, Miller FH, Chen ZE, Merrick L, Mortele KJ, Hoff FL, Hammond NA, Yaghmai V, Nikolaidis P. Diffusion-weighted MR imaging of solid and cystic lesions of the pancreas. Radiographics. 2011;31(3):47–64.
9. Sandrasegaran K, Lin C, Akisik FM, Tann M. State-of-the-Art pancreatic MRI. Am J Roentgenol. 2010;195(1):42–53.
10. Fattahi R, Cem Balci N, Perman WH, Hsueh EC, Alkaade S, Havlioglu N, Burton FR. Pancreatic diffusion-weighted imaging (DWI): comparison between mass-forming focal pancreatitis (FP), pancreatic cancer (PC), and normal pancreas. J Magn Reson Imaging. 2009;29(2):350–6.
11. Rijkers AP, Valkema R, Duivenvoorden HJ, van Eijck CH. Usefulness of F-18-fluorodeoxyglucose positron emission tomography to confirm suspected pancreatic cancer: a meta-analysis. Eur J Surg Oncol. 2014;40(7):794–804.
12. Kwikkeboom DJ, Kam BL, van Essen M, Teunissen JJ, van Eijck CH, Valkema R, de Jong M, de Herder WW, Krenning EP. Somatostatin-receptor-based imaging and therapy of gastroenteropancreatic neuroendocrine tumors. Endocr Relat Cancer. 2010;17(1):53–73.
13. Wiersema MJ. Accuracy of endoscopic ultrasound in diagnosing and staging pancreatic carcinoma. Pancreatology. 2001;1:625–35.
14. Recaldini C, Carpafiello G, Bertolotti E, Angeretti AG, Fugazzola C. Contrast-enhanced ultrasonographic findings in pancreatic tumors. Int J Med Sci. 2008;5:203–8.
15. Jinga M, Gheorghe C, Dumitrescu M, Gheorghe L, Nicolaie T. Endoscopic ultrasound guided fine needle aspiration biopsy in the diagnosis of pancreatic masses. Rom J Gastroenterol. 2004;13(1):49–54.
16. Dimagno EP, Regan PT, Clain JE, et al. Human endoscopic ultrasonography. Gastroenterology. 1982;83:824–9.
17. Hisanaga K, Hisanaga A, Nagata K, et al. High speed rotating scanner for transgastric sonography. AJR Am J Roentgenol. 1980;135:627–9.
18. Tio TL, Tytgat GN. Endoscopic ultrasonography in the assessment of intra-and transmural infiltration of tumours in the oesophagus, stomach and papilla of vater and in the detection of extraoesophageal lesions. Endoscopy. 1984;16:203–10.
19. Vilmann P, Jacobsen GK, Henriksen FW, et al. Endoscopic ultrasonography with guided fine needle aspiration biopsy in pancreatic disease. Gastrointest Endosc. 1992;38:172–3.
20. Wiersema MJ, Hawes RH, Tao LC, et al. Endoscopic ultrasonography as an adjunct to fine needle aspiration cytology of the upper and lower gastrointestinal tract. Gastrointest Endosc. 1992;38:35–9.
21. Wiersema MJ, Kochman ML, Cramer HM, et al. Endosonography-guided real-time fine-needle aspiration biopsy. Gastrointest Endosc. 1994;40:700–7.
22. Giovannini M, Seitz JF, Monges G, et al. Fine-needle aspiration cytology guided by endoscopic ultrasonography: results in 141 patients. Endoscopy. 1995;27:171–7.
23. Binmoeller KF, Jabusch HC, Seifert H, et al. Endosonography-guided fine-needle biopsy of indurated pancreatic lesions using an automated biopsy device. Endoscopy. 1997;29:384–8.
24. Wiersema MJ, Levy MJ, Harewood GC, et al. Initial experience with EUS-guided trucut needle biopsies of perigastric organs. Gastrointest Endosc. 2002;56:275–8.
25. Iglesias-Garcia J, Poley JW, Larghi A, et al. Feasibility and yield of a new EUS histology needle: results from a multicenter, pooled, cohort study. Gastrointest Endosc. 2011;73:1189–96.
26. Mishra G. Equipment in endosonography forth the edition. In: Hawes R, Fockens P, Varadarajulu S, editors. Endosonography. Amsterdam: Elsevier; 2019.
27. McClaine RJ, Lowy AM, Sussman JJ, et al. Neoadjuvant therapy may lead to successful surgical resection and improved survival in patients with borderline resectable pancreatic cancer. HPB (Oxford). 2010;12:73–9.
28. Ngamruengphong S, Swanson KM, Shah ND, et al. Preoperative endoscopic ultrasound-guided fine needle aspiration does not impair survival of patients with resected pancreatic cancer. Gut. 2015;64:1105–10.
29. Polkowski M, Jenssen C, Kaye P, et al. Technical aspects of endoscopic ultrasound (EUS)-guided sampling in gastroenterology: European Society of Gastrointestinal Endoscopy (ESGE) technical guideline - march 2017. Endoscopy. 2017;49(10):989–1006.
30. Machicado JD, Thosani N, Wani S. Will abandoning fine-needle aspiration increase diagnostic yield from tissues collected during endoscopic ultrasound? Clin Gastroenterol Hepatol. 2018;16(8):1203–6.
31. Bunduc S, Iacob R, Costache R, Stoica B, Radu C, Gheorghe C. Very early onset pancreatic adenocarcinoma - clinical presentation, risk factors and therapeutic options. Chirurgia (Bucur). 2018;113(3):405–11.
32. Yu Y, Zheng P, Chen Y, et al. Advances and challenges of neoadjuvant therapy in pancreatic cancer. Asia Pac J Clin Oncol. 2020;17(15):13504. https://doi.org/10.1111/ajco.13504.
33. Krishna SG, Rao BB, Ugbarugba E, Shah ZK, Blaszczak A, Hinton A, Conwell DL, Hart PA. Diagnostic performance of endoscopic ultrasound for detection of pancreatic malignancy following an indeterminate multidetector CT scan: a systemic review and meta-analysis. Surg Endosc. 2017;31(11):4558–67.
34. Harmsen FJ, Domagk D, Dietrich CF, Hocke M. Discriminating chronic pancreatitis from pancreatic cancer: contrast-enhanced EUS and multidetector computed tomography in direct comparison. Endosc Ultrasound. 2018;7(6):395–403.
35. Li X, Xu W, Shi J, Lin Y, Zeng X. Endoscopic ultrasound elastography for differentiating between pancreatic adenocarcinoma and inflammatory masses: a meta-analysis. World J Gastroenterol. 2013;19(37):6284–91.
36. Bang JY, Rosch T. Endoscopic ultrasound and pancreatic tumors. In: Hawes R, Fockens P, Varadarajulu S, editors. Endosonography. 4th ed. Amsterdam: Elsevier; 2019.
37. Madhoun MF, Wani SB, Rastogi A, Early D, Gaddam S, Tierney WM, Maple JT. The diagnostic accuracy of 22-gauge and 25-gauge needles in endoscopic ultrasound-guided fine needle aspiration of solid pancreatic lesions: a meta-analysis. Endoscopy. 2013;45(2):86–92.
38. Rana A, Rana SS. Endoscopic ultrasound-guided tissue acquisition: techniques and challenges. J Cytol. 2019;36(1):1–7.
39. Conti CB, Cereatti F, Grassia R. Endoscopic ultrasound-guided sampling of solid pancreatic masses: the fine needle aspiration or fine needle biopsy dilemma. Is the best needle yet to come? World J Gastrointest Endosc. 2019;11(8):454–71.
40. Facciorusso A, Stasi E, Maso MD, Serviddio G, Ali Hussein MS, Muscatiello N. Endoscopic ultrasound-guided fine needle aspiration of pancreatic lesions with 22 versus 25 gauge needles: a meta-analysis. United European Gastroenterol J. 2017;5(6):846–53.

41. Wang KX, Ben QW, Jin ZD, Du YQ, Zou DW, Liao Z, Li ZS. Assessment of morbidity and mortality associated with EUS-guided FNA: a systematic review. Gastrointest Endosc. 2011;73(2):283–90.
42. Iglesias-Garcia J, de la Iglesia-Garcia D, Olmos-Martinez JM, Lariño-Noia J, Dominguez-Muñoz JE. Differential diagnosis of solid pancreatic masses. Minerva Gastroenterol Dietol. 2020;66(1):70–81.
43. DeWitt J, Jowell P, Leblanc J, McHenry L, McGreevy K, Cramer H, Volmar K, Sherman S, Gress F. EUS-guided FNA of pancreatic metastases: a multicenter experience. Gastrointest Endosc. 2005;61(6):689–96.
44. Raymond SLT, Yugawa D, Chang KHF, Ena B, Tauchi-Nishi PS. Metastatic neoplasms to the pancreas diagnosed by fine-needle aspiration/biopsy cytology: a 15-year retrospective analysis. Diagn Cytopathol. 2017;45(9):771–83.
45. Savari O, Al-Duwal Z, Wang Z, Ganesan S, Danan-Rayes R, Ayub S. Pancreatic lymphoma: a cytologic diagnosis challenge. Diagn Cytopathol. 2020;48(4):350–5.
46. Pishvaian MJ, Blais EM, Brody JR, et al. Overall survival in patients with pancreatic cancer receiving matched therapies following molecular profiling: a retrospective analysis of the know your tumor registry trial. Lancet Oncol. 2020;21(4):508–18.

Enhanced Recovery After Surgery (ERAS): Concept and Purpose

Gregg Nelson and Olle Ljungqvist

Abstract

Enhanced Recovery After Surgery (ERAS) is a global surgical quality improvement initiative started by a group of European surgeons who challenged the evidence surrounding several historical perioperative practices including prolonged fasting (NPO after midnight), and mechanical bowel preparation. With the goal to minimize the stress response to surgery and bring evidence-based practice mainstream, the ERAS® Society was formed, and has now published numerous perioperative practice guidelines including those for pancreatic and liver surgery. This chapter will provide an overview of (i) the philosophy of ERAS, (ii) the pathophysiology and basis of several core ERAS practices, with special attention to those relevant to Hepato-Pancreato-Biliary (HPB) disease, (iii) clinical and financial outcomes associated with ERAS, and (iv) important considerations when starting an ERAS implementation program.

27.1 Introduction

Enhanced Recovery After Surgery (ERAS) is a global surgical quality improvement initiative that was started in the early 2000s by a group of European surgeons [1] who challenged the evidence surrounding several historical perioperative practices including prolonged fasting (NPO after midnight), mechanical bowel preparation, nasogastric drainage and delayed postoperative feeding among others. What they found, in fact, was very little evidence supporting these practices and many were associated with considerable morbidity including dehydration, hypotension, decreased patient satisfaction and prolonged hospital stay. With the goal to minimize the stress response to surgery and bring evidence-based practice mainstream, the ERAS® Society [2] ultimately was formed, and in 2005 the first ERAS consensus guideline was published which provided recommendations for patients undergoing colonic resection [3]. Over the last several years, numerous other ERAS guidelines have been published [4, 5], including guidelines for both pancreatic [6] and liver [7] surgery. This chapter will provide an overview of (i) the philosophy of ERAS, (ii) the pathophysiology and basis of several core ERAS practices, with special attention to those relevant to Hepato-Pancreato-Biliary (HPB) disease (discussed in depth elsewhere in this book), (iii) clinical and financial outcomes associated with ERAS, and (iv) important considerations when starting an ERAS implementation program.

27.2 Philosophy of ERAS

The philosophy of ERAS is based on the idea that care should be developed to coincide with the patient's journey. The surgical care pathway takes the patient through a series of units and departments, where historically the healthcare providers have worked within their silos, not recognizing that what they do may negatively impact the patient further along the continuum. A classic example is the management of fluids where the surgeon orders mechanical bowel preparation which dehydrates the patient and the anesthesiologist orders overnight fasting causing further dehydration. When anesthesia is initiated the blood pressure falls and fluids are administered often in large amounts to counteract hypotension. Intravenous fluid overload leads to several kilograms in weight gain caused by salt and water accumulation when the patient eventually leaves the OR. This will increase the risk of cardiovascular problems and other complications while also delaying return of bowel function. During this scenario, no single person had the complete picture in mind and everyone dealt with their "problem" on their own not appreciating the result of

G. Nelson (✉)
University of Calgary, Calgary, AB, Canada
e-mail: gsnelson@ucalgary.ca

O. Ljungqvist
Örebro University, Örebro, Sweden
e-mail: Olle.Ljungqvist@oru.se

their actions. ERAS principles counteract this by having everyone involved during the entire patient journey to help develop the local ERAS protocol. This work is supported by the efforts of international experts in the ERAS® Society and others who have developed and update current knowledge in the ERAS guidelines (available for free download) [2].

27.3 Pathophysiology and Basis of ERAS Practices

Common ERAS practices, as depicted in Table 27.1, extend across the surgical care continuum including the preadmission, preoperative, intraoperative and postoperative periods. The fundamental goal underlying these practices is to decrease the stress response associated with surgery. Below we highlight several of these practices considered to be central tenets of the ERAS program and which are particularly relevant to patients undergoing HPB surgery.

27.3.1 Pre-Admission Optimization

It is well described that smoking is associated with an increased risk of postoperative complications, and the impacts on the pulmonary system can be improved within 4 weeks of cessation [8]. This is of particular relevance in pancreatic surgery where studies have shown that smoking is a significant predictor of primary delayed gastric emptying and grade C pancreatic fistula [9, 10].

Excessive alcohol consumption has been associated with increased postoperative complications including cardiovascular/pulmonary complications, bleeding episodes, and infections. A meta-analysis has shown that intensive alcohol cessation interventions may reduce postoperative complication rates, however there is no effect on mortality and length of stay [11].

Patients with pancreatic cancer may have significant weight loss and/or cachexia at diagnosis and therefore may benefit from a preoperative nutritional intervention (typically in cases where weight loss is >15% or BMI drop <18.5 kg/m^2) [12].

27.3.2 Avoidance of Prolonged Fasting

The overnight fasting rule (aka NPO after midnight) is a practice that persists to this day despite the fact that it is unsupported by evidence or modern recommendations. Not only is it associated with decreased patient satisfaction secondary to prolonged hunger and thirst, it may also lead to negative metabolic changes that counteract measures to improve recovery. A meta-analysis found no evidence suggesting that a shortened fluid fast resulted in an increased risk of aspiration, regurgitation or morbidity compared with the standard NPO after midnight policy [13]. Furthermore, randomized controlled trials have demonstrated safety with the "6 and 2 rule"—that a light meal up to 6 hours, and clear fluids up to 2 hours, can be given before elective procedures requiring general anesthesia. These recommendations are supported by American [14] and European anesthesiology societies [15] and are applicable to both pancreatic and liver surgery.

27.3.3 Carbohydrate Loading

Administration of oral carbohydrate solutions 2–3 hours before surgery not only have been shown to decrease the catabolic response induced by overnight fasting and surgery [16] but also a Cochrane review reported that preoperative carbohydrate loading was associated with reduced post-operative insulin resistance, enhanced return of bowel function, and shorter hospital stay with no effect on post-operative complication rates [17]. Carbohydrate loading is recommended for both pancreatic [6] and liver surgery [7].

27.3.4 Avoidance of Mechanical Bowel Preparation

Historically, pre-operative mechanical bowel preparation was used prior to colonic resection because the assumption was that the reduction in stool load decreased post-operative infections and anastomotic leak. Level I evidence, however,

Table 27.1 Common ERAS practices

Preadmission	Preoperative	Intraoperative	Postoperative
Preadmission optimization	Carbohydrate loading	Short-acting anesthetics	No nasogastric tubes
Tobacco/alcohol cessation	Avoidance of fasting	Epidural anesthesia/analgesia	Nausea/vomiting prophylaxis
Nutrition screening/treatment	No bowel preparation	No drains	No salt/water overload
Anemia management	Antibiotic prophylaxis	No salt/water overload	Early removal of urinary catheter
Prehabilitation	Nausea/vomiting prophylaxis	Maintenance of normothermia	Early feeding
	Thromboprophylaxis	Minimally invasive surgery (where appropriate)	Narcotic-sparing multimodal analgesia
	No long acting premedication		Stimulation of gut motility
			Early mobilization
			Audit of compliance/outcomes

from the colorectal literature together with the ERAS colorectal guidelines have supported the avoidance of mechanical bowel preparation, particularly due to negative side effects such as hypovolemia and dehydration and the fact that it does not decrease post-operative infectious morbidity [4]. Recently there has been some debate about the role of oral antibiotic preparation given together with mechanical bowel preparation in colorectal surgery [18]. Despite this, it is generally well accepted that there is no role for mechanical bowel preparation in either pancreatic [6, 19] or liver surgery [7].

27.3.5 Avoidance of Nasogastric Drainage

In major abdominal surgery, nasogastric intubation is associated with an increased risk of postoperative pneumonia, poor patient satisfaction, and does not decrease the risk of wound dehiscence or anastomotic leak [20]. Nasogastric drainage in patients undergoing pancreaticoduodenectomy has been shown to be associated with increased length of hospital stay, delayed initiation of diet, and delayed gastric emptying [21]. Level I evidence similarly confirms that there is no role for this practice is liver resection [22]. If a nasogastric tube is inserted during surgery, it should be removed before the end of the case.

27.3.6 Early Feeding

Early introduction of solid diet, as soon as 4 hours after colonic resection, has been shown to be safe and generally well tolerated [4]. In a systematic review of five feeding routes after pancreaticoduodenectomy, there was no evidence supporting routine enteral or parenteral feeding. An oral diet may be safely given in this patient group [23]. This core ERAS practice is similarly acceptable in patients undergoing liver surgery [7].

27.4 Clinical and Financial Outcomes Associated with ERAS

Much of the research to date on outcomes and ERAS stems from the colorectal literature. Implementation of ERAS guidelines in colorectal surgery has been shown to be associated with decreased length of hospital stay and complications, with no concomitant increase in readmissions [1]. There in fact appears to be a dose response relationship between improved compliance to ERAS guidelines and improved outcomes in colorectal surgery [24]. There is also a suggestion of improved survival in patients undergoing ERAS surgery, although this finding requires further validation [25, 26].

ERAS also appears to benefit patients having pancreatic and liver surgery. In a recent multicenter international cohort study of 404 patients undergoing pancreaticoduodenectomy according to an ERAS pathway, protocol compliance ≥70% was significantly associated with a reduction in complications and length of hospital stay [27]. With respect to liver surgery, a recent meta-analysis of six randomized controlled trials and 21 cohort studies found that length of stay and complications were reduced in the ERAS group compared to the standard care group [28].

Improvements in clinical outcomes translate to cost savings for the healthcare system and as such ERAS is considered to be value-based surgery [29]. Savings per patient varies from $1000 USD to $8700 USD depending on the type of surgery [29]; return-on-investment ratios (ROI) have been reported as high as 7.3 [30]. A recent review of cost impact analyses of ERAS programs in colorectal, pancreatic and liver surgery found a mean cost reduction overall of $3010 USD in favor of ERAS, and specific to pancreatic surgery the cost reduction was $7020 USD [31]. This is particularly important given that it is typically hospital administrators who make the decision to invest (or not to invest) in surgical quality improvement programs such as ERAS. Given the substantial cost savings realized, it is no longer acceptable for hospitals to state that they can't afford to implement ERAS.

27.5 ERAS Implementation and Audit

There are several key components that must be considered when beginning an ERAS implementation. The first is translation of the ERAS guideline into a clinical protocol or order set. This is a critical step that can require several iterations, tailoring to the local institutional format and in some cases adjustment for availability of certain medications. Once an ERAS protocol is developed and approved, the next step is formation of the "ERAS team"—specifically those individuals who will be implementing the ERAS protocol. This team is typically multidisciplinary and multi-professional in nature and includes at minimum a surgeon, anesthesiologist, nurse, and other allied health workers where appropriate (physiotherapist, pharmacist, dietitian among others). Once the team is formed, then the final step is to review and audit compliance to the ERAS protocol (know your baseline compliance, i.e. where you are starting from) relative to changes in clinical outcomes (length of stay, complications). It is well established that as the ERAS team reviews their compliance and outcomes regularly (at a frequency of no less than every 2 weeks), and iterates towards improved compliance (through development of plan-do-study-action cycles), they will see commensurate improvements in clinical outcomes. This way of teams coming together to review their data and obtaining complete control over their outcomes is the ERAS® Society way of improving perioperative care for patients [2].

27.6 Conclusion

ERAS is a surgical quality improvement program based on guidelines derived from the best available evidence. The mechanism through which many ERAS practices effect benefit is through attenuation of the surgical stress response. Formal implementation of ERAS guidelines (including audit of protocol compliance) by a dedicated multidisciplinary ERAS team results in significant clinical improvements (decreased length of hospital stay and complications) which translate to cost savings for the healthcare system. While much of the evidence for ERAS to date stems from colorectal surgery, recent evidence demonstrates benefit for patients undergoing pancreatic and liver surgery.

References

1. Ljungqvist O, Scott M, Fearon KC. Enhanced recovery after surgery: a review. JAMA Surg. 2017;152(3):292–8.
2. https://erassociety.org/. Accessed 25 Aug 2020.
3. Fearon KC, Ljungqvist O, Von Meyenfeldt M, et al. Enhanced recovery after surgery: a consensus review of clinical care for patients undergoing colonic resection. Clin Nutr. 2005;24(3):466–77.
4. Gustafsson UO, Scott MJ, Hubner M, et al. Guidelines for perioperative care in elective colorectal surgery: enhanced recovery after surgery (ERAS) society recommendations: 2018. World J Surg. 2019;43(3):659–95.
5. Thorell A, MacCormick AD, Awad S, et al. Guidelines for perioperative care in bariatric surgery: enhanced recovery after surgery (ERAS) society recommendations. World J Surg. 2016;40(9):2065–83.
6. Melloul E, Lassen K, Roulin D, et al. Guidelines for perioperative care for pancreatoduodenectomy: enhanced recovery after surgery (ERAS) recommendations 2019. World J Surg. 2020;44(7):2056–84.
7. Melloul E, Hübner M, Scott M, et al. Guidelines for perioperative care for liver surgery: enhanced recovery after surgery (ERAS) society recommendations. World J Surg. 2016;40(10):2425–40.
8. Sorensen LT. Wound healing and infection in surgery. The clinical impact of smoking and smoking cessation: a systematic review and meta-analysis. Arch Surg. 2012;147(4):373–83. https://doi.org/10.1001/archsurg.2012.5.
9. Eisenberg JD, Rosato EL, Lavu H, et al. Delayed gastric emptying after pancreaticoduodenectomy: an analysis of risk factors and cost. J Gastrointest Surg. 2015;19(9):1572–80.
10. Aoki S, Miyata H, Konno H, et al. Risk factors of serious postoperative complications after pancreaticoduodenectomy and risk calculators for predicting postoperative complications: a nationwide study of 17,564 patients in Japan. J Hepatobiliary Pancreat Sci. 2017;24(5):243–51.
11. Oppedal K, Moller AM, Pedersen B, et al. Preoperative alcohol cessation prior to elective surgery. Cochrane Database Syst Rev. 2012;7:CD008343.
12. Gianotti L, Besselink MG, Sandini M, et al. Nutritional support and therapy in pancreatic surgery: a position paper of the International Study Group on Pancreatic Surgery (ISGPS). Surgery. 2018;164(5):1035–48.
13. Brady M, Kinn S, Stuart P. Preoperative fasting for adults to prevent perioperative complications. Cochrane Database Syst Rev. 2003;2003(4):CD004423.
14. American Society of Anesthesiologists Committee. Practice guidelines for preoperative fasting and the use of pharmacologic agents to reduce the risk of pulmonary aspiration: application to healthy patients undergoing elective procedures: an updated report by the American Society of Anesthesiologists Committee on Standards and Practice Parameters. Anesthesiology. 2011;114(3):495–511.
15. Smith I, Kranke P, Murat I, et al. Perioperative fasting in adults and children: guidelines from the European Society of Anaesthesiology. Eur J Anaesthesiol. 2011;28(8):556–69.
16. Nygren J, Thorell A, Ljungqvist O. Preoperative oral carbohydrate therapy. Curr Opin Anaesthesiol. 2015;28:364–9.
17. Smith MD, McCall J, Plank L, et al. Preoperative carbohydrate treatment for enhancing recovery after elective surgery. Cochrane Database Syst Rev. 2014;2014(8):CD009161.
18. Rollins KE, Lobo DN. The controversies of mechanical bowel and oral antibiotic preparation in elective colorectal surgery. Ann Surg. 2021;273(1):e13–5.
19. Lavu H, Kennedy EP, Mazo R, et al. Preoperative mechanical bowel preparation does not offer a benefit for patients who undergo pancreaticoduodenectomy. Surgery. 2010;148:278–84.
20. Nelson R, Tse B, Edwards S. Systematic review of prophylactic nasogastric decompression after abdominal operations. Br J Surg. 2005;92:673–80.
21. Kunstman JW, Klemen ND, Fonseca AL, et al. Nasogastric drainage may be unnecessary after pancreaticoduodenectomy: a comparison of routine vs selective decompression. J Am Coll Surg. 2013;217(3):481–8.
22. Pessaux P, Regimbeau JM, Dondero F, et al. Randomized clinical trial evaluating the need for routine nasogastric decompression after elective hepatic resection. Br J Surg. 2007;94:297–303.
23. Gerritsen A, Besselink MG, Gouma DJ, et al. Systematic review of five feeding routes after pancreatoduodenectomy. Br J Surg. 2013;100(5):589–98.
24. ERAS Compliance Group. The impact of enhanced recovery protocol compliance on elective colorectal cancer resection: results from an international registry. Ann Surg. 2015;261(6):1153–9.
25. Pisarska M, Torbicz G, Gajewska N, et al. Compliance with the ERAS protocol and 3-year survival after laparoscopic surgery for nonmetastatic colorectal cancer. World J Surg. 2019;43:2552–60.
26. Savaridas T, Serrano-Pedraza I, Khan SK, et al. Reduced medium-term mortality following primary total hip and knee arthroplasty with an enhanced recovery program. A study of 4,500 consecutive procedures. Acta Orthop. 2013;84:40–3.
27. Roulin D, Melloul E, Wellg BE, et al. Feasibility of an enhanced recovery protocol for elective pancreatoduodenectomy: a multicenter international cohort study. World J Surg. 2020;44(8):2761–9.
28. Noba L, Rodgers S, Chandler C, et al. Enhanced recovery after surgery (ERAS) reduces hospital costs and improve clinical outcomes in liver surgery: a systematic review and meta-analysis. J Gastrointest Surg. 2020;24(4):918–32.
29. Ljungqvist O, Thanh NX, Nelson G. ERAS-value based surgery. J Surg Oncol. 2017;116(5):608–12.
30. Thanh NX, Nelson A, Wang X, et al. Return on investment of the enhanced recovery after surgery (ERAS) multi-guideline multi-site implementation in Alberta. Canada Can J Surg. 2020;63(6):E542–50.
31. Joliat GR, Hübner M, Roulin D, et al. Cost analysis of enhanced recovery programs in colorectal, pancreatic, and hepatic surgery: a systematic review. World J Surg. 2020;44(3):647–55.

28. Multidisciplinary Enhanced Recovery After Surgery (ERAS) Pathway for Hepatobiliary and Pancreatic Surgery

Didier Roulin and Nicolas Demartines

Abstract

Enhanced Recovery After Surgery (ERAS) is a multimodal multidisciplinary bundle aiming to provide the best evidence-based care to the patient in order to improve recovery by reducing the surgical stress. The principles of ERAS have been successfully applied in many surgical disciplines, including hepatobiliary and pancreatic surgery. The present chapter will review the current evidence in favor of ERAS for liver and pancreas surgery with focus on the multidisciplinary interaction between healthcare professionals involved in the patient's perioperative care.

28.1 Introduction

Enhanced Recovery After Surgery (ERAS) is a multimodal multidisciplinary pathway aiming to provide the best evidence-based care to the patient with the involvement of a multidisciplinary team [1]. The aim of enhanced recovery is not only to shorten patient's length of stay, which was initially named "fast-track", but mainly to restore patient's preoperative function allowing the patient to get back to his baseline condition early [2]. ERAS focuses on "Enhanced" not on "fast", meaning general improvement of patient's condition is the key that may as secondary (positive) effect speed up the entire perioperative process. The principles of ERAS have been successfully applied in many surgical disciplines, including hepatobiliary and pancreatic surgery. The implementation of ERAS into clinical practice is a new way of conceive the perioperative period with new organization. To apply successfully an ERAS pathway is demanding and requires the full involvement and training of a dedicated multidisciplinary team (MDT), as illustrated on Fig. 28.1.

D. Roulin · N. Demartines (✉)
Department of Visceral Surgery, Lausanne University Hospital, University of Lausanne, Lausanne, Switzerland
e-mail: demartines@chuv.ch

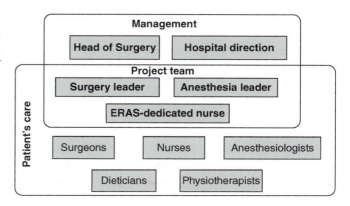

Fig. 28.1 Organization chart of an Enhanced Recovery After Surgery (ERAS) multidisciplinary team

Specific ERAS guidelines were first published in 2016 for liver surgery [3] and were updated in 2019 for pancreatoduodenectomy [4]. These recommendations were based on a systematic review and processed by a modified Delphi process and detailed the associated evidence and recommendation for each ERAS items (23 for liver, 27 for pancreas). The present chapter will go through the practical implementation of an ERAS program and the current evidence supporting ERAS for liver and pancreas surgery, with focus on the multidisciplinary management of the patient and the active involvement of the patient himself.

28.2 ERAS: Moving from Evidence-Based into Clinical Practice

The evidence-based items included in ERAS is a continuous process covering the entire patient's journey, starting from the pre-admission until home-discharge and follow-up. The main areas of focus are preoperative counselling and optimization, normovolemia, multimodal opioid sparing analgesia, as well as early scheduled nutrition and mobilization. According to the latest available guidelines, ERAS items for liver and pancreatic surgery are summarized in Table 28.1. The translation of evidence-based elements of enhancement into clinical practice represent a proper challenge. Simply elaborating and establishing a protocol is not enough [5] and much more efforts and changes in organization are required to improve the perioperative outcome.

Table 28.1 Enhanced Recovery After Surgery (ERAS) items for liver and pancreas surgery

	Liver	Pancreas
Preoperative counselling	Dedicated multimedia preoperative counselling.	
Prehabilitation		Prehabilitation program three to six weeks before surgery.
Biliary drainage		Avoidance of preoperative drainage, only if bilirubin >250 μmol/l, cholangitis, or neoadjuvant treatment.
Smoking and alcohol cessation	Smoking and high alcohol consumption cessation at least four weeks before surgery.	
Preoperative nutrition	Patients at risk (weight loss 10–15% within six months, Body Mass Index (BMI) < 18.5 kg/m² and serum albumin <30 g/l in the absence of liver or renal dysfunction) should receive oral nutritional supplements for seven days prior to surgery.	Preoperative nutritional intervention if severe weight loss. Nutritional status assessment based on BMI and weight loss.
Immunonutrition	Limited evidence for use.	Not recommended.
Oral bowel preparation	Avoidance of oral bowel preparation.	
Fasting and carbohydrate drinks	Clear fluids until two hours, solids six hours before surgery. Carbohydrate loading on evening and two hours before surgery.	
Preanaesthetic medication	No long acting sedative premedication.	No anxiolytics. Acetaminophen and single dose gabapentinoid.
Anti-thrombotic prophylaxis	Concomitant chemical and mechanical thromboprophylaxis.	
Perioperative steroids	Steroids (methylprednisolone) may be used before hepatectomy in normal liver parenchyma, since it decreases liver injury and intraoperative stress. Steroids should not be given in diabetic patients.	
Antimicrobial prophylaxis and skin preparation	Single iv antibiotic 30–60 minutes before incision. Skin preparation with a scrub of chlorhexidine-alcohol.	Single dose iv antibiotic less than 60 min before skin incision. Intraoperative bile culture if preoperative biliary stenting. Therapeutic postoperative antibiotics if positive bile culture. Use of alcohol-based preparations and wound protectors.
Epidural	Not recommended in open liver surgery for ERAS patients. Wound infusion catheter or intrathecal opiates can be good alternatives combined with multimodal analgesia.	Thoracic epidural analgesia (T5–8) for open. If no epidural: Intravenous lidocaine or transversus abdominis plane block/wound infiltration.
Minimally invasive surgery	Laparoscopic liver resection can be performed by hepato-biliary surgeons experienced in laparoscopic surgery, in particular left lateral sectionectomy and resections of lesions located in anterior segments.	Laparoscopic pancreatoduodenectomy (PD) only in highly experienced high-volume center. No recommendation for robotic-assisted PD.
Postoperative analgesia		Multimodal opioid sparing analgesia.
Wound catheter		Preperitoneal wound catheter as alternative to epidural for open PD.
Postoperative Nausea and Vomiting (PONV) prophylaxis	Multimodal PONV prophylaxis adapted to risk factors.	
Hypothermia prevention	Active warming (cutaneous and perfusions warming) to maintain body temperature ≥36 °C.	
Glycaemic control	Glucose levels should be maintained as close to normal as possible without causing hypoglycemia.	
Fluid balance	The maintenance of low central venous pressure (below 5 cmH₂O) with close monitoring during hepatic surgery is advocated. Balanced crystalloid should be preferred.	Avoidance of fluid overload.
Nasogastric intubation	No postoperative gastric tube	

Table 28.1 (continued)

	Liver	Pancreas
Abdominal drains	No routine abdominal drain	Perianastomotic drain removal at 72 hours in low-risk patients
Somatostatin analogues	–	No systematic use of somatostatin
Urinary catheter	Removal on POD 3	Early urinary catheter removal
Delayed gastric emptying (DGE)	An omentum flap to cover the cut surface of the liver reduces the risk of DGE after left-sided hepatectomy	No acknowledged prophylactic strategy. Early diagnosis of intraabdominal complications. Artificial nutrition in case of prolonged DGE.
Stimulation of bowel movement	Stimulation of bowel movement after liver surgery is not indicated.	Use of chewing gum, alvimopan or mosapride.
Diet	Normal diet after surgery according to tolerance.	
Mobilization	Early and active mobilization.	
Audit	Regular and continuous audit.	

A MDT must be gathered first under the initiative of a project leader or "ERAS champion". In our experience, the surgeons in charge of the respective units were designed as leaders of the team and were supported by two to three designated surgeons. In other hospitals anesthesiologists are the champions but the process remain the same: surgeons, anesthesiologists, nurses and patients working together. An optimal MDT should include at least a nurse, an anesthesiologists, an administrator and a surgeon. Other health care workers like physiotherapists or nutritionists as part of the team. A dedicated and specifically trained ERAS nurse is of uttermost importance. The support of the administration is essential from the beginning, to obtain the required resources and monitor the financial benefits. The team should then undergo training to implement an enhanced recovery pathway in their own unit or hospital. ERAS implementation process is a systematic training program provided by ERAS academic experts and conducted over a 8 to 10 months structured period. Following the definition of measurable goals, actions and plans are put into practice, then observation and measurement are taken, and finally adequate adjustments are made. Regular multidisciplinary audit, also including nutritionists and physiotherapists, are conducted in order to monitor compliance and sustainability of changes achieved following the implementation process. The use of a systematic interactive audit system allows standardization of outcomes reporting and continuous data analysis [6]. Long term follow-up studies acknowledged the sustainability of such multidisciplinary implementation and maintenance of ERAS program [7]. With the Covid pandemic, the way to implement ERAS program is about to evolve and e-learning platforms will be used instead of in person meetings.

28.3 ERAS Benefits in Hepato-Biliary and Pancreatic Surgery

Following successful ERAS implementation, clinical benefits in liver surgery were consistently reported. At least five meta-analysis [8–12], with the latest published in 2020 reported a significant reduction in length of stay as well as 30%–50% reduction of postoperative complications, without increasing mortality or readmission. When reported, the functional recovery as well as the quality of life was also improved with ERAS [8]. ERAS compliance was ranging from 65% to 74% [10] and the rate of liver specific complications was not reduced by ERAS implementation [9]. Less than 20% of included studies in the latest metanalysis [10], reported a systematic audit. Therefore, significant improvement in the reporting of compliance as well as the application of systematic audit are awaited in ERAS for hepato-biliary surgery.

Regarding pancreatic surgery, the effect of ERAS on clinical outcome was frequently reported from 2007 until now in many studies. Their results were gathered in five main meta-analysis [13–17], which reported a significant reduction of overall morbidity and length of stay without any increase in readmission rate when an enhanced recovery protocol was applied. Concerning pancreatic surgery specific complications, such as delayed gastric emptying and pancreatic fistula, three of the five abovementioned meta-analysis [14, 15, 17] described a reduction of delayed gastric emptying and a similar rate of clinically significant pancreatic fistula with ERAS compared to historical care. However, the high variability of the number of ERAS items used in each study leads to heterogeneity in the included study.

A recent multicenter cohort study including 404 patients undergoing pancreateoduodenectomy within ERAS assessed the application of the guidelines in daily clinical practice [18]. The number of items applied divided the total number, also called "compliance", was 62%, with the postoperative period being the most challenging part. Each item of an enhanced recovery protocol is of importance, but it is mainly their cumulative proportion, expressed as overall compliance, was a major factor for clinical outcome as an overall compliance of more than 70% was associated with a significant reduction of overall complications and length of stay. When looking at the impact of each element, the avoidance of postoperative nasogastric tube and early mobilization were independent factors associated with improved outcome after pancreatoduodenectomy.

The long-term outcome after pancreatic and liver surgery is also correlated with the multidisciplinary oncological treatment, including adjuvant chemotherapy. As postoperative complications might increase the interval between the surgical procedure and the start of chemotherapy, the potential role of ERAS compliance on this interval was evaluated in a retrospective analysis [19]. An overall compliance equal or more than 67% was associated with a significant decrease of the interval between surgery and chemotherapy for patients >65 years old.

As already mentioned, economical resources are a frequently raised issue when considering implementing ERAS, as it requires specific resources such as an enhanced recovery dedicated nurse, information's booklet and database [20]. These investments may lead to resistance to enhanced recovery implementation [21]. However, these initial costs are quickly overwhelmed by the in-hospital cost reduction induced not only by the reduction of length of stay, but also by the decrease of complications. In hepato-biliary and pancreatic surgery, a recent systematic review [22] described among the five included studies in pancreas surgery, a mean cost reduction in favor of the ERAS of USD 7020. In liver surgery, only three studies were found, which precluded a systematic cost analysis. However, a cost-minimization analysis for liver surgery showed a total mean cost reduction of € 3080 per patient following ERAS implementation [23].

28.4 ERAS as a Multidisciplinary Team Approach

A multidisciplinary team (MDT) approach provides comprehensive patient-centered care by gathering a range of different health care professionals sharing a common objective. As ERAS is a multimodal multidisciplinary approach in order to improve patient outcome, the multidisciplinary work is essential, not only during the implementation period but also in the crucial period of sustainability.

Understanding barriers and enablers to ERAS implementation is a key process to improve collaboration within the MDT. An interesting study assessed qualitative barriers and enables across nurses, surgeons and anesthesiologists [24]. Nurses identified patient's reluctance to early mobilization and feeding, which could be overcome by patient education. Lack of manpower and time was also identified. From the surgeons' perspective, nursing culture and lack of nursing time, as well as personal preferences and resistance to change were potential barriers. Anesthesiologists expressed concerns that changing nursing culture and surgeon's behavior would be difficult, and this could be overwhelmed by improved communication and collaboration. A systematic review [25] included studies with focus on health professionals' experiences of ERAS implementation and identified five main themes: communication and collaboration, resistance to change, role and significance of protocol-based care, and knowledge and expectation. This review concluded that communication among partners and with patients, as well provision of comprehensive information to health professionals and patients, in addition with Identifying a local ERAS champions could improve ERAS implementation.

28.5 Conclusion

ERAS is a powerful improvement tool for the patient's perioperative course. But application of ERAS in hepato-biliary and pancreatic surgery requires multidisciplinary communication and collaboration in order to deliver evidence-based best practice in a setting of patient-centered care. Under these circumstances, ERAS leads to improved patient outcome, with reduced complications and improved functional outcome associated with reduced length of stay for hepato-biliary and pancreatic surgery. In addition, implementation of ERAS pathway is a cost-effective intervention, allowing support from healthcare administration. Patient education and involvement, as well as multidisciplinary communication and collaboration are essential to reach high compliance to ERAS items, resulting in improved outcome.

References

1. Ljungqvist O, Scott M, Fearon KC. Enhanced recovery after surgery a review. JAMA Surg. 2017;152(3):292–8. https://doi.org/10.1001/jamasurg.2016.4952.
2. Ljungqvist O, Young-Fadok T, Demartines N. The history of enhanced recovery after surgery and the ERAS society. J Laparoendosc Adv Surg Tech. 2017;27(9):860–2. https://doi.org/10.1089/lap.2017.0350.
3. Melloul E, Hübner M, Scott M, et al. Guidelines for perioperative care for liver surgery: enhanced recovery after surgery (ERAS) society recommendations. World J Surg. 2016;40:2425–40. https://doi.org/10.1007/s00268-016-3700-1.

4. Melloul E, Lassen K, Roulin D, et al. Guidelines for Perioperative Care for Pancreatoduodenectomy: Enhanced Recovery After Surgery (ERAS) Recommendations 2019. World J Surg. 2020;44(7):2056–84. https://doi.org/10.1007/s00268-020-05462-w.
5. Maessen J, Dejong CHC, Hausel J, et al. A protocol is not enough to implement an enhanced recovery programme for colorectal resection. Br J Surg. 2007;94(2):224–31. https://doi.org/10.1002/bjs.5468.
6. Currie A, Soop M, Demartines N, Fearon K, Kennedy R, Ljungqvist O. Enhanced recovery after surgery interactive audit system: 10 years' experience with an international web-based clinical and research perioperative care database. Clin Colon Rectal Surg. 2019;32(1):75–81. https://doi.org/10.1055/s-0038-1673357.
7. Martin D, Roulin D, Addor V, Blanc C, Demartines N, Hübner M. Enhanced recovery implementation in colorectal surgery-temporary or persistent improvement? Langenbecks Arch Surg. 2016;401(8):1163–9. https://doi.org/10.1007/s00423-016-1518-9.
8. Song W, Wang K, Zhang RJ, Dai QX, Zou SB. The enhanced recovery after surgery (ERAS) program in liver surgery: a meta-analysis of randomized controlled trials. Springerplus. 2016;5(1):1–10. https://doi.org/10.1186/s40064-016-1793-5.
9. Hughes MJ, McNally S, Wigmore SJ. Enhanced recovery following liver surgery: a systematic review and meta-analysis. HPB. 2014;16(8):699–706. https://doi.org/10.1111/hpb.12245.
10. Noba L, Rodgers S, Chandler C, Balfour A, Hariharan D, Yip VS. Enhanced recovery after surgery (ERAS) reduces hospital costs and improve clinical outcomes in liver surgery: a systematic review and meta-analysis. J Gastrointest Surg. 2020;24(4):918–32. https://doi.org/10.1007/s11605-019-04499-0.
11. Wang C, Zheng G, Zhang W, et al. Enhanced recovery after surgery programs for liver resection: a meta-analysis. J Gastrointest Surg. 2017;21(3):472–86. https://doi.org/10.1007/s11605-017-3360-y.
12. Zhao Y, Qin H, Wu Y, Xiang B. Enhanced recovery after surgery program reduces length of hospital stay and complications in liver resection: a PRISMA-compliant systematic review and meta-analysis of randomized controlled trials. Medicine (Baltimore). 2017;96(31):e7628.
13. Coolsen MME, Van Dam RM, Van Der Wilt AA, Slim K, Lassen K, Dejong CHC. Systematic review and meta-analysis of enhanced recovery after pancreatic surgery with particular emphasis on pancreaticoduodenectomies. World J Surg. 2013;37(8):1909–18. https://doi.org/10.1007/s00268-013-2044-3.
14. Xiong J, Szatmary P, Huang W, et al. Enhanced recovery after surgery program in patients undergoing pancreaticoduodenectomy a prisma-compliant systematic review and meta-analysis. Medicine (United States). 2016;95(18):e3497. https://doi.org/10.1097/MD.0000000000003497.
15. Ji HB, Zhu WT, Wei Q, Wang XX, Wang HB, Chen QP. Impact of enhanced recovery after surgery programs on pancreatic surgery: a meta-analysis. World J Gastroenterol. 2018;24(15):1666–78. https://doi.org/10.3748/wjg.v24.i15.1666.
16. Cao Y, Gu HY, Huang ZD, et al. Impact of enhanced recovery after surgery on postoperative recovery for Pancreaticoduodenectomy: pooled analysis of observational study. Front Oncol. 2019;9:687. https://doi.org/10.3389/fonc.2019.00687.
17. Sun Y-M, Wang Y, Mao Y-X, Wang W. The safety and feasibility of enhanced recovery after surgery in patients undergoing pancreaticoduodenectomy: an updated meta-analysis. Biomed Res Int. 2020;2020:1–15. https://doi.org/10.1155/2020/7401276.
18. Roulin D, Melloul E, Wellg BE, et al. Feasibility of an enhanced recovery protocol for elective pancreatoduodenectomy: a multicenter international cohort study. World J Surg. 2020;44(8):2761–9. https://doi.org/10.1007/s00268-020-05499-x.
19. St-Amour P, St-Amour P, Joliat GR, et al. Impact of ERAS compliance on the delay between surgery and adjuvant chemotherapy in hepatobiliary and pancreatic malignancies. Langenbecks Arch Surg. 2020;405(7):959–66. https://doi.org/10.1007/s00423-020-01981-1.
20. Roulin D, Donadini A, Gander S, et al. Cost-effectiveness of the implementation of an enhanced recovery protocol for colorectal surgery. Br J Surg. 2013;100(8):1108–14. https://doi.org/10.1002/bjs.9184.
21. Martin D, Roulin D, Grass F, et al. A multicentre qualitative study assessing implementation of an enhanced recovery after surgery program. Clin Nutr. 2018;37(6 Pt A):2172–7. https://doi.org/10.1016/j.clnu.2017.10.017.
22. Joliat G-R, Hübner M, Roulin D, Demartines N. Cost analysis of enhanced recovery programs in colorectal, pancreatic, and hepatic surgery: a systematic review. World J Surg. 2020;44(3):647–55. https://doi.org/10.1007/s00268-019-05252-z.
23. Joliat GR, Labgaa I, Hübner M, et al. Cost–benefit analysis of the implementation of an enhanced recovery program in liver surgery. World J Surg. 2016;40(10):2441–50. https://doi.org/10.1007/s00268-016-3582-2.
24. Pearsall EA, Meghji Z, Pitzul KB, et al. Qualitative study to understand the barriers and enablers in implementing an enhanced recovery after surgery program. Ann Surg. 2015;261(1):92–6. https://doi.org/10.1097/SLA.0000000000000604.
25. Cohen R, Gooberman-Hill R. Staff experiences of enhanced recovery after surgery: systematic review of qualitative studies. BMJ Open. 2019;9(2):e022259. https://doi.org/10.1136/bmjopen-2018-022259.

ERAS in Pancreatic Surgery

Julie Perinel and Mustapha Adham

Abstract

Pancreatic surgery is associated with a significant morbidity and prolonged length of hospital stay (LOS). In 2012, the Enhanced Recovery After Surgery (ERAS) study group published the first guidelines to implement ERAS program in patients undergoing pancreaticoduodenectomy (PD). These guidelines, updated in 2019, included 27 evidence-based recommendations but also a proper and structured audit system to provide feedback and to report the compliance. Systematic review and meta-analysis reported improved postoperative outcomes in ERAS group, with shorter LOS, lower incidence of delayed gastric emptying and overall complications without increasing readmission rates or mortality. ERAS program represents also a financial issue and is associated with significant cost savings. However, considering the majority of non-randomized studies and the substantial heterogeneity between the studies, more large-scale randomized studies with standardized ERAS program are still needed. Implementation of the ERAS program is a challenging process requiring the commitment of a multidisciplinary team. Compliance is a key element to assess the success of ERAS implementation and also to improve postoperative outcomes.

Enhanced recovery after surgery (ERAS) is a multimodal and multidisciplinary pathway developed to decrease perioperative surgical stress, to reduce postoperative complications and to accelerate postoperative recovery [1]. Initially implemented in colorectal surgery [2], ERAS program was associated with a significant reduction in postoperative morbidity and a shorten length of hospital stay (LOS) [3, 4]. Programs based on enhanced recovery in pancreatic surgery have been developed over a decade [5]. In 2012, the ERAS study group published the first guidelines for pancreaticoduodenectomy (PD) [6]. An updated version has been published in 2019 and included 27 evidence-based recommendations to manage perioperative care after PD [7].

Pancreatic surgery, and especially PD, is considered as a complex and high-risk surgical procedure. While the mortality has significantly decreased to less than 5% with the centralization in high volume centers, the morbidity remains high (30–60%) with prolonged LOS [8]. Postoperative complications such as postoperative pancreatic fistula (POPF), delayed gastric emptying (DGE) and surgical site infections (SSI) contribute to delay the recovery and increase the LOS [9, 10]. Besides, pancreatic surgery remains challenging because several questions remain unsolved considering prophylactic abdominal drainage, preoperative biliary drainage and early feeding in patients at high risk of DGE or ileus. In this context, the implementation of ERAS program could contribute to reduce postoperative complications, to shorten LOS and to standardize the practice in pancreatic surgery.

29.1 ERAS Guidelines in PD

ERAS guidelines for PD included dedicated preoperative counseling and initiation of a prehabilitation program, with physical exercise and nutritional supplements, 3–6 weeks before surgery. Nutritional supports (nasogastric or nasojejunal feeding tube) are recommended in case of malnutrition (15% weight loss or BMI < 18.5 kg/m^2). Immunonutrition is no longer recommended and preoperative fasting is limited to 6 h for solids and 2 h for liquids in absence of contraindication. Carbohydrate loads are given the previous day and up to 2 h before anesthesia. Preoperative biliary drainage should be performed only in the following indications: serum bilirubin level > 250 μmol/L, cholangitis, neoadjuvant treatment. Preoperatively, premedication is avoided and antithrombotic prophylaxis should be started 2–12 h before surgery and continued 4 weeks after surgery in case of can-

J. Perinel (✉) · M. Adham
Department of Digestive Surgery, Edouard Herriot Hospital, Hospices Civils de Lyon, UCBL1, Lyon, France
e-mail: julie.perinel@chu-lyon.fr

cer. Prophylaxis of nausea and vomiting (PONV) is started and consisted of at least two different antiemetics. Antimicrobial prophylaxis is administered less than 60 min before skin incision and repeated according to the duration of procedure. If bile culture is positive, antibiotics should be considered for the postoperative course. Postoperative analgesia is ensured using a thoracic epidural for open PD or preperitoneal wound catheters in case of contraindication to avoid opioid. To prevent hypothermia, a body-bear hugger and warming set for intravenous infusions are used to maintain temperature above 36 °C. Perioperatively, defined protocols are used to maintain normoglycemia and a goal-directed fluid therapy algorithm is used to avoid fluid overload. The nasogastric tube is inserted during the surgery and removed before the reversal of anesthesia. There are still concerns about the safety of minimally invasive PD. Laparoscopic PD should be performed only in high volume and expert centers with selected patients. Robotic PD is not recommended. Management of prophylactic drainage after PD continued to be controversial and the level of evidence is too low to conclude. Guidelines recommend systematic drainage and early removal at 72 h in patients at low risk (i.e., amylase content in drain <5000 U/L on POD1). Systematic use of somatostatin analogues to prevent clinically relevant POPF (CR-POPF) is not recommended due to the lack of evidence. Urinary catheter should be removed on POD1. The patients followed an early oral feeding program according to tolerance. Chewing gums and pharmacological agents (alvimopan and mosapride) may accelerate bowel recovery. Early mobilization is started from day 0. The strength of ERAS program, when compared to other enhanced recovery programs (ERP), is a proper and structured audit system including a prospective database, regular internal and external audits to provide feedback and to report the compliance. Indeed, simply developing evidence-based protocols is not enough to change practice and reporting of adherence to protocol should be a standard practice [11].

29.2 Impact of ERAS on Postoperative Outcomes

During the last few decades, several studies reported the feasibility and the safety of ERAS program in patients undergoing PD [12–23] (Table 29.1). Systematic review and meta-analysis reported improved postoperative outcomes in ERAS group, when compared to traditional care, with shorter LOS, lower incidence of DGE and overall complications without increasing readmission rates or mortality [24, 25]. However, evidence was only based on retrospective case-control studies with limited sample size. More recently, four single-center, prospective randomized controlled trials (RCT) confirmed the benefits of ERAS program to enhance postoperative recovery [26–29] (Table 29.1). While two RCT assessed the effects of ERAS program based on ERAS guidelines [26, 27], one American RCT evaluated an ERP specific to the center [28] and the Korean RCT was a non-inferiority trial on a modified ERAS program [29]. Besides, in three studies, patients were selected, excluding patients over 80 years, with major comorbidities and advanced malignancy. Only open and curative PD were included, without vascular resection or reconstruction [27–29]. Finally, in ERAS group, two studies reported earlier recovery of oral feeding, transit return and mobilization [26, 27], three studies reported shorter LOS [26–28] and only one study reported lower morbidity [27]. In all the RCT, there were no signifi-

Table 29.1 Characteristics of the studies assessing the implementation of ERAS program in pancreatic surgery

Study	Year	Country	Study design	ERAS group[a]	Control group[a]	MINORS score
Abu Hilal et al.	2013	Britain	Case-control study	20	24	14/24
Kobayashi et al.	2014	Japan	Case-control study	100	90	13/24
Braga et al.	2014	Italy	Case-control study	115	115	18/24
Coolsen et al.	2014	Netherlands	Case-control study	86	97	15/24
Shao et al.	2015	China	Case-control study	325	310	14/24
Williamsson et al.	2015	Sweden	Case-control study	50	50	16/24
Joliat et al.	2015	Switzerland	Case-control study	74	87	15/24
Partelli et al.	2015	Italy	Case-control study	22	66	13/24
Bai et al.	2016	China	Case-control study	124	63	15/24
Zouros et al.	2016	Greece	Case-control study	75	50	16/24
Deng et al.	2017	China	RCT	76	83	[b]
Takagi et al.	2019	Japan	RCT	37	37	[b]
Perinel et al.	2019	France	Case-control study	47	30	19/24
Lavu et al.	2019	United States	RCT	37	39	[b]
Hwang et al.	2019	Korea	RCT	123	124	[b]

RCT randomized controlled trial, MINORS methodological index for nonrandomized studies
[a]Sample size
[b]Unconformity to MINORS score criteria

cant difference in term of POPF, mortality and readmission, which confirmed the safety of ERP [26–29]. In 2020, two systematic review and meta-analysis were published including the four RCT. Both reported in ERAS group shorter LOS, lower rate of overall and minor complications, lower incidence of DGE, without increasing POPF rate, 30-day readmission and mortality [30, 31]. However, considering the heterogeneity between the studies, more large-scale RCT are still needed.

ERAS program is also safe for elderly patients. Coolsen et al. reported comparative postoperative outcomes in 55 patients ≥70 years when compared to other 55 younger patients with a good compliance (51–95%) [32]. Partelli et al. reported the feasibility of ERAS program in a cohort of 88 patients ≥75 years [19]. Two RCT evaluated specifically the impact of ERAS program in patients undergoing PD for cancer [26, 29]. In one study, ERAS program was non-inferior to traditional care [29]; in the second one, ERAS program was associated with shorten LOS without increasing morbidity and mortality [26]. In the RCT of Lavu et al., 80% of the patients had cancer and the median time to the initiation of adjuvant therapy was shorter in ERP group [28]. Achieving complete cycles of adjuvant chemotherapy is one of the most important predictor for long-term survival in periampullary cancer. Even if the chemotherapy is delayed after 12 weeks, there is still a benefit on long-term survival [33]. Hence, there is a real benefit to implement ERAS in periampullary cancer. If ERAS favored earlier recovery with shorten LOS, an increasing proportion of patients will be able to achieve chemotherapy. However, further studies are needed to confirm this hypothesis.

29.3 Impact of ERAS on Hospital Costs

Implementation of ERAS program represented also a financial issue. Initially, Kehlet et al. developed ERP to accelerate postoperative recovery but also to reduce overall costs [1]. In pancreatic surgery, most of the studies reported significant cost savings after ERP implementation [16, 17, 22, 34, 35]. Two meta-analysis and systematic review reported data on cost analysis [24, 36]. Xiong et al. reported a significant reduction in in-hospital costs based on the results of four studies [24]. Joliat et al. found a mean difference of USD 7020 (95% CI: 11,600–2430, p = 0.003) in favor of ERP including five studies [36]. In the recent American RCT, the total cost was reduced from USD 31,845 to USD 26,563 (p = 0.011) in ERP group [28]. Cost reduction was interpreted as the results of bed day savings due to shorten LOS, and also as the consequence of the standardization that avoids unnecessary laboratory tests, radiological imaging and medication [35, 36]. However, as mentioned by Joliat et al., the methodology of cost assessment differed between the studies and costs are mostly assessed as a secondary outcome [36]. Specific studies on the subject are needed such as standardization of cost analysis.

29.4 ERAS and Compliance

Measuring the compliance is essential to analyze the success of the implementation of ERAS program into daily practice. In pancreatic surgery, only few studies reported the compliance to ERAS program. While compliance with pre- and intraoperative ERAS items was high (70–100%), the postoperative ERAS items were more difficult to implement with success (30–88%) [14, 20, 21, 27, 37, 38]. In addition, the level of compliance was significantly correlated with postoperative outcomes [14, 21, 37, 38]. In the study of Braga et al., the subgroup analysis showed a higher compliance in uneventful patients, while a lower compliance was found in patients with major complications [14]. In two single-center studies, patients with high compliance had fewer postoperative complications and shorten LOS [21, 37]. Williamson et al. showed that patients with compliance of ≥90% had a median discharge on POD 8 [7–9] and no patient with Clavien–Dindo ≥3a [37]. More recently, in a multicenter study including 404 patients, a level of compliance >70% was associated with a significant shorter LOS and significantly less overall and major complications [38]. Roulin et al. was the first study to assess specifically the impact of each individual ERAS items on postoperative outcomes. Only postoperative items were independent predictors of complications. Avoidance of postoperative nasogastric tube, mobilization on POD0 and more than 6H on the POD2 were significantly associated with decreased overall complications. Early mobilization was the only ERAS item associated with reduced major complications (Clavien Dindo IIIa to IVb) [38]. These results suggest the importance of improving compliance to favor successful postoperative outcomes. In colorectal surgery, a multicenter study has shown that the strongest predictor of optimal recovery was compliance with the postoperative items [39]. Nevertheless, reaching a high level of compliance in the postoperative period is more complex because it is related to the commitment of patients and the occurrence of complications. It is more difficult to mobilize the patient or to start oral feeding in case of surgical complications. Zhang et al. identified in a cohort of 176 patients undergoing PD, that ASA score and nutritional status were independent predictive factors of ERAS success. Besides, postoperative complications including CR-POPF, DGE and SSI were the main reasons for ERAS failure. Among ERAS items, early removal of NGT and intake of oral liquids were closely related to postoperative outcomes and could be early predictors of postoperative complications [10].

29.5 Implementation Strategy and Keys of Success

Implementation of ERAS program is a gradual process that required the commitment of a multidisciplinary team associated to a structured implementation strategy. Regular audits are necessary to identify the facilitators and the barriers to the implementation. In a qualitative study, Lyon et al. reported four key points associated with an effective implementation and a high level of compliance [40]:

- The patient-related factors with patient selection (demographics, comorbidities) and patient expectation;
- The staff-related factors (staff education, change of attitude, and behaviors);
- The practice-related issues (communication, standardized protocol);
- The health system resources (in-hospital and discharge resources).

Successful implementation of ERAS program is also correlated to:

- The medical staff education through regular staff meeting [41];
- The patient education, it is easier to reach a high compliance if the patient has realistic expectations of the care protocol [40];
- The attendance of a dedicated ERAS coordinator who facilitates the communication between the different actors and ensures regular follow up of the patients [41, 42].

Finally, the challenge remained to maintain the sustainability of the ERAS program over years. Only one study reported long-term follow up after ERAS implementation in a cohort of 210 patients undergoing PD [37]. Three years after ERAS implementation, overall compliance increased over time from 65% to 72% without significant change in term of morbidity, LOS, mortality and readmission rate. Continuous change in the process and repeated education were key points to maintain optimal compliance.

29.6 Conclusion

Implementation of ERAS program in pancreatic surgery is a real challenge considering the complexity of the surgical procedures and the high morbidity. Nevertheless, according to the published data, implementation of ERAS is safe and efficient with shorten LOS, lower rate of overall complications and DGE, without increasing POPF rate, 30-day readmission and mortality. It is also feasible with a mean overall compliance of 70%. Lastly, ERAS program induced cost savings, which is also a crucial factor for health care system in the current economic context. However, several potential limitations should be mentioned. First, the majority of the studies are retrospective case-control studies with small sample size, which may lead to limited evidence. Secondly, there is still a substantial heterogeneity between the studies in the number and definition of outcomes and items included in the ERP. Therefore, it is difficult to compare the studies in term of postoperative outcomes and compliance. Finally, compliance level is the key point to improve postoperative outcomes and should be routinely reported in the study. Future RCTs are required with standardized ERAS program to assess the contributions of each ERAS items and to report patients' survival in pancreatic cancer.

References

1. Kehlet H. Multimodal approach to control postoperative pathophysiology and rehabilitation. Br J Anaesth. 1997;78(5):606–17. https://doi.org/10.1093/bja/78.5.606.
2. Anderson AD, McNaught CE, MacFie J, et al. Randomized clinical trial of multimodal optimization and standard perioperative surgical care. Br J Surg. 2003;90(12):1497–504. https://doi.org/10.1002/bjs.4371.
3. Varadhan KK, Neal KR, Dejong CH, et al. The enhanced recovery after surgery (ERAS) pathway for patients undergoing major elective open colorectal surgery: a meta-analysis of randomized controlled trials. Clin Nutr. 2010;29(4):434–40. https://doi.org/10.1016/j.clnu.2010.01.004.
4. Spanjersberg WR, Reurings J, Keus F, et al. Fast track surgery versus conventional recovery strategies for colorectal surgery. Cochrane Database Syst Rev. 2011;2011(2):CD007635. https://doi.org/10.1002/14651858.CD007635.pub2.
5. Coolsen MM, van Dam RM, van der Wilt AA, et al. Systematic review and meta-analysis of enhanced recovery after pancreatic surgery with particular emphasis on pancreaticoduodenectomies. World J Surg. 2013;37(8):1909–18. https://doi.org/10.1007/s00268-013-2044-3.
6. Lassen K, Coolsen MME, Slim K, et al. Guidelines for perioperative care for pancreaticoduodenectomy: enhanced recovery after surgery (ERAS®) society recommendations. World J Surg. 2013;37(2):240–58. https://doi.org/10.1007/s00268-012-1771-1.
7. Melloul L, Lassen K, Roulin D, et al. Guidelines for perioperative care for pancreatoduodenectomy: enhanced recovery after surgery (ERAS) recommendations 2019. World J Surg. 2020;44(7):2056–84. https://doi.org/10.1007/s00268-020-05462-w.
8. Winter JM, Cameron JL, Campbell KA, et al. 1423 pancreaticoduodenectomies for pancreatic cancer: a single-institution experience. J Gastrointest Surg. 2006;10(9):1199–210.; discussion 1210-1. https://doi.org/10.1016/j.gassur.2006.08.018.
9. Eisenberg JD, Rosato EL, Lavu H, et al. Delayed gastric emptying after pancreaticoduodenectomy: an analysis of risk factors and cost. J Gastrointest Surg. 2015;19(9):1572–80. https://doi.org/10.1007/s11605-015-2865-5.
10. Zhang XY, Zhang XZ, Lu FY, et al. Factors associated with failure of enhanced recovery after surgery program in patients undergoing pancreaticoduodenectomy. Hepatobiliary Pancreat Dis Int. 2020;19(1):51–7. https://doi.org/10.1016/j.hbpd.2019.09.006.
11. Maessen J, Dejong CH, Hausel J, et al. A protocol is not enough to implement an enhanced recovery programme for colorectal

resection. Br J Surg. 2007;94(2):224–31. https://doi.org/10.1002/bjs.5468.
12. Abu Hilal M, Di Fabio F, Badran A, et al. Implementation of enhanced recovery programme after pancreatoduodenectomy: a single-centre UK pilot study. Pancreatology. 2013;13(1):58–62. https://doi.org/10.1016/j.pan.2012.11.312.
13. Kobayashi S, Ooshima R, Koizumi S, et al. Perioperative care with fast-track management in patients undergoing pancreaticoduodenectomy. World J Surg. 2014;38(9):2430–7. https://doi.org/10.1007/s00268-014-2548-5.
14. Braga M, Pecorelli N, Ariotti R, et al. Enhanced recovery after surgery pathway in patients undergoing pancreaticoduodenectomy. World J Surg. 2014;38(11):2960–6. https://doi.org/10.1007/s00268-014-2653-5.
15. Coolsen MM, van Dam RM, Chigharoe A, et al. Improving outcomes after pancreaticoduodenectomy: experiences with implementing an enhanced recovery after surgery (ERAS) program. Dig Surg. 2014;31(3):177–84. https://doi.org/10.1159/000363583.
16. Shao Z, Jin G, Ji W, et al. The role of fast-track surgery in pancreaticoduodenectomy: a retrospective cohort study of 635 consecutive resections. Int J Surg. 2015;15:129–33. https://doi.org/10.1016/j.ijsu.2015.01.007.
17. Williamsson C, Karlsson N, Sturesson C, et al. Impact of a fast-track surgery programme for pancreaticoduodenectomy. Br J Surg. 2015;102(9):1133–41. https://doi.org/10.1002/bjs.9856.
18. Joliat GR, Labgaa I, Petermann D, et al. Cost-benefit analysis of an enhanced recovery protocol for pancreaticoduodenectomy. Br J Surg. 2015;102(13):1676–83. https://doi.org/10.1002/bjs.9957.
19. Partelli S, Crippa S, Castagnani R, et al. Evaluation of an enhanced recovery protocol after pancreaticoduodenectomy in elderly patients. HPB (Oxford). 2016;18(2):153–8. https://doi.org/10.1016/j.hpb.2015.09.009.
20. Bai X, Zhang X, Lu F, et al. The implementation of an enhanced recovery after surgery (ERAS) program following pancreatic surgery in an academic medical center of China. Pancreatology. 2016;16(4):665–70. https://doi.org/10.1016/j.pan.2016.03.018.
21. Zouros E, Liakakos T, Machairas A, et al. Improvement of gastric emptying by enhanced recovery after pancreaticoduodenectomy. Hepatobiliary Pancreat Dis Int. 2016;15(2):198–208. https://doi.org/10.1016/s1499-3872(16)60061-9.
22. Dai J, Jiang Y, Fu D. Reducing postoperative complications and improving clinical outcome: enhanced recovery after surgery in pancreaticoduodenectomy - a retrospective cohort study. Int J Surg. 2017;39:176–81. https://doi.org/10.1016/j.ijsu.2017.01.089.
23. Perinel J, Duclos A, Payet C, et al. Impact of enhanced recovery program after surgery in patients undergoing pancreatectomy on postoperative outcomes: a controlled before and after study. Dig Surg. 2020;37(1):47–55. https://doi.org/10.1159/000496510.
24. Xiong J, Szatmary P, Huang W, et al. Enhanced recovery after surgery program in patients undergoing pancreaticoduodenectomy: a PRISMA-compliant systematic review and meta-analysis. Medicine (Baltimore). 2016;95(18):e3497. https://doi.org/10.1097/MD.0000000000003497.
25. Ji HB, Zhu WT, Wei Q, et al. Impact of enhanced recovery after surgery programs on pancreatic surgery: a meta-analysis. World J Gastroenterol. 2018;24(15):1666–78. https://doi.org/10.3748/wjg.v24.i15.1666.
26. Deng X, Cheng X, Huo Z, et al. Modified protocol for enhanced recovery after surgery is beneficial for Chinese cancer patients undergoing pancreaticoduodenectomy. Oncotarget. 2017;8(29):47841–8. https://doi.org/10.18632/oncotarget.18092.
27. Takagi K, Yoshida R, Yagi T, et al. Effect of an enhanced recovery after surgery protocol in patients undergoing pancreaticoduodenectomy: a randomized controlled trial. Clin Nutr. 2019;38(1):174–81. https://doi.org/10.1016/j.clnu.2018.01.002.
28. Lavu H, McCall NS, Winter JM, et al. Enhancing patient outcomes while containing costs after complex abdominal operation: a randomized controlled trial of the Whipple accelerated recovery pathway. J Am Coll Surg. 2019;228(4):415–24. https://doi.org/10.1016/j.jamcollsurg.2018.12.032.
29. Hwang DW, Kim HJ, Lee JH, et al. Effect of enhanced recovery after surgery program on pancreaticoduodenectomy: a randomized controlled trial. J Hepatobiliary Pancreat Sci. 2019;26(8):360–9. https://doi.org/10.1002/jhbp.641.
30. Sun YM, Wang Y, Mao YX, et al. The safety and feasibility of enhanced recovery after surgery in patients undergoing pancreaticoduodenectomy: an updated meta-analysis. Biomed Res Int. 2020;2020:7401276. https://doi.org/10.1155/2020/7401276.
31. Wang XY, Cai JP, Huang CS, et al. Impact of enhanced recovery after surgery protocol on pancreaticoduodenectomy: a meta-analysis of non-randomized and randomized controlled trials. HPB (Oxford). 2020;22(10):1373–83. https://doi.org/10.1016/j.hpb.2020.07.001.
32. Coolsen MM, Bakens M, van Dam RM, et al. Implementing an enhanced recovery program after pancreaticoduodenectomy in elderly patients: is it feasible? World J Surg. 2015;39(1):251–8. https://doi.org/10.1007/s00268-014-2782-x.
33. Mirkin KA, Greenleaf EK, Hollenbeak CS, et al. Time to the initiation of adjuvant chemotherapy does not impact survival in patients with resected pancreatic cancer. Cancer. 2016;122(19):2979–87. https://doi.org/10.1002/cncr.30163.
34. Morgan KA, Lancaster WP, Walters ML, et al. Enhanced recovery after surgery protocols are valuable in pancreas surgery patients. J Am Coll Surg. 2016;222(4):658–64. https://doi.org/10.1016/j.jamcollsurg.2015.12.036.
35. Kagedan DJ, Devitt KS, Tremblay St-Germain A, et al. The economics of recovery after pancreatic surgery: detailed cost minimization analysis of an enhanced recovery program. HPB (Oxford). 2017;19(11):1026–33. https://doi.org/10.1016/j.hpb.2017.07.013.
36. Joliat GR, Hübner M, Roulin D, et al. Cost analysis of enhanced recovery programs in colorectal, pancreatic, and hepatic surgery: a systematic review. World J Surg. 2020;44(3):647–55. https://doi.org/10.1007/s00268-019-05252-z.
37. Williamsson C, Karlsson T, Westrin M, et al. Sustainability of an enhanced recovery program for pancreaticoduodenectomy with pancreaticogastrostomy. Scand J Surg. 2019;108(1):17–22. https://doi.org/10.1177/1457496918772375.
38. Roulin D, Melloul E, Wellg BE, et al. Feasibility of an enhanced recovery protocol for elective pancreatoduodenectomy: a multicenter international cohort study. World J Surg. 2020;44(8):2761–9. https://doi.org/10.1007/s00268-020-05499-x.
39. Aarts MA, Rotstein OD, Pearsall EA, et al. Postoperative ERAS interventions have the greatest impact on optimal recovery: experience with implementation of ERAS across multiple hospitals. Ann Surg. 2018;267(6):992–7. https://doi.org/10.1097/SLA.0000000000002632.
40. Lyon A, Solomon MJ, Harrison JD. A qualitative study assessing the barriers to implementation of enhanced recovery after surgery. World J Surg. 2014;38(6):1374–80. https://doi.org/10.1007/s00268-013-2441-7.
41. Martin D, Roulin D, Grass F, et al. A multicentre qualitative study assessing implementation of an enhanced recovery after surgery program. Clin Nutr. 2018;37(6 Pt A):2172–7. https://doi.org/10.1016/j.clnu.2017.10.017.
42. Bakker N, Cakir H, Doodeman HJ, et al. Eight years of experience with enhanced recovery after surgery in patients with colon cancer: impact of measures to improve adherence. Surgery. 2015;157(6):1130–6. https://doi.org/10.1016/j.surg.2015.01.016.

30. Ultrasound-Guided Anatomic Resection of the Liver

Junichi Shindoh, Kiyoshi Hasegawa, and Masatoshi Makuuchi

Abstract

Anatomic resection of the liver is an important concept to secure the local tumor control for hepatocellular carcinoma (HCC). For patients with primary, solitary HCC, systematic removal of the third-order tumor-bearing portal territories has been shown to be associated with longer time-to-recurrence after surgery and potentially longer overall survival. Although further clinical studies are needed to establish an optimal surgical strategy in management of patients with HCC, anatomic resection of the liver has several clinical advantages, and hepatobiliary surgeons should be familiar with this technique. In this chapter, technical details and clinical advantages of ultrasound-guided anatomic resection of the liver were reviewed.

30.1 Introduction

Liver resection is the first-line treatment in selected patients with primary or metastatic liver tumors. The safety of liver resection has dramatically improved over the decades with refinements of perioperative management and surgical techniques. However, the most important factors influencing on the surgical outcomes are surgeon's knowledge on anatomy and basic principles pertaining to the surgical procedure.

For patients with hepatocellular carcinoma (HCC), systematic removal of the tumor-bearing portal territories, so called "anatomic resection", was proposed in 1980s as a theoretically optimal surgical procedure to expect eradication of potential micrometastases surrounding tumors [1]. To date, a number of studies have reported that anatomic resection may prolong the time-to-recurrence after surgery and potentially improve the overall survival [2–11], with clear evidence of a decrease in the local recurrence rate [6, 8, 10]. A latest study using a Markov model has further clarified that complete removal of the tumor-bearing portal territory at initial hepatectomy delays both recurrence and post-operative stage progression of HCC, yielding improved survival of patients with solitary HCC [11]. Although the optimal choice of surgical procedure for patients with HCC remains under debate, given these encouraging clinical outcomes, hepatobiliary surgeons should be familiar with anatomic resection of the liver as a potentially appropriate surgical procedure in selected cases. In this chapter, we review the basic principles and techniques of ultrasound-guided anatomic resection of the liver.

30.2 Anatomical Principles and Definition of Anatomic Resection of the Liver

Anatomic resection of the liver usually refers to "systematic removal of various combinations of the third-order portal territories". According to the Brisbane 2000 terminology of liver anatomy and resections [12], resection of the first-order portal territory is called hemihepatectomy and resection of the second-order portal area is defined as sectorectomy or sectionectomy. Couinaud's segment is defined as the third-order division of the liver and monosegmentectomy is classified as anatomic resection. However, Couinaud's segment does not always correspond to the third-order portal territory because segment 2 is classified as the second-order portal territory, segment 5 or 8 usually consists of two or three third-order portal territories, and the definition of the caudate lobe (i.e., segment 1) is much more complex. The basic principles are that complete removal of any combination of third-

J. Shindoh (✉)
Hepatobiliary-pancreatic Surgery Division, Department of Gastroenterological Surgery, Toranomon Hospital, Tokyo, Japan
e-mail: shindou-tky@umin.ac.jp

K. Hasegawa
Hepatobiliary-pancreatic Surgery Division, Department of Surgery, Graduate School of Medicine, The University of Tokyo, Tokyo, Japan

M. Makuuchi
Koto Hospital, Tokyo, Japan

order portal territories can be classified as anatomic resection of the liver. Given that segment 5 and 8 usually have two or more third-order branches including ventral and dorsal branches [13], ventral/dorsal part of segment 5 or 8, ventral/dorsal part of the right paramedian sector, or even more complex combination of portal territories [14] can be classified as anatomic resection of the liver as long as systematic removal of the corresponding portal territories is secured.

30.3 Surgical Indication

For liver resection of HCC, strict assessment of hepatic functional reserve is needed because HCC usually develops in an injured liver, and the maximum extent of hepatectomy in patients with chronic hepatitis or cirrhosis is limited to avoid postoperative hepatic insufficiency, compared to those who have healthy livers. Liver resection is indicated only for Child-Pugh class A or B patients with controllable ascites and serum total bilirubin level of <2.0 mg/dL. Maximum extent of resection can be determined based on the measurement of indocyanine green retention rate at 15 min (ICG-R15) as proposed by Makuuchi et al. [4]. In original criteria for the maximum extent of resection, up to 2/3 hepatectomy (right hepatectomy or trisectionectomy) is accepted for patients with ICG-R15 < 10%, up to 1/3 hepatectomy (left hepatectomy or sectorectomy) is indicated for those with ICG-R15 between 10% and 19%, up to 1/6 hepatectomy (monosegmentectomy) is tolerated in those with ICG-R15 between 20% and 29%, and only limited partial hepatectomy or enucleation is indicated for patients with ICG-R15 equal to or greater than 30% (Fig. 30.1). Following strictly this algorithm, no operative mortality due to liver failure was recorded in 1056 consecutive patients at the University of Tokyo Hospital [15]. More recently, our group has adopted more sophisticated criteria based on the estimated ICG disappearing rate and precise three-dimensional volumetry of future liver remnant and it has been reported that the conventional criteria can be expanded safely, avoiding increased risk of postoperative hepatic insufficiency [16, 17].

30.4 Surgical Technique

30.4.1 Exposure

Incision and exposure are key components of the quality of the exploration of the liver and the safety of hepatectomy. Different incisions, including the inverted L incision, the inverted-T incision, the bilateral subcostal (chevron) incision, or the right/left subcostal incisions are used as well as the midline incision to achieve these objectives. Thoracotomy is sometimes required for safe exposure and manipulation of paracaval part of the liver. Meanwhile, recent laparoscopic technique has enabled us to minimize total length of incision through completing mobilization of the liver before opening the abdominal cavity, even in major hepatectomy which is not suitable for pure laparoscopic approach (i.e., laparoscopic-assisted hepatectomy).

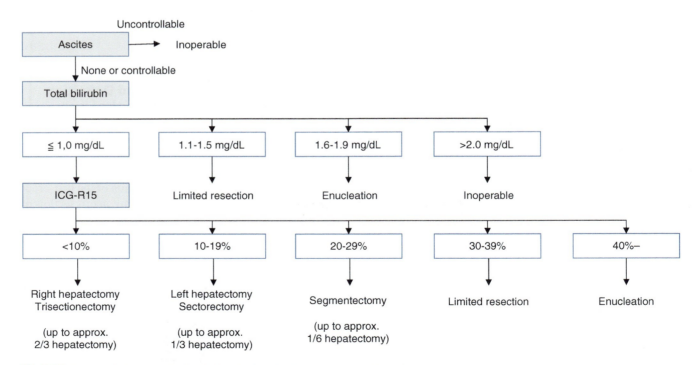

Fig. 30.1 Surgical indication criteria (Makuuchi Criteria) for patients with injured liver

30.4.2 Exploration and Intraoperative Ultrasound

After sufficient exposure of the liver, size, depth, location of tumors, their correlation to the surrounding vascular structures, presence/absence of new lesions, and intrahepatic blood flows are checked by ultrasound with or without contrast enhancement. Final surgical plans were then determined according to the preoperative data and intraoperative findings.

30.4.3 Identification of Segmental Border on the Liver Surface

To confirm the segmental border to be transected, positive or negative staining is then performed. Positive staining (i.e., direct staining of the corresponding portal area) is conventionally performed by injecting a blue dye (indigocarmine, Daiichi Sankyo Co., Ltd. Tokyo, Japan) into portal branches under ultrasound guidance. Tip of the needle is clearly visualized and injected dye can be confirmed as bubbles on ultrasound images. To obtain clear staining, hepatic arteries are needed to be clamped at the hepatic hilum while staining portal branches to delay washout of injected dye. Also, injection point and speed should be adjusted not to stain adjacent portal territories by regurgitation of the dye (Fig. 30.2a). When a tumor is located at the segmental border, corresponding tumor bearing portal branches should be stained respectively (Fig. 30.2b). However, when it is difficult to stain all the portal branches due to presence of multiple branches (e.g., segment 5) or too small size of branches which are difficult to be punctured (e.g., segment 1), negative staining can be used as an alternative method to confirm the segmental border by staining adjacent portal territories.

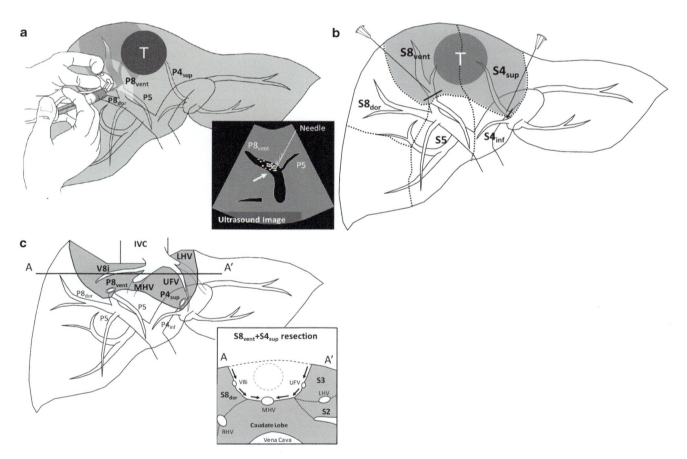

Fig. 30.2 Technical details of anatomic resection of the liver (adapted from Shindoh J, et al. J Hepatol 2016;64(3):594–600 with permission). (**a**) Segmental staining under ultrasound guidance. Tip of the needle and injected dye can be confirmed by ultrasound. (**b**) Staining of contiguous tumor-bearing third-order portal branches. When a tumor is located at the segmental border, corresponding tumor bearing portal branches should be stained respectively. (**c**) Anatomic resection of tumor-bearing segment. Anatomic resection can be achieved by (i) parenchymal transection from the marked segmental border on the liver surface to the land mark veins, (ii) full exposure of the veins on the cut surface of the liver, and (iii) ligation of portal pedicles near the root of the segment. *T* tumor, *P5* segment V portal branch, *P8vent* ventral branch of segment VIII portal branch, *P8dor* dorsal branch of segment VIII portal branch, *P4sup* superior branch of segment IV portal branch, *LHV* left hepatic vein, *MHV* middle hepatic vein, *UFV* umbilical fissure vein, *V8i* intermediate vein for segment VIII, *IVC* inferior vena cava

For sectorectomy/sectionectomy or anatomic resection of left side of the liver, however, portal staining is not always necessary because direct ligation or transient clamp of the corresponding Glissonean pedicle is feasible extrahepatically to visualize demarcation line on the liver surface.

Although these staining methods are relatively easy and can be applicable in most of the cases in actual clinical settings, it is sometimes difficult to obtain a clear staining on liver surface especially in patients with severe cirrhosis or those undergoing repeat hepatectomy requiring extensive lysis of adhesions. For such instances, diluted ICG solution can be used as an alternative material for injection when fluorescent imaging technique can be used [18].

30.4.4 Parenchymal Transection

Parenchymal transection is started along the segmental border confirmed on the liver surface. To secure complete removal of the target part of the liver, the landmark veins are exposed on the cut surface of the liver and the corresponding portal branches are ligated at the root of the segment (Fig. 30.2c). Because the intersegmental planes are not always flat [19], it is important to carry out parenchymal transection under ultrasound guidance (i) from liver surface to the landmark veins and (ii) from the exposed landmark veins to the root of the corresponding portal pedicles. Figure 30.3 demonstrates a typical preoperative evaluation and intraoperative findings of anatomic resection of dorsal part of segment 8.

30.4.5 Hemostasis and Check for Bile Leak

Injury of landmark veins during parenchymal transection can be secured by suture or application of fibrin glue according to the size of injury. Bile leak test [20] should be performed when cholecystectomy is carried out as a part of procedure because the shape of cut surface is relatively complex after anatomic resection of the liver and there is an increased risk of fluid collection compared to those after simple partial hepatectomy.

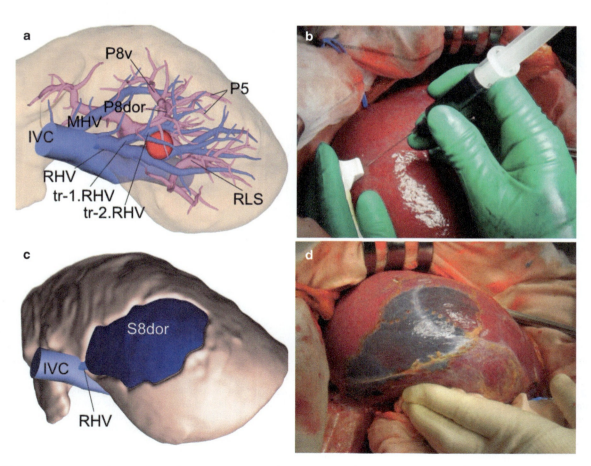

Fig. 30.3 Example of anatomic resection of dorsal part of segment 8 (Adopted from Takamoto T et al. Am J Surg 2013;206(4):530–538 with permission). Anatomic resection of dorsal part of segment 8 is planned (**a**) and corresponding portal branch was punctured under ultrasound guidance (**b**). Stained area visualized on liver surface (**d**) is very similar to the preoperative simulation (**c**). Based on the preoperative three-dimensional simulation (**e**), landmark veins (i.e., right hepatic vein and its tributary) are exposed on the cut surface of the liver (**f**)

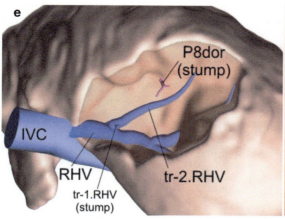
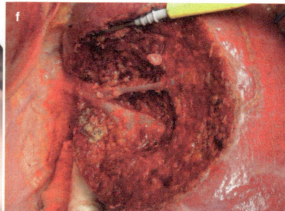

Fig. 30.3 (continued)

30.5 Clinical Advantages

30.5.1 Technical Advantages

From the practical standpoint, anatomic resection has several technical advantages. First, because the intersegmental plane at the watershed of portal territories are usually "avascular" excluding landmark veins, the risk of bile leak and amount of blood loss per area of the transection plane may be decreased [7]. Second, postoperative sustained hepatic dysfunction or disturbance of hepatic regeneration [13, 21, 22] could be avoided because no ischemic area or congested areas is present after complete removal of a portal territory leaving intersegmental venous branches at the cut surface of the liver. Third, branch-based volumetry or meticulous surgical planning is feasible and the option of curative surgery can be proposed based on the objective volumetric data even for patients with a marginal hepatic functional reserve [23–25].

30.5.2 Prognostic Advantages

Potential prognostic advantage of anatomic resection of the liver for primary, solitary HCC has been reported in many studies [2–10]. The University of Tokyo group previously reported that complete removal of tumor-bearing portal territories decreases the risk of local recurrence and death from HCC based on a database established under strict quality control [7] and recent large multi-institutional cohort studies have yielded similar outcomes [2, 9]. Another recent study conducted at a Japanese high-volume center has further clarified the differences in time-to-interventional failure and transition rate from the early recurrence stage to advanced stages according to the choice of surgical maneuver at initial hepatectomy for solitary HCC [11]. Although these results were confirmed only in a specific population with primary, solitary HCC and it remains inconclusive whether or not the same scenario can be applied for recurrent lesions, multiple HCCs, or large HCC occupying two or greater Couinaud's segments, the reported results suggest that initial selection of surgical procedure may have significant influence on subsequent clinical course and survival outcomes of patients with HCC. Therefore, anatomic resection should be considered as a choice of surgical maneuver at initial hepatectomy for patients with solitary HCC.

30.6 Conclusions

Technical details and clinical advantages of anatomic resection of the liver for patients with HCC were reviewed in this chapter. Although further clinical studies are needed to establish an optimal surgical strategy in management of patients with HCC, successful anatomic resection of tumor-bearing portal territory is reportedly delays long-term stage progression of HCC and may prolong survival outcomes. Given that ultrasound-guided anatomic resection of the liver consists of various basic techniques required for more complex liver surgery, hepatobiliary surgeons need to be familiar with this procedure in the era of aggressive surgical management of advanced hepatobiliary malignancies.

References

1. Makuuchi M, Hasegawa H, Yamazaki S. Ultrasonically guided subsegmentectomy. Surg Gynecol Obstet. 1985;161(4):346–50.
2. Kaibori M, Kon M, Kitawaki T, Kawaura T, Hasegawa K, Kokudo N, et al. Comparison of anatomic and non-anatomic hepatic resection for hepatocellular carcinoma. J Hepatobiliary Pancreat Sci. 2017;24(11):616–26.
3. Kakazu T, Makuuchi M, Kawasaki S, Miyagawa S, Hashikura Y, Kosuge T, et al. Repeat hepatic resection for recurrent hepatocellular carcinoma. Hepato-Gastroenterology. 1993;40(4):337–41.

4. Makuuchi M, Kosuge T, Takayama T, Yamazaki S, Kakazu T, Miyagawa S, et al. Surgery for small liver cancers. Semin Surg Oncol. 1993;9(4):298–304.
5. Regimbeau JM, Kianmanesh R, Farges O, Dondero F, Sauvanet A, Belghiti J. Extent of liver resection influences the outcome in patients with cirrhosis and small hepatocellular carcinoma. Surgery. 2002;131(3):311–7.
6. Shindoh J, Hasegawa K, Inoue Y, Ishizawa T, Nagata R, Aoki T, et al. Risk factors of post-operative recurrence and adequate surgical approach to improve long-term outcomes of hepatocellular carcinoma. HPB (Oxford). 2013;15(1):31–9.
7. Shindoh J, Makuuchi M, Matsuyama Y, Mise Y, Arita J, Sakamoto Y, et al. Complete removal of the tumor-bearing portal territory decreases local tumor recurrence and improves disease-specific survival of patients with hepatocellular carcinoma. J Hepatol. 2016;64(3):594–600.
8. Tanaka S, Mogushi K, Yasen M, Noguchi N, Kudo A, Kurokawa T, et al. Surgical contribution to recurrence-free survival in patients with macrovascular-invasion-negative hepatocellular carcinoma. J Am Coll Surg. 2009;208(3):368–74.
9. Vigano L, Procopio F, Mimmo A, Donadon M, Terrone A, Cimino M, et al. Oncologic superiority of anatomic resection of hepatocellular carcinoma by ultrasound-guided compression of the portal tributaries compared with nonanatomic resection: an analysis of patients matched for tumor characteristics and liver function. Surgery. 2018;164(5):1006–13.
10. Wakai T, Shirai Y, Sakata J, Kaneko K, Cruz PV, Akazawa K, et al. Anatomic resection independently improves long-term survival in patients with T1-T2 hepatocellular carcinoma. Ann Surg Oncol. 2007;14(4):1356–65.
11. Shindoh J, Kobayashi Y, Umino R, Kojima K, Okubo S, Hashimoto M. Successful anatomic resection of tumor-bearing portal territory delays long-term stage progression of hepatocellular carcinoma. Ann Surg Oncol. 2021;28(2):844–53.
12. Terminology Committee of the International Hepato-Pancreato-Biliary Association. The Brisbane 2000 terminology of liver anatomy and resections. HPB (Oxford). 2000;2(3):333–9.
13. Shindoh J, Satou S, Aoki T, Beck Y, Hasegawa K, Sugawara Y, et al. Hidden symmetry in asymmetric morphology: significance of Hjortsjo's anatomical model in liver surgery. Hepato-Gastroenterology. 2012;59(114):519–25.
14. Shindoh J, Nishioka Y, Hashimoto M. Bilateral anatomic resection of the ventral parts of the paramedian sectors of the liver with total caudate lobectomy for deeply/centrally located liver tumors: a new technique maximizing both oncological and surgical safety. J Hepatobiliary Pancreat Sci. 2017;24(12):E10–6.
15. Imamura H, Seyama Y, Kokudo N, Maema A, Sugawara Y, Sano K, et al. One thousand fifty-six hepatectomies without mortality in 8 years. Arch Surg. 2003;138(11):1198–206. discussion 206
16. Kobayashi Y, Kiya Y, Nishioka Y, Hashimoto M, Shindoh J. Indocyanine green clearance of remnant liver (ICG-Krem) predicts postoperative subclinical hepatic insufficiency after resection of colorectal liver metastasis: theoretical validation for safe expansion of Makuuchi's criteria. HPB (Oxford). 2020;22(2):258–64.
17. Kobayashi Y, Kiya Y, Sugawara T, Nishioka Y, Hashimoto M, Shindoh J. Expanded Makuuchi's criteria using estimated indocyanine green clearance rate of future liver remnant as a safety limit for maximum extent of liver resection. HPB (Oxford). 2019;21(8):990–7.
18. Kobayashi Y, Kawaguchi Y, Kobayashi K, Mori K, Arita J, Sakamoto Y, et al. Portal vein territory identification using indocyanine green fluorescence imaging: technical details and short-term outcomes. J Surg Oncol. 2017;116(7):921–31.
19. Shindoh J, Mise Y, Satou S, Sugawara Y, Kokudo N. The intersegmental plane of the liver is not always flat--tricks for anatomical liver resection. Ann Surg. 2010;251(5):917–22.
20. Zimmitti G, Vauthey JN, Shindoh J, Tzeng CW, Roses RE, Ribero D, et al. Systematic use of an intraoperative air leak test at the time of major liver resection reduces the rate of postoperative biliary complications. J Am Coll Surg. 2013;217(6):1028–37.
21. Sano K, Makuuchi M, Miki K, Maema A, Sugawara Y, Imamura H, et al. Evaluation of hepatic venous congestion: proposed indication criteria for hepatic vein reconstruction. Ann Surg. 2002;236(2):241–7.
22. Maema A, Imamura H, Takayama T, Sano K, Hui AM, Sugawara Y, et al. Impaired volume regeneration of split livers with partial venous disruption: a latent problem in partial liver transplantation. Transplantation. 2002;73(5):765–9.
23. Mise Y, Hasegawa K, Satou S, Aoki T, Beck Y, Sugawara Y, et al. Venous reconstruction based on virtual liver resection to avoid congestion in the liver remnant. Br J Surg. 2011;98(12):1742–51.
24. Saito S, Yamanaka J, Miura K, Nakao N, Nagao T, Sugimoto T, et al. A novel 3D hepatectomy simulation based on liver circulation: application to liver resection and transplantation. Hepatology. 2005;41(6):1297–304.
25. Takamoto T, Hashimoto T, Ogata S, Inoue K, Maruyama Y, Miyazaki A, et al. Planning of anatomical liver segmentectomy and subsegmentectomy with 3-dimensional simulation software. Am J Surg. 2013;206(4):530–8.

Parenchyma-sparing Hepatic Resection for Multiple Metastatic Tumors

Bruno Branciforte, Flavio Milana, and Guido Torzilli

Abstract

Liver surgery is actually asked to deal with high tumor burden also in case of colorectal metastases. Harming the most diseased part to hypertrophy the future liver remnant remains the mainstream. However, ultrasound guidance has progressively driven to challenge the tumor-vessel detachment (R1vasc), which has proven to be oncologically suitable in term of local control. This finding has boosted the suitability of parenchyma sparing surgery even when tumor burden is extremely high. A further improvement in this sense has been provided in case of hepatic vein tumoral stricture or occlusion: indeed, in these circumstances natural by-pass develop preserving the outflow. Through ultrasound and vessel guidance, parenchyma sparing surgery has entered the complexity. From there, a different way of large tissue deprivation: the meaningful parenchymal sparing major hepatectomies.

31.1 Introduction

Surgical resection is the only potentially curative treatment for metastatic tumors in the liver. Patients with colorectal liver metastases (CLMs) are often addressed to multiple hepatic resections, but initial experiences with major hepatic resection were associated with a high peri-operative mortality. Preservation of an adequate remnant liver volume after resection became recognized as one of the most relevant issue in the prevention of post-hepatectomy liver failure (PHLF), and one of the main cause of post-operative mortality.

To maximize the safety of liver surgery, and expand the suitability of the surgical treatment, surgeons tended to develop operative techniques that limit the extent of parenchymal resection, tailoring the resection to the extent of the pathology without compromising cancer-specific outcomes.

A better understanding of intrahepatic anatomy and tumor biology, as well as advances in imaging technologies, together with improvement in peri- and intraoperative management, allowed expanding indications and performing more aggressive and complex procedures.

The parenchyma-sparing surgery (PSS) philosophy is a part of this perspective and merges the oncologic rules of surgery with minimal sacrifice of liver tissue.

31.2 Multiple Bilobar CLM

Liver surgery represents the standard of treatment for CLMs, even in patients with multiple and/or bilobar lesions. These patients are the most complex to treat because a large parenchyma sacrifice is often needed. Moreover, in patients with underlying liver disease (or even in those who have received multiple cycles of chemotherapy), the risk of developing post hepatectomy liver failure (PHLF) is even higher [1].

Reducing the risk of PHLF whenever a major removal of functioning liver tissue was performed has been the main target of many surgeons. In early 2000 Adam et al. proposed a staged procedure scheduling as first step a debulking surgery, limiting the CLM clearance to one side of the organ, and in a second operation the definitive organ clearance: the so-called 2-stage hepatectomy (TSH) [2]. For improving the efficiency of the approach Jaeck et al. introduced, in between the two step, a portal vein embolization of the right hemiliver for inducing hypertrophy of the left [3]. The main disadvantage

B. Branciforte · F. Milana
Division of Hepatobiliary and General Surgery, Humanitas Clinical and Research Center IRCCS, Milan, Italy

G. Torzilli (✉)
Division of Hepatobiliary and General Surgery, Humanitas Clinical and Research Center IRCCS, Milan, Italy

Department of Biomedical Sciences, Humanitas University, Milan, Italy
e-mail: guido.torzilli@hunimed.eu

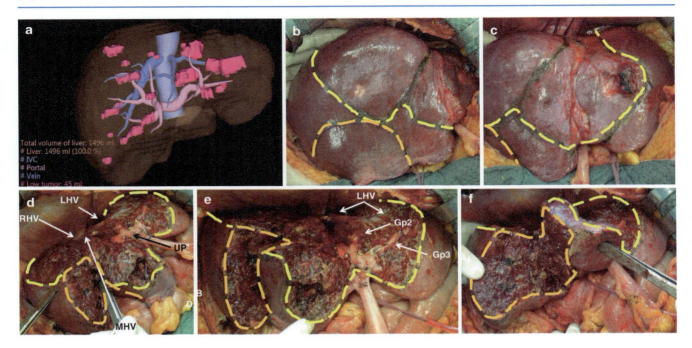

Fig. 31.1 (**a**) virtual liver cast based on CT images of a patient carrier of 19 colorectal liver metastases (dark pink); the glissonean branches in light pink; hepatic veins in dark blue; inferior vena cava in light blue. (**b, c**) resection areas (yellow and orange dotted lines) drawn with electrocautery on the liver surface. (**d–f**) cut surfaces at the end of the tumor removals; the cut surfaces surrounded by the yellow and orange dotted lines refer to the previously highlighted resection areas. *RHV*, Right Hepatic Vein, *MHV* Middle Hepatic Vein, *LHV* Left Hepatic Vein, *IVC* Inferior vena cava, *Gp* glissonean pedicles (numbers refer to the segment fed), *UP* umbilical portion

of TSH is the non-negligible risk of drop-out: about one-third of patients do not receive the second hepatectomy because of disease progression between the 2 stages or inadequate hypertrophy of the future liver remnant (FLR) [4]. More recently, the *associated liver partition and portal vein ligation for staged hepatectomy* (ALPPS) has been proposed: despite, this approach, a sort of fast-track TSH, guarantees a significantly lower drop-out rate compared to TSH, surgical risk and long-term oncological results remain open issues [5–7]. Finally, liver venous deprivation (LVD) followed by major hepatectomy is the last release aiming to empower liver regeneration. Simultaneous occlusion of portal vein inflow and hepatic vein (HV) outflow for harming part of the liver seems safe, and efficient in terms of FLR increase and consequent drastic limitation of patients' drop-out [8, 9]. Anyhow, all these solutions boosting the FLR by means of major vessel amputation reduce the chance of redo surgery in case of relapses. Indeed, it seems somehow obvious that less remnant vascular structures offer lower freedom degrees for finding technical solutions able to clear the organ.

In the last decades, PSS has been increasingly adopted [10]. However, several authors have limited the application of their parenchyma-sparing policy to a "cherry-picking surgery" (limited peripheral resection) or anatomic segmentectomy [11]. In presence of superficial lesions, single-session multiple minor resections are commonly adopted, but in case of deep-located CLMs, staged hepatectomy still remains the preferred option. The authors have extensively demonstrated the feasibility, safety and efficacy of IOUS-guided PSS for CLMs [12–17].

In particular, the possibility to resect in a PSS perspective also deep lesions with complex intrahepatic relations have been explored, namely with the so-called enhanced one-stage hepatectomy (E-OSH) [14, 18] (Fig. 31.1). Minimizing the parenchyma sacrifice, and preserving the liver scaffold were the pillars of an approach devoted to be radical, and conservative. Increased safety and salvageability in case of relapse have been the merits of this policy. In particular, salvageability means better long-term disease control: recent series reported five-year survival rates after surgery of about 50%, despite up to 70–80% of patients having disease recurrence [19, 20].

Intra-operative ultrasound (IOUS) guidance, tumor vessel detachment and the presence of communicating veins (CVs) preserving liver outflow whenever detachment is unfeasible, are the main technical pillars in which advanced PSS relies.

31.2.1 Intraoperative Ultrasound

IOUS, used in hepatic surgery since the early 1980s [21], has been repeatedly advocated as a useful tool for resection guidance both in primary and secondary metastatic tumors, and represents the cornerstone of PSS policy [12]. Despite several reasons may explain decrease in mortality following major hepatic resection reached in the last decades [22], a privileged role should be surely assigned to improved operative techniques which became feasible thanking to IOUS guidance.

Indeed, IOUS makes possible creating complex multiplanar dissection trajectories during liver resection, then really opening to policies alternative to major hepatectomies [23, 24].

The use of IOUS in liver resections could be divided into three main phases: (1) liver exploration for disease staging, (2) planning of the surgical strategy, and (3) surgical maneuvers guidance. Although palpation still plays a fundamental phase, for deep located lesions IOUS exploration represents a crucial intraoperative tool, refined on the possibility of contrast enhancement (CE-IOUS). Despite progress in preoperative imaging, adding CE-IOUS to IOUS exploration showed to modify the operative plan in up to 38% of patients with CLM, with its ability in recognizing new lesions otherwise not visible [25].

Moreover, IOUS allows an accurate estimation of the relationship among the tumor and vessels (both glissonian pedicles and HVs), which is a fundamental step in defining the most appropriate surgical strategy. Indeed, the tumor-vessel relationship represents a crucial point in parenchymal-sparing policy, being informative in discriminating a vascular contact from a vascular infiltration.

31.2.2 Tumor-vessel Detachment

Surgeons have progressively moved from the 1-cm rule to the 1-mm rule, but negative surgical margin (R0) has been considered as the standard while R1 resection as an unfavorable surgical result [26]. Nevertheless, vascular wall may represent a boundary to tumor spread, and vascular detachment could be performed safely. Specifically, R1 vascular (R1vasc) resection is defined as any tumor detachment from first/second-order glissonean pedicles (in contact with up to half of the pedicle circumference) or from HVs (in contact with up to two-thirds of the vein circumference) within their last 4 cm before hepato-caval confluence [23]. R1vasc corresponds to tumor exposure (0-mm margin) along the "detachment area" and it has been demonstrated offering equivalent results to R0 resection in terms of local recurrence and 5-year survival [17, 27]. R1vasc suitability is the crucial finding which could make reliable not just the PSS strategy but the tissue removal preserving the organ scaffold: this could mean resecting conservatively complex presentation otherwise affordable just with major hepatectomies or staged procedure or resulting even unresectable.

To maximize the feasibility of R1vasc resections, IOUS-based criteria have been introduced and validated [12, 13]: the circumferential extent of the contact represents the main driver for deciding to spare or not the vessel.

31.2.3 Communicating Veins

in the event of clear vessel wall infiltration, vascular resection is mandatory. Liver resection for tumors involving the major HVs nearby the hepatocaval junction traditionally requires major anatomical resection with or without venous reconstruction. HVs, when infiltrated, in the majority of situations could be anyhow spared by means of tangential resection with direct reconstruction or seldom patching [17]. In the event this would not be feasible, then in case of more significant infiltration, despite HVs are sacrificed the drained area of liver parenchyma could be almost always spared. Indeed, in such conditions which mimics a Budd-Chiari Syndrome, CVs between major HVs, exist and can be identified in up to 80% of patients with a tumor at the hepatocaval confluence [28]. CVs represent an outflow pathway alternative to major HVs, making suitable to preserve liver venous discharge even when a major HV is resected. This further possibility increases the suitability of conducting PSS.

Preoperative imaging findings can suggest CV patency, by direct visualization or just confirming a uniform enhancement of the liver parenchyma at venous phase for CT or hepato-specific delayed phase for MRI. Anyhow, CV patency is definitively detected by IOUS color-flow analysis. Moreover, HV clamping during surgery may offer additional data: CV patency can be enhanced, and persistent hepatopetal portal inflow, even in the absence of evident CVs, is a permissive condition for PSS [13, 28]. Their presence guarantees otherwise unfeasible technical solutions, thus leading ineligible patients undergoing radical surgery and avoiding major hepatectomies.

31.3 New Procedures

The IOUS indicates the door for entering into the liver, and the vessel guides the surgeon once inside. Following the intrahepatic vessels from the surface to the deep warrantees anyhow an anatomical approach, but with infinite trajectories according to the selected vessel, then infinite solutions. Parenchyma sparing vessel guided hepatectomies (PSVGH) for sculpturing the organ, implementing the portfolio of surgical options, and increasing the salvageability in case of relapse by keeping the major in and out-flow intrahepatic vascular structures [29]. Cornerstone of PSVGH are the following new parenchymal-sparing procedures:

31.3.1 Systematic Extended Right Posterior Sectionectomy (SERPS) [30]

Right posterior sectionectomy (S6-7) extended to part of S5 and S8 with section of the right HV (RHV). The outflow of spared S5 and/or S8 is provided by branches of the middle HV (MHV) (Fig. 31.2).

31.3.1.1 Eligibility Criteria
Patients suitable for SERPS are those with tumors showing:

A. invasion of the RHV close to the hepato-caval confluence (within 4 cm), with other lesions involving segment 6 and eventually segment 7 (Fig. 31.2a).
B. invasion of the RHV close to the hepato-caval confluence (within 4 cm), without other lesions involving segment 6, but without inferior RHV (IRHV), and with hepatofugal portal blood flow at color-flow IOUS in portal branch to segment 6 (P6) when RHV is clamped (Fig. 31.2b).
C. contact with the right anterior glissonean sheat, and a relation with the right posterior having at least one of the following features: contact with dilation of bile ducts of right posterior section, vessel wall invasion, or contact wider than one-third of pedicle circumference (Fig. 31.2c).

31.3.2 Upper Trasversal Hepatectomy (UTH))

Transversal hepatectomies for tumors involving more than one and up to all the HVs at hepato-caval confluence. The following subtypes can be recognized:

31.3.2.1 Mini-Upper Transversal Hepatectomy
Anatomic or limited resection of S7-8 with section of the RHV. The outflow of S5 and S6 is provided by an IRHV [31], by branches of the MHV [20] or by CVs between the RHV and/or left HV (LHV) and the MHV [32].

31.3.2.2 Right Upper Transversal Hepatectomy [33]
Anatomic or limited resection of S7-8-4s with section of the RHV and the MHV. The outflow of S4i-5-6 is provided by the IRHV and/or CVs only, among the RHV, the MHV and the LHV.

31.3.2.3 Left Upper Transversal Hepatectomy [24]
Anatomic or limited resection of S2-4s or of S2-4s-8 with section of the LHV or the LHV and the MHV. The outflow of segments 3-4i-5 is provided by CVs among the RHV, the MHV and the LHV.

31.3.2.4 Total Upper Transversal Hepatectomy [24, 34]
Anatomic or limited resection of S2-4s-7-8 with section of the RHV, the MHV and the LHV in presence of an IRHV and CVs among the liver-side stumps of the HVs, which warrantee the outflow of S3-4i-5-6.

Eligibility Criteria
Tumor at caval confluence invading from one to all HVs at caval confluence in presence of an IRHV, and CVs or just CVs. The tumor could lie over the hilar plate with contact but no invasion of the right and left portal branches, and the segmental portal branches to the antero-inferior segments.

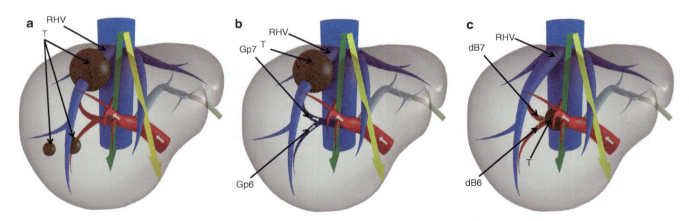

Fig. 31.2 schemas of patterns eligible for Systematic Extended Right Posterior Sectionectomy (SERPS); (**a**) tumor (T) invading the right hepatic vein (RHV) with others involving segment 6; (**b**) T invading the RHV with hepatofugal (white arrows) portal vein blood flow in glissonean pedicles for segments 6 (Gp6) and 7 (Gp7); (**c**) T in contact with the 2nd order right Gp, but with dilated bile duct draining segment 6 (dB6) and 7 (dB7) indicating the invasion of the Gp of the right posterior section. Green arrow = dissection plane of the SERPS. Yellow arrow = dissection plane of the right hepatectomy

31.3.3 Mini-mesohepatectomy (MMH) [35, 36]

This procedure represents an alternative to the conventional meso-hepatectomy in case of tumors invading the MHV at its caval confluence, and consists in a limited resection including the tract of the invaded vein without its reconstruction sparing part of the segment 4 and/or of the right anterior section.

31.3.3.1 Eligibility Criteria
Patients suitable for the MMH are those with tumors having macroscopic signs of vascular invasion (preoperative imaging and IOUS) of the MHV close to the hepato-caval confluence (within 4 cm) in presence of CVs between the MHV and the RHV and/or LHV.

31.3.4 Liver Tunnel [37, 38]

This procedure represents an extension of the MMH, including the total removal of segment 1. The following subtypes can be recognized:

31.3.4.1 Liver Tunnel Without Resection of the Middle Hepatic Vein
Limited or anatomic resection of S8 associated with complete removal of S1 (Fig. 31.3).

31.3.4.2 Liver Tunnel with the Resection of the Middle Hepatic Vein
Limited or anatomic resection of S4s-8 with section of middle HV and complete removal of S1. The outflow of S5 and

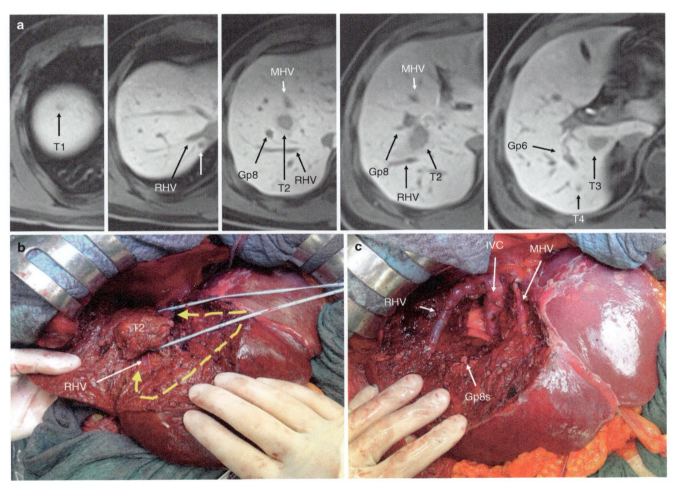

Fig. 31.3 (a) MRI images of a patients carrier of multiple colorectal liver metastases (T); (b) a mid-term phase during liver dissection: yellow arrows represent the directions of the dissections. (c) cut surfaces at the end of the resection representing a liver tunnel without middle hepatic vein (MHV) resection. *RHV* Right Hepatic Vein, *LHV* Left Hepatic Vein, *IVC* Inferior vena cava, *Gp* glissonean pedicles (numbers refer to the segment fed; "s" means stump), *IVC* Inferior vena cava

S4i is provided by CVs between the MHV and the RHV and/or LHV (Fig. 31.4).

Eligibility Criteria

Patients eligible for this approach are those with tumoral involvement of segments 8, 4 superior, and 1, with eventual contact with MHV, and the RHV at caval confluence, the right, and the left 1st and 2nd order portal branches. The MHV could be invaded by the tumor at its caval confluence, in presence of CVs between the MHV, the RHV and/or the LHV.

31.4 Discussion

Sculpturing rather than simply dividing the liver has induced a revision of the concept of minor and major hepatectomy [39], and definitely a new dictionary of liver surgery to be written.

Moreover, other than technical insights and new terminologies, overcoming dogmas as tumor exposure mainly launches new horizons for liver surgery, and more therapeutic options for the patients. In a comparative analysis between E-OSH and TSH, E-OSH shows survivals similar to those of

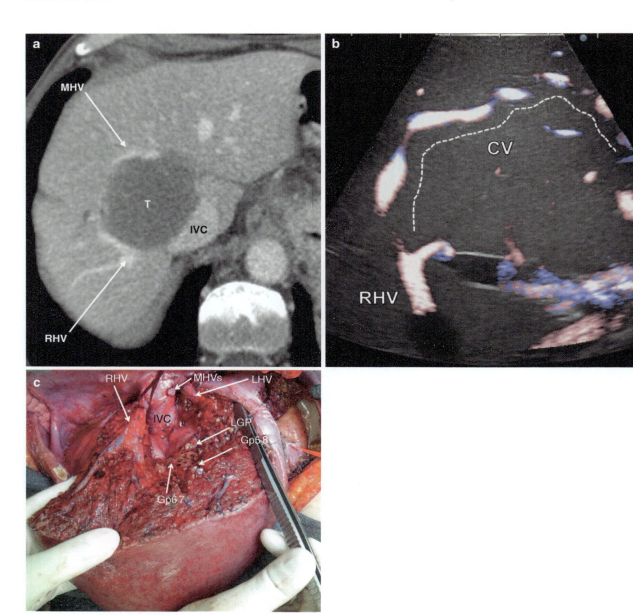

Fig. 31.4 (**a**) CT image of a patients carrier of large colorectal liver metastases (T) in tight relation with the right hepatic vein (RHV) and the middle hepatic vein (MHV); (**b**) at color flow IOUS communicating veins (CV) are evident between the RHV and the MHV; dotted line is highlighting the CV path. (**c**) cut surface at the end of the resection representing a liver tunnel MHV resection. *RHV* Right Hepatic Vein, *LHV* Left Hepatic Vein, *LGP* left glissonean pedicle, *IVC* Inferior vena cava, *Gp* glissonean pedicle (numbers refer to the segment/section fed), *IVC* Inferior vena cava

completed TSH but without the non-negligible 40% rate of dropout, which mainly affected cumulative survival in TSH group in an intention to treat perspective [40]. On the other hand, a more recent multicenter case-match analysis suggests that ALPPS and E-OSH may achieve comparable long-term results in patients affected by bilobar CLM, despite a higher mortality and morbidity rate after ALPPS [41]. A safer clinical outcome after major tissue deprivation in a parenchyma sparing vessel guided fashion compared to that following major resections through conventional vessels amputation should deserve some consideration. On the other hand, ALPPS has shown to be associated with an increment in liver volume which does not translate one to one with liver function [42]. PSVGH keeping the architecture of the organ with its major vessels even in presence of high amount of liver tissue removed as it happens in case of multiple complex resection for bilobar CLM has shown a low risk and in particular a low rate of liver failure: milder regeneration of the liver after PSVGH compared to that evident after major amputation of the organ should be considered as a possibility to be investigated. Through IOUS and vessel guidance, PSS has entered the complexity, and entering the complexity has arrived to a different way of large tissue deprivation: the parenchymal sparing major hepatectomies could be a meaningful and promising paradox.

31.5 Concerns & Future Directions

Despite all these strengths and potentialities, the future of PSVGH in the clinical practice worldwide remains somehow suspended.

PSS can limit the sacrifice of parenchyma; this policy, however, often results in resection margins of 0 mm, which could reach up to 30% of patients [43]. However, PSS and non-PSS had comparable positive margin rates [44]. Furthermore, it has been demonstrated that rather than millimeters, tumor biology is a more important predictor of both intrahepatic or any other site recurrence and overall survival [27]. On the other hand, in patients with CLMs, occult microscopic metastases are definitely uncommon [45, 46]. All of that, supports the concept of performing limited, wedge resections with narrow margins for CLM, rather than non-PSS procedures featured by worse postoperative outcome [47–49].

Technically sophisticated, PSVGH is moreover based on the man-power resources rather than on the availability of a sophisticated technology and dedicated devices: an ultrasound system, a Kelly-clamp, a Metzenbaum scissor, and few more are enough. Therefore, in this viewpoint its cost is low and its applicability wide, which sounds undoubtedly positive on a certain perspective. However, its independence from any highly technological equipment, makes the interest of the health industry relatively low which for sure does not help its diffusion. In this sense, its partial applicability in the minimal access liver surgery (MALS), which attracts most of the investments of the health industry, does not help in terms of visibility within the surgical community. The inability of MALS to address complex a multiplanar dissections, but the possibility to perform even staged procedures [50] for sure does not represent an incentive for the spread of PSVGH. Furthermore, as first impression PSVGH seems a modality requiring an adequate training and for that it should rely on a tutorship which to now is lacking. Inversely, although an isolated experience, learning curve for this approach resulted as long as that of any conventional approach in liver surgery. Indeed, in author's center a team featured by a mean age of 36 years old could cover autonomously up to 80% of surgical procedure carried out on a yearly basis within 5–6 years from his first exposure [51].

31.6 Conclusions

In the 80s Masatoshi Makuuchi introduced the anatomical parenchymal sparing hepatectomy opening to conservative surgery those patients normally operated with risky major anatomical resections [21]. In the 90s Henri Bismuth proposed to "resect the unresectable" introducing the concept of conversion chemotherapy [52]. PSVGH has extended PSS to the high complexity, further challenging to "resect the unresectable" just with a new surgical paradigm: the paradox of parenchyma sparing major hepatectomy.

References

1. Vibert E, Pittau G, Gelli M, et al. Actual incidence and long-term consequences of posthepatectomy liver failure after hepatectomy for colorectal liver metastases. Surgery. 2014;155:94–105.
2. Adam R, Laurent A, Azoulay D, et al. Twostage hepatectomy: a planned strategy to treat irresectable liver tumors. Ann Surg. 2000;232:777–85.
3. Jaeck D, Oussoultzoglou E, Rosso E, Greget M, Weber JC, Bachellier P. A two-stage hepatectomy procedure combined with portal vein embolization to achieve curative resection for initially unresectable multiple and bilobar colorectal liver metastases. Ann Surg. 2004;240(6):1037–49.
4. Wicherts DA, Miller R, de Haas RJ, et al. Long-term results of two-stage hepatectomy for irresectable colorectal cancer liver metastases. Ann Surg. 2008;248:994–1005.
5. Schnitzbauer AA, Lang SA, Goessmann H, et al. Right portal vein ligation combined with in situ splitting induces rapid left lateral liver lobe hypertrophy enabling 2-staged extended right hepatic resection in small-for-size settings. Ann Surg. 2012;255:405–14.
6. De Santibañes E, Clavien PA. Playing Play-Doh to prevent postoperative liver failure: the "ALPPS" approach. Ann Surg. 2012;255:415–7.

7. Schadde E, Ardiles V, Robles-Campos R, et al. Early survival and safety of ALPPS: first report of the International ALPPS Registry. Ann Surg. 2014;260:829–36.
8. Guiu B, Quenet F, Escal L, et al. Extended liver venous deprivation before major hepatectomy induces marked and very rapid increase in future liver remnant function. Eur Radiol. 2017;27(8):3343–52.
9. Laurent C, Fernandez B, Marichez A, et al. Radiological simultaneous portohepatic vein embolization (RASPE) before major hepatectomy: a better way to optimize liver hypertrophy compared to portal vein embolization. Ann Surg. 2020;272(2):199–205.
10. Gold JS, Are C, Kornprat P, Jarnagin WR, Gönen M, Fong Y, DeMatteo RP, Blumgart LH, D'Angelica M. Increased use of parenchymal-sparing surgery for bilateral liver metastases from colorectal cancer is associated with improved mortality without change in oncologic outcome: trends in treatment over time in 440 patients. Ann Surg. 2008;247:109–17.
11. Chouillard E, Cherqui D, Tayar C, Brunetti F, Fagniez PL. Anatomical bi- and trisegmentectomies as alternatives to extensive liver resections. Ann Surg. 2003;238(1):29–34.
12. Torzilli G, Montorsi M, Donadon M, et al. "Radical but conservative" is the main goal for ultrasonography-guided liver resection: prospective validation of this approach. J Am Coll Surg. 2005;201(4):517–28.
13. Torzilli G, Montorsi M, Del Fabbro D, Palmisano A, Donadon M, Makuuchi M. Ultrasonographically guided surgical approach to liver tumours involving the hepatic veins close to the caval confluence. Br J Surg. 2006;93(10):1238–46. https://doi.org/10.1002/bjs.5321.
14. Torzilli G, Procopio F, Botea F, et al. One-stage ultrasonographically guided hepatectomy for multiple bilobar colorectal metastases: a feasible and effective alternative to the 2-stage approach. Surgery. 2009;146(1):60–71.
15. Viganò L, Costa G, Procopio F, Donadon M, Cimino M, Del Fabbro D, Gatti A, Torzilli G. Parenchyma-sparing liver surgery for large segment 1 tumors: ultrasound-guided lateral and superior approaches as safe alternatives to major hepatectomy. J Am Coll Surg. 2015;221(4):e65–73.
16. Torzilli G, Viganò L, Gatti A, Costa G, Cimino M, Procopio F, et al. Twelve-year experience of "radical but conservative" liver surgery for colorectal metastases: impact on surgical practice and oncologic efficacy. HPB. 2017;19:775–84.
17. Torzilli G, Procopio F, Viganò L, Cimino M, Costa G, Del Fabbro D, Donadon M. Hepatic vein management in a parenchyma-sparing policy for resecting colorectal liver metastases at the caval confluence. Surgery. 2018;163(2):277–84.
18. Torzilli G, Cimino MM. Extending the limits of resection for colorectal liver metastases enhanced one stage surgery. J Gastrointest Surg. 2017;21:187–9.
19. Vigano L, Ferrero A, Lo Tesoriere R, et al. Liver surgery for colorectal metastases: results after 10 years of follow-up. Long-term survivors, late recurrences, and prognostic role of morbidity. Ann Surg Oncol. 2008;15:2458–64.
20. Tomlinson JS, Jarnagin WR, DeMatteo RP, et al. Actual 10-year survival after resection of colorectal liver metastases defines cure. J Clin Oncol. 2007;25:4575–80.
21. Makuuchi M, et al. Ultrasonically guided liver surgery. Jpn J Ultrasonics Med. 1980;7:45–9.
22. Kneuertz PJ, Pitt HA, Bilimoria KY, et al. Risk of morbidity and mortality following Hepato-Pancreato-biliary surgery. J Gastrointest Surg. 2012;16:1727–35.
23. Torzilli G, Procopio F, Costa G. Adjuncts to hepatic resection – ultrasound and emerging guidance systems. In: Jarnagin WR, editor. Blumgart's surgery of the liver, pancreas, and biliary tract. 6th ed. Philadelphia: Elsevier Saunders; 2017.
24. Torzilli G. Ultrasound-guided liver surgery: an atlas. 1st ed. Milan: Springer-Verlag; 2014.
25. Torzilli G, et al. Does contrast-enhanced intraoperative ultrasonography impact radicality of hepatectomies for colorectal cancer liver metastases in spite of modern preoperative imaging? Analysis on a prospective cohort. Eur J Cancer. 2008;6:16–23.
26. Pawlik TM, Scoggins CR, Zorzi D, et al. Effect of surgical margin status on survival and site of recurrence after hepatic resection for colorectal metastases. Ann Surg. 2005;241:715–22.
27. Viganò L, Procopio F, Cimino M, et al. Is tumor detachment from vascular structures equivalent to R0 resection in surgery for colorectal liver metastases? An observational cohort. Ann Surg Oncol. 2016;23:1352–60.
28. Torzilli G, Garancini M, Donadon M, Cimino M, Procopio F, Montorsi M. Intraoperative ultrasonographic detection of communicating veins between adjacent hepatic veins during hepatectomy for tumours at the hepatocaval confluence. Br J Surg. 2010;97(12):1867–73.
29. Torzilli G, Viganò L, Gatti A, et al. Twelve-year experience of "radical but conservative" liver surgery for colorectal metastases: impact on surgical practice and oncologic efficacy. HPB (Oxford). 2017;19(9):775–84.
30. Torzilli G, Donadon M, Marconi M, Botea F, Palmisano A, Del Fabbro D, Procopio F, Montorsi M. Systematic extended right posterior sectionectomy: a safe and effective alternative to right hepatectomy. Ann Surg. 2008;247(4):603–11.
31. Makuuchi M, Hasegawa H, Yamazaki S, Takayasu K. Four new hepatectomy procedures for resection of the right hepatic vein and preservation of the inferior right hepatic vein. Surg Gynecol Obstet. 1987;164(1):68–72.
32. Torzilli G, Procopio F, Cimino M, Donadon M, Del Fabbro D, Costa G, Gatti A, Garcia-Etienne CA. Radical but conservative liver resection for large centrally located hepatocellular carcinoma: the mini upper-transversal hepatectomy. Ann Surg Oncol. 2014;21(6):1852.
33. Torzilli G, Procopio F, Donadon M, et al. Upper transversal hepatectomy. Ann Surg Oncol. 2012;19(11):3566.
34. Gentile D, Donadon M, Civilini E, Torzilli G. Total upper transversal hepatectomy with outflow reconstruction for advanced mass-forming cholangiocarcinoma. Updat Surg. 2021; https://doi.org/10.1007/s13304-020-00946-9. Epub ahead of print
35. Torzilli G, Botea F, Donadon M, Cimino M, Del Fabbro D, Palmisano A. Minimesohepatectomy for colorectal liver metastasis invading the middle hepatic vein at the hepatocaval confluence. Ann Surg Oncol. 2010;17(2):483. https://doi.org/10.1245/s10434-009-0728-6. Epub 2009 Oct 23
36. Torzilli G, Palmisano A, Procopio F, et al. A new systematic small for size resection for liver tumors invading the middle hepatic vein at its caval confluence: mini-mesohepatectomy. Ann Surg. 2010;251(1):33–9.
37. Torzilli G, Cimino M, Procopio F, Costa G, Donadon M, Del Fabbro D, Gatti A, Garcia-Etienne CA. Conservative hepatectomy for tumors involving the middle hepatic vein and segment 1: the liver tunnel. Ann Surg Oncol. 2014;21(8):2699.
38. Torzilli G, Procopio F, Viganò L, Costa G, Fontana A, Cimino M, Donadon M, Del Fabbro D. The liver tunnel: intention-to-treat validation of a new type of hepatectomy. Ann Surg. 2019;269(2):331–6.
39. Viganò L, Torzilli G, Troisi R, et al. Minor Hepatectomies: focusing a blurred picture: analysis of the outcome of 4471 open resections in patients without cirrhosis. Ann Surg. 2019;270(5):842–51.
40. Torzilli G, Viganò L, Cimino M, et al. Is enhanced one-stage hepatectomy a safe and feasible alternative to the two-stage hepatectomy in the setting of multiple Bilobar colorectal liver metastases? A comparative analysis between two pioneering centers. Dig Surg. 2018;35(4):323–32.
41. Torzilli G, Serenari M, Viganò L, et al. Outcomes of enhanced one-stage ultrasound-guided hepatectomy for bilobar colorectal liver

metastases compared to those of ALPPS: a multicenter case-match analysis. HPB (Oxford). 2019;21(10):1411–8.
42. Olthof PB, Tomassini F, Huespe PE, et al. Hepatobiliary scintigraphy to evaluate liver function in associating liver partition and portal vein ligation for staged hepatectomy: liver volume overestimates liver function. Surgery. 2017;162(4):775–83.
43. van Dam RM, Lodewick TM, van den Broek MA, et al. Outcomes of extended versus limited indications for patients undergoing a liver resection for colorectal cancer liver metastases. HPB (Oxford). 2014;16(6):550–9.
44. Deng G, Li H, Jia GQ, Fang D, Tang YY, Xie J, et al. Parenchymal-sparing versus extended hepatectomy for colorectal liver metastases: a systematic review and meta-analysis. Cancer Med. 2019;8(14):6165–75.
45. Kokudo N, et al. Genetic and histological assessment of surgical margins in resected liver metastases from colorectal carcinoma: minimum surgical margins for successful resection. Arch Surg. 2002;137(7):833–40.
46. Vigano L, Di Tommaso L, Mimmo A, Sollai M, Cimino M, Donadon M, Roncalli M, Torzilli G. Prospective evaluation of intrahepatic microscopic occult tumor foci in patients with numerous colorectal liver metastases. Dig Surg. 2019;36(4):340–7.
47. Moris D, Ronnekleiv-Kelly S, Rahnemai-Azar AA, Felekouras E, Dillhoff M, Schmidt C, Pawlik TM. Parenchymal-sparing versus anatomic liver resection for colorectal liver metastases: a systematic review. J Gastrointest Surg. 2017 Jun;21(6):1076–85.
48. Even Storli P, Johnsen G, Juel IS, Gronbech JE, Bringeland EA. Impact of increased resection rates and a liver parenchyma sparing strategy on long-term survival after surgery for colorectal liver metastases. A population-based study. Scand J Gastroenterol. 2019;54(7):890–8.
49. Donadon M, Cescon M, Cucchetti A, et al. Parenchymal-sparing surgery for the surgical treatment of multiple colorectal liver metastases is a safer approach than major hepatectomy not impairing Patients' prognosis: a bi-institutional propensity score-matched analysis. Dig Surg. 2018;35(4):342–9.
50. Melandro F, Giovanardi F, Hassan R, et al. Minimally invasive approach in the setting of ALPPS procedure: a systematic review of the literature. J Gastrointest Surg. 2019;23(9):1917–24.
51. Torzilli G, McCormack L, Pawlik T. Parenchyma-sparing liver resections. Int J Surg. 2020;S1743-9191(20):30346.
52. Bismuth H, Adam R, Lévi F, et al. Resection of nonresectable liver metastases from colorectal cancer after neoadjuvant chemotherapy. Ann Surg. 1996;224(4):509–20.

Open and Laparoscopic Liver Hanging Maneuver

Jacques Belghiti and Safi Dokmak

Abstract

In this chapter, we describe the liver hanging maneuver (LHM) as a promising approach to facilitate and guide anatomical liver resection. A blind dissection in the avascular space situated in the central area of the vena cava between the right hepatic vein (RHV) and the middle hepatic vein (MHV) allows the passage of a tape whose traction suspend the liver. This suspension guides the transection plane following anatomical liver resection; allows a better control of the surgical field which become more superficial; decreases blood loss through traction/compression on the vessels especially when associated with pedicle clamping; and facilitates the oncologic "anterior approach". This maneuver is considered as one of the main technical innovations in liver surgery in the past two decades and is commonly adopted as a very useful tool to assist major resection in open surgery and, as practiced by some surgeons, in laparoscopic approach as well.

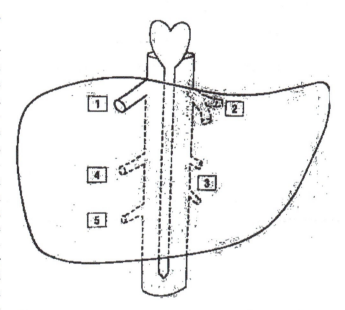

Fig. 32.1 Schema of the avascular plane by Couinaud. *Surgical Anatomy of the Liver, Revisited*. Paris, France: 1989

32.1 Introduction

In 1953, the French anatomist surgeon Claude Couinaud, studying the vascular and bile duct distribution in more than hundred liver casts, demonstrated that the liver parenchyma can be divided into eight autonomous segments [1]. When scrutinizing the position of drainage of hepatic veins, he discovered a "loose cellular space" between the liver and the inferior vena cava describing an avascular space in the central area of the vena cava (Fig. 32.1). We used this space to pass a long dissector along the anterior aspect of the retrohepatic IVC toward the space between the right hepatic vein (RHV) and the middle hepatic vein (MHV), and described this technique as the liver hanging maneuver (LHM) in 2001 [2]. Before any attempts to mobilize the liver, a clamp or a nasogastric tube is introduced in this space permitting the introduction of a tape whose traction suspend the liver. This maneuver which is considered as one of the main technical innovations in liver surgery in the past two decades, facilitate liver transection [3]. Nowadays, LHM is commonly utilized for major liver resection not only in open surgery but also in laparoscopic procedures.

J. Belghiti (✉)
APHP Paris, Paris, France
e-mail: jacques.belghiti@aphp.fr

S. Dokmak
Department of HPB Surgery and Liver Transplantation, Beaujon Hospital, Clichy, France

France University Paris VII, Paris, France

© The Author(s), under exclusive license to Springer Nature Singapore Pte Ltd. 2022
M. Makuuchi et al. (eds.), *The IASGO Textbook of Multi-Disciplinary Management of Hepato-Pancreato-Biliary Diseases*,
https://doi.org/10.1007/978-981-19-0063-1_32

32.2 Advantages of LHM

Advantages of the LHM which were clearly demonstrated in open surgery included (a) better assistance to guide transection plane following anatomical liver resection; (b) improved control of the surgical field which become more superficial; (c) decreased blood loss through traction/compression on the vessels especially when associated with pedicle clamping and (d) facilitation of the oncologic "anterior approach". The oncologic advantage of anterior approach with LHM for patients operated for HCC and CRLM was recently confirmed [4, 5]. Technical advantages of the LHM could impact the surgical procedure allowing smaller incisions (such as midline) when there is no need for right sided liver mobilization [6]. On the opposite side, in the presence of a right-side large liver lesions with adhesions to the diaphragm this maneuver simplified an anterior approach [7]. Some specific situations such as donor liver harvesting and associating liver partition and portal vein ligation for staged hepatectomy (ALPPS) procedures which required parenchymal transection before transection of vascular and biliary structures are facilitated by the LHM [8, 9].

32.3 Anatomical Basis of the LHM

The presence of a longitudinal avascular plane between the IVC described by C. Couinaud was confirmed by several anatomic studies since the first description of our LHM [10, 11]. Some general characteristics of the anatomy of the retro hepatic IVC remain constant including: (a) a constant large caudate vein which is situated in the left of its the middle portion; (b) a frequent right inferior hepatic vein (RIHV) in the right side of the cranial part of the IVC; (c) caudate short hepatic veins are variable in number, position and dimension but most of them are sub millimetric (Fig. 32.2).

32.4 Techniques of LHM

In both open and laparoscopic procedures, the blind dissection can be started either from down to up or from up to down. These two approaches required a short length of dissection of both supra and infra hepatic parts of the IVC.

In open surgery, the "Down to up" LHM was first described (Fig. 32.3). The supra-hepatic IVC is exposed and the space between the right hepatic vein (RHV) and the middle hepatic vein (MHV) is dissected along the IVC axis for approximately 2–3 cm length. The dissection of infra-hepatic IVC is started after a retraction to the left of the hepatic pedicle and the plan between the peritoneal membrane between the anterior aspect of the infra-hepatic IVC and the caudate

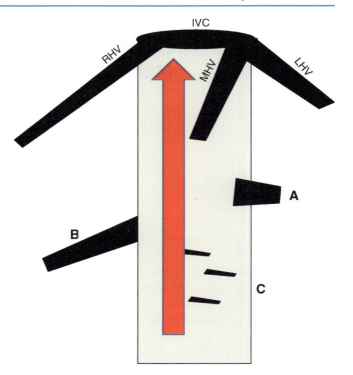

Fig. 32.2 General anatomic characteristics of the avascular plane of retro hepatic IVC. A: constant large caudate vein; B: constant RIHV; C: variables caudate short hepatic veins

capsule is dissected toward the left side of the RIHV. If present some small hepatic veins are ligated and divided. The blind dissection from down to up require a long, lightly curved aortic clamp which is passed cranially along the anterior surface of the IVC between the 10 and 11 o'clock positions towards the space between the previously dissected RHV and MHV. When the dissection is complete, the hepatic parenchyma is looped up with a tape.

The "Up to Down "approach gradually replaced the previous one. The dissection of the space between the right and middle hepatic veins is pushed down for 3–4 cm with a right-angled vascular clamp. A recent anatomical publication of the Glisson capsule emphasized the presence of two capsules delimiting an avascular plan between the liver parenchyma capsule and the capsule covering the vessels (Fig. 32.4). A 16 Fr nasogastric tube is gently introduced and pushed caudally to complete the dissection of the avascular space (Fig. 32.5). The rigidity of the nasogastric tube allows it to be used as a dissector through the avascular space allowing an atraumatic movement. After a dissection between the peritoneal membrane of the anterior aspect of the infra-hepatic IVC and the caudate capsule, the nasogastric tube is collected in front of IVC and can be immediately used as a tape. Very often, the tube spontaneously emerges behind the inferior RHV.

In laparoscopic approach, the steps are broadly the same as in the open approach [12–16]. However, after the creation

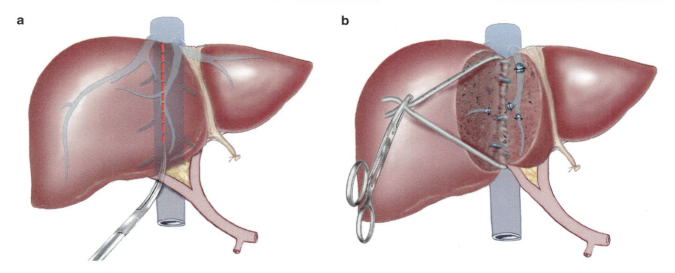

Fig. 32.3 Down to up LHM: (**a**) the blind dissection on the anterolateral surface of the IVC; (**b**) the tape allows traction facilitating liver resection

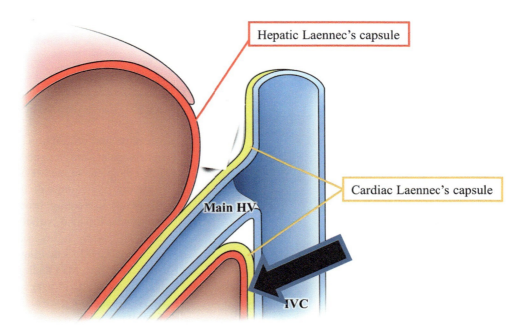

Fig. 32.4 Gilson capsula: the dissection plane of the LHM (arrow) is between the vascular and the parenchymal capsula

of the pneumoperitoneum, a 10 mm trocar is inserted into the epigastric area and the falciform ligament is dissected along the abdominal wall keeping enough tissue for traction [13]. This will enable dissection along the anterior aspect of the supra-hepatic IVC and identification of the MHV and RHV. The plane between the right and middle hepatic veins is blindly dissected with a surgical dissector introduced through the epigastric trocar. Dissection should be vertical, aiming towards the anterior aspect of the IVC, rather than tangentially in order to avoid injury to the right hepatic vein. In larger patients with a big liver, we use a long open surgery vascular clamp introduced through a 10 mm skin incision. The infra-hepatic dissection is similar to that of the open approach. The nasogastric tube is introduced between the MHV and the RHV to finalize the retro-hepatic blind dissection and is replaced by a surgical malleable tape allowing easy manipulation [15]. The "Up-to-down" LHM seems also to be easier and safer for the laparoscopic approach [15]. Although laparoscopy allows better direct visualization of the area to be dissected, some laparoscopic surgeons are reluctant to perform a blind dissection between the anterior surface of the IVC and the liver and they stimulated the "lateral LHM variant" [17]. According to this technique, the upper end of the hanging tape was placed on the lateral side of the right or left hepatic vein and the lower end of the hanging tape between three Glisson's pedicles. The pathway

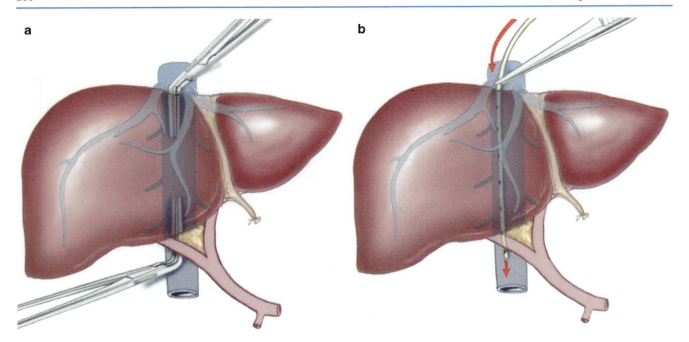

Fig. 32.5 Up to down LHM. (**a**) Dissection is initiated on both sides of the liver. (**b**) A nasogastric tube is introduced in the cranio-caudal direction

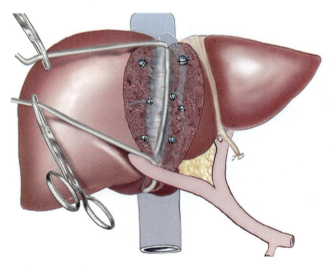

Fig. 32.6 LHM allowing parenchymal transection before transection of both vascular and biliary structures

of the tape was situated along the lateral side of the inferior vena cava in right-sided hepatectomy or the ligamentum venosum in left-sided hepatectomy [17]. When a vascular or biliary reconstruction is required, the use of LHM in laparoscopic liver resection appears to be helpful as illustrated by living donor procedure. LHM allowing parenchymal transection before transection of both vascular and biliary structures (Fig. 32.6).

32.5 Variations of LHM

Since the first description of the LHM aiming to facilitate a right hepatectomy extended to the right part of segment I along the plane of the MHV, this maneuver has been utilized in several indications including a living donor liver transplantation harvesting procedure, native liver resection in transplantation, and partial resection of polycystic liver disease [10]. Many authors have applied the principles of this maneuver LHM to facilitate various anatomical liver resections. The concept of anatomical LHM is defined by the passage of the surgical tape between two hepatic veins with a surgical plane along the plane of a hepatic vein [6]. Depending upon the type of resection required, the technique involves extrahepatic dissection and isolation of the left, right anterior or right posterior Glisson's pedicles. The possibility to use two hanging tapes open several possibilities of central hepatectomies [18]. A concise summary of the various types of anatomic liver resection are shown in Figs. 32.7, 32.8, 32.9, 32.10, 32.11, 32.12, 32.13, 32.14, and 32.15.

32.6 Limits and Contraindications

The only definite contraindication of the blind dissection of the LHM is tumoral invasion of the anterior face of the IVC and particularly the cava-hepatic junction. The presence of

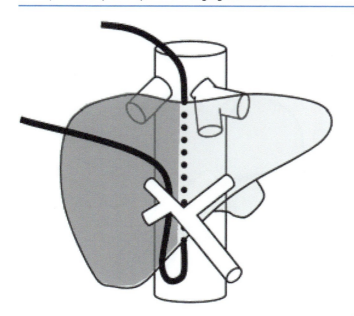

Fig. 32.7 Right Hepatectomy or Left Hepatectomy + S I. Upper end of the tape: Between RHV & MHV, Lower end of the tape: Between Right & Left portal pedicle

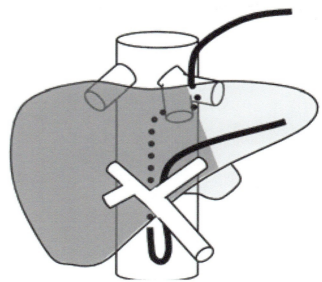

Fig. 32.9 Right trisectionectomy. Tape upper end: Between MHV & LHV, Tape lower end: Between Right & Left portal pedicle

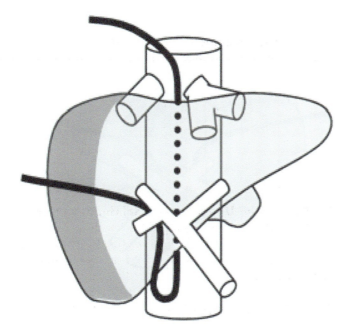

Fig. 32.8 Right posterior sectionectomy or Left trisectionectomy+ S I. Upper end of the tape: Between RHV & MHV, Lower end of the tape: Between Right anterior & Right posterior portal pedicle

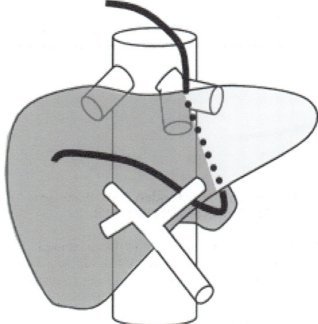

Fig. 32.10 Right trisectioectomy + SI or Left lateral sectionectomy. Tape upper end: Between MHV & LHV, Tape lower end: Between Right & Left portal pedicle

adhesions between the IVC and liver resulting from redo surgery or severe inflammation induced by chemoembolization or portal vein embolization can increase the difficulties [10]. Bleeding which may occur during the bind dissection is usually minimal and related to subcapsular liver dissection. A temporal packing of the dissection area represents an effi-

cient treatment [3]. Severe bleeding from major veins injuries is rare and require an interruption of the maneuver shifting to a classical approach of liver resection [3]. The suppression of the venous outflow induced by the traction on the tape can disturb identification of hepatic veins. Therefore,

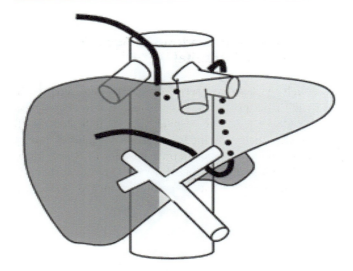

Fig. 32.11 Right hepatectomy + SI or Left hepatectomy. Tape upper end: Between MHV & LHV, Tape lower end: Between Right & Left portal pedicle

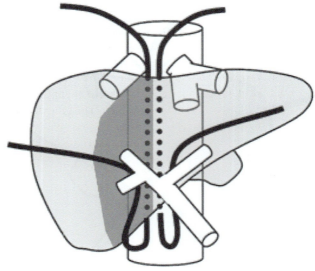

Fig. 32.13 Right anterior sectionectomy. Tape 1 Upper end: Between RHV & MHV—Tape 2 upper end: Between RHV & MHV, Tape 1 lower end: Between right anterior & right posterior portal pedicle—Tape 2 lower end: between Right & Left portal pedicle

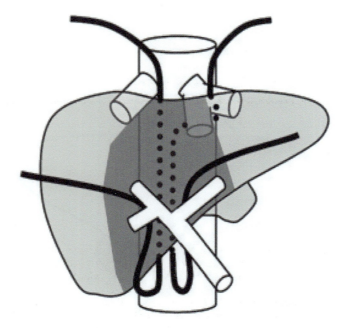

Fig. 32.12 Central bisectionectomy. Tape 1 Upper end: Between RHV & MHV—Tape 2upper end: Between MHV & LHV, Tape 1 Lower end 1: Between Right anterior & Right posterior portal pedicle—Tape 2 Between Right & Left portal pedicle

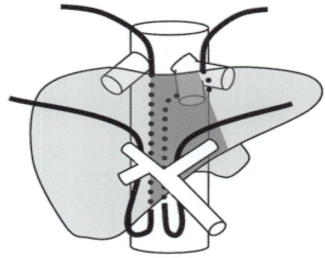

Fig. 32.14 Left medial sectionectomy. Tape 1 upper end: Between RHV & MHV—Tape 2 upper end: Between MHV & LHV, Tape 1 lower end: Between Right & Left portal pedicle—tape 2 lowed end Between Right & Left portal pedicle

this traction should be released from time to time allowing identification of venous tears. In patients with intrahepatic venous collateral circulation, bleeding of the transection parenchyma is exacerbated when the liver remains in anatomic position and therefore, a vertical mobilization of the liver is required in order to reduce the outflow. The presence of this venous collateral circulation is clearly a limitation of LHM with the anterior approach.

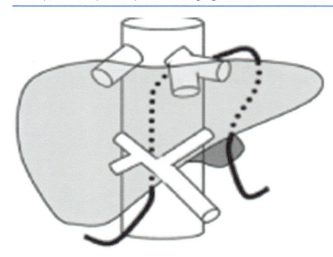

Fig. 32.15 Caudate lobectomy. Upper end: Tape passed between RHV & MHV and then behind MHV and LHV. Lower end: Tape passed behind the Gilson pedicle

References

1. Sutherland F, Harris J. Claude Couinaud: a passion for the liver. Arch Surg. 2002;137:1305–10.
2. Belghiti J, Guevara OA, Noun R, et al. Liver hanging maneuver: a safe approach to right hepatectomy without liver mobilization. J Am Coll Surg. 2001;193(1):109–11.
3. Ogata S, Belghiti J, Varma D, et al. Two hundred liver hanging maneuvers for major hepatectomy: a single-center experience. Ann Surg. 2007;245(1):31–5.
4. Beppu T, Imai K, Okuda K, et al. Anterior approach for right hepatectomy with hanging maneuver for hepatocellular carcinoma: a multi-institutional propensity score-matching study. J Hepatobiliary Pancreat Sci. 2017;24(3):127–36.
5. Llado L, Muñoz A, Ramos E, et al. The anterior hanging-approach improves postoperative course after right hepatectomy in patients with colorectal liver metastases. Results of a prospective study with propensity-score matching comparison. Eur J Surg Oncol. 2016;42(2):176–83.
6. Kim SH, Kim YK. Living donor right hepatectomy using the hanging maneuver by Glisson's approach under the upper midline incision. World J Surg. 2012;36(2):401–6.
7. Liu CL, Fan ST, Cheung ST, et al. Anterior approach versus conventional approach right hepatic resection for large hepatocellular carcinoma: a prospective randomized controlled study. Ann Surg. 2006;244(2):194–203.
8. Shindoh J, Aoki T, Hasegawa K, et al. Donor hepatectomy using hanging maneuvers: Tokyo University experiences in 300 donors. Hepato-Gastroenterology. 2012;59(118):1939–43.
9. Vennarecci G, Levi Sandri GB, Ettorre GM. Performing the ALPPS procedure by anterior approach and liver hanging maneuver. Ann Surg. 2016;263(1):e11. https://doi.org/10.1097/SLA.0000000000001007.
10. Liddo G, Buc E, Nagarajan G, et al. The liver hanging manoeuvre. HPB (Oxford). 2009;11(4):296–305.
11. Kim SH, Park SJ, Lee SA, et al. Various liver resections using hanging maneuver by three Glisson's pedicles and three hepatic veins. Ann Surg. 2007;245(2):201–5.
12. Troisi RI, Montalti R. Modified hanging maneuver using the Goldfinger dissector in laparoscopic right and left hepatectomy. Dig Surg. 2012;29(6):463–7.
13. Dokmak S, Aussilhou B, Rebai W, Cauchy F, Belghiti J, Soubrane O. Up-to-down open and laparoscopic liver hanging maneuver: an overview. Langenbeck's Arch Surg. 2020; https://doi.org/10.1007/s00423-020-01945-5. Epub ahead of print
14. Nitta H, Sasaki A, Fujita T, et al. Laparoscopy-assisted major liver resections employing a hanging technique: the original procedure. Ann Surg. 2010;251(3):450–3.
15. Rhaiem R, Piardi T, Kellil T, et al. The liver hanging maneuver in laparoscopic liver resection: a systematic review. Surg Today. 2018;48(1):18–24.
16. Kim JH, Kim H. Modified liver hanging maneuver in laparoscopic major hepatectomy: the learning curve and evolution of indications. Surg Endosc. 2020;34(6):2742–8.
17. Kim JH. Three-dimensional ventral approach with the modified liver-hanging maneuver during laparoscopic right hemihepatectomy. Ann Surg Oncol. 2019;26(7):2253.
18. Nanashima A, Tobinaga S, Araki M, et al. Double liver hanging manoeuvre for central hepatectomy. HPB (Oxford). 2009;11(6):529–31.

The Glissonean Pedicle Approach: The Takasaki Technique

Shun-ichi Ariizumi and Masakazu Yamamoto

Abstract

Couinaud described three main approaches to control the inflow system at the hepatic hilus in liver surgery: the intrafascial, the extrafascial, and the transfissural with extrafascial approach. The intrafascial approach is the so-called control method. The extrafascial approach and the transfissural with extrafascial approach are considered to be the Glissonean pedicle approach. The Glissonean pedicle approach by extrafascial approach is considered to be the Takasaki technique. The key steps of the Takasaki technique are the following: (1) clamping the Glissonean pedicle, (2) confirming the portal territory which includes the tumor, (3) dissecting the liver parenchyma. When the Glissonean pedicles are ligated at the hepatic hilus prior to liver dissection, various types of anatomical hepatectomy, such as right or left hemihepatectomy and various types of sectionectomy can be carried out. When the tertiary branches of the Glissonean pedicles are ligated extra- or intrahepatically, various types of segmentectomy and cone unit resection can be carried out. This procedure is suitable for patients with hepatocellular carcinoma (HCC), because patients with HCC usually have liver dysfunction and HCC often invades the portal vein. The procedure is also available in laparoscopic hepatectomy, because of its simplicity and safety. The Glissonean pedicle approach is, therefore, considered to be one of the most important procedures in liver surgery which can be achieved safely and has oncological benefit.

33.1 Introduction

Couinaud described three main approaches to the inflow system at the hepatic hilus; the intrafascial, the extrafascial, and the transfissural with extrafascial approach (Fig. 33.1) [1]. The extrafascial approach and the transfissural with extrafascial approach are considered to be the Glissonean pedicle approach. Takasaki et al. successfully performed anatomical anterior sectionectomy with the Glissonean pedicle approach at the hepatic hilus in a patient with hepatocellular carcinoma (HCC) in 1984 and reported the newly developed systematized hepatectomy by Glissonean pedicle transection method in 35 patients with HCC in 1986 (Japanese article) [2]. Therefore, anatomical hepatectomy at the Glissonean pedicle approach is considered to be the Takasaki technique [3–6]. The key steps of the Takasaki technique are the following: (1) clamping the Glissonean pedicle, (2) confirming the portal territory, (3) dissecting the liver parenchyma. Currently, the Glissonean pedicle approach is performed worldwide and is preferred in laparoscopic hepatectomy because of its simplicity and safety.

33.2 Fundamental Concept of Liver Segmentation Based on the Glissonean Pedicle (Takasaki's Liver Anatomy)

The Glissonean pedicle consisting of the portal vein, hepatic artery and bile duct is wrapped in a connective tissue sheath known as Glisson's capsule (Fig. 33.1a). The extrahepatic or Glissonean pedicle branches to form right and left primary Glissonean pedicles (Fig. 33.1a) [3–6]. The left primary Glissonean pedicle continues to form a single secondary pedicle, whilst the right primary Glissonean pedicle branches into two secondary pedicles, namely the middle (right anterior) and right (right posterior) pedicles (Fig. 33.1a). The

S.-i. Ariizumi · M. Yamamoto (✉)
Department of Surgery, Institute of Gastroenterology, Tokyo Women's Medical University, Tokyo, Japan
e-mail: yamamoto.masakazu@twmu.ac.jp

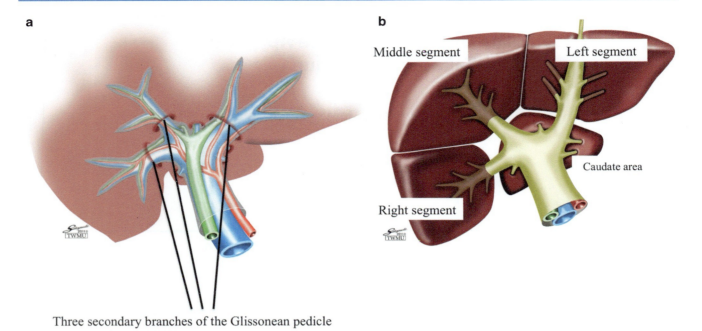

Fig. 33.1 Components of the Glissonean pedicle and Takasaki's liver segmentation. The three secondary Glissonean pedicles divide the liver into 3 segments

three secondary Glissonean pedicles divide the liver into three segments (left, middle and right) according to the ramification of the secondary pedicles (Fig. 33.1b) [3–6].

33.3 Glissonean Pedicle Approach at the Hepatic Hilus (Extrafascial Approach)

The Glissonean pedicles can be detached from the liver parenchyma without liver dissection. The extrafascial approach is to tape the Glissonean pedicles at the hepatic hilus prior to liver dissection. After cholecystectomy, the connective tissue behind Calot's triangle is identified. This connective tissue is referred to as the cystic plate. After dividing the cystic plate, the middle (right anterior) Glissonean pedicle behind the cystic plate can be readily identified (Fig. 33.2a). First, this middle (right anterior) Glissonean pedicle is detached from the liver parenchyma (Fig. 33.2b). The Glissonean pedicle can be detached easily from the liver parenchyma by blunt dissection. After clamping this pedicle, the middle segment (right anterior section) can be recognized by its change of color (Fig. 33.2c). After confirming the demarcation lines between the middle segment (anterior section) and the other segments (sections), the liver parenchyma is dissected along the demarcation lines (Fig. 33.2d). This fundamental technique is useful not only for middle segmentectomy (anterior sectionectomy) but also for right segmentectomy (posterior sectionectomy) or right hemihepatectomy.

For right hepatectomy or right segmentectomy (right posterior sectionectomy), the right (right posterior) Glissonean pedicle can be detached directly from the liver parenchyma. However, the following subtraction method is recommended for taping of the right (right posterior) Glissonean pedicle. At first, the middle (right anterior) Glissonean pedicle is taped (Fig 33.3a). Next, the right primary Glissonean pedicle is taped (Fig 33.3b). The right (right posterior) Glissonean pedicle can then be taped after securing the middle (right anterior) Glissonean pedicle (Fig 33.3c). This technique is useful for right segmentectomy (posterior sectionectomy) and right hemihepatectomy. The left Glissonean pedicle (secondary Glissonean pedicle) can be accessed at the left side of the hilar plate, and the left pedicle can easily be taped prior to liver dissection (Fig 33.3d). Therefore, all three secondary Glissonean pedicles can be taped at the hepatic hilus (Fig 33.3d).

33.4 Ligation of the Glissonean Pedicle

Ligation of the pedicles should be done as close to the liver parenchyma as possible to avoid injury to the remaining bile duct. The pedicle should be doubly ligated with transfixion suture to avoid slipping out (Fig 33.3c). After ligation, the pedicle is divided.

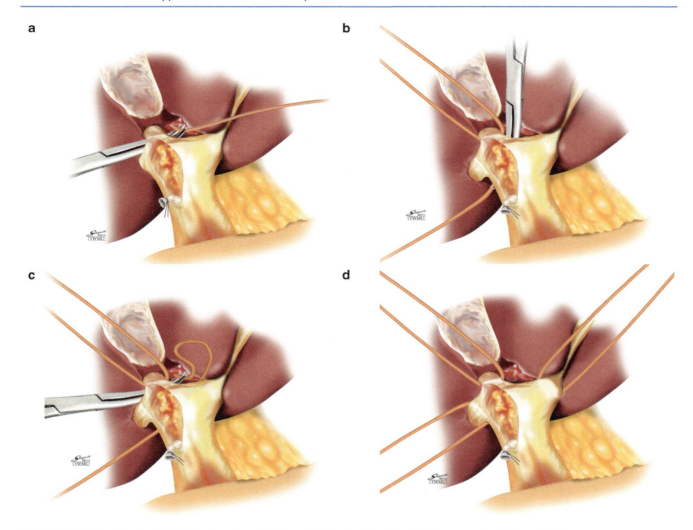

Fig. 33.2 Middle segmentectomy (right anterior sectionectomy) with the Glissonean pedicle approach at the hepatic hilus

33.5 Dissection of the Liver Parenchyma

Dissection should be performed on the demarcated margin line with the crush-clamp method, ultrasonic dissector (CUSA), and energy device. Some branches from the hepatic vein are ligated and cut, but the trunk of the hepatic vein should be maintained intact on the cut surface of the remaining segments. (Fig. 33.4).

33.6 Segmentectomy, Cone Unit Resection

When the tertiary branches of the Glissonean pedicles are ligated extra- or intrahepatically, various types of segmentectomy and cone unit resection can be carried out. A single secondary Glissonean pedicle has six to eight tertiary branches. The territory of a single tertiary branch does not correspond to a Couinaud's segment. We therefore refer to the area fed by one tertiary branch as a cone unit of the liver. For cone unit resection in the middle segment (S5 section), the middle (right anterior) Glissonean pedicle is taped and hepatic dissection is performed along the Rex-Cantlie line. Two tertiary branches from the middle (right anterior) Glissonean pedicle are ligated and divided. For cone unit resection in the middle segment (S8 section), the middle (right anterior) Glissonean pedicle is taped and a test clamp is performed. After confirming the Rex-Cantlie line, liver dissection is performed, and tertiary branches from the middle (right anterior) Glissonean pedicle are taped intrahepatically. The area of S8 can then be identified by demarcation. The tertiary branches are ligated and divided. The middle hepatic vein is identified in the cut surface of the remnant liver.

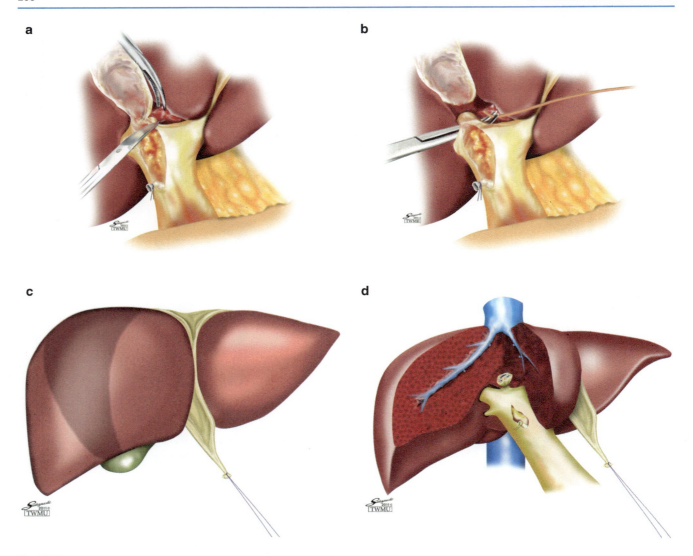

Fig. 33.3 Basic technique to tape the Glissonean pedicle at the hepatic hilus

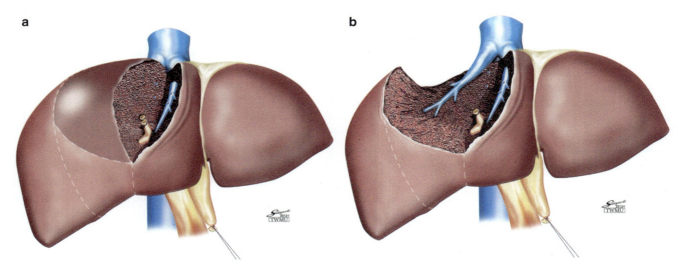

Fig. 33.4 Cone unit resection (segmentectomy No 8) with the Glissonean pedicle approach

33.7 Surgical Outcomes

During a 30-year period, 1953 patients with HCC underwent anatomical hepatectomy with the Glissonean pedicle approach at our institute [7]. The 30-day and 90-day mortality rates decreased gradually in the recent eras (between 2010 and 2014) down to 0.5% and 1.4%, respectively, and the 5-year survival rate increased gradually up to 75% in the recent eras (between 2010 and 2014) [7]. Reducing blood loss and bile leakage are re-recognized as the most important factors in anatomical hepatectomy for patients with HCC.

In conclusion, the Glissonean pedicle approach is suitable for patients with HCC, because patients with HCC usually have liver dysfunction and HCC often invades the portal vein. The procedure is also available in laparoscopic hepatectomy, because of its simplicity and safety. The Glissonean pedicle approach is, therefore, considered to be one of the most important procedures in liver surgery which can be achieved safely and has oncological benefit.

Acknowledgments The authors are indebted to Associate Professor Raoul Breugelmans of the Department of English of Tokyo Medical University for his review of this manuscript.

References

1. Couinaud C. Surgical anatomy of the liver revisited. Paris: Selfprinted; 1989.
2. Takasaki K, Kobayashi S, Tanaka S, et al. New developed systematized hepatectomy by Glissonean pedicle transection method. Syujutsu. 1986;40:7–14. (in Japanese)
3. Takasaki K, Kobayashi S, Tanaka S, Saito A, Yamamoto M, Hanyu F. Highly anatomically systematized hepatic resection with Glissonean sheath cord transection at the hepatic hilus. Int Surg. 1990;75:73–7.
4. Takasaki K. Glissonean pedicle transection method for hepatic resection: a new concept of liver segmentation. J Hepato-Biliary-Pancreat Surg. 1998;5:286–91.
5. Takasaki K. Glissonean pedicle transection method for hepatic resection. Tokyo: Springer; 2007.
6. Yamamoto M, Ariizumi S. Glissonean pedicle approach in liver surgery. Ann Gastroenterol Surg. 2018;13:124–8.
7. Ariizumi S, Katagiri S, Kotera Y, et al. Improved mortality, morbidity and long-term outcome after anatomical hepatectomy with the Glissonean pedicle approach in patients with hepatocellular carcinoma: 30 years' experience at a single institute. Ann Surg. 2020; (in press)

Laparoscopic Major Hepatectomy and Parenchymal-Sparing Anatomical Hepatectomy

34

Kohei Mishima, Go Wakabayashi, Kazuharu Igarashi, and Takahiro Ozaki

Abstract

Although laparoscopic liver resection (LLR) has become recognized as the standard treatment worldwide, laparoscopic major hepatectomy (LMH) has yet to become widespread. LMH was first defined as resection of 3 or more segments or the difficult posterosuperior segments (4a, 7, 8) in 2008. Although the definition is still under debate and is not clearly defined, several studies reported that LMH was associated with less blood loss, shorter hospital stays and fewer complications compared with open surgery. According to a nationwide survey of Japanese National Clinical Database, advanced LLR increased from 3.3% of all resections in 2011 to 10.8% in 2017, with its mortality 3.6% in 2011, and 1.0% in 2017. The IWATE criteria can be used to predict the difficulty of LLR from preoperative variables and to appropriately select patients according to the surgeons' skill level. The learning curve for LMH has been discussed, but conclusive number of cases for the mastery of LMH cannot be decided with variety of studies. Since laparoscopic parenchymal-sparing anatomical liver hepatectomy (Lap-PSAH = segmentectomies and sub-segmentectomies) shares some surgical techniques with LMH, it may help shorten the learning curve of LMH. In conclusion, LMH still remains technically demanding, but it has been gradually developed with the improvement of surgical techniques and the careful expansion of indications.

34.1 Introduction

Although laparoscopic liver resection (LLR) has become recognized as the standard treatment worldwide, laparoscopic major hepatectomy (LMH) has yet to become widespread [1]. This can be attributed to the complexity of the procedures and fear of uncontrolled hemorrhage, combined with high-level technical demands and lack of training opportunities for most surgeons [2]. In this chapter, we reviewed the current status of LMH, referring to the history of LLR and the current surgical techniques that has been standardized in high volume centers.

34.2 Developments of LLR

LLR was first reported in 1991 as laparoscopic excision of benign liver lesions [3]. Since then, LLR has gradually developed with the improvements of surgical techniques and equipment. In 2008, the first international consensus conferences on LLR (ICCLLR) was held in Louisville, USA. Standardized terminologies on LLR were defined and variable technical approaches were introduced by 45 experts [4]. In 2014, the second ICCLLR was held in Morioka, Japan. The summary of expert recommendations covered a novel difficulty scoring system [5, 6], techniques for bleeding control and parenchymal transection, and suitability of energy devices [7]. The conference concluded that LLR had become a standard practice, but LMH was still an innovative procedure in its exploratory phase [1]. After these two ICCLLRs, LLR spread globally with rapidity and the proportion of major LLRs has gradually increased. According to a nationwide survey of the national clinical database of Japan [8], the number of LLRs increased from 1868 (9.9% of all liver resections) in 2011 to 5648 (24.8%) in 2017. The rates of morbidity and 30-day mortality of LLR were 10.8% and 0.5%, respectively, which were better than those of open liver resection (OLR) (19.9% and 0.9%, respectively) in 2017.

K. Mishima · G. Wakabayashi (✉) · K. Igarashi · T. Ozaki
Center for Advanced Treatment of HBP Diseases, Ageo Central General Hospital, Saitama, Japan
e-mail: gowaka@ach.or.jp

34.3 Definitions of LMH

Liver resection has been categorized according to the Brisbane 2000 classification as follows: hemi-hepatectomies, sectionectomies, and segmentectomies [9]. LMH was first defined as resection of 3 or more segments or the difficult posterosuperior segments (4a, 7, 8) in the 1st ICCLLR [4]. Behind this definition is the fact that resections of posterosuperior segments by laparoscopic approach shares some technically difficulties with hemi-hepatectomies [10]. On the other hand, a standard definition of major hepatectomy is resection of four or more segments based on the theory that the extent of resection is most involved in postoperative mortality [11]. Di Fabio et al. divided a total of 156 patients who had undergone LMH according to the Louisville Statement into two subcategories: laparoscopic "traditional" major hepatectomy (LTMH), including hemi-hepatectomies and tri-sectionectomies, and laparoscopic "posterosuperior" major hepatectomy (LPMH), including resection of posterosuperior segments 4a, 7, and 8 [10]. The creation of two subcategories of LMH seemed appropriate to reflect differences in intraoperative and postoperative outcomes between LTMH and LPMH [10]. With improvements in surgical techniques and the innovation of laparoscopic devices over the last decade, the classification of LMH has reached the time of reconsideration based on the technical difficulty and the risk of postoperative mortality [12].

34.4 Difficulty Scoring System (IWATE Criteria) and Learning Curve of LMH

In an effort to estimate the difficulty of LLR appropriately before surgery, a novel difficulty scoring system [5] was created for discussion at the 2nd ICCLLR. After the discussion at the conference, the scoring system was modified and the updated version of the difficulty scoring system (IWATE criteria) has a scale ranging from 0 to 12 [6]. The IWATE criteria can be used to predict the difficulty from preoperative variables and to appropriately select patients according to the surgeons' skill level, ranked as low, intermediate, advanced, or expert. LMH requires a high level of technical skill and has a steep learning curve. A CUSUM analysis of learning curve concluded that 45 standard LMHs are required to overcome the initial learning curve, and expertise in more complex or technically demanding LMHs can be achieved over the next 30 cases [13]. LMH remains challenging as the effective performance of the procedure requires experience; however, it has low mortality rate relative to open major hepatectomy (OMH) (Fig. 34.1).

34.5 Feasibility and Safety of LMH

Since the 2nd ICCLLR Morioka 2014 [1], several studies have described the feasibility of LMH [14–16]. In 2016, Takahara et al. compared LMH and OMH using a propensity score analysis with the national clinical database of Japan, reporting that LMH was associated with less blood loss, shorter hospital stays, and fewer complications [14]. Similar results were obtained from meta-analyses of cases where major LLR was performed for HCC patients [15, 16]. In Japan, the mortality rate of advanced LLRs (tri-sectionenctomy, hemi-hepatectomy, and sectionectomy) improved from 3.6% in 2011 to 1.0% in 2017 [8]. However, it should be noted that these short-term outcomes were from some specialized high volume centers in Japan. Although gradually increasing, the proportion of advanced LLRs is still low (10.8% in 2017) and the dissemination of LMH has yet to be achieved.

34.6 Laparoscopic Parenchymal Sparing Anatomical Hepatectomy (Lap-PSAH)

Anatomical hepatectomy (AH) involves systemic removal of the liver parenchyma confined by tumor-bearing portal tributaries [17, 18], and it has been shown to improve the oncological outcomes in HCC patients [19, 20]. Recently, remnant liver ischemia was noted to be associated with early recurrence and poor survival after hepatectomy in HCC patients [21]. In 2019, we reported a novel technique of laparoscopic parenchymal-sparing AH (Lap-PSAH) (sub-segmentectomies and segmentectomies) [22] with extrahepatic Glissonian approach. The liver segmentation of Lap-PSAH is based on Takasaki's cone unit concept [23]. Our principle of Lap-PSAH is to resect all of the malignant tissue (tumor and possible satellite nodules) while preserving enough liver parenchyma. The extent of

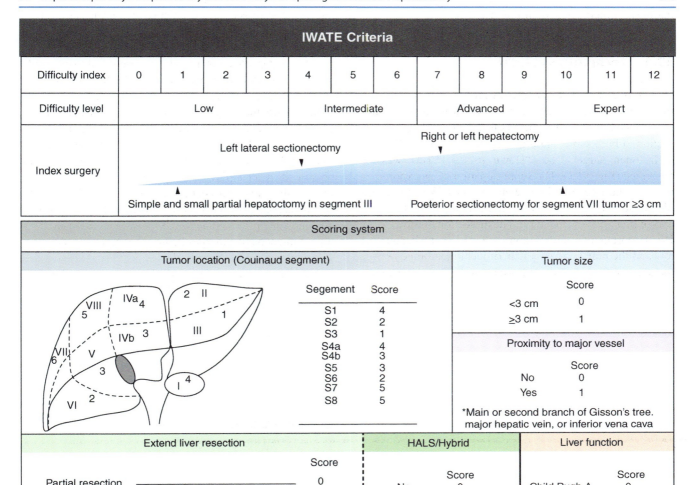

Fig. 34.1 IWATE Criteria [6]

resection is planned prior to surgery by means of CT liver volume calculation. Concordance between preoperative three-dimensional (3D) simulation and intraoperative resection was 98.7% and favorable short-term outcomes were achieved [22]. Precise preoperative planning and a standardized surgical technique enable performing this procedure (Fig. 34.2). Since Lap-PSAH shares some surgical techniques with LMH, it may help shorten the learning curve of LMH. Long-term outcomes should be evaluated in the future.

34.7 Surgical Procedures at Ageo Central General Hospital (ACGH)

Although the first case series of LMHs were reported in 1998 [24], the procedure has been very slow to progress worldwide [12]. At our hospital, LLR is indicated for all liver malignancies except for cases of vascular or biliary reconstruction. Our standard procedure for LLR is extrahepatic Glissonian approach [23] with ICG negative staining. Glissonian pedicles can be safely isolated based on

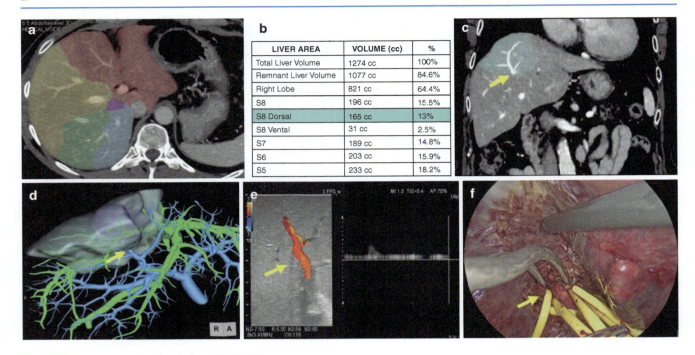

Fig. 34.2 Preoperative planning for Lap-PSAH [22]

Laennec's capsule theory [25]. Clear boundary can be visualized not only liver surface but also in the deep liver parenchyma (=intersegmental plane) during parenchymal transection.

34.7.1 Laparoscopic Left Hemihepatectomy (Fig. 34.3)

1. Mobilization of the left lobe and encircling left hepatic vein (LHV)
2. Encircling and clamping of the Glissonian pedicle (G234)
3. Parenchymal transection along with intersegmental plane after ICG administration
4. Dissection of the G234 and LHV with linear stapler

34.7.2 Lap-PSAH (Segment 7) (Fig. 34.4)

1. Mobilization of the right lobe and dissection of short hepatic veins
2. Cholecystectomy and Encircling and clamping of the Glissonian pedicle (G7)
3. Parenchymal transection after ICG administration
4. Dissection of the G7 and parenchymal transection along with RHV or on the intersegmental plane

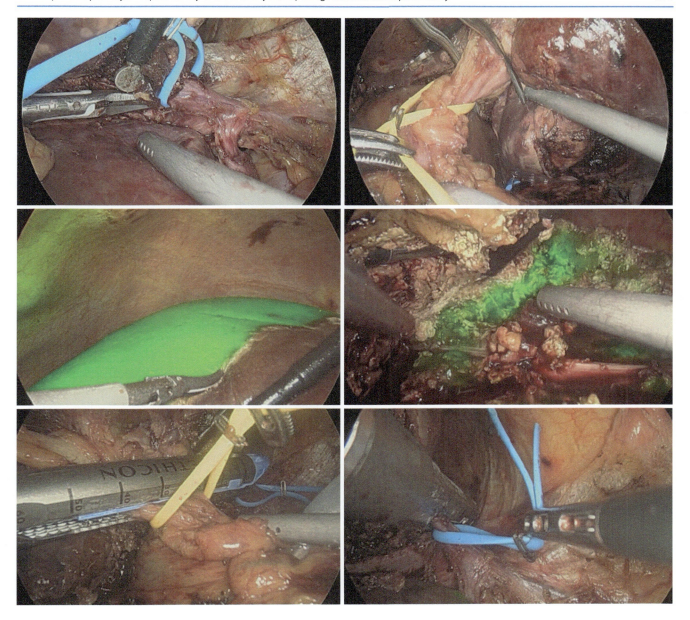

Fig. 34.3 Surgical Procedures of Laparoscopic Left Hemihepatectomy

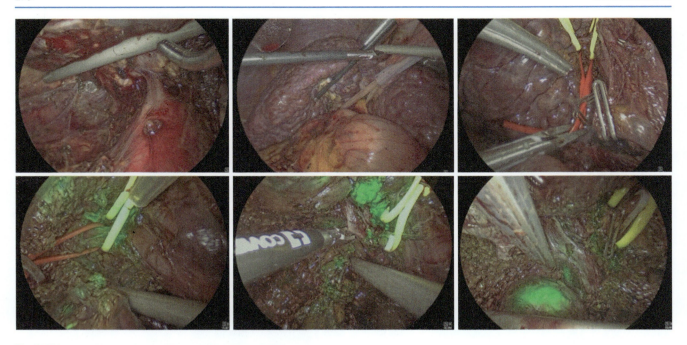

Fig. 34.4 Surgical Procedures of Anatomical Segment 7 Resection

34.8 Conclusion

LMH still remains technically demanding, but it has been gradually developed with the improvement of surgical techniques and the careful expansion of indications. Lap-PSAH shares some surgical techniques with LMH and may help shorten the learning curve of LMH. Long-term outcomes should be evaluated in the future.

Conflicts of Interest The authors have no conflicts of interest to declare.

Ethical Statement The authors are accountable for all aspects of the work in ensuring that questions related to the accuracy or integrity of any part of the work are appropriately investigated and resolved.

References

1. Wakabayashi G, Cherqui D, Geller DA, Buell JF, Kaneko H, Han HS, et al. Recommendations for laparoscopic liver resection: a report from the second international consensus conference held in Morioka. Ann Surg. 2015;261(4):619–29.
2. Dagher I, O'Rourke N, Geller DA, Cherqui D, Belli G, Gamblin TC, et al. Laparoscopic major hepatectomy: an evolution in standard of care. Ann Surg. 2009;250(5):856–60.
3. Reich H, McGlynn F, DeCaprio J, Budin R. Laparoscopic excision of benign liver lesions. Obstet Gynecol. 1991;78(5 Pt 2):956–8.
4. Buell JF, Cherqui D, Geller DA, O'Rourke N, Iannitti D, Dagher I, et al. The international position on laparoscopic liver surgery: the Louisville statement, 2008. Ann Surg. 2009;250(5):825–30.
5. Ban D, Tanabe M, Ito H, Otsuka Y, Nitta H, Abe Y, et al. A novel difficulty scoring system for laparoscopic liver resection. J Hepatobiliary Pancreat Sci. 2014;21(10):745–53.
6. Wakabayashi G. What has changed after the Morioka consensus conference 2014 on laparoscopic liver resection? Hepatobiliary Surg Nutr. 2016;5(4):281–9.
7. Wakabayashi G, Cherqui D, Geller DA, Han HS, Kaneko H, Buell JF. Laparoscopic hepatectomy is theoretically better than open hepatectomy: preparing for the 2nd international consensus conference on laparoscopic liver resection. J Hepatobiliary Pancreat Sci. 2014;21(10):723–31.
8. Ban D, Tanabe M, Kumamaru H, Nitta H, Otsuka Y, Miyata H, et al. Safe dissemination of laparoscopic liver resection in 27, 146 cases between 2011 and 2017 from the National Clinical Database of Japan. Ann Surg. 2020;274(6):1043–50.
9. Strasberg SM. Nomenclature of hepatic anatomy and resections: a review of the Brisbane 2000 system. J Hepato-Biliary-Pancreat Surg. 2005;12(5):351–5.
10. Di Fabio F, Samim M, Di Gioia P, Godeseth R, Pearce NW, Abu HM. Laparoscopic major hepatectomies: clinical outcomes and classification. World J Surg. 2014;38(12):3169–74.
11. Reddy SK, Barbas AS, Turley RS, Steel JL, Tsung A, Marsh JW, et al. A standard definition of major hepatectomy: resection of four or more liver segments. HPB (Oxford). 2011;13(7):494–502.
12. Cheek SM, Sucandy I, Tsung A, Marsh JW, Geller DA. Evidence supporting laparoscopic major hepatectomy. J Hepatobiliary Pancreat Sci. 2016;23(5):257–9.
13. Brown KM, Geller DA. What is the learning curve for laparoscopic major hepatectomy? J Gastrointest Surg. 2016;20(5):1065–71.
14. Takahara T, Wakabayashi G, Konno H, Gotoh M, Yamaue H, Yanaga K, et al. Comparison of laparoscopic major hepatectomy with propensity score matched open cases from the National Clinical Database in Japan. J Hepatobiliary Pancreat Sci. 2016;23(11):721–34.
15. Chen K, Pan Y, Hu GY, Maher H, Zheng XY, Yan JF. Laparoscopic versus open major hepatectomy for hepatocellular carci-

noma: a meta-analysis. Surg Laparosc Endosc Percutan Tech. 2018;28(5):267–74.
16. Wang ZY, Chen QL, Sun LL, He SP, Luo XF, Huang LS, et al. Laparoscopic versus open major liver resection for hepatocellular carcinoma: systematic review and meta-analysis of comparative cohort studies. BMC Cancer. 2019;19(1):1047.
17. Makuuchi M, Hasegawa H, Yamazaki S. Ultrasonically guided subsegmentectomy. Surg Gynecol Obstet. 1985;161(4):346–50.
18. Takasaki K, Kobayashi S, Tanaka S, Saito A, Yamamoto M, Hanyu F. Highly anatomically systematized hepatic resection with Glissonean sheath code transection at the hepatic hilus. Int Surg. 1990;75(2):73–7.
19. Hasegawa K, Kokudo N, Imamura H, Matsuyama Y, Aoki T, Minagawa M, et al. Prognostic impact of anatomic resection for hepatocellular carcinoma. Ann Surg. 2005;242(2):252–9.
20. Zhao H, Chen C, Gu S, Yan X, Jia W, Mao L, et al. Anatomical versus non-anatomical resection for solitary hepatocellular carcinoma without macroscopic vascular invasion: a propensity score matching analysis. J Gastroenterol Hepatol. 2017;32(4):870–8.
21. Cho JY, Han HS, Choi Y, Yoon YS, Kim S, Choi JK, et al. Association of remnant liver ischemia with early recurrence and poor survival after liver resection in patients with hepatocellular carcinoma. JAMA Surg. 2017;152(4):386–92.
22. Berardi G, Igarashi K, Li CJ, Ozaki T, Mishima K, Nakajima K, et al. Parenchymal sparing anatomical liver resections with full laparoscopic approach: description of technique and short-term results. Ann Surg. 2019;273(4):785–91.
23. Takasaki K. Glissonean pedicle transection method for hepatic resection: a new concept of liver segmentation. J Hepato-Biliary-Pancreat Surg. 1998;5(3):286–91.
24. Hüscher CG, Lirici MM, Chiodini S. Laparoscopic liver resections. Semin Laparosc Surg. 1998;5(3):204–10.
25. Sugioka A, Kato Y, Tanahashi Y. Systematic extrahepatic Glissonean pedicle isolation for anatomical liver resection based on Laennec's capsule: proposal of a novel comprehensive surgical anatomy of the liver. J Hepatobiliary Pancreat Sci. 2017;24(1):17–23.

Laparoscopic Anatomical Resection of the Liver: Segmentectomy and Sub-segmentectomy

Boram Lee and Ho-Seong Han

Abstract

Laparoscopic liver resection (LLR) is rapidly increasing, and certain types of resection are considered standard procedures for liver resection. However, laparoscopic anatomical resection (AR) is still challenging procedure, because it requires precise parenchymal liver resection along the anatomic landmark. Operation difficulty varies depending on the location of the resection area. The aim of in this chapter is to provide important technical features of laparoscopic AR for each segment (I-VIII) using Glissonean pedicle approach.

Anatomical liver resection (AR) involves resection of the tumor and entire hepatic parenchymal tissue corresponding to the portal veins draining the tumor [1]. Although the outcomes of AR are still debated, several reports suggested that it is the best way to prevent intrahepatic metastasis occurring via portal tributaries [2, 3]. There are two main types of AR techniques, the Glissonean pedicle approach and transection guided by dye injection into the portal venous branches [4]. The Glissonean pedicle approach is based on the three ramifications of the Glissonean pedicle, namely the left, middle, and right, as initially proposed by Takasaki [5]. According to Takasaki's classification, each segment has one secondary branch of the Glissonean pedicle. Therefore, for resection any one of the segments, the first step is to cut the corresponding segmental branch of the Glissonean pedicle and then dissect the liver parenchyma along the intersegmental plane [5, 6]. Makuuchi et al. [7] propose the anatomical resection with ultrasound-guided dye injection. In this method, the tumor-bearing portal pedicle is punctured and dye is injected under ultrasound guidance [7]. The stained area must be carefully marked with eletrocautery, and transection should gradually proceed from the liver surface towards the portal pedicle stained by dye [1, 7].

Since first report in 1992, laparoscopic liver resection (LLR) is rapidly increasing, and certain types of LLR have become standard procedures. However, laparoscopic AR is still considered challenging procedure, because it usually requires precise parenchymal liver resection using Glissonean approach [8]. Laparoscopic Glissonean pedicle approach is technically difficult because manipulation of laparoscopic instruments for isolation of the pedicles is not easy due to limitation on degree of freedom. Laparoscopic isolation of the Glissonean pedicle before parenchymal liver resection was first reported by HS Han et al. in 2006 [9]. In that study, the authors acknowledged the importance of the Glissonean pedicle approach in laparoscopic AR. Since then, studies of various types of laparoscopic AR through the Glissonean pedicle approach have been reported (Fig. 35.1) [10].

According to practical guidelines for performing LLR, the difficulty is divided by location of the resection area [8]. The peripheral portion of the anterolateral segments of the liver (Segment 2,3,5,6, and the inferior part of segment 4) is considered as safe location for performing LLR [8, 11–13]. Whereas, the posterosuperior portion of the liver (Segment 1, 7, 8, and the superior part of segment 4) is regarded as an unfavorable location for performing LLR [14]. Our aim in this chapter is to describe the operation techniques of Laparoscopic AR for each segment (I-VIII), which is anatomic segementectomy.

35.1 Patient Position and Trocar Placement

The patient's position and trocar placement can vary depending on the location of the tumor. The patient is placed in a supine position or left semi-decubitus position with the surgeon standing on either right or left side, or the patient can be

B. Lee · H.-S. Han (✉)
Department of Surgery, Seoul National University College of Medicine, Seoul National University Bundang Hospital, Seoul, South Korea
e-mail: hanhs@snubh.org

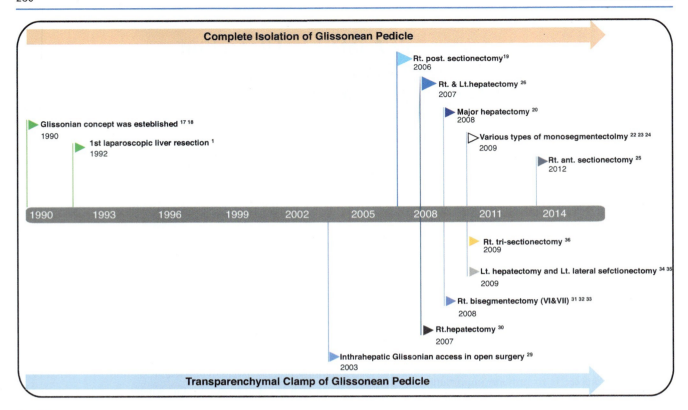

Fig. 35.1 Development of the Glissonean pedicle approach in laparoscopy (HS Han, YR Choi et al. [10])

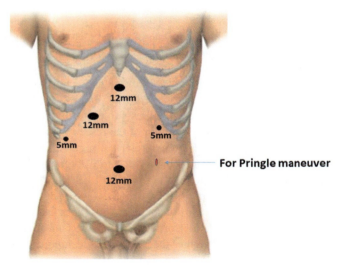

Fig. 35.2 Routine Trocar placement

placed in a lithotomy position with the surgeon standing between the legs of the patient.

The placement of trocar in LLR is important. Usually, five or six trocars are used. Two trocars for operator are placed along the right subcostal line, and two other trocars for assistant are placed at the end of xyphoid process and at the left upper quadrant of the abdomen. Figure 35.2 shows the illustration of routine trocar placement.

35.2 Laparoscopic Segmentectomy I (S1)

Laparoscopic anatomic caudate lobectomy is considered as difficult procedure due to its close proximity to major vessels [15]. Caudate lobe is located in the deep dorsal area of the liver between the portal triad and the inferior vena cava (IVC) [16]. According to Kumon's nomenclature, the caudate lobe consists of three sections; the Spiegel lobe, the paracaval portion (Segment IX), and the caudate process [17]. Trocar placement is shown in Fig. 35.3.

After mobilization of the liver, the left liver is retracted upward and the lesser omentum is opened to expose the S1. Counter-demarcation method is used for S1 segmentectomy in our institution. The right posterior Glissonian pedicle is isolated and temporarily clamped with a bulldog clamp [18]. The counter-demarcated line between caudate process and the right posterior section is marked with electrocautery. The posterior surface of the caudate lobe is freed from the IVC and the short hepatic veins are clipped and cut. During parenchymal dissection, peripheral part of the right hepatic vein (RHV) can be identified and is well exposed meticulously. Dissection of the paracaval portion is continued along the RHV. Resected caudate process and the paracaval portion are retracted to the left side, the middle hepatic vein is identified, and parenchymal transection is performed exposing the vein. With further parenchymal

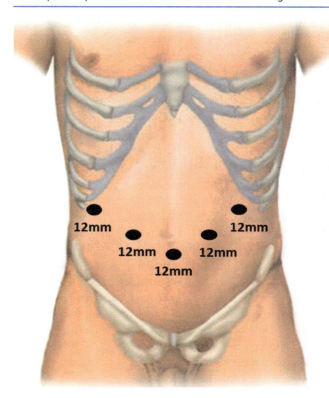

Fig. 35.3 Trocar placement for laparoscopic S1 segmentectomy

dissection and division of the portal branches to the Spigelian lobe, the completely caudate lobe is resected.

35.3 Laparoscopic Segmentectomy II (S2) and Segmentectomy III (S3)

When the tumor is located in S2 or S3, laparoscopic anatomic S2 or S3 segmentectomy can be performed [19]. Segment-oriented hepatic resection on S2 or S3 has the advantage of removing the disease-bearing liver segment, and at the same time, preserving the vascular supply and biliary drainage of the liver remnant [20]. This concept is important in patients with underlying liver disease to prevent postoperative liver failure [21]. With use of the Glissonean approach to control the pedicle, anatomical resection can be achieved.

For laparoscopic S2 segmentectomy, after mobilization of left lateral section, the Glissonean pedicle to S2 is isolated via meticulous dissection. Then, the Glissonean pedicle to S2 is temporarily clamped. The ischemic margin of S2 is marked using electrocautery. Transection of the liver parenchyma is performed thereafter. The liver parenchyma is dissected along the left hepatic vein with the guide of exposing left hepatic vein. The portal pedicle to S2 is divided, and the branches of hepatic veins draining S2 are encountered and clipped along the left hepatic vein.

In laparoscopic S3 segmentectomy, the Glissonean pedicle to S3 is exposed and divided on the left side of the round ligament in the umbilical fossa. Then, the parenchymal dissection is begun along the demarcation line, exposing the left hepatic vein [22]. Parenchymal dissection is performed along the left hepatic vein with the same technique as S2 segmentectomy.

35.4 Laparoscopic Segmentectomy IV (S4) (Subsegmentectomy IVa and IVb)

Left hemihepatectomy is generally performed for tumors located in S4. However, the anatomical S4 segmentectomy has the advantage that the remaining volume of the liver can be preserved as much as possible. This operation is a technically demanding operative procedure because it has two transection planes along two fissures, which are the course of the main hepatic veins [23]. Therefore, it is important to maintain a proper transection line to preserve the vascular structures that supply the remnant liver. S4 can be subdivided into the superior S4a and inferior S4b regions. Anatomical S4a or S4b resection may also be advantages for a tumor that is confined to S4a or S4b [24].

The falciform ligament and coronary ligament are dissected in the cephalic direction until the middle and left hepatic veins are visualized. The medial resection margin is marked along the right side of the falciform ligament, after which transection of the on the medial side is begun. The superficial hepatic parenchyma is transected, and the deeper portion of the parenchyma is dissected, until the inferior vena cava and confluence of left and middle hepatic vein are reached. Intrahepatic approach is used to control the Glissonean pedicle to S4. When performing the subdivisional Glissonean peidcle to S4a or S4b, we have to dissect to more peripherally to enable identification and isolation of each S4a and S4b pedicle. To confirm the correct identification, we have to check for an ischemic color change in the corresponding area after temporarily clamping the S4a or S4b pedicle.

For S4a segmentectomy, the S4a Glissonean pedicle is isolated and ligated. After division of S4a pedicle, the liver parenchyma is dissected along the areas of demarcation on the liver surface, exposing the middle hepatic vein (MHV) toward its confluence with the inferior vena cava (IVC).

For S4b segmentectomy, the S4b Glissonean pedicle is isolated and cut. The liver parenchyma is dissected along the boundary of the demarcated region. Segmentetctomy 4 can be performed by combing the techniques for S4a and S4b. After cutting the S4 Glissonian pedicle, an area of S4 is discolored due to ischemia. For completion of S4 resection, parenchymal transection on right side is performed along ischemic line along the middle hepatic vein.

35.5 Laparoscopic Segmentectomy V (S5)

When the tumor is located in S5, there are several options. One is anatomical major resection such as, right hemihepatectomy, right anterior sectionectomy, and central segmentectomy [25]. Another option is nonanatomical resection such as wedge resection and tumorectomy. The remaining option is anatomical S5 resection.

After cholecystectomy, the Glissonean pedicle to the right anterior section is isolated by meticulous dissection. With a temporary clamp of the right anterior Glissonean pedicle, the ischemic margin of the right anterior section is marked. Transection of the liver parenchyma at the medial margin is started. As the right anterior Glissonean pedicle is further dissected peripherally, the Glissonean pedicle to S5 can be isolated and then, discolored S5 area is marked after temporary clamping of S5 Glissonean pedicle. Selective isolation of the Glissonean pedicle to S5 is crucial in anatomical S5 segmentectomy, as there are no anatomical landmarks for S5 segmentectomy. After the S5 Glissonean pedicle is divided, parenchymal transection at the lateral and superior side of the S5 is performed.

35.6 Laparoscopic Segmentectomy VI (S6)

The small tumor located peripherally in S6 is one of the easily approachable method for LLR like tumorectomy. However, anatomical resection of S6 is complex even in open surgery, thus a laparoscopic resection of S6 is also a challenging procedure [26].

Before the parenchymal dissection, the right liver is mobilized from the diaphragm and right adrenal gland as in the open approach. After cholecystectomy, the Glissonean pedicle to the right posterior section is dissected and isolated. Further hepatic parenchymal dissection is performed until the branches of the Glissonean pedicles of S6 and segment 7 (S7) is identified. Temporary clamping of the Glissonean pedicle of S6 is performed for confirmation the demarcation of S6 based on ischemic line. The S6 Glissonean pedicle is then divided with clips or stapler. After marking of ischemic line of S6, parenchymal transection is performed.

35.7 Laparoscopic Segmentectomy VII (S7)

Laparoscopic liver resection for tumors located in S7 is a challenging procedure [27]. There are several methods for anatomoical S7 resection. First, laparoscopic anatomical S7 segmentectomy via the intrahepatic Gissonean approach [28]. After full mobilization of right liver, the major Glissonean pedicle of the right posterior section is dissected and isolated. Further hepatic parenchymal dissection is performed until the branches of the Glissonean pedicles of S6 and S7 are reached. The S7 Glissonean pedicle is temporarily clamped to confirm demarcation. Dissection is performed until the right hepatic vein (RHV) is exposed. Further dissection is then continued along the RHV. Second, laparoscopic S7 segmentectomy through RHV first approach [29]. After fully mobilization of right liver, rotate the whole liver completely to the left side to approach to the root of RHV. Before the parenchymal dissection, the RHV is encircled by vessel loop to prepare for massive bleeding. Parenchymal transection starts from the confluence of hepatic vein and then, followed along RHV with ligating small branches RHV. Dissection is performed until the Glissonean pedicles of S7 is exposed. Then, the S7 Glissonean pedicle is temporarily clamped to confirm demarcation.

When performing the laparoscopic anatomical S7 segmentectomy, the operative field is difficult to obtain with the use of conventional trocar site. And laparoscope and the instrument need to be advanced backward and forward over a longer distance [30, 31]. Therefore, additional ports inserted through the intercostal space (ICS) will be beneficial in overcoming these difficulties [32]. Additional intercostal ports are placed at the 7th and 9th ICS (Fig. 35.4). When using intercostal trocars, we should be careful to avoid intercostal vessel bleeding. Intercostal trocars can be helpful to easily access the operative field and manipulate the instruments (Fig. 35.5).

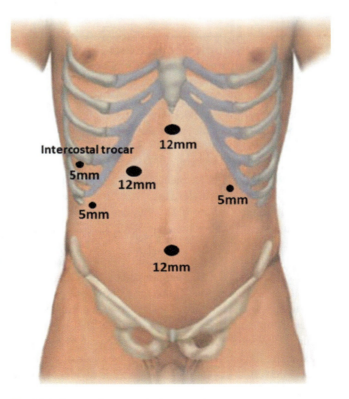

Fig. 35.4 Trocar placement for intercostal space

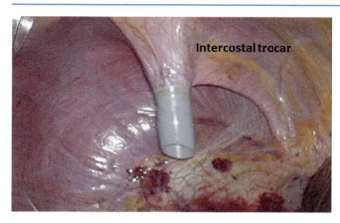

Fig. 35.5 Operative view of laparoscopic segmentectomy VII (S7) using intercostal trocar

35.8 Laparoscopic Segmentectomy VIII (S8)

Laparoscopic anatomical S8 resection is still rarely performed due to its unfavorable location for laparoscopic approach and technical difficulties [32].

After fully mobilization of right liver, the roots of right and middle hepatic vein are identified. After isolation of the right main Glissonean pedicle, the pedicle isolation is continued until the right anterior Glisssonean pedicle is exposed. Then, Glissonean pedicle is further dissected to expose the Glissonean pedicles of S8, and the pedicle is temporarily clamped. After the area of the segment 8 is identified with ischemic discoloration, resection of hepatic parenchyma is started [33]. Once part of MHV (MHV) is exposed, parenchymal resection is proceeded along the plane of the MHV until its root is exposed. Posterior side of the S8 is detached from the IVC with the retraction of S8 to left side. To save the parenchyma as much as possible, the dissection plane is performed along the right hepatic vein. Parenchymal transection is performed until confluence of the right hepatic vein to IVC is reached.

References

1. Makuuchi M. Surgical treatment for HCC--special reference to anatomical resection. Int J Surg. 2013;11(Suppl 1):S47–9.
2. Zhou Y, Xu D, Wu L, Li B. Meta-analysis of anatomic resection versus nonanatomic resection for hepatocellular carcinoma. Langenbeck's Arch Surg. 2011;396:1109–17.
3. Chen J, Hhang K, Wu J, Zhu H, Shi Y, Wang Y, et al. Survival after anatomic resection versus nonanatomic resection for hepatocellular carcinoma: a meta-analysis. Dig Dis Sci. 2011;56:1626–33.
4. Kang KJ, Ahn KS. Anatomical resection of hepatocellular carcinoma: a critical review of the procedure and its benefits on survival. World J Gastroenterol. 2017;23(7):1139–46.
5. Takasaki K. Glissonean pedicle transection method for hepatic resection: a new concept of liver segmentation. J Hepato-Biliary-Pancreat Surg. 1998;5(3):286–91.
6. Yamamoto M, Katagiri S, Ariizumi S, Kotera Y, Takahashi Y. Glissonean pedicle transection method for liver surgery (with video). J Hepatobiliary Pancreat Sci. 2012;19(1):3–8.
7. Makuuchi M, Hasegawa H, Yamazaki S. Ultrasonically guided subsegmentectomy. Surg Gynecol Obstet. 1985;161:346–50.
8. Cho JY, Han HS, Wakabayashi G, Soubrane O, Geller D, O'Rourke N, et al. Practical guidelines for performing laparoscopic liver resection based on the second international laparoscopic liver consensus conference. Surg Oncol. 2018;27:A5–9.
9. Yoon YS, Han HS, Choi YS, et al. Total laparoscopic right posterior sectionectomy for hepatocellular carcinoma. J Laparoendosc Adv Surg Tech A. 2006;16(3):274–7.
10. Choi Y, Han HS, Sultan AM, Yoon YS, Cho JY. Glissonean pedicle approach in laparoscopic anatomical liver resection. Hepato-Gastroenterology. 2014;61(136):2317–20.
11. Kaneko H, Takagi S, Shiba T. Laparoscopic partial hepatectomy and left lateral segmentectomy: technique and results of a clinical series. Surgery. 1996;120:468–75.
12. Cho JY, Han HS, Yoon YS, Shin SH. Experiences of laparoscopic liver resection including lesions in the posterosuperior segments of the liver. Surg Endosc. 2008;22:2344–9.
13. Mosteanu BI, Han HS, Cho JY, Lee B. When should we choose a laparoscopic approach? A high-volume center recommendation score. Surg Oncol. 2020;34:208–11.
14. Guro H, Cho JY, Han HS, Yoon YS, Choi Y, Periyasamy M. Current status of laparoscopic liver resection for hepatocellular carcinoma. Clin Mol Hepatol. 2016;22:212–8.
15. Parikh M, Han HS, Cho JY, et al. Laparoscopic isolated caudate lobe resection. Sci Rep. 2021;11:4328.
16. Oh D, Kwon CH, Na BG, et al. Surgical techniques for totally laparoscopic caudate lobectomy. J Laparoendosc Adv Surg Tech A. 2016;26(9):689–92.
17. Kumon M. Anatomy of the caudate lobe with special reference to portal vein and bile duct. Acta Hepatol Jap. 1985;26:1193–9.
18. Ho KM, Han HS, Yoon YS, et al. Laparoscopic total caudate lobectomy for hepatocellular carcinoma. J Laparoendosc Adv Surg Tech A. 2017;27(10):1074–8.
19. Wakabayashi G, Cherqui D, Geller DA, Buell JF, Kaneko H, O'Rourke N, et al. Recommendations for laparoscopic liver resection: a report from the second international consensus conference held in Morioka. Ann Surg. 2015;261:619–29.
20. Ho KM, Han HS, Yoon YS, et al. Laparoscopic anatomical segment 2 segmentectomy by the Glissonian approach. J Laparoendosc Adv Surg Tech A. 2017;27(8):818–22.
21. Liau KH, Blumgart LH, DeNatteo RP. Segment oriented approach to liver resection. Surg Clin North Am. 2004;84:543–61.
22. Kim SH, Han HS, Sham JG, Yoon YS, Cho JY. Laparoscopic anatomical S3 segmentectomy by the Glissonian approach. Surg Oncol. 2019;28:222.
23. Ishizawa T, Gumbs AA, Kokudo N, Gayet B. Laparoscopic segmentectomy of the liver: from segment I to VIII. Ann Surg. 2012;256:959–64.
24. Kim YK, Han HS, Yoon YS, Cho JY, Lee W. Total anatomical laparoscopic liver resection of segment 4 (S4), extended S4, and subsegments S4a and S4b for hepatocellular carcinoma. J Laparoendosc Adv Surg Tech A. 2015;25(5):375–9.
25. Ahn KS, Han HS, Yoon YS, Cho JY, Kim JH. Laparoscopic anatomical S5 segmentectomy by the Glissonian approach. J Laparoendosc Adv Surg Tech A. 2011;21(4):345–8.
26. Choi H, Han HS, Yoon YS, Cho JY, Choi Y, Jang JY. Laparoscopic anatomic segment 6 liver resection using the Glissonian approach. Surg Laparosc Endosc Percutan Tech. 2017;27(3):e22–5.

27. Ishizawa T, Kokudo N, Makuuchi M. Right hepatectomy for hepatocellular carcinoma: is the anterior approach superior to the conventional approach? Ann Surg. 2008;247:390–1.
28. Kim S, Han HS, Sham JG, Yoon YS, Cho JY. Laparoscopic anatomical S7 segmentectomy by the intrahepatic Glissonian approach. Surg Oncol. 2019;28:158.
29. Lee B, Cho JY, Choi Y, Yoon YS, Han HS. Laparoscopic liver resection in segment 7: hepatic vein first approach with special reference to sufficient resection margin. Surg Oncol. 2019;30:87–9.
30. Cho JY, Han HS, Yoon YS, Shin SH. Experiences of laparoscopic liver resection on including lesions in the posterior segments of the liver. Surg Endosc. 2008;22:2344–9.
31. Reddy SK, Tsung A, Geller DA. Laparoscopic liver resection. World J Surg. 2011;35:1478–86.
32. Lee W, Han HS, Yoon YS, Cho JY, Choi Y, Shin HK. Role of intercostal trocars on laparoscopic liver resection on for tumors in segments 7 and 8. J Hepatobiliary Pancreat Sci. 2014;21(8):E65–8.
33. Jang JY, Han HS, Yoon YS, et al. Three-dimensional laparoscopic anatomical segment 8 liver resection with Glissonian approach. Ann Surg Oncol. 2017;24:1606–9.

Modified ALPPS Procedure

Nobuyuki Takemura, Kyouji Ito, and Norihiro Kokudo

Abstract

In patients with hepatobiliary malignancies located around the hepatic hilum or those with multiple metastatic lesions, a major hepatectomy is the only curative treatment. A major hepatectomy functions to remove tumor cells concomitant with the hemi-liver or liver parenchyma; however, there is a risk of insufficient remnant liver volume, which might cause postoperative morbidity and mortality in these extended hepatectomies. To overcome this problem, Makuuchi et al. first introduced preoperative portal vein embolization (PVE), which increases the volume of the future liver remnant (FLR), allowing extended hepatectomy to be performed safely. However, there is a maximum volume increase in PVE of approximately 40%. The associating liver partition and portal vein ligation for the staged hepatectomy (ALPPS) procedure was first introduced in 2012, and was shown to increase the FLR by up to 80%. Initially, the major problem of the ALPPS procedure was a high morbidity and relatively high mortality compared to these of PVE. To overcome this problem, various modifications of the ALPPS procedure have been proposed, and satisfactory results have been reported. In this section, various modified ALPPS procedures and their results are presented.

36.1 Introduction

A major hepatectomy is the only curative treatment for patients with extensive hepatobiliary malignancies located around the hepatic hilum or with multiple bi-lobular metastatic lesions. A major hepatectomy provides a chance of cure by removing tumor cells concomitant with the hemi-liver or liver parenchyma. However, there is a risk of insufficient remnant liver volume, which may lead to postoperative live failure in these cases with extended hepatectomy. To overcome this problem, Makuuchi et al. first introduced preoperative portal vein embolization (PVE), which increases the volume of the future liver remnant (FLR), allowing extended hepatectomy to be performed safely [1]. However, PVE has a maximum volume increase of approximately 40% [2].

Schnitzbauer et al. introduced combined portal vein ligation and in situ liver partition-induced rapid liver hypertrophy of the liver remnant [3], which was later named associated liver partition and portal vein ligation for staged hepatectomy (ALPPS) [4]. The ALPPS procedure enables a rapid FLR increase of up to 80%; despite this improvement, initial studies reported very high morbidity and mortality [3, 5] in compensation for very rapid hepatic hypertrophy. The majority of the mortality associated with the ALPPS procedures occurred due to bile leakage and septic complications. It is also important to consider the interval to the second operation, with early reports suggesting that the second surgery should be performed within 7 to 9 days after the first operation [3, 5]. In the ALPPS procedure, even with rapid and sufficient liver hypertrophy from the aspect of liver volume only, the presence of immature hepatocytes in the FLR may be one of the reasons for postoperative liver failure after the second operation [6]. Furthermore, Olthof et al. stated that the liver volume overestimates liver function measured by hepatobiliary scintigraphy [7].

Although there are still some problems that need to be overcome, the ALPPS procedure is a novel technique for use in patients with extensive, initially unresectable tumors and very small FLR volumes, especially as a salvage procedure in patients with portal vein embolization/occlusion failure [8]. Various modifications have been proposed to overcome the problems associated with ALPPS procedures. In this section, we introduce the modifications that have led to safer ALPPS procedures and discuss their advantages and disad-

N. Takemura (✉) · K. Ito · N. Kokudo
Department of Surgery, Hepato-Biliary Pancreatic Surgery Division, National Center for Global Health and Medicine, Tokyo, Japan
e-mail: ntakemura@hosp.ncgm.go.jp

vantages with respect to inducing remnant liver hypertrophy in patients with advanced hepatobiliary malignancies with an insufficient FLR.

36.2 Discussion

The ALPPS procedure has been introduced as a new treatment strategy for patients with extensive hepatobiliary malignancies with a small FLR volume [3, 4]. Originally, the ALPPS procedure involved the complete mobilization of the right hemi-liver and total parenchymal transection from the falciform ligament to the inferior vena cava, in addition to the resection of the Glissonian sheath branches of segment 4 and hepatoduodenal ligament dissection for the ligation of the right portal vein (Fig. 36.1). Given the rapid hypertrophy of the FLR, the second stage of the hepatectomy was performed 7 or 9 days after the first hepatectomy [3, 5]. Initial reports on ALPPS procedures demonstrated high morbidity and mortality rates in 12% to 15% of patients, the majority of which were due to biliary and infectious complications and liver failure [3, 5]. Several modifications have been made to reduce these adverse effects, and improved results have been reported.

36.2.1 Parenchymal Transection

Total parenchymal transection from the falciform ligament to the inferior vena cava was performed in the original ALPPS procedure; this had the potential to result in biliary complications of the biliary branches of segment 4, as well as infectious complications of the ischemic area of segment

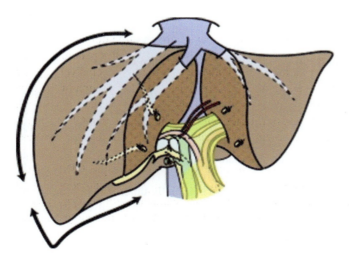

Fig. 36.1 Conventional ALPPS procedure with total parenchymal transection to the inferior vena cava, with resection of the Glissonian branches of segment 4, full mobilization of the right hemiliver, and hepatoduodenal ligament dissection

4. More recent experimental and clinical data has shown that rapid liver hypertrophy is induced by partial transection of at least 50% [9–11]. Furthermore, conducting partial liver transection results in significantly lower morbidity and mortality [9, 10].

36.2.2 Hepatoduodenal Ligament Dissection

Cholecystectomy and the dissection of the hepatoduodenal ligament are essential to correctly approach the right portal vein for ligation; however, this tends to cause dense adhesion around the hepatic hilum and increases the difficulty of the second stage hepatectomy [10]. Another problem with hepatoduodenal ligament dissection is the risk of tumor exposure when the tumor is located close to the hepatic hilum. In order to avoid the skeltonization of the hepatoduodenal ligament, the transhepatic approach or the approach via the mesenteric vein have been proposed for intrahepatic portal vein occlusion [12–15]. If it is difficult to puncture the portal vein because of the presence of multiple bi-lobular tumors, the occlusion approach to the intrahepatic portal vein can be shifted from the transhepatic to the inferior mescenteric or ileocecal portal vein instead.

36.2.3 Interval Between the First and Second Stage Hepatectomy

The main feature of the ALPPS procedure is the rapid hypertrophy of the FLR, which makes it possible to perform a second hepatectomy, even with a short interval. Initial reports advocated that the rapid hypertrophy of the procedure enabled a second hepatectomy within an interval of 7 to 9 days after the first operation [3, 5]. However, there are debates on whether liver hypertrophy truly reflects sufficient functional recovery of the liver. Indeed, microscopic examination and hepatobiliary scintigraphy of the FLR after the ALPPS procedure have highlighted the risk of hepatocyte immaturity and insufficient liver functional recovery [6, 7]; thus, delayed second surgery of the ALPPS procedure is currently recommended [7, 16].

These modifications are shown in Fig. 36.2.

36.2.4 Various Modified Subtypes of the ALPPS Procedure

36.2.4.1 Partial ALPPS

Petrowsky et al. first introduced partial transection (50% to 80% transection of the complete transection plane) in the first stage of the operation. This modification was based on their experimental models and the hypothesis that partial

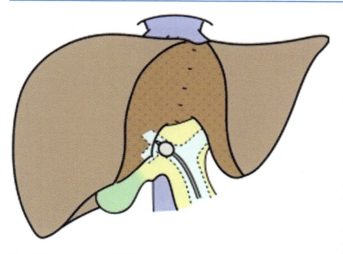

Fig. 36.2 Modified ALPPS procedure with half parenchymal transection without resection of the Glissonian branches of segment 4, without mobilization of the right hemiliver, and without hepatoduodenal ligament dissection. Portal vein occlusion is done transhepatic approach or trans superior/inferior mesenteric vein approach

parenchymal transection triggers a comparable degree of the regeneration of the FLR to complete transection and reduces postoperative complications [9]. This modification, named *Partial ALPPS*, achieved reduced morbidity and mortality and is currently the standard modification of the ALPPS procedure.

36.2.4.2 Hybrid ALPPS

Li et al. suggested an alternative ALPPS method that consisted of three steps: parenchymal splitting, right PVE, and two-stage hepatectomy, named hybrid ALPPS [12]. This method can avoid adhesion around the hepatic hilum, and can be applied even when the tumor is located close to the hepatic hilum. However, this approach is difficult in cases with multiple bi-lobular tumors as it is difficult to ensure an adequate transhepatic puncture line from the body surface.

36.2.4.3 Mini-ALPPS/ALPTIPS

De Santibanes et al. proposed a modification of the ALPPS procedure, known as the "*Mini-ALPPS*" technique, in which partial parenchymal transection combined with intraoperative PVE is performed via the inferior mesenteric vein with minimum liver mobilization [13]. A similar modification was reported by Sakamoto et al., who used the ileocecal vein approach for PVE as an alternative to the inferior mesenteric vein [14, 15]. Both modifications can avoid dense adhesion around the hepatic hilum during the second stage hepatectomy. Furthermore, these procedures can be performed when the tumors are located close to the hepatic hilum without tumor exposure and in cases with multiple bi-lobular tumors where transhepatic puncture of the portal vein may be difficult.

36.2.4.4 Segment 4 Portal Pedicle-spared ALPPS

In five patients, Tanaka et al. reported a modification of the ALPPS procedure that avoids the division of the portal pedicle and prevents parenchymal necrosis due to ischemia. Portal vein ligation was performed using this method; however, the ligation of the Glissonian sheath branches of the additional hepatic area in the future liver removed are preserved [17]. Since the term "*modified ALPPS*" is misleading in this chapter, we have changed it to "*Segment 4 portal pedicle-spared ALPPS*," derived from their procedures. Of course their modification of the preserved portal pedicle were not only segment 4 branch, however, considering the original ALPPS procedure which completely divide portal pedicle of segment 4, this nomenclature seems to be a good reflection of their modification. This modification achieved rapid liver hypertrophies, which were almost identical to those of the original ALPPS procedure without the associated mortality.

36.2.4.5 Tourniquet ALPPS

Robles et al. reported using a tourniquet as an alternative to parenchymal splitting [18]. In this procedure, a tourniquet was placed around the parenchymal transection line using the hanging maneuver, and the right portal vein was ligated and cut. Although this modification is easy to perform during the first stage of the operation, during the second stage, severe adhesion occurs around the hepatic hilum, which requires a longer operation time because parenchymal transection was not performed during the first stage. Furthermore, two mortalities were reported in their initial report, even with the modification.

36.3 Conclusion

The ALPPS procedure provides a potential cure for patients with extensive and initially unresectable hepatobiliary malignancies with a small FLR. Various modifications have been proposed to overcome the high morbidity and mortality associated with the ALPPS procedure; these include reduced hepatic parenchymal transection, no bile duct resection, no dissection of the hepatoduodenal ligament, laparoscopic approach, and avoiding the mobilization of the right hemiliver. However, the safest approach to increase the FLR is PVE, and the indication of the ALPPS procedure should be limited to patients with a very small FLR or failure of PVE. Even with the rapid hepatic hypertrophy associated with the ALPPS procedure, a second hepatectomy should be performed following the maturation of the hepatocytes in the FLR. The modifications mentioned in this section should be selected on a case-by-case basis in order to increase the safety of the ALPPS procedure.

References

1. Makuuchi M, Thai BL, Takayasu K, et al. Preoperative portal embolization to increase safety of major hepatectomy for hilar bile duct carcinoma: a preliminary report. Surgery. 1990;107(5):521–7.
2. Pandanaboyana S, Bell R, Hidalgo E, et al. A systematic review and meta-analysis of portal vein ligation versus portal vein embolization for elective liver resection. Surgery. 2015;157(4):690–8. https://doi.org/10.1016/j.surg.2014.12.009.
3. Schnitzbauer AA, Lang SA, Goessmann H, et al. Right portal vein ligation combined with in situ splitting induces rapid left lateral liver lobe hypertrophy enabling 2-staged extended right hepatic resection in small-for-size settings. Ann Surg. 2012;255(3):405–14. https://doi.org/10.1097/SLA.0b013e31824856f5.
4. de Santibañes E, Clavien PA. Playing Play-Doh to prevent postoperative liver failure: the "ALPPS" approach. Ann Surg. 2012;255(3):415–7. https://doi.org/10.1097/SLA.0b013e318248577d.
5. Schadde E, Ardiles V, Slankamenac K, et al. ALPPS offers a better chance of complete resection in patients with primarily unresectable liver tumors compared with conventional-staged hepatectomies: results of a multicenter analysis. World J Surg. 2014;38(6):1510–9. https://doi.org/10.1007/s00268-014-2513-3.
6. Matsuo K, Murakami T, Kawaguchi D, et al. Histologic features after surgery associating liver partition and portal vein ligation for staged hepatectomy versus those after hepatectomy with portal vein embolization. Surgery. 2016;159(5):1289–98. https://doi.org/10.1016/j.surg.2015.12.004.
7. Olthof PB, Tomassini F, Huespe PE, et al. Hepatobiliary scintigraphy to evaluate liver function in associating liver partition and portal vein ligation for staged hepatectomy: liver volume overestimates liver function. Surgery. 2017;162(4):775–83. https://doi.org/10.1016/j.surg.2017.05.022.
8. Enne M, Schadde E, Björnsson B, et al. ALPPS as a salvage procedure after insufficient future liver remnant hypertrophy following portal vein occlusion. HPB (Oxford). 2017;19(12):1126–9. https://doi.org/10.1016/j.hpb.2017.08.013.
9. Petrowsky H, Györi G, de Oliveira M, et al. Is partial-ALPPS safer than ALPPS? A single-center experience. Ann Surg. 2015;261(4):90–2. https://doi.org/10.1097/SLA.0000000000001087.
10. Alvarez FA, Ardiles V, de Santibañes M, et al. Associating liver partition and portal vein ligation for staged hepatectomy offers high oncological feasibility with adequate patient safety: a prospective study at a single center. Ann Surg. 2015;261(4):723–32. https://doi.org/10.1097/SLA.0000000000001046.
11. Linecker M, Kambakamba P, Reiner CS, et al. How much liver needs to be transected in ALPPS? A translational study investigating the concept of less invasiveness. Surgery. 2017;161(2):453–64. https://doi.org/10.1016/j.surg.2016.08.004.
12. Li J, Kantas A, Ittrich H, et al. Avoid "all-touch" by hybrid ALPPS to achieve oncological efficacy. Ann Surg. 2016;263(1):6–7. https://doi.org/10.1097/SLA.0000000000000845.
13. de Santibañes E, Alvarez FA, Ardiles V, et al. Inverting the ALPPS paradigm by minimizing first stage impact: the mini-ALPPS technique. Langenbeck's Arch Surg. 2016;401(4):557–63. https://doi.org/10.1007/s00423-016-1424-1.
14. Sakamoto Y, Inagaki F, Omichi K, et al. Associating liver partial partition and transileocecal portal vein embolization for staged hepatectomy. Ann Surg. 2016;264(6):21–2. https://doi.org/10.1097/SLA.0000000000001757.
15. Sakamoto Y, Matsumura M, Yamashita S, et al. Partial TIPE ALPPS for perihilar cancer. Ann Surg. 2018;267(2):18–20. https://doi.org/10.1097/SLA.0000000000002484.
16. Lodge JP. ALPPS: the argument for. Eur J Surg Oncol. 2017;43(2):246–8. https://doi.org/10.1016/j.ejso.2016.11.007.
17. Tanaka K, Kikuchi Y, Kawaguchi D, et al. Modified ALPPS procedures avoiding division of portal pedicles. Ann Surg. 2017;265(2):14–20. https://doi.org/10.1097/SLA.0000000000001967.
18. Robles R, Parrilla P, López-Conesa A, et al. Tourniquet modification of the associating liver partition and portal ligation for staged hepatectomy procedure. Br J Surg. 2014;101(9):1129–34. https://doi.org/10.1002/bjs.9547.

37. Artery-First Approach in Pancreaticoduodenectomy

Daisuke Ban and Minoru Tanabe

Abstract

Due to its anatomical characteristics, cancer of the pancreatic head often invades the superior mesenteric vein (SMV), the portal vein (PV), and the plexus surrounding the superior mesenteric artery (SMA). Several different approaches to pancreaticoduodenectomy (PD) have been proposed in order to achieve R0 resection.

37.1 Introduction

Due to its anatomical characteristics, cancer of the pancreatic head often invades the superior mesenteric vein (SMV), the portal vein (PV), and the plexus surrounding the superior mesenteric artery (SMA). Several different approaches to pancreaticoduodenectomy (PD) have been proposed in order to achieve R0 resection.

The mesenteric approach established by Nakao [1] in the 1990s is based on the concept of isolated pancreatectomy, in which the SMA and SMV are first dissected without kocherization. The concept of the artery-first approach to divide the SMA from the pancreatic head by approaching the SMA at an early stage of the PD procedure seems to have originated in the mesenteric approach of Nakao et al. Later, Pessaux et al. reported a comprehensive variety of approaches for the treatment of pancreatic head cancer with suspected SMA invasion [2]. The term "artery-first approach" proposed by Weitz et al. has now become widely used internationally [3].

D. Ban (✉)
Department of Hepatobiliary and Pancreatic Surgery, National Cancer Center Hospital, Tokyo, Japan
e-mail: dban@ncc.go.jp

M. Tanabe
Department of Hepatobiliary and Pancreatic Surgery, Graduate School of Medicine, Tokyo Medical and Dental University, Tokyo, Japan

37.2 Artery-First Approaches in PD

Unlike in artery-first PD, the standard PD procedure is to dissect the gastroduodenal artery, perform a bile duct dissection, perform pancreatic dissection, ligate and dissect the small vessels flowing from the pancreatic head to the SMV, and finally dissect the space between the pancreatic head and the SMA. In contrast, artery-first PD is a procedure to separate the pancreatic head from the SMA by ligating and dissecting the blood vessels feeding the it from the SMA, mainly the first jejunal artery (FJA) and inferior pancreatoduodenal artery (IPDA) at the root, at an early stage of surgery. The advantages of an artery-first approach are that resectability can be determined at an early stage of the procedure and the amount of blood loss during surgery can be reduced because the feeding vessels are blocked [4–11]. The relative anatomical position of the pancreatic head to uncinate is dorsal to the origin of the SMA; bleeding from the SMA or SMV can be fatal. The approach is not always easy, as it is often accompanied by tumor invasion and inflammation. In order to ensure the safety and curative potential of the procedure, various approaches to the SMA from different directions have been proposed, and several names have been given to the same approach. We have modified the terminology summarized by Sanjay et al. [12] and revised it as shown in Fig. 37.1.

37.3 Right-Posterior Approach

For the right-posterior approach, kocherization is performed first. (Fig. 37.2) The duodenum and the head of the pancreas are sufficiently mobilized to dissect the fusion fascia of Treitz, expose the inferior vena cava (IVC) and the origin of the left renal vein, and proceed with dissection to the aorta. The pancreatic head is lifted and the fibrous tissue around the origin of the SMA is dissected to identify and divide the IPDA. The SMA is then separated from the uncinate. Further

postoperative complications [13]. Moreover, the number of lymph nodes dissected and the rate of R0 resection were the same for both procedures in both reports, and the prognosis was not affected.

In laparoscopic PD, some articles described surgical procedure for approaching from the posterior side of the SMA. Wang et al. reported the usefulness of the inferior duodenal approach [14]. This method approaches from behind the SMA. The PV/SMV was also exposed from the posterior side. Honda et al. reported a similar approach that exposed the posterior aspect of the SMA from the caudal side [15].

37.4 Right-Uncinate Approach

There are many reports on approaching from between the ventral side of the pancreatic uncinate and the SMV. (Fig. 37.3) Depending on the structure to be identified first, the name of the approach varies. Reports that focus on the pancreatic uncinate are called "uncinate-first" and those that focus on the first jejunal vein (FJV) that flows into the SMV adjacent to the pancreatic uncinate are called "FJV-first". When dissecting between the pancreatic uncinate and the SMV, it is necessary to dissect several small veins that flow into the FJV [16]. After that vein is divided, the inferior pancreatoduodenal artery (IPDA) is dissected to separate the pancreatic uncinate from the SMA.

In 2007, Shukla et al. reported a complete approach to the SMA/SMV by dissecting the ligament of Treitz and the

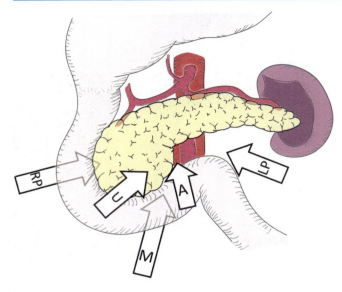

Fig. 37.1 Artery-first approaches for pancreaticoduodenectomy. *RP* right-posterior approach, *U* right-uncinate approach, *M* mesenteric approach, *LP* left-posterior approach

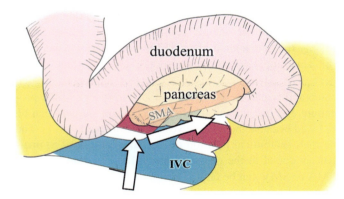

Fig. 37.2 Right posterior artery for pancreaticoduodenectomy

dissection then proceeds in order to expose the PV-SMV. The advantage of this approach is that it allows for early assessment of resectability by determining the extent to which the tumor has invaded the SMA plexus prior to treatment of the intestinal and bile ducts. In addition, appropriate *en bloc* resection of the posterior side of the pancreas can be performed. On the other hand, it is easily affected by adhesions and inflammation around the pancreatic head. It is also easily influenced by body shape, which may make this procedure difficult in obese patients.

Dumitrascu et al. compared artery-first PD with standard PD [9]. They reported that artery-first PD can be completed faster and with less blood loss, and with no difference in postoperative complications. Figueras et al. conducted a similar study and also found that artery-first PD required less time, resulted in less blood loss, again with no difference in

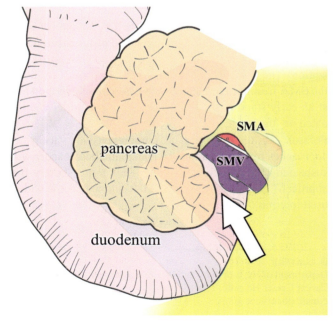

Fig. 37.3 Right posterior artery for pancreaticoduodenectomy. *SMA* superior mesenteric artery, *SMV* superior mesenteric vein

proximal jejunum and passing them to the right under the superior mesenteric vessels [17]. In 2010, Hackert et al. reported an "uncinate-first" approach to first dissect between the pancreatic uncinate and SMA [18]. Nakamura et al. reported that the FJV can be identified first, after which the SMA can be accessed for a safer approach. Shrikhande et al. reported advantages in terms of blood loss, reduced operative time, postoperative complications, lymph node dissection, and margin status.

Although not necessarily artery-first, there are also many reports on approaching from the pancreatic uncinate when performing laparoscopic PD. Zimmitti et al. reported that the right-uncinate approach is useful as an artery-first approach in laparoscopic PD [19, 20]. However, it is also true that the right-uncinate approach often overlaps with the right-posterior approach in some procedural elements, and it is difficult to clearly classify them. The Cattell-Braasch maneuver involves dissecting the right-sided white line of Toldt, dissecting the dorsal side of the ascending colon and the mesentery of the small intestine, and additionally performing sufficient kocherization to elevate it broadly to the left, including the pancreatic head of the duodenum. This method ensures that the root of the SMA can be approached [21, 22]. There is also the derotation technique by Sugiyama et al. to be considered. This is a method to expand the mesopancreas to the right side by generously dissecting the proximal small intestine from the duodenum, releasing the mesenteric rotation, and extensively pulling the mesopancreas to the right side in order to reliably approach the root of the artery branching from the SMA to the pancreatic head [23, 24]. This approach is generally easier to understand anatomically because of the traction deployment of the pancreatic head, and it is easier to determine the resectability between the SMA and the tumor on the ventral side of the pancreatic head.

37.5 Mesenteric Approach

In 1993, Nakao et al. proposed a mesenteric approach to pancreatic head resection using a catheter to bypass SMV blood to the intrahepatic portal vein or systemic circulation as an isolated pancreatectomy. They proposed to call this the mesenteric approach. This method identifies the SMA and SMV through an incision in the fascia over the SMA on the dorsal side of the transverse mesentery without kocherization, with or without portal vein bypass; the middle colonic artery arising from the SMA and the middle colonic vein flowing into the SMV are dissected, and the SMA and SMV are widely separated. (Fig. 37.4) Next, the SMA origin is entered from the right side of the pancreatic uncinate and SMA to widen the space between the SMA and SMV. This technique is basically synonymous with the inferior infracacolic approach proposed by Weitz et al. in 2010. This method can be used to evaluate

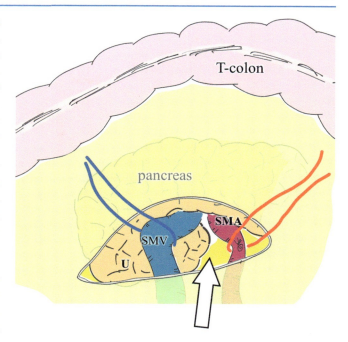

Fig. 37.4 Mesenteric approach. *SMA* superior mesenteric artery, *SMV* superior mesenteric vein, *U* uncinate, *T-colon* transverse colon

resectability by confirming the relationship between the tumor and SMA in the head of the pancreas at an early stage of surgery. It is undoubtedly useful for tumors in the pancreatic uncinate area. Unfortunately, whether there is any oncological benefit has not been established. Currently, a randomized controlled trial of this technique compared with standard PD is underway in Japan, and the results are eagerly awaited [25].

37.6 Left-Posterior Approach

Kurosaki et al. reported data on the left-posterior approach [26]. After the proximal jejunum and duodenum are dissected and innervated from the left side, the proximal jejunum is towed to the left side, exposing the dorsal side of the mesentery and the left to dorsal side of the SMA. (Fig. 37.5) The first jejunal artery arising from the SMA is then dissected at the root. The root of the first jejunal artery or the IPDA branching from the first jejunal artery is also dissected. Once it is confirmed that there is no tumor invasion between the pancreatic uncinate and the SMA, the jejunum is dissected. The SMV is not visible in this field of view, so we approach it again from the right. Kawabata et al. reported the oncological benefit of the mesenteric approach as well as resection of the mesopancreatoduodenum [27]. This approach can be used to reach the SMA without mobilization of the duodenum or colon and may be particularly useful for tumors in the pancreatic uncinate. However, this approach is often difficult by laparoscopy and few cases have been reported [28].

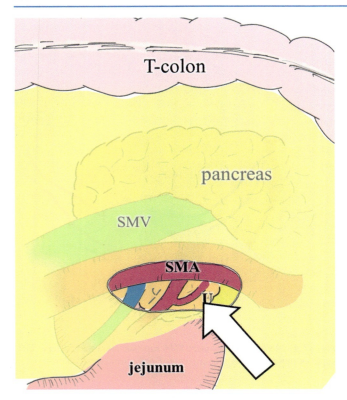

Fig. 37.5 Left-posterior approach. *SMA* superior mesenteric artery, *SMV* superior mesenteric vein, *U* right-uncinate approach, *T-colon* transverse colon

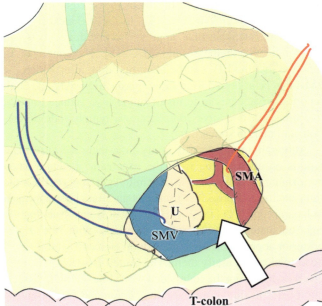

Fig. 37.6 Anterior approach. *SMA* superior mesenteric artery, *SMV* superior mesenteric vein, *U* right-uncinate approach, *T-colon* transverse colon

37.7 Anterior Approach

The SMA/SMV is approached anteriorly from the inferior border of the pancreas, and the SMA secured and pulled to the left side. The SMV is then secured and pulled to the right side. The method is to dissect the SMA and the pancreatic uncinate by extracting the tissue between them. In 2010, Hirota et al. designated this procedure an inferior supracolic approach, and in the original report, the approach was to dissect the stomach at the pylorus and the pancreas at the pancreatic neck, exposing a wide PV-SMV and SMA [29]. The advantage of this method is that it allows for *en bloc* resection by isolating the blood vessels without touching the tumor. However, a disadvantage of the original method as reported by Hirota et al. was that gastrectomy and pancreatic resection are not always necessary to evaluate resectability. In this sense, it is not clear whether the method of Hirota et al. can be called artery-first. In the method reported by Inoue et al., SMA/SMV is approached prior to the dissection of the digestive tract and pancreatic dissection, which is truly an artery-first anterior approach [8]. (Fig. 37.6).

37.8 Mesopancreatic Resection

Although various artery-first techniques have been proposed, the main objective is to resect the pancreatic head from the SMA *en bloc* leaving no residual tumor. Similarly, the concept of resection of the mesopancreas overlaps with the concept of artery-first. However, the definition of mesopancreas is often problematic because it is related to the extent of resection. Gockel et al. referred to the chordae, or fiber bundles, between the blood vessels and the pancreas, as the mesopancreas [30]. It was described as "a vascular-rich connective tissue extending from the dorsal surface of the pancreatic head to the SMV/SMA, histologically containing fat, sparse connective tissue, and nerve fibers". Kawabata et al. proposed the concept of mesopancreatoduodenum for the region including the mesopancreas and the duodenal mesentery up to the left margin of the SMA. They then reported that there was an oncological benefit to be derived from sectioning at the root of the first jejunal artery to resect the mesopancreatoduodenum [27]. Wu et al. suggested dividing the mesopancreas into an anterior part up to the dorsal portal vein and a posterior part between it and the SMA [31]. In contrast, Sharma and Isaji pointed out that the term "meso-" evokes the mesentery (mesorectum, mesocolon, etc.) but is not an appropriate term because it does not meet the definition of mesentery and is better referred to as pseudomesopancreas [32]. However, it is also convincing that it is hard to abandon the idea that this fiber bundle is a membrane-enclosed structure. If viewed dorsally, this is because the celiac plexus and this fiber bundle are separated by Treitz's posterior pancreatic fascia [33]. Muro et al. [34], through anatomical analysis of the pancreatic plexus region, revealed that the fibers are quite intricately intertwined and can be divided into ventral and dorsal portions with different runs. This led to the proposal to call the layered chord-like structures, together with small blood vessels and lymphatic vessels, the P-A ligament that connects the aorta and its main branches to the pancreas. In the area surrounding the pancreas, there are many variations in the trajectories of the arteries, and therefore, the paths of the nerves are also very complicated.

As mentioned above, the extent of resection of the mesopancreas is quite variable among institutions. The artery-first approach is a concept for which it is easier to arrive at a common understanding in respect of the terminology. On the other hand, it should be noted that the details of the extent of resection are fraught with problems such as the issue of the mesopancreas. From this point of view, the Level I, II, and III classification proposed by Inoue et al. is a very realistic stratification that is one step ahead of artery-first [35].

37.9 The Outcome of Artery-First Approaches

Unfortunately, there still appear to be no high-quality reports on the short- and long-term surgical outcomes of artery-first approaches relative to standard PD. Several retrospective comparative studies have reported a reduction in operative time, intraoperative blood loss, and need for blood transfusion [9, 35]. There are reports of improved R0 resection rates, increased number of resected lymph nodes [27], and improved prognosis [26]. However, many others have not been able to show any oncological benefit. There have been several meta-analyses comparing artery-first PD with standard PD. According to some meta-analyses [36–38], intraoperative blood loss and the proportion of patients requiring intraoperative transfusions was significantly lower in the artery-first group. Clearly increased R0 resection rates and overall survival have been reported for artery-first PD. However, there were no differences in mortality, and no differences in tumor pathological factors.

The artery-first approach is considered to improve R0 resection with respect to SMA margins by reliably dissecting the SMA nerve plexus in close proximity to the pancreatic head during dissection from the SMA. The principle that completes margin-negative resection leads to improved survival has facilitated the artery-first approach. It is also hypothesized that the artery-first approach reduces intraoperative circulating tumor cells (CTCs), which may contribute to improved survival. This is based on the theory that the GDA and IPDA are dissected prior to kocherization, and the veins are also dissected to prevent the outflow of CTCs. A recent report showed that CTCs in the portal vein were significantly reduced in 12 patients who underwent artery-first PD, and that the MST of standard PD was 13.0 months, while that of artery-first PD was improved to 16.7 months [39]. Because of the small size of this cohort, we have to be careful in the interpretation of these results. In fact, according to a report by Yamamoto et al., among the reports of artery-first approaches, kocherization is often preceded by arterial dissection, and the order of intestinal dissection and pancreatic dissection varies [40].

There are many reports that the surgical advantage of the artery-first approach is that early dissection of the IPDA prior to dissection of the veins in the outflow tract prevents congestion in the pancreatic head and reduces intraoperative bleeding. Intraoperative bleeding is a risk factor for postoperative complications, which may have led to a reduction in postoperative complications in artery-first PD.

Here, it should be mentioned that there are some limitations to the reports so far, all of which are on non-randomized and retrospective studies. One of the advantages of the artery-first approach is that resectability is determined early in the surgery, which may result in a relative increase in survival due to the exclusion of advanced cases and hence act as a selection bias. It is unfortunate that there are few reports on negative laparotomy; and there seem to be no reports at all describing the rate of failure to undergo PD after an artery-first approach. On the other hand, it is also possible that these reports show biased results reflecting the enhanced ability of the experts in high-volume centers to implement the artery-first approach. Even though the artery-first approach is not a new technique, it is difficult to collate high-quality evidence. This is due to the heterogeneity in patient backgrounds and the technical demands made on the surgeons who perform the procedures. However, an RCT of the mesenteric versus standard approach is currently underway in Japan, and the results are eagerly awaited [25].

37.10 Summary

In performing PD for pancreatic head cancer, especially for advanced pancreatic head cancer, it is essential to consider (1) curative resection, (2) appropriate evaluation of resectability, and (3) safe resection. Therefore, the approach to the SMA, which is the most critical stage of the procedure, is the key. How to evaluate the status of SMA and tumor in the pancreatic head at the early stage of surgery and how to surely and safely proceed are important issues for the performance of safe and curative surgery. Various approaches that have been proposed have been described in the literature, all of which have their strengths and weaknesses depending on the individual condition of the tumor in the pancreatic head cancer patient. These variables include the size of the tumor, whether it is ventral or dorsal to the pancreatic head, and whether it is in the pancreatic uncinate. I believe that most experts do not stick to a single approach, but rather combine and use several approaches depending on the situation with the individual patient. I would like to encourage surgeons who are learning PD to benefit from the approaches that experts have developed so far, and to become familiar with multiple approaches to ensure a reliable artery-first approach.

Conflict of Interest Statement There are no conflicts of interests for any of the authors.

References

1. Nakao A, Takagi H. Isolated pancreatectomy for pancreatic head carcinoma using catheter bypass of the portal vein. Hepato-Gastroenterology. 1993;40(5):426–9.
2. Pessaux P, Varma D, Arnaud JP. Pancreaticoduodenectomy: superior mesenteric artery first approach. J Gastrointest Surg. 2006;10(4):607–11.
3. Weitz J, Rahbari N, Koch M, Buchler MW. The "artery first" approach for resection of pancreatic head cancer. J Am Coll Surg. 2010;210(2):e1–4.
4. Kawai M, Tani M, Ina S, et al. CLIP method (preoperative CT image-assessed ligation of inferior pancreaticoduodenal artery) reduces intraoperative bleeding during pancreaticoduodenectomy. World J Surg. 2008;32(1):82–7.
5. Hirono S, Kawai M, Okada KI, et al. Mesenteric approach during pancreaticoduodenectomy for pancreatic ductal adenocarcinoma. Ann Gastroenterol Surg. 2017;1(3):208–18.
6. Nakamura M, Nakashima H, Tsutsumi K, et al. First jejunal vein oriented mesenteric excision for pancreatoduodenectomy. J Gastroenterol. 2013;48(8):989–95.
7. Kawabata Y, Nishi T, Tanaka T, Tajima Y. Safety and feasibility of a pancreaticoduodenectomy with total meso-pancreatoduodenum excision: analysis in various periampullary disorders. Hepato-Gastroenterology. 2014;61(131):821–7.
8. Inoue Y, Saiura A, Tanaka M, et al. Technical details of an anterior approach to the superior mesenteric artery during pancreaticoduodenectomy. J Gastrointest Surg. 2016;20(10):1769–77.
9. Dumitrascu T, David L, Popescu I. Posterior versus standard approach in pancreatoduodenectomy: a case-match study. Langenbeck's Arch Surg. 2010;395(6):677–84.
10. Gundara JS, Wang F, Alvarado-Bachmann R, et al. The clinical impact of early complete pancreatic head devascularisation during pancreatoduodenectomy. Am J Surg. 2013;206(4):518–25.
11. Shah OJ, Gagloo MA, Khan IJ, Ahmad R, Bano S. Pancreaticoduodenectomy: a comparison of superior approach with classical Whipple's technique. Hepatobiliary Pancreat Dis Int. 2013;12(2):196–203.
12. Sanjay P, Takaori K, Govil S, Shrikhande SV, Windsor JA. 'Artery-first' approaches to pancreatoduodenectomy. Br J Surg. 2012;99(8):1027–35.
13. Figueras J, Codina-Barreras A, Lopez-Ben S, et al. Cephalic duodenopancreatectomy in periampullary tumours. Dissection of the superior mesenteric artery as aninitial approach. Description of the technique and an assessment of our initial experience. Cir Esp. 2008;83(4):186–93.
14. Wang XM, Sun WD, Hu MH, et al. Inferoposterior duodenal approach for laparoscopic pancreaticoduodenectomy. World J Gastroenterol. 2016;22(6):2142–8.
15. Honda G, Kurata M, Okuda Y, Kobayashi S, Sakamoto K, Takahashi K. Laparoscopic pancreaticoduodenectomy: taking advantage of the unique view from the caudal side. J Am Coll Surg. 2013;217(6):e45–9.
16. Nakata K, Higuchi R, Ikenaga N, et al. Precision anatomy for safe approach to pancreatoduodenectomy for both open and minimally invasive procedure: a systematic review. J Hepatobiliary Pancreat Sci. 2022;29(1):99–113.
17. Shukla PJ, Barreto G, Pandey D, et al. Modification in the technique of pancreaticoduodenectomy: supracolic division of jejunum to facilitate uncinate process dissection. Hepato-Gastroenterology. 2007;54(78):1728–30.
18. Hackert T, Werner J, Weitz J, Schmidt J, Buchler MW. Uncinate process first--a novel approach for pancreatic head resection. Langenbeck's Arch Surg. 2010;395(8):1161–4.
19. Morales E, Zimmitti G, Codignola C, et al. Follow "the superior mesenteric artery": laparoscopic approach for total mesopancreas excision during pancreaticoduodenectomy. Surg Endosc. 2019;33(12):4186–91.
20. Zimmitti G, Manzoni A, Addeo P, et al. Laparoscopic pancreatoduodenectomy with superior mesenteric artery-first approach and pancreatogastrostomy assisted by mini-laparotomy. Surg Endosc. 2016;30(4):1670–1.
21. Akita M, Yamasaki N, Miyake T, et al. Cattell-Braasch maneuver facilitates the artery-first approach and complete excision of the mesopancreas for pancreatoduodenectomy. J Surg Oncol. 2020;121(7):1126–31.
22. Del Chiaro M, Segersvard R, Rangelova E, et al. Cattell-Braasch Maneuver combined with artery-first approach for superior mesenteric-portal vein resection during pancreatectomy. J Gastrointest Surg. 2015;19(12):2264–8.
23. Sugiyama M, Suzuki Y, Nakazato T, et al. Vascular anatomy of mesopancreas in pancreatoduodenectomy using an intestinal derotation procedure. World J Surg. 2020;44(10):3441–8.
24. Sugiyama M, Suzuki Y, Nakazato T, et al. Intestinal derotation procedure for facilitating pancreatoduodenectomy. Surgery. 2016;159(5):1325–32.
25. Hirono S, Kawai M, Okada KI, et al. MAPLE-PD trial (mesenteric approach vs. conventional approach for pancreatic cancer during pancreaticoduodenectomy): study protocol for a multicenter randomized controlled trial of 354 patients with pancreatic ductal adenocarcinoma. Trials. 2018;19(1):613.
26. Kurosaki I, Minagawa M, Takano K, Takizawa K, Hatakeyama K. Left posterior approach to the superior mesenteric vascular pedicle in pancreaticoduodenectomy for cancer of the pancreatic head. JOP. 2011;12(3):220–9.
27. Kawabata Y, Tanaka T, Nishi T, Monma H, Yano S, Tajima Y. Appraisal of a total meso-pancreatoduodenum excision with pancreaticoduodenectomy for pancreatic head carcinoma. Eur J Surg Oncol. 2012;38(7):574–9.
28. Nagakawa Y, Watanabe Y, Kozono S, et al. Surgical approaches to the superior mesenteric artery during minimally invasive pancreaticoduodenectomy: a systematic review. J Hepatobiliary Pancreat Sci. 2022;29(1):114–23.
29. Hirota M, Kanemitsu K, Takamori H, et al. Pancreatoduodenectomy using a no-touch isolation technique. Am J Surg. 2010;199(5):e65–8.
30. Gockel I, Domeyer M, Wolloscheck T, Konerding MA, Junginger T. Resection of the mesopancreas (RMP): a new surgical clas-

sification of a known anatomical space. World J Surg Oncol. 2007;5:44.
31. Wu W, Wang X, Wu X, et al. Total mesopancreas excision for pancreatic head cancer: analysis of 120 cases. Chin J Cancer Res. 2016;28(4):423–8.
32. Sharma D, Isaji S. Mesopancreas is a misnomer: time to correct the nomenclature. J Hepatobiliary Pancreat Sci. 2016;23(12):745–9.
33. Yi S, Nagakawa Y, Ren K, et al. The mesopancreas and pancreatic head plexus: morphological, developmental, and clinical perspectives. Surg Radiol Anat. 2020;42(12):1501–8.
34. Muro S, Sirirat W, Ban D, Nagakawa Y, Akita K. What comprises the plate-like structure between the pancreatic head and the celiac trunk and superior mesenteric artery? A proposal for the term "P-A ligament" based on anatomical findings. Anat Sci Int. 2021;96(3):370–7.
35. Inoue Y, Saiura A, Yoshioka R, et al. Pancreatoduodenectomy with systematic mesopancreas dissection using a supracolic anterior artery-first approach. Ann Surg. 2015;262(6):1092–101.
36. Ironside N, Barreto SG, Loveday B, Shrikhande SV, Windsor JA, Pandanaboyana S. Meta-analysis of an artery-first approach versus standard pancreatoduodenectomy on perioperative outcomes and survival. Br J Surg. 2018;105(6):628–36.
37. Jiang X, Yu Z, Ma Z, et al. Superior mesenteric artery first approach can improve the clinical outcomes of pancreaticoduodenectomy: a meta-analysis. Int J Surg. 2020;73:14–24.
38. Negoi I, Hostiuc S, Runcanu A, Negoi RI, Beuran M. Superior mesenteric artery first approach versus standard pancreaticoduodenectomy: a systematic review and meta-analysis. Hepatobiliary Pancreat Dis Int. 2017;16(2):127–38.
39. Gall TM, Jacob J, Frampton AE, et al. Reduced dissemination of circulating tumor cells with no-touch isolation surgical technique in patients with pancreatic cancer. JAMA Surg. 2014;149(5):482–5.
40. Yamamoto J, Kudo H, Kyoden Y, et al. An anatomical review of various superior mesenteric artery-first approaches during pancreatoduodenectomy for pancreatic cancer. Surg Today. 2021;51(6):872–9.

38

Organ- and Parenchyma-sparing Pancreatic Surgery

Calogero Iacono, Mario De Bellis, Andrea Ruzzenente, and Alfredo Guglielmi

Abstract

Conventional pancreatectomies, such as pancreaticoduodenectomy and distal and total pancreatectomy, result in an important loss of normal pancreatic parenchyma and the nearby organs (spleen, upper digestive tract, and common bile duct). In addition, these procedures involve significant mortality, high morbidity, and long-term disorders, including infections, thromboembolic complications, digestive disorders, pancreatic exocrine insufficiency, and diabetes. Although conventional pancreatectomies are mandatory for malignant tumor, they are an overtreatment for benign tumors as healthy functional pancreatic parenchyma is sacrificed, especially in young patients with long life expectancy. Unfortunately, enucleation is not always advisable in lesions of uncertain histology or those deeply located in the pancreatic gland owing to the risk of a positive surgical margin or injury to the main pancreatic duct, respectively. Since the 1980s, the prospects for pancreatic resection have widened with the development of organ- and parenchyma-sparing pancreatic surgery (OPSPS) for benign or low-grade malignant tumors involving isolated or multiple segments of the pancreas. New operations, such as spleen-preserving distal pancreatectomy, duodenum-sparing pancreas head resection, dorsal pancreatectomy, resection of the ventral or uncinate process of the pancreas, middle-preserving pancreatectomy, and central pancreatectomy (the Dagradi-Serio-Iacono operation), aim to preserve pancreatic exocrine and endocrine function, spare the nearby organs, ensure oncological radicality, and achieve better quality of life after surgery. In fact, according to vascular anatomy and embryological development, the pancreatic gland is divided in four segments and each of these can be resected independently. In experienced hands, OPSPS is technically feasible and can be performed with low mortality. Early morbidity is greater than that achieved using standard resection owing to the high rate of postoperative pancreatic fistula. However, most of these pancreatic leakages are managed conservatively. Furthermore, possible poor short-term outcomes are counterbalanced by the preservation of pancreatic endocrine and exocrine function and the low rate of reoperations for tumor recurrence. Currently, OPSPS can also be performed by laparoscopic or robotic approach achieving better results in term of blood loss, operative time, hospital stay, recovery and scarring. Careful case selection, accurate pre- and intraoperative evaluation of the lesion, and experience in pancreatic surgery are required for optimal results.

38.1 Introduction

Conventional pancreatic resections for malignant and benign tumors are pancreaticoduodenectomy (PD), distal pancreatectomy (DP), and total pancreatectomy (TP). Severe morbidity remains high despite advances in decreasing postoperative mortality below 4%, as reported by high-volume centers. In addition, these standard surgical procedures are associated with long-term disorders, including infections, thrombotic complications, digestive disorders, pancreatic exocrine insufficiency, and diabetes.

Conventional pancreatectomies are mandatory for malignant tumors; however, they are considered an overtreatment of benign tumors as the healthy functional pancreatic parenchyma is sacrificed, especially in young patients with long life expectancy. In fact, standard pancreatic resections are burdened by disappointing results in terms of deficit in endocrine and exocrine function in the long term. This has a negative impact on quality of life (QOL) and increases the cost of pancreatic enzyme replacement therapy and anti-diabetic drugs. Furthermore, because overall survival after pancreatic resections continues to improve, postoperative pancreatic

C. Iacono (✉) · M. De Bellis · A. Ruzzenente · A. Guglielmi
Department of Surgery, Unit of HPB Surgery, University of Verona Medical School, Verona, Italy
e-mail: calogero.iacono@univr.it

insufficiency has become increasingly important to consider as may lead eventually to malnutrition, maldigestion, and nutritional deficiencies. The frequency, degree, and long-term persistence of endocrine and exocrine dysfunction varies depending on pre-existing conditions, benign or malignant diseases, the amount of pancreatic parenchyma saved, the pancreatic resection type, and follow-up duration. Roughly, the incidence of new-onset diabetes mellitus (NODM) and exocrine pancreatic insufficiency after PD is 22% and 53%, respectively [1]. Likewise, the incidence of NODM in patients undergoing DP ranges 14–39% [2]. Many patients subsequently develop insulin-dependent diabetes mellitus.

In theory, pancreatic enucleation (EN) is the most optimal surgical option used to preserve the maximum amount of normal parenchyma and reduce the risk of endocrine and exocrine insufficiency. Surgeons also favor this method because it does not require digestive tract reconstruction. Nevertheless, the benefits of this approach could be jeopardized by an increase in tumor recurrence and postoperative morbidity. In fact, EN is contraindicated in malignant cases, and it is not advisable in tumors of uncertain histology since it does not ensure an adequate surgical margin nor facilitate systematic regional lymph node dissection. Moreover, EN can only be performed when the lesion fulfills anatomic and technical considerations. The relationship between the lesion and the main pancreatic duct (MPD) is the most important and limiting factor. Indeed, duct injury can lead to high-output and prolonged pancreatic fistula (PF), a source of severe postoperative complications. Thus, EN can be performed in a minority of patients diagnosed with pancreatic lesions; the selection is based on the biological behavior and localization of the tumor within the pancreatic parenchyma.

Since the 1980s, the prospects for pancreatic resection have widened owing to the development of organ- and parenchyma-sparing pancreatic surgery for tumors involving isolated or multiple segments of the pancreas. In fact, according to vascular anatomy and embryological development, the pancreatic gland can be divided into four segments (i.e., the anterior head, body, and tail [originating from dorsal pancreas] and the posterior head [ventral pancreas]), and each one can be resected independently [3]. These new operations, such as spleen-preserving DP (SPDP), duodenum-preserving pancreatic head resection (DPPHR), central pancreatectomy (CP), dorsal pancreatectomy, the resection of the ventral or uncinate process of the pancreas, and middle-preserving pancreatectomy (MPP), aim to preserve pancreatic exocrine and endocrine function, spare the nearby organs, ensure oncological radicality, and achieve better QOL after surgery.

The main indications for OPSPS are: (1) benign or low-grade malignant tumors (neuroendocrine tumors, serous and mucinous cystadenomas, noninvasive branch duct type intraductal papillary mucinous neoplasms (IPMN) [4], and small solid pseudopapillary tumors, (2) non-neoplastic cysts (simple lymphoepithelial or hydatid cysts) not suitable for EN, and (3) isolated pancreatic metastases (especially from renal cancer).

38.2 Organ-Sparing Techniques

38.2.1 Spleen-Preserving Distal Pancreatectomy

SPDP should always be considered when patients have non-malignant disease. Several middle- and long-term complications, such as abdominal abscesses, thrombocytosis, pulmonary hypertension, venous and arterial thrombosis, and overwhelming infection, have been described after splenectomy. Furthermore, splenectomized patients should be vaccinated against pneumococcus, *Haemophilus influenzae* type b, and meningococcus at additional cost to the national health system. On the contrary, SPDP is associated with a low rate of postoperative complications, especially infectious ones.

SPDP can be carried out in two different ways, either by splenic vessels resection, as proposed by Warshaw, or by splenic vessels preservation, as proposed by Kimura (Fig. 38.1). The resection of splenic vessels reduces blood supply to the spleen, along with the risk of splenic infarction, which requires a subsequent splenectomy. Moreover, an increased blood flow through the short gastric veins may cause gastric varices, with a consequent small risk of bleeding. Both procedures can be performed using a minimally invasive [5] or open approach; however, splenic vessels preservation ensures better outcomes. Some surgeons have expressed concerns about Warshaw's procedure and would rather perform a splenectomy if splenic vessels preservation is unfeasible.

38.2.2 Duodenum-Preserving Pancreatic Head Resection

Growing evidence supports the use of DPPHR to remove benign lesions located in the pancreatic head. Nonetheless, the use of the DPPHR involves two major challenges: oncological radicality and having to avoid ischemic duodenal lesions.

Radical extirpation necessitates segmental resection of the duodenal wall in the peripapillary region. Although dissection of the pancreatic head from the duodenal wall (i.e., roughly 3 cm on both sides of the papilla major) is easy to perform, total resection of the pancreatic head can result in devascularization of the duodenal segment, with the risk of ischemic lesions.

Blood supply to the duodenum is provided by the anterior and posterior branches of the gastroduodenal artery

38 Organ- and Parenchyma-sparing Pancreatic Surgery

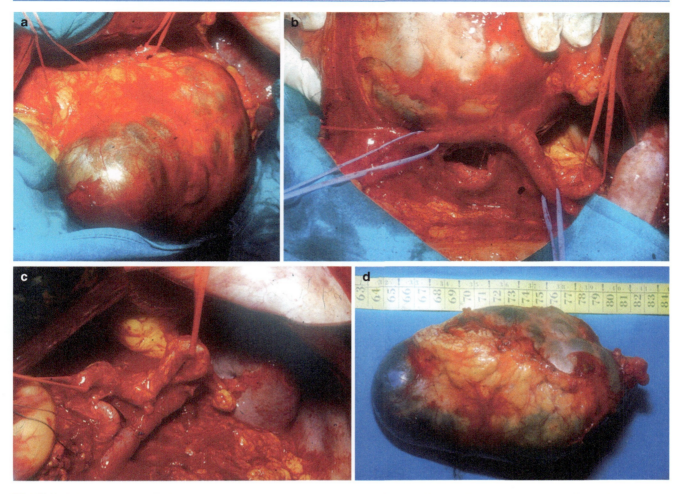

Fig. 38.1 Spleen preserving distal pancreatectomy with splenic vessels preservation for a mucinous cystadenoma of the pancreatic body/tail. Intraoperative image showing a large pancreatic cystic lesion of the body/tail (**a**). Isolation of the pancreatic body/tail from splenic vein (**b**). Preservation of splenic artery and vein (**c**). Pancreatic specimen (**d**)

(GDA) and the corresponding branches of the inferior pancreaticoduodenal arcades and the supraduodenal artery. The papilla of Vater maintains the blood supply derived from the posterior GDA and the posterior branches of the inferior pancreaticoduodenal artery. Dissection of the pancreatic head results in an interruption to the arterial blood and nerve supply to the papilla area and surrounding duodenal wall.

To avoid ischemic lesions in the duodenal segment, preservation of the anterior inferior pancreaticoduodenal arcade, which runs along the duodenal wall, and the anterior superior pancreaticoduodenal arcade from the GDA, is necessary. Conversely, the posterior superior and inferior pancreatoduodenal arcades may be completely divided without negatively impacting regarding duodenal wall perfusion.

DPPHR and conventional PD outcomes compare favorably. Notably, the DPPHR procedure preserves pancreatic endocrine and exocrine function and is characterized by low rates of surgery-related morbidity, clinically relevant PF, reinterventions, and hospital mortality [6].

38.3 Parenchyma-Sparing Techniques

38.3.1 Central Pancreatectomy (The Dagradi-Serio-Iacono Operation)

CP is a segmental pancreatic resection that is indicated for the removal of benign or low-grade malignant isthmus tumors and proximal part of the pancreas body (Fig. 38.2). It is also known as middle pancreatectomy, medial pancreatectomy, intermediate pancreatectomy, limited conservative pancreatectomy, and the Dagradi-Serio-Iacono operation [7]. This technique was first performed for an insulinoma of the

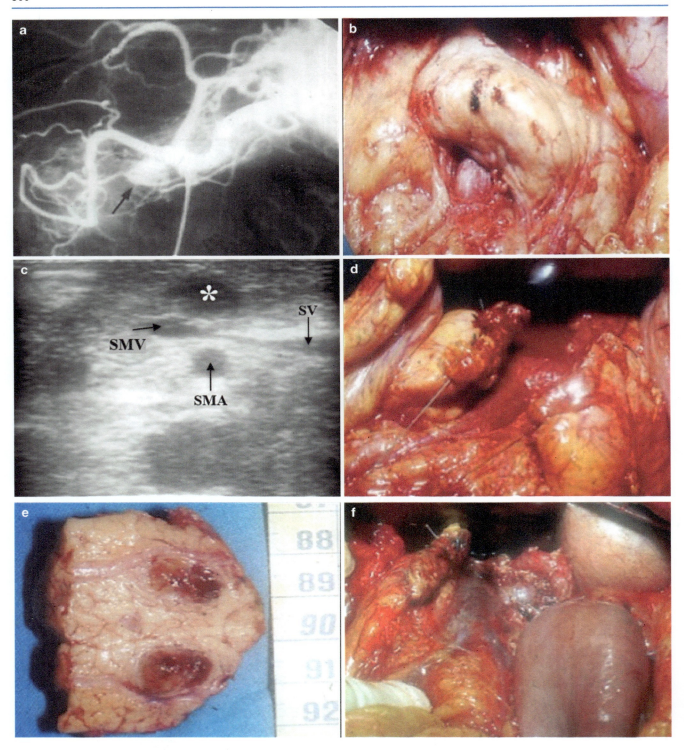

Fig. 38.2 Central pancreatectomy for an insulinoma of the pancreatic isthmus. Small hypervascular lesion in the neck of the pancreas (black arrow) showed by angiography (**a**). Intraoperative image of the pancreas with no visible lesion (**b**). Intraoperative ultrasonography shows the tumor (*) deeply located in the pancreatic parenchyma, superior mesenteric vein (SMV), superior mesenteric artery (SMA), and splenic vein (SV) (**c**). Proximal and distal pancreatic stumps after resection of the pancreatic isthmus (**d**). Pancreatic specimen cut open to show the relationship between the insulinoma and the Wirsung's duct (**e**). The proximal pancreatic stump can be closed with "mattress" stitches after selective closure of the main pancreatic duct with a figure-of-eight stitch and the distal pancreatic stump can be anastomosed with the jejunum by a Roux-en-Y end to end pancreaticojejunostomy (**f**)

pancreatic isthmus in 1982. A few years later, it was described in the *Enciclopedia Medica Italiana* by Dagradi and Serio. Subsequently, Iacono validated it using functional endocrine and exocrine tests, popularizing it worldwide [8].

Incisions are made in the posterior peritoneum along the superior and inferior margins of the central segment of the pancreas. After passing a vessel loop around the isthmus, the spleno-mesenteric axis is dissected free from the posterior surface of the gland dividing some pancreatic veins. Another vessel loop is passed around the splenic artery, and its collaterals, including the dorsal pancreatic artery, are divided.

Surgeons should be aware that a large dorsal pancreatic artery raises a high index of suspicion of a pancreatic vascularization of the body/tail maintained exclusively by the transverse pancreatic artery (i.e., the left branch of the dorsal pancreatic artery). This vascular variant (type III, according to Mellière and Moullè) means that CP is contraindicated owing to the risk of necrosis in the left pancreas (Fig. 38.3).

The transection limit of the gland is the GDA on the cephalic side, while on the caudal side the authors suggest sparing at least 5 cm of pancreatic tail with no signs of atrophy. The specimen should be sent to the pathologist for the

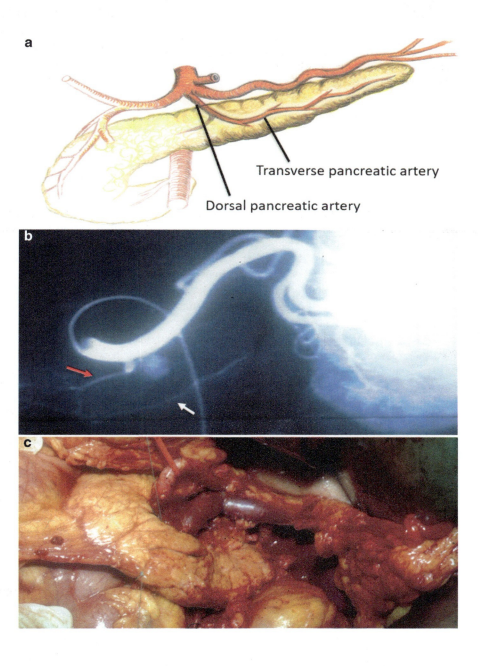

Fig. 38.3 Anatomical vascular contraindication to central pancreatectomy. Schematic representation of the Mellière and Moullè type III vascularity of the pancreas (**a**). Angiography shows pancreatic vascularization of the body/tail maintained exclusively by the transverse pancreatic artery (white arrow), that is the left branch of the dorsal pancreatic artery (red arrow) (**b**). Spleen-preserving distal pancreatectomy with splenic vessel preservation can be performed instead of central pancreatectomy (**c**)

frozen section procedure to confirm the diagnosis and determine if the resection margin is tumor-free. In the case of a positive surgical margin, the resection can be extended further, but if the pathologist diagnoses malignant disease, the operation has to switch to PD or DP with extended lymphadenectomy, depending on extension of the lesion toward the pancreatic head or body/tail.

If IPMN are identified, pancreatoscopy can be performed, just after resection, through MPD in both stumps to rule out other ductal lesions. The cephalic stump can be closed with "mattress" stitches after separate closure of the MPD with a figure-of-eight stitch. The distal pancreatic stump should be separated from the splenic vessels by two centimeters to easily carry out the anastomosis of the digestive tract.

Reconstruction can be performed using either Roux-en-Y pancreaticojejunostomy or pancreaticogastrostomy. *Pancreaticojejunostomy* can be conducted in different ways, for example, end to end (simple or telescopic invagination), end to side, duct to mucosa, and side to side (Puestow procedure or Partington-Rochelle technique if the duct of Wirsung is dilated, for example, in the case of chronic pancreatitis). Some authors also perform an anastomosis of the cephalic stump using the same jejunal loop (double pancreaticojejunostomy). Pancreaticogastrostomy is usually performed by the implantation of the open end of the pancreas directly into the gastric pouch through a 2–3 cm opening in the posterior surface.

The disadvantages of this type of reconstruction primarily relate to alterations to the digestive enzymes, particularly lipase, caused by gastric acid, which results in exocrine function impairment. In our opinion, alterations to exocrine pancreatic function signify the failure of this conservative surgical technique. Closure of the distal pancreatic stump can be performed in exceptional cases as atrophy of the remnant pancreas or MPD not evident. Instead, closure of the MPD of the distal stump, using injected synthetic glue, causes pancreatic atrophy and diabetes; therefore, we do not recommend this technique. End-to-end anastomosis of the MPD and parenchyma, with or without stent placement for internal or external pancreatic juice drainage, is another type of reconstruction [9]. The key benefit of this kind of reconstruction is complete mobilization of the distal pancreatic remnant achieved through peripancreatic ligament transection, which, in turn, pulls the two pancreatic stumps together. In the past, this technique was used to repair traumatic pancreatic neck transections with minimal loss of parenchyma. Notably, the MPD of most patients who undergo CP is too thin (not dilatated) to confidently perform duct-to-duct anastomosis.

The aim of CP is to preserve the functional tissue of the pancreatic body/tail segment where there are numerous islet cells; however, compared with DP and PD, this technique is associated with higher rates of postoperative PF. In fact, CP has two points of "weakness", the proximal head stump and the distal one, which is anastomosed to the digestive tract. Furthermore, since CP is indicated for benign or low-grade malignant tumors, the anastomosis is usually performed on a soft pancreas with a nondilated MPD and this entails a high risk of fistula. However, PF following CP is classified as a biochemical leak or postoperative PF grade B according to the international study group of PF and it usually heals spontaneously with drainage management, parenteral nutrition, and the administration of somatostatin analog drugs. In fact, the leak from the proximal stump or from the pancreaticojejunostomy is not subject to the enzymatic activation of bile, as is the case of a PF after PD [10].

38.3.2 Dorsal Pancreatectomy

Dorsal pancreatectomy is a conservative surgical technique that allows for complete removal of the dorsal portion of the pancreatic head, along with the pancreatic neck, body, and tail.

The pancreas comprises two embryological segments, the dorsal and ventral primordia. During the sixth week of embryonic development, the ventral primordium, along with the developing bile duct, rotates clockwise behind the duodenum and the dorsal primordium. The differences in embryologic origin reflect the histological characteristics. In fact, compared with the dorsal pancreas, the ventral pancreas is characterized by smaller and densely packed lobuli, irregular islets of Langerhans, and rich immunostaining with antipancreatic polypeptide. The dorsal pancreas comprises the pancreatic neck, body, and tail, as well as the anterior segment of the head. The ventral pancreas makes up the majority of the uncinate process and the posterior segment of the head. Autoptic pancreatic anatomical studies have demonstrated that the pancreas head can be removed while preserving the vascular arcades and branches to the duodenum, the common bile duct (CBD), and the papilla of Vater and that there is an anatomical fusion plane between the dorsal and ventral pancreas that contains small pancreatic ducts and vascular collateral branches. The embryological fusion plane contains a few communicating vessels or ducts (except for the junction of the dorsal and ventral duct systems, present in over 90% of cases). The presence of pancreas divisum, namely the lack of fusion between the dorsal and ventral pancreas during embryological development, is a favorable anatomical condition that promotes easier pancreatic segmental resection. Nevertheless, the procedure is still technically feasible and safe when the normal pancreatic fusion plane is present.

Dorsal pancreatectomy avoids the need to perform biliary and digestive tract resection and reconstruction, while preserving pancreatic endocrine and exocrine function. In selected cases, this operation represents the only alternative to TP and difficulties managing the ensuing "fragile" diabetes. Although postoperative diabetes is commonly observed after dorsal pancreatectomy, it is easier to control than that resulting from TP because the glucose-stabilizing effect of glucagon can be maintained.

To identify the intrapancreatic tract of the CBD in the ventral segment, a catheter can be inserted through the cystic duct to the duodenum. Alternatively, preoperative endoscopic biliary and/or pancreatic stent placement can be performed to facilitate the intraoperative identification of CBD and MPD. Pancreatic resection is conducted from the left (tail) to the right (head). At the head of the pancreas, the dorsal segment is dissected stepwise from the duodenal wall toward the CBD plane, while preserving the GDA and the anterior superior pancreaticoduodenal artery. Sparing the anterior and posterior pancreaticoduodenal arcades enables mobilization of the duodenum without ischemic risk. Santorini's duct is identified, dissected, and ligated at its outlet into the duodenum, followed by dissection of the pancreatic parenchyma along the anterior surface of the CBD. To complete the dorsal pancreatectomy, the fusion plane between the dorsal and ventral segments is identified and carefully dissected. The MPD in the ventral segment of the dissected parenchymal surface is identified and ligated using an unabsorbable monofilament suture. Frozen sections of the pancreatic parenchymal margin should be collected and analyzed in all cases. Branch ducts identified on the surface of the ventral segment can be sutured in an interrupted pattern. A methylene blue injection or intraoperative cholangiography through the trans-cystic catheter can be performed to exclude damage to the CBD. If necessary, a T-tube can be placed [11].

Head dorsal pancreatectomy, a segmental pancreatic resection, performed to spare the pancreatic neck, body, and tail, is a conservative form of total dorsal pancreatectomy. Unlike total dorsal pancreatectomy, head dorsal pancreatectomy includes a reconstructive phase. The authors usually perform an end-to-side, duct-to-mucosa pancreatojejunostomy with a Roux-en-Y method with transmesocolic transposition. The pancreatic duct is sutured to the jejunal mucosa with interrupted stitches using 5-0 absorbable monofilament sutures and a plastic stent in the MPD. The pancreatojejunostomy is completed with interrupted stitches placed between the seromuscular layer of the jejunum and the capsule of the pancreas using 4-0 absorbable monofilament sutures in both the posterior and anterior layers. End-to-side, two-layer jejunum–jejunum anastomosis, approximately 50 cm from the pancreatico-jejunum anastomosis, completes the reconstruction [12].

38.3.3 Resection of the Ventral or Uncinate Process of the Pancreas

Isolated resection of the ventral pancreas is reserved for benign or low-grade malignant tumors exclusively impacting the uncinate process. The preservation of maximal pancreatic parenchyma and the flow of normal pancreatic juice through the duct of Wirsung are the main benefits. In addition, the duodenum and the CBD are preserved, thereby avoiding digestive anastomoses and reducing the morbidity typically associated with extensive pancreatic resection.

Despite the clear advantages of this procedure, compared to PD, isolated resection of the uncinate process of the pancreatic is rarely reported in the literature as it is a complex operation that requires accurate knowledge of pancreatic anatomy [13]. The uncinate process of the pancreas is merged to the head, and its limits are not easy to identify, especially its upper margin, which maintains a close relationship with MPD which must be preserved. Usually, when using an open or laparoscopic approach, the use of intraoperative ultrasound can assist with the identification of the MPD. However, the MPD is frequently small and difficult to visualize. Therefore, intraoperative cholangiography is recommended in these situations.

In the absence of a gallbladder, the preoperative endoscopic placement of biliary and pancreatic plastic stents should be considered to facilitate the intraoperative identification of the CBD and MPD. The uncinate process is dissected away from the superior mesenteric vein on its left border; attention should be paid to the venous branches as they can cause massive bleeding if the dissection plain is inaccurate. In addition, in the lower and right limits of the uncinate process an arterial arcade, formed by the inferior pancreatic artery, is responsible for duodenal perfusion and must be preserved. The dissection plane should preserve the inferior pancreatic artery, while controlling its arterial branches attached to the uncinate process. While performing parenchymal transection, steps are taken to preserve the MPD.

38.3.4 Middle-Preserving Pancreatectomy

Many diseases manifest as multiple lesions in the pancreas, including IPMN, multiple endocrine neoplasia type I, von Hippel-Lindau syndrome, and metastatic pancreatic cancer. TP is currently regarded as the standard surgical treatment for multiple lesions involving the entire pancreas. However, pancreatic insufficiency after TP leads to complex glucose metabolism disorders and altered nutritional balance, significantly compromising postoperative QOL. The postoperative incidence of diabetes directly relates to the extent of pancreatic resection. Clinically, significant malabsorption does not occur until 85–90% of pancreatic enzyme output is lost. In terms of endocrine function, there is usually little change to glycemic control unless more than 80% of the pancreas is resected in patients with a previously normal pancreas. The pancreatic middle segment volume corresponds to approximately 25% of the entire gland, measured using computed tomography (CT)-based pancreatic volumetry. Theoretically, this implies that the use of MPP could preserve enough parenchyma to reduce the risk of the patient developing endocrine and exocrine insufficiency [14]. MPP also preserves the glucagon-secreting alpha cells in the pancreatic body, the loss of which is responsible for postoperative hypoglycemic episodes, a major challenge after TP.

The objective of performing MPP is to combine right resection of the head lesions with left resection of the body/tail lesions, while preserving the pancreatic body segment and its blood supply from the pancreatic dorsal artery. MPP can be performed either by simultaneous PD and SPLP or as a two-stage approach. First, the distal pancreatic parenchyma must be resected; if this margin is negative at the frozen section, selective suture ligation of the MPD must be performed on the transection plane on the raw surface of the distal remnant. Thereafter, a PD is performed, and the proximal margin of the body is checked by a second frozen section. MPP results in a pancreatojejunostomy and a blunt transection margin, which, has the potential to double the risk of PF developing. A high PF incidence may also be caused by ischemia of the pancreatic remnant. However, the limited use of MPP does not permit definitive conclusions to be drawn.

Other types of multiple pancreatic resections in the field of parenchyma-sparing surgery have been reported anecdotally (e.g., resection of the uncinate process combined with CP as well as head dorsal pancreatectomy combined with DP).

38.4 Conclusion

Recent advances in high-resolution multi-slice CT and magnetic resonance imaging for diagnosis and screening have resulted in the incidental discovery of many benign, low-grade, small-sized tumors of the pancreas in young and middle-aged patients with long life expectancy. In these patients, OPSPS could ensure a better QOL compared to conventional pancreatectomies. In experienced hands, both surgical strategies have a similar rate of low mortality. Instead, early morbidity is higher with OPSPS due to the high rate of PF. Nonetheless, most of these pancreatic leakage can be managed conservatively, and possible poor short-term outcomes are counterbalanced by the preservation of pancreatic endocrine and exocrine function.

Presently, OPSPS can be performed either by traditional open resection or using a minimally invasive approach [15]. Laparoscopic and robotic surgery achieves similar outcomes yielding lower blood loss, reduced operative time, shorter hospital stay, faster recovery, and reduced scarring. Although minimally invasive OPSPS requires a long learning curve, we believe its implementation will enables to perform increasingly complex resections, thereby ensuring enhanced outcomes.

OPSPS is technically demanding and requires specific surgical experience, so it is performed less frequently compared with conventional pancreatectomies, and it is mainly conducted mainly in specialized centers. Hopefully, increased confidence in the treatment of PF and improvements in pancreatic neoplasm natural history knowledge will encourage surgeons to preserve as much pancreatic parenchyma as possible. Careful case selection, accurate pre- and intraoperative evaluations of the lesions, and thorough knowledge of pancreas anatomy are recommended to obtain optimal results.

References

1. Beger HG, Poch B, Mayer B, Siech M. New onset of diabetes and pancreatic exocrine insufficiency after pancreaticoduodenectomy for benign and malignant tumors: a systematic review and meta-analysis of long-term results. In: Annals of surgery, vol. vol 267. Lippincott Williams and Wilkins; 2018. p. 259–70. https://doi.org/10.1097/SLA.0000000000002422.
2. De Bruijn KMJ, Van Eijck CHJ. New-onset diabetes after distal pancreatectomy: a systematic review. Ann Surg. 2015;261(5):854–61. https://doi.org/10.1097/SLA.0000000000000819.
3. Suda K, Nobukawa B, Takase M, Hayashi T. Pancreatic segmentation on an embryological and anatomical basis. J Hepato-Biliary-Pancreat Surg. 2006;13(2):146–8. https://doi.org/10.1007/s00534-005-1039-3.
4. Sauvanet A, Gaujoux S, Blanc B, et al. Parenchyma-sparing pancreatectomy for presumed noninvasive intraductal papillary mucinous neoplasms of the pancreas. Ann Surg. 2014;260(2):364–71. https://doi.org/10.1097/SLA.0000000000000601.
5. Yongfei H, Javed AA, Burkhart R, et al. Geographical variation and trends in outcomes of laparoscopic spleen-preserving distal pancreatectomy with or without splenic vessel preservation: a meta-analysis. Int J Surg. 2017;45:47–55. https://doi.org/10.1016/j.ijsu.2017.07.078.
6. Beger HG, Rau BM, Gansauge F, Poch B. Duodenum-preserving subtotal and total pancreatic head resections for inflammatory and cystic neoplastic lesions of the pancreas. J Gastrointest Surg. 2008;12(6):1127–32. https://doi.org/10.1007/s11605-008-0472-4.
7. Iacono C, Bortolasi L, Facci E, et al. The Dagradi-Serio-Iacono operation central pancreatectomy. J Gastrointest Surg. 2007;11(3):364–76. https://doi.org/10.1007/s11605-007-0095-1.
8. Iacono C, Ruzzenente A, Bortolasi L, Guglielmi A. Central pancreatectomy: the Dagradi Serio Iacono operation. Evolution of a surgical technique from the pioneers to the robotic approach. World J

Gastroenterol. 2014;20(42):15674–81. https://doi.org/10.3748/wjg.v20.i42.15674.
9. Wang ZZ, Zhao GD, Zhao ZM, et al. An end-to-end pancreatic anastomosis in robotic central pancreatectomy. World J Surg Oncol. 2019;17(1):1–8. https://doi.org/10.1186/s12957-019-1609-5.
10. Iacono C, Verlato G, Ruzzenente A, et al. Systematic review of central pancreatectomy and meta-analysis of central versus distal pancreatectomy. Br J Surg. 2013;100(7):873–85. https://doi.org/10.1002/bjs.9136.
11. Conci S, Ruzzenente A, Bertuzzo F, Campagnaro T, Guglielmi A, Iacono C. Total dorsal pancreatectomy, an alternative to total pancreatectomy: report of a new case and literature review. Dig Surg. 2019;36(5):363–8. https://doi.org/10.1159/000490198.
12. Iacono C, Ruzzenente A, Conci S, Xillo L, Guglielmi A. Head dorsal pancreatectomy: an alternative to the pancreaticoduodenectomy for not enucleable benign or low-grade malignant lesions. Pancreatology. 2014;14(5):419–24. https://doi.org/10.1016/j.pan.2014.07.014.
13. Machado MAC, Surjan R, Basseres T, Makdissi F. Robotic resection of the uncinate process of the pancreas. J Robot Surg. 2019;13(5):699–702. https://doi.org/10.1007/s11701-018-0898-y.
14. Okano K, Murakami Y, Nakagawa N, et al. Remnant pancreatic parenchymal volume predicts postoperative pancreatic exocrine insufficiency after pancreatectomy. Surgery (United States). 2016;159(3):885–92. https://doi.org/10.1016/j.surg.2015.08.046.
15. Kuroki T, Eguchi S. Laparoscopic parenchyma-sparing pancreatectomy. J Hepatobiliary Pancreat Sci. 2014;21(5):323–7. https://doi.org/10.1002/jhbp.29.

# Isolated Pancreatoduodenectomy with Portal Vein Resection Using the Nakao Mesenteric Approach

Akimasa Nakao

Abstract

The ideal surgical approach for pancreatic head cancer is isolated pancreatoduodenectomy (PD); that is, en bloc resection using non-touch isolation technique. However, this approach is difficult because of the complex peripancreatic vascular anatomy. In 1981, we developed an antithrombogenic bypass catheter for the portal vein (PV) to prevent portal congestion or hepatic ischemia during PV resection and facilitate simultaneous resection of the hepatic artery. In 1992, we developed a mesenteric approach for PD. The mesenteric approach allows dissection from the non-cancer infiltrating side and determination of cancer-free surgical margins and resectability, followed by systematic lymphadenectomy around the superior mesenteric artery. This approach enables early ligation of the inferior pancreatoduodenal artery and excision of the second portion of pancreatic head nerve plexus. Through this development of the mesenteric approach and antithrombogenic catheter-bypass procedure of the PV, establishment of isolated PD was completed in 1992. This is the ideal surgery for pancreatic head cancer from both surgical and oncological viewpoints. The precise surgical techniques of isolated PD, using the Nakao mesenteric approach are herein introduced.

39.1 Introduction

The ideal surgical approach for cancer in the head of the pancreas is isolated pancreatoduodenectomy (PD); that is, en-bloc resecstion using a non-touch isolation technique. However, this approach is difficult because of the complex peripancreatic vascular anatomy. PD combined with portal vein (PV) resection is sometimes necessary to complete curative surgery for cancer in the head of the pancreas.

In 1981, we developed an antithrombogenic bypass catheter for the PV to prevent portal congestion during resection and reconstruction [1–5]. This was accomplished by bypassing portal blood through a branch of the superior mesenteric vein (SMV), either to the femoral vein or the intrahepatic PV through the umbilical vein in the hepatic round ligament, preventing both portal congestion and hepatic ischemia during simultaneous resection and reconstruction of the PV and hepatic artery. This method circumvented the time constraints on portal occlusion during surgery. We have since successfully resected pancreatic cancer with portal invasion using PV catheter bypass [6–9].

Typically, the first step in PD is Kocher's maneuver [10]. When we first performed PD combined with PV resection in the 1980s, Kocher's maneuver was routinely used as the first step in PD. However, pancreatic cancer with PV obstruction and well-developed collateral veins is sometimes observed when resecting such cancer using Kocher's maneuver, and massive bleeding was observed, even when PV catheter bypass was applied. We noticed that the first step in PD is clearance of the mesenteric root instead of Kocher's maneuver. Thus, we named this procedure the "mesenteric approach" and non-touch isolation PD isolated PD [11–20].

In cancer surgery, the term "isolated" refers to en-bloc resection using a non-touch isolation technique. In PD, all arteries that supply the pancreatic head and all drainage veins in this region are ligated and divided before manipulation of cancer in the pancreatic head.

The first step we take when performing PD is the mesenteric approach; we do not perform Kocher's maneuver. The mesenteric approach involves clearing the connective tissues around the SMV and superior mesenteric artery (SMA) in the mesenteric root, which includes systematic lymphadenectomy around the SMA [21]. Resection starts from the non-cancerous side and cancer-free surgical margin, and

A. Nakao (✉)
Professor Emeritus, Nagoya University, Nagoya, Japan

Nagoya Central Hospital, Nagoya, Japan

Department of surgery, Nagoya Central Hospital, Nagoya, Japan
e-mail: akimasa.nakao@jr-central.co.jp

resectability can be diagnosed at the beginning of surgery. The inferior pancreatoduodenal artery (IPDA), which arises from the SMA, is first ligated and divided; thus, it is an artery-first operation. This approach makes it possible to perform total excision of the mesopancreas [22]; in other words, the second portion of the pancreatic head nerve plexus (PLph II) is completely excised, which is the so-called SMA margin [23]. This is the most important technique with which to obtain a cancer-free surgical margin in PD for cancer in the pancreatic head. The mesenteric approach also makes it easy to reconstruct the PV using an end-to-end anastomosis after PV resection.

The development of PV catheter bypass and the mesenteric approach have made it possible to easily and safely perform isolated PD with PV resection.

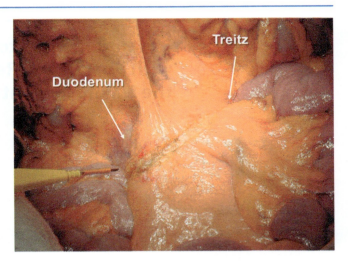

Fig. 39.1 Mesenteric incision from the Treitz ligament to the lower border of the second portion of the duodenum

39.2 Surgical Techniques Used in the Nakao Mesenteric Approach

39.2.1 Laparotomy

Laparotomy is performed with an upper midline skin incision. The abdominal cavity is examined by washing cytology and ultrasound.

39.2.2 Supramesocolic Approach

The supramesocolic approach is usually indicated for cancer of the distal bile duct or the duodenal papilla of Vater. After laparotomy via an upper midline skin incision, the gastrocolic ligament is divided and the lesser peritoneal cavity is opened. The middle colic artery (MCA) and middle colic vein (MCV) are visible on the anterior surface of the mesocolon. The SMV and SMA are exposed along the roots of the MCV and MCA. The SMV and SMA are then taped. The connective tissues, including the lymph nodes along the SMA, are dissected. The first jejunal artery (JA1) and the IPDA are exposed in this procedure. Preoperative multidetector computed tomography is very important to detect the location of the IPDA. Total mesopancreas excision is usually unnecessary for cancer of the distal bile duct or papilla of Vater. The supramesocolic mesenteric approach makes it easy to perform systematic lymph node dissection around the SMA and to achieve early ligation of the IPDA.

39.2.3 Inframesocolic Approach

The inframesocolic approach is usually indicated for ductal adenocarcinoma of the pancreatic head. This is the typical Nakao mesenteric approach.

39.3 Mesenteric Incision

The first step in isolated PD is the mesenteric approach, and the first step of the mesenteric approach is incision of the mesentery from the ligament of Treitz to the lower border of the second portion of the duodenum using electrocautery (Fig. 39.1). The surface of the mesentery is incised until the anterior walls of the SMV and SMA are exposed. With this approach, Kocher's maneuver is not performed.

39.4 Connective Tissue Clearance around the SMV and SMA

All of the connective tissues, including the lymph nodes around the SMV and SMA (No. 14d lymph nodes) [23], are dissected to the lower border of the pancreatic head (Fig. 39.2). If no cancer invasion of the PLph II is observed, the nerve plexus around the SMA (PLsma) is completely preserved to avoid severe postoperative diarrhea (Fig. 39.2). If cancer invasion into the PLph II or the PLsma is detected, the PLsma is resected together with the PLph II to obtain a cancer-free surgical margin. If it is difficult or impossible to obtain cancer-free surgical margins, radical resection is terminated. Radical resection is also terminated when reconstruction of the SMV is determined impossible because of severe cancer invasion into the peripheral branches of the SMV.

39.5 Division of the MCA and MCV

The MCA and MCV are exposed on the anterior side of the SMA and SMV. They are generally ligated and divided at the root. This makes it easier to perform connective tissue clear-

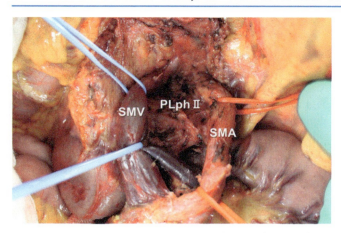

Fig. 39.2 Connective tissue clearance around the SMV and SMA. The PLph II between the uncinate process and the SMA is exposed. *SMA* superior mesenteric artery, *SMV* superior mesenteric vein, *PLph II* second portion of the pancreatic head nerve plexus

ance around the root of the SMA (No. 14 lymph nodes) compared with preservation of the MCA and MCV.

39.6 Division of the Gastrocolic Ligament and Incision of the Mesocolon

The gastrocolic ligament is incised near the transverse colon and the lesser abdominal cavity is opened. The mesocolon can therefore be examined from both the anterior and posterior sides, and the anterior surface of the pancreas can be visualized.

The root of the mesocolon is horizontally incised and resected, preserving the arcade of the MCA. Generally, no ischemic changes occur in the transverse colon when the arcade of the MCA is preserved. This makes it easier and safer to perform connective tissue clearance around the root of the SMA through the large opening in the mesocolon.

39.7 Connective Tissue Clearance Around the Root of the SMA and Exposure of the Mesopancreas (PLph II)

Connective tissue clearance around the SMV and SMA proceeds to the roots of the SMV and SMA. All connective tissues of the mesenteric root are dissected, including the lymph nodes (No. 14d, p lymph nodes). The PLsma is preserved if cancer invasion to the PLph II or PLsma is not observed. The mesopancreas is exposed between the uncinate process of the pancreatic head and the SMA (Fig. 39.2).

The term "mesopancreas" was first used in 2007 by Gockel et al. [22] However, there is no precise anatomical definition for the mesopancreas. In the Japanese classification of pancreatic cancer [23, 24], extrapancreatic nerve plexus anatomy is precisely described. I propose that "mesopancreas" refers to the PLph II. During radical PD for cancer of the pancreatic head, the first portion of the pancreatic head nerve plexus (PLph I) and the PLph II are completely excised using the mesenteric approach.

39.8 Exposure of the Jejunal Arteries and the IPDA and Total Mesopancreas Excision

The first and second branches of the jejunal artery generally reside behind the SMA. The IPDA is usually a branch of the JA1 and lies within the region of the PLph II. There are many anatomical variations of the IPDA. Ligation and division of the IPDA (Fig. 39.3) and total excision of the PLph II (Fig. 39.4) from the attachment of the SMA complete the mesenteric approach; in other words, total excision of the mesopancreas is accomplished. Early ligation of the dorsal pancreatic artery from the SMA also reduces intraoperative bleeding [25]. In patients with locally advanced cancer, excision of the JA1, the second branches of the jejunal artery, and total excision of PLsma may be necessary. If it is difficult to expose the IPDA or JA1 using the mesenteric approach, these vessels can be exposed by dividing the pancreas along

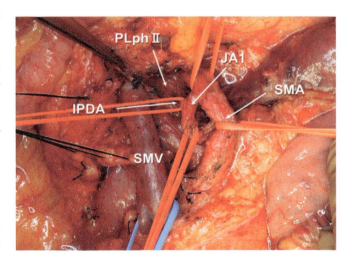

Fig. 39.3 Exposure of the IPDA in the PLph II. *SMA* superior mesenteric artery, *SMV* superior mesenteric vein, *PLph II* second portion of the pancreatic head nerve plexus, *JA1* first jejunal artery, *IPDA* inferior pancreatoduodenal artery

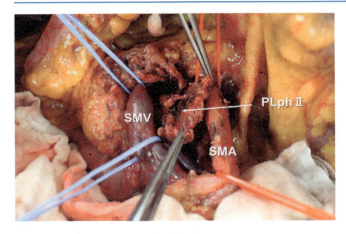

Fig. 39.4 Excision of the PLph II and completion of the mesenteric approach. *PLph II* second portion of the pancreatic head nerve plexus, *SMA* superior mesenteric artery, *SMV* superior mesenteric vein

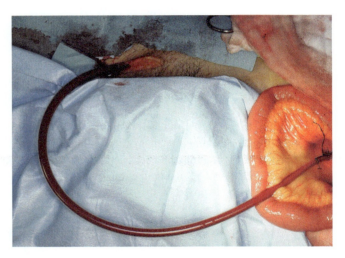

Fig. 39.5 Portal vein catheter bypass between a branch of the superior mesenteric vein and the femoral vein

the line of the SMA because the root of the SMA can be visualized easily. The mesenteric approach is completed using these procedures (Fig. 39.4).

39.9 Antithrombogenic PV Catheter Bypass

When resection and reconstruction of the PV and SMV are possible even if the PV and SMV are severely stenosed or obstructed due to cancer invasion, the antithrombogenic PV catheter bypass procedure can be applied to reduce PV congestion and operative bleeding (Fig. 39.5). When it will be time-consuming to resect and reconstruct the PV and the SMV during surgery. The catheter bypass procedure is a good indication.

39.10 Typical Procedures After the Mesenteric Approach to Perform Isolated PD

After completion of the mesenteric approach, the operative field moves to the hepatic hilum. The gallbladder is resected along with the common hepatic duct. Clearance of the hepatoduodenal ligament and lymph nodes (No. 12a, b, p) is performed, and the gastroduodenal artery is ligated and divided. The stomach is divided at the pre-pylorus, and lymph node dissection around the common hepatic artery (CHA; No. 8a, p) and celiac artery (No. 9) is performed. The dorsal pancreatic artery from the CHA, celiac artery, or splenic artery is ligated and divided by these lymph node dissection procedures [24]. The PLph I is also dissected.

39.11 Portal Vein Resection and Reconstruction

If cancer invasion into the PV or SMV is observed, the PV or SMV can be resected and reconstructed. End-to-end anastomosis in portal reconstruction is easily performed by the mesenteric approach without tension. During resection of the SMV–PV confluence, splenic vein reconstruction is generally unnecessary and left gastric vein preservation is very important to reduce left-sided portal hypertension [26, 27] (Fig. 39.6). Simultaneous resection of the PV and CHA can be performed safely using PV catheter bypass. When we use antithrombogenic PV catheter bypass, the catheter is

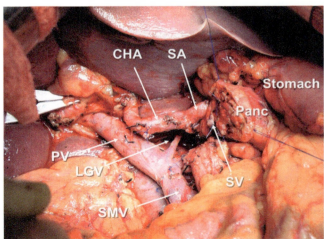

Fig. 39.6 Resection of the SMV–PV confluence and end-to-end anastomosis between the PV and SMV. The SV was not reconstructed. The LGV was preserved in this case to reduce left-sided portal hypertension. *LGV* left gastric vein, *PV* portal vein, *SMV* superior mesenteric vein, *SV* splenic vein, *CHA* common hepatic artery, *SA* splenic artery, *Panc* pancreas

extracted after vascular reconstruction. These procedures conclude isolated PD with the mesenteric approach.

39.12 Reconstruction of the Alimentary Canal

After completion of isolated PD, alimentary tract reconstruction is performed.

39.13 Discussion

Previously, Kocher's maneuver was the first step in PD. Based on our extensive experience with vascular resection using antithrombogenic PV catheter bypass in PD [1–5], we developed a mesenteric approach [11, 12]. In our opinion, isolated PD using this mesenteric approach and antithrombogenic PV catheter bypass is the ideal surgery to treat cancer of the pancreatic head from both surgical and oncological viewpoints.

No randomized controlled trials have compared the surgical and oncological merits of the Nakao mesenteric approach with Kocher's conventional approach to PD. However, in patients with resectable cancer of the pancreatic head, isolated PD using the Nakao mesenteric approach is suspected to result in higher survival compared with conventional PD using Kocher's maneuver [28]. Therefore, a randomized controlled trial is being undertaken in Japan to compare the surgical and oncological benefits of these two procedures [29].

The mesenteric approach allows dissection from the non-cancer-infiltrated side and initial determination of cancer-free margins and resectability, followed by systematic lymphadenectomy around the SMA [21]. This approach also enables early ligation of the IPDA, which reduces venous congestion in the pancreatic head along with ligation of the gastroduodenal artery and total mesopancreas excision, which makes it an artery-first operation.

The term "mesopancreas" has no precise anatomical definition [22]. We propose that the mesopancreas can be defined as the PLph II according to the classification of pancreatic carcinoma described by the Japan Pancreas Society [23, 24]. Additionally, it is better to use the PLph I or PLph II instead of the mesopancreas.

Compared with the recent developments in chemotherapy and chemoradiotherapy for pancreatic cancer, conversion surgery for unresectable locally advanced pancreatic cancer has been indicated for some time. The mesenteric approach and PV catheter bypass are essential techniques in conversion surgery. The Nakao mesenteric approach has been gradually adapted throughout Japan. By mastering this mesenteric approach and PV catheter bypass, surgeons can successfully perform isolated PD.

References

1. Nakao A, Horisawa M, Suenaga M, et al. Temporal portosystemic bypass with the use of the heparinized hydrophilic catheter. Jpn J Artif Organs. 1982;11:962–5. (In Japanese with English abstract)
2. Nakao A, Hirosawa M, Kondo T, et al. Total pancreatectomy accompanied by portal vein resection using catheter–bypass of the portal vein. Shujutsu (Operation). 1983;37:1–6. (In Japanese)
3. Nakao A, Kondo T. New technique of radical pancreatectomy with the use of the heparinized hydrophilic bypass catheter of the portal vein. Jpn J Artif Organs. 1983;12:697–700. (In Japanese with English abstract)
4. Nakao A, Kano T, Nonami T, et al. Application of an antithrombogenic Anthron bypass tube to experimental orthotopic liver transplantation. Studies on blood coagulation and fibrinolysis. ASAIO Trans. 1986;32:503–7.
5. Nakao A, Nonami T, Harada A, Kasuga T, Takagi H. Portal vein resection with a new antithrombogenic catheter. Surgery. 1990;108:913–8.
6. Nakao A, Harada A, Nonami T, Takagi H. Clinical experience of 107 cases with portal vein resection using catheter bypass of the portal vein. Artif Organs Today. 1993;3:107–12.
7. Nakao A, Harada A, Nonami T, Kaneko T, Inoue S, Takagi H. Clinical significance of portal invasion by pancreatic head carcinoma. Surgery. 1995;117:50–5.
8. Nakao A, Harada A, Nonami T, Kaneko T, Takagi H. Regional vascular resection using catheter bypass procedure for pancreatic cancer. Hepato-Gastroenterology. 1995;42:734–9.
9. Nakao A, Kanzaki A, Fujii T, et al. Correlation between radiographic classification and pathological grade of portal vein wall invasion in pancreatic head cancer. Ann Surg. 2012;255:103–8.
10. Kocher T. Mobilisierung des duodenum und gastroduodenostomie. Zentralbl Chir. 1903;2:33–40. (In German)
11. Nakao A, Takagi H. Pancreatoduodenectomy, non-touch isolation technique using catheter-bypass of the portal vein and Imanaga method. Shujutsu (Operation). 1992;46:1457–63. (In Japanese)
12. Nakao A, Takagi H. Isolated pancreatectomy for pancreatic head carcinoma using catheter bypass of the portal vein. Hepato-Gastroenterology. 1993;40:426–9.
13. Nakao A, Takeda S, Inoue S, et al. Indications and techniques of extended resection for pancreatic cancer. World J Surg. 2006;30:976–82.
14. Nakao A. Selection and outcome of portal vein resection in pancreatic cancer. Cancers. 2010;2010:1990–2000.
15. Nakao A. Isolated pancreatoduodenectomy combined with portal vein resection. In: Nakao A, editor. Isolated pancreatoduodenectomy. Nagoya: Takeda Printing; 2014. p. 3–11.
16. Nakao A. Extended resection for pancreatic cancer: risks and benefits. In: Beger HG, Nakao A, Neoptolemos JP, Peng SY, Sarr MG, editors. Pancreatic cancer, cystic neoplasms and endocrine tumors: diagnosis and management. Oxford: Wiley-Blackwell; 2015. p. 47–53.
17. Nakao A. The mesenteric approach in pancreatoduodenectomy. Dig Surg. 2016;33:308–13.
18. Nakao A. Mesenteric approach in pancreatoduodenectomy. J Digestive Cancer Report. 2016;4:77–82.
19. Nakao A. Concepts in isolated pancreatectomy for pancreatic cancer using Nakao mesenteric approach and catheter bypass of the portal vein. In: Kim SW, Yamaue H, editors. Pancreatic cancer: with special focus on topical issue and surgical techniques. Springer; 2017. p. 225–30.
20. Nakao A. Nakao mesenteric approach in pancreatotduodenectomy for pancreatic head cancer. J Pnactreatol. 2019;2:117–22.

21. Nakao A, Harada A, Nonami T, Kaneko T, Murakami H, Inoue S, et al. Lymph node metastases in carcinoma of the head of the pancreas region. Br J Surg. 1995;82:399–402.
22. Gockel I, Domeyer M, Wolloscheck T, Konerding MA, Junginger T. Resection of the mesopancreas (RMP): a new surgical classification of a known anatomical space. World J Surg Oncol. 2007;5:44.
23. Japan Pancreas Society. Classification of pancreatic carcinoma. 3rd English ed. Tokyo: Kanehara; 2011.
24. Yoshioka H, Wakabayashi T. Therapeutic neurotomy on head of pancreas for relief of pain due to chronic pancreatitis: a new technical procedure and its results. Arch Surg. 1958;76:546–54.
25. Iede K, Nakao A, Oshima K, et al. Early ligation of the dorsal pancreatic artery with a mesenteric approach reduces intraoperative blood loss during pancreatoduodenectomy. J Hepatobiliary Pancreatic Sci. 2018;25:329–34.
26. Tanaka H, Nakao A, Oshima, et al. Splenic vein reconstruction is unnecessary in pancreatoduodenectomy combined with resection of the superior mesenteric vein-portal vein confluence according to short-term outcomes. HPB. 2017;19(9):785–92.
27. Nakao A, Yamada S, Fujii T, et al. Gastric venous congestion and bleeding in association with total pancreatectomy. J Hepatobiliary Pancreatic Sci. 2018;25:150–4.
28. Hirono S, Kawai M, Okada K, et al. Mesenteric approach during pancreaticoduodenectomy for pancreatic ductal adenocarcinoma. Ann Gastroenterol Surg. 2017;1:208–18.
29. MAPLE –PD trial: mesenteric approach vs. conventional approach for pancreatic cancer during pancreaticoduodenectomy. UMIN000029615.

Pancreaticoduodenectomy with Hepatic Artery Resection

Atsushi Oba, Tomotaka Kato, Marco Del Chiaro, Y. H. Andrew Wu, Yosuke Inoue, and Yu Takahashi

Abstract

With the development of novel and effective multidrug chemotherapy, several pancreatic centers have reported that the combination of preoperative chemotherapy and arterial resection can provide a favorable long-term prognosis for T4-stage (i.e., major artery infiltration) pancreatic cancer (PC) patients. A recent nomogram formulated to predict the post-resection prognosis of PC found that neoadjuvant treatment was an independent prognostic factor, whereas T4 stage was not a factor of poor prognosis. This implies that systemic control is the most important factor for improving the prognosis of PC and local progression has less impact on the prognosis in the era of useful multidrug regimens. However, even if favorable control of PC is achieved with neoadjuvant chemotherapy, pancreatectomy with hepatic artery (HA) resection is technically challenging. This approach requires a high expertise that is characterized with detailed preoperative image preparation, planning several options of HA reconstruction, meticulous intraoperative resection, and appropriate postoperative management. This chapter examines the innovative surgical approach and management in the pancreaticoduodenectomy with HA resection and reconstruction.

40.1 Introduction

T4-stage pancreatic cancer (PC) implies a tumor that involves the hepatic artery (HA), superior mesenteric artery (SMA), or the celiac axis and is classified as "unresectable" or "locally advanced" PC (LAPC) according to the National Comprehensive Cancer Network guidelines [1, 2]. Despite the challenges of some excellent surgeons including Dr. Fortner, the outcomes after resection were poor when surgery was initially performed on these tumors [3, 4]. However, in recent years, with the advent of novel and effective multidrug chemotherapy, several high-volume centers have reported that the combination of preoperative chemotherapy and arterial resection can provide a favorable long-term prognosis for the T4-stage PC patients [5–9]. In addition, a recently reported National-Cancer-Database-based study that predict the post-resection prognosis of PC found that neoadjuvant treatment was an independent prognostic factor, whereas T4 stage was not a factor of poor prognosis [10]. The results of this study, which was limited by a relatively new cohort starting in 2010, suggest that in the era of useful multidrug regimens, systemic control is of paramount importance for improving the prognosis of PC after resection and that local progression has less impact on prognosis [10].

Even if favorable control of PC is achieved with preoperative chemotherapy, pancreatectomy with arterial resection is technically challenging [11]. In particular, HA and SMA reconstructions are critical and can be life-threatening. These procedures require careful perioperative management and needs to be performed at an institution with adequate experience. In this chapter, we will introduce our innovative surgical approach and management in the pancreaticoduodenectomy (PD) with HA resection and reconstruction.

A. Oba (✉)
Division of Hepatobiliary and Pancreatic Surgery, Cancer Institute Hospital, Japanese Foundation for Cancer Research, Tokyo, Japan

Division of Surgical Oncology, Department of Surgery, University of Colorado, Anschutz Medical Campus, Denver, CO, USA
e-mail: atsushi.oba@jfcr.or.jp

T. Kato · Y. Inoue · Y. Takahashi
Division of Hepatobiliary and Pancreatic Surgery, Cancer Institute Hospital, Japanese Foundation for Cancer Research, Tokyo, Japan

M. Del Chiaro · Y. H. A. Wu
Division of Surgical Oncology, Department of Surgery, University of Colorado, Anschutz Medical Campus, Denver, CO, USA

40.2 Indication and Preparation

Tumors located at the head or neck of the pancreas that contact or invade the HA at 180 degrees or more are eligible for the preparation for PD with HA resection. After giving enough neoadjuvant treatment for a borderline resectable PC or LAPC based on the institutional strategy [12, 13], multidetector Computed Tomography (MDCT), magnetic resonance imaging, positron emission tomography-CT, preoperative blood testing, including tumor markers, (and, if necessary for high-risk PC, staging laparoscopy) need to be performed to evaluate the current status and biology of the tumor [14, 15]. Due to invasive surgery, conditional factors including neutrophil-to-lymphocyte ratio, modified Glasgow prognostic score (a combination of C-reactive protein and albumin levels), or Charlson-Dayo-Comorbidity-index could also be utilized to evaluate the indication of resection [10, 16]. A detailed understanding of the anatomy of abdomen on MDCT is of utmost importance. Preoperative sketching of the anatomy is highly recommended to check arterial and venous branching anatomy and vascular anomalies. If transposition of artery (i.e., middle colic artery [MCA], gastroduodenal artery [GDA], splenic artery [SpA], or left gastric artery, etc.) or autologous vein graft (i.e., internal jugular vein, saphenous vein, left renal vein or external iliac vein, etc.) is considered as an option for HA reconstruction, the anatomy and vessel diameters of these vessels must be recognized preoperatively [17–19].

40.3 The Dissection or Resection of HA

Resection for PC that involves major vessels is challenging. The procedure is often complicated with increased intraoperative blood loss and longer operative time due to the tumor invasion of organs such as the mesentery, colon, vena cava, the development of cavernous transformation or left-side collaterals [20, 21]. Minimal blood loss can be achieved with precise dissection. Several high-volume centers have recently reported good short-term results with the artery first approach [22–24]. The HA and super mesenteric vein (SMV)/portal vein (PV) are vital for the liver's blood supply and are only cut and reconstructed at the end of the resection. The key to safely complete PD with arterial reconstruction is dissecting out the tissue around the SMA or pancreas and completing the resection promptly with minimal blood loss.

Inoue et al. recently classified the extent of HA dissection during PD into three levels: Level 1 (lymph node and plexus dissection is not required for the case such as benign disease or low-grade malignancy); Level 2 (*en bloc* lymph nodes dissection preserving the nerve plexus around HA for the malignancy case without the involvement around HA); and Level 3 (*en bloc* dissection of lymph nodes and the nerve plexus close to tumor invasion). Level 3 dissection is planned for PCs that contact or invade HA [25]. The adventitia of the common HA root and that of the peripheral branches (the right or left HA, or proper HA) needs to be exposed and taped. The nerve plexus is peeled off circumferentially from both proximal and peripheral sides toward the common HA close to the tumor. When a solid invasion of the artery is encountered, dissection needs to be terminated immediately, and the dissected nerve plexus closest to the tumor needs to be taken for intraoperative frozen section to confirm negative for cancer. After completing other PD procedures, HA resection and reconstruction can be performed where it is confirmed to be negative for cancer.

Many experienced institutions that actively perform arterial reconstruction often question whether periadventitial dissection (PAD) or pancreatectomy with arterial resection (PAR) is a better procedure for approaching the border between the tumor infiltration and the adventitia of the artery [5, 26]. Loos et al. from Heidelberg group evaluated 190 patients with PAD and 195 patients with PAR (including 102 patients with HA resection; 52.3%) for LAPC. Although the patients with PAR had more advanced PC that is characterized with higher rate of lymph node positivity and lower rate of neoadjuvant chemotherapy induction, PAD was associated with lower morbidity and mortality after resection and more favorable long-term prognosis [5]. Based on these results, they concluded PAD may be the first choice for LAPC patients with arterial involvement after neoadjuvant chemotherapy and if PAD was not technically feasible, PAR can be performed in experienced centers. Although it is difficult to conclude whether PAD or PAR is better due to the possible selection bias in this retrospective study in which PAD was performed whenever possible, it must be recognized that arterial reconstruction is a hurdle in surgery.

40.4 HA Reconstruction

40.4.1 Simple Reconstruction Case

If a curative resection cannot be performed by sharp dissection along HA's periadventitial layer, HA reconstruction can be performed. In most cases, the tumor may infiltrate the root of the GDA. The most optimal approach in these situations is to resect a short segment of HA around the root of the GDA and perform a direct end-to-end anastomosis of the common HA with the proper HA (Fig. 40.1). With the dissection of PD and that of HA, the central and peripheral sides of HA is clamped by the small vascular clip, respectively, and cut with sharp scissors, and the specimen is extracted. End-to-end microvascular anastomosis of the common HA and the

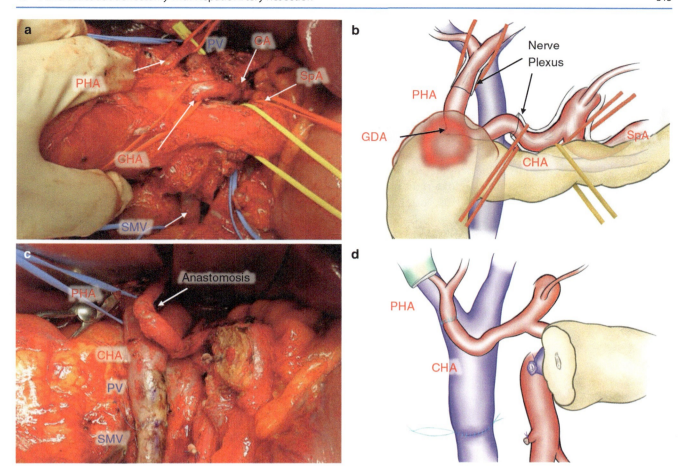

Fig. 40.1 Simple reconstruction case. (**a** and **b**) A tumor infiltrating the common hepatic artery (CHA) and the proper hepatic artery (PHA) around the root of the gastric duodenal artery (GDA). The adventitia of the CHA and the PHA were exposed and taped. The nerve plexus was peeled off circumferentially toward the HA close to the tumor. When a solid invasion of the artery was encountered, dissection was terminated. The dissected nerve plexus closest to the tumor was taken for intraoperative frozen section to confirm negative for cancer. (**c** and **d**) The CHA and the PHA were clamped by the small vascular clip, respectively, and cut with sharp scissors, and the specimen was extracted. End-to-end microvascular anastomosis of the CHA and the PHA was performed with interrupted sutures. *CA* celiac axis, *SpA* splenic artery, *PV* portal vein, *SMV* superior mesenteric vein

proper HA is performed with interrupted 9-0 (or 8-0) Polypropylene sutures. After reconstruction, HA blood flow is checked with Doppler ultrasonography and palpation.

40.4.2 Complicated Reconstruction Case

Although the above method to perform direct end-to-end anastomosis for HA could achieve unanimous agreement according to current literature [5, 9, 18], in a case wherein it is not feasible due to longer defect or resected root of HA, we have to consider other ways to reconstruct the HA. Transposition of artery (MCA, GDA, SpA, etc), autologous artery/vein graft, artificial graft (polytetrafluoroethylene or polyethylene terephthalate), or cryopreserved homologous vessels are considered as an option for HA reconstruction, but the risk of anastomotic bleeding, infection, and obstruction due to exposure to postoperative pancreatic fistula (POPF) should be well recognized [7, 17–19]. Del Chiaro et al. actively adopt total pancreatectomy in such cases to avoid the risk of POPF and arterial anastomotic problems after resection. In this sense, the use of SpA for HA reconstruction and total pancreatectomy is highly applicable [19, 27, 28]. However, for the institutions where total pancreatectomy is avoided whenever possible in consideration of the risk of decreased quality of life and postoperative insulin dependence, the usage of SpA is not a priority due to preservation of the distal pancreas and the spleen [28].

In contrast, transposition of other arteries is highly promoted due to its high patency rate and simplicity of procedure [18]. As we have introduced the new procedure of distal pancreatectomy with celiac axis resection and left gastric artery reconstruction, we are also actively using MCA for HA reconstruction [8, 29]. Figure 40.2 shows the representative case of HA and MCA reconstruction. Exposure of the proper HA was not feasible as the tumor has extended to the right HA and left HA. In response, right HA-MCA reconstruction was planned, and the MCA was exposed before HA resection. The root of the MCA and the bifurcation of the right and left branches within the transverse mesocolon should be thoroughly identified. The MCA needed to be dissected carefully to avoid injury to the marginal arterial arcade of transvers colon. In most of the time, the right branch of MCA is suitable for reconstruction for its vessel diameter and ability to achieve tension-free anastomosis. The right branch of MCA was clamped temporarily, and the arterial blood flow of the arcade was checked by palpation (indocyanine green-fluorescence imaging can be done in unsure situations) [29]. After prompt extraction of the specimen and the direct end-to-end anastomosis of PV and SMV, the MCA was cut and reconstructed to the right HA by end-to-end microvascular anastomosis with interrupted 9-0 Polypropylene sutures. Although some surgeons demonstrated that the left HA can be sacrificed if the right HA blood flow and intrahepatic blood flow between both right and left lobes were sufficient [18], we prefer reconstructing the left HA whenever possible to avoid postoperative liver abscess complications. In this case, the right inferior phrenic artery was exposed and reconstructed to the left HA (segment 2 and 3 artery). Doppler ultrasonography showed a better arterial pulse on the left-side intrahepatic artery after the reconstruction of the left HA. Concomitant left lateral sectionectomy can also be performed as an alternative option.

40.4.3 Concomitant Vein Resection

Since PC is more likely to invade the PV/SMV, many cases of HA reconstruction require concomitant vein resection and reconstruction. To minimize the total liver ischemic period,

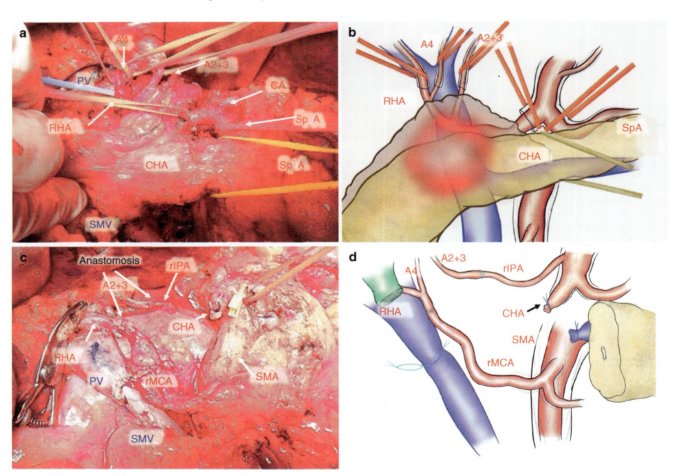

Fig. 40.2 Complicated reconstruction case. (**a** and **b**) Exposure of the PHA was not feasible as a tumor infiltrating the right HA (RHA) and the left HA (LHA). (**c** and **d**) The right branch of the middle colic artery (rMCA) was dissected and RHA—rMCA reconstruction was performed. We prefer reconstructing the LHA whenever possible to avoid postoperative liver abscess complications. In this case, the right inferior phrenic artery (rIPA) was exposed and reconstructed to the LHA (segment 2 and 3 artery [A2+3]). Doppler ultrasonography showed a better arterial pulse on the left-side intrahepatic artery after the LHA reconstruction. *A4* segment 4 artery, *SMA* superior mesenteric artery

either HA reconstruction or PV reconstruction could be performed prior to the extraction of the specimen whenever possible. At this time point, it is important to complete the dissection of the pancreas, relevant organs, lymph nodes, and peripancreatic nerve plexus, except for the HAs and PV/SMV. Cattell-Braasch Maneuver and the resection of portomesenterico-splenic confluence could also be used to achieve tension-free anastomosis [30, 31].

40.4.4 Management after HA Reconstruction

Doppler ultrasonography and blood tests need to be routinely performed within the first 3 postoperative days to detect possible thrombotic complications promptly. If there are any signs or concerns of liver problem, MDCT is immediately performed. Antiplatelet or anticoagulation therapy has rarely been used.

40.5 Conclusions

The recommendations for HA reconstruction were presented. Detailed preoperative image preparation, planning of several options of HA reconstruction, precise intraoperative resection, and postoperative Doppler ultrasonography are necessary. Although there are promising reports from limited centers, the technique of PD with HA resection and reconstruction requires higher expertise [5, 7, 9, 18]. With the advancement of chemotherapy and the increase in the number of PC patients, HA reconstruction will be required in many cases in the near future. It is important to accumulate experience, share observations, and improve the techniques through international and multicenter collaborations.

Declaration of Interests Dr. Del Chiaro has received grants from Haemonetics, Inc., and is the principal investigator of the study sponsored by Boston Scientific, which is not directly associated with the submitted work. The remaining authors have declared no competing interests.

References

1. Tempero MA, Malafa MP, Al-Hawary M, Asbun H, Bain A, Behrman SW, et al. Pancreatic adenocarcinoma, version 2.2017, NCCN clinical practice guidelines in oncology. J Natl Compr Cancer Netw. 2017;15(8):1028–61.
2. NCCN clinical practice guidelines in oncology: pancreatic adenocarcinoma, version 1.2020. 2020.
3. Fortner JG, Kim DK, Cubilla A, Turnbull A, Pahnke LD, Shils ME. Regional pancreatectomy: en bloc pancreatic, portal vein and lymph node resection. Ann Surg. 1977;186(1):42–50.
4. Oba A, Bao QR, Barnett CC, Al-Musawi MH, Croce C, Schulick RD, et al. Vascular resections for pancreatic ductal adenocarcinoma: vascular resections for PDAC. Scand J Surg. 2020;109(1):18–28.
5. Loos M, Kester T, Klaiber U, Mihaljevic AL, Mehrabi A, Muller-Stich BM, et al. Arterial resection in pancreatic cancer surgery: effective after a learning curve. Ann Surg. 2020; https://doi.org/10.1097/SLA.0000000000004054.
6. Westermark S, Rangelova E, Ansorge C, Lundell L, Segersvard R, Del Chiaro M. Cattell-Braasch maneuver combined with local hypothermia during superior mesenteric artery resection in pancreatectomy. Langenbeck's Arch Surg. 2016;401(8):1241–7.
7. Truty MJ, Colglazier JJ, Mendes BC, Nagorney DM, Bower TC, Smoot RL, et al. En bloc celiac axis resection for pancreatic cancer: classification of anatomical variants based on tumor extent. J Am Coll Surg. 2020;231(1):8–29.
8. Sato T, Inoue Y, Takahashi Y, Mise Y, Ishizawa T, Tanakura K, et al. Distal pancreatectomy with celiac Axis resection combined with reconstruction of the left gastric artery. J Gastrointest Surg. 2017;21(5):910–7.
9. Bachellier P, Addeo P, Faitot F, Nappo G, Dufour P. Pancreatectomy with arterial resection for pancreatic adenocarcinoma: how can it be done safely and with which outcomes?: a single Institution's experience with 118 patients. Ann Surg. 2020;271(5):932–40.
10. Oba A, Croce C, Hosokawa P, Meguid C, Torphy RJ, Al-Musawi MH, et al. Prognosis based definition of resectability in pancreatic cancer: a road map to new guidelines. Ann Surg. 2022;275(1):175–81.
11. Oba A, Wu YA, Schulick RD, Del Chiaro M. Pancreatic surgery with arterial resections. Textbook of pancreatic cancer. Springer; 2021. p. 877–89.
12. Inoue Y, Saiura A, Oba A, Ono Y, Mise Y, Ito H, et al. Neoadjuvant gemcitabine and nab-paclitaxel for borderline resectable pancreatic cancers: intention-to-treat analysis compared with upfront surgery. J Hepatobiliary Pancreat Sci. 2021;28(2):143–55.
13. Rangelova E, Wefer A, Persson S, Valente R, Tanaka K, Orsini N, et al. Surgery improves survival after neoadjuvant therapy for borderline and locally advanced pancreatic cancer: a single institution experience. Ann Surg. 2021;273(3):579–86.
14. Oba A, Inoue Y, Ono Y, Irie S, Sato T, Mise Y, et al. Radiologically occult metastatic pancreatic cancer: how can we avoid unbeneficial resection? Langenbeck's Arch Surg. 2020;405(1):35–41.
15. Oba A, Inoue Y, Ono Y, Ishizuka N, Arakaki M, Sato T, et al. Staging laparoscopy for pancreatic cancer using intraoperative ultrasonography and fluorescence imaging: the SLING trial. Br J Surg. 2021;108(2):115–8.
16. Ushida Y, Inoue Y, Ito H, Oba A, Mise Y, Ono Y, et al. High CA19-9 level in resectable pancreatic cancer is a potential indication of neoadjuvant treatment. Pancreatology. 2021;21(1):130–7.
17. Sato T, Saiura A, Inoue Y, Takahashi Y, Arita J, Takemura N. Distal pancreatectomy with en bloc resection of the celiac axis with preservation or reconstruction of the left gastric artery in patients with pancreatic body cancer. World J Surg. 2016;40(9):2245–53.
18. Otsuka S, Kaneoka Y, Maeda A, Takayama Y, Fukami Y, Onoe S. Hepatic artery reconstruction with a continuous suture method for hepato-biliary-pancreatic surgery. World J Surg. 2016;40(4):951–7.
19. Hackert T, Weitz J, Büchler MW. Splenic artery use for arterial reconstruction in pancreatic surgery. Langenbeck's Arch Surg. 2014;399(5):667–71.
20. Kinny-Koster B, van Oosten F, Habib JR, Javed AA, Cameron JL, Lafaro KJ, et al. Mesoportal bypass, interposition graft, and mesocaval shunt: surgical strategies to overcome superior mesenteric vein involvement in pancreatic cancer. Surgery. 2020;168(6):1048–55.
21. Ito H, Takahashi Y, Saiura A. Commentary: complex venous resection and reconstruction for locally advanced pancreatic cancer: our approach. Surgery. 2020;168(6):1056–7.
22. Inoue Y, Saiura A, Yoshioka R, Ono Y, Takahashi M, Arita J, et al. Pancreatoduodenectomy with systematic mesopancreas dissection using a supracolic anterior artery-first approach. Ann Surg. 2015;262(6):1092–101.

23. Del Chiaro M, Segersvärd R, Rangelova E, Coppola A, Scandavini CM, Ansorge C, et al. Cattell-Braasch Maneuver combined with artery-first approach for superior mesenteric-portal vein resection during pancreatectomy. J Gastrointest Surg. 2015;19(12):2264–8.
24. Sanjay P, Takaori K, Govil S, Shrikhande S, Windsor J. 'Artery-first' approaches to pancreatoduodenectomy. Br J Surg. 2012;99(8):1027–35.
25. Inoue Y, Saiura A, Takahashi Y. A novel classification and staged approach for dissection along the celiac and hepatic artery during pancreaticoduodenectomy. World J Surg. 2018;42(9):2963–7.
26. Del Chiaro M, Schulick RD. Commentary on: divestment or skeletonization of the SMA or the hepatic artery for locally advanced pancreatic ductal cancer after neoadjuvant therapy. Surgery. 2021;169(5):1039–40.
27. Del Chiaro M, Schulick RD. Use of total pancreatectomy and preoperative radiotherapy in patients undergoing pancreatectomy with artery resection. J Am Coll Surg. 2019;228(1):131.
28. Stoop TF, Ateeb Z, Ghorbani P, Scholten L, Arnelo U, Besselink MG, et al. Surgical outcomes after total pancreatectomy: a high-volume center experience. Ann Surg Oncol. 2021;28(3):1543–51.
29. Oba A, Inoue Y, Sato T, Ono Y, Mise Y, Ito H, et al. Impact of indocyanine green-fluorescence imaging on distal pancreatectomy with celiac axis resection combined with reconstruction of the left gastric artery. HPB. 2019;21(5):619–25.
30. Del Chiaro M, Segersvard R, Rangelova E, Coppola A, Scandavini CM, Ansorge C, et al. Cattell-Braasch Maneuver combined with artery-first approach for superior mesenteric-portal vein resection during pancreatectomy. J Gastrointest Surg. 2015;19(12):2264–8.
31. Oba A, Ito H, Ono Y, Sato T, Mise Y, Inoue Y, et al. Regional pancreatoduodenectomy versus standard pancreatoduodenectomy with portal vein resection for pancreatic ductal adenocarcinoma with portal vein invasion. BJS open. 2020;4(3):438–48.

Pancreaticoduodenectomy with Splenic Artery Resection for Tumors of the Pancreatic Head and/or Body Invading the Splenic Artery

Shugo Mizuno, Kazuyuki Gyoten, and Motonori Nagata

Abstract

Background: We have developed a new surgical technique, pancreaticoduodenectomy (PD) with splenic artery (SA) resection (PD-SAR), for tumors of the pancreatic head and/or body with SA invasion. In PD with portal vein (PV)/superior mesenteric vein (SMV) confluence resection, splenic vein (SV) division may cause left-sided portal hypertension (LPH).

Methods: Ninety-five patients with pancreatic ductal adenocarcinoma who underwent PD with PV/SMV resection after chemoradiotherapy were classified into three groups: PD-SVP (SV and SA were preserved, $n = 23$), PD-SVR (SV was divided and SA was preserved, $n = 55$), and PD-SAR (SV and SA were divided, $n = 17$). We evaluated the influence of SV and/or SA resection on LPH after PD with PV/SMV resection.

Results: Postoperative computed tomography demonstrated remnant pancreas enhancement in all patients in PD-SAR. The incidence of postoperative variceal formation in PD-SVP, PD-SVR, and PD-SAR was 4.3%, 60.9%, and 41.2%, respectively ($p < 0.001$), and variceal bleeding occurred only in PD-SVR ($n = 4$, 7.3%). The platelet counts ($\times 10^3/\mu L$) at postoperative 6 months were 185, 138, and 154 in PD-SVP, PD-SVR, and PD-SAR, respectively (PD-SVP vs. PD-SVR, $p < 0.001$), and spleen volume (mL) at 6 months was 91.8, 160, and 115 in PD-SVP, PD-SVR, and PD-SAR, respectively (PD-SVP vs. PD-SVR, $p < 0.001$). No significant differences in overall survival were observed among all groups.

Conclusion: In PD with PV-SMV confluence resection, SV division causes LPH; however, concomitant division of the SV and SA may attenuate this risk.

41.1 Introduction

In 2014, we developed and reported a new surgical technique for proximal subtotal pancreatectomy with splenic artery (SA) and splenic vein (SV) resection, so-called pancreaticoduodenectomy (PD) with SA resection (PD-SAR), for tumors of the pancreatic head and/or body invading the SA [1]. Although insufficient blood flow to the remnant pancreas was a concern, we have not experienced any postoperative complications related to lack of blood supply to the pancreatic parenchyma in patients who underwent PD-SAR. In addition, we have revealed that PD-SAR could achieve curative resection of tumors and prevent total pancreatectomy, which inevitably leads to diabetes mellitus and poor quality of life.

In cases of PD with combined resection of the portal vein (PV)/superior mesenteric vein (SMV) confluence, left-sided portal hypertension (LPH) resulting in variceal bleeding and thrombocytopenia due to hypersplenism has been a focus of recent studies [2–4]. In patients undergoing PD-SAR, the tumors frequently involve the PV and/or SMV or the PV-SMV confluence, and patients need to undergo combined resection of the PV/SMV and/or SV, with a risk of LPH development.

With respect to the splenic circulation, it has been considered that PD with SA resection could reduce the portal venous pressure because SA embolization/ligation or splenectomy is proven to reduce portal hyperperfusion, resulting in improvement of small-for-size syndrome in living-donor liver transplant patients [5]. PD-SAR is expected to reduce the portal venous pressure, resulting in improvement of LPH after PD.

S. Mizuno (✉) · K. Gyoten
Department of Hepatobiliary Pancreatic and Transplant Surgery, Mie University Graduate School of Medicine, Tsu, Mie, Japan
e-mail: mizunos@clin.medic.mie-u.ac.jp

M. Nagata
Department of Radiology, Mie University Graduate School of Medicine, Tsu, Mie, Japan

The aim of the present study was to introduce the surgical technique of PD-SAR and to evaluate its efficacy by examining the surgical outcomes, prognosis, and incidence of LPH after PD-SAR in comparison with conventional PD, with attention to the development of variceal formation and bleeding, as well as postoperative changes in platelet count and spleen volume.

41.2 Surgical Procedures of PD-SAR

The conventional PD for pancreatic ductal adenocarcinoma (PDAC) has been standardized as an anterior approach to the superior mesenteric artery at our institution [6, 7]. When the tumor is invading the PV/SMV, we perform resection and reconstruction of the PV and SMV using 6-0 nonabsorbable running sutures. In cases of tumors involving the SV or inferior mesenteric vein (IMV), these veins are divided and not reconstructed. When tumor involvement of the SA is identified, PD-SAR is employed [1]. Pancreaticojejunostomy is performed using the pair-watch suturing technique, as described in our previous report [8].

The surgical procedures of PD-SAR are similar to those of PD, except for combined resection of the SA and SV (Fig. 41.1a, b). Focusing on the arterial anatomy around the pancreas and the cutting sites of the artery, the blood supply of the remnant pancreas is provided by the short gastric arteries, left gastroepiploic artery, and posterior epiploic artery [9]. During surgery, sufficient blood supply of the remnant pancreas and spleen is confirmed with Doppler ultrasonography and/or by the color of the remnant pancreas and the spleen. When the tumor is invading both the left gastric artery (LGA) and the SA, we perform combined resection of the LGA followed by total gastrectomy and splenectomy if curative-intent resection is possible. In such cases, the blood supply of the remnant pancreas is provided by posterior epiploic artery alone [1].

41.3 Patients and Methods

41.3.1 Patients

Between April 2005 and July 2017, a total of 361 patients who had a cytological or histological diagnosis of localized PDAC, determined using 64-slice multidetector computed tomography (MDCT), underwent our chemoradiotherapy (CRT) protocol, as previously reported [10–12] (Fig. 41.2). We retrospectively reviewed the electronic medical records of 172 patients who underwent PD after CRT. Among them, 158 (91.8%) patients underwent combined resection of the PV and SMV. The present study finally included 95 patients after excluding 63 patients for the following reasons: concomitant splenectomy ($n = 4$), postoperative PV/SMV anastomotic stricture ($n = 8$), preoperative portal hypertension ($n = 7$), PV-SV anastomosis ($n = 1$), insufficient follow-up ($n = 6$), death within 30 days after the surgery ($n = 1$), concomitant colectomy ($n = 7$), and SA ligation ($n = 29$). These 95 patients were classified into three groups: PD-SVP (both SV and SA were preserved, $n = 23$), PD-SVR (SV was divided and SA was preserved, $n = 55$), and PD-SAR (both SV and SA were divided, $n = 17$).

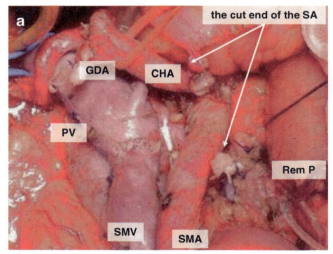
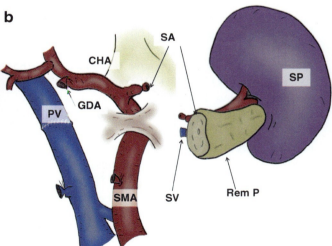

Fig. 41.1 (a) Intraoperative findings after pancreaticoduodenectomy with SA resection (PD-SAR). (b) Schema of reconstruction after PD-SAR. *PV* portal vein, *SMA* superior mesenteric artery, *SA* splenic artery, *CHA* common hepatic artery, *GDA* gastroduodenal artery, *SV* splenic vein, *Rem P* remnant pancreatic parenchyma, *SP* spleen

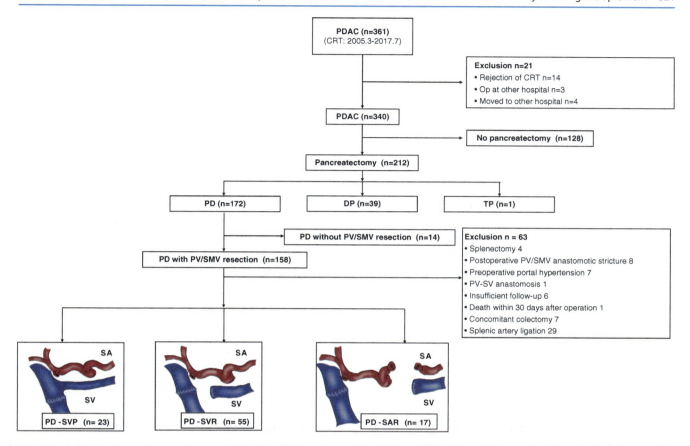

Fig. 41.2 Flow diagram of the enrollment of 361 patients who underwent PD with combined PV/SMV resection for PDAC after CRT. Between March 2005 and December 2018, 158 patients with PDAC underwent PD with PV resection after CRT. After excluding 63 patients, the present study enrolled 95 patients: PD-SVP (n = 23), PD-SVR (n = 55), and PD-SAR (n = 17). *PDAC* pancreatic ductal adenocarcinoma, *CRT* chemoradiotherapy, *PD* pancreaticoduodenectomy, *DP* distal pancreatectomy, *TP* total pancreatectomy, *PV* portal vein, *SMV* superior mesenteric vein, *SV* splenic vein, *SVP* splenic vein preservation, *SAR* splenic artery resection, *SVR* splenic vein resection

41.3.2 Preoperative Treatments

Our treatment protocols for gemcitabine-based chemotherapy (G-CRT) and gemcitabine plus gemcitabine-based CRT (GS-CRT) have been reported previously [11, 13]. Between February 2005 and October 2011, patients were administered an infusion of gemcitabine at a dose of 800 mg/m^2 on days 1, 8, 22, and 29 for one cycle (G-CRT). From November 2011, patients were administered S1 orally twice daily at a dose of 60 mg/m^2 per day on days 1 through 21 of a 28-day cycle, and an infusion of gemcitabine at a dose of 600 mg/m^2 on days 8 and 22 for one cycle (GS-CRT). Patients were treated with three-dimensional conformal radiotherapy using the four-field box technique from directions that avoided exposure of the kidney, which is an organ at risk. The total radiation dose delivered was 45–50.4 Gy in 25–28 fractions (5 fractions/week). The patients underwent reassessment at 4–6 weeks after CRT. When we determined that curative-intent resection was possible, the patients were scheduled to undergo pancreatectomy.

41.3.3 Preoperative Characteristics and Surgical Outcomes

We compared various variables among the three groups, including preoperative characteristics such as age, sex, body mass index, maximum tumor size on computed tomography (CT), performance status, tumor marker (carcinoembryonic antigen and carbohydrate antigen 19-9) levels, presence of preoperative CRT including regimens, T and N factors according to the Union for International Cancer Control eighth classification, and tumor resectability (classified as resectable, borderline resectable, and unresectable according to the National Comprehensive Cancer Network guideline) [14] based on the findings of MDCT, as previously reported. We also collected data on surgical outcomes, including intraoperative blood loss, operative duration, degree of postoperative complications according to the Clavien-Dindo classification [15], and pancreatic fistula according to the International Study Group on Pancreatic Fistula [16].

41.3.4 Assessment of LPH: Incidence of Variceal Formation, Serial Changes of Platelet Count, Spleen Volume, and Hemodynamics in the Left-Side Area

To assess the development of LPH, a radiologist (N.M.) who was blinded to the patients' characteristics and outcomes evaluated enhanced MDCT images for any newly developed varices and collateral pathways at 6 months after PD. Esophageal, gastric, pancreatic, and colonic varices were diagnosed when dilated and beaded veins were detected within the submucosal layer of each organ compared with before the surgery. Collateral pathways from the divided SV were diagnosed when the diameter of the splenosystemic or splenoportal routes was 1.5 times larger than that before surgery. The splenosystemic route was defined as a splenorenal shunt, a gastrorenal shunt, and others. Splenoportal routes were classified as superior and inferior routes according to the definition of Strasberg et al. [17]. The superior route was defined as a pathway starting in the divided SV; following a superior and rightward direction through gastric, coronary, and/or perigastric veins; and finally ending in the PV. The inferior route was defined as a pathway starting in the divided SV, joining the venous routes in the mesocolon through the gastrocolic ligament and/or the IMV, and proceeding in an inferior and rightward direction to end in the SMV. Blood supply to the spleen after PD-SAR was evaluated using enhanced MDCT within 10 days postoperatively. Platelet count data were collected before and 6 months after PD. The total spleen volume was estimated by tracing the spleen on each transverse CT image obtained at 2.0-mm intervals. Spleen volume was measured before and 6 months after PD. We withdrew the evaluation of LPH when PV/SMV occlusion or patient mortality occurred. The study protocol was approved by the Medical Ethics Committee of Mie University Hospital (no. H2019–070), and the study was performed in accordance with the ethical standards established in the 1964 Declaration of Helsinki.

41.3.5 Statistical Analyses

Continuous variables are expressed as medians and ranges. Statistical significance was determined using the Mann-Whitney U test for comparison between two groups and the Kruskal–Wallis test for comparison among multiple groups. Categorical variables were compared using Pearson's chi-square test. Overall survival (OS) was calculated using the Kaplan-Meier method and tested using the log-rank test. Statistical analysis was performed using SPSS version 24.0 (SPSS, Chicago, IL, USA). A p value of <0.05 was considered statistically significant.

41.4 Results

41.4.1 Patients' Background and Surgical Outcomes

Table 41.1 shows a comparison of background characteristics and surgical outcomes between PD-SVP, PD-SVR, and PD-SAR. The intraoperative blood loss was significantly higher in PD-SVR than in PD-SVP and PD-SAR (464 vs. 1160 vs. 578 mL, $p = 0.004$). The incidence rates of coronary vein division and IMV division were as follows (PD-SVP vs. PD-SVR vs. PD-SAR): 60.9% vs. 89.1% vs. 82.4% ($p = 0.015$) and 13.0% vs. 60.0% vs. 94.1% ($p < 0.001$), respectively. No significant differences were observed in postoperative complications of Clavien-Dindo grade IIIa or higher and in pancreatic fistula of grade B or C between the two groups. The incidence rates of pathological PV invasion were 8.7% in PD-SVP, 25.5% in PD-SVR, and 47.1% in PD-SAR ($p = 0.022$). The incidence rates of postoperative variceal formation and splenosystemic shunt development were as follows (PD-SVP vs. PD-SVR vs. PD-SAR): 4.3% vs. 70.9% vs. 41.2% ($p < 0.001$) and 4.3% vs. 45.5% vs. 5.9% ($p < 0.001$), respectively. Variceal bleeding was identified in four patients (7.3%), all in PD-SVR ($p = 0.212$).

41.4.2 Arterial Blood Supply to the Left-Sided Area after PD-SAR

Blood supply to the spleen after PD-SAR ($n = 17$) was secured from the LGA and subphrenic artery (SubPA), which passed through the stomach and joined to the distal SA and spleen. On dynamic CT imaging performed within 10 days after PD-SAR, blood supply from the LGA and SubPA was identified in 100% (17/17) and 94.1% (16/17), respectively. PD-SAR did not cause any severe complications, such as spleen necrosis and abscess. Partial splenic infarction was identified in 11.8% (2/17) of the patients, although all of them improved within 1 month.

41.4.3 Serial Changes of Platelet Count and Spleen Volume

Figure 41.3a shows the change in platelet counts. At postoperative 6 months, the median platelet count ($\times 10^3/\mu L$) in the PD-SVR group was significantly lower than that in the PD-SVP group (138 vs. 185, $p < 0.001$). The postoperative platelet counts ($\times 10^3/\mu L$) significantly decreased compared with the preoperative counts only in PD-SVR (138 vs. 205, $p < 0.001$). Figure 41.3b shows the change in spleen volume. At 6 months postoperatively, the median spleen volume in PD-SVR was significantly larger than that in PD-SVP (160

Table 41.1 Background and surgical outcomes

Perioperative variables	PD-SVP n = 23	PD-SVR n = 55	PD-SAR n = 17	p
Age	68 (52~84)	66 (48~84)	69 (53~82)	0.344
Man/female	10/13	39/16	8/9	0.038
BMI, kg/m^2	20.6 (15.2~27.1)	20.6 (15.2~28.3)	21.5 (17.3~25.6)	0.848
Maximum tumor size on CT (mm)	25.3 (13.1~38.7)	25.7 (11.2~45.9)	25.4 (12.3~72.6)	0.894
Performance status 0/1/2	15/6/2	31/23/1	13/4/0	0.208
CEA, ng/mL	3.4 (1.0~8.4)	4.2 (1.0~13.2)	2.8 (1.4~369)	0.166
CA19-9, U/mL	28.9 (0.1~497)	34.2 (0.1~1690)	43.1 (0.1~1475)	0.981
TNM classification (UICC 8th) T factor (T1/T2/T3/T4)	4/8/0/11	10/19/3/23	1/3/0/13	0.244
TNM classification (UICC 8th) N factor (N0/N1/N2)	17/6/0	41/13/1	14/3/0	0.885
Resectability, R: BR: UR	10/7/6	20/20/15	1/9/7	0.128
Preoperative chemotherapy regimen G: GS	7/16	26/29	6/11	0.532
Platelet counts, ×1000/uL	214 (150~447)	205 (87.0~423)	190 (83.0~298)	0.088
Spleen volume, mL	121 (43.2~416)	118 (28.8~277)	104 (57.9~223)	0.850
Operative procedures (PD/SSPPD)	0/23	6/51	3/42	0.246
Operative duration (min)	533 (345~818)	552 (351~780)	604 (384–804)	0.680
Blood loss (mL)	**464 (103~2500)**	**1160 (110~5089)**	**578 (80~4000)**	**0.004**
CV division, yes/no (%)	**14/9 (60.9%)**	**49/6 (89.1%)**	**14/3 (82.4%)**	**0.015**
IMV division, yes/no (%)	**3/20 (13.0%)**	**33/22 (60.0%)**	**16/1 (94.1%)**	**<0.001**
C-D >/= IIIa, yes/no (yes %)	2/21 (8.7%)	15/40 (27.3%)	2/15 (11.8%)	0.112
Pancreatic fistula (Grade B or C), yes/no (yes %)	0/23	3/52 (5.5%)	0/17	0.324
pPV positive, yes/no (yes%)	**2/21 (8.7%)**	**14/41 (25.5%)**	**8/9 (47.1%)**	**0.022**
R0 resection, yes/no (yes %)	21/2 (91.3%)	50/5 (90.9%)	12/5 (70.6%)	0.071
Postoperative chemotherapy, yes/no (yes %)	23/0 (100%)	45/10 (81.8%)	13/4 (76.5%)	0.056
Postoperative variceal formation, yes/no (%)	**1/22 (4.3%)**	**39/16 (70.9%)**	**7/10 (41.2%)**	**<0.001**
Esophageal varices	**0/23 (0.0%)**	**18/37 (32.7%)**	**3/14 (17.6%)**	**0.006**
Gastric varices	**0/23 (0.0%)**	**19/36 (34.5%)**	**5/12 (29.4%)**	**0.005**
Pancreatic varices	**0/23 (0.0%)**	**15/40 (27.3%)**	**2/15 (11.8%)**	**0.013**
Colonic varices	**1/22 (4.3%)**	**25/30 (45.5%)**	**1/16 (5.9%)**	**<0.001**
The development of spleno-systemic shunt, yes/no (yes %)	**0/23**	**11/44 (20.0%)**	**1/16 (5.9%)**	**0.035**
Spleno-renal shunt	0/23	3/52 (5.5%)	0/17 (0.0%)	0.324
Gastro-renal shunt	0/23	7/48 (12.7%)	1/16 (5.9%)	0.167
Others	0/23	2/53 (3.6%)	0/17 (0.0%)	0.476
The development of superior collateral route, yes/no (yes %)	0/23 (0.0%)	0/57 (0.0%)	0/45 (0.0%)	–
The development of inferior collateral route, yes/no (yes %)	3/20 (13.0%)	15/40 (27.3%)	3/14 (17.6%)	0.342
Variceal bleeding, yes/no (%)	0/23	4/51 (7.3%)	0/17 (0.0%)	0.219

vs. 91.8 mL, $p < 0.001$). In PD-SVR, spleen volume significantly increased compared with that before the surgery (160 vs. 118 mL, $p < 0.001$).

41.4.4 OS Rates After the Initial Treatment

A significant difference in median survival time and OS rates was observed among the three groups (PD-SVP vs. PD-SVR vs. PD-SAR): median survival time, 36 vs. 26 vs. 26 months; 3-year OS, 46.5% vs. 32.7% vs. 34.0% ($p = 0.272$).

41.5 Discussion

In this paper, we described the surgical techniques of PD-SAR and revealed the following insights: (1) PD-SAR can be safely performed without any major complications related to this procedure. (2) PD-SAR decreases variceal formations due to LPH after SV division compared with PD-SVR. (3) We have never experienced cases of variceal bleeding caused by LPH in patients who underwent PD-SAR.

To justify the PD-SAR procedure, sustained blood supply to the spleen and remnant pancreas is mandatory. The arterial blood supply to the spleen after PD-SAR was secured from the LGA (100%) and the left SubPA (94.1%) through and around the stomach without causing any major complications. In addition to the arterial blood flow on dynamic CT images within 10 days, MDCT clearly demonstrated enhancement of the remnant pancreas at 1 and 6 months postoperatively in all the examined patients (data not shown). The secondary point is the oncological validity of PD-SAR. With respect to the R0 resection rates, no significant differences were observed among the three groups (PD-SVP, PD-SVR, and PD-SAR) regardless of tumor extension. Additionally, surgical outcomes such as degree of

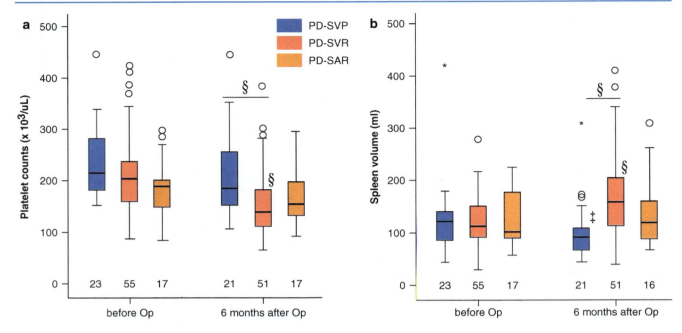

Fig. 41.3 Changes of platelet counts and spleen volume. (**a**) At 6 months postoperatively, the median platelet count in the PD-SVR group was significantly lower than that in the PD-SVP group. Only in PD-SVR, platelet counts significantly decreased compared with the preoperative counts. (**b**) Change of spleen volume. At 6 months postoperatively, the median spleen volume in the PD-SVR group was significantly larger than that in the PD-SVP group. Only in PD-SVR, the spleen volume significantly increased compared with before the surgery. ‡ $p < 0.01$, § $p < 0.001$. *Op* operation

postoperative complications and pancreatic fistula did not differ among the three groups. The OS of the PD-SAR group was very similar to that of the PD-SVP and PD-SVR groups.

As previously reported [18], LPH is a clinical syndrome due to outflow obstruction of the SV when the SV is ligated and not reimplanted, leading to the development of varices with hemorrhage and splenomegaly with thrombocytopenia. Although rare, LPH-related gastrointestinal bleeding is a life-threatening complication, and it can be managed depending on the situation with endoscopic procedures, radiologic procedures, or surgical intervention, with a low mortality. We experienced four patients who developed variceal bleeding and required treatments at 6, 6, 18, and 96 months after PD, respectively [19]. All four patients underwent PD-SVR, and LPH did not occur in patients who underwent PD-SAR.

In summary, we have developed a PD-SAR procedure for pancreatic head and body tumors invading the SA without attempting to prevent LPH after PV/SMV confluence resection; however, unexpectedly, this procedure was observed to attenuate the development of LPH. Consequently, SA ligation or division may be a useful and simple procedure to prevent LPH when PV/SMV confluence resection is performed. Nevertheless, further studies with a large number of cases are required to clarify its efficacy.

Acknowledgments We are grateful to Dr. Takehiro Fujii, Department of Hepatobiliary Pancreatic and Transplant Surgery, Mie University Graduate School of Medicine, Mie, Japan, for help in creating the schema.

Disclosure The authors of this manuscript have no conflicts of interest to disclose.

References

1. Desaki R, Mizuno S, Tanemura A, et al. A new surgical technique of pancreaticoduodenectomy with splenic artery resection for ductal adenocarcinoma of the pancreatic head and/or body invading splenic artery. Biomed Res Int. 2014;2014:219038.
2. Mizuno S, Kato H, Yamaue H, et al. Left-sided portal hypertension after pan- creaticoduodenectomy with resection of the portal vein/superior mesenteric vein confluence in patients with pancreatic cancer: a project study by the Japanese Society of Hepato-Biliary-Pancreatic Surgery. Ann Surg. 2021;274(1):e36–44. https://doi.org/10.1097/sla.0000000000003487.
3. Tanaka H, Nakao A, Oshima K, et al. Splenic vein reconstruction is unnecessary in pancreatoduodenectomy combined with resection of the superior mesen- teric vein-portal vein confluence according to short-term outcomes. HPB (Oxford). 2017;19:785–92.
4. Ono Y, Matsueda K, Koga R, et al. Sinistral portal hypertension after pancreaticoduodenectomy with splenic vein ligation. Br J Surg. 2017;102(3):219–28.

5. Ikegami T, Shimada M, Imura S, et al. Current concept of small-for-size grafts in living donor liver transplantation. Surg Today. 2008;38:971–82.
6. Isaji S, Usui M, Sakurai H, et al. Antegrade proximal pancreatectomy for lower bile duct adenocaricinoma and ampulla of Vater carcinoma. Operation. 2007;61:821–7. (In Japanese)
7. Mizuno S, Isaji S, Tanemura A, et al. Anterior approach to the superior mesenteric artery by using nerve plexus hanging maneuver for borderline resectable pancreatic head carcinoma. J Gastrointest Surg. 2014;18(6):1209–15.
8. Azumi Y, Isaji S, Kato H, Nobuoka Y, Kuriyama N, Kishiwada M, Hamada T, Mizuno S, Usui M, Sakurai H, Tabata M. A standardized technique for safe pancreaticojejunostomy: pair-watch suturing technique. World J Gastrointest Surg. 2010;2:260–4.
9. Mizuno S, Isaji S, Ohsawa I, et al. Pancreaticoduodenectomy with resection of the splenic artery and splenectomy for pancreatic double cancers after total gastrectomy. Preservation of the pancreatic function via the blood supply from the posterior epiploic artery: report of a case. Surg Today. 2012;42:482–8.
10. Yamada R, Mizuno S, Uchida K, et al. Human equilibrative nucleoside transporter 1 expression in endoscopic ultrasonography–guided fine-needle aspiration biopsy samples is a strong predictor of clinical response and survival in the patients with pancreatic ductal adenocarcinoma undergoing gemcitabine-based chemoradiotherapy. Pancreas. 2016;45:761–71.
11. Kobayashi M, Mizuno S, Murata Y, et al. Gemcitabine-based chemoradiotherapy followed by surgery for borderline resectable and locally unresectable pancreatic ductal adenocarcinoma. Pancreas. 2014;43:350–60.
12. Isaji S, Kishiwada M, Kato H. Surgery for borderline pancreatic cancer: the Japanese experience. In: Katz MD, Ahmad SA, editors. Multimodality management of borderline resectable pancreatic cancer. Cham: Springer International Publishing Switzerland; 2016. p. 265–87.
13. Takeuchi T, Mizuno S, Murata Y, et al. Comparative study between gemcitabine-based and gemcitabine plus S1–based preoperative chemoradiotherapy for localized pancreatic ductal adenocarcinoma, with special attention to initially locally advanced unresectable T tumor. Pancreas. 2019;48:281–91.
14. National Comprehensive Cancer Network. Pancreaticadenocarcinoma. NCCN clinical practice guidelines in oncology. Version 2. 2016. http://www.nccn.org/professionals/physician_gls/pdf/pancreatic.pdf. Accessed 14 Jun 2018.
15. Dindo D, Demartines N, Clavien PA. Classification of surgical complications. Ann Surg. 2004;240:205–13.
16. Bassi C, Dervenis C, Butturini G, et al. International Study Group on Pancreatic Fistula Definition. Postoperative pancreatic fistula: an international study group (ISGPF) definition. Surgery. 2005;138:8–13.
17. Strasberg SM, Bhalla S, Sanchez LA, Linehan DC. Pattern of venous collateral development after splenic vein occlusion in an extended Whipple procedure: comparison with collateral vein pattern in cases of sinistral portal hypertension. J Gastrointest Surg. 2011;15(11):2070–9.
18. Petrucciani N, Debs T, Rosso E, et al. Left-sided portal hypertension after pancreatoduodenectomy with resection of the portal/superior mesenteric vein confluence. Results of a systematic review. Surgery. 2020;168(3):434–9.
19. Gyoten K, Mizuno S, Nagata M, Ogura T, Usui M, Isaji S. Significance of simultaneous splenic artery resection in left-sided portal hypertension after pancreaticoduodenectomy with combined portal vein resection. World J Surg. 2017;41(8):2111–20.

Pancreaticoduodenectomy with Superior Mesenteric Resection and Reconstruction for Locally Advanced Tumors

Philippe Bachellier and Pietro Addeo

Abstract

Pancreatectomies with arterial resections were initially characterized by high postoperative mortality and poor long-term survival as reported by Fortner et al. and then abandoned. The introduction of new efficacious chemotherapy regimens (FOLFIRINOX) along with the extensive experience in venous resection for borderline pancreatic tumors has brought renewed interest in extended pancreatic resection for locally advanced malignancy. The experience needed for performing such complex resections goes beyond pancreatic surgery alone and entails skills in vascular surgery. Reconstructing arterial vessels might need autologous and/or heterologous vascular substitutes which should be available immediately and accurate preoperative planning and simulation on the basis of cross-sectional imaging should be the rule. Resection of the superior mesenteric artery could be seen as one of the most challenging arterial resection at the time of pancreatectomy because of: (1) the frequent presence of an associated venous invasion; (2) the variable degree of tumoral infiltration downward through the mesentery; (3) the necessity of a mesenteric approach and complete mesenteric dissection; (4) the need for reconstructing several jejunal and ileal branches; (5) the high mortality rates (20%) reported so far. In this chapter we will describe step-by-step the surgical technique of our standardized approach for superior mesenteric artery resection during pancreaticoduodenectomy.

P. Bachellier (✉) · P. Addeo
Hepato-Pancreato-Biliary Surgery and Liver Transplantation, Pôle des Pathologies Digestives, Hépatiques et de la Transplantation, Hôpital de Hautepierre-Hôpitaux Universitaires de Strasbourg, Université de Strasbourg, Strasbourg, France
e-mail: Philippe.Bachellier@chru-strasbourg.fr

42.1 Introduction

The introduction of new efficacious chemotherapy regimens (FOLFIRINOX) along with the extensive experience in venous resection for borderline pancreatic tumors has led to the development of extended pancreatic resection for locally advanced malignancy [1–4]. In these procedures the arterial vessels of the coeliac and superior mesenteric axes are resected and reconstructed simultaneously with pancreatectomy in order to achieve local control for locally advanced pancreatic malignancy. Pancreatectomies with arterial resections were initially characterized by high postoperative mortality and poor long-term survival as reported by Fortner et al. and then abandoned [5, 6]. The establishment of high volume center for pancreatic resection along with experience in vascular resection during HPB surgery and liver and pancreas transplant let some centers to revisit these procedures for patients with locally advanced disease [7–10]. The experience needed for performing such complex resections goes beyond pancreatic surgery alone and entails skills in vascular surgery which can need a multidisciplinary approach including eventually vascular surgeons. Reconstructing arterial vessels might need autologous and/or heterologous vascular substitutes which should be available immediately. For these reasons accurate preoperative planning and simulation on the basis of cross-sectional imaging should be the rule when planning these procedures. The occurrence of pancreatic leak into the postoperative period could be very often a lethal event by causing erosion and thrombosis of reconstructed vessels and consequent death. These highlights such as arterial resections should be reserved to very high volume centers to surgeons well beyond their learning curve with standard pancreatic resections [8]. Arterial resections are now gradually centralized in very high volume centers and as a matter of fact the largest series of arterial resection are now reported by few European, American and Asian centers [4, 11–14]. Such as every surgical procedure some type of arterial resection with simultaneous pancreatectomy are more challenging than other. Resection of the superior mesenteric artery could be seen as one of the most challenging arterial resection at the time of pancreatectomy because of: (1) the frequent presence of an associated venous invasion; (2) the variable degree of tumoral infiltration downward through the mesentery; (3) the necessity of a mesenteric approach and complete mesenteric dissection; (4) the need for reconstructing more jejunal and ileal branches; (5) the high mortality rates (20%) reported so far [15]. In this chapter we will present the surgical technique of our standardized approach for SMA resection during pancreaticoduodenectomy (PD).

42.1.1 Preoperative Planning

Our standardized protocol for managing patients with locally advanced pancreatic cancers has been previously described in detail [9–11, 16–21]. Briefly every patients presenting with a superior mesenteric artery involvement is considered as a locally advanced tumor independently from the presence of venous invasion and candidate for induction chemotherapy [11]. More often SMA involvement is seen (1) in patients having tumors located at the uncinated process along with a variable degree of venous invasion; (2) in tumors located at the proximal part of the pancreatic body invading the SMA, the splenoportal venous confluence and the coeliac trunk; (3) in bulky tumors of the pancreatic head associated with venous invasion and invasion of both the coeliac trunk and the SMA. When considering the presence of SMA involvement for surgery three factors should be considered. First the longitudinal extent of SMA invasion with three types easily recognized: (1) Type 1 invasion limited to the retro pancreatic tract of the SMA trunk: (2) type 2 invasion extended to the origin of the first jejunal branches; (3) type 3 invasion reaching the origin of the ileocolic branches and of the secondary or third jejunal branches (Fig. 42.1). Secondly it

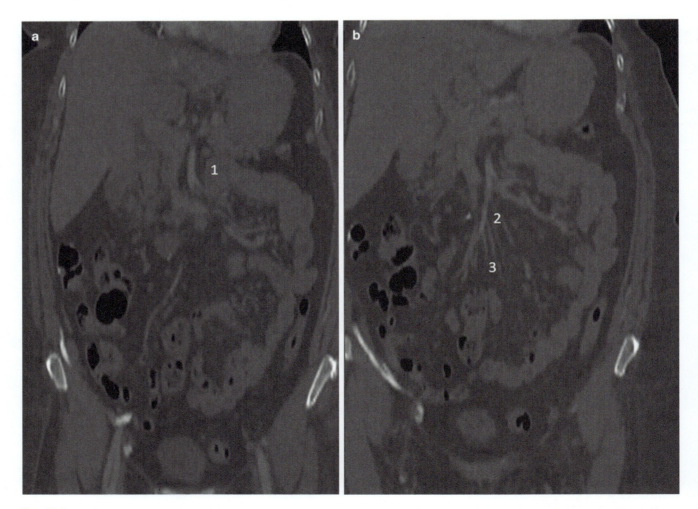

Fig. 42.1 Strasbourg's classification of Superior mesenteric artery invasion pattern: (**a**) Type 1 invasion limited to the retropancreatic tract of the SMA trunk: (**b**) type 2 invasion extended to the origin of the first jejunal branches and type 3 invasions reaching the origin of the ileocolic branches and/or of the secondary or third jejunal branches

should be remarked: (1) the presence and the extent of an associated venous invasion (superior mesenteric vein versus splenomesentericoportal confluence) as well the presence of thrombosis (superior mesenteric vein, portal vein, splenic vein) and venous cavernoma transformation. Thirdly, the coexistence of coeliac trunk invasion should be remarked. Intuitively, the presence of CT invasion, a longitudinal invasion beyond the SMA trunk and the presence of venous infiltration increases the technical difficulties of SMA resection and indicate more aggressive disease. As a general suggestion preoperative planning is of paramount importance and all these three factors have been extensively planned before scheduling surgery. The need for autologous and /or heterologous graft should be planned. Usually we schedule surgery 4 weeks after the last chemotherapy cycle and preoperative nutrition is also encouraged to prepare patients for surgery. Rehabilitation should be the rule and regular daily physical activity is also strongly encouraged.

42.2 Surgical Technique

42.2.1 Basic Preliminary Maneuvers

A bilateral subcostal incision with midline extension up to the xiphoidal process is usually performed. The groins are also systematically included in the operative field in case of need for saphenous grafts. Preliminary exploration included systematic search for liver metastases and peritoneal carcinomatosis. The right colon and the mesenteric root are sectioned during a Cattel–Braasch maneuver. A large Kocher maneuver is then performed up to the left border of the aorta. The interaorticocaval area is cleared from lymphatic tissues which are sent for pathological examination. The origin of the SMA is cleared at the superior border of the left renal vein and isolated. Infiltration of the origin of the SMA on the aorta indicates not resectable disease. The dissection is moved toward the mesentery in order to delineate the longitudinal extent of SMA infiltration. The insertion of the transverse mesocolon is sectioned right-to-left by ligating the superior right colonic and the middle colonic pedicles. These sections are performed far from the colonic wall in order to preserve the communicating arterial and venous arcades. Now the mesentery is sectioned right-to-the-left perpendicularly to the axis of the SMA and the SMV. This dissection goes downward 1–2 cm beyond the macroscopic venous/ arterial tumoral infiltration. The SMV and/or its branches and the SMA and/or its branches are isolated and looped into the mesentery (Mikado's technique). Infiltration of the SMA trunk needing more than two branches distal reconstruction can be particularly challenging especially in older and obese patients and could eventually discouraged.

42.2.2 Management of the Mesenteric Venous System

In our experience management of the superior mesenteric venous system is of a paramount importance when performing SMA resection for several reasons. First, frequently there is a variable degree of venous obstruction related to the tumoral infiltration which goes from right to the left in cancers of the uncinated process. Dissection of the mesentery and of the hepatic pedicle progressively interrupts all the collateral circulations which drains the bowel and supplies the liver in patients with venous obstruction. The section of these venous collaterals increases difficulties in dissection and might cause profuse bleeding and liver hypoperfusion. We therefore systematically advocate early section of the SMV or its branches and derivation into the portal system at the beginning of the dissection. This is achieved by a transitory mesenterico-portal shunt using Gore-Tex ringed prosthesis interposed between the SMV and the right lateral side of the portal vein (Fig. 42.2). Indeed, the SMV previously isolated is directly sectioned over a clamp and anastomosed on one end to a 20-cm long Gore-Tex ringed prosthesis which is then anastomosed to the lateral wall of the PV just below its bifurcation. The use of this shunt achieves immediate decompression of the bowel venous flow into the portal system which is of great importance in patients with cavernoma. Furthermore it provides superior dexterity for the dissection of the mesentery and provides continuous venous drainage into the portal vein though the entire operation [11, 20]. The advantages of this transitory shunt include (1) greater mobility of the mesenteric root because of the extra-length provided by the prosthesis which avoids completely the risk of venous disruption (2) the need for combined arterial and venous clamping; (3) provides superior exposure for the arterial resection and reconstruction (4) maintains portal venous inflow to the liver which is very often damaged by the preoperative chemotherapy.

42.2.3 Dissection of the Superior Mesenteric Artery and of the Hepatic Pedicle

Once the transitory mesentericoportal shunt has been unclamped, attention is directed toward the different branches of the SMA which are isolated and looped. In presence of SMA infiltration the section of the inferior pancreaticoduodenal artery and the first jejunal artery is not possible. The SMA trunk is currently only isolated on the future transection point. Dissection proceeds on the hepatic pedicle which is completely dissected. The pyloric and the gastroduodenal artery are sectioned; the portal vein trunk is looped such as the common bile duct. The dissection is pursued downward

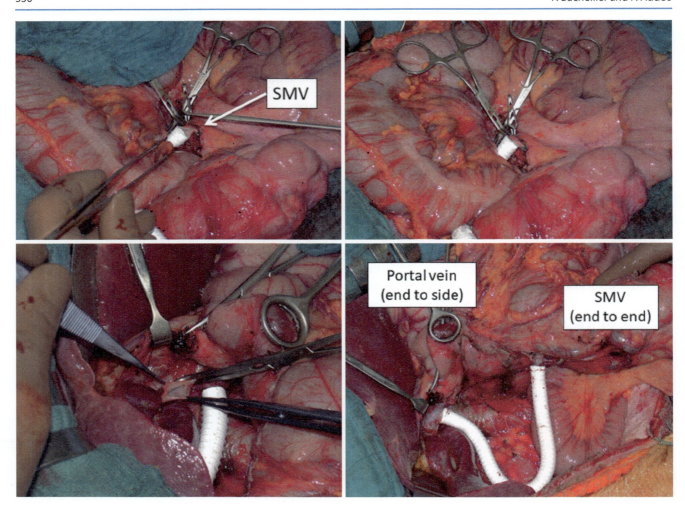

Fig. 42.2 The management of the venous system is achieved by a transitory mesentericoportal shunt interposed between the right side of the portal vein and the SMV as showed

on the coeliac trifurcation. The common hepatic artery, the splenic artery and the left gastric artery are looped. The coeliac trunk is dissected circumferentially, and the diaphragmatic arteries are sectioned.

42.2.4 Section of the Pancreas and Vascular Resection

A tunnel is created beyond the pancreatic body at the level of entry of the splenic artery or at the confluence of the inferior mesenteric vein into the splenic vein depending on the degree of tumoral spreading toward the left pancreas. The pancreatic body is progressively dissected from the splenic vein and sectioned. The pancreas is then dissected over 6-cm from the splenic artery and vein. The splenic vein is then sectioned and this will provide superior view on the superior mesenteric artery trunk on its origin. With this exposure a clamp is positioned on the origin of the SMA and another on the trunk or the branches of the SMA. After systemic heparin administration, the proximal and the distal SMA trunk and the distal branches are sectioned. Arterial replacement is performed either end-to-end (resection up to 3-cm length) (Fig. 42.3) or using a saphenous graft which is anatomized between the two ends using running 8/0 sutures (Figs. 42.4 and 42.5). The attention is now directed toward the venous system with sequential removal of the shunt and direct anastomoses between the SMV and the Portal Vein. The management of the splenic vein includes either a distal splenorenal shunt on the left renal vein or preservation of the natural confluence between the inferior mesenteric vein and the splenic vein [16] (Fig. 42.6). Digestive reconstruction is performed with a telescoped pancreaticogastrosotmy [22], hepaticojejunostomy and gastroenterostomy.

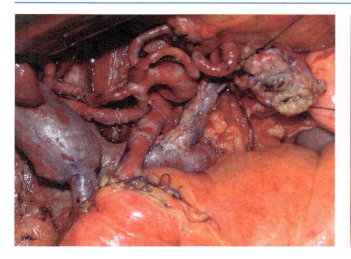
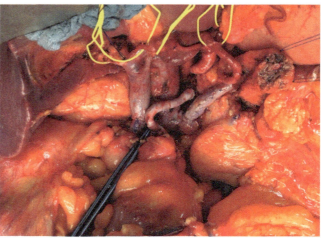

Fig. 42.3 Intraoperative view of a PD with SMA resection. A direct end-to-end without graft interposition is generally possible in case of short (<3 cm) SMA resection

Fig. 42.4 Intraoperative view of a PD with SMA resection. A saphenous graft is interposed between the origin of the SMA on the aorta and the stump of SMA into the mesentery

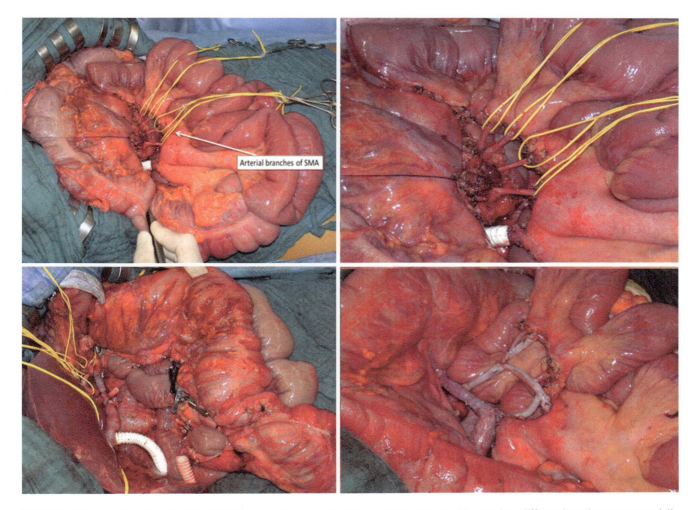

Fig. 42.5 Intraoperative view of a PD with SMA resection using the Mikado's technique. In this case four different branches are sequentially reconstructed by using several saphenous grafts. While feasible this type of resection remains very challenging

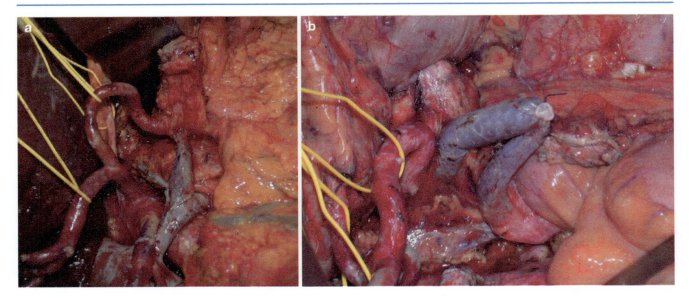

Fig. 42.6 Intraoperative view of splenic vein management either by a splenorenal shunt (**a**) or ligation of the splenic vein with preservation of its confluence with the inferior mesenteric vein (**b**)

42.3 Postoperative Management

Intravenous heparin is administered during the first 7 days. A computed tomography scan is performed at postoperative days one and tenth to control vascular permeability. Long-term anti-aggregant therapy by aspirin is maintained in all patients (3 months). An oral feeding is restarted beginning from postoperative day 7. Postoperative diarrhea is frequent after such extended dissection of the SMA and is managed with codeine. Adjuvant chemotherapy administration is indicated according to the presence of prognostic factors given by pathology.

42.4 Conclusions

Herein we have described a standardized technique for resecting locally advanced pancreatic cancers invading the SMA. The technique presented entails extensive bowel mobilization, management of the venous system by temporary shunting, resection of the artery and reconstruction by direct anastomosis or by interposing autologous saphenous graft according to segment resected.

The performance of PD with SMA requires extensive experience in vascular and pancreatic resection and should be reserved to high volume center.

References

1. Conroy T, Hammel P, Hebbar M, et al. FOLFIRINOX or gemcitabine as adjuvant therapy for pancreatic cancer. N Engl J Med. 2018;379:2395–406.
2. Janssen QP, Buettner S, Suker M, et al. Neoadjuvant FOLFIRINOX in patients with borderline resectable pancreatic cancer: a systematic review and patient-level meta-analysis. J Natl Cancer Inst. 2019;111:782–94.
3. Hackert T, Sachsenmaier M, Hinz U, et al. Locally advanced pancreatic cancer: neoadjuvant therapy with Folfirinox results in resectability in 60% of the patients. Ann Surg. 2016;264:457–63.
4. Rangelova E, Wefer A, Persson S, et al. Surgery improves survival after neoadjuvant therapy for borderline and locally advanced pancreatic cancer: a single institution experience. Ann Surg. 2021;273(3):579–86.
5. Fortner JG. Regional resection of cancer of the pancreas: a new surgical approach. Surgery. 1973;73:307–20.
6. Fortner JG, Kim DK, Cubilla A, Turnbull A, Pahnke LD, Shils ME. Regional pancreatectomy: en bloc pancreatic, portal vein and lymph node resection. Ann Surg. 1977;186:42–50.
7. de Wilde RF, Besselink MG, van der Tweel I, et al. Impact of nationwide centralization of pancreaticoduodenectomy on hospital mortality. Br J Surg. 2012;99:404–10.
8. Panni RZ, Panni UY, Liu J, et al. Re-defining a high volume center for pancreaticoduodenectomy. HPB (Oxford). 2021;23(5):733–8.
9. Bachellier P, Nakano H, Oussoultzoglou PD, et al. Is pancreaticoduodenectomy with mesentericoportal venous resection safe and worthwhile? Am J Surg. 2001;182:120–9.
10. Bachellier P, Rosso E, Lucescu I, et al. Is the need for an arterial resection a contraindication to pancreatic resection for locally advanced pancreatic adenocarcinoma? A case-matched controlled study. J Surg Oncol. 2011;103:75–84.
11. Bachellier P, Addeo P, Faitot F, Nappo G, Dufour P. Pancreatectomy with arterial resection for pancreatic adenocarcinoma: how can it be done safely and with which outcomes?: a single institution's experience with 118 patients. Ann Surg. 2020;271:932–40.
12. Christians KK, Pilgrim CH, Tsai S, et al. Arterial resection at the time of pancreatectomy for cancer. Surgery. 2014;155:919–26.
13. Kwon J, Shin SH, Yoo D, et al. Arterial resection during pancreatectomy for pancreatic ductal adenocarcinoma with arterial invasion: a single-center experience with 109 patients. Medicine (Baltimore). 2020;99:e22115.
14. Truty MJ, Kendrick ML, Nagorney DM, et al. Factors predicting response, perioperative outcomes, and survival following total neoadjuvant therapy for borderline/locally advanced pancreatic cancer. Ann Surg. 2021;273(2):341–9.
15. Jegatheeswaran S, Baltatzis M, Jamdar S, Siriwardena AK. Superior mesenteric artery (SMA) resection during pancreatectomy for

malignant disease of the pancreas: a systematic review. HPB (Oxford). 2017;19:483–90.
16. Addeo P, De Mathelin P, Averous G, et al. The left splenorenal venous shunt decreases clinical signs of sinistral portal hypertension associated with splenic vein ligation during pancreaticoduodenectomy with venous resection. Surgery. 2020;168:267–73.
17. Addeo P, Nappo G, Felli E, Oncioiu C, Faitot F, Bachellier P. Management of the splenic vein during a pancreaticoduodenectomy with venous resection for malignancy. Updat Surg. 2016;68:241–6.
18. Addeo P, Rosso E, Fuchshuber P, et al. Resection of borderline resectable and locally advanced pancreatic adenocarcinomas after neoadjuvant chemotherapy. Oncology. 2015;89:37–46.
19. Addeo P, Velten M, Averous G, et al. Prognostic value of venous invasion in resected T3 pancreatic adenocarcinoma: depth of invasion matters. Surgery. 2017;162:264–74.
20. Bachellier P, Rosso E, Fuchshuber P, et al. Use of a temporary intraoperative mesentericoportal shunt for pancreatic resection for locally advanced pancreatic cancer with portal vein occlusion and portal hypertension. Surgery. 2014;155:449–56.
21. Fukuda S, Oussoultzoglou E, Bachellier P, et al. Significance of the depth of portal vein wall invasion after curative resection for pancreatic adenocarcinoma. Arch Surg. 2007;142:172–9; discussion 80.
22. Addeo P, Rosso E, Fuchshuber P, et al. Double purse-string telescoped pancreaticogastrostomy: an expedient, safe, and easy technique. J Am Coll Surg. 2013;216:e27–33.

Robotic Pancreaticoduodenectomy

Thilo Hackert

Abstract

Robotic or robotic assisted surgery can be regarded as an advancement of minimally invasive surgery and has been implemented in various field of surgery including pancreatic surgery in recent years. Acceptance worldwide is increasing—also for complex surgical procedures—and nearly all types of pancreatic resections have been performed robotically in the meantime. Although robotic pancreas surgery is potentially burdened by a long learning curve and increased procedure costs, standardized resections such as distal pancreatectomy and partial pancreatico-duodenectomy (PD) are well established in specialized centers today. The first robotic PD has been reported by Giulianotti in 2001, yet, due to the complex reconstruction technique required, this has not been adopted in the following years before larger case series were published. The robotic technology advancements offer a three-dimensional movement of minimally-invasive instruments as well as a high-definition view, however, tissue handling and manipulation during resection and especially reconstruction require a high level of training and expertise to achieve good results. During the learning curve, increased morbidity has to be accepted, including high conversion rates. Based on experiences of the pioneers of this technique, approximately 80 procedures are required to achieve a sufficient level of expertise and consequently surpass the learning curve. Yet, no randomized controlled trials (RCTs) on the perioperative and long-term outcomes of robotic PD compared to open or laparoscopic PD have been published, leaving a low level of evidence to support this technique today. Despite this situation, which is commonly observed when new techniques are introduced, a number of observational studies with promising results in terms of morbidity, mortality and oncological outcomes have been published. Practically, no absolute contraindications to choose a robotic approach for standard PD exist. In addition, the robotic technique may also be suitable for challenging pancreatic anastomoses with a high risk of postoperative pancreatic fistula (POPF) without the need to convert to an open procedure in such situations. Presumed advantages of robotic PD include faster postoperative mobilization and return to activity of the patients as well as shorter hospital stay without an increased need for readmission when compared to open PD. Considering the low methodological quality of the currently available studies, these results have to be considered with caution due to the observational character of the published series and a potential bias of underreporting morbidity which may especially be a risk of bias during the learning curve of this procedure.

43.1 Background

Since the mid-1980s minimally-invasive surgery (MIS) has been established in various surgical fields, starting with gynecological operations and extending to other disciplines including visceral surgery in the 1990s [1]. After initial skepticism, "small" procedures like appendectomy or cholecystectomy were accepted and finally regarded as the standard of care, yet, it took several years to establish more complex procedures adopting this technique. The first MIS-PD was performed in 1994 [2] demonstrating that this was generally feasible in highly specialized centers, however, no widespread acceptance occurred. Regarding MIS for PD, the debate is still ongoing today which is based on the data from non-observational studies, but RCTs that have reported conflicting results. Today, there are three RCTs available, two of them reporting favorable outcomes, one showing that MIS for PD may be potentially dangerous when brought into wide-spread practice [3–5]. Systematically analyzing these results, a potential thread for the patient is not reproducible

T. Hackert (✉)
Department of General, Visceral and Transplantation Surgery,
University of Heidelberg, Heidelberg, Germany
e-mail: Thilo.Hackert@med.uni-heidelberg.de

[6], however, a high level of specialization as well as case load seems to be required when offering MIS for PD and the potential problem is the generalizability of results which may limit the acceptance of MIS for PD in daily practice as only few centers will be able to overcome the learning curve and offer a MIS-PD program on a high level of expertise [5]. Considering this, MIS-PD does not seem to be a promising alternative approach to open PD today. In this situation, the application of the robotic technology may be the key to facilitate minimally-invasive procedures and help to spread this approach in PD as especially the phase of reconstruction can be performed much more easily than in conventional MIS.

Regarding the development of robotic surgery, after its establishment as a small start-up joint-venture between academic institutions and industry as well as the US army, in 1995 the company Intuitive Surgical© was founded and introduced the DaVinci® system as a robotic platform in 1999, receiving FDA approval for MIS procedures in 2000. Today, the company has achieved a nearly exclusive worldwide monopolistic market position and the DaVinci® system is by far the most commonly used device. In pancreatic surgery, robotic distal pancreatectomies and enucleations were performed as early as 2001 [7]. Giulianotti pioneered the first robotic PD in the same year [8] but mainly due to the complex reconstruction, it took several before larger patient series were published, mainly from the Pittsburgh center [9]. With this increase of utilization, other centers introduced robotic PD increasing the number of procedures worldwide and establishing or adopting the standards published before. For any type of robotic surgery, there are mainly observational studies to date, yet, a large number of RCTs are planned or already recruiting with the aim to compare either robotic vs. conventional MIS or open procedures [10]. Consequently, more data on the safety and oncological feasibility are awaited within the next 3–5 years. The present review summarizes the currently available data on robotic PD.

43.2 Robotic PD

Robotic PD is the most complex procedure among all types of robotic pancreas resections. Despite the advantages of the robotic platform compared to conventional MIS—especially the possibilities of three-dimensional instrument movement and high-definition view—tissue handling and manipulation during resection as well as reconstruction requires a high level of expertise as the tactile feedback is still lacking which limits the surgeon's ability to adjust his technique to certain challenging situations including vascular involvement during resection or very soft tissue conditions during reconstruction. This implies that a very accurate diagnostic workup is mandatory to recognize potential venous or arterial involvement by pancreatic tumors preoperatively and estimate the suitability of a patient for a robotic procedure. Vascular resection and reconstruction is well possible during robotic PD, however, it has to be planned and requires an adequate level of experience and technical kills when attempted. Otherwise, conversion to an open procedure—also in an emergency setting—is inevitable. This also implies that every surgeon doing robotic PD has to be trained not only in this procedure but also in open PD to be able to convert and fix any occurring problem by an open approach if required—a merely robotic training seems to be inadequate in such a setting, especially as during the learning curve of robotic PD, an increased morbidity caused by intraoperative challenges may occur and high conversion rates are possible. Regarding the implementation of robotic PD, some preconditions have to be respected. Firstly, a center needs to have a level of experience in open pancreatic surgery and handling the potential complications; secondly, a certain case load has to be guaranteed—although there is no clear consensus on the minimal number of annal procedures, it seems to be reasonable to have a volume of at least 50 PDs per year to select proper patients for robotic PD and to surpass the learning curve for this procedure in a reasonable time frame. Thirdly, an environment of experienced open—an ideally—laparoscopic surgeons has to be present, who are able and willing to go through training (including simulator skills, tissue training, visiting experienced centers), on-site proctoring and teaching of robotic PD. Presumed these preconditions are fulfilled, a patient selection is absolutely mandatory to start a robotic PD program. This implies to select clearly resectable cases of any type of pancreatic tumors to start and assure quality monitoring, which can be realized within a prospective database or a clinical study setting. Especially with regard to resectability of any pancreatic pathology, a certain selection bias is inherent during the learning curve of robotic PD. As it is common knowledge that during PD easy resection (small—potentially benign or borderline lesions, no duct dilation) is usually associated with rather difficult reconstruction (small pancreatic/bile duct, soft pancreatic remnant tissue), this may initially lead to an increase of postoperative morbidity, underlining the importance of complication management to avoid any failure to rescue and endanger patients undergoing robotic PD. Furthermore, the standardization of all operative steps of PD is not only possible but also helpful to achieve good outcomes. Giulianotti et al. published a 17-step procedure line for robotic PD including all key points of resection and reconstruction [11]. Although this is only a guide to perform the procedure and every patient may require individual adoption, a certain standardization is certainly helpful and defined steps of the operation can be standardized very well, i.e. positioning of the patient, trocar placement and positioning of the instruments on the respective arms of the robot [12]. A basic consideration is the decision to perform robotic PD as a "one-surgeon" procedure in which the console surgeon basically does all steps of the procedure himself and the table-site assistant is only helping with exposition, suction and instrument changes. Alternatively, robotic PD may be performed in a "two-surgeon" approach if the table-site surgeon also actively participated in the operative steps, i.e. by using a sealing/cutting device, dividing structures by scissor or applying clips. Both approaches have advantages, the first guarantees a high grade of independence for the console surgeon and allows to perform the procedure also with less qualified or changing table-site personnel. The disadvantage is a potentially high frequency of instrument changes that are required. The second approach may allow a faster procedure with less instrument changes if the team is well-practiced. This approach however, requires a steady team composed of two experienced surgeons and may be therefore difficult to realize in some centers.

Regarding technical aspects of robotic PD, the common principles of radical resection should be respected. This implies the common standard of required lymphadenectomy during PD including the lymph nodes on the right side of the superior mesenteric artery, celiac axis and the hepatoduodenal ligament [13]. Furthermore, soft tissue in the "triangle" between superior mesenteric artery, celiac axis and portal vein should be cleared [14]. As resection is technically easier if all preparation can be done from the right side of the mesenteric root without changing perspective and the field of preparation to the left side of the Treitz ligament, the first jejunal loop needs to pulled through after dividing Treitz ligament and after skeletonizing the loop, an "uncinate-first approach" is a very convenient procedure for resection during robotic PD [15]. Division of the pancreatic neck can be done by stapler or by monopolar cautery as well as by sealing/cutting devices.

After completion of the resection, pancreatic anastomosis reconstruction can be done by pancreatico-jejunostomy (PJ) or pancreatico-gastrostomy, however, most surgeons prefer PJ in a modified Blumgart fashion using an internal pancreatic stent as this is technically the easiest way of reconstruction (Fig. 43.1) [16]. Hepatico-jejunostomy can be done by one-layer running sutures for dilated bile ducts (Fig. 43.2) or by monofilament single stitches in case of small bile ducts, comparably to hepato-jejunostomy in open PD. For gastro-jejunostomy, side-to side stapling with suture closure of the stapler introducing incision is the quickest possibility of reconstruction, but all other types of sutured anastomoses are possible, depending on the surgeon's preference.

With regard to outcomes of robotic PD, these have to be weighed against open PD as the gold standard as well as conventional MIS-PD. No RCTs have yet compared these procedures and data are mainly retrieved from a number of case series as well as mono-and multicenter comparative observational studies [17–21]. Overall, these studies confirm technical feasibility and promising results regarding morbidity, mortality and oncological outcomes.

The largest observational study includes 500 robotic PD performed over a 10-year period and reports an improvement of operative performance with a reduction of operating room time during the first 240 procedures with a plateau phase afterwards [22]. This impressively underlines the duration of the learning curve, furthermore the study shows

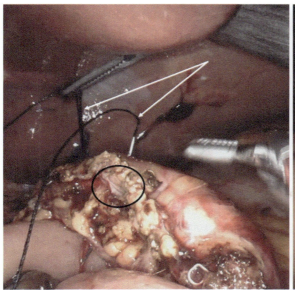 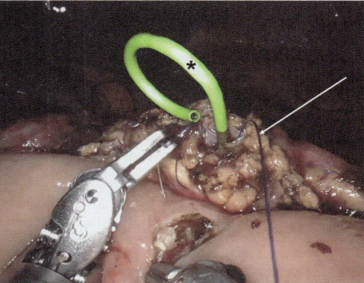

Fig. 43.1 Pancreatico-jejunostomy, modified Blumgart technique. Left side: preparation of the transparenchymal stitches (white arrows), pancreatic duct (black circle). Right side: duct-to-mucosa stitches (white arrow), inserted pancreatic duct stent (black asterisk)

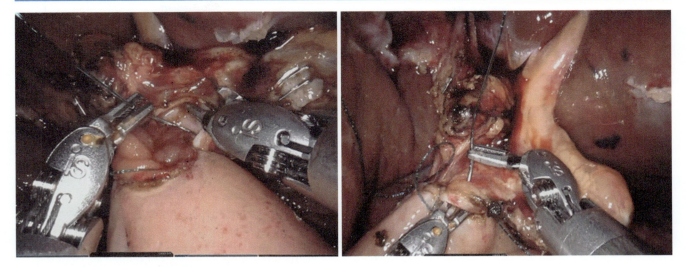

Fig. 43.2 Hepatic-jejunostomy, running sutures. Left side: single-layer backwall suture Right side: single-layer frontwall suture

that during the last 100 cases in this series operation time remained stable although an increasing proportion of vascular resections were performed and more patients undergoing neoadjuvant therapy—with presumably more difficult conditions during resection—were selected. A comparative series from the US includes eight centers and 211 post learning-curve robotic PD vs. 817 open PD [17]. This study shows that a high BMI or a history of previous abdominal surgery are no basic contraindications to choose a robotic approach, overall conversion rate was 4.7%. For malignant indications, surgeons tended to prefer an open approach as 55% of open vs. 33% of robotic PDs were performed for cancerous lesions. This may well be explained by basic concerns regarding radicality of the robotic procedures, results remain unclear in this respect. The proportion of R1 resections was higher for the robotic group (50% vs. 33%) whereas the number of retrieved lymph nodes favored the robotic resection ($n = 27.5$ vs. $n = 19$ harvested lymph nodes) without results on long-term outcomes. Perioperative outcomes were comparable, especially clinically relevant POPF (robotic 13.8% vs. open 9.0%). With a similar length of hospital stay, robotic patients were readmitted more frequently (31% robotic PD vs. 24% open PD).

A definitive evaluation especially regarding long-term oncological outcomes is not possible from these data. A recent systematic review [19] includes 11 non-randomized studies comparing robotic and open PD. The number of robotic procedures in the underlying studies accounts to overall $n = 514$ robotic PD vs. $n = 1263$ open PD. The results show significant differences in operation time (robotically +1.5 h) and blood loss (robotically −200 mL) with similar transfusion rate. In the subgroup of oncological patients, robotic PD showed a lower rate of R1 resections with a similar number of retrieved lymph nodes. The data favor robotic PD in terms of lower overall morbidity (especially surgical site infections) and faster postoperative mobilization of the patients, although this does not turn into shorter length of hospital stay.

Long-term oncological outcome as the potentially most important variable for pancreatic cancer surgery has recently been investigated in an analysis of the US National Cancer Database [23]. Stage I–III pancreatic cancer patients who underwent either robotic PD ($n = 626$) or open PD ($n = 17.205$) showed no relevant differences in baseline data regarding tumor characteristics. In the short-term outcomes, robotic PD was superior with regard to lymph node yield whereas R0 resection status was similar in both groups. Robotic PD resulted in a shorter hospital stay (−1 day) at similar readmission and 90-day mortality rates (9% vs. 8% readmission and 4% vs. 6% mortality, respectively). Median overall survival was 22.0 months (robotic PD) vs. 21.8 months (open PD) with 1-, 3- and 5-year survival rates of 74% vs. 73%, 33% vs. 31% and 19% vs. 19%, respectively. Based on such data, there should not be a general restrictive attitude towards robotic PD in malignant indications, even if results have to be considered with caution to the retrospective nature of this registry study.

Beyond standard PD, extended procedures, namely vascular resections have been performed in a few centers worldwide [24–26]. Principally, such operations are possible using the robotic system for venous as well as arterial reconstructions. Due to the very limited reported number of patients undergoing extended robotic PD it is not possible to give a valid estimation about potential advantages. In addition, considerable morbidity (up to 80%) and mortality rates (up to 14%) may burden these approaches which certainly require an even longer learning curve than that for standard robotic PD [27, 28].

43.3 Conclusion

Robotic procedures have changed all fields of surgery including visceral and pancreatic surgery in the last two decades. Today, robotic PD has gained acceptance in many centers, mainly for standard PD, although also extended PD resections are possible after passing a considerable learning curve. Due to the currently available mostly observational studies, the level of evidence regarding short- and long-term results of robotic PD compared to open PD is still low. The present studies confirm the feasibility of robotic PD and postulate potential advantages associated with the minimally-invasive nature of the operation. These include less blood loss, earlier mobilization and shorter hospital stay. To confirm such conclusions, RCTs are warranted and currently being planned or already recruiting to create more high-level evidence in the near future.

References

1. Mack MJ. Minimally invasive and robotic surgery. JAMA. 2001;285:568–72.
2. Gagner M, Pomp A. Laparoscopic pylorus-preserving pancreatoduodenectomy. Surg Endosc. 1994;8(5):408–10.
3. Poves I, Burdio F, Morato O, et al. Comparison of perioperative outcomes between laparoscopic and open approach for pancreatoduodenectomy: the PADULAP randomized controlled trial. Ann Surg. 2018;268(5):731–9.
4. Palanivelu C, Senthilnathan P, Sabnis SC, et al. Randomized clinical trial of laparoscopic versus open pancreatoduodenectomy for periampullary tumours. Br J Surg. 2017;104(11):1443–50.
5. van Hilst J, de Rooij T, Bosscha K, et al. Laparoscopic versus open pancreatoduodenectomy for pancreatic or periampullary tumours (LEOPARD-2): a multicentre, patient-blinded, randomised controlled phase 2/3 trial. Lancet Gastroenterol Hepatol. 2019;4(3):199–207.
6. Nickel F, Haney CM, Kowalewski KF, et al. Laparoscopic versus open pancreatoduodenectomy: a systematic review and meta-analysis of randomized controlled trials. Ann Surg. 2020;271(1):54–66.
7. Joyce D, Morris-Stiff G, Falk GA, El-Hayek K, Chalikonda S, Walsh RM. Robotic surgery of the pancreas. World J Gastroenterol. 2014;20(40):14726–32.
8. Giulianotti PC, Coratti A, Angelini M, Sbrana F, Cecconi S, Balestracci T, Caravaglios G. Robotics in general surgery: personal experience in a large community hospital. Arch Surg. 2003;138(7):777–84.
9. Zureikat AH, Moser AJ, Boone BA, Bartlett DL, Zenati M, Zeh HJ 3rd. 250 robotic pancreatic resections: safety and feasibility. Ann Surg. 2013;258(4):554–9; discussion 559–62.
10. Kirchberg J, Weitz J. Evidence for robotic surgery in oncological visceral surgery. Chirurg. 2019;90(5):379–86.
11. Giulianotti PC, Mangano A, Bustos RE, et al. Educational step-by-step surgical video about operative technique in robotic pancreaticoduodenectomy (RPD) at University of Illinois at Chicago (UIC): 17 steps standardized technique-lessons learned since the first worldwide RPD performed in the year 2001. Surg Endosc. 2020;34(6):2758–62.
12. Liu R, Wakabayashi G, Palanivelu C, et al. International consensus statement on robotic pancreatic surgery. Hepatobiliary Surg Nutr. 2019;8(4):345–60.
13. Tol JA, Gouma DJ, Bassi C, et al. Definition of a standard lymphadenectomy in surgery for pancreatic ductal adenocarcinoma: a consensus statement by the international study group on pancreatic surgery (ISGPS). Surgery. 2014;156(3):591–600.
14. Hackert T, Strobel O, Michalski CW, et al. The TRIANGLE operation - radical surgery after neoadjuvant treatment for advanced pancreatic cancer: a single arm observational study. HPB (Oxford). 2017;19(11):1001–7.
15. Hackert T, Werner J, Weitz J, et al. Uncinate process first--a novel approach for pancreatic head resection. Langenbeck's Arch Surg. 2010;395(8):1161–4.
16. Kim AC, Rist RC, Zureikat AH. Technical detail for robot assisted pancreaticoduodenectomy. J Vis Exp. 2019;(151) https://doi.org/10.3791/60261.
17. Zureikat AH, Postlewait LM, Liu Y, et al. A multi-institutional comparison of perioperative outcomes of robotic and open pancreaticoduodenectomy. Ann Surg. 2016;264(4):640–9.
18. van Oosten AF, Ding D, Habib JR, et al. Perioperative outcomes of robotic pancreaticoduodenectomy: a propensity-matched analysis to open and laparoscopic pancreaticoduodenectomy. J Gastrointest Surg. 2021;25(7):1795–804. https://doi.org/10.1007/s11605-020-04869-z.
19. Zhao W, Liu C, Li S, Geng D, Feng Y, Sun M. Safety and efficacy for robot-assisted versus open pancreaticoduodenectomy and distal pancreatectomy: a systematic review and meta-analysis. Surg Oncol. 2018;27(3):468–78.
20. Baimas-George M, Watson M, Murphy KJ, et al. Robotic pancreaticoduodenectomy may offer improved oncologic outcomes over open surgery: a propensity-matched single-institution study. Surg Endosc. 2020;34(8):3644–9.
21. Guerra F, Checcacci P, Vegni A, et al. Surgical and oncological outcomes of our first 59 cases of robotic pancreaticoduodenectomy. J Visc Surg. 2019;156(3):185–90.
22. Zureikat AH, Beane JD, Zenati MS, et al. 500 minimally invasive robotic pancreatoduodenectomies: one decade of optimizing performance. Ann Surg. 2021;273(5):966–72. https://doi.org/10.1097/SLA.0000000000003550.
23. Nassour I, Winters SB, Hoehn R, et al. Long-term oncologic outcomes of robotic and open pancreatectomy in a national cohort of pancreatic adenocarcinoma. J Surg Oncol. 2020;122(2):234–42. https://doi.org/10.1002/jso.25958.
24. Kauffmann EF, Napoli N, Menonna F, et al. Robotic pancreatoduodenectomy with vascular resection. Langenbeck's Arch Surg. 2016;401(8):1111–22.
25. Giulianotti PC, Addeo P, Buchs NC, et al. Robotic extended pancreatectomy with vascular resection for locally advanced pancreatic tumors. Pancreas. 2011;40(8):1264–70.
26. Marino MV, Giovinazzo F, Podda M, et al. Robotic-assisted pancreaticoduodenectomy with vascular resection. Description of the surgical technique and analysis of early outcomes. Surg Oncol. 2020;35:344–50.
27. Rice MK, Hodges JC, Bellon J, et al. Association of mentorship and a formal robotic proficiency skills curriculum with subsequent generations' learning curve and safety for robotic pancreaticoduodenectomy. JAMA Surg. 2020;155(7):607–15.
28. Schmidt CR, Harris BR, Musgrove KA, et al. Formal robotic training diminishes the learning curve for robotic pancreatoduodenectomy: implications for new programs in complex robotic surgery. J Surg Oncol. 2021;123(2):375–80. https://doi.org/10.1002/jso.26284.

44

Duodenum-Preserving Pancreatic Head Resection

Elena Usova

Abstract

Duodenum-preserving pancreatic head resection (DPPHR) remains a rare procedure even for high volume centers since its clinical implementation in 1979. Reports on this surgery are scattered and present mostly as sporadic systematic reviews and case reports/case series. Terminology for those procedures varies among authors. Present chapter aims to pool current knowledge and give an idea of anatomical and surgical fundamentals of DPPHR. Latter one needs meticulous knowledge of vascular anatomy of pancreatic head and adjacent organs and might become technically more challenging when compared to pancreaticoduodenectomy. Postoperative complication rate and location of the lesion are other contributing factors to limited use of DPPHR. Limited pancreatic resection is useful mostly for benign focal pancreatic lesions and chronic pancreatitis. Exposure of main pancreatic duct and/or common bile duct and their subsequent management require large experience in hepatopancreatobiliary surgery that feels to be never enough. Author is hoping to expand the knowledge of the reader on DPPHR and promote organ-sparing technique for benign lesions just like it has become in regard to liver surgery of last decade. Any further comments and suggestions will be appreciated.

Duodenum-preserving pancreatic head resection (DPPRH) has not been precisely defined or classified in the literature or existing guidelines. Roughly, it can be defined as the procedure with either total or partial resection of the pancreatic head parenchyma and with preservation of the duodenum or its segmental resection. According to the pioneer of DPPHR, Hans Beger, a total DPPHR involves resection of the pancreatic head conserving the pancreatic neck. Peripapillary segment of the duodenum and the intrapancreatic common bile duct segment might be either resected or preserved [1]. In case of the former, three anastomoses are required; i.e., end-to-end duodenum to duodenum, end-to-side common bile duct (CBD) to postpyloric duodenum and end-to-side pancreaticointestinal anastomoses, in addition to Roux-en-Y jejuno-jejunostomy.

Unlike the total one, a partial DPPHR includes limited resection of the pancreatic head parenchyma with preservation of the duodenum and common bile duct and parts of the ventral or dorsal pancreatic head tissue or resection only of the tumour bearing tissue of the uncinate process [2]. An anastomosis between the pancreatic head and an excluded jejunal loop is necessary in either case.

44.1 History of DPPHR

Role of the pioneer of DPPHR may belong to Beger. In 1972 he started his dog experiments on subtotal pancreatic head resection. First report on in-human use of this procedure has been done in 1980 by the same author [1]. Surgery was performed in 12 patients: nine of them experienced chronic pancreatitis (CP) and three underwent DPPHR for suspected malignancy and pathology showed benign lesions. Author reported no clinical lethality with 75% rate of complete recovery 3 years after surgery. A total DPPHR removing pancreatic head parenchyma completely was suggested by Imaizumi in 1990 [3]. Later on, Nakao argued that blood supply to the duodenum and common bile duct is compromised significantly during a total DPPHR to cause ischemic necrosis of them and that a segmental duodenectomy is required to avoid this complication [4]. He proposed this procedure as a pancreatic head resection with segmental duodenectomy (PHRSD) and distinguished PHRSD from DPPHR.

DPPHR for CP became a standard of care soon after its implementation into clinical practice [5]. The most likely

E. Usova (✉)
International Association of Surgeons, Gastroenterologists and Oncologists, Kyoto, Japan

reason is that surgery has been done to patients with fibrotic changes of pancreatic tissue thus mostly giving the sense of safety to the surgeon in light of postoperative pancreatic fistula. Recent systematic review and meta-analysis includes 797 patients with DPPHR for CP in 15 studies [6].

However, DPPHR for focal lesions of pancreatic head remains of limited use even in high volume centers partly because it demands meticulous technique to dissect along the mostly intact pancreatic parenchyma. Thus, further in this chapter author wants to focus specifically on DPPHR for focal lesions. To date, as of last review by Beger et al., totally 523 cases of DPPHR for benign and low-grade malignant pancreatic neoplasms within 26 cohort studies have been identified [7]. Minimally invasive or robotic-assisted approach has been used in 37 of 523 (7.1%) patients.

Progress in technologies for minimally invasive surgery and advanced techniques made it possible to perform a laparoscopic DPPHR as performed in 2004 and published in 2007 by Takaori [8]. In his first laparoscopic DPPHR, however, the case was converted into open for reconstruction, specifically for pancreaticojejunostomy, using a small laparotomy incision. As of nowadays, a totally laparoscopic DPPHR including laparoscopic reconstruction has been performed sporadically by several surgeons including the present author and this minimally invasive procedure has been indicated for IPMN, neuroendocrine tumors and other non-invasive neoplasms of the pancreatic head.

Robotic pancreatic surgery became notable for DPPHR in 2012 [9]. Peng et al. presented four cases of DPPHR: one for CP and three for benign pancreatic neoplasms. As of 2018, he reported 34 patients to undergo this procedure while currently it remains the largest single center experience [10].

44.2 Classification

As for now, DPPHR can be classified as total, subtotal, and partial ones. In the first scenario, the duodenum can be either totally preserved or resected segmentally. Subtotal DPPHR presumes to spare duodenum and to either spare common bile duct (CBD) or perform its resection along with resection of the pancreatic head leaving only the thin layer of pancreatic tissue along the duodenum. Partial DPPHR usually spares all the above structures.

44.3 Blood Supply to Pancreatic Head and Pertinent Adjacent Organs

It is well known that pancreatic head blood supply goes from celiac axis (CA) and superior mesenteric artery (SMA). Likewise, there is no need for expert pancreatic surgeons to recall where all the pancreaticoduodenal arteries (PDAs) arise from. Nonetheless, some aspects of blood supply to pertinent segments of the pancreas, CBD and duodenum, especially those vulnerable for ischemia, need to be mentioned.

Description of vascular anatomy of the pancreas goes back to 1748 when Haller described anterior and posterior arches (arcades between CA and SMA) [11]. Since then, not many studies have been done on this specific issue using post-mortem specimens. Falconer and Griffiths investigated 50 specimens (27 dissections and 23 injection-corrosion preparations) [12]. In all the cases, gastroduodenal artery (GDA) gave rise to the anterior vessel, the anterior superior pancreaticoduodenal artery (ASPDA), which went over the head of the pancreas inferiorly toward duodenopancreatic sulcus and then medially in the groove, and posteriorly along the gland. Anastomosis was present behind the uncinate process with an anterior inferior pancrearticoduodenal artery (AIPDA). Posterior superior pancreaticoduodenal artery (PSPDA) was present in 25 dissections. In all but two cases (when it was arising from hepatic branch of SMA) PSPDA originated 1.5 cm distally to the origin of GDA. Then PSPDA went backwards over the upper border of the pancreas in front of the CBD along the posterior pancreaticoduodenal sulcus followed by leaving the latter shortly and going medially across the posterior surface of the pancreatic head and creating an anastomosis with the posterior inferior pancreaticoduodenal artery (PIPDA).

Bertelli et al. did summarize anatomy and nomenclature of pancreas blood supply over past two centuries based on over 1000 angiographic studies [13–16]. This is the classic anatomy we use nowadays. Typically, blood supply to the head of the pancreas goes from CA (via ASPDA and PSPDA as its terminal branches) and SMA (via AIPDA and PIPDA as its terminal branches) with arcade formation anteriorly and posteriorly. Authors also emphasize on the dorsal pancreatic artery (known also as Haller's artery) as a source of blood supply to pancreatic head originating from either splenic artery (most commonly), or CHA, or CA, or SMA, or other smaller visceral artery [17]. Its right terminal branch goes behind the superior mesenteric vein and then passes along anterior surface of pancreatic head. Before supplying pancreatic head, it forms prepancreatic arch, anastomosing with branch of the GDA, AS PDA or right gastroepiploic artery.

Furukawa et al. highlighted in their study blood supply to the pancreatic head taking into consideration its embryogenesis by computed tomography during arteriography, specifically its derivation from the ventral (smaller) and dorsal (larger) buds [18]. The former one corresponds to caudal part of pancreatic head and equals to uncinate process and gets blood supply from SMA (inferior PDAs, respectively) while the latter one is supplied by CA (superior PDAs, respectively) and equals to cephalic part of the head of the pancreas. Blood supply to CBD and ampulla of Vater is provided by CA, specifically by PSPDA, which is located along the intrapancreatic bile duct. Proximal part of the duodenum gets supply from CA, while distal part gets the one from SMA. According to the study, the boundary between those two areas was in the second part of the duodenum in 56%, in the third in 40%, and in fourth part in 4% of cases, respectively. Duodenum, mainly its first portion and proximal part of the second portion, also gets blood supply from the supraduodenal artery arising from GDA, and from retroduodenal artery arising from the PSPDA [19]. Those two are especially important to be preserved during DPPHR. Another study from Japan showed the presence of arcade formation between the ASPDA and the AIPDA in 100% of cases as well as between PSPDA and PIPDA in 88%, consequently. There was also found the membrane on the posterior aspect of the pancreas head where all of the PDAs were situated. One of the important details depicted in the study was that ASPDA eventually turns to the posterior aspect of the pancreas and joins there AIPDA [20]. Authors emphasize on the crucial role of the above membrane preservation to spare the blood supply to duodenum as well as PDAs themselves.

44.4 Technical Aspects of Total DPPHR

A total DPPHR is a procedure which requires removing all the pancreatic head tissue. In order to approach head of the pancreas, transection of gastrocolic ligament should be done along with access to lesser sac regardless of type of DPPHR.

Major pitfall of this procedure is how to preserve duodenal blood supply to avoid its ischemia. Given the description by Imaizumi, Kocher's maneuver should not be done [3, 21]. Nonetheless, author recommends ligation of GDA and right gastroepiploic artery along with sparing mesoduodenal vessels, especially when resecting uncinate process. Main pancreatic duct (MPD) and CBD are ligated extramurally followed by end-to-side pancreaticoduodenostomy and cholodochoduodenostomy, both with second part of duodenum. For the above procedure duodenum is totally preserved.

Nakao suggested 3–4 cm segmental duodenectomy along with both papilla resection for PHRSD to avoid duodenal ischemia [4]. Conservation of right gastric artery and AIPDA is required. Surgery is completed with pancreaticogastrostomy, end-to-end duodenoduodenostomy and end-to-side choledochoduodenostomy.

Takaori emphasized on preservation of PSPDA and PIPDA while ASPDA was divided at the origin of GDA. Hence, blood supply to the duodenum was preserved [8].

Hirata et al. when describing their technique of pylorus-preserving pancreaticoduodenectomy emphasize that preservation of retroduodenal artery arising from PSPDA and supplying first and proximal portion of second part of duodenum is critical, and ligation site should be after its root [18]. Likewise, Takada et al. claimed that PSPDA to be preserved while they avoided Kocher's maneuver [22].

Kim et al. demonstrated feasibility of total DPPHR with CBD preservation, however long-term outcomes as incidence of bile duct stenosis have not been reported but one during early postoperative course [23]. Authors advocate on sparing of all but ASPDA.

In general, type of anastomosis for pancreas remnant with gut as well as bile duct anastomosis is not a matter of discussion. None of the technique has been demonstrated as being safer [24]. The techniques highlighted above are preferences of each author. Aspects that matter are extent of parenchyma resection and preservation of blood supply to adjacent organs.

44.5 Technical Aspects of Subtotal DPPHR

A subtotal DPPHR, described as a typical Beger procedure, presumes preservation of thin layer of the pancreatic tissue of about 5–8 mm adjacent to the duodenum along with complete parenchyma transection followed by Roux-en-Y pancreaticojejunostomy [25]. The authors advocated that there is no need to preserve GDA. In turn, blood supply through supraduodenal vessels and dorsal duodenopancreatic arcade along with mesoduodenal vessels blood flow should be spared.

Unlike Beger procedure, its Bern modification leaves bridge of pancreatic tissue in front of superior mesenteric vein as well as opened both MPD and CBD followed by end-to-side anastomosis of pancreatic head with the jejunum including both ducts [26]. Kocher's maneuver and preservation of the entire duodenum is performed in both cases. Both procedures have become useful for CP with occasional use for benign or low-grade focal pancreatic lesions.

44.6 Technical Aspects of Partial DPPHR

A partial DPPHR is a procedure designed for benign and low-grade focal pancreatic lesions [27]. However, due to numerous technical aspects and sometimes being unsure about malignant potential of the lesion, surgeons tend to prefer Whipple procedure over DPPHR. In young patients with benign/low-grade pancreatic head lesions Whipple procedure seems to be excessive while removing organs not pertinent to the disease itself.

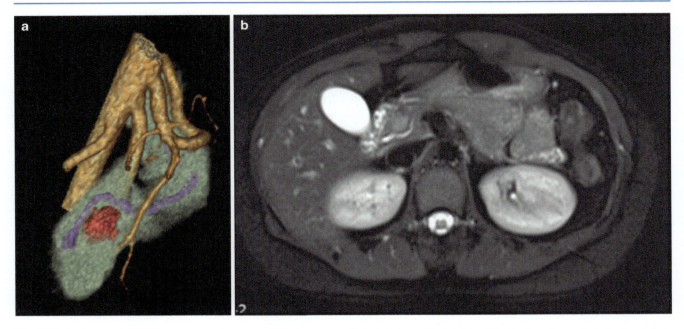

Fig. 44.1 (a) Abdominal 3D CT measured a 3 mm distance of pancreatic head mass (red) to MPD (purple) as well as demonstrated aberrant vascular anatomy of CA (yellow) giving rise to right hepatic artery, left hepatic artery, splenic artery, left gastric artery, and transverse pancreatic artery. (b) Abdominal MRI. Hyperintense pancreatic head mass in close proximity to MPD on its posterior surface

Extent of pancreatic head parenchyma resection can be defined as partial by extrapolating extent of pancreatic parenchyma resection for other types of surgery when comparing pancreatic function during long-term follow-up [28]. In order to get satisfactory endocrine and exocrine function in most cases resection of no more than 50% of pancreatic head parenchyma is recommended. Enucleation cannot be included into partial DPPHR as it doesn't presume resection of pancreatic tissue. In contrast, uncinatectomy represents a typical partial DPPHR. We recommend to avoid MPD exposure when possible during partial DPPHR. This is usually feasible with tumor distance to MPD of more than 2 mm.

Here is an example of partial DPPHR. Approach to pancreatic head was the same as described above. Surgery became a challenge due to intraparenchymal location of the tumor and its close proximity to MPD (Fig. 44.1a, b). Pancreatic lesion had been additionally visualized using intraoperative US (Fig. 44.2). Kocherization of duodenum has been done given that PDA arcades (between both anterior and both posterior PDAs) were preserved. Patient underwent partial DPPHR with preservation of MPD integrity. Lesion was excised with small portion of pancreatic parenchyma followed by Roux-en-Y pancreaticojejunostomy using simple interrupted suture (Fig. 44.3a, b). Pathology revealed proinsulin-only secreting tumor.

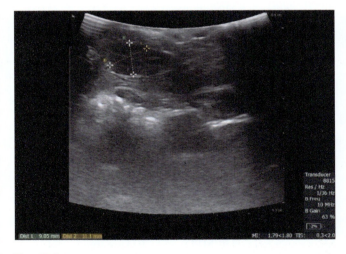

Fig. 44.2 Intraoperative US revealed hypovascular pancreatic head lesion close to MPD

44.7 Outcomes of DPPHR

For CP there is a sufficient number of studies highlighting short- and long-term outcomes. First randomized trial has been published by authors from Ulm and Bern [29]. The authors compared patients randomly assigned to either pylorus-preserving Whipple group or DPPHR group.

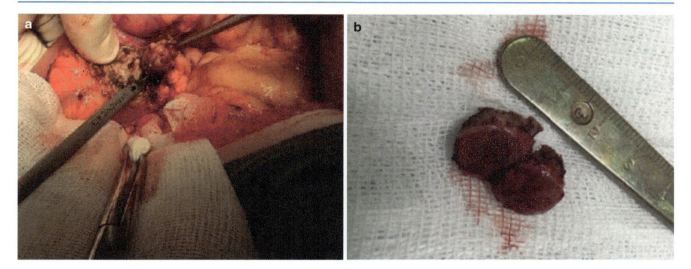

Fig. 44.3 (a) Pancreatic head bed after resection. (b) Macroscopic specimen of pancreatic head lesion

There was no postoperative mortality in both groups. Postoperative complication rate was 20% and 15%, respectively. However, patients who underwent DPPHR showed favourable long-term outcomes as less pain, greater weight gain, a better glucose tolerance, and a higher insulin secretion capacity. Authors also emphasize on preservation of duodenum as crucial factor for further intact glucose metabolism.

About two decades later, the same authors published multicentre, randomised, controlled, double-blind trial focusing mostly on long-term outcomes of surgery for CP comparing DPPHR vs partial pancreatectomy [30]. There was no difference in morbidity, mortality, and quality of life 24 months after surgery in DPPHR vs partial pancreaticoduodenectomy group. However, being a more definitive treatment, a partial pancreaticoduodenectomy was associated with fewer readmissions due to ongoing or recurrent pancreatitis.

Another meta-analysis on CP demonstrated that DPPHR has been shown to have more benefits over conventional pancreaticoduodenectomy/pylorus-preserving pancreaticoduodenectomy in reducing prevalence of endocrine insufficiency, delayed gastric emptying, and duration of postoperative stay, as well as increasing quality of life for patients, consequently. However, there was no significant differences between two groups in prevalence of pain relief, development of pancreatic fistula, wound infection, or exocrine insufficiency, as well as mortality rate [6].

As for DPPHR for focal premalignant and low-grade malignant neoplasms with IPMN as being the most frequent, according to meta-analysis, severe complication rate has been reported as 8.9% for total DPPHR and 13.9% for subtotal DPPHR. Overall in-hospital and late mortality with mean follow-up over 47 months were 0.6% and 1.5%, respectively [7].

As for long-term outcomes, single center study on functional results after various types of pancreas resection for neuroendocrine neoplasms found body mass index (BMI) to be the strongest predictor of postoperative diabetes mellitus (DM) with greater BMI being the greater risk for development of DM [28]. In addition, patients with advanced age, male gender, and non-functioning tumor were more prone to develop postoperative DM. Multivariate logistic regression analysis of predictors of postoperative pancreatic exocrine insufficiency showed that the extent of pancreatic parenchyma resection was the only independent predictor of postoperative pancreatic exocrine insufficiency.

Sporadic single center studies done before ChroPac presumed that quality of life and some other long-term variables after DPPHR for CP are above those after pancreaticoduodenectomy [30, 31]. However, non-randomized nature and other disadvantages like possible experimenter expectancy bias do not allow to support this hypothesis.

ChroPac study showing the outcomes of DPPHR for CP made it clear that most of those patients present with latent or prominent impairment of pancreatic function before surgery. In contrast, there are no similar studies yet for focal pancreatic lesions with intact parenchyma surrounding the tumors. This might cause a major argument over the organ-preserving surgery, especially in young patients. Our experience of DPPHR favors this procedure for specific patients as mentioned above.

References

1. Beger HG, Witte C, Krautzberger W, et al. Erfahrung mit einer das Duodenum erhaltenden Pankreaskopfresektion bei chronischer Pankreatitis. Chirurg. 1980;51:303–7.
2. Beger HG, Siech M, Poch B, Mayer B, Schoenberg MH. Limited surgery for benign tumours of the pancreas: a systematic review. World J Surg. 2015;39(6):1557–66.
3. Imaizumi T, Hanyu F, Suzuki M, et al. A new procedure: duodenumpreserving total resection of the head of the pancreas with pancreaticocholedocho-duodenostomy. J Bil Tract Pancreas. 1990;11:621–6. (In Japanese)
4. Nakao A. Pancreatic head resection with segmental duodenectomy and preservation of the gastroduodenal artery. Hepato-Gastroenterology. 1998;45(20):533–5.
5. Büchler MW, Friess H, Müller MW, Beger HG. Die duodenumerhaltende Pankreaskopfresektion: Eine neue Standardoperation bei chronischer Pankreatitis [Duodenum preserving resection of the head of the pancreas: a new standard operation in chronic pancreatitis]. Langenbecks Arch Chir Suppl Kongressbd. 1997;114:1081–3.
6. Zhao Y, Zhang J, Lan Z, et al. Duodenum-preserving resection of the pancreatic head versus pancreaticoduodenectomy for treatment of chronic pancreatitis with enlargement of the pancreatic head: systematic review and meta-analysis. Biomed Res Int. 2017;2017:3565438.
7. Beger HG, Mayer B, Poch B. Parenchyma-sparing, local pancreatic head resection for premalignant and low-malignant neoplasms - a systematic review and meta-analysis. Am J Surg. 2018;216(6):1182–91.
8. Takaori K, Tanigawa N. Laparoscopic pancreatic resection: the past, present, and future. Surg Today. 2007;37:535–45.
9. Peng CH, Shen BY, Deng XX, Zhan Q, Han B, Li HW. Early experience for the robotic duodenum-preserving pancreatic head resection. World J Surg. 2012;36(5):1136–41.
10. Jiang Y, Jin JB, Zhan Q, Deng XX, Peng CH, Shen BY. Robot-assisted duodenum-preserving pancreatic head resection with pancreaticogastrostomy for benign or premalignant pancreatic head lesions: a single-centre experience. Int J Med Robot. 2018;14(4):e1903.
11. von Haller A. Elementa physiologiae corporis humani, Tome VI. Societatistipographicae, Bemae; 1764. pp. 431–432.
12. Falconer CW, Griffiths E. The anatomy of the blood-vessels in the region of the pancreas. Br J Surg. 1950;37(147):334–44.
13. Bertelli E, Di Gregorio F, Bertelli L, Mosca S. The arterial blood supply of the pancreas: a review. I. The superior pancreaticoduodenal and the anterior superior pancreaticoduodenal arteries. An anatomical and radiological study. Surg Radiol Anat. 1995;17(2):97–3.
14. Bertelli E, Di Gregorio F, Bertelli L, Civeli L, Mosca S. The arterial blood supply of the pancreas: a review. II. The posterior superior pancreaticoduodenal artery. An anatomical and radiological study. Surg Radiol Anat. 1996;18(1):1–9.
15. Bertelli E, Di Gregorio F, Bertelli L, Civeli L, Mosca S. The arterial blood supply of the pancreas: a review. III. The inferior pancreaticoduodenal artery. An anatomical review and a radiological study. Surg Radiol Anat. 1996;18(2):67–74.
16. Bertelli E, Di Gregorio F, Bertelli L, Orazioli D, Bastianini A. The arterial blood supply of the pancreas: a review. IV. The anterior inferior and posterior pancreaticoduodenal aa., and minor sources of blood supply for the head of the pancreas. An anatomical review and radiologic study. Surg Radiol Anat. 1997;19(4):203–12.
17. Bertelli E, Di Gregorio F, Mosca S, et al. The arterial blood supply of the pancreas: a review. V. The dorsal pancreatic artery. Surg Radiol Anat. 1998;20:445–52.
18. Furukawa H, Iwata R, Moriyama N, Kosuge T. Blood supply to the pancreatic head, bile duct, and duodenum: evaluation by computed tomography during arteriography. Arch Surg. 1999;134(10):1086–90.
19. Hirata K, Mukaiya M, Kimura M, et al. The anatomy of the parapancreaticoduodenal vessels and the introduction of a new pylorus-preserving pancreatoduodenectomy with increased vessel preservation. J Hep Bil Pancr Surg. 1994;1:335–41.
20. Kimura W, Nagai H. Study of surgical anatomy for duodenum-preserving resection of the head of the pancreas. Ann Surg. 1995;221(4):359–63.
21. Imaizumi T, Hanyu F, Suzuki M. A new procedure for duodenum-preserving total resection of the head of the pancreas with pancreaticocholedochoduodenostomy. In: Beger HG, Büchler M, Malfertheiner P, editors. Standards in pancreatic surgery. Berlin, Heidelberg: Springer; 1993.
22. Takada T, Yasuda H, Uchiyama K, Hasegawa H. Duodenum-preserving pancreatoduodenostomy. A new technique for complete excision of the head of the pancreas with preservation of biliary and alimentary integrity. Hepato-Gastroenterology. 1993;40(4):356–9.
23. Kim SW, Kim KH, Jang JY, Park S, Park YH. Practical guidelines for the preservation of the pancreaticoduodenal arteries during duodenum-preserving resection of the head of the pancreas: clinical experience and a study using resected specimens from pancreaticoduodenectomy. Hepato-Gastroenterology. 2001;48(37):264–9.
24. Yeo CJ, Cameron JL, Maher MM, et al. A prospective randomized trial of pancreaticogastrostomy versus pancreaticojejunostomy after pancreaticoduodenectomy. Ann Surg. 1995;222(4):580–92.
25. Büchler M, Friess H, Jseumann R, Bittner R, Beger HG. Duodenum-preserving resection of the head of the pancreas: the Ulm experience. In: Beger HG, Büchler M, Malfertheiner P, editors. Standards in pancreatic surgery. Berlin, Heidelberg: Springer; 1993.
26. Gloor B, Friess H, Uhl W, Büchler MW. A modified technique of the Beger and Frey procedure in patients with chronic pancreatitis. Dig Surg. 2001;18(1):21–5.
27. Beger HG, Mayer B, Rau BM. Parenchyma-sparing, limited pancreatic head resection for benign tumors and low-risk periampullary cancer--a systematic review. J Gastrointest Surg. 2016;20(1):206–17.
28. Andreasi V, Partelli S, Capurso G, et al. Long-term pancreatic functional impairment after surgery for neuroendocrine neoplasms. J Clin Med. 2019;8(10):1611.
29. Büchler MW, Friess H, Müller MW, Wheatley AM, Beger HG. Randomized trial of duodenum-preserving pancreatic head resection versus pylorus-preserving Whipple in chronic pancreatitis. Am J Surg. 1995;169(1):65–70.
30. Diener MK, Hüttner FJ, Kieser M, et al. Partial pancreatoduodenectomy versus duodenum-preserving pancreatic head resection in chronic pancreatitis: the multicentre, randomised, controlled, double-blind ChroPac trial. Lancet. 2017;390(10099):1027–37.
31. Witzigmann H, Max D, Uhlmann D, et al. Quality of life in chronic pancreatitis: a prospective trial comparing classical whipple procedure and duodenum-preserving pancreatic head resection. J Gastrointest Surg. 2002;6:173–80.

# Artery-First Approaches to Distal Pancreatectomy

Kyoichi Takaori, Yosuke Kasai, and Kenji Yoshino

Abstract

Artery-first approaches to pancreatic resections have been widely practiced in the setting of a pancrearticoduodenectomy or Whipple procedure for pancreatic cancer. The purposes of artery-first approaches are to determine the resectability in the early phase of operation, to perform more oncologic resection by isolation of the tumor from the blood flow and to reduce the intraoperative blood loss. Until recently, however, artery approaches to a distal pancreatectomy (DP) have been scarcely performed due to the difficulty in approaching the origin of the splenic artery before the transection of the pancreas especially in open surgery. In contrast, by laparoscopic approaches, a surgeon can enter the retroperitoneal space behind the pancreatic body taking advantage of the caudo-cranial angle view through a laparoscope and explore the origin of the celiac artery from the aorta and the origin of the splenic artery without dividing the pancreas. The same approaches can be carried out in open surgery also with techniques, so-called "Tiger Den" approach, as follows. First, we divide the ligament of Treitz and mobilize the fourth portion of the duodenum and proximal jejunum. The adipose tissue in the retroperitoneal space is dissected and the inferior vena cava (IVC) is exposed. The mesentery of the transverse colon is also divided along the posterior border of the pancreatic body, the dissection over the IVC is extended to the left and the left renal vein is exposed. By careful dissections over the aorta, a surgeon can identify the origin of superior mesenteric artery (SMA) and that of the celiac artery. Large Kelly forceps can be passed through the retroperitoneal space behind the pancreatic body toward the left side of the left gastric artery. A Penrose drain is passed thorough the retroperitoneal space and the pancreatic body is lifted upward by the Penrose drain as this procedure is called a hanging maneuver of the pancreas. By the hanging maneuver, the origin of the celiac artery is well visualized. The splenic artery is temporally occluded to isolate the specimen from blood inflow. In cases that en bloc resection of the celiac artery is required due to the extension of the tumor, the celiac artery occluded with bulldog clamps, the blood flow of intrahepatic arteries evaluated with Doppler ultrasonography, the celiac artery is to be ligated or clipped after the confirmation of sufficient arterial blood flow to the liver. After the occlusion of the splenic artery or celiac artery for a conventional DP or distal pancreactectomy with celiac artery resection (DP-CAR), respectively, the pancreas is divided at the designated part, typically in front of the superior mesenteric vein (SMV). The splenic vein is divided and the pancreatic body is flapped to the left side. The pancreatic body is dissected together with posterior tissue. The splenic artery, which had been already occluded, is now divided for DP, while the celiac artery and common hepatic artery are divided for DP-CAR. During DP-CAR, the left gastric artery is also divided if the origin of the left gastric artery is involved by the tumor. When needed, the left adrenal gland is resected en bloc and the tail of the pancreas and the spleen are dissected to complete DP or DP-CAR. In conclusion, the Tiger Den approach and the hanging maneuver of the pancreas are useful for artery-first approaches to DP and DP-CAR.

45.1 Introduction

Prognosis of pancreatic cancer remains bleak even after curative-intent resections [1]. As a multi-disciplinary approach to the treatment of pancreatic cancer, there is a trend toward neoadjuvant therapy for patient with resectable and borderline resectable pancreatic cancer worldwide. Even for locally advanced pancreatic cancer, enthusiasms for conversion surgery after chemotherapy or chemoradiation therapy exist. This means that surgeons have to encounter more and more advanced disease at the operation room and there are technical challenges for surgeons, in particular due to

K. Takaori (✉) · Y. Kasai · K. Yoshino
Department of Surgery, Nagahama City Hospital
Nagahama, Japan

Department of Surgery, Graduate School of Medicine,
Kyoto University, Kyoto, Japan
e-mail: takaori@iasgo.org

fibrosis after chemoradiation therapy. Under such circumstances, artery-first approaches to pancreatic resections have become widely practiced in the setting of a pancrearticoduodenectomy (PD) or Whipple procedure in specialized centers. According to the literature, the advantages of artery-first approaches include; (1) determination of the resectability in the early phase of operation, (2) higher ratio of negative surgical margins, (3) oncological rationale by isolation of the tumor from the blood flow before extensive mobilization of the tumor, and (4) less amount of intraoperative blood loss [2]. However, until the report by Takaori, artery approaches to a distal pancreatectomy (DP) have been scarcely performed [3]. In open surgery, it had been considered very difficult to approach the origin of the splenic artery before the transection of the pancreas. On the other hand, in the setting of laparoscopic surgery, a surgeon can enter the retroperitoneal space behind the pancreatic body taking advantage of the caudo-cranial angle view through a laparoscope and explore the origin of the celiac artery from the aorta and the origin of the splenic artery without dividing the pancreas [4]. The same approaches can be carried out in open surgery as well by using specific techniques [5]. The two technical elements of importance are dissection behind the pancreatic body after the wide division of the ligament of Treitz and the hanging maneuver of the pancreas. In this chapter, these technical aspects of artery-first approaches to DP and a distal pancreatectomy with celiac artery resection (DP-CAR) are described.

45.2 Surgical Technique

45.2.1 Dissection Behind the Pancreatic Body

The surgeons stand around the operation table as shown in the Fig. 45.1. The third assistant lift the transvers colon upward (or you may use a retractor if the third assistant is not available) and the operator divide the ligament of Treitz along the lateral margin of the upper jejunum (the arrow in Fig. 45.2a). The retroperitoneal space behind the fourth portion of the duodenum and proximal jejunum is entered and the adipose tissue behind the pancreatic head is dissected until the inferior vena cava (IVC) is exposed (Fig. 45.2b). Do not try to dissect over the hilum of the left kidney at this point or you may end up with unexpected injury of the left renal artery. The mesentery of the transverse colon is divided widely along the posterior inferior border of the pancreatic body (the full-line arrow in Fig. 45.3a) and the retroperitoneal tissues including the hilum of the left kidney are well visualized (Fig. 45.3b). The inferior mesenteric vein (IMV) is also divided during the division of the mesentery. The dissection over the IVC is extended to the left side and the left renal vein is exposed.

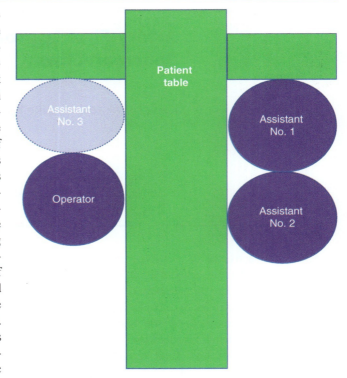

Fig. 45.1 Positions of surgeons for artery first approaches to a distal pancreatectomy

Thus, the retroperitoneal space behind the pancreatic body can be well developed though the gaping hole created by the techniques described above. We call the gaping hole "Tiger Den", or "Tora-no-Ana" in Japanese, which derives from a Chinese proverb; "one may not catch a tiger cub without entering tiger den".

45.2.2 Partial Resection of the Mesentery of Transverse Colon

The gastrocolic ligament is divided and the lesser sac is entered. The left gastro-epiploic artery and short gastric arteries are divided with a vessel sealer and the stomach is mobilized upward. The transvers colon is also lifted upward and the mesentery of the transverse colon is divided along the anterior inferior margin of the pancreas (the full-line arrow in Fig. 45.4), while the middle colic artery is preserved. In this way, a part of the mesentery of transverse colon covering the pancreatic body and tail can be resected en bloc. This part of the mesentery in patients with invasive cancer of the pancreatic body and tail is often involved by the tumor and we routinely resect this portion regardless of the presence or absence of macroscopic involvement. Although one may concern about ischemia of the colon after this procedure, we have never experienced any problem as far as we can preserve the arcade of vessels along the transverse colon.

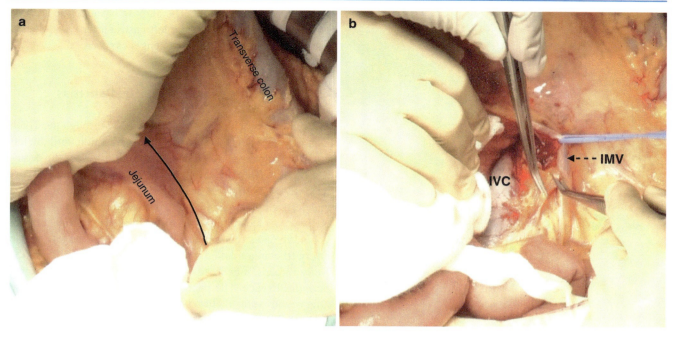

Fig. 45.2 Tiger Den approach. The ligament of Treitz is divided along the lateral margin of the upper jejunum (the full line arrow in **a**). The jejunum is retracted to the left side and the inferior vena cava (IVC) is well exposed (**b**). The inferior mesenteric vein (IMV) is taped and to be transected later on

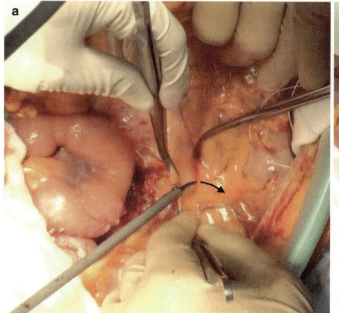

Fig. 45.3 Division of the mesentery of the transverse colon along the posterior inferior border of the pancreas. The mesentery of the transvers colon is divided along the posterior inferior border of the pancreatic body (the full line arrow in **a**). The division of the mesentery is widely extended while the arcade vessels along the transvers colon is preserved (**b**)

However, when the tumor involves the vessels along the transverse colon, a resection of the affected part of the colon may be required.

45.2.3 Dissection on the Left Side of the Left Gastric Artery

The stomach body is retracted upward and the left gastric

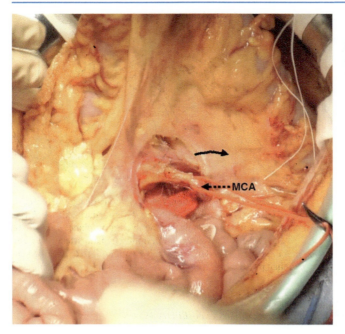

Fig. 45.4 Division of the mesentery of the transverse colon along the anterior inferior border of the pancreas. The mesentery of the transvers colon is divided along the anterior inferior border of the pancreatic body (the full line arrow). Thus, a part of the mesentery covering the inferior side of the pancreatic body is resected en bloc. The middle colic artery (MCA) is preserved unless it is involved by the tumor

artery is extended straight. The adipose tissue in the avascular area on the left side of the left gastric artery is dissected until a part of the left crus ligament is exposed.

45.2.4 Hanging Maneuver of the Pancreas

The dissection behind the pancreatic body through the Tigen Den is further developed to the cranial direction until the left crus is encountered. In case that the tumor invades the posterior tissue, a deep dissection plane, which represents the posterior RAMPS [6, 7], is developed so that the Gerota's fascia and left adrenal gland should be resected en bloc. Large Kelly forceps can be passed from the retroperitoneal space behind the pancreatic body to the left side of the left gastric artery (the area marked with #1 in Fig. 45.5a). Utilizing the Kelly forceps, a Penrose drain is passed thorough the retroperitoneal space. The pancreatic body including the splenic artery and vein is lifted upward by the Penrose drain (Fig. 45.5b). After the hanging maneuver of the liver as proposed by Belghiti [8], we call this procedure a hanging maneuver of the pancreas. By the hanging maneuver, the retroperitoneal space is widely opened and the surgeon can visualize the anatomical structures in this area through the Tiger Den.

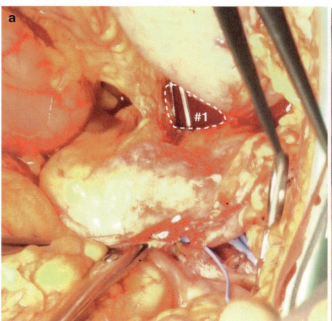 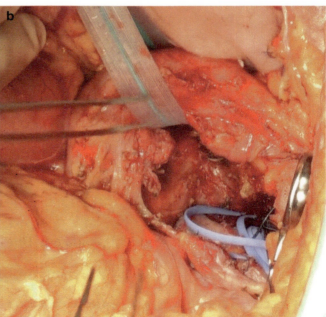

Fig. 45.5 Hanging maneuver. The avascular area on the left side of the left gastric artery is first dissected. Large Kelly forceps is passed from the retroperitoneal space behind the pancreatic body to this area (marked with #1 in **a**). A Penrose drain is passed with the large Kelly's forceps and hanged upward (**b**)

45.2.5 Dissection Around the Superior Mesenteric Artery (SMA) and Celiac Artery

Taking advantage of the good exposure of the retroperitoneal space by the hanging maneuver, the surgeon can dissect over the aorta safely and identify the origin of superior mesenteric artery (SMA) and that of the celiac artery. Be aware that the left renal artery may be located more anteriorly than anticipated in some patients. Once the celiac artery is identified, we usually remove the left celiac ganglion in order to expose the left-side wall of the celiac artery for patient with pancreatic cancer. The surrounding tissue around the celiac artery is dissected from the proximal origin toward distal direction until the takeoff of the splenic artery is exposed (Fig. 45.6). For DP, the origin of the splenic artery is occluded with bulldog clumps if the surgeon is not 100% sure that it is the splenic artery. For DP-CAR, the celiac artery is occluded provisionally with bulldog clumps or with an atraumatic tourniquet. Then the surgeon can measure arterial blood flow in the liver with intraoperative Doppler ultrasonography in order to determine the feasibility of DP-CAR.

45.2.6 Division of the Pancreas and Splenic Vein

The neck of the pancreas is divided, most commonly with a linear stapler. However, if the pancreatic parenchyma is thicker than 12 mm or of very hard texture, we prefer division of the pancreatic parenchyma with a cautery and manual ligation of the main pancreatic duct. The splenic vein is also divided by a vascular stapler. For DP-CAR, once sufficient arterial blood flow is confirmed with Doppler sonography after occlusion of the celiac artery, the common hepatic artery is divided.

45.2.7 Division of the Splenic Artery and Completion of Resection

The splenic artery is divided close to its origin after positive identification of the common hepatic artery (Fig. 45.7). We prefer Hem-o-lok clips to suture ligations so that we might be able to avoid collapsing the intima completely. Especially, after chemoradiation therapy for the tumor involving the splenic artery, the wall of splenic artery is often fragile. In such a case, we do not use ligations or clips but treat the stump of the splenic artery with a running suture of 6-0

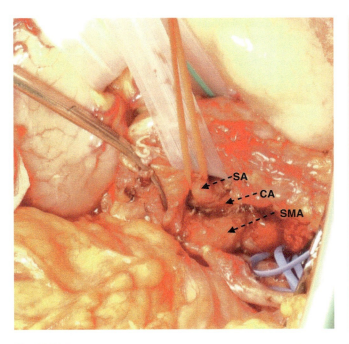

Fig. 45.6 Dissection around the proximal origin of the splenic artery. The celiac artery (CA) and superior mesenteric artery (SMA) are well visualized after the hanging maneuver. By dissecting around CA starting at its origin from the aorta toward distal direction, the takeoff of the splenic artery (SA) can be identified. SA is taped near the origin from CA

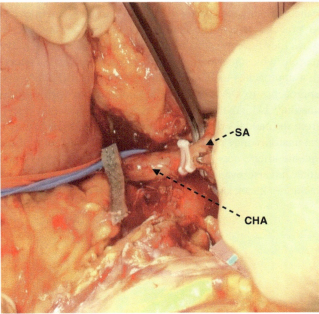

Fig. 45.7 Division of the splenic artery. While the splenic artery (SA) is temporally occluded with bulldog clumps after the hanging maneuver of the pancreas, division of SA may be carried out at a later stage of the operation usually after the transection of the pancreas. We recommend to divide SA after positive identification of the common hepatic artery (CHA) in order to prevent misidentification of these vessels

Prolene in order to prevent pseudo-aneurysm and to maximize the surgical margin. The pancreatic body and spleen are dissected free from the posterior tissue and radical resection is completed. For DP-CAR, the celiac artery is divided in the same fashion as that for the splenic artery during DP. The site of division of the celiac artery depends on the extent of the tumor involvement. If the tumor extends close to the aorta, the celiac artery should be divided at the takeoff and the surgeon may have to stitch the aortic wall around the takeoff of the celiac artery. On the contrary, when the tumor extension is confined to the distal part of the celiac artery, one may be able to preserve the left gastric artery and the proximal part of the celiac artery. For the details of preservation of the left gastric artery, please refer to the "Modified DP-CAR" by Okada and Yamaue in this IASGO Textbook.

45.3 Discussion

We have used the technique of artery-first approaches to DP routinely in patients with pancreatic cancer since 2010 and Takaori published the details of the technique in Japanese language in 2014 [5] and for the first time in the English literature to our knowledge in 2016 [3]. Although this technique is useful especially in the setting of laparoscopic surgery, it is practiced only in a limited number of specialized centers of excellence to date. In contrast, artery-first approaches to PD has become popular among expert pancreatic surgeons partly because the surgeons are impelled to practice artery-first approaches or similar approaches when they have to resect portal vein and/or SMV. One of the reasons why some surgeons, even those who practice artery-first approaches to PD, are reluctant to perform artery-first approaches to DP is that they are not familiar with surgical anatomy behind the pancreas especially when they see it from the caudal side. It is true that unfamiliar view of surgical anatomy may potentially lead to misidentification of the splenic artery, accidental injury of the left renal artery and other adverse events. However, by utilizing the techniques including knack and pitfalls described in the present chapter, one can avoid such adverse events and carry out artery-first approaches to DP safely and securely.

DP-CAR is another challenging operation for locally advanced pancreatic cancer which involves the celiac artery. It is imperative to determine the resectability before the "point of no return" in such cases. By applying the artery first approaches to DP-CAR, one can evaluate the extent of the tumor along the celiac artery before the transection of the pancreas.

In conclusion, by paying attention to knack and pitfalls including the Tiger Den approach and hanging maneuver of the pancreas described herein, artery-first approaches to DP and DP-CAR are feasible and safe in all settings of open, laparoscopic and robotic surgery.

Conflict of Interest The authors have no conflicts of interest to disclose.

References

1. Kamisawa T, Wood LD, Itoi T, Takaori K. Pancreatic cancer. Lancet. 2016;388:73–85.
2. Sanjay P, Takaori K, Govil S, Shrikhande SV, Windsor JA. 'Artery-first' approaches to pancreatoduodenectomy. Br J Surg. 2012;99:1027–35.
3. Takaori K, Uemoto S. Artery-first distal pancreatectomy. Dig Surg. 2016;33(4):314–9.
4. Nagai K, Kiguchi G, Yogo A, Anazawa T, Yagi S, Taura K, Takaori K, Masui T. Left-posterior approach for artery-first en bloc resection in laparoscopic distal pancreatectomy for left-sided pancreatic cancer. Langenbeck's Arch Surg. 2020;405:1251–8.
5. Takaori K, Masui T, Kawaguchi M, Iwanaga Y, Mizumoto M, Uemoto S. Distal pancreatectomy with celiac artery resection by artery-first approach. Shujutsu. 2014;68:581–68. (In Japanese)
6. Strasberg SM, Drebin JA, Linehan D. Radical antegrade modular pancreatosplenectomy. Surgery. 2003;133:521–7.
7. Strasberg SM, Linehan DC, Hawkins WG, et al. Radical antegrade modular pancreatosplenectomy procedure for adenocarcinoma of the body and tail of the pancreas: ability to obtain negative tangential margins. J Am Coll Surg. 2007;204:244–9.
8. Belghiti J, Guevara OA, Noun R, Saldinger PF, Kianmanesh R. Liver hanging maneuver: a safe approach to right hepatectomy without liver mobilization. J Am Coll Surg. 2001;193:109–11.

46. Spleen-Preserving Distal Pancreatectomy

Kohei Nakata and Masafumi Nakamura

Abstract

Concomitant splenectomy has traditionally been performed during conventional distal pancreatectomy because of the anatomic proximity of the pancreas and splenic vessels. Spleen-preserving distal pancreatectomy has been proposed however, subsequent to a more detailed understanding of the function of the spleen and various complications after splenectomy, including severe post-splenectomy infections, thrombocytosis, and increased cancer risk (Di Sabatino et al., The Lancet 378:86–97, 2011; Mellemkjoer et al., Cancer 75:577–583, 1995). Splenic preservation can be performed with splenic vessel preservation (Kimura et al., Surgery 120:885–890, 1996) or Warshaw's technique (Warshaw, Arch Surg 123:550–553, 1988). Indications, technical methods, and potential pitfalls of spleen-preserving distal pancreatectomy are introduced in this chapter.

46.1 Introduction

Traditionally, concomitant splenectomy has been performed during conventional distal pancreatectomy because of the anatomic proximity of the pancreas and splenic vessels. Spleen-preserving distal pancreatectomy (SPDP) has been proposed however, following a more detailed understanding of the function of the spleen and various complications after splenectomy, including overwhelming post-splenectomy infections (OPSI), thrombocytosis, and increased risk of cancer [1, 2]. Splenic preservation can be performed with splenic vessel preservation [3] or Warshaw's technique [4]. Laparoscopic distal pancreatectomy has become increasingly popular since it was first reported in 1996 [5–7], and it is currently used to treat lesions in the distal pancreas. We have previously reported that laparoscopic SPDP yields significantly better outcomes than DPS for laparoscopic procedures [8]. Notably however, spleen preservation in laparoscopic procedures is technically difficult. In this chapter, indications, technical methods, and potential pitfalls of laparoscopic SPDP are introduced.

46.2 Indications

Laparoscopic SPDP is indicated for benign tumors located in the body or the tail of the pancreas. We perform a splenic vessel preservation procedure and if the tumor is substantially adhered to the splenic vein or artery, and Warshaw's technique may be considered before the operation.

46.3 Patient Positioning and Setup

The positions of the equipment and surgical team for laparoscopic SPDP are shown in Fig. 46.1a. The patient is placed in a supine position with their legs apart and both arms spread. The surgeon stands to the right of the patient, the camera operator stands between the legs, and the assistant stands to the left of the patient. Two visual display units are used, one placed near each of the patient's shoulders. We usually use the "open Hasson" technique to safely insert the first cannula through the umbilicus. If the width between the xiphoid process and the umbilicus is short, the camera port is placed under the umbilicus. Ports are then placed in the following order: right lower abdominal region (12 mm), right abdominal region (5 mm), left lower abdominal region (12 mm), left abdominal region (5 mm). If the patient is large and instruments inserted from the right side would not reach the splenic hilum, the ports placed on the right side are inserted toward the left side (Fig. 46.1a).

K. Nakata · M. Nakamura (✉)
Department of Surgery and Oncology, Graduate School of Medical Sciences, Kyushu University, Fukuoka, Japan
e-mail: nakamura.masafumi.861@m.kyushuu.ac.jp

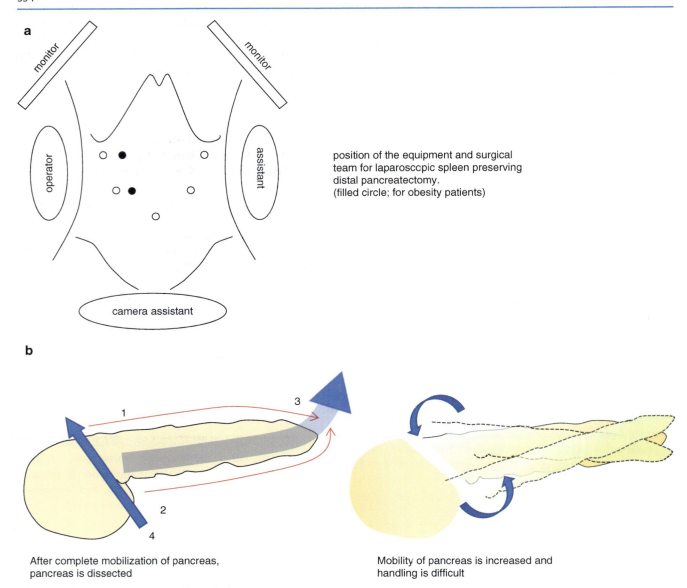

Fig. 46.1 (**a**) Positions of the equipment and surgical team for laparoscopic spleen-preserving distal pancreatectomy (filled circle; for obese patients). (**b**) Operation procedure. Transection of the pancreas is performed after the completion of mobilization

46.4 Technique

The procedure is divided into three parts; (1) dissecting the omentum and exposing the entire pancreas; (2) isolating the common hepatic artery (CHA) and splenic artery (SPA); and (3) mobilizing the pancreas and isolating the splenic vein (SPV). We prefer to dissect the pancreas after the completion of mobilization, because if there is too much mobility of the pancreas it makes it difficult to handle during operation, and we prefer to dissect it from the medial side to the lateral side (Fig. 46.1b).

On the surface of the pancreas the gastrocolic ligament is divided using an ultrasonic coagulating system or a vessel-sealing device. Although the arcade of gastroepiploic vessels should be preserved, the omentum is divided near the arcade along the greater curvature to prevent the omentum from hanging down from the stomach side during the procedure (Fig. 46.2a). The lesser sac is accessed via the outside of the gastroepiploic arcade. The omentum is first dissected toward to the left side of the patient, the dissection is stopped before the left gastroepiploic vessels, and the vessels should be preserved to the greatest extent possible. The omentum is then dissected toward the right side and the dissection should reach the duodenum to facilitate a wide clear view of the entire surface of the pancreas. Usually the posterior wall of the stomach is adhered to the surface of the pancreas due to

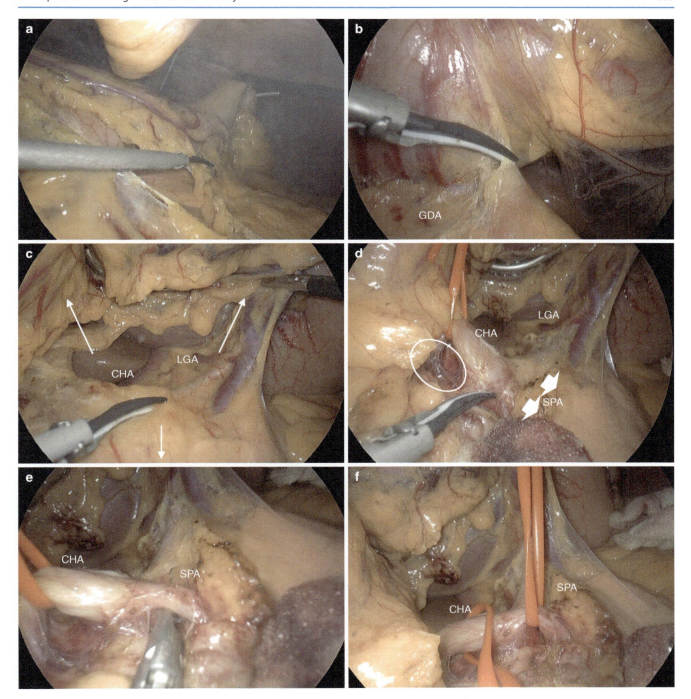

Fig. 46.2 (**a**) The omentum is divided near the arcade along the greater curvature. (**b**) The posterior wall of the antrum is adhered to the head of the pancreas and dissected to identify the gastroduodenal artery. (**c**) A liver retractor is used to push up the stomach, and the pancreas is pulled down with gauze by the assistant to facilitate a clear view of the suprapancreatic region (arrow). (**d**) The root of the splenic artery is covered by the pancreas and difficult to isolate. The common hepatic artery (white circle) is retracted after a wide space is created around it, then it is retracted and the root of splenic artery is bluntly dissected (arrow) to expose it clearly. (**e, f**) The root of the SPA is adequately dissected for isolation. *CHA* common hepatic artery, *SPA* splenic artery, *SPV* splenic vein

concomitant pancreatitis, and the stomach is separated from the pancreas via sharp and blunt dissection to move the posterior gastric wall away from the pancreas. The region of the antrum is also adhered to the head of the pancreas, and it is dissected to enable identification of the gastroduodenal artery (Fig. 46.2b). After exposure of the entire surface of the pancreas the tumor location is confirmed via intraoperative ultrasonography.

A liver retractor is used to push up the stomach, and the pancreas is pulled down with gauze by an assistant to facilitate a clear view of the supra-pancreatic region (Fig. 46.2c). We usually isolate the common hepatic artery (CHA). Identifying the CHA can be easy, but it is sometimes difficult if it is covered by the pancreas or lymph nodes, especially in obese patients. Therefore, we routinely identify the gastroduodenal artery and dissect the surface of that artery toward its root, then identify the CHA (Fig. 46.2b, c). To isolate the CHA the tissues between it and the cranial edge of the pancreas should be widely dissected to prevent injury during isolation. After isolating the CHA with tape, it is retracted with tape and dissection is continued toward the root of the SPA (Fig. 46.2d).

Isolating the root of the SPA is an important step during laparoscopic distal pancreatectomy, and the root of the SPA is sometimes buried behind the pancreas. We classify the root of the SPA as either "buried" or "non-buried" based on its relationship with the pancreas. If the root of the SPA is buried and covered by the pancreas it can be difficult to identify, therefore a wide space between the CHA and pancreas should be created (Fig. 46.2d). The root of the SPA and the pancreas are then dissected bluntly and the root of the SPA is exposed. After the creation of a wide space, the root of the SPA can be identified and dissected from the pancreas to ensure sufficient space to isolate the root of the SPA (Fig. 46.2e, f).

The next step is preservation of the SPA. The SPA runs along the cranial side of the pancreas and is usually covered by the pancreas, but it is also usually free from the pancreas on the distal side. Therefore, we prefer to isolate it with tape and retract tape on both the proximal and distal sides to straighten the SPA, which makes it easier to dissect the SPA from the pancreas (Fig. 46.3a). There are several branches to the pancreas, including the dorsal pancreatic artery, and the SPA should be dissected in the center of the artery to prevent injury to these branches (Fig. 46.3b). We dissect the SPA from surrounding tissues with forceps, and create space and dissect tissues with an ultrasonic coagulation system or vessel sealing system to prevent injury to the adventitia by these devices. After exposure of the SPA, several branches to the pancreas are detected, tied, and cut (Fig. 46.3c, d). The SPA has branches to the pancreatic tail, and these branches should be carefully dissected and ligated. The SPA is then completely freed from the pancreas (Fig. 46.3e). Although the SPV runs to the center of the pancreas, at the pancreatic tail it runs around the cranial side of it, therefore we usually isolate and tape it from the cranial side (Fig. 46.3f).

The transverse mesocolon is appropriately retracted toward the inferior side by the assistant to make the mesocolon form a plane, and the inferior border of the pancreas is clearly identified (Fig. 46.4a). The anterior surface of the mesocolon is then cut and moved behind the retropancreatic fascia (the anterior side of Toldt's fusion fascia). This layer is easily divided via blunt dissection, and the pancreatic body and tail are smoothly mobilized (Fig. 46.4b). Although only a few blood vessels are encountered in this procedure, the inferior mesenteric vein and duodenum should be identified. After complete mobilization of the body to tail of the pancreas, the body to tail is flipped to the ventral side and the SPV covered by the retropancreatic fascia is visualized (Fig. 46.4b). The retroperitoneum is dissected at the center of the SPV to avoid injury to the branches from the pancreas (Fig. 46.4c). The SPV is exposed and the small branches are tied and cut (Fig. 46.4d). Retracting the tape isolating the SPV at the tail of the pancreas is useful for isolating the SPV. After sufficient surgical margins are attained the pancreas is transected with a 60-mm stapler via the prolonged peri-firing compression method [9] (Fig. 46.4e). If bleeding occurs after stapling at the stump, hemostasis is achieved via clipping, not by coagulation. Lastly, a pancreatic specimen is recovered in the bag and pulled out through an extended umbilical port site incision (Fig. 46.4f).

46.4.1 Warshaw's Technique

When using Warshaw's technique most of the procedure is the same as that for SPDP. The root of the SPA is triply transected with transfixing suturing. Before ligating the SPA, the clump test should be performed to confirm blood flow of the CHA after ligation of the SPA. At the tail of the pancreas the SPA and SPV are branched, therefore the distal sides of the SPA and SPV are double-ligated. The left gastroepiploic vessels should definitely be preserved.

46.5 Postoperative Follow-Up

Postoperative computed tomography is performed 7 days after the operation to confirm blood flow to the spleen.

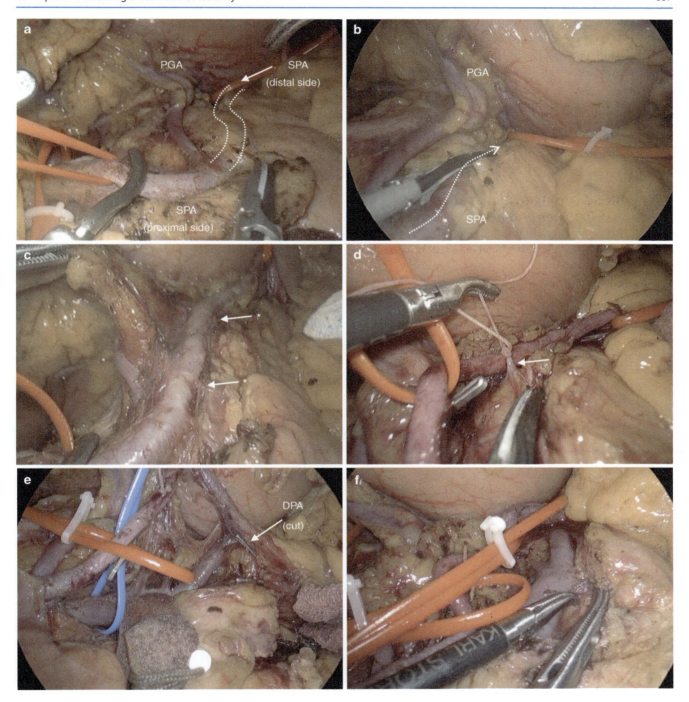

Fig. 46.3 (a) The splenic artery (SPA) runs along the cranial side of the pancreas and is covered by the pancreas (dotted line). The proximal and distal sides of the SPA that are free of the pancreas are taped. (b) The SPA is dissected at its center to prevent injury to the branches. (c) The SPA is completely exposed and several branches to the pancreas are detected (*). (d) Branches to the pancreas are tied (white arrow). (e) The SPA is completely freed from the pancreas. (f) The splenic vein runs around the cranial side of the pancreas at its tail side. *SPA* splenic artery, *SPV* splenic vein

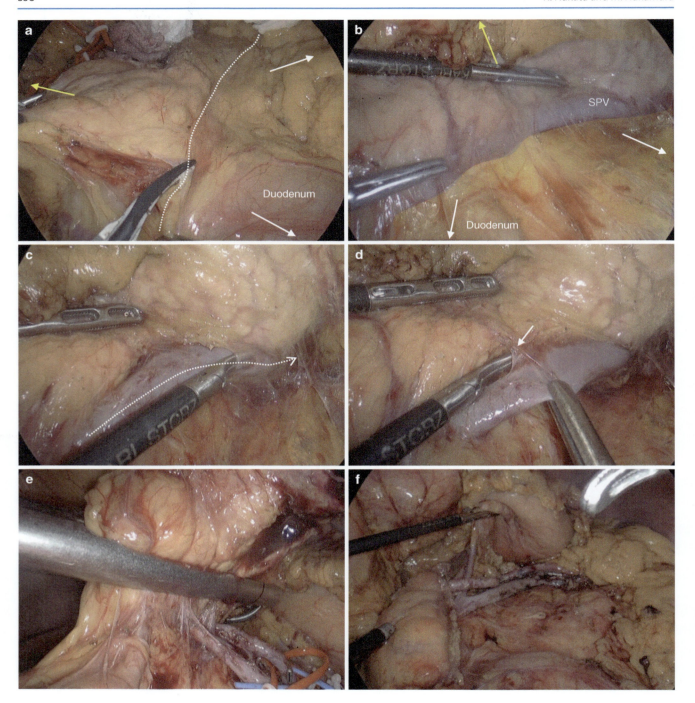

Fig. 46.4 (a) The mesocolon is appropriately retracted by the surgeon (yellow arrow) and the assistant (white arrow). The inferior border of the pancreas is clearly identified (dotted line). (b) The anterior side of Toldt's fusion fascia is dissected (yellow), and the splenic vein (SPV) covered by the retropancreatic fascia (blue) is identified. Retraction is appropriately performed by the surgeon (yellow arrow) and the assistant (white arrow). (c) The retroperitoneum is dissected at the center of the SPV to avoid injury to the branches from the pancreas (dotted line). (d) The SPV is exposed and the small branches are identified. (e) After complete mobilization of the pancreas with sufficient surgical margins, it is transected with a 60-mm stapler. (f) Surgical view after resection. *SPV* splenic vein

References

1. Di Sabatino A, Carsetti R, Corazza GR. Post-splenectomy and hyposplenic states. Lancet. 2011;378(9785):86–97.
2. Mellemkjoer L, Olsen JH, Linet MS, Gridley G, McLaughlin JK. Cancer risk after splenectomy. Cancer. 1995;75(2):577–83.
3. Kimura W, Inoue T, Futakawa N, Shinkai H, Han I, Muto T. Spleen-preserving distal pancreatectomy with conservation of the splenic artery and vein. Surgery. 1996;120(5):885–90.
4. Warshaw AL. Conservation of the spleen with distal pancreatectomy. Arch Surg. 1988;123(5):550–3.
5. Cuschieri A, Jakimowicz JJ, van Spreeuwel J. Laparoscopic distal 70% pancreatectomy and splenectomy for chronic pancreatitis. Ann Surg. 1996;223(3):280–5.
6. Gagner M, Pomp A, Herrera MF. Early experience with laparoscopic resections of islet cell tumors. Surgery. 1996;120(6):1051–4.
7. Shiroshita H, Inomata M, Bandoh T, Uchida H, Akira S, Hashizume M, et al. Endoscopic surgery in Japan: the 13th national survey (2014-2015) by the Japan Society for Endoscopic Surgery. Asian J Endosc Surg. 2019;12(1):7–18.
8. Nakata K, Shikata S, Ohtsuka T, Ukai T, Miyasaka Y, Mori Y, et al. Minimally invasive preservation versus splenectomy during distal pancreatectomy: a systematic review and meta-analysis. J Hepatobiliary Pancreat Sci. 2018;25(11):476–88.
9. Nakamura M, Ueda J, Kohno H, Aly MY, Takahata S, Shimizu S, et al. Prolonged peri-firing compression with a linear stapler prevents pancreatic fistula in laparoscopic distal pancreatectomy. Surg Endosc. 2011;25(3):867–71.

47. Distal Pancreatectomy with *En Bloc* Celiac Axis Resection

Satoshi Hirano, Toru Nakamura, and Toshimichi Asano

Abstract

Distal pancreatectomy with en bloc celiac axis resection (DP-CAR), which is an extended surgical procedure for locally advanced cancer of the pancreatic body, is performed for complete resection of tumors with invasion to the celiac, and/or the common hepatic artery, and/or their plexuses. Although the procedure of DP-CAR is technically demanding, a high rate of negative surgical margin resection can be achieved with cautious selection of candidates and with appropriate systematic techniques. A relatively high morbidity rate due to postoperative pancreatic fistula and ischemic gastropathy has been reported. A recent report on the long-term outcomes following DP-CAR in 80 patients has described a 5-year overall survival (OS) rate of 32.7% and median survival time of 30.9 months. It was revealed that OS for the patients who underwent preoperative therapy were significantly better than for those who underwent upfront surgery.

47.1 Concepts of Distal Pancreatectomy with Celiac Axis Resection (DP-CAR)

Locally advanced cancer of the body of the pancreas often involves the common hepatic artery (CHA) and/or the celiac axis (CA), with perineural invasion of the nerve plexuses surrounding these arteries. Although these tumors are regarded as borderline resectable or locally advanced diseases according to the NCCN guidelines® Version 1.2021 [1], distal pancreatectomy with celiac axis resection (DP-CAR) may be the only surgical option for treatment of such advanced diseases [2]. An advantage of DP-CAR is reduction in the likelihood of a positive retroperitoneal margin by complete *en bloc* resection of the distal pancreas, together with the entire surrounding structures, especially the CHA, CA, and the circumferential nerve plexus along with the superior mesenteric artery (SMA), without the need for either arterial, pancreatobiliary or gastrointestinal reconstruction (Fig. 47.1).

This procedure was originally designed as *en bloc* lymphadenectomy combined with total gastrectomy and resection of the celiac axis for advanced gastric cancer by Appleby in 1953 [3]. It was first adopted by Nimura in 1976 [4] for patients with advanced pancreatic body cancer with invasion of the celiac axis. A modification to the procedure with preservation of the entire stomach was made by Ogata and his colleagues [5] in 1991 (in Japanese with English abstract) and Kondo [6] in 2001, which resulted in better postoperative nutritional status. The first report regarding the long-term outcome of DP-CAR was published by Kondo and Hirano in 2007 [7], which included the results of 24 consecutive patients with favorable postoperative survival. Since then, the procedure and the term "DP-CAR" have been widely

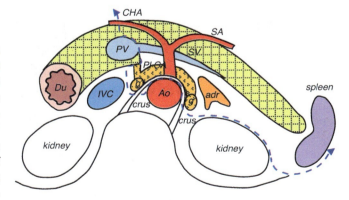

Fig. 47.1 Schematic cross-sectional view demonstrating the resection area of distal pancreatectomy with en bloc celiac axis resection (DP-CAR). The dotted line indicates the dissection plane. *adr* adrenal gland, *Ao* aorta, *CA* celiac axis, *CHA* common hepatic artery, *crus* crus of the diaphragm, *Du* duodenum, *g* celiac ganglion, *IVC* inferior vena cava, *pl* celiac plexus, *PV* portal vein, *SA* splenic artery, *SV* splenic vein

acknowledged. Nowadays, several pancreatic surgeons have performed this procedure for carcinoma of the body and tail of the pancreas.

47.2 Resected and Preserved Organs in DP-CAR

Perineural invasion in patients with pancreatic body cancer can spread towards the celiac plexus and ganglions directly or via the nerve plexuses surrounding the splenic and the common hepatic arteries. Although DP-CAR includes *en bloc* resection of these arteries and plexuses, reconstruction of the arterial system is not required because of early development of a collateral arterial circulation via the pancreatoduodenal arcades from the superior mesenteric artery. The entire alimentary tract, including the stomach and bile duct, which are not invaded by the cancer, is preserved. Cholecystectomy is, however, performed for preventing postoperative ischemic rupture of the gallbladder. If the tumor of the pancreatic body invades other organs directly, concomitant resection of the organs, including the alimentary tract, could be performed. In case that a tumor has invaded the stomach to a depth that necessitates full-thickness resection, total gastrectomy should be considered because healing of the anastomosis might be disturbed by an insufficient collateral arterial flow. As far as possible, the entire stomach should be preserved in cases without cancer invasion of the stomach, to maintain the patient's nutritional status and tolerance of oral anticancer agents. SMA preservation, even with complete eradication of the surrounding plexus, is the key feature of this procedure, which maintains arterial supply to the hepatobiliary system and the stomach. Resection of the portal vein is an optional procedure.

47.3 Arterial Supply to the Liver and the Stomach After DP-CAR

After division of the CA with the CHA and splenic artery (SA), the hepatic and the gastric arterial flow depend on the flow from the gastroduodenal artery (GDA), which should, therefore, definitely be preserved with the pancreatic head during DP-CAR. The collateral pathways via the SMA, pancreatoduodenal arcades, and GDA maintain the arterial blood supply to the hepatobiliary system. Since the collateral pathways also ensure arterial flow to the right gastroepiploic artery, the entire stomach can be preserved (Fig. 47.2).

In the past, preoperative coil embolization of the CHA had routinely performed to enlarge the collateral arterial pathway, so as to reduce ischemia-related complications such as ischemic gastropathy, liver abscess, and perforation of the biliary system. However, the usefulness of the CHA

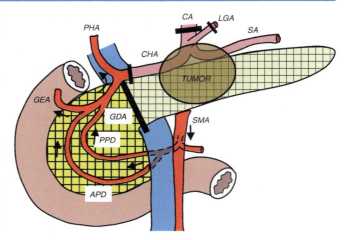

Fig. 47.2 Schematic drawing of collateral arterial pathways via the pancreatoduodenal arcades from the superior mesenteric artery following DP-CAR. The arrows show the direction of arterial flow from the superior mesenteric artery to the liver and stomach via the pancreatoduodenal arcades. *APD* anterior pancreatoduodenal arcade, *CA* celiac axis, *CHA* common hepatic artery, *GDA* gastroduodenal artery, *GEA* right gastroepiploic artery, *LGA* left gastric artery, *PHA* proper hepatic artery, *PPD* posterior pancreatoduodenal arcade, *SA* splenic artery, *SMA* superior mesenteric artery

embolization has been reported to be negative [8]. The procedure has been no longer essential.

47.4 Selection of Candidates for DP-CAR

Tumor progression is cautiously evaluated mainly with preoperative multi-detector row computed tomography (MDCT), with supplemental use of magnetic resonance imaging (MRI) and endoscopic ultrasonography (EUS). The indication for DP-CAR is locally advanced ductal adenocarcinoma of the body of the pancreas, such as that involving or abutting the CHA, the root of the SA, and/or the CA, without involvement of the GDA, SMA, and inferior pancreatoduodenal artery (IPDA). Patients with involvement of less than approximately half the circumference of the SMA plexus should be considered candidates for DP-CAR because complete dissection of the SMA plexus without exposing the cancer can be achieved by dividing the plexus on the opposite side of the tumor. For oncologically safe ligation and division of the root of the CA in front of the aorta, a 5–7 mm non-cancerous length of the CA from the adventitia of the aorta is required.

47.5 Surgical Procedure of DP-CAR

DP-CAR usually includes resection of the distal pancreas and the spleen, together with *en bloc* resection of the celiac, common hepatic and left gastric arteries, the celiac plexus

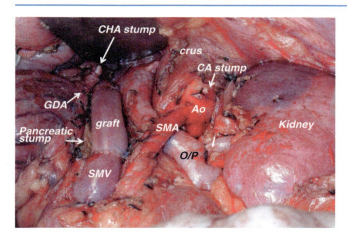

Fig. 47.3 Post-resection view during distal pancreatectomy with en bloc celiac axis resection (DP-CAR). *Ao* aorta, *CA* celiac axis, *CHA* common hepatic artery, *crus* crus of the diaphragm, *GDA* gastroduodenal artery, *graft* interposed iliac vein graft, *IVC* inferior vena cava, *RV* renal vein, *SMA* superior mesenteric artery, *SMV* superior mesenteric vein

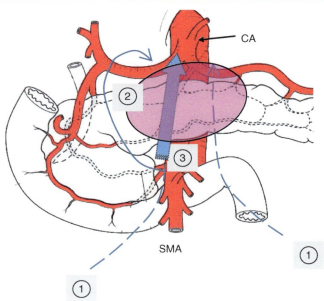

Fig. 47.4 A systematic procedure for achieving negative surgical margin in DP-CAR. The procedure is composed with 3 steps; the first step (①) is Rt. and Lt. dorsal approach, the second (②) is ventral approach, and final step (③) is medial approach

and bilateral ganglions, and the circumferential nerve plexus around the SMA. Left perirenal fat tissue, the left adrenal gland, the entire retroperitoneal fat tissue containing lymph nodes cranial to the left renal vein, the transverse mesocolon covering the body of the pancreas, and the inferior mesenteric vein are also resected (Fig. 47.3).

To achieve R0 resection, a systematic procedure of DP-CAR, which consisted of right and left dorsal (first step), ventral (second step), and medial (third step) approaches, is recommended (Fig. 47.4). In the first step (dorsal approach), the lower parts of the SMA are exposed following Kocher's maneuver, with complete eradication of the right celiac ganglion by exposing the right crus of the diaphragm. The plexus of the SMA is first divided at the dorsal end (opposite side of the tumor), and the excision is extended by 4–5 cm in the longitudinal direction. The median arcuate ligament has to be divided to expose just the root of the CA where it should be divided. Then, after moving to the left side, en bloc resection of the retroperitoneal fat, together with the upper part of the perirenal fat, including the left adrenal gland cranial to the left renal vessels are performed in exposing the left crus. In this approach, bilateral para-aortic nodes and ganglions are completely dissected. In the second step (ventral approach), transection of the pancreas is performed after dividing the common hepatic artery. When a tumor is located near the GDA, it should be mobilized laterally in order to obtain a cancer-free margin at the site of division of the pancreatic parenchyma. Reconstruction of the portal and/or superior mesenteric vein should be performed in this step, if necessary. In the third step (medial approach), division of the SMA plexus that was performed in the first step is extended longitudinally to just proximal to the IPDA to achieve complete resection of the plexus. The procedure is completed after dissecting between the SMA plexus and the uncinate process of the pancreas.

Accidental injury to the IPDA or GDA compromises collateral blood flow and leads to fatal complications, such as gastric necrosis and/or liver infarction. If this occurs, microscopic anastomosis between the proper hepatic artery and middle colic artery (MCA) [9], or the right gastroepiploic artery and MCA [10] could be a possible option for maintaining arterial flow to both the stomach and the liver.

47.6 Postoperative Course Following DP-CAR

The most frequent morbidity after DP-CAR is pancreatic fistula, which occurs relatively easily because the pancreatic parenchyma needs to be divided at the pancreatic head in patients with a tumor extending to the proximal end of the pancreas, beyond the portal vein. In such cases, the cut surface of the pancreas becomes wider than that after usual distal pancreatectomy, in which the pancreatic parenchyma is divided at the neck of the pancreas. It is rather important to insert an indwelling drain at an appropriate position beside the pancreatic stump during surgery, so as to avoid postoperative hemorrhage from a pseudoaneurysm in the stump of the CHA. The second most common morbidity is ischemic gastropathy due to decreased gastric blood flow [11]. According to data from 80 consecutive patients who underwent DP-CAR [12], the major complications defined as grade 3 or higher in the Clavien-Dindo classification occurred in 33 (41.3%) patients; pancreatic fistula and ischemic gastropathy occurred in 47 (57.5%) and 23 (28.8%) patients, respectively. Four patients out of 80 (5%) died in the hospital. Postoperative hospital stays ranged from 12 to 208 days, with a median of 38 days [12].

One of the other postoperative complications is stubborn diarrhea due to complete dissection of the nerve system around the SMA, CA, and bilateral ganglions. From a published data, approximately half of the patients regularly required anti-diarrheal agents, and the remaining half only occasionally required or never used the agents over a median follow-up period of 39 months [13].

Contrary to the adverse effects of resection of nerve tissues, patients enjoy the complete disappearance of pain, even if it has been controlled by opioids just before surgery [6].

Since both the incidence of morbidity and poor quality of life postoperatively are major factors influencing the tolerance of adjuvant treatment, surgeons should make greater efforts to improve these factors following DP-CAR.

47.7 Long-Term Outcomes Following DP-CAR

In 2007, the long-term outcomes of DP-CAR were first reported in a series of 23 patients with locally advanced pancreatic body cancer who underwent DP-CAR under a policy of "surgery first" [7]. With R0 resectability in 91% of the cases and a median follow-up time of 27.4 months, the estimated 5-year survival rate was 42% and the median survival was 21 months. Nine years after the first report, a recent report that included 80 patients was published from the same institute, which indicated estimated disease-specific 1-, 3-, and 5-year overall survival rates of 81.1%, 56.9%, and 32.7%, respectively, and a median survival time of 30.9 months after a median follow-up period of 63.5 months [12].

Despite the excellent local control with an R0 resection rate of 92.5% in the report, early recurrence (predominantly in the liver) occurred after surgery, which resulted in poor survival time. It was also revealed that the survival time of the patients who underwent preoperative therapy were significantly better than for those who underwent upfront surgery [12]. The findings show DP-CAR should be performed as part of multidisciplinary treatment.

Although DP-CAR could be used to treat locally advanced pancreatic body cancer, future prospective studies with a large patient cohort for ensuring adequate patient selection, and perioperative treatments are necessary to demonstrate the effectiveness of this innovative surgery.

References

1. NCCN Clinical Practice Guidelines in Oncology (NCCN Guidelines®). Pancreatic adenocarcinoma version 1. 2021. https://www.nccn.org/professionals/physician_gls/pdf/pancreatic.pdf
2. Kondo S, Katoh S, Hirano S, Ambo Y, Tanaka E, Okushiba S, Morikawa T, Kanai M, Yano T. Results of radical distal pancreatectomy with en bloc resection of the celiac artery for locally advanced cancer of the pancreatic body. Langenbeck Arch Surg. 2003;388:101–6.
3. Appleby LH. The coeliac axis in the expansion of the operation for gastric carcinoma. Cancer. 1953;6:707.
4. Nimura Y, Hattori T, Miura K, Nakajima N, Hibi M. A case of advanced carcinoma of the body and tail of the pancreas resected by the Appleby operation. Operation. 1976;30:885–9. (In Japanese)
5. Hishinuma S, Ogata Y, Matsui J, Ozawa I, Inada T, Shimizu H, Kobu K, Ikeda T, Koyama Y. Two cases of cancer of the pancreatic body undergoing preservation with distal pancreatectomy combined with resection of the celiac axis. Jap J Gastroenterol Surg. 1991;24:2782–6. (In Japanese with English abstract)
6. Kondo S, Katoh H, Omi M, Hirano S, Ambo Y, Tanaka E, Okushiba S, Morikawa T, Kanai M, Yano T. Radical distal pancreatectomy with en bloc resection of the celiac artery, plexus, and ganglions for advanced cancer of the pancreatic body: a preliminary report on perfect pain relief. JOP. 2001;2:93–7.
7. Hirano S, Kondo S, Hara T, Ambo Y, Tanaka E, Shichinohe T, Suzuki O, Hazama K. Distal pancreatectomy with en bloc celiac axis resection for locally advanced pancreatic body cancer: long-term results. Ann Surg. 2007;246:46–51.
8. Ueda A, Sakai N, Yoshitomi H, Furukawa K, Takayashiki T, Kuboki S, Takano S, Suzuki D, Kagawa S, Mishima T, Nakadai E, Miyazaki M, Ohtsuka M. Is hepatic artery coil embolization useful in distal pancreatectomy with en bloc celiac axis resection for locally advanced pancreatic cancer? World J Surg Oncol. 2019;17:124.
9. Suzuki H, Hosouchi Y, Sasaki S, Araki K, Kubo N, Watanabe A, Kuwano H. Reconstruction of the hepatic artery with the middle colic artery is feasible in distal pancreatectomy with celiac axis resection: a case report. World J Gastrointest Surg. 2013;5:224–8.
10. Kondo S, Ambo Y, Katoh H, Hirano S, Tanaka E, Okushiba S, Morikawa T, Igawa H, Yamamoto Y, Sugihara T. Middle colic artery-gastroepiploic artery bypass for compromised collateral flow in distal pancreatectomy with celiac artery resection. Hepato-Gastroenterology. 2003;50:305–7.
11. Kondo S, Katho H, Hirano S, Ambo Y, Tanaka E, Maeyama Y, Morikawa T, Okushiba S. Ischemic gastropathy after distal pancreatectomy with celiac axis resection. Surg Today. 2004;34:337–40.
12. Nakamura T, Hirano S, Noji T, Asano T, Okamura K, Tsuchikawa T, Murakami S, Kurashima Y, Ebihara Y, Nakanishi Y, Tanaka K, Shichinohe T. Distal pancreatectomy with en bloc celiac axis resection (modified Appleby procedure) for locally advanced pancreatic body cancer: a single-center review of 80 consecutive patients. Ann Surg Oncol. 2016;23:969–75.
13. Hirano S, Kondo S, Tanaka E, Shichinohe T, Tsuchikawa T, Kato K, Matsumoto J. Postoperative bowel function and nutritional status following distal pancreatectomy with en-bloc celiac axis resection. Dig Surg. 2010;27:212–6.

Modified Distal Pancreatectomy with Celiac Axis En-bloc Resection

48

Ken-ichi Okada and Hiroki Yamaue

Abstract

Since most pancreatic adenocarcinomas recur systemically, and tumor involving arterial structures recur rapidly even after the radical resection. In the era of neoadjuvant therapy, surgeon should re-consider whether the presence of just an R0 resection should be the primary issue of cure in borderline resectable and locally advanced pancreatic adenocarcinoma. By safer modification of the Appleby operation, this procedure attract the attention of pancreatic surgeon again as a radical pancreatectomy for borderline resectable or locally advanced pancreatic body/tail carcinoma. The roles of the Appleby operation and arterial resection are the ability to take a wide surgical margin in pancreatic body/tail carcinoma, and to relieve the cancer pain by celiac axis en-bloc resection combined with removal of the tumor infiltrating nerve plexuses. The modified Appleby operation, a synonym for "distal pancreatectomy with celiac axis en-bloc resection"; DP-CAR was feasible and safe compared with standard distal pancreatectomy when it was performed at high-volume center. In the era of stronger regimen of chemotherapy for pancreatic carcinoma, there will be increased frequency of the chance to consider the indication of this procedure. The procedure may be justified in highly selected patients owing to the potential survival benefit in sophisticated institutions. In this chapter, we particularly describe about the technique and impact of preservation of the left gastric artery in DP-CAR.

48.1 Introduction

The application of distal pancreatectomy with celiac axis en-bloc resection; DP-CAR [1], so-called the modified Appleby operation, for pancreatic carcinoma still remains controversial because of the lack of large number of study. One of the advantages of this procedure is the surgical radicality of deep dissection behind of tumor by the division of the root of the celiac axis, and another is the impact to resolve the preoperative cancer pain according to the tumor invasion into nerve plexus. There are surely several prior reports suggesting that an R0 resection is an essential requirement for long survival. In contrast, an R0 resection is not the only consideration for the impact of survival in advanced pancreatic carcinoma. Recently, in an international multicenter analysis for 174 patients with pancreatic ductal adenocarcinoma who underwent DP-CAR, the R0 resection rate was 60%, neoadjuvant and adjuvant therapies were applied for respectively 69% and 67% of the patients, and the median overall survival period was 19 months [2]. Despite these reports, the indications for DP-CAR remain controversial with regard to the curability and survival benefit. This procedure can provide a clinical benefit for the patients with borderline resectable or locally advanced pancreatic body/tail carcinoma after the strategy of neoadjuvant therapy. Furthermore stronger and adequate preoperative therapy prior to surgery is required to improve their survival.

48.2 History, Background, and Modification of Appleby Operation for Pancreatic Cancer

In 1973, Fortner introduced the regional resection of pancreatic cancer with major vascular en-bloc resection as a new approach [3]. In this literature, actual survival by Kaplan-Meier estimate was 62% at one year, compared with a 36% one year survival rate for 17 patients undergoing pancreati-

K.-i. Okada (✉) · H. Yamaue
Second Department of Surgery, Wakayama Medical University, Wakayama, Japan
e-mail: okada@wakayama-med.ac.jp

coduodenectomy for less advanced cancer at same institution from 1959–1969 [4]. This approach was described that the greatest potential benefit of regional pancreatectomy would appear to be in patients with a small pancreatic cancer where regional resection would give a wide margin. Appleby operation was firstly reported as resection of celiac axis for complete lymphadenectomy in radical resection of gastric carcinoma in 1953 [5, 6]. Nimura et al. reported the adaptation the Appleby operation for resection of pancreatic body/tail carcinoma involving celiac axis and/or common hepatic artery in 1976 [7]. In 1991, Hishinuma et al. modified this procedure with preservation of the entire stomach, which improved postoperative nutritional status and quality of life [8]. Konishi et al. reported reconstruction of the hepatic artery when pulsation in the proper hepatic artery was weak after test occlusion of the celiac axis in 2000 [9]. Since then, several institutions have reported their experienced with the modified Appleby operation for advanced pancreatic body/tail carcinoma, i.e., distal pancreatectomy combined with celiac axis en-bloc resection, which was named DP-CAR by Kondo et al. [10]. Despite reports of a few long-term survivors, the overall survival benefit and the risks of this challenging operation are unknown because previous reports have included only a small number of patients. In the era of safer modification and innovation of the Appleby operation and the transition of the concept of borderline resectable pancreatic carcinoma, this procedure attract pancreatic surgeon's attention again as a radical pancreatectomy for borderline resectable or locally advanced pancreatic body/tail carcinoma. In 2014, we have firstly introduced the preservation of the left gastric artery (LGA) on the basis of anatomical features in DP-CAR (modified DP-CAR) [11].

48.3 The Anatomical Features About Celiac Trunk and Its Branches

Although there are many reports on the classification of celiac artery anatomy, the classification that can be applied to variations of past papers is relatively simple and easy to understand is the classification described by Marco-Clement et al. in 2016 (Fig. 48.1) [12]. In this paper, almost 90% are Type I called complete celiac trunk, Type Ia: complete bifurcated celiac trunk (LGA arises first) is 57.6%, Type Ib: complete trifurcated celiac trunk is 32.1%, and incomplete celiac trunk is the Type IIa called hepatosplenic trunk is Type IIa

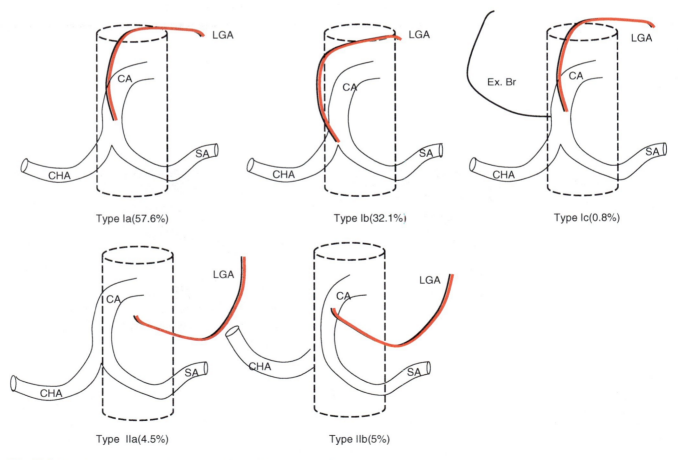

Fig. 48.1 Classification of celiac branches by Marco-Clement et al. [12]

4.5%, and the gastrosplenic trunk Type IIb is 5%. From the viewpoint of anatomical factors, LGA cannot preserved in Type Ib cannot preserve in pancreatic body cancer with positive invasion of the roots of the celiac artery, common hepatic artery, and splenic artery. For other are examined for each individual case, and the LGA can be preserved without microscopic cancer residual (R0). The planned surgical method and planned dissection layer should be planned in consideration of the distance from the tumor to the LGA and the site of the LGA root [11].

48.4 The Organs and Tissues Resected by the Modified Appleby Operation (DP-CAR)

Hirano and Kondo et al. described [1] the resected organ and tissues by this procedure were as follows, the procedures routinely included en bloc resection of the celiac, common hepatic, and LGA, the celiac plexus and ganglions, the nerve plexus around the superior mesenteric artery, a part of the crus of the diaphragm and the Gerota's fascia, the left adrenal gland, the retroperitoneal fat tissues bearing lymph nodes above the left renal vein, the transverse mesocolon covering the body of the pancreas, and the inferior mesenteric vein. Resection of the portal vein and the middle colic vessels was optional. In general, no reconstruction of the arterial system was required because of early development of the collateral arterial pathways via the pancreatoduodenal arcades from the superior mesenteric artery. In addition, with preservation of the stomach, no reconstruction of the alimentary tract was required. Sato et al. reported about the feasibility of middle colic artery—LGA bypass in patients who undergo LGA resecting DP-CAR [13]. Based on the anatomical features and the relationship between the tumor and artery, the LGA and inferior phrenic arteries can be preserved. Table 48.1 shows the list of organs, vessels, and other tissues which is resected and preserved in this procedure.

48.5 The Indication of Modified Appleby Operation (DP-CAR) in Patient with Pancreatic Body/Tail Carcinoma

First, this procedure should be performed in the selected institutions where well-trained and skillful staffs [2]. Regarding the tumor status, in the early period of the adaptation of the modified Appleby operation (DP-CAR), this procedure was indicated for patients with pancreatic body/tail carcinoma involving celiac axis and/or common hepatic artery. Recent literature reported this procedure is indicated for the patients whose pancreatic body/tail tumors involved or touched at least one of the common hepatic artery, the root of the splenic artery, or the celiac axis [1], which means

Table 48.1 The organs, vessels, and other tissues that are resected or preserved in the modified Appleby operation

	Resection	Preservation	Optional resection
Organ	Pncreas (body/tail), left adrenal gland, gallbladder[a], spleen	Stomach, duodenum	
Vessels	Celiac artery, common hepatic artery, splenic artery, dorsal pancreatic artery, short gastric vessels, posterior gastric artery, inferior mesenteric vein.	inferior pancreaticoduodenal artery, gastroduodenal artery (pancreatoduodenal arcades), proper hepatic artery, the right gastric and right gastroepiploic vessels, gastrocolic trunk.	Portal vein, middle colic vessels. Left gastric artery[a] and inferior phrenic arteries can be preserved based on the anatomical features.
Other tissues	Part of the crus of the diaphragm, the Gerota's fascia, the celiac plexus and ganglions, the nerve plexus around the superior mesenteric artery, the retroperitoneal fat tissues bearing lymph nodes above the left renal vein, the transverse mesocolon covering the body of the pancreas.	Right adrenal gland, bilateral kidneys.	

[a]Several institutions resect gallbladder, left gastric artery routinely, and others preserve under definite condition or reconstruct it

a parts of resectable pancreatic body/tail carcinomas situated near the root of the splenic artery also indicated for this procedure as well. Our investigation regarding the relationship between curability and the distance between the edge of the tumor and the splenic artery root in patients who underwent standard DP revealed that the microscopically positive margins were detected more frequently in the patients with tumors situated ≤10 mm from the splenic artery than those with a distance of >10 mm from the splenic artery [14]. Therefore, we suggest that DP-CAR should be performed to obtain an R0 resection in those patients with potentially resectable pancreatic body/tail carcinoma who would otherwise receive a standard DP. In addition to that, our study demonstrated the overall survival rate in patients with pathologically negative invasion for portal venous system and artery (double negative invasion) was greater than that of the other patients. Moreover, extended pancreatectomy with major arterial resection did not result in any long-term survivors in many previous reports. Therefore, we evaluate carefully the patients with double negative invasion into portal venous system and artery on preoperative imaging study for indication of DP-CAR.

48.6 Risk Score for the Modified Appleby Operation (DP-CAR)

From an international multicenter analysis for 191 DP-CAR patients, the 90-day mortality rate was 5.5% at 5 high-volume (≥1 DP-CAR/year) and 18% at 18 low-volume DP-CAR centers ($P = 0.015$). A risk score with age, sex, body mass index, American Society of Anesthesiologists score, multivisceral resection, open versus minimally invasive surgery, and low- versus high-volume center performed well in both the design and validation cohorts ($P = 0.642$). The main finding is that annual DP-CAR case volume is the most important predictor for 90-day mortality. The investigators of this study concluded that future studies should aim at (prospectively) validating the clinical risk score, which was made available online at www.pancreascalculator.com [2].

48.7 Preoperative Preparation for the Modified Appleby Operation (DP-CAR)

The necessity of the preoperative coil embolization still remains controversial. Several investigators have performed the modified Appleby operation without preoperative coil embolization of the common hepatic artery (CHA). The safety and efficacy is still needed to be evaluated in the clinical trials. Although, there is no evidence of decreased risk of these ischemia related complication by preoperative embolization of the CHA, preoperative angiography should be carried out and variations of the inferior pancreaticoduodenal artery (IPDA) were examined to safely perform this procedure. The preoperative coil embolization of the CHA should be performed as collaborative work between the surgeons and the interventional radiologist. The surgeons should request the planned ligation/division site precisely to them, and the radiologist was requested to place the coil in hopeful position without coil migration into the preserving planned arteries in a safe manner. The diameter of the IPDA usually increase about 1.5–2 times by the procedure.

48.8 The Procedure and Pitfalls of Modified Appleby Operation (DP-CAR)

The specific procedure for DP-CAR was as follows: firstly, right gastroepiploic artery/vein, right gastric artery/vein are encircled by vessel tape and preserved. Before the transection of the neck of the pancreas, firstly the bifurcation of the gastroduodenal artery (GDA) and the common hepatic artery (CHA) was exposed, followed by exposure of the origin of the proper hepatic artery (PHA). Confirming the negative for cancer cell infiltration of frozen section by harvesting the periarterial nerve plexus around the bifurcation should be performed to evaluate the resectability in patients whose tumor is adjacent this region. Kocher's maneuver should be performed in case of accidental bleeding from portal venous system. The gastrocolic trunk was preserved for venous return from the stomach. Transection of the pancreas was performed with enough margin from the tumor to confirm the negative for cancer cell infiltration. In patient whose tumor involves the portal vein, the resection and reconstruction of the portal vein was performed antecedently. After pancreatic transaction, the dissection of the retroperitoneum must be performed from the right side to the left side in the manner of radical antegrade modular pancreatosplenectomy procedure, because the surgical field of this procedure is better and safer for surgeon and assistant in case of accidental bleeding. By en-bloc dissecting the lymph nodes around the CHA, the right celiac ganglion and celiac nerve plexus, the origin of the celiac axis was exposed. Then, blood flow through the PHA, the right gastric artery, and the right gastroepiploic artery was confirmed by palpation, and intrahepatic arterial flow was also checked by intraoperative Doppler ultrasonography after clamping the end of the CHA in the patients who had undergone preoperative embolization of the CHA. The CHA was divided just proximal to the origin of the GDA. In the cases with dog-leg branching of PHA and GDA, great care was taken to preserve both arteries by avoiding the ligation of bifurcation site. Lifting up the cut end of the distal pancreas and the CHA into the left caudal side, the superior mesenteric artery (SMA) was dissected from the surrounding lymph node and nerve plexus toward its origin. Great care was taken to preserve the inferior pancreaticoduodenal artery (IPDA) arising from the SMA or the first jejunal artery. The dissecting layer around the SMA is connected to that of the celiac axis (CA) from the caudal side to dorsal side. The origin of the celiac axis was identified circumferentially just above the aorta and as divided. The origin and the direction of inferior phrenic arteries should be taken care in dissecting around the CA in front of the aorta.

48.9 Preservation of the Left Gastric Artery on the Basis of Anatomical Features

Despite the recent favorable surgical outcomes, delayed gastric emptying (DGE) or ischemic gastropathy after the modified Appleby operation (DP-CAR) is a continuous and frustrating complication. DGE induced by ischemic gastropathy, with had an incidence varying from 13.0% to 30.8% in previous series [1, 14], is not a life-threatening complication, but results in a prolonged hospital stay and leads to a decreased quality of life (QOL), poorer nutritional status and delayed administration of postoperative adjuvant chemotherapy. In the past studies, several patients underwent combined total gastrectomy to prevent gastric ischemic complications during the modified Appleby operation (DP-CAR) [1, 14]. The left gastric artery (LGA) develops as the first branch of the celiac trunk embryologically, and it was reported to branch antecedently in 68% to 72% of cases as a first branch of trifurcation described as above [12]. However, the procedures used for the modified Appleby operation (DP-CAR) routinely included en-bloc resection of the LGA [1], although pancreas body cancer requiring DP-CAR does not always involve the LGA or the nerve plexus surrounding the LGA. We prospectively tried to preserve the LGA with enough margins in patients whose LGA branched antecedently and in whom the distance between the LGA and carcinoma was more than 10 mm to clarify whether LGA preservation in DP-CAR (modified DP-CAR) could reduce the incidence of DGE and other postoperative complications [11] (Fig. 48.2). The medical records of 37 consecutive patients who underwent DP-CAR were evaluated for the incidence of DGE in 23 patients (62%) with LGA-resecting DP-CAR (conventional DP-CAR) and compared it with 14 patients (38%) who underwent distal pancreatectomy with resection of the common hepatic artery and splenic artery, with preservation of the LGA (modified DP-CAR) for pancreatic carcinoma. The patients with tumors situated more than 10 mm away from the antecedent branching LGA underwent modified DP-CAR. The antecedent branching of the LGA was found in 19 patients (51%) in this study. In the conventional DP-CAR group, the LGA were involved in 20 patients (87.0%). Clinically relevant DGE according to the ISGPS grades were: 30% in the conventional DP-CAR group, and 0% in the modified DP-CAR group ($P = 0.035$). The R0 rate was higher in the modified DP-CAR group (79%) compared to the conventional DP-CAR group (43%) ($P = 0.048$). Multivariate analysis demonstrated that resection of the LGA was an independent risk factor for increased incidence of DGE. Therefore, modified DP-CAR significantly reduced the incidence of DGE in comparison to conventional DP-CAR. In this series, distal stomach blood/nerve supply including right gastric, right gastroepiploic arteries and antral nerve branch were preserved, but proximal stomach blood supply including, left gastroepiploic and short gastric arteries were resected in all cases. The LGA preservation can reduce the ischemic gastropathy after DP-CAR, and this approach (preservation of the LGA when feasible) provides another option for surgeons performing DP-CAR. Furthermore, in patients whose collateral flow had injured or proved to be insufficient during the surgery, arterial reconstruction would compromise collateral flow [13].

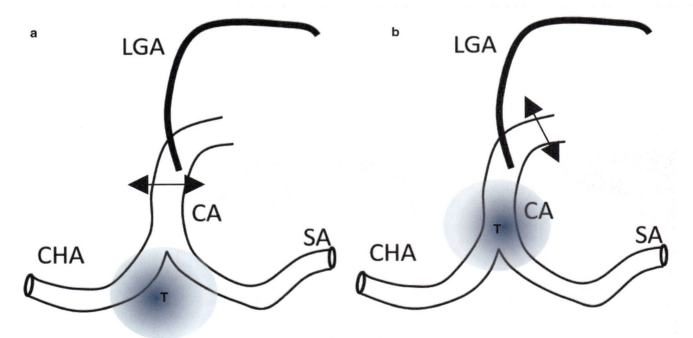

Fig. 48.2 The patients with tumors situated more than 10 mm away from the antecedent branching left gastric artery (LGA) underwent modified DP-CAR. A schematic drawing showing the relationship between the division site and the branching site of the LGA (a) in conventional DP-CAR and (b) in distal pancreatectomy with resection of the common hepatic and splenic artery, with preservation of the LGA (modified DP-CAR). Double-headed arrows indicating the site of the division. *CA* celiac axis, *SA* splenic artery, *CHA* common hepatic artery, *LGA* left gastric artery, *T* tumor

48.10 Surgical Technique Preserving Left Gastric Artery

Even when we intent to preserve left gastric artery (LGA) preoperatively, right gastroepiploic artery/vein, right gastric artery/vein are also firstly encircled by vessel tape and preserved, and we rule out the cancer cell infiltration into the periarterial nerve plexuses around GDA or CHA as soon as possible to evaluate resectability. We check the pulsation of GDA and PHA before clamping. After clamping the CHA, we confirmed the pulsation again, and the CHA was ligated and divided at the distal part described as above. We encircled the LGA by vessel tape to preserve in the early phase of surgery as a destination of dissection. Lifting up the CHA by en-bloc dissecting of lymph nodes around the CHA from the pancreas, the celiac axis was exposed. After confirming that the patients were negative for cancer cell infiltration into the nerve plexus surrounding the LGA by an intraoperative histopathological diagnosis of several frozen sections, the celiac artery was divided just after the branching of the LGA. The resection and reconstruction of the portal vein is performed antecedently before radical antegrade modular pancreatosplenectomy procedure. The depth of dissecting layer of retroperitoneum was controlled with wide margin according to the tumor position. Figure 48.3 shows the surgical field after modified DP-CAR.

48.11 Postoperative Complications After Modified Appleby Operation (DP-CAR)

The rates of morbidity after this procedure is not low [2]. The presence of postoperative hemorrhage from the resected stump of the common hepatic artery due to a pancreatic fistula after DP-CAR is difficult to rescue by interventional radiology (IVR) techniques because of the resection of the common hepatic artery. In addition, DP-CAR is associated with significant morbidities such as ischemic gastropathy or hepatic ischemia [15]. Total gastrectomy was added if severe ischemia of the stomach was observed during operation and if surgeon could not exclude the possibility of future necrosis of the remnant stomach in several institutions. Unplanned arterial reconstruction was required in patients with accidental injury [1]. The possible ischemic gastropathy includes irregular, shallow, and wide ulcerations usually in cardia of the stomach thought to be ischemic in origin and delayed gastric emptying after surgery. The issue would directly affect the postoperative recovery and the schedule of adjuvant chemotherapy. As regarding the hepatic ischemia, the recent studies reported the low incidence of clinically relevant hepatic infarction as a case requiring drainage of abscess, and usually abnormal liver function recovered after several days. Necrotic cholecystitis is also reported which could occur postoperatively probably due to the spasm of the gastroduodenal artery and/or proper hepatic artery reported in several studies. The most concern is diarrhea after the removal of the plexus around the celiac axis and the superior mesenteric artery, because the diarrhea would influence the nutritional status and quality of life after surgery. In many studies, diarrhea after this procedure is reported as controllable degree to maintain quality of life and nutritional status by medication, usually with loperamide hydrochloride, and rarely with tincture of opium [1].

48.12 Conclusions

The modified Appleby operation (DP-CAR) may be justified in highly selected patients owing to the potential survival benefit compared with patients without resection, and these patients should be treated in multimodal therapy. Recent additional modification by preservation of LGA, i.e. "modified DP-CAR" can lead the procedure to be a safer option.

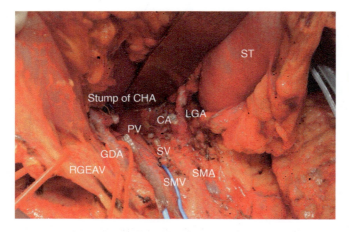

Fig. 48.3 The surgical field after modified DP-CAR. *ST* stomach, *PV* portal vein, *SMV* superior mesenteric vein, *SV* splenic vein, *RGEAV* right gastroepiploic artery/vein, *GDA* gastroduodenal artery, *CA* celiac artery, *LGA* left gastric artery, *SMA* superior mesenteric artery, *CHA*, common hepatic artery

References

1. Hirano S, Kondo S, Hara T, et al. Distal pancreatectomy with en bloc celiac axis resection for locally advanced pancreatic body cancer: long-term results. Ann Surg. 2007;246:46–51.
2. Klompmaker S, Peters NA, van Hilst J, et al. Outcomes and risk score for Distal Pancreatectomy with Celiac Axis Resection (DP-CAR): an international multicenter analysis. Ann Surg Oncol. 2019;26:772–81.
3. Fortner JG. Regional resection of cancer of the pancreas: a new surgical approach. Surgery. 1973;73:307–20.
4. Fortner JG, Kim DK, Cubilla A, et al. Regional pancreatectomy: en bloc pancreatic, portal vein and lymph node resection. Ann Surg. 1977;186:42–50.
5. Appleby LH. The coeliac axis in the expansion of the operation for gastric carcinoma. Cancer. 1953;6:704–7.

6. Appleby LH. Removal of the celiac axis in gastrectomy for carcinoma of the stomach in selected cases: a ten-year assessment. J Int Coll Surg. 1960;34:143–7.
7. Nimura Y, Hattori T, Miura K, et al. Experience of Appleby's operation for advanced carcinoma of the pancreatic body and tail (in Japanese). Shujutsu. 1976;30:885–9.
8. Hishinuma S, Ogata Y, Matsui J, et al. Two cases of cancer of the pancreatic body undergoing gastric preservation with distal pancreatectomy combined with resection of the celiac axis. Jpn J Gastroenterol Surg. 1991; 24: 2782–2786 (in Japanese with English abstract).
9. Konishi M, Kinoshita T, Nakagori T, et al. Distal pancreatectomy with resection of the celiac axis and reconstruction of the hepatic artery for carcinoma of the body and tail of the pancreas. J Hepato-Biliary-Pancreat Surg. 2000;7:183–7.
10. Kondo S, Katoh H, Hirano S, et al. Results of radical distal pancreatectomy with en bloc resection of the celiac artery for locally advanced cancer of the pancreatic body. Langenbeck's Arch Surg. 2003;388:101–6.
11. Okada K, Kawai M, Tani M, et al. Preservation of the left gastric artery on the basis of anatomical features in patients undergoing distal pancreatectomy with celiac axis en-bloc resection (DP-CAR). World J Surg. 2014;38:2980–5.
12. Marco-Clement I, Martinez-Barco A, Ahumada N, et al. Anatomical variations of the celiac trunk: cadaveric and radiological study. Surg Radiol Anat. 2016;38:501–10.
13. Sato T, Saiura A, Inoue Y, et al. Distal pancreatectomy with en bloc resection of the celiac axis with preservation or reconstruction of the left gastric artery in patients with pancreatic body cancer. World J Surg. 2016;40:2245–53.
14. Okada K, Kawai M, Tani M, et al. Surgical strategy for patients with pancreatic body/tail carcinoma: who should undergo distal pancreatectomy with en-bloc celiac axis resection? Surgery. 2013;153:365–72.
15. Okada KI, Kawai M, Hirono S, et al. Ischemic gastropathy after distal pancreatectomy with en bloc celiac axis resection for pancreatic body cancer. Langenbeck's Arch Surg. 2018;403:561–71.

Robotic Distal Pancreatectomy

Marco Vito Marino, Marco Ramera, and Alessandro Esposito

Abstract

Since its first description in 1994 by Cuschieri (J R Coll Surg Edinb 39:178–84, 1994), laparoscopic left pancreatectomy has been increasingly performed by hepato-pancreato-biliary surgeons worldwide. Despite reported benefits of less blood loss, faster recovery and shorter hospital stay over the classic open procedure (de Rooij et al. Ann Surg 269(1):2–9, 2019; Bjornsson et al. Br J Surg 2020), the first International Survey on Minimally Invasive Pancreatic Resection reported the minimally invasive distal pancreatectomy median lifetime case volume was quite low even for expert pancreatic surgeons (van Hilst et al. HPB (Oxford) 19:190–204, 2017). The technical expertise required for tissue manipulation, vascular dissection and control of bleeding while ensuring adequate oncological outcome remains a significant hindrance to widespread adoption. The lack of specific training program, the poor ergonomics definitively limited the widespread of the laparoscopic distal pancreatectomy. The da Vinci robotic system (Intuitive Surgical, Sunnyvale, CA, USA) with its microsuturing and microdissection capabilities associated to an enhanced visualization may potentially provide several advantages over the laparoscopic approach. Early reports show encouraging results over the laparoscopic distal pancreatectomy in terms of reduced blood loss (Chen et al. Surg Endosc 29:3507–18, 2015), increased splenic preservation rate (Hong et al. Surg Endosc 34:2465–2473, 2020), reduced conversion to open with comparable short term oncological efficacy (Marino et al. Dig Surg 37:229–239, 2020). There is a lack to technical standardization of approach and patient selection via novel difficulty scoring needs to be validated in larger cohorts. The prevention of clinically significant pancreatic fistula continues to be a challenge and long term oncological outcomes for malignancy remains unclear. Limitations of cost and learning curve especially with the adoption of more complex procedures will need to be overcome for wider application of the robotic approach.

M. V. Marino (✉)
General Surgery Department, Azienda Ospedaliera Ospedali Riuniti Villa Sofia-Cervello, Palermo, Italy

General Surgery Department, Istituto Villa Salus, Siracusa, Italy

M. Ramera
General Surgery Department, Fondazione Poliambulanza, Brescia, Italy

A. Esposito
General and Pancreatic Surgery Department, University Hospital of Verona, Verona, Italy

49.1 Surgical Technique

49.1.1 Instruments and Tools

For robotic-assisted distal pancreatectomy we personally use the following instrumentations which should be available in the operating room before starting the operation. Four robotic ports and one 12 mm laparoscopic ports are employed, sometimes a 5 mm laparoscopic port is used when the exposure of the operative field is challenging.

A 30° robotic camera is preferred instead of the 0° scope for the opportunity to switch from up to down during the dissection around the pancreas, a Tip-Up Fenestrated Grasper is preferred as retractor instrument for the longer length of the tips, a Monopolar Curved Scissors and a Fenestrated Bipolar Forceps as energy device, finally the Harmonic ACE®Curved Shears (Ethicon Endo-Surgery, Inc., Cincinnati, OH, USA) as advanced energy device. In case of obese patients, we employ the Vessel Sealer Extend that has a higher hemostatic effect than Harmonic ACE®, conversely the latter has in our opinion a better dissecting capability which are crucial in case of smooth and meticulous dissection.

Medium-large and large robotic Hem-o-lok® clips and Horizon™ small-wide titanium clips (Teleflex Medical Ltd., RTP Durham, NC, USA) should be available as well as a 45 mm Laparoscopic stapler (Purple or Black load) for the pancreatic transection. We do not recommend the utilization of a robotic stapler for the pancreatic transection due to the lack of tactile feedback and the difficulties in modulating the closure of the jaws. Monofilament sutures of 3–0 Prolene® and a 25 cm cotton tape complete the armamentarium. Two atraumatic laparoscopic instruments are available.

49.1.2 Operating Room Configuration

The patient under general anesthesia is located in supine position, with legs apart and arms tucked to the body. The robotic cart is docked over the right flank of the patient, while the surgeon console is located at the inferior left corner of the operating theater. The bed assistant is located between the patient's legs, while the scrub nurse stands at the lower left side of the patient.

The pneumoperitoneum is established by using a Veress needle. The bed is tilted in reverse-Trendelenburg position (15–20°) and right lateral decubitus (10°). A total of five trocars are inserted. The four 8 mm robotic ports are placed in a straight line at the umbilical line as following:

- in the right flank for arm number 1 (R1),
- in the right pararectal area for arm number 2 (R2),
- in the periumbilical area for arm number 3 (R3),
- in the left flank for arm number 4 (R4) (Fig. 49.1).

A 12 mm laparoscopic port connected to the AirSeal® system is placed between R3 and R4 in the left pararectal area.

A Tip-Up Fenestrated Grasper, a Monopolar Curved Scissors and a Fenestrated Bipolar Forceps are used as initial instruments for arm number 1, 2 and 4 respectively.

49.1.3 Distal Splenopancreatectomy

The operation starts by inspecting the abdominal cavity, an intraoperative ultrasound is performed with the aims to exclude liver metastasis and to assess the tumor location. The gastrocolic ligament is then opened preserving the gastroepiploic arcade by the Monopolar Scissors while the stomach is retracted cephalad by the arm number 1. The posterior wall of the stomach is fixed to the anterior abdominal wall by a running suture of 3–0 V-loc™ thus freeing the arm number 1 which is used for the tissue retraction. The spleno-gastric ligament is transected, and the short gastric vessels are completely cut by the Harmonic ACE®.

The splenic flexure is routinely taken down through a supramesocolic approach or by mobilizing the left colon from its lateral attachments. The pancreatic gland is entirely exposed, and its inferior margin is progressively dissected free from the transverse mesocolon.

The splenic vein is visualized and dissected towards the confluence with the superior mesenteric vein, finally it is encircled by a vessel-loop. Similarly, the superior margin of the pancreas is incised and the splenic artery is dissected at its origin and encircled by a vessel-loop. A retropancreatic tunnel is started and the pancreas is suspended by a cotton-tape which is handled by the arm number 1. The splenic artery and next the splenic vein are clipped by the Hem-o-lok® and divided (Fig. 49.2).

The distal pancreas is transected at the level of the neck with a laparoscopic stapler (Endo GIA™ Medtronic, Minneapolis, MN, USA) purple (3–4 mm) or black (4–5 mm) load or alternatively with the Harmonic ACE® depending on the thickness of pancreatic gland (Fig. 49.3). Prior to division, 2 stay sutures of 3–0 Prolene® are placed, one proximally and one distally the transection point, at the inferior

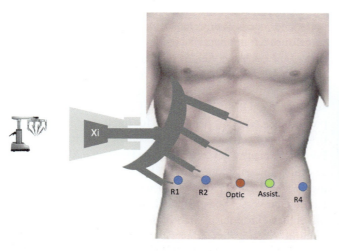

Fig. 49.1 Trocart layout

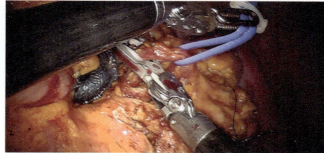

Fig. 49.2 Splenic artery control

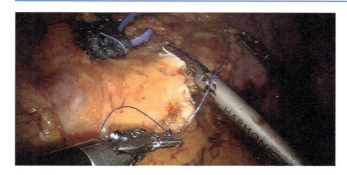

Fig. 49.3 Pancreatic transection

border of the pancreas for retraction. The distal pancreas is dissected from the retroperitoneum.

The phrenocolienal ligament is cut and the spleen is freed from its lateral attachments.

49.1.4 Spleen-Preserving Distal Pancreatectomy

Once the gastrocolic ligament is opened the left gastroepiploic and the short gastric vessels are preserved. The inferior and the superior margins of the pancreas are dissected and The splenic artery and veins are both isolated and encircled by two vessel-loops. The level of pancreatic transection is assessed by an IOUS and tunnelized by a cotton tape.

If a Kimura technique was attempted, the distal pancreas is dissected and mobilized in a medial to lateral fashion the splenic vessels are skeletonized from the isthmus toward the hilum of the spleen, ligating and dividing all pancreatic branches trough Harmonic ACE® scalpel or small titanium clips.

If a Warshaw technique was performed the splenic vessels (artery first) are controlled and divided between Hem-o-lok® clips or sectioned through a white stapler load application. In particular the artery is isolated clipped proximally at its origin and distally at the level of splenic hilum preserving the origin of the left gastroepiploic artery. The splenic vein was controlled at the splenic hilum preserving the left gastroepiploic vein.

No fibrin glue was placed on the pancreatic stump. An intraoperative frozen section of the pancreatic remnant was sent for pathological examination to confirm negative margins when appropriate. A single suction drain is placed close to the pancreatic remnant. The specimen, inserted in endoscopic bag, is retrieved through a Pfannenstiel incision or through the incision of the 12-mm trocar in case of spleen preservation and for non-bulky lesions.

49.2 Results

A total of 45 patients (25 males, 20 females) underwent robotic distal pancreatectomy since October 2016 up to now. In Thirty-five cases a distal pancreatectomy with splenectomy was carried out, while in ten cases a spleen-preserving approach was pursued.

The mean age was 58.5 years. The BMI was 27.4. Ten out of 45 (22.2%) had a previous abdominal surgery and the majority (30 out of 45) suffered by a malignant pancreatic pathology. The leading indication for surgery was pancreatic ductal adenocarcinoma (22) followed by chronic pancreatitis [1] and neuroendocrine tumors [2]. The mean operative time was 225 min (range 150–655 min), the spleen preserving procedures were associated to a longer operative time (255 vs 190 min). The overall estimated blood loss was 115 ml (5–300 ml). In case of benign conditions, a spleen preserving procedures was completed in 100% of cases. Only 2 patients were converted to open due to the difficulties in bleeding control and concerns regarding the oncologic adequacy. Eleven patients experimented post-operative complications, seven were classified as minor, while four were major (8.9%). Only three patients developed a postoperative pancreatic fistula (2 grade B and 1 grade C according ISGPS classification [3]). Two patients were reoperated the first for a peripancreatic fluid collection associated to a grade C pancreatic fistula, the second for a colon perforation. The mean length of hospital stay was 9 days (range 6–21 days). The 90-day mortality rate was one due to postoperative pulmonary embolism. An R0 resection rate was achieved in 100% of cases. The mean nodal harvested was 19.5 nodes (range 7–25 nodes). The recurrence rate at a mean follow-up of 16 months was 15%. The disease-free survival at 3-year was 57.8% while the overall-free survival was 70.2%.

49.3 Discussion

The robotic pancreatic surgery is progressively gaining momentum as it is applied both for pancreatoduodenectomy or enucleation [4, 5].

Spleen preserving distal pancreatectomy (SPDP) is an important organ preservation technique for pancreatic body/tail non-malignant tumors that offers several hematological and immunological benefits, as proven in several studies [6, 7]. Two techniques are commonly applied for this purpose and differ in the preservation or not of the splenic vessels [8]. With the advent of the minimally invasive approach and in particular of the robotic platform, there was great interest in evaluating the contribution that this technology could bring in the preservation of the spleen.

Three recent meta-analyses [9, 10] have evaluated the spleen preservation rate between RDP and LDP with controversial results. All of these studies actually report that spleen preservation rates were less than 50%. In almost all of the series included in these meta-analyses, the parameter "spleen preservation rate" actually refers to the ratio between the number of operations in which the spleen has been preserved and the total number of minimally invasive procedures performed for any pathology. Other retrospective studies have carefully evaluated this issue. A Korean single-center and single-surgeon analysis conducted on more than 200 patients undergoing MIDP has the laparoscopic and robotic approach (about one fifth of cases) [11]. Although the nature of the study is retrospective, the authors report the number of cases where there was an intent to preserve the spleen. RDP was associated with a higher preservation success rate (96.8% vs 82.5%; $P = 0.02$). another study carefully considered this question. From the retrospective analysis of all patients undergoing SPDP for low-grade benign or malignant tumors at the Shanghai hospital, a propensity score matching was obtained compared RDP and ODP [12]. The RDP cohort showed a significantly higher spleen preservation rate (63.5% vs 26.5%, $P < 0.001$), less estimated blood loss and, interestingly, shorter operative time. In logistic regression analysis, the open approach, together with increasing age, tumor size, and blood loss, such as the pathological type of inflammatory neoplasm, were independent predictors of spleen preservation failure.

It is possible that the surgeon's and/or patient's preference for a particular approach has still limited the design of randomized prospective trails.

Another widely debated point is the adequacy of the robotic approach for malignant tumors, especially PDAC. Three systematic reviews and meta-analyses suggested comparable oncological outcomes in terms of resection margin, 30-day mortality, disease-free survival, and overall survival between MIDP and ODP [13–15]. Once again, the currently available data could suffer from retrospective selection bias. Results from 2 ongoing randomized controlled trials, the European multicenter DIPLOMA trial (ISRCTN44897265), and the Chinese multicenter "Study of Laparoscopic Versus Open Distal Pancreatectomy in Patients with Pancreatic Cancer at the Body and Tail" (NCT03792932), should increase the level of evidence available on this topic.

References

1. Marino MV, Mirabella A, Gomez Ruiz M, et al. Robotic-assisted versus laparoscopic distal pancreatectomy: the results of a case-matched analysis from a tertiary care center. Dig Surg. 2020;37(3):229–39.
2. Chen S, Zhan Q, Chen JZ, et al. Robotic approach improves spleen-preserving rate and shortens postoperative hospital stay of laparoscopic distal pancreatectomy: a matched cohort study. Surg Endosc. 2015;29(12):3507–18.
3. Bassi C, Marchegiani G, Dervenis C, et al. The 2016 update of the International Study Group (ISGPS) definition and grading of postoperative pancreatic fistula: 11 Years After. Surgery. 2017;161(3):584–91.
4. Liu R, Wakabayashi G, Palanivelu C, et al. International consensus statement on robotic pancreatic surgery. Hepatobiliary Surg Nutr. 2019;8(4):345–60.
5. Marino MV, Podda M, Gomez Ruiz M, Fernandez CC, Guarrasi D, Gomez FM. Robotic-assisted versus open pancreaticoduodenectomy: the results of a case-matched comparison. J Robot Surg. 2020;14(3):493–502.
6. Benoist S, Dugue L, Sauvanet A, et al. Is there a role of preservation of the spleen in distal pancreatectomy? J Am Coll Surg. 1999;188(3):255–60.
7. Shoup M, Brennan MF, McWhite K, et al. The value of splenic preservation with distal pancreatectomy. Arch Surg. 2002;137(2):164–8.
8. Esposito A, Casetti L, De Pastena M, et al. Robotic spleen-preserving distal pancreatectomy: the Verona experience. Updat Surg. 2020;
9. Hu YH, Qin YF, Yu DD, et al. Meta-analysis of short-term outcomes comparing robot-assisted and laparoscopic distal pancreatectomy. J Comp Eff Res. 2020;9(3):201–18.
10. Kamarajah SK, Sutandi N, Robinson SR, et al. Robotic versus conventional laparoscopic distal pancreatic resection: a systematic review and meta-analysis. HPB (Oxford). 2019;21(9):1107–18.
11. Hong S, Song KB, Madkhali AA, et al. Robotic versus laparoscopic distal pancreatectomy for left-sided pancreatic tumors: a single surgeon's experience of 228 consecutive cases. Surg Endosc. 2020;34(6):2465–73.
12. Weng Y, Jin J, Huo Z, et al. Robotic-assisted versus open distal pancreatectomy for benign and low-grade malignant pancreatic tumors: a propensity score-matched study. Surg Endosc. 2020;
13. van Hilst J, Korrel M, de Rooij T, et al. Oncologic outcomes of minimally invasive versus open distal pancreatectomy for pancreatic ductal adenocarcinoma: a systematic review and meta-analysis. Eur J Surg Oncol. 2019;45(5):719–27.
14. Riviere D, Gurusamy KS, Kooby DA, et al. Laparoscopic versus open distal pancreatectomy for pancreatic cancer. Cochrane Database Syst Rev. 2016;4(CD011391)
15. Nakamura M, Nakashima H. Laparoscopic distal pancreatectomy and pancreatoduodenectomy: is it worthwhile? A meta-analysis of laparoscopic pancreatectomy. J Hepatobiliary Pancreat Sci. 2013;20(4):421–8.

Total Pancreatectomy

Aleksandar Karamarkovic, Jovan Juloski, and Vladica Cuk

Abstract

Total pancreatectomy (TP) plays an important role in the treatment of some pancreatic disorders for several reasons: (I) TP is the only surgery for a radical resection of pancreatic cancer with extensive tumors for which complete removals cannot be achieved by means of pancreatoduodenectomy (PD) or distal pancreatectomy (DP). (II) TP is helpful to the dissection of surrounding lymph nodes and nerves, and may improve the long-term prognosis of pancreatic cancer. (III) Pancreatic cancer involving multi segments extensively, as well as main-duct IPMN and multifocal branch-duct IPMN involving the entire pancreas, require TP. (IV) Anastomotic leak, postoperative pancreatic fistula (POPF), and postoperative pancreatic hemorrhage (PPH) as the consequence of POPF can be prevented by performing TP.

In order to achieve better local control for borderline resectable pancreatic cancer (BRPC) and locally advanced pancreatic cancer (LAPC), especially after neoadjuvant treatment, we recommend adding TRIANGLE operation to TP as a key procedure.

50.1 Introduction

The first successful TP for pancreatic adenocarcinoma was performed by Rockey [1] in 1943. After advances made in the surgical techniques and glycemic monitoring as well as the development of synthetic insulin and pancreatic enzymes, the medical management after TP has improved. Some studies have demonstrated acceptable QOLs after TP for neoplastic disease [2–4]. With growing experience, technical improvement and perioperative care advancement, we now have mortality less than 3% and morbidity rates around 40% in high-volume centers [5, 6].

50.2 Indications

Indications for TP can be classified into four "T" groups [7, 8]:

1. Tumors of advanced stage or specific localization
2. Technical problems due to soft pancreatic tissue or small pancreatic duct
3. Troubles due to perioperative surgical complications
4. Therapy refractory pain due to chronic pancreatitis

The most frequent indication for TP is advanced or multifocal pancreatic tumors [8]. Recurrent pancreatic carcinoma, IPMN and extensive neuroendocrine tumors are also tumor related indications for total pancreatectomy [9–11]. TP for cases of main-duct IPMN and mixed-type IPMN is conducted either as a primary en block resection, when IPMN extends throughout the entire pancreas, or as a sequential operation, when frozen section analysis reveals IPMN on the resection margin after partial resection [12]. Management of multifocal branch-duct IPMN is a bit more challenging, and still a matter of controversies, regarding indication, correct timing, and extent of surgical interventions [12]. Based on the "Fukuoka" criteria, the risk of malignancy in these lesions have been described [13]. According to these guidelines, resection of lesion greater than 3 cm in diameter should be resected. Smaller ones should be resected, but only if "high risk" stigmata are present (mural nodules, positive cytology, symptoms, or a synchronously dilated main duct). Still remaining concerns are, among all IPMN smaller than 3 cm, that are resected, about 25% were shown to be malignant [13]. Standard approach for all suspected malignant branch-duct IPMN is adequate resection with lymphadenectomy, similar to the approach in main-duct IPMN [12].

A. Karamarkovic (✉) · J. Juloski · V. Cuk
Department of HPB Surgery, Surgical Clinic "Nikola Spasic", University Clinical Center Zvezdara, Belgrade, Serbia

Faculty of Medicine University of Belgrade, Belgrade, Serbia
e-mail: alekara@sbb.rs

In the case of chronic pancreatitis without dilation of pancreatic duct in patients resistant to medical treatment, TP has been proposed [14]. The procedure is also proposed for patients with hereditary pancreatitis who are at elevated risk for pancreatic cancer development [15].

Technical problems due to soft pancreatic tissue represent not so uncommon indication for TP. In cases when reconstructions of the common hepatic (CHA) and superior mesenteric arteries (SMA) are undertaken, TP is generally performed and recommended [16, 17]. The complete resection of pancreas reduces the rate of morbidity and mortality by eliminating completely the incidence of POPF and its potentially fatal effect on the arterial anastomosis [15].

Following "partial" pancreatic resection, complications such as POPF complicated by acute bleeding, sepsis, can occur. In these cases, TP is indicated as a salvage procedure [7].

In patients undergoing pancreatectomy for PDAC, TP provides chances of R0 resection in isolated neck margin-positive patients and was associated with a survival benefit. TP is recommended for patients having cancer spread from the head to the left part of the pancreas [15, 18].

The definition of BRPC and LAPC is based on the relationship of tumor and its nearby main blood vessels [19]. Previous classification made by AHPBA/SSO/SSAT was further clarified by the National Comprehensive Cancer Network (NCCN), and International Study Group of Pancreatic Surgery (ISGPS) also [20, 21].

While neoadjuvant therapy is necessary in LAPC to achieve a chance of conversion surgery afterwards, its use in BRPC and especially resectable pancreatic cancer is currently still under debate. Surgical resection of BRPC is still controversial; i.e., Whether or not to resect the tumor largely depends on preoperative imaging diagnosis, which unfortunately cannot always provide real resectability [22] or distinguish tumor invasion from fibrosis caused by inflammation [23].

Despite the wide application of MDT in the treatment of pancreatic cancer [24], there is still a dilemma where the patient may lose the opportunity of surgery for a resectable tumor or the surgeon may end up by excising an unresectable tumor for which R0 resection cannot be achieved. For example, especially those patients who are considered unresectable because of CA, CHA or SMA encasement (no more than half in circumference) can get R0 resection with surgeon's effort. For the treatment of BRPC, neoadjuvant therapy is highly recommended in guidelines especially in Europe and US [25]. Some treatment reported has greatly improved the resection rate and prognosis of BRPC and LAPC [26, 27].

The TRIANGLE operation (Fig. 50.1) was proposed by Heidelberg group in 2017 [28] as novel approach for the patients with LAPC after the neoadjuvant therapy. The rationale of this procedure is the observation that after neoadju-

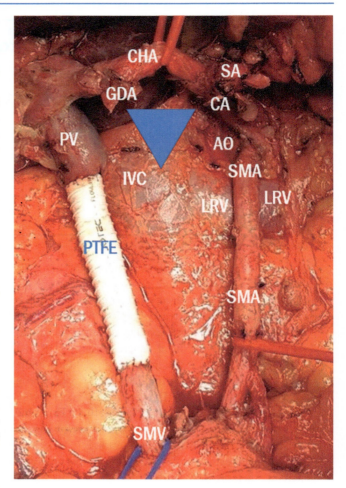

Fig. 50.1 TRIANGLE total pancreatectomy with en block portomesenteric vein resection. Intraoperative view after complete dissection of the TRIANGLE region including circumferential skeletonization of the CA/CHA, SMA (red tape) and PV/SMV (blue tape) resection and reconstruction with ringed PTFE allograft interposition

vant therapy conventional imaging fails to differentiate between actual tumor encasement or abutment and only fibrotic residual tissue mainly to the arterial structures [28].

However, some patients, whose tumor fails to down-stage but develops after neoadjuvant therapy, lose the opportunity to undergo radical resection of the tumor. For those patients with artery encasement, upfront surgery with extensive dissection of the TRIANGLE region including celiac axis (CA), CHA, SMA portal vein (PV) and superior mesenteric vein (SMV), as well as complete skeletonization of these vessels, may allow R0 resection and decrease the local recurrence. In fact, those patients in the study of Zhai et al., do not appear local recurrence after surgery [29]. Some studies described that the TRIANGLE operation for BRPC was safe and efficient [29, 30]. TRIANGLE operation should be added to TP as a key procedure, which will help to increase the number of lymph nodes examined, reduce complications rate and have better radical treatment efficacy for BRPC [29].

50.3 Surgical Procedure

TP can be performed in two different situations, namely:

1. *TP as a second step after* PD.

This is the situation, which takes place after PD due to technical reasons, early septic and bleeding complications or neoplastic infiltration of the pancreatic resectional margin found at frozen section. In such cases, left pancreatectomy is performed after PD.

2. *TP as an "at once" procedure.*

In this case, an en-bloc resection is performed of the entire pancreas, part of the stomach, duodenum, jejunum, common bile duct, gallbladder, and spleen.

Resectability was evaluated according to NCCN guidelines (version 3. 2017.) [31].

1. Kocher's Maneuver to Lift the Head of the Pancreas and the Duodenum.

After the exposure of left renal vein and the abdominal aorta leftwards, expose the root of SMA (Artery First approach). The origin of SMA isolated from a right posterior approach [32] just above the aorta and left renal vein; after that, infrapancreatic portion of SMA taped using Mesenteric approach, proposed by Nakao [33] (Fig. 50.2). The concept of this Artery First strategy, is to evaluate any potential tumor adherence to the SMA or replacing RHA origin at the beginning of the operation and either stop resection or plan an arterial resection if required and indicated.

2. Skeletonizing the Hepatoduodenal Ligament.

The elements of the hepatic pedicle are skeletonized, according to technique for PD.

3. Mobilization of the Spleen and the Body and Tail Portion of Pancreas.

The body and tail of the pancreas are mobilized from left to right, in order to dissect and isolate the spleno-pancreatic complex from distal to proximal till meet the pancreatic isthmus and head.

4. Clearance of TRIANGLE.

Technique comprises dissection of all soft tissue along the CA, SMA, SMV, and PV in association with a radical tumor removal. During the resection process, if must be proven that the specific periarterial tissue does not include viable tumor by frozen section; afterwards a radical artery-sparing approach can be conducted [34]. Complete skeletonization of the regional vasculature is required. Arterial circumferential skeletonization is obligatory, which include complete clearance of the sheath of the proper vasculature, on the adventitial level.

This results in an anatomic TRIANGLE bordered by the CA/CHA, SMA and PV/SMV revealed by the dissection and finally resection indicating the comprehensive removal of all soft tissue contained within these borders - usually fibrotic, neural, and lymphatic tissue (Fig. 50.3).

The resection and reconstruction of SMV or PV could be done when either of them was invaded by tumor, vein reconstruction including direct anastomosis or artificial vascular graft (Fig. 50.3). TRIANGLE TP exerts great impact on the radical resection the negative rate of surgical margin and long-time survival of patients of pancreatic cancer [28, 29].

The coronary vein is usually divided during the procedure when TP is performed and a re-insertion is not possible in most patients due to the extent of resection. Therefore, stomach perfusion has to be critically evaluated at the end of the operation and a distal or even subtotal stomach resection may be required to avoid congestion-related ischemia [35].

5. Detachment of the Cephalic duodenopancreatic complex, Dividing the Gastric Antrum, Transecting Jejunum.

Once the left splenopancreatic complex has been entirely mobilized and the retropancreatic vessels have been freed,

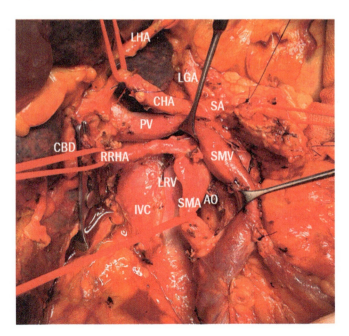

Fig. 50.2 Pancreatectomy with complete circumferential vascular clearance and total mesopancreas excision (mesenteric approach)

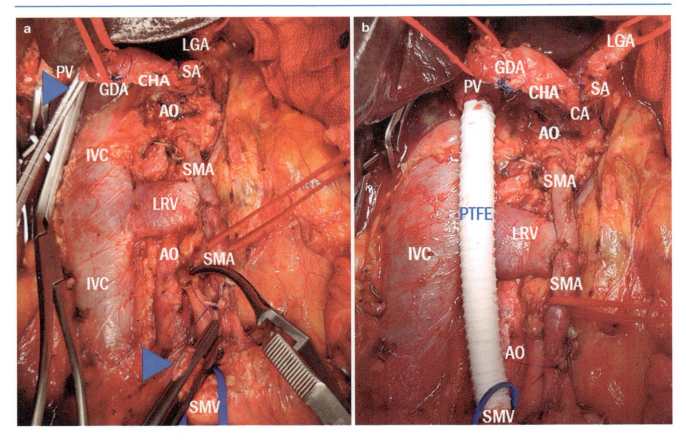

Fig. 50.3 Radical total pancreatectomy with vascular resection: Clearance of TRIANGLE with en block porto-mesenteric venous trunk resection (proximal and distal stumps of PV/SMV are clamped with vascular clamps—marked with blue arrowhead, while SMA is clamped with vascular bulldog in order to reduce intestinal congestion) (**a**); dissection of all soft tissue (TRIANGLE) between CA/CHA and SMA (red tapes) as well as the reconstructed PV/SMV with PTFE ringed allograft interposition (blue tape) (**b**)

the procedure completed with detachment of the cephalic duodenopancreatic complex, as in extended PD.

6. Bilio-digestive Reconstruction.

Include jejunal loop to perform transmesocolic biliodigestive anastomosis and, subsequently, transmesocolic gastrojejunal anastomosis.

50.4 Vascular Resection

TRIANGLE TP can be combined with arterial resection and reconstruction, while venous resection is frequently required in this situation. The most recent meta-analysis described that patients with pancreatectomy plus venous resection seemed to attain a larger tumor size, positive lymph nodes and R1 resection rates and higher 30-day mortality [36]. Controversially to the reported impaired survival after venous resection, a recent propensity score-matched analysis showed similar survival among the patients with venous resection and pancreatectomy alone groups [37].

In contrast to vein resection, artery resection is more debatable for its increased morbidity and mortality and mostly considered as an individual decision in selected patients [34, 38]. Furthermore, during recent years, the techniques of replacement applied for the hepatic artery or the superior mesenteric artery have been improved and procedures such as SA use (Fig. 50.4) have been described for restoration of hepatic or small-intestine perfusion [16].

According to our policy, we have performed arterial resection, only if replacing right hepatic artery (RRHA) origin from the SMA, was infiltrated by the tumor (Fig. 50.5).

Regarding specific complications and outcomes, the postoperative complications and the length of hospital stay and non-R0 rate were not significantly different compared to those without artery resection. Another recent study, covering nearly 40 years of experience confirmed the safety and efficacy of arterial resection for patients with LAPC, additionally suggesting preoperative neoadjuvant therapy with artery resection as a useful concept for LAPC [39].

A single-center cohort study reported that pancreatectomy with artery resection can obtain better one-, three-, and five-year survival rates compared to palliation for patients with LAPC [40].

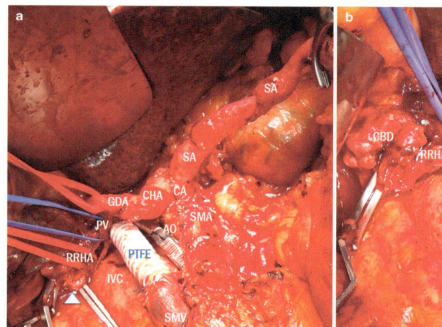
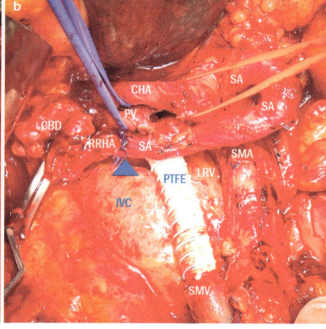

Fig. 50.4 TRIANGLE total pancreatectomy with combined vascular resections (PTFE graft interposition with SA transposition in reconstruction): Venous resection of PV/SMV trunk and arterial RRHA from SMA resection (SA prepared for transposition and RRHA reconstruction) (**a**); PTFE ringed allograft interposition used for PV/SMV reconstruction while SA transpositioned and anastomosed for the RRHA reconstruction (SA-RRHA end to end anastomosis marked with blue arrowhead) (**b**)

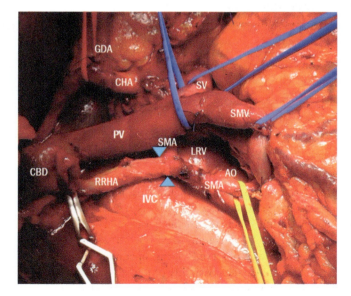

Fig. 50.5 TRIANGLE total pancreatectomy with arterial resection: Clearance of TRIANGLE space with concomitant resection of RRHA arising from SMA: direct "side to end" SMA-RRHA arterial reconstruction (anastomotic line marked with blue arrowheads). *PV* portal vein, *SMV* superior mesenteric vein, *IVC* inferior vena cava, *LRL* left renal vein, *AO* aorta, *SMA* superior mesenteric artery, *CA* celiac axis, *CHA* common hepatic artery, *SA* splenic artery, *LGA* left gastric artery, *GDA* gastroduodenal artery, *RRHA* replacing right hepatic artery from SMA; *CBD* common bile duct

50.5 Comment

Use of TP is supported for the treatment of PDAC in appropriately selected patients because the long-term survival rates of patients who underwent TP for pancreatic cancer were comparable to those for patients who underwent PD [41]. The similar 3- and 5-year survival rates in patients who underwent TP vs. those who underwent PD suggested that the glycemic issues were not major determinants of death in the long term [42]. TRIANGLE operation is a possible method to achieve the radical resection of BRPC in patients who have not received neoadjuvant therapy or in LAPC patients after neoadjuvant treatment. With TRIANGLE TP, artery sparing resection can be achieved and the postoperative risk of POPF and PPH can be reduced. However, more studies are needed to further assess the reliability, feasibility and long-term effect of this operation [29].

Acknowledgements The authors have no conflicts of interest to disclose.

References

1. Rockey EW. Total pancreatectomy for carcinoma: case report. Ann Surg. 1943;118(4):603–11.
2. Barbier L, Jamal W, Dokmak S, et al. Impact of total pancreatectomy: short- and long-term assessment. HPB (Oxford). 2013;15(11):882–92.
3. Müller MW, Friess H, Kleeff J, et al. Is there still a role for total pancreatectomy? Ann Surg. 2007;246(6):966–74; discussion 74–5.
4. Casadei R, Monari F, Buscemi S, et al. Total pancreatectomy: indications, operative technique, and results: a single centre experience and review of literature. Updat Surg. 2010;62(1):41–6.
5. Büchler MW, Wagner M, Schmied BM, et al. Changes in morbidity after pancreatic resection: toward the end of completion pancreatectomy. Arch Surg (Chicago, IL: 1960). 2003;138(12):1310–4; discussion 5.
6. Cameron JL, Riall TS, Coleman J, et al. One thousand consecutive pancreaticoduodenectomies. Ann Surg. 2006;244(1):10–5.
7. Janot MS, Belyaev O, Kersting S, et al. Indications and early outcomes for total pancreatectomy at a high-volume pancreas center. HPB Surg. 2010;2010.
8. Coco D, Leanza S, Guerra F. Total pancreatectomy: indications, advantages and disadvantages – a review. Maedica. 2019;14(4):391–6.
9. Cuillerier E, Cellier C, Palazzo L, et al. Outcome after surgical resection of intraductal papillary and mucinous tumors of the pancreas. Am J Gastroenterol. 2000;95(2):441–5.
10. Norton JA, Kivlen M, Li M, et al. Morbidity and mortality of aggressive resection in patients with advanced neuroendocrine tumors. Arch Surg (Chicago, IL: 1960). 2003;138(8):859–66.
11. Crippa S, Tamburrino D, Partelli S, et al. Total pancreatectomy: indications, different timing, and perioperative and long-term outcomes. Surgery. 2011;149(1):79–86.
12. Hackert T, Fritz S, Büchler MW. Main- and branch-duct intraductal papillary mucinous neoplasms: extent of surgical resection. Viszeralmedizin. 2015;31(1):38–42.
13. Tanaka M, Fernández-Del Castillo C, Kamisawa T, et al. Revisions of international consensus Fukuoka guidelines for the management of IPMN of the pancreas. Pancreatology. 2017;17(5):738–53.
14. Sutherland DE, Radosevich DM, Bellin MD, et al. Total pancreatectomy and islet autotransplantation for chronic pancreatitis. J Am Coll Surg. 2012;214(4):409-424; discussion 24–6.
15. Liu X-SWY-B. Total pancreatectomy. In: Liu Y-B, editor. Surgical Atlas of pancreatic cancer. Singapore: Springer Nature Singapore; 2020.
16. Hackert T, Weitz J, Büchler MW. Splenic artery use for arterial reconstruction in pancreatic surgery. Langenbeck's Arch Surg. 2014;399(5):667–71.
17. Del Chiaro M, Segersvärd R, Rangelova E, et al. Cattell-Braasch Maneuver combined with artery-first approach for superior mesenteric-portal vein resection during pancreatectomy. J Gastrointest Surg. 2015;19(12):2264–8.
18. Schmidt CM, Glant J, Winter JM, et al. Total pancreatectomy (R0 resection) improves survival over subtotal pancreatectomy in isolated neck margin positive pancreatic adenocarcinoma. Surgery. 2007;142(4):572–8; discussion 8–80.
19. Sabater L, Muñoz E, Roselló S, et al. Borderline resectable pancreatic cancer. Challenges and controversies. Cancer Treat Rev. 2018;68:124–35.
20. Bockhorn M, Uzunoglu FG, Adham M, et al. Borderline resectable pancreatic cancer: a consensus statement by the International Study Group of Pancreatic Surgery (ISGPS). Surgery. 2014;155(6):977–88.
21. Tempero MA, Malafa MP, Chiorean EG, et al. Pancreatic Adenocarcinoma, Version 12019 Journal of the National Comprehensive Cancer Network: JNCCN. 2019;17(3):202–210.
22. Joo I, Lee JM, Lee ES, et al. Preoperative MDCT assessment of resectability in borderline resectable pancreatic cancer: effect of neoadjuvant chemoradiation therapy. AJR Am J Roentgenol. 2018;210(5):1059–65.
23. Tosolini C, Michalski CW, Kleeff J. Response evaluation following neoadjuvant treatment of pancreatic cancer patients. World J Gastrointest Surg. 2013;5(2):12–5.
24. Kumar R, Herman JM, Wolfgang CL, et al. Multidisciplinary management of pancreatic cancer. Surg Oncol Clin N Am. 2013;22(2):265–87.
25. Shaib WL, Ip A, Cardona K, et al. Contemporary management of borderline resectable and locally advanced unresectable pancreatic cancer. Oncologist. 2016;21(2):178–87.
26. Hackert T, Sachsenmaier M, Hinz U, et al. Locally advanced pancreatic cancer: neoadjuvant therapy with folfirinox results in resectability in 60% of the patients. Ann Surg. 2016;264(3):457–63.
27. Murakami Y, Uemura K, Sudo T, et al. Survival impact of neoadjuvant gemcitabine plus S-1 chemotherapy for patients with borderline resectable pancreatic carcinoma with arterial contact. Cancer Chemother Pharmacol. 2017;79(1):37–47.
28. Hackert T, Strobel O, Michalski CW, et al. The triangle operation – radical surgery after neoadjuvant treatment for advanced pancreatic cancer: a single arm observational study. HPB (Oxford). 2017;19(11):1001–7.
29. Zhai S, Huo Z, Wang Y, et al. Triangle operation for borderline resectable pancreatic cancer in total pancreatectomy. Transl Cancer Res. 2019;8(6):2416–24.
30. Rosso E, Zimmitti G, Iannelli A, et al. The 'triangle operation' by laparoscopy: radical pancreaticoduodenectomy with major vascular resection for borderline resectable pancreatic head cancer. Ann Surg Oncol. 2020;27(5):1613–4.
31. Tempero MA, Malafa MP, Al-Hawary M, et al. Pancreatic Adenocarcinoma, Version 2.2017, NCCN Clinical Practice Guidelines in Oncology. J Natl Compreh Cancer Netw JNCCN. 2017;15(8):1028–1061.
32. Pessaux P, Varma D, Arnaud JP. Pancreaticoduodenectomy: superior mesenteric artery first approach. J Gastrointest Surg. 2006;10(4):607–11.
33. Nakao A. The mesenteric approach in pancreatoduodenectomy. Dig Surg. 2016;33(4):308–13.
34. Wei K, Hackert T. Surgical treatment of pancreatic ductal adenocarcinoma. Cancers 2021;13(8).
35. Hackert T, Weitz J, Büchler MW. Reinsertion of the gastric coronary vein to avoid venous gastric congestion in pancreatic surgery. HPB (Oxford). 2015;17(4):368–70.
36. Fancellu A, Petrucciani N, Porcu A, et al. The impact on survival and morbidity of portal-mesenteric resection during pancreaticoduodenectomy for pancreatic head adenocarcinoma: A systematic review and meta-analysis of comparative studies Cancers 2020;12(7).
37. Xie ZB, Li J, Gu JC, et al. Pancreatoduodenectomy with portal vein resection favors the survival time of patients with pancreatic ductal adenocarcinoma: a propensity score matching analysis. Oncol Lett. 2019;18(5):4563–72.
38. Klaiber U, Mihaljevic A, Hackert T. Radical pancreatic cancer surgery-with arterial resection. Transl Gastroenterol Hepatol. 2019;4:8.
39. Sonohara F, Yamada S, Takami H, et al. Novel implications of combined arterial resection for locally advanced pancreatic

cancer in the era of newer chemo-regimens. Eur J Surg Oncol. 2019;45(10):1895–900.
40. Del Chiaro M, Rangelova E, Halimi A, et al. Pancreatectomy with arterial resection is superior to palliation in patients with borderline resectable or locally advanced pancreatic cancer. HPB (Oxford). 2019;21(2):219–25.
41. Suzuki S, Kajiyama H, Takemura A, et al. The clinical outcomes after total pancreatectomy. Dig Surg. 2017;34(2):142–50.
42. Billings BJ, Christein JD, Harmsen WS, et al. Quality-of-life after total pancreatectomy: is it really that bad on long-term follow-up? J Gastrointest Surg. 2005;9(8):1059-1066; discussion 66–7.

Pancreatic Resection for Solid Pseudopapillary Neoplasms

Wenming Wu, Qiang Xu, and Rui Jiang

Abstract

Pancreatic solid pseudopapillary neoplasms (SPNs) are rare and relatively benign tumors, with a malignancy ratio of 10–15%. The utility of multiple imaging modalities, combining with age and gender profile, is crucial for the diagnosis of SPNs. At present, surgery remains the only curative method for SPNs. While opinions towards surgical procedures are highly divided due to its rarity, minimally invasive procedures for SPNs are gradually recommended, whether extent of resection or surgical path. Although patients with SPNs always have a favorable prognosis, postoperative follow-ups remain essential. In general, we mainly discussed the diagnosis, treatment, and follow-up for patients with SPNs.

Pancreatic solid-pseudopapillary neoplasms (SPNs) are rare, accounting for 1–2% and 5% of pancreatic exocrine neoplasms and pancreatic cystic neoplasms, respectively [1]. SPNs are relatively benign neoplasms with a malignancy rate of 10–15% [2]. The mutation of *CTNNB1*, present in over 90% of cases, is a molecular hallmark of the disease, leading to the activation of Wnt/β-catenin signaling pathway [3, 4]. SPNs are mostly found in younger women [5], with a female to male ratio of 10:1 [6]. The symptoms are not well-defined, but the most common symptom is abdominal discomfort, which is present in over half of patients [7]. In addition, about a third of patients are asymptomatic. There is no significant difference in presentation between men and women [8], nor in symptom and tumor characteristics between children and adults [9, 10].

W. Wu (✉) · Q. Xu · R. Jiang
Department of General Surgery, State Key Laboratory of Complex Severe and Rare Diseases, Peking Union Medical College Hospital, Chinese Academy of Medical Science and Peking Union Medical College, Beijing, China
e-mail: wuwm@pumch.cn

Radiological examinations are important for SPNs diagnosis. Computed tomography (CT) is the most commonly used imaging modality, followed by ultrasound (US) and magnetic resonance imaging (MRI) [7]. The combination of imaging manifestations of US, CT, and MRI is crucial for the diagnosis of SPNs [11]. However, the CT imaging features of SPNs are different between males and females, such as tumor shape and tumor composition. Tumor imaging in male patients always features a solid mass with lobulated margin and progressive enhancement [12]. Compared to symptomatic SPNs, asymptomatic ones have significantly smaller tumor size and may lack the typical features [13, 14]. The characteristic imaging manifestation combined with age and gender profile may be sufficient for most SPNs diagnosis [15]. EUS-guided fine-needle aspiration (FNA) is a accurate diagnosis method with sensitivity and specificity as high as 91% and 94%, respectively. However, the procedure of FNA may entail certain risks, such as hemorrhage, pancreatitis, pancreatic fistula, gastrointestinal perforation, and even tumor cells dissemination [15]. Previous studies recommended that laparoscopic biopsy should be avoided due to the risk of tumor recurrence and peritoneal dissemination [16–18]. In addition to diagnosis, the preoperative imaging workups are helpful for discriminating between potentially malignant and benign tumors to guide clinical treatment options. Previous studies have indicated that preoperative CT imaging may be helpful to discriminate aggressive SPNs from non-aggressive tumors [12]. Incomplete capsule, ill-defined margin, and absence of bleeding feature in CT imaging are risk factors for aggressive SPNs, which could be used to guide the preoperative selection of surgical procedure. In addition to radiographic results, researchers have also found that preoperative neutrophil-to-lymphocyte ratio (NLR) is predictive of malignant SPNs [19].

At present, surgical resection remains the mainstay of treatment for SPNs, which is recommended by the 2017 International Association of Pancreatology (IAP) and the 2018 European Pancreatic Club guidelines [20–22]. The common surgical procedures for SPNs generally include enucleation, segmental pancreatectomy, and pancreaticoduodenectomy, which depend on the location of the tumor [23]. Tumors located in the head or uncinate of the pancreas require enucleation, or pancreaticoduodenectomy with or without pylorus-preserving. For tumors located in the neck or body of the pancreas, surgeons could resect the midportion of the pancreas or perform enucleation. Distal pancreatectomy (DP) with or without splenectomy is often performed for SPNs located in the body or tail of the pancreas [2, 15, 24]. However, there is currently no uniform standard on the selection of surgical procedures. The procedure may be performed either laparoscopically or by open surgery and could be aggressive or function-preserving. The lack of a golden standard is partially due to the rarity of SPNs, and that the current experience is mostly based on the small-scale studies or case reports.

Due to the favorable prognosis and low-grade malignancy of SPNs, pancreatic function and adjacent organ preserving surgery has been proposed by multiple studies [25]. Deficient residual volume of the pancreas is correlated with pancreatic functional deficiency [26]. Previous studies have shown that enucleation could be performed for SPNs located within the head, neck, or body of the pancreas, especially with no indications of dilated pancreatic duct and/or common bile duct [23]. However, opinions regarding such a surgical procedure are highly divided. Some studies maintained that enucleation is indicated for smaller tumors [24], while others considered that it should not be performed because of the increased risk of dissemination, recurrence, and pancreatic fistula [2, 27]. For SPNs in children, enucleation may be a safe and effective surgical procedure if taking tumor size and location into consideration, but it correlates with increased risk of prolonged fasting times and development of pancreatic fistula [28]. Enucleation may be more beneficial for children than adults with SPNs, because it could preserve the exocrine and endocrine functions of the pancreas to the greatest extent. However, because age < 13.5 is associated with a higher risk of recurrence [29], surgeons should balance the benefits and risks of enucleation. Whether enucleation should be performed on patients with SPNs and the selection of patients for enucleation require future researches.

Patients undergoing Whipple's procedure experience significantly longer postoperative hospitalization and increased unadjusted mortality than segmental pancreatectomy, while with no significant difference in postoperative complication rates [30]. Compared to conventional DP, spleen-preserving distal pancreatectomy (SPDP) may reduce the risk of overwhelming post-splenectomy infection, without increasing the complication rate and prolonging postoperative hospitalization [31, 32]. It appears that function or organs preserving surgery is superior to invasive surgery. The function or organ preserving surgery could preserve the function of digestive system, pancreas, or spleen to a large extent, which is crucial for the life quality of patients, especially for younger ones. However, some studies have indicated that parenchyma-preserving surgical procedure is associated with an increased risk for postoperative recurrence due to the incomplete resection [33].

When it comes to the surgical path, laparoscopic surgery is recently becoming more prevalent with the improvement of surgical techniques. Shorter time to diet and postoperative hospitalization, lower intraoperative blood loss and transfusion requirement, and lower complication rates have been previously observed in minimally invasive pancreatectomy (MIP) for SPNs than open groups [34, 35]. However, laparoscopic management may be correlated with a higher risk of local or disseminated recurrence than open laparotomy [36].

There is a growing body of literature that recommends function-preserving and laparoscopic surgery for SPNs due to low-grade malignancy, but routine lymphadenectomy is not indicated because of the rarity of metastasis [15]. However, patients with preoperative imaging workups or histopathological examination showing high-grade malignancy, such as locally advanced tumors or distant metastasis, require more aggressive surgical procedures [37, 38]. For instance, patients with portal-superior mesenteric vein (PV/SMV) and/or adjacent organ involvement, who underwent en bloc primary tumor excision with synchronous PV/SMV and/or adjacent organ resection could obtain a good prognosis [39]. The principle of surgical management for patients with distant metastasis is to resect both the primary and metastatic tumors as completely as possible [40]. But for patients with unresectable tumors of SPNs, adjuvant radiation, chemotherapy, vascular resection and reconstruction, and liver transplantation may be acceptable options, but the evidence level is relatively low [41–44].

Although patients with SPNs always have a favorable prognosis, with the 5-year survival rate of more than 95% [15, 45], postoperative follow-ups remain essential. The majority of recurrences or metastases occur within 5 years after surgery. However, in a small but significant number of patients, recurrence or metastasis has been seen between 5 and 10 years. Long-term follow-ups are needed to examine the outcome of surgery for patients with SPNs. About 2% of patients who underwent surgical resection experience recurrence after surgery [46]. Over the last decades, the factors suggesting malignant potential of SPNs have been broadly explored, which could predict surgical outcome and guide postoperative follow-ups. Extensive researches have shown that tumor size and microscopic malignant features are significant prognostic factors for postoperative recurrence [47–49]. Besides, multiple large-scale studies have demonstrated that blood vessel invasion and larger tumor size may be associated with high-grade malignancy [48, 50, 51]. However, previous studies have shown differences in predictive ability and cut-off value of tumor size to predict recurrence [52, 53]. Recently, Yang et al. have shown that the combination of Ki-67 and tumor size is helpful to predict postoperative recurrence, superior to the current American Joint Committee on Cancer (AJCC) and European Neuroendocrine Tumor Society (ENETS) staging systems [54]. Negative surgical margins are essential to avoid recurrence, and the intraoperative frozen section could be used for validation [55, 56]. On the other hand, a meta-analysis study that summarized the studies analyzing the relationships between clinicopathological factors and SPNs malignancy has found no reliable factor [57]. In addition to the clinicopathological characteristics, Cohen et al. analyzed the miRNA patterns among normal pancreas, primary tumors, and metastatic tumors through miRNA array. They found that lower expression of miR-375, miR-217, and miR-200c and higher expression of miR-184, miR-10a, and miR-887 are associated with metastasis [58]. However, even if patients relapsed at follow-up, reoperation could still result in long-term survival [24].

We herein summarize the diagnosis, treatment, and postoperative follow-up for patients with SPNs. Yet, the current literature regarding SPNs mostly come from case reports and studies by an isolated center with low levels of evidence. Regardless, minimally invasive procedures are increasingly being recommended for the treatment of SPNs, not only for the extent of resection but also as surgical path. Meanwhile, future studies should establish methods for more accurate preoperative diagnosis and malignant markers. Large-scale multicenter studies are urgently needed to verify and update the current understanding of SPNs.

References

1. Klöppel G, Basturk O, Klimstra D, Lam A, Notohara K. Solid pseudopapillary neoplasm of the pancreas. In: Carneiro Fatima CJ, NYA C, et al., editors. Digestive system tumours, vol. 1. 5th ed. Lyon: IARC Press; 2019. p. 340–2.
2. Naar L, Spanomichou DA, Mastoraki A, Smyrniotis V, Arkadopoulos N. Solid pseudopapillary neoplasms of the pancreas: a surgical and genetic enigma. World J Surg. 2017;41(7):1871–81.
3. Springer S, Wang Y, Dal Molin M, et al. A combination of molecular markers and clinical features improve the classification of pancreatic cysts. Gastroenterology. 2015;149(6):1501–10.
4. Audard V, Cavard C, Richa H, et al. Impaired E-cadherin expression and glutamine synthetase overexpression in solid pseudopapillary neoplasm of the pancreas. Pancreas. 2008;36(1):80–3.
5. Stark A, Donahue TR, Reber HA, Hines OJ. Pancreatic cyst disease: a review. JAMA. 2016;315(17):1882–93.
6. Papavramidis T, Papavramidis S. Solid pseudopapillary tumors of the pancreas: review of 718 patients reported in English literature. J Am Coll Surg. 2005;200(6):965–72.
7. Law JK, Ahmed A, Singh VK, et al. A systematic review of solid-pseudopapillary neoplasms: are these rare lesions? Pancreas. 2014;43(3):331–7.
8. Wang P, Wei J, Wu J, et al. Diagnosis and treatment of solid-pseudopapillary tumors of the pancreas: a single institution experience with 97 cases. Pancreatology. 2018;18(4):415–9.
9. Leraas HJ, Kim J, Sun Z, et al. Solid pseudopapillary neoplasm of the pancreas in children and adults: a national study of 369 patients. J Pediatr Hematol Oncol. 2018;40(4):e233–6.
10. Waters AM, Russell RT, Maizlin, II, Group C, Beierle EA. Comparison of pediatric and adult solid pseudopapillary neoplasms of the pancreas. J Surg Res. 2019;242:312–317.
11. Cheng DF, Peng CH, Zhou GW, et al. Clinical misdiagnosis of solid pseudopapillary tumour of pancreas. Chin Med J. 2005;118(11):922–6.
12. Park MJ, Lee JH, Kim JK, et al. Multidetector CT imaging features of solid pseudopapillary tumours of the pancreas in male patients: distinctive imaging features with female patients. Br J Radiol. 2014;87(1035):20130513.
13. Hu S, Zhang H, Wang X, et al. Asymptomatic versus symptomatic solid pseudopapillary tumors of the pancreas: clinical and MDCT manifestations. Cancer Imaging. 2019;19(1):13.
14. Inoue T, Nishi Y, Okumura F, et al. Solid pseudopapillary neoplasm of the pancreas associated with familial adenomatous polyposis. Intern Med. 2015;54(11):1349–55.
15. Yang F, Fu DL, Jin C, et al. Clinical experiences of solid pseudopapillary tumors of the pancreas in China. J Gastroenterol Hepatol. 2008;23(12):1847–51.
16. Petrosyan M, Franklin AL, Jackson HT, McGue S, Reyes CA, Kane TD. Solid pancreatic pseudopapillary tumor managed laparoscopically in adolescents: a case series and review of the literature. J Laparoendosc Adv Surg Tech A. 2014;24(6):440–4.
17. Butte JM, Brennan MF, Gonen M, et al. Solid pseudopapillary tumors of the pancreas. Clinical features, surgical outcomes, and long-term survival in 45 consecutive patients from a single center. J Gastrointest Surg. 2011;15(2):350–7.
18. Cavallini A, Butturini G, Daskalaki D, et al. Laparoscopic pancreatectomy for solid pseudo-papillary tumors of the pancreas is a suitable technique; our experience with long-term follow-up and review of the literature. Ann Surg Oncol. 2011;18(2):352–7.
19. Yang F, Bao Y, Zhou Z, Jin C, Fu D. Preoperative neutrophil-to-lymphocyte ratio predicts malignancy and recurrence-free survival of solid pseudopapillary tumor of the pancreas. J Surg Oncol. 2019;120(2):241–8.
20. van Huijgevoort NCM, Del Chiaro M, Wolfgang CL, van Hooft JE, Besselink MG. Diagnosis and management of pancreatic cystic neoplasms: current evidence and guidelines. Nat Rev Gastroenterol Hepatol. 2019;16(11):676–89.
21. Vege SS, Ziring B, Jain R, Moayyedi P, Committee CG, Association AG. American gastroenterological association institute guideline on the diagnosis and management of asymptomatic neoplastic pancreatic cysts. Gastroenterology. 2015;148(4):819–822; quize812–813.
22. Pancreas ESGoCTot. European evidence-based guidelines on pancreatic cystic neoplasms. Gut. 2018;67(5):789–804.
23. Chang H, Gong Y, Xu J, Su Z, Qin C, Zhang Z. Clinical strategy for the management of solid pseudopapillary tumor of the pancreas: aggressive or less? Int J Med Sci. 2010;7(5):309–13.
24. Cai Y, Ran X, Xie S, et al. Surgical management and long-term follow-up of solid pseudopapillary tumor of pancreas: a large series from a single institution. J Gastrointest Surg. 2014;18(5):935–40.
25. Liu M, Liu J, Hu Q, et al. Management of solid pseudopapillary neoplasms of pancreas: a single center experience of 243 consecutive patients. Pancreatology. 2019;19(5):681–5.
26. DiNorcia J, Ahmed L, Lee MK, et al. Better preservation of endocrine function after central versus distal pancreatectomy for mid-gland lesions. Surgery. 2010;148(6):1247–1254; discussion 1254–1246.

27. Vassos N, Agaimy A, Klein P, Hohenberger W, Croner RS. Solid-pseudopapillary neoplasm (SPN) of the pancreas: case series and literature review on an enigmatic entity. Int J Clin Exp Pathol. 2013;6(6):1051–9.
28. Cho YJ, Namgoong JM, Kim DY, Kim SC, Kwon HH. Suggested indications for enucleation of solid pseudopapillary neoplasms in pediatric patients. Front Pediatr. 2019;7:125.
29. Irtan S, Galmiche-Rolland L, Elie C, et al. Recurrence of solid pseudopapillary neoplasms of the pancreas: results of a nationwide study of risk factors and treatment modalities. Pediatr Blood Cancer. 2016;63(9):1515–21.
30. Manuballa V, Amin M, Cappell MS. Clinical presentation and comparison of surgical outcome for segmental resection vs. Whipple's procedure for solid pseudopapillary tumor: Report of six new cases & literature review of 321 cases. Pancreatology. 2014;14(1):71–80.
31. Lee SE, Jang JY, Lee KU, Kim SW. Clinical comparison of distal pancreatectomy with or without splenectomy. J Korean Med Sci. 2008;23(6):1011–4.
32. He Z, Qian D, Hua J, Gong J, Lin S, Song Z. Clinical comparison of distal pancreatectomy with or without splenectomy: a meta-analysis. PLoS One. 2014;9(3):e91593.
33. Tjaden C, Hassenpflug M, Hinz U, et al. Outcome and prognosis after pancreatectomy in patients with solid pseudopapillary neoplasms. Pancreatology. 2019;19(5):699–709.
34. Hao EIU, Rho SY, Hwang HK, et al. Surgical approach to solid pseudopapillary neoplasms of the proximal pancreas: minimally invasive vs. open. World J Surg Oncol. 2019;17(1):160.
35. Tan HL, Syn N, Goh BKP. Systematic review and meta-analysis of minimally invasive pancreatectomies for solid pseudopapillary neoplasms of the pancreas. Pancreas. 2019;48(10):1334–42.
36. Fais PO, Carricaburu E, Sarnacki S, et al. Is laparoscopic management suitable for solid pseudo-papillary tumors of the pancreas? Pediatr Surg Int. 2009;25(7):617–21.
37. Kumar NAN, Bhandare MS, Chaudhari V, Sasi SP, Shrikhande SV. Analysis of 50 cases of solid pseudopapillary tumor of pancreas: aggressive surgical resection provides excellent outcomes. Eur J Surg Oncol. 2019;45(2):187–91.
38. Kim CW, Han DJ, Kim J, Kim YH, Park JB, Kim SC. Solid pseudopapillary tumor of the pancreas: can malignancy be predicted? Surgery. 2011;149(5):625–34.
39. Cheng K, Shen B, Peng C, Yuan F, Yin Q. Synchronous portal-superior mesenteric vein or adjacent organ resection for solid pseudopapillary neoplasms of the pancreas: a single-institution experience. Am Surg. 2013;79(5):534–9.
40. Wang WB, Zhang TP, Sun MQ, Peng Z, Chen G, Zhao YP. Solid pseudopapillary tumor of the pancreas with liver metastasis: clinical features and management. Eur J Surg Oncol. 2014;40(11):1572–7.
41. Sperti C, Berselli M, Pasquali C, Pastorelli D, Pedrazzoli S. Aggressive behaviour of solid-pseudopapillary tumor of the pancreas in adults: a case report and review of the literature. World J Gastroenterol. 2008;14(6):960–5.
42. Sumida W, Kaneko K, Tainaka T, Ono Y, Kiuchi T, Ando H. Liver transplantation for multiple liver metastases from solid pseudopapillary tumor of the pancreas. J Pediatr Surg. 2007;42(12):e27–31.
43. Ward HC, Leake J, Spitz L. Papillary cystic cancer of the pancreas: diagnostic difficulties. J Pediatr Surg. 1993;28(1):89–91.
44. Maffuz A, Bustamante Fde T, Silva JA, Torres-Vargas S. Preoperative gemcitabine for unresectable, solid pseudopapillary tumour of the pancreas. Lancet Oncol. 2005;6(3):185–6.
45. Yu PF, Hu ZH, Wang XB, et al. Solid pseudopapillary tumor of the pancreas: a review of 553 cases in Chinese literature. World J Gastroenterol. 2010;16(10):1209–14.
46. Yepuri N, Naous R, Meier AH, et al. A systematic review and meta-analysis of predictors of recurrence in patients with Solid Pseudopapillary Tumors of the Pancreas. HPB (Oxford). 2020;22(1):12–9.
47. Kang CM, Choi SH, Kim SC, et al. Predicting recurrence of pancreatic solid pseudopapillary tumors after surgical resection: a multicenter analysis in Korea. Ann Surg. 2014;260(2):348–55.
48. Kim MJ, Choi DW, Choi SH, Heo JS, Sung JY. Surgical treatment of solid pseudopapillary neoplasms of the pancreas and risk factors for malignancy. Br J Surg. 2014;101(10):1266–71.
49. Gao H, Gao Y, Yin L, et al. Risk factors of the recurrences of pancreatic solid pseudopapillary tumors: a systematic review and meta-analysis. J Cancer. 2018;9(11):1905–14.
50. Wu JH, Tian XY, Liu BN, Li CP, Zhao M, Hao CY. Clinicopathological features and prognostic factors of solid pseudopapillary neoplasms of pancreas. Pak J Pharm Sci. 2019;32(1(Special)):459–64.
51. Estrella JS, Li L, Rashid A, et al. Solid pseudopapillary neoplasm of the pancreas: clinicopathologic and survival analyses of 64 cases from a single institution. Am J Surg Pathol. 2014;38(2):147–57.
52. Kang CM, Kim KS, Choi JS, Kim H, Lee WJ, Kim BR. Solid pseudopapillary tumor of the pancreas suggesting malignant potential. Pancreas. 2006;32(3):276–80.
53. Machado MC, Machado MA, Bacchella T, Jukemura J, Almeida JL, Cunha JE. Solid pseudopapillary neoplasm of the pancreas: distinct patterns of onset, diagnosis, and prognosis for male versus female patients. Surgery. 2008;143(1):29–34.
54. Yang F, Wu W, Wang X, et al. Grading solid pseudopapillary tumors of the pancreas: the Fudan prognostic index. Ann Surg Oncol. 2020.
55. Canzonieri V, Berretta M, Buonadonna A, et al. Solid pseudopapillary tumour of the pancreas. Lancet Oncol. 2003;4(4):255–6.
56. Ng KH, Tan PH, Thng CH, Ooi LL. Solid pseudopapillary tumour of the pancreas. ANZ J Surg. 2003;73(6):410–5.
57. You L, Yang F, Fu DL. Prediction of malignancy and adverse outcome of solid pseudopapillary tumor of the pancreas. World J Gastrointest Oncol. 2018;10(7):184–93.
58. Cohen SJ, Papoulas M, Graubardt N, et al. Micro-RNA expression patterns predict metastatic spread in solid pseudopapillary neoplasms of the pancreas. Front Oncol. 2020;10:328.

Pancreatic Resection for Neuroendocrine Neoplasms of the Pancreas

Yosuke Kasai, Toshihiko Masui, Kyoichi Takaori, Kenji Yoshino, and Eric K. Nakakura

Abstract

Pancreatic resection is the mainstay treatment of pancreatic neuroendocrine neoplasm (PNEN) for curative intent or symptom control. In this chapter, we describe the indication of pancreatic resection for PNENs and procedures based on the need for systematic lymph node dissection (LND). Recent guidelines accept initial observation for incidentally discovered small non-functional PNEN (NF-PNEN) without malignant signs. Otherwise, formal pancreatic resection with systematic LND is recommended (pancreatoduodenectomy for head/uncinate tumor and distal pancreatectomy for body/tail tumor). For hormone-secreting functional PNENs, pancreatic resection is generally recommended because hormonal symptoms severely impair the patients' quality of life. Tumor enucleation without systematic LND can be indicated for insulinoma, whereas formal pancreatectomy with systematic LND is recommended for gastrinoma. When systematic LND is omitted, sampling peritumoral lymph nodes should be performed for accurate staging. In the setting of unresectable distant metastasis, the significance of resection of the primary tumor has been controversial. For patients with resectable pancreatic head tumor and liver metastasis, staged operation of liver metastasectomy followed by pancreatoduodenectomy is recommended to avoid biliary infection after bilioenteric anastomosis. Survival benefit of resection of poorly-differentiated pancreatic neuroendocrine carcinoma has not been demonstrated due to the extremely poor prognosis.

Y. Kasai (✉)
Department of Surgery, Nagahama City Hospital, Nagahama, Shiga, Japan

Department of Surgery, Graduate School of Medicine, Kyoto University, Kyoto, Japan

Department of Surgery, University of California, San Francisco, CA, USA
e-mail: yokasai@kuhp.kyoto-u.ac.jp

T. Masui
Department of Surgery, Graduate School of Medicine, Kyoto University, Kyoto, Japan

K. Takaori
Department of Surgery, Nagahama City Hospital, Nagahama, Shiga, Japan

Department of Surgery, Graduate School of Medicine, Kyoto University, Kyoto, Japan

K. Yoshino
Department of Surgery, Nagahama City Hospital, Nagahama, Shiga, Japan

Department of Surgery, Graduate School of Medicine, Kyoto University, Kyoto, Japan

E. K. Nakakura
Department of Surgery, University of California, San Francisco, CA, USA

Abbreviations

CP	central pancreatectomy
DP	distal pancreatectomy
ENETS	European Neuroendocrine Tumor Society
EUS-FNA	endoscopic ultrasound-guided fine needle aspiration
LND	lymph node dissection
LNM	lymph node metastasis
MEN1	multiple endocrine neoplasia type 1
MPD	main pancreatic duct
NANETS	North American Neuroendocrine Tumor Society
NCCN	National Comprehensive Cancer Network
NF-PNEN	non-functional pancreatic neuroendocrine neoplasm
PD	pancreatoduodenectomy
PNEC	pancreatic neuroendocrine carcinoma
PNEN	pancreatic neuroendocrine neoplasm
PNET	pancreatic neuroendocrine tumor
SASI	selective arterial secretagogue injection
SPDP	spleen-preserving distal pancreatectomy
WHO	World Health Organization

52.1 Introduction

Pancreatic neuroendocrine neoplasm (PNEN) accounts for 3% of malignancies arising in the pancreas [1]. The incidence has increased four folds over the past two decades, with an age-adjusted annual incidence of 0.8 per 100,000 population in the United States [2]. Although most PNENs behave benignly compared to pancreatic ductal adenocarcinoma, the prognosis of patients with metastatic or high-grade PNEN is poor [2]. Pancreatic resection is the mainstay treatment of PNENs for curative intent or symptom control. The operative indication and procedure depend on various factors, including the tumor size, World Health Organization (WHO) grade [3], tumor location, functionality, inherited syndrome, and the presence or absence of metastasis.

In this chapter, we describe the indication of pancreatic resection for PNENs and procedures based on the need for systematic lymph node dissection (LND).

52.2 Indication of Pancreatic Resection for PNENs

52.2.1 Non-Functional PNEN (NF-PNEN)

For patients with NF-PNEN, the tumor is not accompanied by hormonal symptoms, accounting for 60–90% of all PNENs [4, 5]. The incidental discovery of small NF-PNENs is increasing due to improvements in diagnostic modalities. Because such NF-PNENs usually exhibit indolent phenotypes [6], guidelines of the National Comprehensive Cancer Network (NCCN), the European Neuroendocrine Tumor Society (ENETS), and the North American Neuroendocrine Tumor Society (NANETS) accept initial observation for patients with small NF-PNEN (≤2 cm for NCCN and ENETS, and <1 cm for NANETS guidelines) under certain conditions [7–9]. Although endoscopic ultrasound-guided fine needle aspiration (EUS-FNA) is a useful tool for the diagnosis of PNEN, grading by EUS-FNA is underestimated in 20–30% of cases due to intratumor heterogeneity [10, 11]. Therefore, radiological signs of malignancy, as shown in Table 52.1, should be carefully evaluated to determine resection versus observation. Any finding suggesting malignancy should direct patients toward pancreatic resection. Figure 52.1 summarizes the indication of pancreatic resection for NF-PNEN.

52.2.2 Functional PNEN

Functional PNENs are hormone-secreting tumors, including insulinoma, gastrinoma, glucagonoma, and VIPoma.

Table 52.1 Reported radiological signs of malignancy

Radiological factors
Tumor size >4 cm [12]
Tumor size >2 cm [13, 14]
Tumor size >1.5 cm [15–17]
Tumor size (continuous) [18, 19]
Absence of early enhancement [20]
Calcification [18]
MPD involvement/dilatation [21, 22]
Lymphadenopathy [12]
^aCystic component [23–25]

^aCystic component has been reported as a benign sign

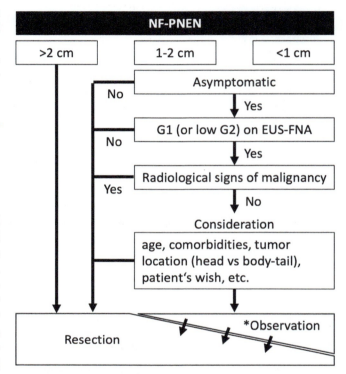

Fig. 52.1 Indication of pancreatic resection for NF-PNEN based on the recommendations of NCCN, ENETS, and NANETS guidelines [7–9]. *Patients should be followed up every 6–12 months. If the tumor progresses over time, patients should proceed to operation

Because hormonal symptoms severely impair the patients' quality of life, resection of functional PNENs is generally recommended [7–9]. Some functional PNENs are too small to be detected on conventional imaging modalities. The selective arterial secretagogue injection (SASI) test has been used to identify the feeding artery and localize functional tumors [26]. Somatostatin receptor imaging (^{68}Ga DOTA TATE or DOTA TOC positron emission tomography/computed tomography) is highly sensitive for detecting PNENs, including insulinoma [27, 28]. Although most PNENs are sporadic and solitary, nearly 10% of insulinomas and 20% of gastrinomas are associated with inherited syndrome, including multiple endocrine neoplasia type 1 (MEN1), and most of them are multiple [29]. In such cases, all lesions do not need to be resected, but excising only the dominant lesions >2 cm and those responsible for the hormone secretion based on SASI test is enough [8, 9].

52.2.3 PNEN with Distant Metastasis

Curative or even debulking resection of neuroendocrine liver metastasis provides favorable long-term outcomes in select cases, with a 5-year survival rate of 70–80% [30–33]. Therefore, candidates for metastasectomy should benefit from resection of the primary tumor. For patients with resectable pancreatic head tumor and liver metastasis, staged operation of liver metastasectomy followed by pancreatoduodenectomy (PD) is recommended to reduce the risk of biliary infection and liver abscess after bilioenteric anastomosis [7, 34]. In the setting of unresectable distant metastasis, several registry-based studies showed that resection of the primary tumor was associated with prolonged survival compared to non-surgical management [35, 36]. However, these studies had potential selection biases, including metastatic tumor burden and patients' comorbidities of which the registry does not cover the data [9]. Therefore, it is inconclusive whether resection of the primary tumor is truly beneficial in the setting of unresectable distant metastasis. For functional PNEN with distant metastasis, resection of the primary tumor with or without debulking metastasectomy may be beneficial for symptom control, if evidence suggests that the primary tumor is responsible for hormone secretion.

52.2.4 High-grade PNEN

In the WHO Classification 2017, high-grade PNENs (G3: Ki-67 index >20% and/or >20 mitoses/10 high-power fields) were reclassified to well-differentiated pancreatic neuroendocrine tumor (PNET) and poorly-differentiated pancreatic neuroendocrine carcinoma (PNEC) based on the histological morphology [3]. PNET-G3 is completely different from PNEC in the genetic backgrounds (*MEN1*, *ATRX*, and *DAXX* mutations versus *TP53*, *RB*, and *KRAS* mutations) [37], response to platinum-based regimens (low versus high) [38], and the prognosis (years versus months) [39]. Based on these points, locoregional PNET-G3 is indicated for pancreatic resection as well as PNET-G1/2, whereas survival benefit of resection for PNEC is yet to be determined due to the extremely poor prognosis [9].

52.3 Procedures Based on the Need for Systematic LND

Lymph node metastasis (LNM) is present in 18–39% of patients with PNENs without distant metastasis [40–42]. Prognostic significance of LNM and regional LND is controversial for PNEN [15, 40–43], possibly because the indication and extent of LND have not been unified. The site and frequency of LNM by the location of the primary tumor, reported by Izumo, et al. [44], are described in Fig. 52.2, which guides the regions of lymph nodes to be dissected systematically for accurate staging and R0 resection. Based on this finding, the standard procedure for PNEN should be PD

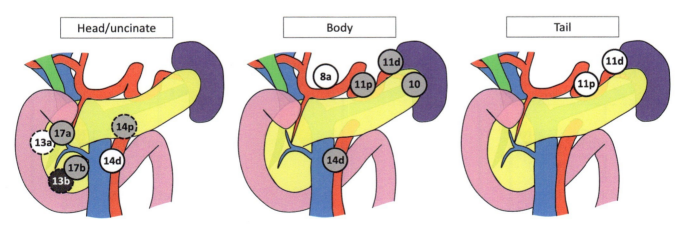

Fig. 52.2 Site and frequency of lymph node metastasis by the location of the primary tumor. The proportion of patients with metastasis in each lymph node to those who had the lymph node dissected was classified to ≥20% (thick grey circle), 10–20% (thin grey circle), and 0%<, <10% (white circle): data referenced from the report by Izumo, et al. [44] Nodes with dotted line represent those located on the posterior surface of the pancreas. The lymph node numbers are in accordance with the Classification of Pancreatic Carcinoma by Japan Pancreas Society [45]

for head/uncinate tumors and distal pancreatectomy (DP) with splenectomy for body/tail tumors.

The risk of LNM varies depending on tumor size [16, 40], functionality (non-functional vs gastrinoma vs insulinoma) [46, 47], and WHO grade [12, 48]. Patients at low risk of LNM can be offered a limited resection [enucleation, partial pancreatectomy, or central pancreatectomy (CP)] without systematic LND to preserve pancreatic endocrine and exocrine function [9, 49]. In NF-PNEN, the candidates for observation (≤2 cm, G1, and no radiological signs of malignancy) are at low risk of LNM, and limited resection without systematic LND may be considered, especially for head/uncinate tumors [7]. Most insulinomas are benign, so enucleation without LND is sufficient, unless the tumor is proximal to the main pancreatic duct (MPD) or there is a sign of local invasion [7, 8]. A spleen-preserving distal pancreatectomy (SPDP) should be considered for patients with body/tail insulinoma in whom enucleation is not feasible due to involvement of the MPD. In contrast, gastrinoma is generally malignant with an LNM rate of >40%, and systematic LND should be performed [7–9, 47, 50]. Nevertheless, enucleation remains optional for head/uncinate gastrinoma away from the MPD as an alternative to PD. [7] Even if systematic LND can be omitted, sampling peritumoral lymph nodes is required for staging. Procedures of pancreatic resection for sporadic PNENs are summarized in Fig. 52.3. For experienced surgeons at high-volume centers, a laparoscopic approach may be consid-

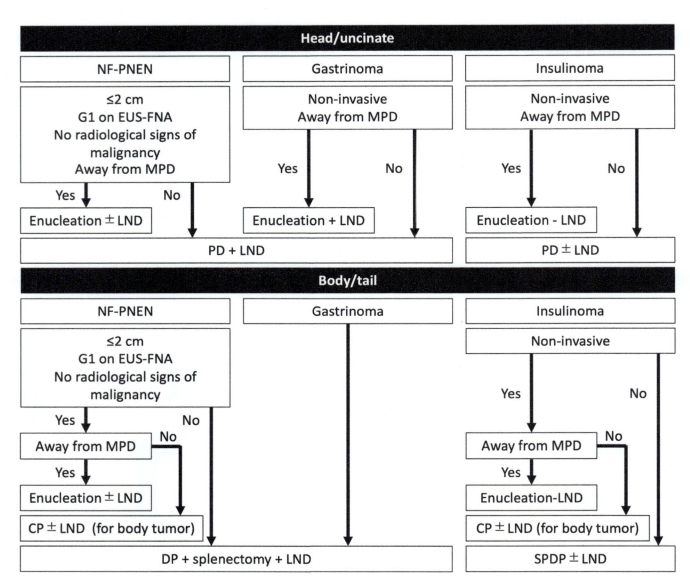

Fig. 52.3 Procedures of pancreatic resection for sporadic PNENs based on the recommendations of NCCN, ENETS, and NANETS guidelines [7–9]

ered for resection of insulinoma and DP for PNENs without signs of local invasion [7, 9].

52.4 Conclusions

Indication and procedures of pancreatic resection for PNENs are determined by tumor size, tumor location, functionality, inherited syndrome, malignant potential, and the presence or absence of metastasis. Systematic LND or sampling peritumoral lymph nodes according to the risk of LNM is required for accurate staging and R0 resection.

Conflict of interest None.

References

1. Fesinmeyer MD, Austin MA, Li CI, De Roos AJ, Bowen DJ. Differences in survival by histologic type of pancreatic cancer. Cancer Epidemiol Biomark Prev. 2005 Jul;14(7):1766–73. https://doi.org/10.1158/1055-9965.EPI-05-0120.
2. Dasari A, Shen C, Halperin D, et al. Trends in the incidence, prevalence, and survival outcomes in patients with neuroendocrine tumors in the United States. JAMA Oncol. 2017;3(10):1335–42. https://doi.org/10.1001/jamaoncol.2017.0589.
3. Lloyd R, Osamura R, Klöppel G, Rosai J. Neoplasms of the neuroendocrine pancreas. *WHO classification of tumours of endocrine organs*. 4th ed. IARC Press; 2017:209–240: Chap 6.
4. Halfdanarson TR, Rabe KG, Rubin J, Petersen GM. Pancreatic neuroendocrine tumors (PNETs): incidence, prognosis and recent trend toward improved survival. Ann Oncol. 2008;19(10):1727–33. https://doi.org/10.1093/annonc/mdn351.
5. Ito T, Igarashi H, Nakamura K, et al. Epidemiological trends of pancreatic and gastrointestinal neuroendocrine tumors in Japan: a nationwide survey analysis. J Gastroenterol. 2015;50(1):58–64. https://doi.org/10.1007/s00535-014-0934-2.
6. Sadot E, Reidy-Lagunes DL, Tang LH, et al. Observation versus resection for small asymptomatic pancreatic neuroendocrine tumors: a matched case-control study. Ann Surg Oncol. 2016;23(4):1361–70. https://doi.org/10.1245/s10434-015-4986-1.
7. NCCN Clinical Practice Guidelines in Oncology. Neuroendocrine and adrenal tumors. Ver 2.2020. https://www.nccn.org
8. Falconi M, Eriksson B, Kaltsas G, et al. ENETS consensus guidelines update for the management of patients with functional pancreatic neuroendocrine tumors and non-functional pancreatic neuroendocrine tumors. Neuroendocrinology. 2016;103(2):153–71. https://doi.org/10.1159/000443171.
9. Howe JR, Merchant NB, Conrad C, et al. The North American neuroendocrine tumor society consensus paper on the surgical management of pancreatic neuroendocrine tumors. Pancreas. 2020;49(1):1–33. https://doi.org/10.1097/MPA.0000000000001454.
10. Hasegawa T, Yamao K, Hijioka S, et al. Evaluation of Ki-67 index in EUS-FNA specimens for the assessment of malignancy risk in pancreatic neuroendocrine tumors. Endoscopy. 2014;46(1):32–8. https://doi.org/10.1055/s-0033-1344958.
11. Boutsen L, Jouret-Mourin A, Borbath I, van Maanen A, Weynand B. Accuracy of pancreatic neuroendocrine tumour grading by endoscopic ultrasound-guided fine needle aspiration: analysis of a large cohort and perspectives for improvement. Neuroendocrinology. 2018;106(2):158–66. https://doi.org/10.1159/000477213.
12. Partelli S, Gaujoux S, Boninsegna L, et al. Pattern and clinical predictors of lymph node involvement in nonfunctioning pancreatic neuroendocrine tumors (NF-PanNETs). JAMA Surg. 2013;148(10):932–9. https://doi.org/10.1001/jamasurg.2013.3376.
13. Bettini R, Partelli S, Boninsegna L, et al. Tumor size correlates with malignancy in nonfunctioning pancreatic endocrine tumor. Surgery. 2011;150(1):75–82. https://doi.org/10.1016/j.surg.2011.02.022.
14. Postlewait LM, Ethun CG, Baptiste GG, et al. Pancreatic neuroendocrine tumors: preoperative factors that predict lymph node metastases to guide operative strategy. J Surg Oncol. 2016;114(4):440–5. https://doi.org/10.1002/jso.24338.
15. Hashim YM, Trinkaus KM, Linehan DC, et al. Regional lymphadenectomy is indicated in the surgical treatment of pancreatic neuroendocrine tumors (PNETs). Ann Surg. 2014;259(2):197–203. https://doi.org/10.1097/SLA.0000000000000348.
16. Dong DH, Zhang XF, Poultsides G, et al. Impact of tumor size and nodal status on recurrence of nonfunctional pancreatic neuroendocrine tumors ≤2 cm after curative resection: a multi-institutional study of 392 cases. J Surg Oncol. 2019;120(7):1071–9. https://doi.org/10.1002/jso.25716.
17. Kishi Y, Shimada K, Nara S, Esaki M, Hiraoka N, Kosuge T. Basing treatment strategy for non-functional pancreatic neuroendocrine tumors on tumor size. Ann Surg Oncol. 2014;21(9):2882–8. https://doi.org/10.1245/s10434-014-3701-y.
18. Poultsides GA, Huang LC, Chen Y, et al. Pancreatic neuroendocrine tumors: radiographic calcifications correlate with grade and metastasis. Ann Surg Oncol. 2012;19(7):2295–303. https://doi.org/10.1245/s10434-012-2305-7.
19. Pulvirenti A, Javed AA, Landoni L, et al. Multi-institutional development and external validation of a nomogram to predict recurrence after curative resection of pancreatic neuroendocrine tumors. Ann Surg. 2019; https://doi.org/10.1097/SLA.0000000000003579.
20. Mizumoto T, Toyama H, Terai S, et al. Prediction of lymph node metastasis in pancreatic neuroendocrine tumors by contrast enhancement characteristics. Pancreatology. 2017 Nov–Dec 2017;17(6):956–961. https://doi.org/10.1016/j.pan.2017.08.003.
21. Nanno Y, Matsumoto I, Zen Y, et al. Pancreatic duct involvement in well-differentiated neuroendocrine tumors is an independent poor prognostic factor. Ann Surg Oncol. 2017;24(4):1127–33. https://doi.org/10.1245/s10434-016-5663-8.
22. Zhou B, Zhan C, Xiang J, Ding Y, Yan S. Clinical significance of the preoperative main pancreatic duct dilation and neutrophil-to-lymphocyte ratio in pancreatic neuroendocrine tumors (PNETs) of the head after curative resection. BMC Endocr Disord. 2019;19(1):123. https://doi.org/10.1186/s12902-019-0454-4.
23. Singhi AD, Chu LC, Tatsas AD, et al. Cystic pancreatic neuroendocrine tumors: a clinicopathologic study. Am J Surg Pathol. 2012;36(11):1666–73. https://doi.org/10.1097/PAS.0b013e31826a0048.
24. Koh YX, Chok AY, Zheng HL, Tan CS, Goh BK. A systematic review and meta-analysis of the clinicopathologic characteristics of cystic versus solid pancreatic neuroendocrine neoplasms. Surgery. 2014;156(1):83–96.e2. https://doi.org/10.1016/j.surg.2014.03.026.
25. Cloyd JM, Kopecky KE, Norton JA, et al. Neuroendocrine tumors of the pancreas: degree of cystic component predicts prognosis. Surgery. 09 2016;160(3):708–13. https://doi.org/10.1016/j.surg.2016.04.005.
26. Imamura M, Takahashi K, Adachi H, et al. Usefulness of selective arterial secretin injection test for localization of gastrinoma in the Zollinger-Ellison syndrome. Ann Surg. 1987;205(3):230–9. https://doi.org/10.1097/00000658-198703000-00003.
27. Sadowski SM, Neychev V, Millo C, et al. Prospective study of 68Ga-DOTATATE positron emission tomography/computed

28. Nockel P, Babic B, Millo C, et al. Localization of insulinoma using 68Ga-DOTATATE PET/CT Scan. J Clin Endocrinol Metab. 01 2017;102(1):195–199. https://doi.org/10.1210/jc.2016-3445.
29. Krampitz GW, Norton JA. Pancreatic neuroendocrine tumors. Curr Probl Surg. 2013;50(11):509–45. https://doi.org/10.1067/j.cpsurg.2013.08.001.
30. Mayo SC, de Jong MC, Pulitano C, et al. Surgical management of hepatic neuroendocrine tumor metastasis: results from an international multi-institutional analysis. Ann Surg Oncol. 2010;17(12):3129–36. https://doi.org/10.1245/s10434-010-1154-5.
31. Maxwell JE, Sherman SK, O'Dorisio TM, Bellizzi AM, Howe JR. Liver-directed surgery of neuroendocrine metastases: What is the optimal strategy? Surgery. 2016;159(1):320–33. https://doi.org/10.1016/j.surg.2015.05.040.
32. Morgan RE, Pommier SJ, Pommier RF. Expanded criteria for debulking of liver metastasis also apply to pancreatic neuroendocrine tumors. Surgery. 2018;163(1):218–225. https://doi.org/10.1016/j.surg.2017.05.030.
33. Kasai Y, Hirose K, Corvera CU, et al. Residual tumor volume discriminates prognosis after surgery for neuroendocrine liver metastasis. J Surg Oncol. 2019; https://doi.org/10.1002/jso.25811.
34. De Jong MC, Farnell MB, Sclabas G, et al. Liver-directed therapy for hepatic metastases in patients undergoing pancreaticoduodenectomy: a dual-center analysis. Ann Surg. 2010;252(1):142–8. https://doi.org/10.1097/SLA.0b013e3181dbb7a7.
35. Hüttner FJ, Schneider L, Tarantino I, et al. Palliative resection of the primary tumor in 442 metastasized neuroendocrine tumors of the pancreas: a population-based, propensity score-matched survival analysis. Langenbeck's Arch Surg. 2015;400(6):715–23. https://doi.org/10.1007/s00423-015-1323-x.
36. Ye H, Xu HL, Shen Q, Zheng Q, Chen P. Palliative resection of primary tumor in metastatic nonfunctioning pancreatic neuroendocrine tumors. J Surg Res. 2019;11(243):578–87. https://doi.org/10.1016/j.jss.2019.04.002.
37. Tang LH, Basturk O, Sue JJ, Klimstra DS. A practical approach to the classification of WHO grade 3 (G3) Well-differentiated Neuroendocrine Tumor (WD-NET) and Poorly Differentiated Neuroendocrine Carcinoma (PD-NEC) of the pancreas. Am J Surg Pathol. 2016;40(9):1192–202. https://doi.org/10.1097/PAS.0000000000000662.
38. Hijioka S, Hosoda W, Matsuo K, et al. Rb Loss and KRAS mutation are predictors of the response to platinum-based chemotherapy in pancreatic neuroendocrine neoplasm with grade 3: a Japanese multicenter pancreatic NEN-G3 study. Clin Cancer Res. 2017;23(16):4625–32. https://doi.org/10.1158/1078-0432.CCR-16-3135.
39. Tang LH, Untch BR, Reidy DL, et al. Well-differentiated neuroendocrine tumors with a morphologically apparent high-grade component: a pathway distinct from poorly differentiated neuroendocrine carcinomas. Clin Cancer Res. 2016;22(4):1011–7. https://doi.org/10.1158/1078-0432.CCR-15-0548.
40. Conrad C, Kutlu OC, Dasari A, et al. Prognostic value of lymph node status and extent of lymphadenectomy in pancreatic neuroendocrine tumors confined to and extending beyond the pancreas. J Gastrointest Surg. 2016;20(12):1966–1974. https://doi.org/10.1007/s11605-016-3243-7.
41. Genç CG, Jilesen AP, Partelli S, et al. A new scoring system to predict recurrent disease in grade 1 and 2 nonfunctional pancreatic neuroendocrine tumors. Ann Surg. 2018;267(6):1148–1154. https://doi.org/10.1097/SLA.0000000000002123.
42. Assi HA, Mukherjee S, Kunz PL, et al. Surgery versus surveillance for well-differentiated, nonfunctional pancreatic neuroendocrine tumors: an 11-year analysis of the national cancer database. Oncologist. 2020;25(2):e276–83. https://doi.org/10.1634/theoncologist.2019-0466.
43. Mao R, Zhao H, Li K, et al. Outcomes of lymph node dissection for non-metastatic pancreatic neuroendocrine tumors: a propensity score-weighted analysis of the national cancer database. Ann Surg Oncol. 2019;26(9):2722–9. https://doi.org/10.1245/s10434-019-07506-5.
44. Izumo W, Higuchi R, Furukawa T, et al. Evaluation of the site and frequency of lymph node metastasis with non-functioning pancreatic neuroendocrine tumor. Eur Surg Res. 2019;60(5–6):219–28. https://doi.org/10.1159/000504410.
45. Japan Pancreas Society. Classification of pancreatic carcinoma. Fourth English ed Kanehara & Co, Ltd; 2017.
46. Zhao YP, Zhan HX, Zhang TP, et al. Surgical management of patients with insulinomas: result of 292 cases in a single institution. J Surg Oncol. 2011;103(2):169–74. https://doi.org/10.1002/jso.21773.
47. Tsutsumi K, Ohtsuka T, Mori Y, et al. Analysis of lymph node metastasis in pancreatic neuroendocrine tumors (PNETs) based on the tumor size and hormonal production. J Gastroenterol. 2012;47(6):678–85. https://doi.org/10.1007/s00535-012-0540-0.
48. Lopez-Aguiar AG, Ethun CG, Zaidi MY, et al. The conundrum of < 2-cm pancreatic neuroendocrine tumors: A preoperative risk score to predict lymph node metastases and guide surgical management. Surgery. 07 2019;166(1):15–21. https://doi.org/10.1016/j.surg.2019.03.008.
49. Xiao W, Zhu J, Peng L, Hong L, Sun G, Li Y. The role of central pancreatectomy in pancreatic surgery: a systematic review and meta-analysis. HPB (Oxford). 2018;20(10):896–904. https://doi.org/10.1016/j.hpb.2018.05.001.
50. Bartsch DK, Waldmann J, Fendrich V, et al. Impact of lymphadenectomy on survival after surgery for sporadic gastrinoma. Br J Surg. 2012;99(9):1234–40. https://doi.org/10.1002/bjs.8843.

53. International Consensus Guidelines for the Management of Intraductal Papillary Mucinous Neoplasms

Brian K. P. Goh

Abstract

The management algorithm for pancreatic cystic neoplasms (PCN) has evolved with rapid advancements in the knowledge of the diagnostic features, natural history and biology of these neoplasms together with the introduction of new and improvement in diagnostic modalities and tests. Over time, the management of PCNs has gradually trended from an aggressive resection approach in the past towards a more conservative approach with surveillance at present. Due to controversy in the management of intraductal papillary mucinous neoplasms (IPMN) especially with regards to branch duct (BD)-IPMN over the past 2 decades, several international consensus guidelines have been formulated to guide clinicians on the management of these neoplasms. These guidelines in general serve 2 main objectives: (1) diagnostic workup and clinical decision making and (2) surveillance protocol including methods, interval and duration. The present consensus guidelines' are useful in in guiding clinicians in decision making for the management of IPMNs by utilizing widely and easily available clinical parameters and morphological features from conventional cross-sectional imaging. Nevertheless, present guidelines remain far from ideal and are still associated with various limitations.

53.1 Introduction

Over the past three decades, the management algorithm for pancreatic cystic neoplasms (PCN) has evolved with rapid advancements in the knowledge of the diagnostic features, natural history and biology of these neoplasms together with the introduction of new and improvement in diagnostic modalities and tests [1–3]. In general, management of PCNs has gradually trended from an aggressive resection approach in the past towards a more conservative approach with surveillance at present [3–5]. Today, with the widespread use of cross-sectional imaging; there is an exponential increase in the number of incidental asymptomatic PCNs detected worldwide [3, 4, 6]. However, numerous investigators have demonstrated that the vast majority of these lesions have an indolent nature and a benign natural history [3–6].

The main pathological types of PCNs are intraductal papillary mucinous neoplasms (IPMN), serous cystic neoplasms (SCN), mucinous cystic neoplasms (MCN) and solid pseudopapillary neoplasms (SPPN) [7, 8]. At present, it is widely accepted that SCNs are almost universally benign and can be managed conservatively unless they grow to a large size resulting in local compressive symptoms [1, 8]. SPPNs on the other hand are potentially malignant neoplasms which occur in children and young adults especially females and hence, aggressive surgery when technically feasible is almost always warranted [1, 8, 9]. Similarly, surgical resection is usually indicated for MCNs as these premalignant neoplasms usually occur in middle-aged females [10]. Nonetheless, selected cases of small (<4 cm) MCN [8] may be observed especially in older patients with a shorter life-expectancy.

However, unlike the management of SCN, SPPN and MCN; the management approach towards IPMN remains controversial and debatable [1, 5]. Depending on the site of involvement of the pancreatic duct, IPMNs are classified into main-duct (MD), branch-duct (BD) and mixed-duct IPMNs (MT-IPMNs) [11, 12]. At present, there is uniform consensus among experts that most MD-IPMN and MT-IMPNs should be surgically removed due to the high-risk (>50%) of harboring malignancy or progressing to malignancy. On the other hand, most BD-IPMNs can be treated conservatively due to their indolent biology and only selected cases require surgical resection [8, 11, 12]. At present, several clinical and radiological criteria are now widely-accepted and have been well-

B. K. P. Goh (✉)
Department of Hepatopancreatobiliary and Transplant Surgery, Singapore General Hospital, Singapore, Singapore

Duke-National University of Singapore Medical School, Singapore, Singapore

validated to be associated with malignancy in IPMN. These include parameters such as main pancreatic duct dilatation, larger cyst size, enhancing mural nodule/solid component, positive cytology, pancreatitis, jaundice and elevated serum carbohydrate antigen (CA) 19-9 which are utilized in most management guidelines for IPMN [8, 11–14].

Due to controversy in the management of IPMNs especially with regards to BD-IPMN over the past 2 decades, several international consensus guidelines have been formulated to guide clinicians on the management of these neoplasms. These guidelines in general serve 2 main objectives: (1) diagnostic workup and clinical decision making and (2) surveillance protocol including methods, interval and duration [1, 15]. In 2006, international experts convened in Sendai and formulated the first widely-accepted expert guidelines for IPMN and MCN which came to be widely known as the Sendai Guidelines (SG06) [11]. SG06 (Table 53.1) was a

Table 53.1 Summary of international consensus guidelines criteria for the management pancreatic cystic neoplasms

Guideline	Criteria	Management
Sendai 2006		
MCN	NA	Surgery
IPMN	Symptoms MPD >6 mm Size >3 cm Mural nodule Positive cytology	Surgery
Fukuoka Guidelines 2012, revised 2017—IPMN only[a]		
IPMN	High risk – Proximal lesion with obstructive jaundice – *Enhancing mural nodules ≥ 5 mm*[a] (enhancing solid component) – Dilated main duct ≥10 mm	Surgery
	Worrisome risk – Size ≥3 cm – Pancreatitis – *Enhancing mural nodule < 5 mm*[a] (non-enhanced mural nodule) – Thickened, enhancing cyst walls – Dilated main duct 5 to 9 mm – Abrupt change in duct caliber with distal atrophy – Lymphadenopathy – *Elevated Ca 19-9 > 37 U/ml*[a] – *Rapid growth rate > 5 mm/2 years*[a]	EUS: mural nodule, main duct involvement, positive or suspicious cytology – surgery Size >3 cm—strongly consider surgery in young fit patients
	Low risk	Surveillance Size 2–3 cm: consider surgery in young fit patients
MCN	NA	Surgery
European Guidelines 2018		
IPMN	Absolute indication – Jaundice – Enhancing mural nodule ≥5 mm – Solid component – Dilated main duct ≥10 mm – Positive cytology for HGD or carcinoma	Surgery
	Relative indication – Size ≥4 cm – Pancreatitis – New onset diabetes – Dilated main duct 5 to 9.9 mm – Growth rate ≥ 5 mm/year – Enhancing mural nodule <5 mm – Elevated Ca 19-9 ≥ 37 U/ml	Surgery: no significant comorbidities; significant comorbidities/≥2 RI Intensive surveillance: significant comorbidities/1 RI
	No indication	Surveillance
MCN	– Symptomatic – Size ≥4 cm – Mural nodule – Growth rate	Surgery
SCN	– Compressive symptoms	Surgery
SPPN	NA	Surgery
PNEN	– >20 mm, symptoms	Surgery
American Gastroenterological Association 2015		
Asymptomatic IPMN/MCN	– Dilated main duct ≥5 mm and solid component/positive cytology for malignancy – At last 2 high-risk features: Size ≥3 cm, Dilated pancreatic duct, solid component – < 3 cm, no solid component, no dilated duct	Surgery EUS-FNA Surveillance
American College of Gastroenterologists 2018		

(continued)

Table 53.1 (continued)

Guideline	Criteria	Management
IPMN/MCN	– Jaundice – Acute pancreatitis – Elevated Ca 19-9 – Mural nodule/solid component – Dilated main duct >5 mm – Concerning focal dilatation of main duct – Change in main duct caliber with upstream atrophy – Size ≥3 cm – Cytology showing HGD or carcinoma	EUS and/or referral to MDT for consideration of resection
	– New onset or worsening diabetes – Increase in cyst size ≥3 mm/year	Short interval MRI/EUS-FNA

[a]2017 revisions

2-tier system which proposed that in addition to MCNs; all MD-IPMNs and BD-IPMNs with features such as size >3 cm, symptoms or main pancreatic duct diameter > 6 mm be considered for surgical resection. These guidelines were adopted in clinical practice world-wide for over 5 years but numerous studies subsequently performed to validate the utility of these guidelines [12, 13] demonstrated several major limitations. The main criticism of the guideline was its "over-aggressive" recommendation for surgical resection of BD-IPMN. The SG06 was demonstrated to have a low positive predictive value (PPV) of only about 33% for predicting malignant IPMN and adherence to the guideline resulted in overtreatment of patients whereby many benign BD-IPMNs were resected [16, 17]. The risks associated with the overtreatment of patients with IPMN should not be underestimated as despite advances in pancreatic surgery today, it remains a major operation associated with a significant morbidity and mortality even in high volume centers [16]. Hence, bearing the limitations of SG06 in mind, international experts convened in Fukuoka and proposed a new revised guideline termed the Fukuoka Consensus Guidelines in 2012 (FG12) [12]. Similar to SG06 the FG12 recommended resection for all MCN but revisions were made to the management guidelines for IPMN. The main objective was of the FG12 was to reduce the number of "unnecessary" surgical interventions and overtreatment of BD-IPMN [12].

53.1.1 Fukuoka Guidelines 2012 (Revised 2017)

Unlike the original SG06 guideline, the FG12 was a 3-tier system which categorized IPMNs into high risk, worrisome risk (WR^{FG12}) and low risk groups (Table 53.1) [12]. High risk lesions (HR^{FG12}) were to be managed via surgical resection whereas those which were low-risk could be conservatively managed via close surveillance [12]. The revised guidelines also recognized the role of endoscopic ultrasound (EUS) which had been increasingly utilized in the diagnostic evaluation of PCNs. In general, the use of EUS was recommended for IPMNs with WR^{FG12} although upfront surgical resection could be considered for selected WR^{FG12} such as young healthy patients with cysts ≥3 cm [12]. Notably, some of the major revisions in the FG12 to highlight was that cyst size ≥3 cm and pancreatic duct dilatation between 5-9 mm were no longer regarded as high risk indications for immediate surgical intervention but were only considered as worrisome risks. Furthermore, the need for enhancement on imaging was included to confirm that a mural nodule/solid component was suspicious as it was recognized that mucin within the cyst could mimic a non-enhancing nodule on cross-sectional imaging [1]. Systematic reviews [17–19] summarizing the literature have been performed to evaluate the utility of both the SG06 and FG12 and both guidelines have been shown to be associated with a low PPV but high NPV. Nonetheless, the FCG seemed to have a better PPV than the SCG (47% vs 33%) albeit at the expense of a slightly lower NPV [18].

In 2017, further refinements were made to the FG12 with regards to the management of IPMN (Table 53.1) [16, 20]. This included demoting enhancing mural nodules <5 mm to the WR^{FG12} and adding features such as elevated Ca 19-9 and cyst growth rate to WR^{FG12}. To date, these revisions remain the most recent updates to the guidelines (FG17) [20].

53.1.2 European Guidelines 2018 (EG18)

The EG18 [8] represents an update to the previous European guidelines published in 2013 [21]. It was formulated by a multidisciplinary expert panel from several European associations and unlike the FG12/17 which focused on IPMN, treatment recommendations for different pathological types of PCNs were included. Of note, whereas the FG12 recommended resection for all MCNs, the EG18 was more conservative than its predecessors and proposed surgical resection only for MCNs with worrying features such as presence of mural nodules or a cyst size >4 cm [8].

Similar to the FG12/17, the EG18 was a 3-tier system (Table 53.1) which classified IPMN into three categories according to the indication for surgery: absolute indication (AI^{EG18}), relative indication (RI^{EG18}) and no indication for surgery (Table 53.1). These were in general very similar to the FG17 with a few notable differences [1]. Upfront resection was recommended for patients in the absolute AI^{EG18} group like the HR^{FG17} group. Similarly, patients were conservatively managed in the no indication group like the FG17 low risk group. Notably, for the RI^{EG18} group, EG18 was more aggressive in proposing upfront surgery. Surgery was recommended for patients without significant comorbidity and 1 RI^{EG18} and for patients with significant comorbidity and 2/more RI^{EG18}. This differed from the WR^{FG17} which recommended further investigation via EUS-FNA and to only consider surgery in young healthy patients with cyst ≥3 cm. Unlike FG17, the EG18 also took into account the number of worrisome features and patients' comorbidities in their recommendations [1].

Several other minor differences between the EG18 and FG17 worth highlighting include the inclusion of new onset diabetes, using a cyst growth rate of ≥5 mm/year rather than 2 years and notably the change in cyst size cut-off from 3 to 4 cm in the RI^{EG18} [1]. The obvious impact of the change in the size cut-off is that this would result in a larger group of patients which can be managed conservatively via surveillance. However, more studies are needed to confirm if patients with BD-IPMN within the 3 to 4 cm size range can be observe safely. Due to its recency, not surprisingly, there are remain relatively few studies to date [22, 23] validating the EG18. The PPV for HGD/IC of AI^{EG18} and RI^{EG1} has been reported to range from 48.3% to 72.7% and 40.5% to 47.4% within the limitations of surgical series'. Of note, the false negative rate for malignancy of the EG18 was reported to be 1.9% [22].

Thus far the 3 guidelines discussed (SG06, FG12/17 and EG18) are the most common guidelines used to date (Table 53.1). In addition to these 3 guidelines, other guidelines less commonly used outside the United States include the American Gastroenterological Association (AGA) 2015 guidelines [13] and the American College of Gastroenterology (ACG) 2018 guidelines [14] which will not be discussed here. It is interesting to note that the EG18, AGA, ACG were formulated based on the evidence-based GRADE framework [16] whereas the SG06 and FG12 was developed based on expert opinion.

53.1.3 Surgery for IPMN

The objective of surgical resection in IPMN is complete removal of the tumor with negative margins (FG17) [20]. Depending on the tumor location, this may require a proximal or distal pancreatectomy. However, it is important to add that the exact type of resection may not always be easy to determine such as for diffuse type MD-IPMN without a definite focal lesion. This may also be difficult to distinguish from chronic pancreatitis. In such cases, ERCP or EUS may be useful to identify features of IPMN such as visualization of a mural nodule or mucin extrusion from a dilated papilla. A formal pancreatectomy with lymphadenectomy such as a pancreatoduodenectomy, left-sided pancreatectomy or total pancreatectomy should be the standard treatment when surgery is performed for suspected malignancy. However, more limited resections [20, 24] such as enucleation, middle pancreatectomy or spleen-saving pancreatectomy may be considered in selected cases of BD-IPMN when preoperative suspicion of malignancy is low. Frozen section should be routinely performed on parenchyma transection margins [20]. In the event of the presence of invasive cancer or high grade dysplasia at the transection margin, further resection should be performed and all patients should be counselled on the possibility of a total pancreatectomy. The presence of IPMN with low grade dysplasia does not warrant further resection of the margins.

53.1.4 Surveillance for IPMN

Based on present knowledge, all patients with IPMN managed conservatively should continue life-long surveillance (until deemed unfit for surgery) as the risk of progression does not diminish over time. It is also important to be cognizant of the development of concomitant pancreatic ductal adenocarcinoma especially in patients with a significant family history of pancreatic cancer and these patients would require more intensive surveillance. Similarly, patients who had undergone complete resection of non-invasive IPMN should undergo life-long surveillance for similar reasons due to the field-change effect associated with IPMN [25].

53.2 Discussion

The ideal guideline for the management IPMN should not only identify current risk of harboring HGD or invasive cancer but also future risk of developing malignancy. This would enable early intervention and avoid prolong surveillance. It must be emphasized that patients with IPMN on surveillance should undergo resection before the development of invasive carcinoma due to the poor prognosis of invasive IPMN which is similar to pancreatic ductal adenocarcinoma [26]. It is also imperative to add that an ideal guideline should also avoid surgical overtreatment resulting in unnecessary operations in patients who have little or no risk of developing malignancy during their lifetime [1, 2]. At present, it may be assumed that the optimal timing for surgery in IPMN in most patients would be when lesions harbor HGD as surgical resection will result in cure.

Management of patients with IPMN should be individualized and tailored according to a patient's risk-benefit profile for surveillance versus resection [1, 27]. In addition to the malignancy risk of the IPMN, other important factors to consider in the clinical decision-making process include the patient's projected life expectancy which would be determined by his/her age and presence of comorbidities, operative risk which is determined by the type of resection and patient's overall fitness; and even cost-effectiveness. Unfortunately, most guidelines today do not take into consideration these other important factors other than the recent EG18 which has included presence of comorbidities into the guidelines [1].

The present consensus guidelines' are useful in in guiding clinicians in decision making for the management of IPMNs. These guidelines utilize widely and easily available clinical parameters and morphological features from conventional cross-sectional imaging [1, 8, 12, 20], However present guidelines remain far from ideal and are still associated with various limitations. More robust scientific evidence is needed to support many of their recommendations [4]. Moreover, the added difficulty in accurately distinguishing IPMN from other PCNs preoperatively, frequently further diminishes the accuracy and hence, utility of these guidelines [1]. Several promising parameters which have been shown to be associated with malignancy in IPMN include inflammatory indices such as neutrophil lymphocyte ratio or platelet lymphocyte ratio [28] and the additive effect of increasing number of worrisome or high risk features on the malignancy risk. These should be considered in future updates of the guidelines [29]. Pathological subtypes of IPMN such as gastric, intestinal and pancreatobiliary subtypes have also been shown to be associated with the malignancy risk of IPMN and may have a major role in future guidelines [30].

Development of novel prognostic nomograms [31, 32] may also enable better prediction of the risk of malignancy of IPMN. The use of these nomograms when coupled with mathematical tools predicting an individual patient's surgical risk and estimated life expectancy would enable clinicians to determine the most appropriate management option for an individual patient with greater precision.

Moreover, recent advancements in imaging and diagnostic modalities such as confocal laser endomicroscopy [16], micro-forceps biopsy and identification of novel cyst fluid DNA-based, micro-RNA-based or protein-based biomarkers are showing great promise in the future management of IPMN and PCNs in general [4, 16]. Together these developments may potentially be used to improve future IPMN guidelines.

References

1. Wash RM, Perlmutter BC, Adsay V, Reid MD, Baker ME, Stevens T, Hue JJ, Hardacre JM, Shen GQ, Simon R, Aleassa EM, Augustin T, Eckhoff A, Allen PJ, Goh BK. Advances in the management of pancreatic cystic neoplasms. Current Prob Surg. 2020.
2. Goh BK, Tan Y, Thng C, et al. How useful are clinical, biochemical, and cross-sectional imaging features in predicting potentially malignant or malignant cystic lesions of the pancreas? Results from a single institution experience with 220 surgically treated patients. J Am Coll Surgeons. 2008;206(1):17–27.
3. Goh BK, Tan Y, Cheow PC, et al. Cystic lesions of the pancreas: an appraisal of an aggressive resectional policy adopted at a single institution during 15 years. Am J Surg. 2006;192:148–54.
4. DiMaio CJ. Current guideline controversies in the management of pancreatic cystic neoplasms. Gastrointest Endosc Clin N Am. 2018;28:529–47.
5. Goh BK. International guidelines for the management of pancreatic intraductal papillary mucinous neoplasms. World J Gastroenterol. 2015;21:9833–7.
6. Heckler M, Michalski CW, Schaefle S, Kaiser J, Buchler MW, Hackert T. The Sendai and Fukuoka consensus criteria for the management of branch duct IPMN – a meta-analysis on their accuracy. Pancreatology. 2017;17:255–62.
7. Goh BK, Tan DM, Thng CH, Lee SY, Low AS, Chan CY, et al. Are the Sendai and Fukuoka Consensus Guidelines for cystic mucinous neoplasms of the pancreas useful in the initial triage of all suspected pancreatic cystic neoplasms? A single institution experience with 317 surgically treated patients. Ann Surg Oncol. 2014;21:1919–26.
8. European Study Group on Cystic Tumours of the Pancreas. European evidence-based guidelines on pancreatic cystic neoplasms. Gut. 2018;67:789–804.
9. Goh BK, Tan YM, Cheow PC, Chung AY, Chow PK, Wong WK, Ooi LL. Solid pseudopapillary neoplasms of the pancreas: an updated experience. J Surg Oncol. 2007;15(95):640–4.
10. Goh BK, Tan YM, Chung YF, et al. A review of mucinous cystic neoplasms of the pancreas defined by ovarian-type stroma: clinicopathological features of 344 patients. World J Surg. 2006;30(12):2236–45.
11. Tanaka M, Chari S, Adsay V, et al. International consensus guidelines for management of intraductal papillary mucinous neoplasms and mucinous cystic neoplasms of the pancreas. Pancreatology. 2006;6:17–2.
12. Tanaka M, Fernandez-del Castillo C, Adsay V, et al. International consensus guidelines 2012 for the management of IPMN and MCN of the pancreas. Pancreatology. 2012;12:183–97.
13. Vege SS, Ziring B, Jain R, Moayyedi P. Clinical Guidelines committee; American Gastroenterology Association. American gastroenterological association institute guideline on the diagnosis and management of asymptomatic neoplastic pancreatic cysts. Gastroenterology. 2015;148:819–22.
14. Elta GH, Enestvedt BK, Sauer BG, Lennon AM. ACG clinical guideline: diagnosis and management of pancreatic cysts. Am J Gastroenterol. 2018;113:464–79.
15. Hasan A, Visrodia K, Farrel JJ, Gonda TA. Overview and comparison of guidelines for management of pancreatic cystic neoplasms. World J Gastronterol. 2019;25:4405–13.
16. Vilas-Boas F, Macedo G. Management guidelines for pancreatic cystic lesions: should we adopt or adapt current roadmaps? J Gastrointestin Liver Dis. 2019;28:495–501.
17. Goh BK, Tan DM, Ho MM, et al. Utility of the sendai consensus guidelines for branch-duct intraductal papillary mucinous neoplasms: a systematic review. J Gastrointest Surg. 2014;18:1350–7.
18. Srinivasan N, Teo JY, Chin YK, Hennedige T, Tan DM, Low AS, Thng CH, Goh BK. Systematic review of the clinical utility and validity of the Sendai and Fukuoka Consensus guideliens for the management of intraductal papillary mucinous neoplasms of the pancreas. HPB. 2018;20:497–504.
19. Goh BK, Lin Z, Tan DM, et al. Evaluation of the Fukuoka Consensus Guidelines for intraductal papillary mucinous neoplasms of the pancreas: results from a systematic review of 1,382 surgically resected patients. Surgery. 2015;158(5):1192–202.
20. Tanaka M, Fernandez-del Castillo C, Kamisawa T, et al. Revisions of international consensus Fukuoka guidelines for the management of IPMN of the pancreas. Pancreatology. 2017;17:738–53.

21. Del Chiaro M, Verbeke C, Salvia R, et al. European expert consensus statement on cystic tumours of the pancreas. Dig Liver Dis. 2013;45:703–11.
22. Jan IS, Chang MC, Yang CY, Tien YW, Jeng YM, Wu CH, Chen BB, Chang YT. Validation of indications for surgery of European evidence-based guidelines for patients with pancreatic intraductal papillary mucinous neoplasms. J Gastronintest Surg. 2019.
23. Sun L, Wang W, Wang Y, Jiang F, Peng L, Jin G, Jin Z. Validation of European evidence-based guidelines and American College of Gastroenterology guidelines as predictors of advanced neoplasia in patients with suspected mucinous pancreatic cystic neoplasms. J Gastroenterol Hepatol. 2019.
24. Sauvanet A, Gaujoux S, Blanc B, Couverlard A, Dokmak S, Vullierme MP, et al. Parenchyma-sparing pancreatectomy for presumed noninvasive intraductal papillary mucinous neoplasms of the pancreas. Ann Surg. 2014;260:364–71.
25. Tamura K, Ohtsuka T, Ideno N, et al. Treatment strategy for main duct IPMN of the pancreas based on the assessment of recurrence in the remnant pancreas after resection: a systematic review. Ann Surg. 2014.
26. Koh YX, Chok AY, Zheng HL, Tan CS, Goh BK. Systematic review and meta-analysis comparing the surgical outcomes of invasive intraductal papillary mucinous neoplasms and conventional pancreatic ductal adenocarcinoma. Ann Surg Oncol. 2014;21(8):2782–800.
27. Goh BK. Sendai consensus guidelines for branch-duct IPMN: guidelines are just guidelines. Ann Surg. 2015;262(2):e65.
28. Goh BK, Tan DM, Chan CY, et al. Are preoperative blood neutrophil-to-lymphocyte ratio useful in predicting malignancy in surgically-treated mucin-producing pancreatic cystic neoplasms. J Surg Oncol. 2015;112:366–71.
29. Goh BK, Thng CH, Tan DM, et al. Evaluation of the Sendai and 2012 International Consensus Guidelines based on cross-sectional imaging findings performed for the initial triage of mucinous cystic lesions of the pancreas: a single institution experience with 114 surgically treated patients. Am J Surg. 2014;208:202–9.
30. Koh YX, Zheng HL, Chok AY, et al. Systematic review and meta-analysis of different histologic subtypes of noninvasive and invasive IPMN. Surgery. 2015;157:496–509.
31. Jang JY, Park T, Lee S, Kim Y, Lee SY, Kim SW, Kim SC, et al. Proposed nomogrm predicting the individual risk of malignancy in patients with branch duct type intraductal papillary mucinous neoplasms of the pancreas. Ann Surg. 2017;266:1062–8.
32. Han Y, Jang JY, Oh MY, et al. Natural history and optimal treatment strategy of intraductal papillary mucinous neoplasm of the pancreas: analysis using a nomogram and Markov decision model. J Hepatobiliary Pancreat Sci. 2021;28:131–42.

Remnant Pancreatic Cancer After Surgical Resection for Pancreatic Cancer

Yoshihiro Miyasaka and Masafumi Nakamura

Abstract

Improvements in multidisciplinary treatment and diagnostic modalities for pancreatic cancer have increased the number of long-term survivors after surgical resection for pancreatic cancer. Consequently, reports of patients who developed cancer in the remnant pancreas have also increased. Two possible mechanisms underlie the development of cancer in the remnant pancreas after resection for pancreatic cancer: local recurrence of the initial pancreatic cancer and the metachronous development of a new primary lesion. Genetic analyses may help distinguish between local recurrence and new primary cancer. The identification of predictive factors may facilitate the early detection of remnant pancreatic cancer. The presence of concomitant intraductal papillary mucinous neoplasms may predict the development of remnant pancreatic cancer. Surgical resection for remnant pancreatic cancer may provide favorable short- and long-term outcomes. Life-long surveillance focusing on remnant pancreatic cancer is recommended after surgical resection for pancreatic cancer.

54.1 Introduction

Pancreatic cancer (PC) is the most lethal digestive malignancy, with a 5-year overall survival rate of 9% [1]. In addition, it is expected to become the second leading cause of cancer-related death by 2030 [2]. The only curative treatment is surgical resection. Owing to advances in multidisciplinary approaches, including neoadjuvant and adjuvant therapy, the outcomes of surgical resection for PC have improved. Although the median overall survival after surgical resection alone for resectable PC is approximately 20 months, that after resection followed by the administration of recently reported adjuvant chemotherapy regimens (S-1 or FOLFIRINOX) exceeds 45 months [3–5]. In addition, progress in the development of diagnostic modalities has facilitated the detection of early-stage PC, which carries better prognostic outcomes after surgery than advanced-stage PC [6]. The improved outcomes of surgical resection have increased the number of long-term PC survivors. However, the prolonged survival of patients may also increase the risk of PC in the remnant pancreas (Fig. 54.1).

Since the beginning of this century, several case reports of remnant pancreatic cancer (RPC) after surgical resection for PC have been published [7–20]. In the last decade, several investigators reported cohort studies regarding RPC after surgical resection for PC [21–34]. Some of the studies focused on the treatment of RPC, and others focused on the developmental mechanisms of RPC. Furthermore, Japanese Clinical Practice Guidelines for Pancreatic Cancer 2019 recommend long-term regular surveillance after surgical resection for PC to detect RPC [35]. These factors imply that the incidence of RPC has increased and that considerable attention should be paid to this pathology. To improve our understanding of RPC after surgical resection for PC, current information regarding the developmental mechanism, designations, incidence, predictive factors, and treatment of RPC is summarized in this chapter.

54.1.1 Developmental Mechanism

There are two possible mechanisms of the development of RPC after pancreatic resection for PC: local recurrence of the initial lesion within the remnant pancreas and the meta-

---

Y. Miyasaka
Department of Surgery, Fukuoka University Chikushi Hospital, Chikushino, Fukuoka, Japan

Department of Surgery and Oncology, Graduate School of Medical Sciences, Kyushu University, Higashi-ku, Fukuoka, Japan

M. Nakamura (✉)
Department of Surgery and Oncology, Graduate School of Medical Sciences, Kyushu University, Higashi-ku, Fukuoka, Japan
e-mail: mnaka@surg1.med.kyushu-u.ac.jp

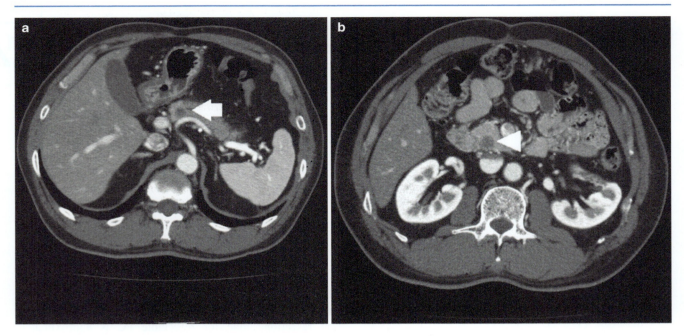

Fig. 54.1 A case of remnant pancreatic cancer after resection for pancreatic cancer. (**a**) Enhanced CT at initial presentation revealed a low-density mass in the pancreatic body (arrow). Distal pancreatectomy with splenectomy was performed. The postoperative course was uneventful. The pathological examination revealed ductal adenocarcinoma (pT1, pN0, R0). (**b**) Thirty months after initial pancreatic resection, routine follow-up CT revealed a low-density mass in the pancreatic head (arrowhead). Total remnant pancreatectomy was performed. The postoperative course was uneventful. The pathological examination revealed ductal adenocarcinoma (pT3, pN0, R0)

chronous development of a new primary lesion in the remnant pancreas [21, 22, 26].

Recurrence after surgical resection occurs in approximately 80% of patients of PC [36–38]. Along with liver metastasis, local recurrence is a common recurrence pattern of PC [36–38]. Although local PC recurrence usually occurs in the pancreas bed, regional lymph nodes, or adjacent structures (e.g., SMA or SMV), it can occur within the remnant pancreas. In previous cohort studies, several investigators considered cancer lesions that arose in the remnant pancreas after PC resection to represent recurrence [29, 30, 33]. There are several possible pathways through which cancer cells move from the initial lesion to the remnant pancreas. First, a positive pancreatic cut margin can lead to recurrence. In this situation, the secondary tumor arises near the pancreatic stump. Second, intraparenchymal metastasis may occur via blood or lymphatic vessels. Another possible pathway is intraductal dissemination. Genetic analyses of multiple lesions of intraductal papillary mucinous neoplasm (IPMN) revealed that genetic mutation patterns were similar among different lesions in some cases and suggested that neoplastic cells might metastasize through the pancreatic duct [39–41]. In addition, Makohon-Moore et al. [42] proposed that even precancerous neoplastic cells of the pancreas could be disseminated through the pancreatic ductal system. In the second and third situations, the secondary tumor can arise distantly from the pancreatic stump.

Synchronous multifocal lesions are occasionally observed in patients with PC. Histopathological examination of the pancreas of patients who underwent total pancreatectomy for PC revealed multifocal cancer lesions in 20–32% of patients [43, 44]. Therefore, it is logical that multifocal PC lesions appear after the surgical resection of initial PC as new primary lesions.

Several researchers have attempted to classify RPC as recurrent lesions and new primary lesions. Hashimoto et al. [22] compared the KRAS mutation status and immunohistochemical MUC1 and MUC2 staining between the initial lesion and remnant pancreatic lesion. Gotoh et al. [21] divided RPC into local recurrence and metachronous multifocal lesions (new primary lesions) using KRAS mutational analyses and immunohistochemical analyses of TP53, CDKN2A, and SMAD4. Luchini et al. [26] employed histopathological analysis and mutation analysis using next-generation sequencing to differentiate "true" recurrence and independent lesions (new primary lesions).

It is expected that prognosis of recurrence is generally worse than that of a new primary lesion. Gotoh et al. [21] reported that local recurrence was associated with a shorter interval between the initial and secondary cancer, a greater cumulative recurrence rate, and shorter disease-specific survival than metachronous multifocal lesions. They also reported that the disease-specific survival of patients with local recurrence after second resection was comparable to that of patients with unresectable RPC or patients with extrapancreatic recurrence.

54.1.2 Designations

In previous reports, various designations were used to describe RPC, including 'remnant pancreatic cancer' [10, 28, 32], 'pancreatic cancer (ductal adenocarcinoma) in the remnant pancreas' [22, 27], 'pancreatic cancer arising in the remnant pancreas' [26], 'carcinoma developing in the remnant pancreas' [7, 11, 18], 'metachronous pancreatic cancer' [12], 'second primary pancreatic ductal carcinoma' [24], 'recurrent peancreatic cancer' [31, 34], '(isolated) local recurrence in the remnant pancreas' [29, 30, 33], and 'high-risk lesions in the remnant pancreas' [21]. The use of different designations for RPC may be attributable to the fact that this malignancy was recently recognized and it includes lesions with different developmental mechanisms. For further research on this pathology, unification of the designation is desirable.

54.1.3 Incidence

According to previous cohort studies, the proportions of patient who developed RPC among those who underwent pancreatic resection for PC ranged 0.7–26.7% (Table 54.1). Ishida et al. [24] calculated the cumulative incidence rates of RPC using the Kaplan–Meier method and reported a 5-year cumulative incidence rate of 17.7%. Although the proportions of patients with RPC were less than 6% in most studies, two studies of early-stage PC reported much higher proportions (26.7% and 15.5%) [23, 25]. Our recent study found that the cumulative incidence of RPC after pancreatic resection was comparable between patients with early- and advanced-stage PC, whereas proportion of patients who developed RPC were significantly higher in early-stage PC than advanced-stage PC [28]. It is suggested that the higher proportion of patients who developed RPC after early-stage PC was attributable to the higher number of long-term survivors in this cohort. Therefore, it is expected that the number of patients who develop RPC after surgical resection for PC will further increase if further improvements in the prognosis of PC are achieved.

The interval between the initial resection of PC and development of RPC ranged from 6 to 240 months (Table 54.1). It is suggested that RPC can develop more than 5 years after the initial resection of PC.

54.1.4 Predictive Factors

Identification of the predictive factors of RPC may facilitate the early detection of RPC and assist in the creation of postoperative surveillance schedules. Matsuda et al. analyzed the long-term outcomes of 379 patients who underwent partial pancreatectomy for pancreatic ductal adenocarcinoma (PDAC) and identified 14 patients (3.96%) who developed RPC [27]. According to multivariate analysis, concomitant IPMN was an independent predictive factor for RPC after partial pancreatic resection for PDAC. In addition, they microscopically compared background pancreatic parenchyma between patients with PDAC concomitant with IPMN and those with PDAC without IPMN, observing that the den-

Table 54.1 Cohort studies of the development of remnant pancreatic cancer after resection for pancreatic cancer

Author	Year	Number of cases of initial pancreatic resection for pancreatic cancer	Number of cases of remnant pancreatic cancer	Proportion of cases with remnant pancreatic cancer (%)	Margin status of the initial resection (R0/R1)	Median interval (range) between the initial resection and appearance of remnant pancreatic lesions (months)	Number of cases of resection for remnant pancreatic cancer
Thomas et al. [33]	2012	700	5	0.7	NA	68 (7–81)	5
Miyazaki et al. [29]	2014	284	11	3.9	9/2	32 (7–89)	11
Hashimoto et al. [22]	2014	227	8	3.5	7/1	23.5 (17–39)	6
Shima et al. [31]	2015	185	6	3.2	6/0	25 (12–60)	6
Ishida et al. [24]	2016	130	6	4.6	6/0	43.5 (14–60)	4
Suzuki et al. [32]	2016	826	23	2.8	23/0	53.6 (15–240)	12
Nakayama et al. [30]	2018	194	11	5.7	11/0	24 (6–41)	11
Ikemoto et al. [23]	2018	30	8	26.7	NA	56.5 (16–85)	5
Kanno et al. [25]	2018	200	31	15.5	NA	NA	NA
Gotoh et al. [21]	2019	411	22	5.4	NA	NA	12
Matsuda et al. [27]	2020	379	14	3.7	12/2	42.5 (20–160)	10
Miyasaka et al. [28]	2020	321	19	5.9	17/2	51 (20–160)	13

sity of pancreatic intraepithelial neoplasia was significantly higher in patients with PDAC and concomitant IPMN. Careful postoperative surveillance focusing on the development of RPC is recommended for patients who undergo partial pancreatectomy for PDAC concomitant with IPMN.

54.1.5 Treatment

Similar to initial PC, surgery, chemotherapy, and radiotherapy are used to treat RPC. For lesions restricted to the remnant pancreas, surgical resection is often performed. Although surgery for RPC may be difficult because of adhesion and anatomical changes and RPC possibility of recurrence of the initial cancer, it has been reported that the short- and long-term outcomes of surgical resection for RPC after initial resection for PC were relatively favorable. Yamada et al. [34] conducted a multicenter study of patients who developed RPC after pancreatic resection for PC. Among the 90 patients who underwent surgical resection for RPC, postoperative complications (Clavien–Dindo classification III or greater) were observed in eight patients (9%), and the 30- and 90-day mortality rates were 0 and 1%, respectively. Zhou et al. [45] performed a pooled analysis of 19 studies of second pancreatectomy for RPC and found no perioperative mortality. Several authors compared the prognosis of patients who underwent resection for RPC with that of patients who underwent nonsurgical treatment and observed significantly better prognosis among patients who underwent resection [27, 29, 30, 32, 34]. Suzuki et al. [32] reviewed publications on RPC and collected data for 49 patients who underwent completion pancreatectomy for RPC after resection for initial PC. According to their analysis, the median survival time after resection for RPC was 32 months. A pooled analysis by Zhou et al. [45] reported a 5-year overall survival rate of 40.6% for patients after second pancreatectomy. Although surgery for RPC was performed in selected patients, their outcomes appeared to be more favorable than those of patients who underwent initial pancreatic resection for PC. The most common surgical procedure for RPC is total remnant pancreatectomy (completion pancreatectomy). The long-term outcomes of total pancreatectomy including total remnant pancreatectomy have been improved by progress in the management of endocrine and exocrine insufficiency [46–48]. Hashimoto et al. reported that total remnant pancreatectomy after distal pancreatectomy was linked to a longer operative time and greater blood loss than total remnant pancreatectomy after pancreaticoduodenectomy [49]. In addition, several reports described laparoscopic and robotic total remnant pancreatectomy [50–52].

Adjuvant chemotherapy after resection for PC became a standard treatment after several studies highlighted its efficacy [3–5]. However, the efficacy of adjuvant chemotherapy after surgery for RPC is not certain. Nakayama et al. [30] analyzed 11 patients with resected RPC and found that patients who underwent adjuvant chemotherapy exhibited significantly longer survival than their counterparts. Conversely, a pooled analysis by Zhou et al. [45] reported that adjuvant chemotherapy did not have a significant effect on overall survival. Although neoadjuvant therapy was also performed for RPC in some cases, detailed analysis of its efficacy was not performed. Similar to primary PC, chemotherapy or chemoradiotherapy is indicated for locally advanced or metastatic RPC [22, 24, 32, 53].

54.2 Conclusion

To date, attention has been paid to the development of local recurrence or metastasis during postoperative surveillance after surgery for PC. Although most cases of recurrence or metastasis occur within 5 years after the resection of PC, RPC can develop a long time after surgery. Surgeons should pay attention to this condition and provide life-long surveillance for patients who undergo partial pancreatic resection for PC.

References

1. Siegel RL, Miller KD, Jemal A. Cancer statistics, 2020. CA Cancer J Clin. 2020;70:7–30.
2. Rahib L, Smith BD, Aizenberg R, Rosenzweig AB, Fleshman JM, Matrisian LM. Projecting cancer incidence and deaths to 2030: the unexpected burden of thyroid, liver, and pancreas cancers in the United States. Cancer Res. 2014;74:2913–21.
3. Conroy T, Hammel P, Hebbar M, Ben Abdelghani M, Wei AC, Raoul JL, et al. FOLFIRINOX or gemcitabine as adjuvant therapy for pancreatic cancer. N Engl J Med. 2018;379:2395–406.
4. Oettle H, Post S, Neuhaus P, Gellert K, Langrehr J, Ridwelski K, et al. Adjuvant chemotherapy with gemcitabine vs observation in patients undergoing curative-intent resection of pancreatic cancer: a randomized controlled trial. JAMA. 2007;297:267–77.
5. Uesaka K, Boku N, Fukutomi A, Okamura Y, Konishi M, Matsumoto I, et al. Adjuvant chemotherapy of S-1 versus gemcitabine for resected pancreatic cancer: a phase 3, open-label, randomised, non-inferiority trial (JASPAC 01). Lancet. 2016;388:248–57.
6. Egawa S, Toma H, Ohigashi H, Okusaka T, Nakao A, Hatori T, et al. Japan pancreatic cancer registry; 30th year anniversary: Japan Pancreas Society. Pancreas. 2012;41:985–92.
7. Akabori H, Shiomi H, Naka S, Murakami K, Murata S, Ishida M, et al. Resectable carcinoma developing in the remnant pancreas 7 years and 10 months after distal pancreatectomy for invasive ductal carcinoma of the pancreas: report of a case. World J Surg Oncol. 2014;12:224.
8. Bauer TM, Dhir T, Strickland A, Thomsett H, Goetz AB, Cannaday S, et al. Genetic drivers of pancreatic cancer are identical between the primary tumor and a secondary lesion in a long-term (>5 years) survivor after a whipple procedure. J Pancreat Cancer. 2018;4:81–7.

9. Dalla Valle R, Mancini C, Crafa P, Passalacqua R. Pancreatic carcinoma recurrence in the remnant pancreas after a pancreaticoduodenectomy. JOP. 2006;7:473–7.
10. Eriguchi N, Aoyagi S, Imayama H, Okuda K, Hara M, Fukuda S, et al. Resectable carcinoma of the pancreatic head developing 7 years and 4 months after distal pancreatectomy for carcinoma of the pancreatic tail. J Hepato-Biliary-Pancreat Surg. 2000;7:316–20.
11. Frei L, Stieger R, Bayerl C, Breitenstein S, Staerkle RF. Resectable adenocarcinoma developing in the remnant pancreas 7 years after partial pancreatoduodenectomy for invasive ductal adenocarcinoma of the pancreas: a case report. J Med Case Rep. 2017;11:194.
12. Hamner JB, White M, Crowder C, Singh G. Resection of metachronous pancreatic cancer 4 years after pancreaticoduodenectomy for stage III pancreatic adenocarcinoma. World J Surg Oncol. 2015;13:290.
13. Ikematsu Y, Tamura H, Nakata Y, Hayashi T, Kanai T, Hirayama K, et al. Metachronous multiple adenocarcinomas of the pancreas. Int J Clin Oncol. 2011;16:726–31.
14. Kinoshita H, Yamade N, Nakai H, Sasaya T, Matsumura S, Kimura A, et al. Successful resection of pancreatic carcinoma recurrence in the remnant pancreas after a pancreaticoduodenectomy. Hepato-Gastroenterology. 2011;58:1406–8.
15. Koizumi M, Sata N, Kasahara N, Morishima K, Sasanuma H, Sakuma Y, et al. Remnant pancreatectomy for recurrent or metachronous pancreatic carcinoma detected by FDG-PET: two case reports. JOP. 2010;11:36–40.
16. Ogino T, Ueda J, Sato N, Takahata S, Mizumoto K, Nakamura M, et al. Repeated pancreatectomy for recurrent pancreatic carcinoma after pylorus-preserving pancreatoduodenectomy: report of two patients. Case Rep Gastroenterol. 2010;4:429–34.
17. Shonaka T, Inagaki M, Akabane K, Yanagida N, Shomura H, Yanagawa N, et al. Total pancreatectomy for metachronous mixed acinar-ductal carcinoma in a remnant pancreas. World J Gastroenterol. 2014;20:11904–9.
18. Tajima Y, Kuroki T, Ohno T, Furui J, Tsuneoka N, Adachi T, et al. Resectable carcinoma developing in the remnant pancreas 3 years after pylorus-preserving pancreaticoduodenectomy for invasive ductal carcinoma of the pancreas. Pancreas. 2008;36:324–7.
19. Takamatsu S, Ban D, Irie T, Noguchi N, Kudoh A, Nakamura N, et al. Resection of a cancer developing in the remnant pancreas after a pancreaticoduodenectomy for pancreas head cancer. J Gastrointest Surg. 2005;9:263–9.
20. Wada K, Takada T, Yasuda H, Amano H, Yoshida M. A repeated pancreatectomy in the remnant pancreas 22 months after pylorus-preserving pancreatoduodenectomy for pancreatic adenocarcinoma. J Hepato-Biliary-Pancreat Surg. 2001;8:174–8.
21. Gotoh Y, Ohtsuka T, Nakamura S, Shindo K, Ohuchida K, Miyasaka Y, et al. Genetic assessment of recurrent pancreatic high-risk lesions in the remnant pancreas: metachronous multifocal lesion or local recurrence? Surgery. 2019;165:767–74.
22. Hashimoto D, Chikamoto A, Ohmuraya M, Sakata K, Miyake K, Kuroki H, et al. Pancreatic cancer in the remnant pancreas following primary pancreatic resection. Surg Today. 2014;44:1313–20.
23. Ikemoto J, Hanada K, Minami T, Okazaki A, Abe T, Amano H, et al. Prospective follow-up study of the recurrence of pancreatic cancer diagnosed at an early stage: the value of endoscopic ultrasonography for early diagnosis of recurrence in the remnant pancreas. Pancreas. 2018;47:482–8.
24. Ishida J, Toyama H, Matsumoto I, Asari S, Goto T, Terai S, et al. Second primary pancreatic ductal carcinoma in the remnant pancreas after pancreatectomy for pancreatic ductal carcinoma: high cumulative incidence rates at 5 years after pancreatectomy. Pancreatology. 2016;16:615–20.
25. Kanno A, Masamune A, Hanada K, Maguchi H, Shimizu Y, Ueki T, et al. Multicenter study of early pancreatic cancer in Japan. Pancreatology. 2018;18:61–7.
26. Luchini C, Pea A, Yu J, He J, Salvia R, Riva G, et al. Pancreatic cancer arising in the remnant pancreas is not always a relapse of the preceding primary. Mod Pathol. 2019;32:659–65.
27. Matsuda R, Miyasaka Y, Ohishi Y, Yamamoto T, Saeki K, Mochidome N, et al. Concomitant intraductal papillary mucinous neoplasm in pancreatic ductal adenocarcinoma is an independent predictive factor for the occurrence of new cancer in the remnant pancreas. Ann Surg. 2020;271:941–8.
28. Miyasaka Y, Ohtsuka T, Kimura R, Matsuda R, Mori Y, Nakata K, et al. Is remnant pancreatic cancer after pancreatic resection more frequent in early-stage pancreatic cancer than in advanced-stage cancer? Ann Gastroenterol Surg. 2020;4:448–54.
29. Miyazaki M, Yoshitomi H, Shimizu H, Ohtsuka M, Yoshidome H, Furukawa K, et al. Repeat pancreatectomy for pancreatic ductal cancer recurrence in the remnant pancreas after initial pancreatectomy: is it worthwhile? Surgery. 2014;155:58–66.
30. Nakayama Y, Sugimoto M, Gotohda N, Konishi M, Takahashi S. Efficacy of completion pancreatectomy for recurrence of adenocarcinoma in the remnant pancreas. J Surg Res. 2018;221:15–23.
31. Shima Y, Okabayashi T, Kozuki A, Sumiyoshi T, Tokumaru T, Saisaka Y, et al. Completion pancreatectomy for recurrent pancreatic cancer in the remnant pancreas: report of six cases and a review of the literature. Langenbeck's Arch Surg. 2015;400:973–8.
32. Suzuki S, Furukawa T, Oshima N, Izumo W, Shimizu K, Yamamoto M. Original scientific reports: clinicopathological findings of remnant pancreatic cancers in survivors following curative resections of pancreatic cancers. World J Surg. 2016;40:974–81.
33. Thomas RM, Truty MJ, Nogueras-Gonzalez GM, Fleming JB, Vauthey JN, Pisters PW, et al. Selective reoperation for locally recurrent or metastatic pancreatic ductal adenocarcinoma following primary pancreatic resection. J Gastrointest Surg. 2012;16:1696–704.
34. Yamada S, Kobayashi A, Nakamori S, Baba H, Yamamoto M, Yamaue H, et al. Resection for recurrent pancreatic cancer in the remnant pancreas after pancreatectomy is clinically promising: results of a project study for pancreatic surgery by the Japanese Society of Hepato-Biliary-Pancreatic Surgery. Surgery. 2018;164:1049–56.
35. Okusaka T, Nakamura M, Yoshida M, Kitano M, Uesaka K, Ito Y, et al. Clinical practice guidelines for pancreatic cancer 2019 from the Japan pancreas society: a synopsis. Pancreas. 2020;49:326–35.
36. Groot VP, Gemenetzis G, Blair AB, Ding D, Javed AA, Burkhart RA, et al. Implications of the pattern of disease recurrence on survival following pancreatectomy for pancreatic ductal adenocarcinoma. Ann Surg Oncol. 2018;25:2475–83.
37. Sperti C, Pasquali C, Piccoli A, Pedrazzoli S. Recurrence after resection for ductal adenocarcinoma of the pancreas. World J Surg. 1997;21:195–200.
38. Van den Broeck A, Sergeant G, Ectors N, Van Steenbergen W, Aerts R, Topal B. Patterns of recurrence after curative resection of pancreatic ductal adenocarcinoma. Eur J Surg Oncol. 2009;35:600–4.
39. Nagai K, Mizukami Y, Omori Y, Kin T, Yane K, Takahashi K, et al. Metachronous intraductal papillary mucinous neoplasms disseminate via the pancreatic duct following resection. Mod Pathol. 2020;33:971–80.
40. Pea A, Yu J, Rezaee N, Luchini C, He J, Dal Molin M et al. Targeted DNA sequencing reveals patterns of local progression in the pancreatic remnant following resection of Intraductal Papillary Mucinous Neoplasm (IPMN) of the pancreas. Ann Surg. 2016.
41. Tamura K, Ohtsuka T, Ideno N, Aso T, Shindo K, Aishima S, et al. Treatment strategy for main duct intraductal papillary mucinous neoplasms of the pancreas based on the assessment of recurrence in the remnant pancreas after resection: a retrospective review. Ann Surg. 2014;259:360–8.

42. Makohon-Moore AP, Matsukuma K, Zhang M, Reiter JG, Gerold JM, Jiao Y, et al. Precancerous neoplastic cells can move through the pancreatic ductal system. Nature. 2018;561:201–5.
43. Launois B, Franci J, Bardaxoglou E, Ramee MP, Paul JL, Malledant Y, et al. Total pancreatectomy for ductal adenocarcinoma of the pancreas with special reference to resection of the portal vein and multicentric cancer. World J Surg. 1993;17:122–126; discussion 126–127.
44. Tryka AF, Brooks JR. Histopathology in the evaluation of total pancreatectomy for ductal carcinoma. Ann Surg. 1979;190:373–81.
45. Zhou Y, Song A, Wu L, Si X, Li Y. Second pancreatectomy for recurrent pancreatic ductal adenocarcinoma in the remnant pancreas: a pooled analysis. Pancreatology. 2016;16:1124–8.
46. Crippa S, Tamburrino D, Partelli S, Salvia R, Germenia S, Bassi C, et al. Total pancreatectomy: indications, different timing, and perioperative and long-term outcomes. Surgery. 2011;149:79–86.
47. Müller MW, Friess H, Kleeff J, Dahmen R, Wagner M, Hinz U et al. Is there still a role for total pancreatectomy? Ann Surg. 2007;246:966–974; discussion 974–965.
48. Watanabe Y, Ohtsuka T, Matsunaga T, Kimura H, Tamura K, Ideno N, et al. Long-term outcomes after total pancreatectomy: special reference to survivors' living conditions and quality of life. World J Surg. 2015;39:1231–9.
49. Hashimoto D, Chikamoto A, Taki K, Arima K, Yamashita Y, Ohmuraya M, et al. Residual total pancreatectomy: short- and long-term outcomes. Pancreatology. 2016;16:646–51.
50. Kyaw PPP, Goh BKP. Robotic assisted laparoscopic completion pancreatectomy for recurrent intraductal papillary mucinous neoplasm after previous open pancreatoduodenectomy: a case report and literature review. Ann Hepatobiliary Pancreat Surg. 2019;23:206–9.
51. Sahakyan MA, Yaqub S, Kazaryan AM, Villanger O, Berstad AE, Labori KJ, et al. Laparoscopic completion pancreatectomy for local recurrence in the pancreatic remnant after pancreaticoduodenectomy: case reports and review of the literature. J Gastrointest Cancer. 2016;47:509–13.
52. Sunagawa H, Mayama Y, Orokawa T, Oshiro N. Laparoscopic total remnant pancreatectomy after laparoscopic pancreaticoduodenectomy. Asian J Endosc Surg. 2014;7:71–4.
53. Groot VP, van Santvoort HC, Rombouts SJ, Hagendoorn J, Borel Rinkes IH, van Vulpen M, et al. Systematic review on the treatment of isolated local recurrence of pancreatic cancer after surgery; re-resection, chemoradiotherapy and SBRT. HPB (Oxford). 2017;19:83–92.

Benign Biliary Diseases

Abdel Hadi S. Al Breizat, Salam S. Daradkeh, and Ali A. Al-Sarira

Abstract

Most of the benign biliary diseases are consequences of cholelithiasis and its treatment. Weight reduction interventions have increased the incidence and added a new category of patients. Biliary injuries and strictures remain a big challenge and become more challenging because of liver transplant biliary complications. Different diagnostic modalities are used including intraoperative color Doppler ultrasound, intraoperative contrast studies, and fluorescence using indocyanine green to delineate the biliary and vascular anatomy. Liver transplant is increasingly used to treat primary sclerosing cholangitis. One-stage laparoscopic management of cholelithiasis and choledocholithiasis decreased the likelihood of complications resulting from interventions on sphincter of Oddi. Total excision of choledochal cysts with hepaticojejunostomy presenting in adults withstood the proof of time.

Multidisciplinary team approach including surgeon, radiologist, and endoscopist with properly timed usage of different diagnostic and therapeutic modalities in a specialized centers is the key for successful management.

55.1 Introduction

Most of benign biliary diseases are consequences of cholelithiasis and its treatment. Weight reduction interventions have increased the incidence and added a new category of patients. Biliary injuries and strictures remain a big challenge and become more challenging because of liver transplant biliary complications. Different diagnostic modalities are used including intraoperative color Doppler ultrasound, intraoperative contrast studies, and fluorescence using indocyanine green to delineate the biliary and vascular anatomy. Liver transplant is increasingly used to treat primary sclerosing cholangitis. One-stage laparoscopic management of cholecystolithiasis and choledocholithiasis decreased the likelihood of complications resulting from interventions on sphincter of Oddi. Total excision of choledochal cysts with hepaticojejunostomy presenting in adults withstood the proof of time. Multidisciplinary team approach including surgeon, radiologist, and endoscopist with properly timed usage of different diagnostic and therapeutic modalities in a specialized center is the key for successful management.

55.2 Congenital Anomalies

55.2.1 Biliary Atresia

Biliary atresia (BA) is a neonatal disease with progressive obstructive cholangiopathy of the extrahepatic biliary tree as well as fibrosis of the liver parenchyma that occurs in 1 per 10,000 live births. Although the etiology and pathogenesis remain unknown, there is experimental evidence for a primary perinatal infection as well as cellular and humoral autoimmunity. Presentation is usually in the early neonatal period with prolongation of neonatal jaundice. Kasai hepatoportoenterostomy (HPE) achieves restoration of bile flow in about 50%–70% of infants depending on the age at time of surgery. Successful HPE is not curative but it is necessary for transplant free survival [1]. BA remains the leading indication for liver transplant in pediatric recipients accounting for 32.3% of pediatric liver transplants. Better outcomes reported following maternal liver-related liver transplantation [2].

55.2.2 Choledochal Cyst

Choledochal cyst (CC) is believed to be congenital cystic dilatation of the biliary tree with a frequency of 1 in 150,000 in western countries and has a female to male ratio of 4:1. Pathogenesis of CC is unknown. However, anomalous pancreaticobiliary junction (APBJ) leading to chronic pancreatobiliary reflux may explain it as 70% of patients with CC have APBJ [3]. While children usually have symptoms and signs, adults tend to be asymptomatic. The classical triad of presentation (jaundice, abdominal pain, and mass) is rare to be present all together and most cases still diagnosed incidentally. According to the refined Todani classification, Type I and Type IV are the most common and frequently associated with APBJ, whereas Types II, III, and V are less frequent [4].

55.3 Diagnosis

Liver function tests may be useful but not specific. Abdominal ultrasound is a useful preliminary test. Endoscopic ultrasonography (EUS) helps to differentiate between choledochal and pancreatic cysts. Computed tomography (CT) detects CC and associated malignancy with an accuracy >90%. Magnetic resonance cholangiopancreatography (MRCP) is the most sensitive and specific (90–100%) noninvasive modality [5]. Endoscopic retrograde cholangiopancreatography (ERCP) is the gold standard but it is reserved for delineating biliary anatomy when MRCP fails or for relieving biliary obstruction [5].

55.4 Complications

Adult patients may develop the following complications: hepatic abscesses, cirrhosis, portal hypertension, recurrent pancreatitis, cystolithiasis, hepatolithiasis, and cholelithiasis. There is an increased risk of biliary tract malignancy in patients with CC (10–20%) which increases significantly with age and presence of APBJ [4, 6]. Malignancy occur not only in the cyst wall but also in the remainder of the hepatobiliary and pancreatic tree with gallbladder cancer being reported more frequently (67%) in patients with CC [4]. Risk of malignancy is higher for types I and IV CCs, whereas it is negligible for other types [6].

55.5 Management

Surgery is the mainstay, not only because of the risk of malignancy but also to prevent recurrent complications. Complete excision of the extrahepatic biliary tree to the level of the pancreaticobiliary junction with cholecystectomy and Roux-en-Y hepaticojejunostomy is the standard therapy in Types I and IV [6]. Type II CC is treated with simple cyst excision and primary repair. Small type III CC can be managed effectively with endoscopic sphincterotomy, while lesions >3 cm need surgical excision. For type V, partial hepatectomy is indicated for confined CC or liver transplant if the entire intrahepatic biliary tree involved. In the absence of malignancy, the 5-year overall survival is more than 90%. But it is poor if malignancy coexists [6]. Patients need lifelong follow-up as the rest of the pancreaticobiliary tree is still at risk of subsequent cancer development (about 11%) 25 years post resection and for early detection of anastomotic stricture [7].

55.5.1 Gallstones

Gallstones (GS) affect 10–20% of adult Caucasians with variable prevalence throughout the world. The highest prevalence is in North American Indians, whereas it is the lowest among Asia and sub-Saharan Africa. In addition to ethnicity, female sex, increasing age, and overnutrition are the main risk factors. Only 1–2% develop GS related complications requiring surgery. The prevalence overall was 7.9% of men and 16.6% of women [8].

55.6 Pathogenesis

Gallstones are classified as cholesterol (80–85%) that forms mainly in the gallbladder or pigment stones. The mechanisms contributing to the formation of cholesterol gallbladder stones are cholesterol supersaturation of bile, gallbladder hypomotility, and destabilization of bile by kinetic protein factors [9]. Stasis of bile in the gallbladder favors stone formation, as indicated by stone formation during pregnancy, rapid weight loss, or total parenteral nutrition. Gallbladder hypomotility is probably due to absorption of cholesterol from supersaturated bile by the gallbladder wall that paralyzing gallbladder contractile function [9].

Black pigment stones consist mainly of polymerized calcium bilirubinate. Hemolytic anemias or ineffective erythropoiesis are the most common sources of excess unconjugated bilirubin. Another pathway involves ileal disease or resection causing spillage of bile salts into the colon that results in increased enterohepatic cycling and biliary secretion of bilirubin [9].

Brown pigment stones are mostly formed within the bile ducts as a consequence of bacterial infection and hydrolysis of glucuronic acid from bilirubin by bacterial b-glucuronidase. Intrahepatic brown pigment stones are related to infestation with the parasites *Clonorchis sinensis* and *Ascaris lumbricoides* [9].

55.7 Natural History of Gallstones

Over 80% of GS are asymptomatic [9]. Around 30% of people with asymptomatic GS will require surgical intervention in their lifetime [10]. So, prophylactic cholecystectomy is not recommended for this group of asymptomatic patients [8].

Biliary pain "colic" is a constant dull aching pain in the epigastrium or right upper quadrant for more than half an hour radiating to the back or right shoulder that might be associated with nausea and vomiting but not fever [11]. GS can also cause nonspecific abdominal symptoms [8]. Abdominal ultrasonography is the imaging method of choice with diagnostic accuracy for the detection of GS exceeds 95% [8]. EUS or MRCP can detect microlithiasis [9].

55.8 Complications

Complications of gallstone disease include: acute cholecystitis, Mirizzi syndrome, biliary pancreatitis, acute ascending cholangitis, and gallstone ileus.

55.9 Bile Duct Stones

Common bile duct stones (CBDS) are estimated to be present in 10–20% of patients with symptomatic GS [11]. Symptoms of CBDS are mainly epigastric and/or right upper quadrant abdominal pain and obstructive jaundice can be the presentation [9]. CBDS are usually characterized by elevation of liver enzymes and dilatation of the diameter of the common bile duct. The most reliable method of diagnosis is MRCP or EUS [11].

55.10 Management

Symptomatic GBS are managed by laparoscopic cholecystectomy (LC) which represents the gold standard. Asymptomatic GS should be observed and until now there are no randomized controlled trials performed on whether asymptomatic GS should be managed in the general population [9].

Symptomatic CBDS represent around 10% [11]. ERCP with endoscopic sphincterotomy and extraction of the stone is one option of treatment although there is a risk of complications like acute pancreatitis, bleeding, and perforation. Open or laparoscopic common bile duct exploration depending on the experience of the surgeon is performed when ERCP is failed. There is strong evidence in the literature now that laparoscopic one-stage surgery for both the GBS and CBDS is the preferred treatment [11].

55.11 Intrahepatic Stones

Prevalent but decreasing in south east Asia, rare in the west, represent a challenging problem because usually associated with biliary stricture, recurrent cholangitis, secondary biliary cirrhosis and may progress to cholangiocarcinoma. Four factors seem to contribute to its pathogenesis (stasis, infection, anatomic biliary variation, and bile metabolic defect). Liver resection is the ideal treatment for isolated unilateral disease. Minimally invasive procedures like percutaneous or endoscopic lithotripsy may be the ideal treatment for diffuse bilateral disease [12].

55.12 Gallstones in Pregnancy

Cholecystitis is considered the second most common surgical emergency in pregnancy that ranges from 0.05–0.8%. Conservative management versus LC has the same morbidity and mortality on the mother and fetus. LC proved its safety in all trimesters of pregnancy, but if possible, to be done during the second trimester [13, 14].

55.13 Gallbladder Stones and Biliary Cancer

Evidence from cohort studies suggest an increased incidence of gallbladder cancer and intra and extrahepatic cholangiocarcinoma in patients with GS, this risk diminishes several years after cholecystectomy [15].

55.13.1 Benign Biliary Strictures (BBS)

BBS most often arise from postoperative or inflammatory etiologies. Surgery-related BBS most frequently results from LC (0.4–0.6%), bile duct surgery, and liver transplant [16, 17]. BBS are iatrogenic (80%) related to LC while chronic pancreatitis-related are the most common nonsurgical BBS (13–21%) [18].

55.14 Iatrogenic Biliary Injury

Iatrogenic biliary injury occurs when surgeons fail to appropriately avoid the main bile duct (MBD) and its blood supply during cholecystectomy [19]. It causes significant patient morbidity, mortality, and decreased survival rate, requiring complex and costly management [20, 21].

Adequate dissection to achieve the critical view of safety described by Strasberg, Rouviere's sulcus as the first landmark and using indocyanine green fluorescence contrast are widely believed to decrease the risk of MBD injury in LC [22–24]. Also, indication for LC and presence of anatomical variation are considered risk factors. Routine use of intraoperative cholangiogram (IOC) does not prevent MBD injury but has the ability to intraoperatively recognize it [25].

The outcome of reconstruction depends on the type of injury, associated vascular injury, and the anatomical location. Bismuth and Strasberg classifications are the most commonly used systems to describe iatrogenic bile duct injuries [26, 27].

Injuries are recognized intraoperatively only in approximately one third of patients and in 70–80% of cases with true partial injury or transection of the MBD. It should be considered if more than a single duct is seen or suspected and if bile is observed to be leaking from the area of the porta hepatis and hepatoduodenal ligament [28]. A majority of these unrecognized injuries involve bile leaks from the cystic duct and rarely small ducts of Luschka and may present early with a postoperative biliary fistula, symptoms of biliary peritonitis or jaundice but they can be vague and the diagnosis can be challenging. Ligation of the bile duct will present early with jaundice; however, later presentation may occur as a result of stricture formation from a partial injury, localized inflammation, or ischemic insult [28]. In many patients there is a delay until referral and this delay is not inconsequential as the opportunity for an early repair is lost and results in poor outcome [28, 29].

Work up for patients depends on patient status. Abdominal ultrasound may visualize fluid collection. Doppler imaging can aid in diagnosis of concomitant vascular injury [30]. CT scan should be done in patient with diffuse abdominal pain and tenderness. MRCP allows for confirmation and delineation of the anatomy proximal and distal to the injury [31]. Although ERCP can only assess biliary tree anatomy distal to an injury, it can be of therapeutic value at the time of diagnosis [32]. Hepatobiliary iminodiacetic acid (HIDA) scan has increased sensitivity compared with MRCP for demonstrating ongoing bile leak particularly in the early postoperative period [33].

Controlling biliary injury and associated sepsis is the first treatment aim which can be achieved by: percutaneous transhepatic cholangiography (PTC) and drainage in case of cholangitis with MBD occlusion, percutaneous drainage in case of intra-abdominal abscess or biloma, or prompt emergent operative exploration in case of biliary peritonitis. Establishing bile flow from the biliary tree to the alimentary tract is the next step.

Who, when, and where? are important factors to determine the outcome of the repair [34, 35]. Early referral to a tertiary care center with a multidisciplinary team management is the standard of care. Timing of repair can be challenging and remains controversial [35]. Repairs performed early, within 72 hours of injury, or late, more than 6 weeks after the injury with limited number of concomitant vascular injuries had significantly fewer long-term strictures compared with intermediate repairs [36]. No difference in the outcome was noticed with intermediate repairs compared with late repair provided it is done by hepatobiliary surgeons. But worse outcome in all categories when repair was performed early by the primary surgeon [35, 37].

Nonoperative management in the form of percutaneous and ERCP therapy for biliary injury can be used as a definitive treatment or as a temporary management. ERCP, sphincterotomy, balloon dilatation, and stenting were a successful definitive treatment in about 82% of patients with bile duct injury but without transection and 80% of patients with postcholecystectomy MBD stricture [32]. Definitive operative reconstruction should be performed under optimal conditions [21]. Operative management remains the gold standard for repair of iatrogenic biliary injury when complete MBD transections and occlusions present and injury cannot be managed with ERCP. Simple repair over a T tube is appropriate for non-thermal injuries involving less than 50% of the diameter of the CBD and for small lateral sidewall injuries [38]. Primary end to end tension free anastomosis is possible in case of sharp transection injury without involvement of hepatic duct confluence and no significant tissue loss [39]. The gold standard for operative repair of iatrogenic MBD injury is a hepaticojejunostomy with 70 cm Roux limb to minimize the risk of enteric reflux. Lowering the hilar plate allows easier identification of the left and right hepatic ducts [40]. Anastomotic strictures are reported in 4%–38% of patients who underwent hepaticojejunostomy with a revision rate of 20–25% [19, 29]. Liver resection and transplantation may be necessary [29]. Concomitant vasculo-biliary injury and lesions proximal to the hepatic duct confluence are the significant risk factors for such sequalae [28].

55.15 Mirizzi Syndrome (MS)

MS is a rare complication of symptomatic gallstone. It is due to impacted gallstone in the infundibulum causing compression on the bile duct and chronic inflammation of the gallbladder wall. Type I is external compression of the bile duct only while other types are associated with cholecystobiliary fistula. They present most commonly with obstructive jaundice or picture of acute cholecystitis. ERCP is the gold standard for diagnosis and therapeutic intervention. As it is most commonly diagnosed during surgery and carries a high risk for biliary injury (17%), conversion to open cholecystectomy is still the standard of care. For type I, classical open cholecystectomy or subtotal cholecystectomy is recommended. For types II and III, subtotal cholecystectomy is recommended leaving a small remnant of gallbladder wall over the cholecystobiliary fistula. But if the defect is large and for type IV, it is recommended to do bilioenteric anastomosis [41].

55.16 Liver Transplantation Related BBS

BBS after liver transplantation occurs at an incidence of 10%–40% most commonly at the anastomotic site [17]. Anastomotic strictures are typically single focal stricture and more frequently associated with living-donor livers. Endoscopic therapy is an effective first-line treatment with high stricture resolution rate of 66.7–100%. Late-onset strictures (≥6 months post transplantation) are likely to require more endoscopic interventions than those presenting in the early post-transplant period [42].

Non-anastomotic strictures are defined as those occurring ≥5 mm proximally to the anastomosis and are associated with ischemic events. They are characterized by multiple extrahepatic and/or intrahepatic strictures with recurrent sludge or stone formation. Late-onset non-anastomotic strictures (≥1 year post transplantation) are more resistant to endoscopic therapy than anastomotic types with higher rates of stricture recurrence [42].

55.17 Primary Sclerosing Cholangitis (PSC)

PSC is a progressive, immune-mediated, obliterative inflammatory process of intrahepatic and extrahepatic biliary ducts. Patients usually present between 35 and 47 years of age, with male predilection. It is highly associated with inflammatory bowel disease and highly regarded as a premalignant lesion for hepatobiliary and colorectal malignancy. The gold standard for the diagnosis of PSC is cholangiography that shows short annular strictures alternating between normal and dilated intervening segments resulting in the classical appearance of "beads on a string." MRCP is routinely recommended as the initial imaging study of choice while ERCP is recommended because of the likelihood of requiring intervention [43]. Ursodeoxycholic acid is used to treat pruritus and is associated with improvement in biochemical and histological appearance. Liver transplantation remains the only curative therapy at present [43].

55.17.1 Biliary Dyskinesia

Biliary dyskinesia is a functional disorder of gallbladder and biliary sphincter of Oddi (SOD). As it is a diagnosis of exclusion, it is recommended to follow Rome IV consensus criteria when investigating patients with biliary type pain to exclude stones or microlithiasis within the gallbladder or biliary tree or any other structural abnormalities [44].

In case of functional gallbladder disorder, a low ejection fraction on gallbladder scintigraphy (<40%) is no longer required for diagnosis, but remains an important supportive criterion [50]. Cholecystectomy is considered the mainstay of management with reported symptomatic relief of (91–98%).

Functional biliary SOD is incompletely understood. In the current Rome IV criteria, the classical types of SOD (types I, II, and III) are no longer used. Previous type I (papillary stenosis) is a pure mechanical obstruction. The diagnosis of SOD relies on clinical suspicion, exclusion of functional and organic mimickers. In the EPISOD trial, patients diagnosed with type III SOD (normal laboratory studies, normal bile duct) did not benefit from ERCP and sphincterotomy. Also, no benefit was observed in the limited number of patients with type II [45]. In view of procedure-related complications and unsatisfactory results, ERCP and sphincterotomy should only be performed for carefully selected patients at specialized centers.

References

1. Shneider BL, Abel B, Haber B, et al. Portal hypertension in children and young adults with biliary atresia. J Pediatr Gastroenterol Nutr. 2012;55(5):567–73.
2. Kim WR, Lake JR, Smith JM, et al. OPTN/SRTR 2016 annual data report: liver. Am J Transplant. 2018;18(Suppl 1):172–253.
3. Japanese Study Group on Pancreaticobiliary Maljunction (JSPBM). Sum of registered cases. In: Komi N, Funabiki T (eds) Pancreaticobiliary maljunction. Its consensus and controversy (in Japanese). Igakutosho, Tokyo, 1997; pp 409–425.
4. Todani T, Watanabe Y, Narusue M, Katsusuke T, Okajima K. Congenital bile duct cysts: classification, operative procedures, and review of thirty-seven cases including cancer arising from choledochal cyst. Am J Surg. 1997;134:263–9.
5. Itoh S, Fukushima H, Takada A, et al. Assessment of anomalous pancreaticobiliary ductal junction with high-resolution multiplanar reformatted images in MDCT. Am J Roentgenol. 2006;187:668–75.
6. Huang CS, Huang CC, Chen DF. Choledochal cysts: differences between pediatric and adult patients. J Gastrointest Surg. 2010;14:1105–10.
7. Soares KC, Arnaoutakis DJ, Kamel I, et al. Choledochal cysts: presentation, clinical differentiation, and management. J Am Coll Surg. 2014;219(6):1167–80.
8. Ohashi T, Wakai T, Kubota M, et al. Risk of subsequent biliary malignancy in patients undergoing cyst excision for congenital choledochal cysts. J Gastroenterol Hepatol. 2013;28(2):243–7.
9. Paumgartner G, Sauerbruch T. Gallstones: pathogenesis. Lancet. 1991;338:1117e1121.
10. Grunhage F, Lammert F. Nature Reviews | Disease Primers, Best Practice & Research Clinical. Gastroenterology. 2006;20(6):997e1015.
11. S.daradkeh: Laparoscopic cholecystectomy:analytical study of 1208 cases. Hepatogastroenterology 2005;52:1011–1014.
12. Xi Ran, Baobing Yin, and Baojin Ma. Four major factors contributing to intrahepatic stones. Gastroenterol Res Pract Volume 2017, Article ID 7213043, 5 pages.

13. Date RS, Kaushal M, Ramesh A. A review of the management of gallstone disease and its complications in pregnancy. Am J Surg. 2008;196:599–608.
14. Daradkeh S, Sumrein I, Daoud F, et al. Management of gallbladder stones during pregnancy: conservative treatment or laparoscopic cholecystectomy? Hepato-Gastroenterology. 1999;46:3074–6.
15. Nordenstedt H, et al. Gallstones and cholecystectomy in relation to risk of intra- and extrahepatic cholangiocarcinoma. Br J Cancer. 2012;106:1011–5.
16. Fong ZV, Pitt HA, Strasberg SM, et al. Diminished survival in patients with bile leak and ductal injuries: management strategy and outcomes. J Am Coll Surg 2018; 226(4):568–76. e1.
17. Chan CH, Donnellan F, Byrne MF, et al. Response to endoscopic therapy for biliary anastomotic strictures in deceased versus living donor liver transplantation. Hepatobiliary Pancreat Dis Int. 2013;12(5):488–93.
18. Lévy P, Barthet M, Mollard BR, Amouretti M, Marion-Audibert AM, Dyard F. Estimation of the prevalence and incidence of chronic pancreatitis and its complications. Gastroentérol Clin Biol. 2006;30(6–7):838–44.
19. Kholdebarin R, Boetto J, Harnish JL, et al. Risk factors for bile duct injury during laparoscopic cholecystectomy: a case-control study. Surg Innov. 2008;15(2):114–9.
20. Halbert C, Altieri MS, Yang J, et al. Long-term outcomes of patients with common bile duct injury following laparoscopic cholecystectomy. Surg Endosc. 2016;30(10):4294–9.
21. Sarno G, Al-Sarira AA, Ghaneh P, Fenwick SW, Malik HZ, Poston GJ. Cholecystectomy-related bile duct and vasculobiliary injuries. Br J Surg. 2012;99(8):1129–36.
22. Pucher PH, Brunt LM, Fanelli RD, et al. SAGES expert Delphi consensus: critical factors for safe surgical practice in laparoscopic cholecystectomy. Surg Endosc. 2015;29(11):3074–8.
23. Singh M, Prasad N. The anatomy of Rouviere's sulcus as seen during laparoscopic cholecystectomy: a proposed classification. J Minim Access Surg. 2017;13(2):89–95.
24. Ankersmit M, van Dam DA, van Rijswijk AS, van den Heuvel B, Tuynman JB, Meijerink WJHJ. Fluorescent imaging with indocyanine green during laparoscopic cholecystectomy in patients at increased risk of bile duct injury. Surg Innov. 2017;24(3):245–52.
25. Ragulin-Coyne E, Witkowski ER, Chau Z, et al. Is routine intraoperative cholangiogram necessary in the twenty-first century? a national view. J Gastrointest Surg. 2013;17(3):434–42.
26. Bismuth H, Majno PE. Biliary strictures: classification based on the principles of surgical treatment. World J Surg. 2001;25:1241–4.
27. Schmidt SC, Settmacher U, Langrehr JM, et al. Management and outcome of patients with combined bile duct and hepatic arterial injuries after laparoscopic cholecystectomy. Surgery. 2004;135(6):613–8.
28. Li J, Frilling A, Nadalin S, et al. Timing and risk factors of hepatectomy in the management of complications following laparoscopic cholecystectomy. J Gastrointest Surg. 2011;16(4):815–20.
29. Johnson SR, Koehler A, Pennington LK, Hanto DW. Long-term results of surgical repair of bile duct injuries following laparoscopic cholecystectomy. Surgery. 2000;128(4):668–77.
30. McPartland KJ, Pomposelli JJ. Iatrogenic biliary injuries: classification, identification, and management. Surg Clin North Am. 2008;88(6):1329–43.
31. Ragozzino A, De Ritis R, Mosca A, et al. Value of MR cholangiography in patients with iatrogenic bile duct injury after cholecystectomy. AJR Am J Roentgenol. 2004;183(6):1567–72.
32. Rainio M, Lindström O, Udd M, et al. Endoscopic therapy of biliary injury after cholecystectomy. Dig Dis Sci. 2017;63(2):474–80.
33. Bujanda L, Calvo MM, Cabriada JL, et al. MRCP in the diagnosis of iatrogenic bile duct injury. NMR Biomed. 2003;16(8):475–8.
34. Fischer CP, Fahy BN, Aloia TA, et al. Timing of referral impacts surgical outcomes in patients undergoing repair of bile duct injuries. HPB (Oxford). 2009;11(1):32–7.
35. Felekouras E, Petrou A, Neofytou K, et al. Early or delayed intervention for bile duct injuries following laparoscopic cholecystectomy? A dilemma looking for an answer. Gastroenterol Res Pract. 2015;1–10.
36. Sahajpal AK, Chow SC, Dixon E, et al. Bile duct injuries associated with laparoscopic cholecystectomy: timing of repair and long-term outcomes. Arch Surg. 2010;145(8):757–63.
37. Perera MTPR, Silva MA, Hegab B, et al. Specialist early and immediate repair of post laparoscopic cholecystectomy bile duct injuries is associated with an improved long-term outcome. Ann Surg. 2011;253(3):553–60.
38. Brunicardi FC, Anderson DK, Billiar TR, et al. Schwartz's principles of surgery. 10th ed. New York: McGraw-Hill; 2015. p. 1332–4.
39. Jablonska B. End-to-end ductal anastomosis in biliary reconstruction: indications and limitations. Can J Surg. 2014;57(4):271–7.
40. Moris D, Papalampros A, Vailas M, et al. The hepaticojejunostomy technique with intra-anastomotic stent in biliary diseases and its evolution throughout the years: a technical analysis. Gastroenterol Res Pract. 2016:1–7.
41. Beltran MA, Csendes A, Cruces KS. The relationship of Mirizzi syndrome and cholecystoenteric fistula: validation of a modified classification. World J Surg. 2008;32(10):2237–43.
42. Ryu CH, Lee SK. Biliary strictures after liver transplantation. Gut Liver. 2011;5(2):133–42.
43. Chapman R, Fevery J, Kalloo A, et al. Diagnosis and management of primary sclerosing cholangitis. Hepatology. 2010;51(2):660–78.
44. Cotton PB, Elta GH, Carter CR, et al. Gallbladder and sphincter of Oddi disorders. Gastroenterology. 2016;150(6):1420–9. e2.
45. Cotton PB, Durkalski V, Romagnuolo J, et al. Effect of endoscopic sphincterotomy for suspected sphincter of Oddi dysfunction on pain-related disability following cholecystectomy: the EPISOD randomized clinical trial. JAMA. 2014;311(20):2101–9.

Major Hepatic Resection for Peri-hilar Biliary Cancers

Fabio Bagante, Marzia Tripepi, Alfredo Guglielmi, Calogero Iacono, and Andrea Ruzzenente

Abstract

Surgical resection remains the only potentially curative treatment for pCC but, given the tumor anatomical position and advances stage at diagnosis, surgery is still demanding with high risk of postoperative morbidity and unsatisfactory long term outcomes.

Preoperative management of pCC patients includes biliary drainage and modulation of future liver volume, mainly by using portal vein embolization (PVE).

The type of surgical resection is related to tumor extension according to the Bismuth-Corlette classification, and in most cases is a major liver resection associated with caudate resection, extra hepatic bile duct. In addition, an adequate regional lymph-node dissection is required to achieve a curative surgery.

Extended liver resections (of more than 5 liver segments) associated with portal and/or arterial resections has been proposed to increase the radicality of surgery and improve long term results, however results of aggressive surgery are still under evaluation in Western Countries.

Among factors related with long term results, surgical margins and lymph node status are those with higher prognostic value.

An improvement of short- and long-term result of surgery for pCC is desirable, enhanced preoperative patients' management and improvements of technical aspects of surgical resection are nowadays under evaluation.

56.1 Introduction

Cholangiocarcinoma (CCA) is the second most common primary liver tumor. CCA is usually classified based on the anatomical location in intrahepatic (iCC) and extrahepatic (eCC) which can be further classified in perihilar (pCC) and distal (dCC) cholangiocarcinoma [1]. While pCC includes tumor arising from the U point (the umbilical portion of the left portal vein) and the P point (the bifurcation of the anterior branch and the posterior branch of the right portal vein) to the common hepatic duct above the cystic duct, iCC comprises tumor arising more distally along the intrahepatic bile ducts. Conversely, dCCA includes tumors from the common bile duct to ampulla of Vater [2]. pCC is the most frequent biliary cancer representing approximately 60–70% of all CCA [3]. Currently, surgical resection remains the only potentially curative treatment for pCC but, given the tumor anatomical position close to the hilum, the majority of pCCA patients present at diagnosis an advanced disease [4, 5]. Even though liver resection for pCCA has been associated with a high incidence of morbidity and 90-day mortality, a careful staging, and perioperative and multidisciplinary management as well as an optimal surgical approach could improve short-term outcomes [6].

56.2 Preoperative Evaluation

Preoperatively, the majority of pCC patients have varying degrees of malnutrition, requiring a precise assessment of the nutritional status [7]. Moreover, accurate preoperative patients imaging (computer tomography, magnetic resonance imaging) studies are required to evaluate the suitability of surgical resection, to estimate the longitudinal and circumferential extension, to identify individual anatomic variations as well as to plan the most precise surgical approach [2, 8]. Importantly, an accurate estimation of the

F. Bagante · M. Tripepi · A. Guglielmi (✉) · C. Iacono · A. Ruzzenente
Department of Surgery, Dentistry, Gynecology and Pediatrics, Division of General and Hepato-Biliary Surgery, University of Verona, Verona, Italy
e-mail: alfredo.guglielmi@univr.it

future liver remnant (FLR) volume and function is essential in the management of pCC and should be carefully done in order to plan the surgical resection.

56.2.1 Preoperative Biliary Drainage

The vast majority of patients with pCC have jaundice at presentation requiring a prompt management. In particular, a prolonged obstructive jaundice due to pCC might cause hepatic dysfunction and increase the risk of postoperative mortality in patients undergoing major/extended liver resection [9]. Even though Farges et al. reported that patients undergoing left-sided hepatectomy should not undergo preoperative biliary drainage, pCC patients undergoing right-side major hepatectomies should undergo biliary drainage to reduce the post-operative complications [10]. While there is a general consensus on the bile drainage of the FLR, the optimal type of biliary drainage (i.e., percutaneous transhepatic biliary drainage [PTBD] or endoscopic biliary drainage [EBD]) is still being debated [11]. In particular, while Eastern authors have reported that PTBD might increases the incidence of metastasis and EBD is recommended as the optimal method for preoperative biliary drainage, several Western authors did not identify any difference when comparing PTBD and EBD [12, 13]. A recent randomized clinical trial comparing PTBD and EBD for resectable pCC patients was prematurely stopped because of higher all-cause mortality in the PTBD group [14]. Interestingly, post-drainage complications were similar between the two groups indicating the need of more evidence to identify the optimal strategy for biliary drainage for pCC patients [14]. Finally, even though Eastern surgeons suggest to perform an endoscopic nasobiliary drainage (ENBD) for pCC patients undergoing liver surgery based on studies reporting a low incidence of preoperative cholangitis, currently, ENBD is rarely performed in Western centers [15].

56.2.2 Portal Vein Embolization

The most common complication following major/extended liver resection for pCC is post-hepatectomy liver failure (PHLF) strongly associated with the volume of the FLR. To reduce the risk of PHLF, the limits for a safe resection the FLR should be greater than 30% of total liver volume (TLV) among patients with normal liver. Conversely, among patients with injured livers (i.e., cirrhosis, cholestasis), the FLR should be 30–40% of TLV [16]. Portal vein embolization (PVE) aims to interrupt the portal circulation in the territory to be resected and to initiate a compensatory liver hypertrophy in the FLR. Using a cohort of 1667 patients, the Perihilar Cholangiocarcinoma Collaboration Group performed a propensity score matching to compare 98 patients who underwent PVE versus 98 patients who did not underwent PVE with similar characteristics [17]. The authors reported that the group of patients who underwent PVE had a lower incidence of PHLF (8% vs. 36%, $p < 0.001$), biliary leakage (10% vs. 35%, $p < 0.01$), intra-abdominal abscesses (19% vs. 34%, $p = 0.01$), and 90-day mortality (7% vs. 18%, $p = 0.03$) compared to the other group demonstrating the importance of PVE as an fundamental part of the surgical treatment of pCC [17]. Several techniques, including associating liver partition with portal vein ligation for staged hepatectomy (ALPPS), and mini-ALPPS has been proposed as an alternative to PVE. Currently, the application of the ALPPS technique in the treatment of pCC resulted in a high incidence of in-hospital morality (up to 48%), appeared inferior compared to standard extended resections in high-risk patients, and ALPPS is no recommended in patients with pCC by the most current guideline [18, 19]. Interestingly, hybrid technique as percutaneous radiofrequency-assisted liver partition with portal vein embolization in staged liver resection (PRALPPS) and laparoscopic mini-ALPPS have been providing encouraging results and might be safe techniques to achieve hypertrophy of FRL more rapidly than PVE [20, 21].

56.3 Principles of Surgical Resection

Curative liver surgery for pCC aims to obtain negative margins (R0) without residual tumor often requiring the resection of bile duct and frequently associated with a major (≥ 3 segments) or extended (≥ 5 segments) hepatectomy, including resection of caudate lobe (S1) and a regional lymphadenectomy [6, 19, 22].

56.3.1 Major Hepatectomy and Concomitant Resection of Segment 1

Several studies have investigated the best surgical approach to achieve a curative resection (R0) for patients with pCC including left hepatectomy (LH), left trisectionectomy (LT), right hepatectomy (RH), and right trisectionectomy (RT) extended to segment 1 with extrahepatic bile duct resection (Fig. 56.1) [23].

In particular, the type of resection depends on location of the tumor, tumor radial and longitudinal extent, its association with the vascular hilar structures as well as patient's biliary anatomy and the FLR [19]. Currently, major hepatectomies are the standard procedures for Bismuth Corlette (BC) type III and IV pCC while the type of liver resection in the treatment of BC type I and II pCC remains controversial [24].

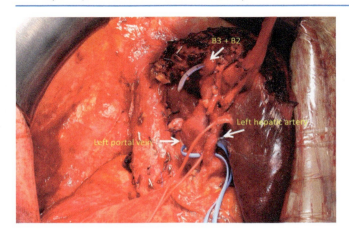

Fig. 56.1 Right trisectionectomy. Red and blue elastic band identify left hepatic artery and main portal vein. Plastic tube in the bile ducts for the 2 and 3 segments

Recently, Chen et al. conducted a systematic review and meta-analysis to compare the incidence of R0 resection and long-term survival outcomes between biliary duct resection and hepatic resection for BC type I and II pCC. The authors showed that hepatic resection was associated with an increased incidence of R0 resection (OR 4.45) and a prolonged overall survival (HR 2.15) compared with isolated biliary duct resection suggesting that BC type I and II pCC patients might benefit from an aggressive surgical approach even with a limited extent of disease [25].

For patients with BC type III and IV pCC, major (≥3 segments) and extended (≥5 segments) hepatectomies represent the best surgical treatments able to achieve a curative treatment (R0). While for pCC involving the right ductal system (BC IIIa or IV) RH/RT are often preferred and LH/LT are done for BC IIIb or IV with a left predominance pCC, RH/RT are often considered the best curative options for patients with BC type III and IV pCC because the right hepatic artery and the right portal vein are more frequently involved and close to the tumor [26, 27]. First proposed by Nimura et al. in 1990, the resection of the caudate segment (S1) has been reported as an important part of the major hepatectomies for pCC to increase the possibility to achieve an R0 status given that the S1 bile ducts join the biliary confluence [28].

56.3.2 Hilar No Touch "En-bloc" Technique

Despite an aggressive surgical approach, pCC is still associated with a significant incidence of local recurrence which strongly impacts the prognosis of pCC patients [29]. Based on these considerations, Neuhaus et al. have proposed a hilar *"en bloc"* resection including RT, extrahepatic bile ducts resection with the portal vein bifurcation, right hepatic artery, and liver segments 1 and 4 to 8 in an effort to avoid spilling neoplastic cells during liver resection. Comparing 50 patients who underwent RT and hilar *"en bloc"* resection versus 50 patients who underwent conventional major/extended hepatectomies for pCC, Neuhaus et al. reported that 5-year overall survival for *"en bloc"* resection was 58% compared with 29% for conventional surgery (p = 0.021) [30]. Despite these encouraging results, several authors have reported doubts about the surgical oncological significance of portal vein resection in patients without tumor vascular infiltration [19, 31, 32].

56.3.3 Vascular Resection

Japanese surgeons were the first to show that an aggressive approach including vascular resection could provide an increased incidence of curative resection in the surgical treatment of pCC [32]. Chen et al. investigated 1921 pCC patients in a systematic review and meta-analysis and reported that even though patients who had portal vein resection showed a poor prognosis compared with patients who did not undergo portal vein resection (HR = 1.90; p < 0.001), patients with a portal vein resection had a significant better prognosis compared with patients who did not undergo liver resection (HR = 0.33; p < 0.001) (Fig. 56.2 and 56.3) [33]. Moreover, the role of hepatic artery resection is still being debated in the treatment of pCC, even though recent studies support the idea that artery resection might save a large number of patients who have a locally advanced pCC otherwise unresectable [34].

56.3.4 Margin Status

Even though there is a general consensus on the importance of a complete resection of the tumor at the surgical margin (R0 resection), the role of intraoperative analysis of frozen section of the bile duct margins to perform an additional resection in case of an R1 margins remains unclear [35]. In particular, several authors have showed that patients who had a R0 surgical margin after an additional resection of previous R1 margin status had a prolonged long-term survival compared with patients with an R1 surgical margin [36]. Conversely, Shingu et al., investigated 303 patients undergoing surgery for pCC and reported that limited resection (<5 mm) of positive margin was not associated with prolonged survival even when a negative (R0) margin can be achieved [37]. Moreover, the clinical implication of the presence of high-grade dysplasia/carcinoma in situ at the surgical margins of pCC is still controversial and some authors reported that it has no clinical implications in terms of recur-

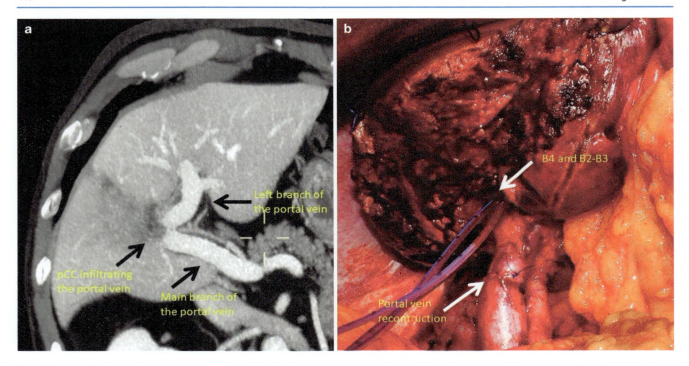

Fig. 56.2 (**a**) CT scan showing perihilar cholangiocarcinoma infiltrating the right and the origin of the left portal vein. (**b**) Right hepatectomy with portal vein reconstruction. Plastic tubes in the bile ducts for the 4 and 2–3 segments

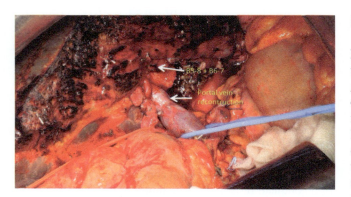

Fig. 56.3 Left hepatectomy with portal vein reconstruction. White arrow indicating the anterior (B 5–8) and posterior (B 6–7) right bile ducts stumps

rence and overall survival [38–40]. Recently, Shinohora et al. investigated the incidence and prognostic role of radial margin status for pCC patients undergoing curative resection rather than only distal margin status. The authors reported that among 478 patients analyzed, the incidence of positive radial margin was the most common cause of R1 resection and that radial margin status would impact the prognosis of pCC patients as positive distal margin [41]. In Eastern series, several authors have proved the survival benefit of hepato-pancreato-duodenectomy in patients with distal/intra-pancreatic bile duct involvement [42].

56.3.5 Lymph Node Dissection

Even though lymph node status has been reported as one of the most important predictor of survival for patients undergoing liver surgery for pCC, the role of lymphadenectomy during surgery for pCC is still debated with significant differences comparing Western and Eastern centers [43, 44]. Recently, the eighth edition of the American Joint Committee on Cancer (AJCC) staging system for pCC has underlined the importance of the nodal status for pCC patients defining stage N1 as patients with 1–3 metastatic lymph nodes, and stage N2 as patients with >3 lymph nodes [45]. Ruzzenente et al. investigated the long-term outcomes of 214 patients who underwent curative-intent surgery at two Italian major hepatobiliary centers (University of Verona and Catholic University of Rome) reporting a 5-year OS was of 33.5% for N1 patients compared with a 5-year OS of 19.1% for N1 patients. Interestingly, none of the patients with stage N2 disease survived for five years after surgery [46].

56.3.6 Minimally Invasive Surgery

Even though in the last decade, minimally invasive surgery (MIS) – laparoscopic and robot-assisted surgery – has played a key role in the surgical treatment of malignant and benign liver disease, there are few data available regarding the application of this surgical approach for pCC patients [47]. In a recent study, Ratti et al. analyzed the outcome of 16 patients with pCC who underwent laparoscopic surgery compared with a group of patients operated by open technique. The authors showed that laparoscopic resections resulted in longer operative time (360 vs 275 min, p = 0.048) while a lower blood loss (380 vs 470, p = 0.048) a lower intraoperative blood transfusion (12.5% vs 21.9%, p = 0.032) and a shorter hospital stay. No differences were found in incidence of R0 resection and in number of lymph node harvested [48]. The laparoscopic approach for pCC is still in a preliminary phase and further studies are needed to validate the results of this surgical approach in pCC patients.

56.4 Short-term Results

The incidence of post-operative morbidity and mortality after major surgery for pCC is still high. In a recent systematic review and meta-analysis, Franken et al. analyzed the short-term outcomes after major liver resection in patients with pCC reported in 51 studies for a total of 4634 patients [49]. The authors reported a pooled overall morbidity and severe morbidity of 57% and 40%, respectively. Interestingly, Western studies reported an a significantly higher overall morbidity (63%) compared with Eastern studies (54%, p = 0.048) [49]. Moreover, pooled incidence of 30-day and 90-day mortality was 5% and 9%, respectively. Similarly, Western studies reported an a significantly higher incidence of 30-day (8%) and 90-day (12%) mortality compared with Eastern studies (30-day: 2%, p < 0.001; 90-day: 3%, p < 0.001) [49]. These results are comparable with those reported by Bagante et al. investigating the US National Surgery Quality Improvement Program (NSQIP) database to identify benchmark values for liver surgery [50]. The authors reported that among the patients undergoing major/extended resection and bile duct resection the benchmark value was 72% as the 75th percentile of the distribution of the probability to have a complication [50].

56.5 Long-term Results

In a recent systematic review and meta-nalysis by Tang et al. on the prognosis of patients with resectable perihilar cholangiocarcinoma, a comparison between the long-term results of Eastern and Western centers revealed a significant difference [51]. While the median incidence of resectability in Eastern (74.9%) and Western (41.2%) countries was significant different (p = 0.025), the difference in terms of R0 resection comparing Eastern (70.7%) and Western (75.9%) centers was comparable (p = 0.98) [51]. Importantly, the median overall survival (OS) at 5-year for Eastern centers was 33.0% was significantly higher compared with the median 5-year OS at Western centers 25.5% (p = 0.001) [51]. Interestingly, in a recent systematic review and meta-analysis, Bird et al. analyzed 24 articles including 4599 pCC patients undergoing curative surgery to identify the most significant prognostic factors. In the pooled analyses, age (HR = 1.16), AJCC T category (HR = 1.49), positive lymph node (HR = 1.78), microvascular invasion (HR = 1.49), perineural invasion (HR = 1.54), and tumor differentiation (HR 1.54) were all associated with patients' prognosis.

56.6 Conclusions

Curative surgery of pCC remains the treatment of choice to achieve long term results, in order to obtain an R0 resection extended liver resections including S1 resection are often required. Although recent advances in preoperative optimizations of liver function with biliary drainage and future liver volume modulation with PVE improved significantly results, surgery for pCC is still a demanding procedure, associated with a high risk of postoperative morbidity and mortality.

An improvement of short- and long-term result of surgery for pCC is desirable, and enhanced preoperative patients' management and improvements of technical aspects of surgical resection are nowadays under evaluation.

Bibliography

1. Cholangiocarcinoma Working G: Italian Clinical Practice Guidelines on Cholangiocarcinoma – Part I: Classification, diagnosis and staging. Dig Liver Dis. 2020;52(11):1282–1293.
2. Endo I, Matsuyama R, Mori R, Taniguchi K, Kumamoto T, Takeda K, Tanaka K, Kohn A, Schenk A. Imaging and surgical planning for perihilar cholangiocarcinoma. J Hepatobiliary Pancreat Sci. 2014;21(8):525–32.
3. Khan SA, Thomas HC, Davidson BR, Taylor-Robinson SD. Cholangiocarcinoma. Lancet. 2005;366(9493):1303–14.
4. Nagino M. Perihilar cholangiocarcinoma: a surgeon's viewpoint on current topics. J Gastroenterol. 2012;47(11):1165–76.
5. Kimbrough CW, Cloyd JM, Pawlik TM. Surgical approaches for the treatment of perihilar cholangiocarcinoma. Expert Rev Anticancer Ther. 2018;18(7):673–83.
6. Mizuno T, Ebata T, Nagino M. Advanced hilar cholangiocarcinoma: an aggressive surgical approach for the treatment of advanced hilar cholangiocarcinoma: perioperative management, extended procedures, and multidisciplinary approaches. Surg Oncol. 2020;33:201–6.
7. Braga M, Gianotti L, Nespoli L, Radaelli G, Di Carlo V. Nutritional approach in malnourished surgical patients: a prospective randomized study. Arch Surg. 2002;137(2):174–80.
8. Lee DH, Kim B, Lee ES, Kim HJ, Min JH, Lee JM, Choi MH, Seo N, Choi SH, Kim SH, et al. Radiologic evaluation and structured reporting form for extrahepatic bile duct cancer: 2019 consensus recommendations from the Korean Society of abdominal radiology. Korean J Radiol. 2021;22(1):41–62.

9. Nuzzo G, Giuliante F, Ardito F, Giovannini I, Aldrighetti L, Belli G, Bresadola F, Calise F, Dalla Valle R, D'Amico DF, et al. Improvement in perioperative and long-term outcome after surgical treatment of hilar cholangiocarcinoma: results of an Italian multicenter analysis of 440 patients. Arch Surg. 2012;147(1):26–34.
10. Farges O, Regimbeau JM, Fuks D, Le Treut YP, Cherqui D, Bachellier P, Mabrut JY, Adham M, Pruvot FR, Gigot JF. Multicentre European study of preoperative biliary drainage for hilar cholangiocarcinoma. Br J Surg. 2013;100(2):274–83.
11. Iacono C, Ruzzenente A, Campagnaro T, Bortolasi L, Valdegamberi A, Guglielmi A. Role of preoperative biliary drainage in jaundiced patients who are candidates for pancreatoduodenectomy or hepatic resection: highlights and drawbacks. Ann Surg. 2013;257(2):191–204.
12. Komaya K, Ebata T, Yokoyama Y, Igami T, Sugawara G, Mizuno T, Yamaguchi J, Nagino M. Verification of the oncologic inferiority of percutaneous biliary drainage to endoscopic drainage: a propensity score matching analysis of resectable perihilar cholangiocarcinoma. Surgery. 2017;161(2):394–404.
13. Wiggers JK, Groot Koerkamp B, Coelen RJ, Doussot A, van Dieren S, Rauws EA, Schattner MA, van Lienden KP, Brown KT, Besselink MG, et al. Percutaneous preoperative biliary drainage for resectable perihilar cholangiocarcinoma: no association with survival and no increase in seeding metastases. Ann Surg Oncol. 2015;22(Suppl 3):S1156–63.
14. Coelen RJS, Roos E, Wiggers JK, Besselink MG, Buis CI, Busch ORC, Dejong CHC, van Delden OM, van Eijck CHJ, Fockens P, et al. Endoscopic versus percutaneous biliary drainage in patients with resectable perihilar cholangiocarcinoma: a multicentre, randomised controlled trial. Lancet Gastroenterol Hepatol. 2018;3(10):681–90.
15. Maeda T, Ebata T, Yokoyama Y, Mizuno T, Yamaguchi J, Onoe S, Watanabe N, Kawashima H, Nagino M. Preoperative course of patients undergoing endoscopic nasobiliary drainage during the management of resectable perihilar cholangiocarcinoma. J Hepatobiliary Pancreat Sci. 2019;26(8):341–7.
16. Guglielmi A, Ruzzenente A, Conci S, Valdegamberi A, Iacono C. How much remnant is enough in liver resection? Dig Surg. 2012;29(1):6–17.
17. Olthof PB, Aldrighetti L, Alikhanov R, Cescon M, Groot Koerkamp B, Jarnagin WR, Nadalin S, Pratschke J, Schmelze M, Sparrelid E, et al. Portal vein embolization is associated with reduced liver failure and mortality in high-risk resections for perihilar cholangiocarcinoma. Ann Surg Oncol. 2020;27(7):2311–8.
18. Olthof PB, Coelen RJS, Wiggers JK, Groot Koerkamp B, Malago M, Hernandez-Alejandro R, Topp SA, Vivarelli M, Aldrighetti LA, Robles Campos R, et al. High mortality after ALPPS for perihilar cholangiocarcinoma: case-control analysis including the first series from the international ALPPS registry. HPB (Oxford). 2017;19(5):381–7.
19. Cholangiocarcinoma Working G: Italian Clinical Practice Guidelines on Cholangiocarcinoma – Part II: Treatment. Dig Liver Dis. 2020;52(12):1430–1442.
20. Melekhina O, Efanov M, Alikhanov R, Tsvirkun V, Kulezneva Y, Kazakov I, Vankovich A, Koroleva A, Khatkov I. Percutaneous radiofrequency-assisted liver partition versus portal vein embolization before hepatectomy for perihilar cholangiocarcinoma. BJS Open. 2020;4(1):101–8.
21. de Santibanes E, Alvarez FA, Ardiles V, Pekolj J, de Santibanes M. Inverting the ALPPS paradigm by minimizing first stage impact: the Mini-ALPPS technique. Langenbeck's Arch Surg. 2016;401(4):557–63.
22. Rassam F, Roos E, van Lienden KP, van Hooft JE, Klumpen HJ, van Tienhoven G, Bennink RJ, Engelbrecht MR, Schoorlemmer A, Beuers UHW, et al. Modern work-up and extended resection in perihilar cholangiocarcinoma: the AMC experience. Langenbeck's Arch Surg. 2018;403(3):289–307.
23. Nagino M, Ebata T, Yokoyama Y, Igami T, Sugawara G, Takahashi Y, Nimura Y. Evolution of surgical treatment for perihilar cholangiocarcinoma: a single-center 34-year review of 574 consecutive resections. Ann Surg. 2013;258(1):129–40.
24. Miyazaki M, Kimura F, Shimizu H, Yoshidome H, Otsuka M, Kato A, Hideyuki Y, Nozawa S, Furukawa K, Mituhashi N, et al. Extensive hilar bile duct resection using a transhepatic approach for patients with hepatic hilar bile duct diseases. Am J Surg. 2008;196(1):125–9.
25. Chen RX, Li CX, Luo CH, Zhang H, Zhou T, Wu XF, Wang XH, Li XC. Surgical strategies for the treatment of bismuth type I and II Hilar cholangiocarcinoma: bile duct resection with or without hepatectomy? Ann Surg Oncol. 2020;27(9):3374–82.
26. Uesaka K. Left hepatectomy or left trisectionectomy with resection of the caudate lobe and extrahepatic bile duct for hilar cholangiocarcinoma (with video). J Hepatobiliary Pancreat Sci. 2012;19(3):195–202.
27. Bismuth H. Surgical anatomy and anatomical surgery of the liver. World J Surg. 1982;6(1):3–9.
28. Nimura Y, Hayakawa N, Kamiya J, Kondo S, Shionoya S: Hepatic segmentectomy with caudate lobe resection for bile duct carcinoma of the hepatic hilus. World J Surg. 1990;14(4):535–543; discussion 544.
29. Zhang XF, Beal EW, Chakedis J, Chen Q, Lv Y, Ethun CG, Salem A, Weber SM, Tran T, Poultsides G, et al. Defining early recurrence of hilar cholangiocarcinoma after curative-intent surgery: a multi-institutional study from the US extrahepatic biliary malignancy consortium. World J Surg. 2018;42(9):2919–29.
30. Neuhaus P, Thelen A, Jonas S, Puhl G, Denecke T, Veltzke-Schlieker W, Seehofer D. Oncological superiority of hilar en bloc resection for the treatment of hilar cholangiocarcinoma. Ann Surg Oncol. 2012;19(5):1602–8.
31. Tamoto E, Hirano S, Tsuchikawa T, Tanaka E, Miyamoto M, Matsumoto J, Kato K, Shichinohe T. Portal vein resection using the no-touch technique with a hepatectomy for hilar cholangiocarcinoma. HPB (Oxford). 2014;16(1):56–61.
32. Nagino M. Fifty-year history of biliary surgery. Ann Gastroenterol Surg. 2019;3(6):598–605.
33. Chen W, Ke K, Chen YL. Combined portal vein resection in the treatment of hilar cholangiocarcinoma: a systematic review and meta-analysis. Eur J Surg Oncol. 2014;40(5):489–95.
34. Mizuno T, Ebata T, Yokoyama Y, Igami T, Yamaguchi J, Onoe S, Watanabe N, Kamei Y, Nagino M: Combined vascular resection for locally advanced perihilar cholangiocarcinoma. Ann Surg. 2020.
35. Komaya K, Ebata T, Yokoyama Y, Igami T, Sugawara G, Mizuno T, Yamaguchi J, Nagino M. Recurrence after curative-intent resection of perihilar cholangiocarcinoma: analysis of a large cohort with a close postoperative follow-up approach. Surgery. 2018;163(4):732–8.
36. Zhang XF, Squires MH 3rd, Bagante F, Ethun CG, Salem A, Weber SM, Tran T, Poultsides G, Son AY, Hatzaras I, et al. The impact of intraoperative re-resection of a positive bile duct margin on clinical outcomes for Hilar cholangiocarcinoma. Ann Surg Oncol. 2018;25(5):1140–9.
37. Shingu Y, Ebata T, Nishio H, Igami T, Shimoyama Y, Nagino M. Clinical value of additional resection of a margin-positive proximal bile duct in hilar cholangiocarcinoma. Surgery. 2010;147(1):49–56.
38. Matthaei H, Lingohr P, Strasser A, Dietrich D, Rostamzadeh B, Glees S, Roering M, Mohring P, Scheerbaum M, Stoffels B, et al. Biliary intraepithelial neoplasia (BilIN) is frequently found in surgical margins of biliary tract cancer resection specimens but has no clinical implications. Virchows Arch. 2015;466(2):133–41.

39. Otsuka S, Ebata T, Yokoyama Y, Mizuno T, Tsukahara T, Shimoyama Y, Ando M, Nagino M. Clinical value of additional resection of a margin-positive distal bile duct in perihilar cholangiocarcinoma. Br J Surg. 2019;106(6):774–82.
40. Sasaki R, Takeda Y, Funato O, Nitta H, Kawamura H, Uesugi N, Sugai T, Wakabayashi G, Ohkohchi N. Significance of ductal margin status in patients undergoing surgical resection for extrahepatic cholangiocarcinoma. World J Surg. 2007;31(9):1788–96.
41. Shinohara K, Ebata T, Shimoyama Y, Mizuno T, Yokoyama Y, Yamaguchi J, Onoe S, Watanabe N, Nagino M. A study on radial margin status in resected perihilar cholangiocarcinoma. Ann Surg. 2021;273(3):572–8.
42. Endo I, Hirahara N, Miyata H, Yamamoto H, Matsuyama R, Kumamoto T, Homma Y, Mori M, Yasuyuki S, Wakabayashi G et al. Mortality, morbidity and failure to rescue in hepatopancreatoduodenectomy: an analysis of 422 patients registered in the National Clinical Database in Japan. J Hepatobiliary Pancreat Sci. 2021.
43. Guglielmi A, Ruzzenente A, Bertuzzo F, Iacono C. Assessment of nodal status for perihilar cholangiocarcinoma location, number, or ratio of involved nodes. Hepatobiliary Surg Nutr. 2013;2(5):281–3.
44. Bagante F, Tran T, Spolverato G, Ruzzenente A, Buttner S, Ethun CG, Groot Koerkamp B, Conci S, Idrees K, Isom CA, et al. Perihilar cholangiocarcinoma: number of nodes examined and optimal lymph node prognostic scheme. J Am Coll Surg. 2016;222(5):750–759 e752.
45. Chun YS, Pawlik TM, Vauthey JN. 8th Edition of the AJCC cancer staging manual: pancreas and hepatobiliary cancers. Ann Surg Oncol. 2018;25(4):845–7.
46. Ruzzenente A, Bagante F, Ardito F, Campagnaro T, Scoleri I, Conci S, Iacono C, Giuliante F, Guglielmi A. Comparison of the 7th and 8th editions of the American Joint Committee on Cancer Staging Systems for perihilar cholangiocarcinoma. Surgery. 2018;164(2):244–50.
47. Franken LC, van der Poel MJ, Latenstein AEJ, Zwart MJ, Roos E, Busch OR, Besselink MG, van Gulik TM. Minimally invasive surgery for perihilar cholangiocarcinoma: a systematic review. J Robot Surg. 2019;13(6):717–27.
48. Ratti F, Fiorentini G, Cipriani F, Catena M, Paganelli M, Aldrighetti L. Perihilar cholangiocarcinoma: are we ready to step towards minimally invasiveness? Updat Surg. 2020;72(2):423–33.
49. Franken LC, Schreuder AM, Roos E, van Dieren S, Busch OR, Besselink MG, van Gulik TM. Morbidity and mortality after major liver resection in patients with perihilar cholangiocarcinoma: a systematic review and meta-analysis. Surgery. 2019;165(5):918–28.
50. Bagante F, Ruzzenente A, Beal EW, Campagnaro T, Merath K, Conci S, Akgul O, Alexandrescu S, Marques HP, Lam V, et al. Complications after liver surgery: a benchmark analysis. HPB (Oxford). 2019;21(9):1139–49.
51. Tang Z, Yang Y, Zhao Z, Wei K, Meng W, Li X. The clinicopathological factors associated with prognosis of patients with resectable perihilar cholangiocarcinoma: a systematic review and meta-analysis. Medicine (Baltimore). 2018;97(34):e11999.

57

Surgical Management of Intrahepatic Cholangiocarcinoma

Mohamed Abdel-Wahab and Ahmed Shehta

Abstract

Intrahepatic cholangiocarcinoma (ICC) is the second most common primary liver cancer, accounting for 10–15% of primary hepatic malignancy. Currently, liver resection is still the most effective treatment for ICC patients to achieve adequate long-term survival, although its overall efficacy may not be as good as that for hepatocellular carcinoma (HCC) patients due to the unique pathogenesis and clinical-pathological profiles of ICC.

Adequate preoperative evaluation of the patients is essential and it mainly focuses on establishing the diagnosis of ICC, rather than other metastatic adenocarcinoma from other primary tumors, and assessment of the suitability of the patient and the tumor for operation. Thorough evaluation should include a detailed history, physical examination, assessment of comorbid conditions, assessment of hepatic function, measurement of tumor markers, and radiologic imaging to assess the extent of disease.

57.1 Introduction

Intrahepatic cholangiocarcinoma (ICC) is the second most common primary liver cancer, accounting for 10–15% of primary hepatic malignancy [1]. Currently, liver resection is still the most effective treatment for ICC patients to achieve adequate long-term survival, although its overall efficacy may not be as good as that for hepatocellular carcinoma (HCC) patients due to the unique pathogenesis and clinical-pathological profiles of ICC [2].

Adequate preoperative evaluation of the patients is essential and it mainly focuses on establishing the diagnosis of ICC, rather than other metastatic adenocarcinoma from other primary tumors, and assessment of the suitability of the patient and the tumor for operation. Thorough evaluation should include a detailed history, physical examination, assessment of comorbid conditions, assessment of hepatic function, measurement of tumor markers, and radiologic imaging to assess the extent of disease [3].

57.2 Clinical Presentation

ICC often present as asymptomatic hepatic mass detected during physical examination or on cross-sectional imaging examinations. Abdominal pain is the most frequent presentation for symptomatic patients. Most patients also present with nonspecific symptoms such as weight loss of appetite. Jaundice can be present in centrally located ICC that compresses or invades the biliary confluence [4].

57.3 Serum Tumor Markers

Serum tumor markers are an attractive method for diagnosing and monitoring treatment response in patients with ICC. To be effective, a marker must be accurate in detecting the presence of malignancy (sensitivity) and defining the presence of benign disease (specificity).

Carcinoembryonic antigen (CEA) is widely used because of its availability but is elevated in only one third of patients with ICC [5]. Carbonic anhydrase 19-9 (CA19-9) is also widely used in the diagnosis of cancers of the upper digestive tract and is elevated in gastric, pancreatic, biliary, and gallbladder cancers, as well as in smokers, cholangitis, and conditions causing cholestasis [6]. Another marker which is commonly used is interleukin-6 (IL-6).

M. Abdel-Wahab (✉) · A. Shehta
Department of Surgery, Liver Transplantation Unit, Gastrointestinal Surgery Center, Mansoura University, Mansoura, Egypt

Serum levels of IL-6 correlate with tumor burden in ICC, but it is also elevated in HCC, metastatic disease, and benign biliary lesions [7].

57.4 Imaging

Accurate cross-sectional imaging is required to diagnose and stage the tumors as well as plan resection or other possible treatments. Most patients will be imaged with a number of modalities.

Transabdominal ultrasound is often used as a screening examination for patients with upper abdominal pain, palpable mass, or jaundice. ICC has a nonspecific appearance as a hypoechoic hepatic mass. Ultrasound is useful for defining the presence of satellite nodules, lymphadenopathy, and associated biliary dilation or portal venous invasion [8].

Triphasic computed tomography (CT) scan is the single most effective investigation in diagnosing and staging ICC. ICC presents as hypodense lesions with irregular, infiltrative margins and a variable degree of delayed enhancement in the portal venous phase (Fig. 57.1a). CT scan can also detect the presence of intrahepatic biliary dilation, portal or hepatic venous involvement, and lobar atrophy. CT scan is also useful in detecting metastatic disease affecting regional lymph nodes, peritoneum, or lung fields. Also, CT volumetry can provide accurate assessment of hepatic remnant volume and the risk of postoperative liver failure [9].

On magnetic resonance imaging (MRI), ICCs appear as hypointense lesions on T1-weighted images and hyperintense on T2-weighted images, with pooling of contrast within the lesions on delayed images. It is also useful in evaluating venous and arterial involvement by tumor. It also allows obtaining a noninvasive cholangiopancreatography [10].

57.5 Treatment

The treatment protocols for ICC are in the development phase when compared to other intrahepatic tumors, owing to the rarity of the tumor. Surgical resection is the most effective treatment for ICC at the present time, but its resectability and curability remain low. Less commonly, liver transplantation has also been applied. The current roles of neoadjuvant and adjuvant chemotherapy, both systemic and regional; conformal radiation therapy; and ablative therapies are under investigation. We aim to review the surgical aspects of the management of ICC including major hepatic resection.

57.6 Surgical Management

57.6.1 Liver Resection

Liver resection is the most effective treatment for ICC at the present time, but its resectability and curability remain low. Only 20–40% of patients with ICC are eligible for potential curative liver resection at the time of the diagnosis. Adjuvant

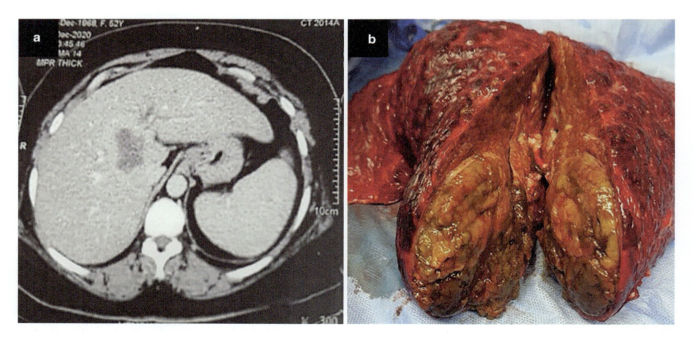

Fig. 57.1 (a) Abdominal computed tomography showing hypodense focal lesion in segment IV of the liver with dilatation of the segmental biliary radicles. (b) Operative specimen after left hemi-hepatectomy for intrahepatic cholangiocarcinoma

chemotherapy and/or radiotherapy has failed to improve survival in most patients of ICC [11].

57.7 Aim of Surgical Resection

The main goal of surgical resection for ICC is to perform R0 margin negative resection with preservation of an adequate future liver remnant (FLR), which means two or more contiguous liver segments with adequate arterial and portal inflow, biliary drainage, and venous outflow [11]. Unlike HCC, most ICC cases have poor blood supply and rare liver cirrhosis, thus extended hepatectomy is often required, including bloc resection with resection of the vessel, bile duct, and adjacent tissue invaded by the tumor in some cases. The extent of resection should be determined by the size and location of the lesion, satellite situation, and the degree of tumor infiltration [2].

57.8 Indications for Surgical Resection

R0 surgical resection of ICC is the most effective treatment modality and the only therapy associated with improved survival outcomes. There is no general agreement on the current indications for surgical resection of ICC. It is generally recommended that R0 resection is best achieved in patients with solitary tumor, negative lymph nodes, and resectable hepatic safety margin of 1 cm or more. With application of these restrictive criteria, excellent survival rates could be accomplished with 2- and 5-years overall survival of 100% and 42%, respectively [12, 13]. On the other hand, ICC patients with one or more negative prognostic factors will not be allowed to undergo surgical resection of ICC and will receive only palliative and supportive care. Therefore, it is evident that the precise indications for surgical resection of ICC require further analysis by future studies.

While negatively affecting outcomes, tumor size, multicentric tumors, and vascular invasion should not be considered absolute contra-indications if negative margins can be achieved. Even patients with advanced complex tumors requiring extensive hepatic resections and major vascular and biliary reconstruction should be considered for curative-intent surgery [14].

57.9 Strategies to Improve the Future Liver Remnant

As previously mentioned, the main goal of surgical resection for ICC is to perform R0 margin resection with preservation of an adequate future liver remnant (FLR), which means two or more contiguous liver segments with adequate arterial and portal inflow, biliary drainage, and venous outflow [11].

A FLR size of at least 20% is generally recommended for patients without underlying liver disease. For patients with underlying hepatic steatosis, the FLR size should be at least 30%. For patients with liver cirrhosis and fibrosis with preserved hepatic function (Child A patients), at least 40% are required to avoid the risk for the development of posthepatectomy liver dysfunction and failure [15]. For patients with marginal expected FLR volume, measures to improve the FLR volume had been applied. Preoperative portal vein embolization (PVE) is usually employed to cause hypertrophy of the contralateral lobe and achieve greater FLR volume. It is applied under radiologic guidance where selective embolization of the target branches of the portal vein is performed. If PVE is properly selected and managed, patients with Child A cirrhosis may achieve similar long-term oncologic outcomes compared to patients with no underlying liver disease [16, 17]. Improvement of FLR with the application of preoperative PVE had been reported to be around 30%–50% after 4–8 weeks from preoperative PVE. The FLR volume increase caused by PVE ranges between 30% and 50% after 4–8 weeks; however, it also may increase the risk of drop-out by up to 30% [18].

A more recently introduced, associating liver partition and portal vein ligation (ALPPS) procedure helps to induce faster improvement of FLR volume compared to PVE (more than 60% in 7 days). It is performed in two stages. In stage 1, the appropriated main branch of the portal vein is ligated together with liver partition at the planned transection line by the anterior approach. In stage 2, division of the remaining inflow and outflow structures of the planned portion to be resected is done. However, outcomes of ALPPS for primary liver tumors are actually discouraging. The procedure is associated with high perioperative morbidity and mortality rates [19, 20]. PVE remains the gold-standard procedure when FLR hypertrophy is needed [21].

57.10 Staging Laparoscopy and Intraoperative Assessment of Resectability

At the time of diagnosis, patients with ICC are frequently found to have a disease burden beyond the limits of surgical intervention. The presence of locally advanced solitary tumors involving either inflow or outflow bilaterally, multiple intrahepatic tumors, extrahepatic disease, including involvement of lymph nodes beyond the regional lymph nodes such as celiac and the para-aortic nodes are considered contraindication to hepatic resection [22, 23].

Staging laparoscopy can be useful in ruling out small peritoneal implants or distant LN disease. When associated with intraoperative ultrasound, it can evaluate the extent of intrahepatic disease, vascular invasion and reveal intraparenchymal metastasis. Therefore, it has a potential role in detecting unresectable disease and avoiding unessential laparotomy, which has been reported to happen in 25–36% of patients [11, 24]. Staging laparoscopy is essentially important in high-risk patients especially those patients with suspected multifocal ICC, suspected peritoneal implants or major vascular invasion, and those with high preoperative tumor markers. The routine use of laparoscopic ultrasound in these cases is therefore advocated.

Also, it is important to carefully evaluate the condition of the hepatic parenchyma, especially the presence of chronic liver disease or cirrhosis which could limit or contraindicate the surgical resection [25].

57.11 Surgical Resection Procedure

Surgical therapy for ICC is based on the surgical principles applied to resection for any hepatic malignancy. Anatomical liver resection with wide margins is generally recommended for ICC if adequate functional liver remnant with adequate venous and biliary drainage remains.

ICC usually develops on a background of non-cirrhotic liver; thus, extended resections can be safely performed (Fig. 57.1b). Advanced stages of ICC can be treated by extended hepatic resection with extension of the resection to the extrahepatic biliary tree, vascular hilar structures, hepatic veins, inferior vena cava, and diaphragm [11, 26]. Studies addressing surgical resection for ICC are summarized in Table 57.1.

The intraductal growth type of ICC is associated with intraductal growth with intraductal tumor thrombus. In these patients, the biliary duct margin should be evaluated by intraoperative frozen section after major hepatic resection. If neoplastic invasion of the bile duct margin is found, extended resection of the extrahepatic biliary tree should be performed [40].

The mass forming type of ICC is associated with high incidence of satellite nodules. It is essential to perform intraoperative ultrasonography in order to identify the presence of metastatic nodules and a radical transection plane [26].

Vascular invasion may be found in about 27%–85% of patients with ICC [46]. Previous studies had shown that the survival outcomes of patients who underwent surgical resection are better than those who did not underwent surgical resection [47]. Vascular resection in combination with hepatectomy increases not only the probability to achieve negative surgical margins, but also the incidence of postoperative

Table 57.1 Short- and long-term outcomes of surgical resection for intrahepatic cholangiocarcinoma

Study	Year	N	Morbidity (%)	30 days mortality (%)	Median survival (month)	Survival (%) 1 Y	3 Ys	5 Ys
Cherqui et al. [12]	1995	14	28	7	27	100		
Pichlmayr et al. [27]	1995	32		10.5	12.8			
Casavilla et al. [28]	1997	34				60	37	31
Madariaga et al. [29]	1998	34	32	14	19	67	40	25
Chu et al. [30]	1999	39	41.7	16.7	12.2	57.3	23.9	15.9
Weber et al. [31]	2001	33			37			31
Kawarada et al. [32]	2002	37	21.6	0	31.5	54.1	34	23.9
Ohtsuka et al. [33]	2002	48	50	8		62	38	23
Lang et al. [24]	2005	16	52	6	46	94	82	
Nakagawa et al. [34]	2005	44	69	5.7	22	66		26
De Oliveira et al. [35]	2007	34	35	4	28			63
Endo et al. [2]	2008	82			36			
Guglielmi et al. [36]	2009	62	32	3.8	41			26
Lang et al. [37]	2009	83	58	7	26	71		21
Nathan et al. [38]	2009	598			21			18
Shen et al. [39]	2009	429			12	51		17
De Jong et al. [40]	2011	449			27	78		31
Farges et al. [41]	2011	212			28	77		28
Saiura et al. [42]	2011	44	35	0	41	87	56	43
Sriputtha et al. [43]	2013	73			12.4	52.1	21.7	11.2
Luo et al. [44]	2014	1333	11.5	0.6	30	79.1	42.6	28.7
Ali et al. [45]	2015	150			44	84		43
Tabrizian et al. [3]	2015	82			16	60	24	16

N, patient number; Ys, years

major complications. Therefore, liver resection in combination with inferior vena cava and portal vein partial resection plus reconstruction or hepatic artery resection may be considered in adequately assessed cases to achieve a R0 resection. Therefore, vascular invasion does not represent an absolute contraindication for surgical resection.

Patients with untreated IHCC have a median survival of less than 12 months. Resection with positive margins or residual macroscopic disease is associated with median survival of 1.8–3 months, indicating that a cytoreductive approach is ineffective at prolonging survival. In contrast, 5-year survival rates after complete resection range between 13% and 43% [26].

57.12 Status of Lymphadenectomy

Although the importance of achieving an R0 resection is clear, the role of routine lymph node dissection is debated. The presence and extent of nodal metastatic disease are important prognostic factors. Current National Comprehensive Cancer Network (NCCN, 2012) guidelines suggest that regional lymphadenectomy should be considered in patients to provide staging information, but that resection should be carefully considered in patients with bulky nodal disease in the porta hepatis [48].

With respect to staging, uniform agreement is lacking on the optimal number of nodes harvested per patient. Usually, three or less are harvested [40], although up to seven nodes are suggested for patients with hilar cholangiocarcinoma [49]. This has led Guglielmi and associates to suggest that the lymph node ratio (LNR) is an important prognostic factor, with an LNR of greater than 0.25 associated with worse survival (19 months, compared to 43 months with LNR of zero) [36].

Currently, there is no clear therapeutic benefit attributable to routine nodal dissection accompanying hepatectomy for ICC. Thorough assessment of all intraabdominal nodal basins should be undertaken before hepatic resection, and sampling of suspicious nodes is indicated to stage disease accurately, which may direct postoperative treatment.

Major lymphatic spread of ICC follows three routes. First, through the hepatoduodenal ligament. Second, through the paracardial, lesser curvature, and left gastric artery. Third, through the inferior phrenic artery to the para-aortic group. Consequently, the extent of radical lymphadenectomy should include the hepatoduodenal ligament with hepatic artery, para-aortic, retro-pancreatic, and left gastric lymph nodes [36, 50].

57.13 Results of Surgery

57.13.1 Morbidity and Mortality

Surgical resection for ICC is a complex surgical procedure. Despite the improvement of surgical techniques and perioperative patients' care, extended liver resection still entails significant perioperative morbidities and mortality.

The rate of postoperative complications following surgical resection for ICC is variable between 11.5% and 58%, as shown in Table 57.1. The incidence is comparable to that reported following liver resection in non-cirrhotic patients. Posthepatectomy liver failure is less frequent among this group of patients when compared to liver resection for hepatocellular carcinoma. Other complications include bile leakage, abdominal infection, pulmonary embolism, and respiratory complications [24, 43].

The postoperative complications rate is also related to the extent of surgical resection. Lang et al. reported higher incidence among ICC patients who underwent extended hepatic resection with vascular and hilar resection (56%), when compared to simple liver resections (45%) [24].

On the other hand, postoperative mortality following surgical resection for ICC is variable between 0% and 16.7%, as shown in Table 57.1. The most common causes of postoperative mortality are liver failure, septic shock, and multiple organ dysfunction [40].

57.13.2 Long-Term Outcomes

The prognosis after surgical resection of ICC is still unsatisfactory. The s-years overall survival rate after surgical resection of ICC varies from 0% to 43% in the most recent series as shown in Table 57.1. The main reasons for these outcomes are the late diagnosis due to lack of specific symptoms or risk factors for screening, and spread of ICC through the intrahepatic and lymphatic metastasis [2]. A better survival rate as high as 63% could be achieved in ICC patients with negative margins (R0 resections) and negative lymph node involvement [31, 51].

Several prognostic factors for long-term survival after liver resection for ICC had been identified. A propensity score matching **analysis** showed that the use of nomograms is a good way to predict survival after resection. Wang et al. developed a nomogram for ICC, including tumor (T) and nodal (N) classifications, tumor size, the number of tumor nodules, preoperative level of serum tumor markers, and presence of vascular invasion [52].

57.14 Recurrence

Recurrence after R0 resection is frequent ranging between 38% and 82%. Most of recurrences occur early postoperative and most commonly in the first two years after surgical resection [3, 53]. Local recurrence is the most common recurrence pattern after radical surgical resection [54], although other patterns such as lymph nodes, abdominal wall, and extrahepatic distant recurrences were also observed [55]. A study utilizing an international database investigated 563 patients underwent curative-intent resection for ICC with a median follow-up of 19 months and found that the most common recurrence site was intrahepatic only (59.8%), extrahepatic only (14.5%), or both intra- and extrahepatic (25.7%) [56].

Management of recurrence has not been established in literature. Most of these patients receive only palliative therapy. Salvage surgery for intrahepatic recurrence or metastasectomy is usually not indicated, because it is destined to be followed by further rapid recurrences [31, 57].

57.14.1 Liver Transplantation

The role of transplantation in ICC will continue to be limited by the lack of a truly effective adjuvant systemic treatment regimen. This is in contrast to the emerging protocol of neoadjuvant chemoradiation before transplantation for hilar cholangiocarcinoma [58].

The first significant report regarding liver transplantation for ICC is that of Pichlmayr et al. in 1995. They reported a median survival of 5 months in 18 patients treated with liver transplantation, with a 1-year survival rate of 13.9% [59]. Several studies confirmed these findings afterwards [60, 61]. Cherqui et al. reported two long-term survivors and concluded that a patient with an intrahepatic tumor with no extrahepatic spread that cannot be resected for anatomic reasons may be a candidate for liver transplantation [12]. More recent experience has resulted in improved survival, with disease-free survival at 5 and 10 years of 27% and 23%, respectively, reported in 23 patients with IHCC treated with orthotopic liver transplantation [62]. However, liver transplantation remains a controversial issue due to the controversial indications and low cost-effectiveness which limit its use in treatment of ICC.

References

1. Wang K, Zhang H, Xia Y, et al. Surgical options for intrahepatic cholangiocarcinoma. Hepatobil Surg Nutr. 2017;6(2):79.
2. Endo I, Gonen M, Yopp AC, et al. Intrahepatic cholangiocarcinoma: rising frequency, improved survival, and determinants of outcome after resection. Ann Surg. 2008;248:84–96.
3. Tabrizian P, Jibara G, Hechtman JF, et al. Outcomes following resection of intrahepatic cholangiocarcinoma. HPB (Oxford). 2015;17:344–51.
4. Brown KM, Parmar AD, Geller DA, et al. Intrahepatic cholangiocarcinoma. Surg Oncol Clin N Am. 2014;23:231–46.
5. Patel T, Singh P. Cholangiocarcinoma: emerging approaches to a challenging cancer. Curr Opin Gastroenterol. 2007;23:317–23.
6. Alvaro D. Serum and bile biomarkers for cholangiocarcinoma. Curr Opin Gastroenterol. 2009;25:279–84.
7. Cheon YK, Cho YD, Moon JH, et al. Diagnostic utility of interleukin-6 (IL-6) for primary bile duct cancer and changes in serum IL-6 levels following photodynamic therapy. Am J Gastroenterol. 2007;102:2164–2170.
8. Slattery JM, Sahani DV. What is the current state-of-the-art imaging for detection and staging of cholangiocarcinoma? Oncologist. 2006;11:913–22.
9. Asayama Y, Yoshimitsu K, Irie H, et al. Delayed-phase dynamic CT enhancement as a prognostic factor for mass-forming intrahepatic cholangiocarcinoma. Radiology. 2006;238:150–5.
10. Ringe KI, Wacker F. Radiological diagnosis in cholangiocarcinoma: application of computed tomography, magnetic resonance imaging, and positron emission tomography. Best Pract Res Clin Gastroenterol. 2015;29:253–65.
11. Weber SM, Ribero D, O'Reilly EM, et al. Intrahepatic cholangiocarcinoma: expert consensus statement. HPB (Oxford). 2015;17:669–80.
12. Cherqui D, Tantawi B, Alon R, et al. Intrahepatic cholangiocarcinoma. Results of aggressive surgical management. Arch Surg. 1995;130(10):1073–8.
13. Harrison LE, Fong Y, Klimstra DS, et al. Surgical treatment of 32 patients with peripheral intrahepatic cholangiocarcinoma. Br J Surg. 1998;85(5):1068–70.
14. Waisberg DR, Pinheiro RS, Nacif LS, et al. Resection for intrahepatic cholangiocellular cancer: new advances. Transl Gastroenterol Hepatol. 2018;3(60).
15. Thirunavukarasu P, Aloia TA. Preoperative assessment and optimization of the future liver remnant. Surg Clin North Am. 2016;96:197–205.
16. Nagino M, Kamiya J, Nishio H, et al. Two hundred forty consecutive portal vein embolizations before extended hepatectomy for biliary cancer: surgical outcome and long-term follow-up. Ann Surg. 2006;243:364–72.
17. Sulpice L, Rayar M, Boucher E, et al. Intrahepatic cholangiocarcinoma: impact of genetic hemochromatosis on outcome and overall survival after surgical resection. J Surg Res. 2013;180:56–61.
18. Shindoh J, Vauthey JN, Zimmitti G, et al. Analysis of the efficacy of portal vein embolization for patients with extensive liver malignancy and very low future liver remnant volume, including a comparison with the associating liver partition with portal vein ligation for staged hepatectomy approach. J Am Coll Surg. 2013;217:126–33.
19. Tanaka K, Matsuo K, Murakami T, et al. Associating liver partition and portal vein ligation for staged hepatectomy (ALPPS): short-term outcome, functional changes in the future liver remnant, and tumor growth activity. Eur J Surg Oncol. 2015;41:506–12.
20. López-López V, Robles-Campos R, Brusadin R, et al. Tourniquet-ALPPS is a promising treatment for very large hepatocellular carcinoma and intrahepatic cholangiocarcinoma. Oncotarget. 2018;9:28267–80.
21. Aloia TA. Associating liver partition and portal vein ligation for staged hepatectomy: portal vein embolization should remain the gold standard. JAMA Surg. 2015;150:927–8.
22. Squires MH, Cloyd JM, Dillhoff M, et al. Challenges of surgical management of intrahepatic cholangiocarcinoma. Expert Rev Gastroenterol Hepatol. 2018;12:671–81.
23. Baron TH, Harewood GC, Rumalla A, et al. A prospective comparison of digital image analysis and routine cytology for the identifi-

cation of malignancy in biliary tract strictures. Clin Gastroenterol Hepatol. 2004;2:214–9.
24. Lang H, Sotiropoulos GC, Fruhauf NR. Extended hepatectomy for intrahepatic cholangiocarcinoma in 50 patients over a 5 year period. Ann Surg. 2005;241(1):134–43.
25. Isaji S, Kawarada Y, Taoka H, et al. Clinicopathological features and outcomes of hepatic resection for intrahepatic cholangiocarcinoma Japan. J Hepato-Biliary-Pancreat Surg. 1999;6(2):108–16.
26. Mavros MN, Economopoulos KP, Alexiou VG, et al. Treatment and prognosis for patients with intrahepatic cholangiocarcinoma: systematic review and meta-analysis. JAMA Surg. 2014;149:565–74.
27. Pichlmayr R, Weimann A, Klempnauer J, et al. Surgical treatment in proximal bile duct cancer. A single-center experience. Ann Surg. 1996;224(5):628.
28. Casavilla FA, Marsh JW, Iwatsuki S, et al. Hepatic resection and transplantation for peripheral cholangiocarcinoma. J Am Coll Surg. 1997;185(5):429–36.
29. Madariaga JR, Iwatsuki S, Todo S, et al. Liver resection for hilar and peripheral cholangiocarcinomas: a study of 62 cases. Ann Surg. 1998;227(1):70.
30. Chu KM, Fan ST. Intrahepatic cholangiocarcinoma in Hong Kong. J Hepato-Biliary-Pancreat Surg. 1999;6(2):149–53.
31. Weber SM, Jarnagin WR, Klimstra D, et al. Intrahepatic cholangiocarcinoma: resectability, recurrence pattern and outcomes. J Am Coll Surg. 2001;193:384–91.
32. Kawarada Y, Yamagiwa K, Das BC. Analysis of the relationships between clinicopathologic factors and survival time in intrahepatic cholangiocarcinoma. Am J Surg. 2002;183(6):679–85.
33. Ohtsuka MH, Ito H, Kimura F, et al. Results of surgical treatment for intrahepatic cholangiocarcinoma and clinicopathological factors influencing survival. Br J Surg. 2002;89(12):1525–31.
34. Nakagawa T, Kamiyama T, Kurauchi N, et al. Number of lymph node metastases is a significant prognostic factor in intrahepatic cholangiocarcinoma. World J Surg. 2005;29(6):728–33.
35. DeOliveira ML, Cunningham SC, Cameron JL, Kamangar F, Winter JM, Lillemoe KD, Choti MA, Yeo CJ, Schulick RD. Cholangiocarcinoma: thirty-one-year experience with 564 patients at a single institution. Ann Surg. 2007;245(5):755.
36. Guglielmi A, Ruzzenente A, Campagnaro T, et al. Intrahepatic cholangiocarcinoma: prognostic factors after surgical resection. World J Surg. 2009;33(6):1247–54.
37. Lang H, Sotiropoulos GC, Sgourakis G, et al. Operations for intrahepatic cholangiocarcinoma: single-institution experience of 158 patients. J Am Coll Surg. 2009;208(2):218–28.
38. Nathan H, Aloia TA, Vauthey JN, et al. A proposed staging system for intrahepatic cholangiocarcinoma. Ann Surg Oncol. 2009;16(1):14–22.
39. Shen WF, Zhong W, Xu F, et al. Clinicopathological and prognostic analysis of 429 patients with intrahepatic cholangiocarcinoma. World J Gastroenterol: WJG. 2009;15(47):5976.
40. de Jong MC, Nathan H, Sotiropoulos GC, et al. Intrahepatic cholangiocarcinoma: an international multi-institutional analysis of prognostic factors and lymph node assessment. J Clin Oncol. 2011;29:3140–5.
41. Farges O, Fuks D, Le Treut YP, et al. AJCC 7th edition of TNM staging accurately discriminates outcomes of patients with resectable intrahepatic cholangiocarcinoma: by the AFC-IHCC-2009 study group. Cancer. 2011;117(10):2170–7.
42. Saiura A, Yamamoto J, Kokudo N, et al. Intrahepatic cholangiocarcinoma: analysis of 44 consecutive resected cases including 5 cases with repeat resections. Am J Surg. 2011;201(2):203–8.
43. Sriputtha S, Khuntikeo N, Promthet S, Kamsaard S. Survival rate of intrahepatic cholangiocarcinoma patients after surgical treatment in Thailand. Asian Pac J Cancer Prev. 2013;14(2):1107–10.
44. Luo X, Yuan L, Wang Y, et al. Survival outcomes and prognostic factors of surgical therapy for all potentially resectable intrahepatic cholangiocarcinoma: a large single-center cohort study. J Gastrointest Surg. 2014;18(3):562–72.
45. Ali SM, Clark CJ, Mounajjed T, et al. Model to predict survival after surgical resection of intrahepatic cholangiocarcinoma: The Mayo Clinic experience. HPB. 2015;17(3):244–50.
46. Weinbren K, Mutum SS. Pathological aspects of cholangiocarcinoma. J Pathol. 1983;139(2):217–38.
47. Inoue K, Makuuchi M, Takayama T, et al. Long-term survival and prognostic factors in the surgical treatment of mass-forming type cholangiocarcinoma. Surgery. 2000;127(5):498–505.
48. National Comprehensive Cancer Network (NCCN) guidelines, V 2, 2012. http://www.nccn.org.
49. Ito K, Ito H, Gonen M, Allen PJ, et al. Adequate lymph node assessment for extrahepatic bile duct cancer: do the data support the current AJCC recommendations?. J Clin Oncol. 2009;27(15_suppl):4576.
50. Tsuji T, Hiraoka T, Kanemitsu K, et al. Lymphatic spreading pattern of intrahepatic cholangiocarcinoma. Surgery. 2001;129(4):401–7.
51. Paik KY, Jung JC, Heo JS, et al. What prognostic factors are important for resected intrahepatic cholangiocarcinoma? J Gastroenterol Hepatol. 2008;23:766–70.
52. Wang Y, Li J, Xia Y, et al. Prognostic nomogram for intrahepatic cholangiocarcinoma after partial hepatectomy. J Clin Oncol. 2013;31:1188–95.
53. Huang JL, Biehl TR, Lee FT, et al. Outcomes after resection of cholangiocellular carcinoma. Am J Surg. 2004;187(5):612–7.
54. Hasegawa S, Ikai I, Fujii H, et al. Surgical resection of hilar cholangiocarcinoma: analysis of survival and postoperative complications. World J Surg. 2007;31:1256–63.
55. Zhu AX, Knox JJ. Adjuvant therapy for intrahepatic cholangiocarcinoma: the debate continues. Oncologist. 2012;17:1504–7.
56. Spolverato G, Kim Y, Alexandrescu S, et al. Management and outcomes of patients with recurrent intrahepatic cholangiocarcinoma following previous curative-intent surgical resection. Ann Surg Oncol. 2016;23:235–43.
57. Chu KM, Fan ST. Intrahepatic cholangiocarcinoma in Hong Kong. J Hepato-Biliary-Pancreat Surg. 1999;6(2):149–53.
58. Fu B, Zhang T, Li H, et al. The role of liver transplantation for intrahepatic cholangiocarcinoma: a single-center experience. Eur Surg Res. 2011;47:218–21.
59. Pichlmayl R, Lamesch P, Weimann A, et al. Surgical treatment of cholangiocellular carcinoma. World J Surg. 1995;19(1):83–8.
60. Ismail T, Angrisani L, Gunson BK, et al. Primary hepatic malignancy: the role of liver transplantation. Br J Surg. 1990;77(9):983–7.
61. O'Grady JG, Polson RJ, Rolles KE, et al. Liver transplantation for malignant disease. Results in 93 consecutive patients. Ann Surg. 1988;207(4):373.
62. Robles R, Figueras J, Turrión VS, Margarit C, Moya A, Varo E, Calleja J, Valdivieso A, Valdecasas JC, López P, Gómez M. Spanish experience in liver transplantation for hilar and peripheral cholangiocarcinoma. Ann Surg. 2004;239(2):265.

58

Hepatopancreatoduodenectomy (HPD) for Biliary Tract Cancers

Tomoki Ebata, Takashi Mizuno, and Shunsuke Onoe

Abstract

Biliary tract cancers exhibit various modes of local extension, and some can only be resected by hepatopancreatoduodenectomy (HPD), which is defined as the resection of the whole extrahepatic biliary system with the adjacent liver and pancreatoduodenum. Early experiences with HPD were frequently associated with liver failure and subsequent mortality. However, with improvements in surgical techniques and perioperative patient care, the mortality rate after HPD has gradually reduced. Recent studies on HPD, although limited, have demonstrated a favorable survival in cholangiocarcinoma; whereas, controversial benefit in gallbladder cancer because of the extremely poor survival. HPD is a standard approach for laterally-spreading cholangiocarcinoma that is otherwise unresectable.

58.1 Introduction

Biliary tract cancers (cholangiocarcinomas and gallbladder cancer) often exhibit an extensive ductal spread invading from the hepatic hilus to the lower bile duct, a bulky tumor mass invading the liver, pancreas, and duodenum, and an evident nodal metastasis around the pancreatic head [1, 2]. Such extensive tumor spread represents a difficult local aggressiveness because typical resection procedures, including hepatectomy or pancreatoduodenectomy (PD), cannot offer R0 resection. However, as only a complete resection potentially provides an improved long-term survival in biliary tract cancers [3–6], hepatectomy combined with pancreatoduodenectomy (i.e., hepatopancreatoduodenectomy [HPD]) can be theoretically considered a definitive surgery for advanced biliary tract cancers. Even today, however, HPD for biliary cancer remains challenging and controversial because of rarity, very high-risk nature, and uncertain survival benefit.

58.1.1 Terminology Associated with HPD

HPD is a multivisceral resection that is defined as resection of the extrahepatic bile duct, the liver, the pancreatic head, and the duodenum (Figs. 58.1 and 58.2). HPD is anatomically characterized as complete removal of the entire extrahepatic biliary system denoting the duct from the ampulla of Vater up to the hilar bile duct and the gallbladder, thereby suiting resection for biliary tract cancer (Fig. 58.3). Therefore, most HPDs include a hemihepatectomy or more extended hepatectomy. Occasionally, hepatectomy with pancreatoduodenectomy or hepatectomy with pancreatectomy has been used as a synonym for HPD [7, 8]. For instance, PD and simultaneous partial liver resection is performed for pancreatic endocrine tumor with hepatic metastasis [9–13] or for gallbladder cancer with peripancreatic node involvement [8, 14, 15]. The authors emphasize that this procedure is not labeled as HPD (even if the right hepatectomy is combined) because the hilar bile duct remains in situ, which does not meet the above requirement of extirpation of the whole extrahepatic biliary system (Fig. 58.4). Again, genuine HPD attempts to remove the entire extrahepatic biliary system with the adjacent liver and the pancreatoduodenum, representing the most challenging procedure in the hepatobiliary field.

58.1.2 Surgical Techniques

HPD has several variations in terms of types of hepatectomy and pancreatoduodenectomy. Here, we describe right hemihepatectomy with subtotal stomach-preserving PD as a common example of HPD. Laparotomy is performed by a right

T. Ebata (✉) · T. Mizuno · S. Onoe
Division of Surgical Oncology, Department of Surgery, Nagoya University Graduate School of Medicine, Nagoya, Japan
e-mail: tomoki@med.nagoya-u.ac.jp

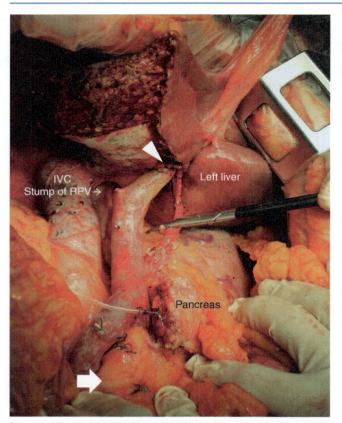

Fig. 58.1 Intraoperative photo of hepatopancreatoduodenectomy. Right hemihepatectomy, caudate lobectomy, and pancreatoduodenectomy were performed for diffusely infiltrating cholangiocarcinoma. Regional lymphadenectomies in the hepatoduodenal ligament (scissors indicate) and around the superior mesenteric artery (arrow) were completed. The proximal bile duct was transected at the right side of the left portal vein (arrow head). IVC, inferior vena cava; RPV, right portal vein

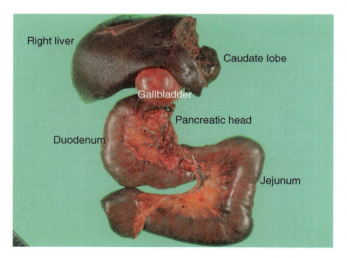

Fig. 58.2 Typical resected specimen after hepatopancreatoduodenectomy. The right liver, caudate lobe, extrahepatic biliary tree, duodenopancreas were removed en bloc

subcostal incision with the midline upward extension. When peritoneal seeding, hepatic metastasis, or periaortic node metastasis (M1 disease) is confirmed by gross inspection or by frozen section histologic examination, HPD is absolutely contraindicated.

HPD is basically performed using the following steps. First, the common, proper, or left hepatic arteries, which feed the future liver remnant, are carefully dissected and preserved. The left hepatic artery is further dissected toward the liver entry. When these major arteries cannot be isolated, the tumor is considered far-advanced local disease beyond the scope of resection. Otherwise, the right hepatic artery and the gastroduodenal artery are ligated and divided. The stomach is divided approximately 2 cm proximal from the pylorus, and the superior mesenteric vein is exposed above and below the pancreatic neck.

Second, the jejunum is divided approximately 10–20 cm distal from the ligament of Treitz. For lymphadenectomy along the superior mesenteric artery, the mesentery of the jejunum was resected along the second jejunal artery keeping in situ. The resection line is set upward along the left side of superior mesenteric artery; the root of the first jejunal artery and infrapancreatoduodenal artery is divided. The upper jejunum and the fourth part of the duodenum are passed posterior to the superior mesenteric vessels toward the right side of the operative field. The pancreatic nerve plexus intervening between the uncinate process and the superior mesenteric artery (i.e., the retroperitoneal soft tissue margin) is divided step-by-step along the right lateral border of the superior mesenteric artery. Tiny anonymous arteries are carefully divided. Then, the pancreas neck is sharply divided with a surgical knife, and a drainage tube is introduced into the main pancreatic duct after hemostasis. The remaining retropancreatic tissue and the posterior suprapancreatic duodenal vein are divided. The phase of pancreatoduodenectomy is completed.

Third, the lymph node clearance of the hepatoduodenal ligament is continued in the upward direction. The right portal vein is divided with vascular clamps, and the stump is oversewn with a monofilament suture. The variable-sized portal branches of the caudate lobe are carefully divided, and the canal of Arantius is divided at its origin to the left portal elbow. As the vascular inflow of the right liver is completely controlled, the right hemiliver and caudate lobe are fully mobilized by dividing the right and short hepatic veins. Liver transection is initiated along the ischemic demarcation (the main portal fissure) using Pringle's maneuver, advancing along the middle hepatic vein that leaves on the transection surface. When the liver transection is completed, the left hepatic duct is circumferentially exposed. After the clamp is placed on the distal side to minimize bile spillage, the intra-

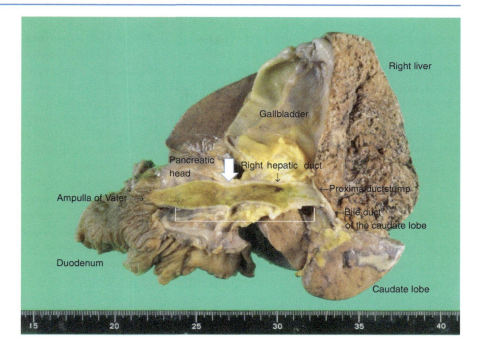

Fig. 58.3 Resected specimen after hepatopancreatoduodenectomy. The bile duct was opened longitudinally. Although the tumor was located mainly at the level of the pancreatic entry (arrow head), indicating distal cholangiocarcinoma, the photo visualized a laterally-spreading cholangiocarcinoma (bracket)

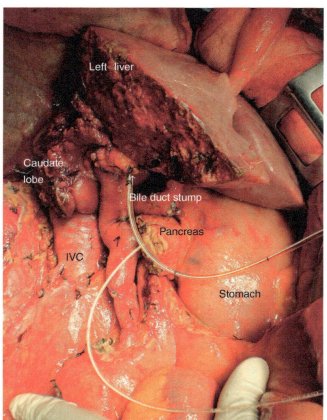

Fig. 58.4 Completion photo of pancreatoduodenectomy combined with hepatectomy. Pancreatoduodenectomy was performed for gallbladder cancer with extensive nodal involvement, followed by right hepatectomy for hepatocellular carcinoma. The common bile duct was divided and the hilar bile duct remained in situ. This procedure is not categorized as hepatopancreatoduodenectomy. *IVC* inferior vena cava

hepatic bile duct is divided with scissors. The stump of the intrahepatic duct is located at the right side of the left portal elbow.

Finally, the pancreatic remnant, intrahepatic bile duct, and stomach are reconstructed with a Roux-en Y jejunal limb in the order listed (modified Child method). We usually perform duct-to-mucosa anastomosis followed by a seromuscular envelope (Blumgart method) for end-to-side pancreatojejunostomy, and a single-layer interrupted end-to-side hepaticojejunostomy. Our perioperative management has been previously described [16].

58.1.3 Pioneers of HPD

In 1976, Kasumi et al. [17] reported a surgical strategy for advanced gallbladder cancer in a Japanese article, in which one of the 11 patients received a right hepatectomy, PD, and bile duct resection. Although the detailed information of this patient was not given, this procedure was the first successful HPD in Japan. In 1980, Takasaki et al. [18] reported 5 case series of HPD for locally advanced gallbladder cancer in detail. These patients had bulky tumors measuring 3 to 10 cm in diameter; direct involvement of the pancreatic head or the duodenum, and extensive nodal metastasis. For curative intent, all patients underwent HPD including extended right hepatectomy, and one patient received combined portal vein resection and reconstruction. Unfortunately, 3 of the 5 patients died within 30 days after surgery, signifying a mortality rate up to 60%; the remaining 2 patients were alive without disease 5 and 16 months after surgery. Takasaki's report clearly showed a technical feasibility of HPD; however, the optimal indication, safety assessment, and survival benefit of HPD remained equivocal at that time. Thus, HPD was initiated against far-advanced gallbladder cancer in Japan approximately 40 years ago, and patients, if unresected, just had to receive best supportive care, ending in a very short survival time of 4 months. Considering these difficult backgrounds, HPD would be unsatisfactory but at least better than untreated option. At present, the following over 30 years' history of HPD [19–21] says that such patients fail to get a survival benefit from HPD.

58.1.4 Outcomes After HPD

Although not many, some specific centers have continued to perform HPD in selected patients. Because portal vein embolization has been widely used in the preoperative management, the incidence of liver failure has decreased gradually in patients undergoing HPD [22]. Accordingly, nearly zero mortality is often reported in high-volume centers [13, 23, 24]. Nonetheless, a few authors have reported a high mortality, 13% to 21% [25–27], indicating a high-risk nature of HPD.

A favorable survival rate was observed in cholangiocarcinoma. Kaneoka et al. [25] and Miwa et al. [28] demonstrated 5-year survival rates of 52% (n = 9) and 64% (n = 10), respectively. In addition, Ebata et al. [16] reported 85 patients with cholangiocarcinoma who underwent HPD between 1992 and 2011; the reported overall survival rate was 37% at 5 years. Together, these results show that HPD provides a survival benefit in selected patients with cholangiocarcinoma.

As for gallbladder cancer, most studies [25–29] consistently showed a poor survival. Mizuno et al. [19] recently observed a median survival time of only 10 months after HPD in 38 gallbladder cancer patients, which equals to a survival time in patients with unresectable disease who received the first-line chemotherapy [30]. This finding clearly suggests a decreased oncologic value of up-front HPD in gallbladder cancer. However, they identified that patients with cystic duct cancer may be a potential beneficiary [19]. This disease is now categorized in gallbladder tumor, but behaves similar to cholangiocarcinoma due to its anatomical approximation to the common bile duct.

58.1.5 Practical Management During Surgery

HPD is indicated as a treatment for the following modes of spread in cholangiocarcinoma that otherwise can be completely removed: (1) a diffusely infiltrating tumor of the whole extrahepatic bile duct; (2) a perihilar tumor exhibiting downward superficial spreading [4, 31], or inversely; (3) a distal tumor exhibiting upward superficial spreading; (4) a middle tumor infiltrating both the right hepatic artery and the pancreatic head at the advancing margin; (5) a perihilar tumor with bulky nodal metastasis of the pancreatoduodenal region; and finally, (6) multiple bile duct tumors. Recently, Toyoda et al. [32] investigated cholangiographic findings in 100 patients who underwent HPD, and found that patients with localized type (the above 2 and 3 types tumor) had a better survival than those with diffuse type: 59.0% vs 26.3% at 5 years.

During hepatobiliary resection, a frozen section histologic examination often reveals cancer involvement at the distal ductal stump. Surgical management in this setting is controversial because the biologic aggressiveness of the remnant tumor depends on its histology (i.e., invasive versus non-invasive cancer). Margin involvement with invasive cancer significantly reduced rate of survival [4, 33, 34]; therefore, PD should be performed when the distal ductal margin is involved with invasive cancer, provided that the other surgical margins are tumor-free [35]. In contrast, several practical options can be employed for the treatment of a positive distal ductal margin with non-invasive cancer because remnant non-invasive foci show a slow progressive nature with a mild survival impact [36]. Therefore, it works as a significant prognostic indicator in the subset with T1-2N0 disease (early-stage disease); whereas, it does not in the subset with advanced disease or in the whole resected cohort [4, 33, 34]. Considering these findings, the additional resection of the intrapancreatic duct alone is first recommended [37]. When the margin is still positive after addition ductal resection, then PD should be considered unless the patient has other adverse prognostic factors representing nodal metastasis, pancreatic invasion, or vascular invasion [3, 5, 16, 38, 39].

Conflict of interest None.

References

1. Sakamoto E, Nimura Y, Hayakawa N, et al. The pattern of infiltration at the proximal border of hilar bile duct carcinoma: a histologic analysis of 62 resected cases. Ann Surg. 1998;227:405–11.
2. Ebata T, Watanabe H, Ajioka Y, Oda K, Nimura Y. Pathological appraisal of lines of resection for bile duct carcinoma. Br J Surg. 2002;89:1260–7.
3. Ebata T, Kamiya J, Nishio H, Nagasaka T, Nimura Y, Nagino M. The concept of perihilar cholangiocarcinoma is valid. Br J Surg. 2009;96:926–34.
4. Igami T, Nagino M, Oda K, et al. Clinicopathologic study of cholangiocarcinoma with superficial spread. Ann Surg. 2009;249:296–302.
5. Nagino M, Nimura Y, Nishio H, et al. Hepatectomy with simultaneous resection of the portal vein and hepatic artery for advanced perihilar cholangiocarcinoma: an audit of 50 consecutive cases. Ann Surg. 2010;252:115–23.
6. Nagino M, Ebata T, Yokoyama Y, et al. Evolution of surgical treatment for perihilar cholangiocarcinoma: a single-center 34-year review of 574 consecutive resections. Ann Surg. 2013;258:129–40.

7. Miyagawa S, Makuuchi M, Kawasaki S, et al. Outcome of major hepatectomy with pancreatoduodenectomy for advanced biliary malignancies. World J Surg. 1996;20:77–80.
8. Shirai Y, Ohtani T, Tsukada K, Hatakeyama K. Combined pancreaticoduodenectomy and hepatectomy for patients with locally advanced gallbladder carcinoma: long term results. Cancer. 1997;80:1904–9.
9. D'Angelica M, Martin RC 2nd, Jarnagin WR, Fong Y, DeMatteo RP, Blumgart LH. Major hepatectomy with simultaneous pancreatectomy for advanced hepatobiliary cancer. J Am Coll Surg. 2004;198:570–6.
10. Gleisner AL, Assumpcao L, Cameron JL, et al. Is resection of periampullary or pancreatic adenocarcinoma with synchronous hepatic metastasis justified? Cancer. 2007;110:2484–92.
11. McKay A, Sutherland FR, Bathe OF, Dixon E. Morbidity and mortality following multivisceral resections in complex hepatic and pancreatic surgery. J Gastrointest Surg. 2008;12:86–90.
12. Hartwig W, Hackert T, Hinz U, et al. Multivisceral resection for pancreatic malignancies: risk-analysis and long-term outcome. Ann Surg. 2009;250:81–7.
13. Hemming AW, Magliocca JF, Fujita S, et al. Combined resection of the liver and pancreas for malignancy. J Am Coll Surg. 2010;210(808–14):14–6.
14. Nakamura S, Nishiyama R, Yokoi Y, et al. Hepatopancreatoduodenectomy for advanced gallbladder carcinoma. Arch Surg. 1994;129:625–9.
15. Sasaki R, Takahashi M, Funato O, et al. Hepatopancreatoduodenectomy with wide lymph node dissection for locally advanced carcinoma of the gallbladder—long-term results. Hepato-Gastroenterology. 2002;49:912–5.
16. Ebata T, Yokoyama Y, Igami T, et al. Hepatopancreatoduodenectomy for cholangiocarcinoma: a single-center review of 85 consecutive patients. Ann Surg. 2012;256:297–305.
17. Kasumi F, Takagi K, Konishi T, Sakamoto G. Surgical treatment of carcinoma of the gallbladder, analysing its modes of spread (in Japanese). Jpn J Gatroenterol Surg. 1976;9:170–7.
18. Takasaki K, Kobayashi S, Mutoh H, et al. Our experiences (5 cases) of extended right lobectomy combined with pancreatoduodenectomy for the carcinoma of the gall bladder (in Japanese). Tan to Sui. 1980;1:923–32.
19. Mizuno T, Ebata T, Yokoyama Y, et al. Major hepatectomy with or without pancreatoduodenectomy for advanced gallbladder cancer. Br J Surg. 2019;106:626–35.
20. Higuchi R, Ota T, Araida T, et al. Surgical approaches to advanced gallbladder cancer: a 40-year single-institution study of prognostic factors and resectability. Ann Surg Oncol. 2014;21:4308–16.
21. Araida T, Yoshikawa T, Azuma T, Ota T, Takasaki K, Hanyu F. Indications for pancreatoduodenectomy in patients undergoing lymphadenectomy for advanced gallbladder carcinoma. J Hepato-Biliary-Pancreat Surg. 2004;11:45–9.
22. Ebata T, Nagino M, Nishio H, Arai T, Nimura Y. Right hepatopancreatoduodenectomy: improvements over 23 years to attain acceptability. J Hepato-Biliary-Pancreat Surg. 2007;14:131–5.
23. Kaneoka Y, Yamaguchi A, Isogai M, Kumada T. Survival benefit of hepatopancreatoduodenectomy for cholangiocarcinoma in comparison to hepatectomy or pancreatoduodenectomy. World J Surg. 2010;34:2662–70.
24. Aoki T, Sakamoto Y, Kohno Y, et al. Hepatopancreaticoduodenectomy for biliary cancer: strategies for near-zero operative mortality and acceptable long-term outcome. Ann Surg. 2018;267:332–7.
25. Kaneoka Y, Yamaguchi A, Isogai M. Hepatopancreatoduodenectomy: its suitability for bile duct cancer versus gallbladder cancer. J Hepato-Biliary-Pancreat Surg. 2007;14:142–8.
26. Lim CS, Jang JY, Lee SE, Kang MJ, Kim SW. Reappraisal of hepatopancreatoduodenectomy as a treatment modality for bile duct and gallbladder cancer. J Gastrointest Surg. 2012;16:1012–8.
27. Wakai T, Shirai Y, Tsuchiya Y, Nomura T, Akazawa K, Hatakeyama K. Combined major hepatectomy and pancreaticoduodenectomy for locally advanced biliary carcinoma: long-term results. World J Surg. 2008;32:1067–74.
28. Miwa S, Kobayashi A, Akahane Y, et al. Is major hepatectomy with pancreatoduodenectomy justified for advanced biliary malignancy? J Hepato-Biliary-Pancreat Surg. 2007;14:136–41.
29. Sakamoto Y, Nara S, Kishi Y, et al. Is extended hemihepatectomy plus pancreaticoduodenectomy justified for advanced bile duct cancer and gallbladder cancer? Surgery. 2013;153:794–800.
30. Valle J, Wasan H, Palmer DH, et al. Cisplatin plus gemcitabine versus gemcitabine for biliary tract cancer. N Engl J Med. 2010;362:1273–81.
31. Nakamura S, Suzuki S, Serizawa A, et al. Hepatopancreatoduodenectomy for superficially spreading bile duct carcinoma: a report of two 5 year survivals. Hepato-Gastroenterology. 1996;43:138–42.
32. Toyoda Y, Ebata T, Mizuno T, et al. Cholangiographic tumor classification for simple patient selection prior to hepatopancreatoduodenectomy for cholangiocarcinoma. Ann Surg Oncol. 2019;26:2971–9.
33. Wakai T, Shirai Y, Moroda T, Yokoyama N, Hatakeyama K. Impact of ductal resection margin status on long-term survival in patients undergoing resection for extrahepatic cholangiocarcinoma. Cancer. 2005;103:1210–6.
34. Shingu Y, Ebata T, Nishio H, Igami T, Shimoyama Y, Nagino M. Clinical value of additional resection of a margin-positive proximal bile duct in hilar cholangiocarcinoma. Surgery. 2010;147:49–56.
35. Otsuka S, Ebata T, Yokoyama Y, et al. Clinical value of additional resection of a margin-positive distal bile duct in perihilar cholangiocarcinoma. Br J Surg. 2019;106:774–82.
36. Tsukahara T, Ebata T, Shimoyama Y, et al. Residual carcinoma in situ at the ductal stump has a negative survival effect: an analysis of early-stage cholangiocarcinomas. Ann Surg. 2017;266:126–32.
37. Kondo S, Hirano S, Ambo Y, et al. Pancreas-preserving biliary amputation with pancreatic diversion: a new surgical technique for complete resection of the intrapancreatic biliary system. Hepato-Gastroenterology. 2004;51:1255–8.
38. Ebata T, Nagino M, Kamiya J, Uesaka K, Nagasaka T, Nimura Y. Hepatectomy with portal vein resection for hilar cholangiocarcinoma: audit of 52 consecutive cases. Ann Surg. 2003;238:720–7.
39. Aoba T, Ebata T, Yokoyama Y, et al. Assessment of nodal status for perihilar cholangiocarcinoma: location, number, or ratio of involved nodes. Ann Surg. 2013;257:718–25.

Hepato-biliary Injuries

Ender Dulundu

Abstract

Hepatobiliary surgery has become a safer as a result of considerable progress in equipment, technology, perioperative management, and surgical techniques. However, hepato-biliary surgical complications still remain as a serious problem.

Laparoscopic cholecystectomy is one of the most commonly performed abdominal surgical procedures through the world, and as a result hepato-biliary injuries are encountered after this procedure. Iatrogenic hepatobiliary injuries occur after various types of procedures such as surgical, interventional, and endoscopic interventions, and may needs surgical managements to overcome.

These injuries may be identified during, subsequently after, or in the late after the procedure, and may result in substantial morbidity and mortality. Hepato-biliary injuries are categorized into vascular, parenchymal or biliary injuries such as arteriovenous fistulas, bleeding, haematoma, fluid collection-abscesses, biliary leak or stricture. These injuries can manifest themselves with some clinical findings and laboratory results.

Although numerous imaging modalities such as ultrasound, computed tomography, magnetic resonance imaging, and digital subtraction angiography are critical for proper diagnosis and have facilitated management hepatobiliary injuries especially bile duct injury which is usually occur after simple cholecystectomy can be one of the most difficult challenges for the surgeons to overcome.

As new technologies became available (i.e. fluorescence guided surgery), physicians must follow the developments and adapt them to a daily practice to achieve more secure results. There are several pathological conditions that predispose to hepatobiliary injury (etc.; scleroatrofic gallbladder, Mirrizi's syndrome, hepatic neoplasm, obesity), surgeon should be aware and take into account of all these conditions preoperatively.

Multidisciplinary treatment strategies and team work especially with interventional radiologists are crucial to the management of these complications.

Hepatobiliary system injuries are an important cause of morbidity and mortality that can occur after surgery such as cholecystectomy, liver resections, pancreatic surgery, gastrointestinal surgery, and non surgical procedures (i.e. ERCP, PTHC, or percutaneous biopsy) [1–3].

These injuries can be noticed during surgery, or they can manifest themselves in the early period following the surgery, months or even years later. Frequently they result in additional surgeries, long recovery time, as well as an increase in hospital costs of up to 126% [4, 5].

Hepatobiliary injuries should be evaluated by a multidisciplinary team including hepatobiliary surgeon, gastroenterologist, and preferably an experienced interventional radiologist [6].

59.1 Etiology

Cholecystectomy is one of the most common causes of iatrogenic biliary injuries. Incidence of bile duct injury (BDI) is widely reported at 0.4% to 0.6% in laparoscopic cholecystectomy, and 0.2–0.3% with open surgery [2, 5, 7–9].

Traumatic injury to the biliary tree and gallbladder is a rare occurrence typically seen in the setting of blunt trauma, and injury to the biliary tree is seen in only 0.1% of trauma cases [10]. Especially in hilar tumors following radiofrequency ablation bile duct injuries can be seen in 0.1% to 12% [11].

E. Dulundu (✉)
Department of General Surgery, HPB Unit, Director of Liver Transplantation Unit, Istanbul University-Cerrahpasa, Cerrahpasa Medical School, Istanbul, Turkey
e-mail: ender.dulundu@iuc.edu.tr

59.2 Risk Factors for Biliary Injury

There are a number of risk factors that make cholecystectomy more challenging. These factors can be patient related, disease related, or extrinsic.

Cognitive factors play an important role in bile duct injury (BDI). An analysis examining biliary injuries during laparoscopic cholecystectomy found that 97% of injuries were caused by visual-perceptual illusion or inadequate visualization [12].

Disease-related risk factors include severity of inflammation, hemorrhage, and presence of abscess. Acute cholecystitis, impacted large gallstones, Mirizzi syndrome, or fistulas to neighboring organs can all complicate standard surgical plans, making dissection plans questionable, difficult and sometimes impossible [13–17].

Patient-related factors include male sex, prior operations, obesity, skeletal deformity, advanced age, and variation in the biliary tract anatomy [13, 18–20].

In spite of many surgeons accept the Luschka ducts as a small bile duct which directly connected with the gallbladder (hepaticocholecystic ducts), according to recent literature it would be more correct to describe those structures that are thought to cause bile leakage from the gallbladder bed after cholecystectomy as subvesicular bile ducts which is a different entities form hepaticocholecystic ducts [21–23].

Examples of extrinsic factors increasing the risk include equipment failure, operating room distractions, and fitness or training level of operative personnel [24]. Inadvertent thermal injury to the common bile duct may not cause immediate injury but can result in delayed structuring [13].

59.3 Strategies to Avoid Biliary Injury

Despite their efficacy, routine preoperative MRCP, and contrast-enhanced multislice computed tomography cholangiography are expensive tools and should be reserved for select cases [25, 26].

Injury prevention theories have suggested that strategies to prevent injuries would be most effective at the time of anatomical identification and orientation, and prior to dissection.

The Critical View of Safety (CVS) has been shown to be a good way of getting secure anatomical identification; once the calot triangle and the cystic plate have been exposed, it should be confirmed that no structures other than the cystic artery and cystic duct enter the gallbladder [27, 28]. If the infundibular structures of the gallbladder cannot be dissected safely operation can be stopped and patient can be referred to a hepatobiliary specialist, another options cholecystostomy tube can be inserted and operation postponed, or subtotal cholecystectomy can be performed [29, 30].

If the biliary tree has been transected retrograde catheter can be placed using for controlling the bile leak and allowing access for cholangiography to facilitate placement of percutaneous transhepatic biliary catheters in the postoperative period [31]. In addition, a closed-suction drain should be placed in the gallbladder bed and patient can be referred to a hepatobiliary specialist.

59.3.1 Classification Systems

A number of classification systems have been proposed to describe biliary injuries. The first reported was the Bismuth system (Table 59.1) [32]. This system categorizes strictures based on anatomical level of injury, but not more complex injuries often seen with laparoscopic cholecystectomies.

Strasberg proposed expansion of the Bismuth classification system (Table 59.2) [27]. This system can accurately describe the location of leak, full or partial transection, and complete occlusions. It has the advantage of guiding operative repair based on level of injury but does not account for concomitant vascular injury.

In Stewart-Way classification system patients divided into 4 classes according to the mechanism and anatomy of the injury [12].

Table 59.1 Bismuth classification system

Type	Criteria
I	Transection >2 cm from the confluence of the hepatic ducts
II	Transection <2 cm from the confluence of the hepatic ducts
III	Transection involving the confluence of the hepatic ducts with continued right and left ductal communication
IV	Transection resulting in the destruction of the hepatic confluence (disruption of the confluence ceiling)
V	Aberrant right hepatic duct stricture ± Common hepatic duct stricture

Table 59.2 Strasberg classification system

Type	Criteria
A	Leakage from cystic duct or minor duct in gallbladder fossa
B	Occlusion of abberant hepatic duct
C	Transection of aberrant hepatic duct (without concomitant occlusion)
D	Injury to the common hepatic duct or common bile duct (CBD) lateral wall without transection
E1	Transection >2 cm from the confluence of the hepatic ducts
E2	Transection <2 cm from the confluence of the hepatic ducts
E3	Transection involving the confluence of the hepatic ducts with continued right and left ductal communication
E4	Transection resulting in the destruction of the hepatic confluence (disruption of the confluence ceiling)
E5	Aberrant right hepatic duct injury ± Common hepatic duct injury

The Hanover classification is extremely descriptive considering that defining the level of vascular damage and biliary injury but due to its complexity can be hard to use in a clinical setting [33].

59.4 Diagnosis

59.4.1 Clinical Presentation

Only one-third of injuries from the ductus cysticus or small bile ducts in the liver bed are noticed during surgery [34]. On the other hand, partial or complete transections of CBD can be noticed in 70–80% of cases during surgery [14, 19, 35].

Peritonitis, abdominal pain, tenderness and fever are the most common complaints due to bile leakage in most of the patients. In addition, cholangitis, hyperbilirubinemia, high alkaline phosphatase and transient liver enzyme elevations are encountered in 30–50% of patients due to CBD obstruction. Liver enzyme elevations are more pronounced in the presence of accompanying vascular injury [34, 36, 37].

59.4.2 Imaging

Recently studies has shown no difference in CBD injury rate with surgeons who routinely used intraoperative cholangiography (IOC) compared with those who only selectively used it [38, 39].

If the anatomy is not clear (i.e. severe inflammation or different biliary anatomy), or there is a suspicion of biliary injury surgeon should not hesitate to use of IOC [15, 30].

Bile ductal blue staining or water injection test, intraoperative choledochoscopy can be used to determine the details of BDI [40].

Intraoperative ultrasonography is used in some centers for evaluation of choledocholithiasis with assuming to less expense, lower failure rate, no exposure to ionizing radiation for the patient and staff and reducing the bile duct injury [41].

One of the more contemporary techniques being investigated to reduce bile duct injury during cholecystectomy is near infrared cholangiography, but current evidence comparing near infrared cholangiography for identification of biliary anatomy during cholecystectomy to IOC is insufficient [30].

59.4.3 Evaluation of Bile Duct Injury

The rate of intraoperative diagnosis of BDI ranges between 15% and 80%, and manifest in a delayed fashion as a leakage or obstruction [42–44]. In the postoperative period, if there is an extensive peritonitis and hemodynamic instability, urgent surgical exploration may be required. For patient with stable condition initial imaging modality can be the doppler ultrasonography which can be helpful to detect obstructive findings of the bile duct, abdominal fluid collection, and concomitant vascular injury of the hepatic arterial circulation [15, 19, 45]. Contrast enhanced computed tomography (CT) is useful imaging modality to confirm ultrasonographic findings if any, and can show biloma, ascites, abscess, vascular injuries [15, 19, 33]. When bile duct injury is considered with abdominal ultrasonography and computed tomography, diagnosis can be confirmed with MRCP and HIDA scan [46, 47].

Although ERCP is useful tool in diagnosis, it is an invasive, and should be preferred to use its therapeutic advantages [19, 36, 46].

Placement of a percutaneous transhepatic biliary drainage catheter in a patient with signs of cholangitis and obstructive jaundice is of great importance in terms of both therapeutic drainage and delineation of biliary tract anatomy [37].

59.4.4 Management of Bile Duct Injuries

The success rate of bile duct injury repair in hepatobiliary surgeon's hands versus the primary surgeon is significantly higher (79% vs 27%) [42]. And, many authors agree that intraoperative recognition of BDI with immediate repair by specialized HPB surgeons offers the best results [44, 48].

All injuries must first be adequately characterized by the location, the degree of injury, and presence of concomitant vascular injury. The experience of the operating team, the stability of the patient, the severity of acute inflammation, as well as the extent of vasculobiliary injury all play an important part in determining the success of a repair [36, 49].

If a patient is unstable, septic, or has peritonitis then the repair should be delayed. Recent systematic review and meta-analysis has shown that; repair delayed for 4–6 weeks is associated with substantially decreased rates of repair failure, stricture, and postoperative complication [50, 51]. Strasberg et al. generally waited for 3 months from the time of injury before performing repair [52].

The blood supply to the bile ducts is derived from the right hepatic artery and rarely from the left at the level of the confluence. These superior branches will travel at the 3-and 9-o'clock positions inferiorly where they form an anastomosis with a blood supply derived from the gastroduodenal artery. Concomitant vascular injury occurs in 12% to 61% of biliary injury cases and will involve the right hepatic artery or its branches 90% of the time [53, 54].

Although the benefit of repairing the injured hepatic artery is controversial, some authors argue that with this repair, potential hepatic parenchymal ischemia, necrosis and atrophy can be avoided, and risk of ischemic stricture of reconstructed bile duct can be reduced [55].

If the right hepatic artery injury does not extend to the liver hilum, a significant liver ischemia is rare, due to existing shunts in the hilum and preserved portal vein flow [53].

On the other hand, it is the primary blood supply to the common hepatic bile duct and its transection may contribute to delayed bile duct stricturing secondary to bile duct ischemia.

Minor injury such a small leak from the cystic duct stump or from a segmental or accessory duct less than 3 mm can be ligated. Small lateral injuries (Strasberg type D) can be repaired over a T-tube or after inserting a thin cystic tube into the cystic duct instead of the T tube. Small lateral injuries can also be managed endoscopically or with a percutaneous transhepatic biliary drainage (PTBD). If the injured segment of the bile duct is short (<1 cm), an end-to-end anastomosis can be performed over a T-tube. However end-to-end repair is not recommended as it is associated with a 50% failure rate and postoperative stricture [56].

More complex injuries such as Strasberg type E4 or type E5 injuries often require complex procedures, and attempted repair of complex injuries by an inexperienced surgeon should be avoided as it is associated with an 80% failure rate [30, 57].

Other than this, patients with severe concomitant vascular injury, or in the setting of severe inflammation, a delayed repair is often advisable. Nearly one third of patients undergoing early repair of Strasberg type E injuries (Fig. 59.1) will develop an anastomotic stricture requiring intervention [58].

In patients who are planned to undergo surgery, it is very important to perform the Roux-en-Y anastomosis in a tension free fashion in the form of mucosa-to-mucosa. Since the area with the richest blood supply is at biliary confluence,

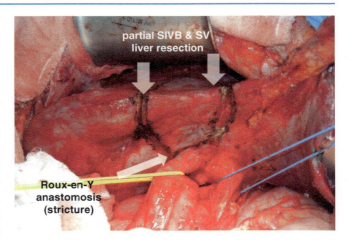

Fig. 59.2 Stricture of Roux-en-Y anastomosis after biliary injury

anastomosis should be attempted to be made proximally as possible.

Bilioenteric stenting following reconstruction is controversial. In current practice, stents are preferred in cases where the duct is small, the tissues are inflamed or when there is a concern about the viability of anastomosis. Potential risks of stents include pressure necrosis, scar formation, or bleeding via arteriobiliary fistula [59]. If patient has PTBD this can be aid in visualization of the duct, allow more secure anastomosis and help to obtain a cholangiography postoperatively to evaluate the integrity of the anastomosis. For some Strasberg type E4 and E5 injury or main hepatic duct is injured within the parenchyma of the liver, it may be necessary to perform a limited 4B/5 liver resection to gain enough length of bile duct and have adequate room for creating the bilioenteric anastomosis (Fig. 59.2).

If the injury is so high that an anastomosis to third order biliary radicles is required for repair, then an anatomical liver resection may be preferable because the stricture rate with these small anastomoses is very high. Resection may also be required in patients with severe concomitant vascular injury leading to parenchymal necrosis, delayed stricture, or recurrent abscesses in the injured liver [60]. In rare cases patients may need transplantation especially due to severe vasculobiliary injury, subsequent acute fulminant liver failure or secondary biliary cirrhosis [61].

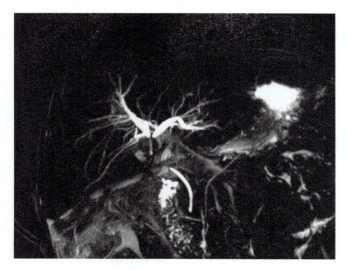

Fig. 59.1 MRI imaging of Strasberg E bile duct injury

References

1. Dixon JA, Morgan KA, Adams DB. Management of common bile duct injury during partial gastrectomy. Am Surg. 2009;75(3):719–21.
2. Fragulidis G, Marinis A, Polydorou A, et al. Managing injuries of hepatic duct confluence variants after major hepatobiliary surgery: an algorithmic approach. World J Gastroenterol. 2008;14(19):3049.
3. Kholdebarin R, Boetto J, Harnish JL, et al. Risk factors for bile duct injury during laparoscopic cholecystectomy: a case-control study. Surg Innov. 2008;15(2):114–9.

4. Melton GB, Lillemoe KD, Cameron JL, Sauter PA, Coleman J, Yeo CJ. Major bile duct injuries associated with laparoscopic cholecystectomy: effect of surgical repair on quality of life. Ann Surg. 2002;235:888–95.
5. Fong ZV, Pitt HA, Strasberg SM, et al. Diminished survival in patients with bile leak and ductal injuries: management strategy and outcomes. J Am Coll Surg. 2018;226(4):568–76.
6. Nuzzo G, Giuliante F, Giovannini I, et al. Advantages of multidisciplinary management of bile duct injuries occurring during cholecystectomy. Am J Surg. 2008;195(6):763–9.
7. Murray AC. An observational study of the timing of surgery, use of laparoscopy and outcomes for acute cholecystitis in the USA and UK. Surg Endosc. 2018;32(7):3055–63.
8. Roslyn JJ, Binns GS, Hughes EF, Saunders-Kirkwood K, Zinner MJ, Cates JA. Open cholecystectomy. A contemporary analysis of 42,474 patients. Ann Surg. 1993;218(2):129–37.
9. Kohn JF, Trenk A, Kuchta K, et al. Characterization of common bile duct injury after laparoscopic cholecystectomy in a high-volume hospital system. Surg Endosc. 2018;32(3):1184–91.
10. Thomson NK, Nardino B, Gumm K, et al. Management of blunt and penetrating biliary tract trauma. J Trauma Acute Care Surg. 2012;72:1620–5.
11. Fonseca AZ, Santin S, Gomes LGL, Waisberg J, Ribeiro MAF Jr. Complications of radiofrequency ablation of hepatic tumors: frequency and risk factors. World J Hepatol. 2014;6(3):107–13.
12. Way LW, Stewart L, Gantert W, et al. Causes and prevention of laparoscopic bile duct injuries: analysis of 252 cases from a human factors and cognitive psychology perspective. Ann Surg. 2003;273:460–9.
13. Rose JB, Hawkins WG. Diagnosis and management of biliary injuries. Curr Probl Surg. 2017;54:406–35.
14. Lillemoe KD, Martin SA, Cameron JL, et al. Major bile duct injuries during laparoscopic cholecystectomy. Ann Surg. 1997;225:459–71.
15. McPartland KJ, Pomposelli JJ. Iatrogenic biliary injuries: classification, identification, and management. Surg Clin North Am. 2008;88(6):1329–43.
16. Tornqvist B, Waage A, Zheng Z, et al. Severity of acute cholecystitis and risk of iatrogenic bile duct injury during cholecystectomy, a population-based case–control study. World J Surg. 2015;40(5):1060–7.
17. Yokoe M, Hata J, Strasberg SM, et al. Tokyo Guidelines 2018: diagnostic criteria and severity grading of acute cholecystitis. J Hepatobiliary Pancreat Sci. 2018;25:41–54.
18. Waage A, Nilsson M. Iatrogenic bile duct injury: a population based study of 152 776 cholecystectomies in the Swedish Inpatient Registry. Arch Surg. 2006;141(12):1207–13.
19. Jablonska B, Lampe P. Iatrogenic bile duct injuries: etiology, diagnosis and management. World J Gastroenterol. 2009;15(33):4097–104.
20. Meyers WC, Peterseim DS, Pappas TN, et al. Low insertion of hepatic segmental duct VII–VIII is an important cause of major biliary injury or misdiagnosis. Am J Surg. 1996;171(1):187–91.
21. Doumenc B, Boutros M, Dégremont R, Bouras AF. Biliary leakage from gallbladder bed after cholecystectomy: Luschka duct or hepatocholecystic duct? Morphologie. 2016;100:36–40.
22. Kocabiyik N, Yalcin B, Kilbas Z, Karadeniz SR, Kurt B, Comert A, et al. Anatomical assessment of bile ducts of Luschka in humanfetuses. Surg Radiol Anat SRA. 2009;31:517–21.
23. Schnelldorfer T, Sarr MG, Adams DB. What is the duct of Luschka? A systematic review. JOGS. 2012;16(3):656–62.
24. Yaghoubian A, Saltmarsh G, Rosing DK, Lewis RJ, Stabile BE, de Virgilio C. Decreased bile duct injury rate during laparoscopic cholecystectomy in the era of the 80-hour resident work week. Arch Surg. 2008;143(9): 847–851. [discussion851].
25. Chung YH, Kim DJ, Kim I-G, et al. Relationship between the risk of the bile duct injury during laparoscopic cholecystectomy and types of preoperative magnetic resonance cholangiopancreaticography. Korean J Hepato-Biliary-Pancreat Surg. 2012;16(1):17–23.
26. Alibrahim E, Gibson RN, Vincent J, Speer T, Collier N, Jardine C. Spiral computed tomography-intravenous cholangiography with three-dimensional reconstructions for imaging the biliary tree. Australas Radiol. 2006;50(2):136–42.
27. Strasberg SM, Hertl M, Soper NJ. An analysis of the problem of biliary injury during laparoscopic cholecystectomy. J Am Coll Surg. 1995;180:101–25.
28. Izwashita Y, Hibi T, Ohyama T, Umezawa A, Takada T, Strasberg SM, et al. Delphi consensus on bile duct injuries duringlaparoscopic cholecystectomy: an evolutionary cul-de-sac or the birth pangs of a new technical framework? J Hepatobiliary Pancreat Sci. 2017;24:591–602.
29. Strasberg SM, Pucci MJ, Brunt LM, Deziel DJ. Subtotal cholecystectomy-"Fenestrating" vs "reconstituting" subtypes and the prevention of bile duct injury:definition of the optimal procedure in difficult operative conditions. J Am Coll Surg. 2016;222(1):89–96.
30. L. Michael Brunt, Y Daniel J. Deziel, Dana A. Telem, et al. safe cholecystectomy multi-society practice guideline and state of the art consensus conference on prevention of bile duct injury during cholecystectomy and the Prevention of Bile Duct Injury Consensus Work Group. Ann Surg. 2020;272(1):3–23.
31. Mercado MA, Chan C, Jacinto JC, Sanchez N, Barajas A. Voluntary and involuntary ligature of the bile duct in iatrogenic injuries: a nonadvisable approach. J Gastrointest Surg. 2008;12:1029.
32. Bismuth H. Postoperative strictures of the bile duct. In: Blumgart L, editor. The biliary tract. Edinburgh: Churchill Livingstone Inc; 1982. p. 209–18.
33. Bektas H, Schrem H, Winny M, et al. Surgical treatment and outcome of iatrogenic bile duct lesions after cholecystectomy and the impact of different clinical classification systems. Br J Surg. 2007;94(9):1119–27.
34. Maddah G, Mashhadi MTR, Mashhadi MP, et al. Iatrogenic injuries of the extrahepatic biliary system. J Surg Res. 2015;213:215–21.
35. Tornqvist B, Stromberg C, Persson G, et al. Effect of intended intraoperative cholangiography and early detection of bile duct injury on survival after cholecystectomy: population based cohort study. BMJ. 2012;345(1):1–10.
36. Sicklick JK, Camp MS, Lillemoe KD, et al. Surgical management of bile duct injuries sustained during laparoscopic cholecystectomy. Ann Surg. 2005;241(5):786–95.
37. Cohen JT, Charpentier KP, Beard RE. An update on iatrogenic biliary injuries identification, classification, and management. Surg Clin N Am. 2019;99:283–99.
38. Giger U, Ouaissi M, Schmitz SF, et al. Bile duct injury and use of cholangiography during laparoscopic cholecystectomy. Br J Surg. 2011;98:391–6.
39. Ragulin-Coyne E, Witkowski ER, Chau Z, et al. Is routine intraoperative cholangiogram necessary in the twenty-first century? A national view. J Gastrointest Surg. 2013;17(3):434–42.
40. Feng X, Dong J. Surgical management for bile duct injury. Biosci Trends. 2017;11(4):399–405.
41. Jamal KN, Smith H, Ratnasingham K, Siddiqui MR, Mc Lachlan G, Belgaumkar AP. Meta-analysis of the diagnostic accuracy of laparoscopic ultrasonography and intraoperative cholangiography in detection of common bile duct stones. Ann R Coll Surg Engl. 2016;98:244–9.
42. Carroll BJ, Birth M, Phillips EH. Common bile duct injuries during laparoscopic cholecystectomy that result in litigation. Surg Endosc. 1998;12(4):310–4.
43. Lee CM, Stewart L, Way LW. Postcholecystectomy abdominal bile collections. Arch Surg. 2000;135(5):538–44.
44. Silva M, Coldham C, Mayer A, et al. Specialist outreach service for on-table repair of iatrogenic bile duct injuries a new kind of "traveling surgeon". Ann R Coll Surg Engl. 2008;90:243–6.

45. Stewart L, Way LW. Bile duct injuries during laparoscopic cholecystectomy. Arch Surg. 1995;130:1123–9.
46. Copelan A, Bahoura L, Tardy F, et al. Etiology, diagnosis, and management of bilomas: a current update. Tech Vasc Interv Radiol. 2015;18(4):236–43.
47. Kalayci C, Aisen A, Canal D, et al. Magnetic resonance cholangiopancreatography documents bile leak site after cholecystectomy in patients with aberrant right hepatic duct where ERCP fails. Gastrointest Endosc. 2000;52(2):277–81.
48. Pekolj J, Alvarez FA, Palavecino M, Claria RS, Mazza O, de Santibanes E. Intraoperative management and repair of bile duct injuries sustained during 10,123 laparoscopic cholecystectomies in a high-volume referral center. J Am Coll Surg. 2013;216(5):894–901.
49. Bachellier P, Nakano H, Weber J-C, Lemarque P, Oussoultzoglou E, Candau C, et al. Surgical repair after bile duct and vascular injuries during laparoscopic cholecystectomy: when and how? World J Surg. 2001;25:1335–45.
50. Xiang Wang, MD, Wen-Long Yu, MD, Xiao-Hui Fu, MD, Bin Zhu, MD, Teng Zhao, MD, and Yong-Jie Zhang. Early versus delayed surgical repair and referral for patients with bile duct injury a systematic review and meta-analysis. Ann Surg. 2020;271(3):449–459.
51. Bismuth H, Majno PE. Biliary strictures: classification based on the principles of surgical treatment. World J Surg. 2001;25(10):1241–4.
52. Strasberg SM, Picus DD, Drebin JA. Results of a new strategy for reconstruction of biliary injuries having an isolated right-sided component. J Gastrointest Surg. 2001;5:266–74.
53. Strasberg SM, Helton WS. An analytical review of vasculobiliary injury in laparoscopic and open cholecystectomy. HPB. 2011;13:1–14.
54. Koffron A, Ferrario M, Parsons W, Nemcek A, Saker M, Abecassis M. Failed primary management of iatrogenic biliary injury: incidence and significance of concomitant hepatic arterial disruption. Surgery. 2001;130(4):722–31.
55. Schmidt SC, Settmacher U, JanM. Langrehr, and P. Neuhaus. Management and outcome of patients with combined bile duct and hepatic arterial injuries after laparoscopic cholecystectomy. Surgery. 2004;135:613–8.
56. De Reuver PR, Busch ORC, Rauws EA, Lameris JS, Van Gulik TM, Gouma DJ. Long-term results of a primary end-to-end anastomosis in peroperative detected bile duct injury. JOGS. 2007;11(3):296–302.
57. Stewart L, Way LW. Bile duct injuries during laparoscopic cholecystectomy. Arch Surg. 1995;130:1123–9.
58. Stilling NM, Fristrup C, Wettergren A, et al. Long-term outcome after early repair of iatrogenic bile duct injury. A national Danish multicenter study. HPB. 2015:394–400.
59. Mercado MA, Chan C, Orozco H, et al. To stent or not to stent bilioenteric anastomosis after iatrogenic injury: a dilemma not answered? Arch Surg. 2002;137(1):60–3.
60. Perini MV, Herman P, Montagnini AL, et al. Liver resection for the treatment of post-cholecystectomy biliary stricture with vascular injury. World J Gastroenterol. 2015;21(7):2102–7.
61. Thomson BNJ, Parks RW, Madhavan KK, Garden OJ. Liver resection and transplantation in the management of iatrogenic biliary injury. World J Surg. 2007;31(12):2363–9.

Surgical Treatment for Severe Liver Injuries

Florin Botea, Alexandru Barcu, and Irinel Popescu

Abstract

Traumatic injuries represent the third cause of death world-wide, with over five million deaths each year. Because of its anterior location in the abdomen and its fragility, the liver is one of the most frequently injured organs in abdominal trauma. The advancements in diagnosis and interventional therapy shifted the approach of liver injury towards a non-operative management (NOM). In high-grade liver injuries, surgical treatment remains the main option; surgical approach is mandatory in hemodynamically unstable patients, while debatable in stable ones: some authors support the surgical approach, others advocate the NOM. As in any trauma, for optimal results, the emergency centers, emergency medical services transport and the tertiary centers must effectively cooperate in order to maximize the therapeutic efficiency.

60.1 Background

Traumatic injuries represent the third cause of death worldwide, with over five million deaths each year [1]. Blunt abdominal trauma accounts for 13% of all emergencies and 80% of abdominal injuries [2], 75% being related to motor vehicle collision or auto versus pedestrian accidents [3], while blows and falls are responsible for 15% and 6–9%, respectively [4]; occult trauma may occur with domestic violence and child abuse.

The liver and spleen are the most commonly injured solid organs [3, 4]. Other organs are often injured in patients with liver injury (LI). LI usually occur after blunt trauma of the upper abdomen and lower thorax, but also in penetrating trauma (the second most injured organ) [5, 6]. LI is more common in young men, with a male/female ratio of 3:1 [1]. In blunt LI, organs like spleen, pancreas, kidney, lung, heart, ribs, pelvic bones, vertebras and spinal cord are injured in approximately 80% of cases [7, 8]. Blunt LI is usually caused by motor vehicle collision [6], the right posterior section (segments 6 and 7) being the most common site of trauma [9]. In penetrating LI, structures like inferior vena cava, liver hilum (main bile duct, portal vein, hepatic artery), mesentery, colon, diaphragm, right lung, duodenum, right kidney and abdominal aorta may be injured. Also, association between various potential lesions are to be always considered.

The advancements in diagnosis and interventional therapy shifted the approach of LI towards a non-operative management (NOM). Indeed, many studies reported better outcome after conservative management [10, 11]. Nevertheless, in high-grade LI, surgical treatment remains the main option; surgical approach is mandatory in hemodynamically unstable patients, while debatable in stable ones: some authors support the surgical approach [12], others advocate the NOM [13]. As in any trauma, for optimal results, the emergency centers, emergency medical services transport and the tertiary centers must effectively cooperate in order to maximize the therapeutic efficiency.

60.2 Diagnostics

The evaluation of the trauma patient is based on historical data (trauma to the right and middle upper quadrant, right rib cage, or right flank), mechanism of injury, prehospital vital signs and its fluctuations, examination findings (pain in the right upper abdomen, right chest wall, or right shoulder due to diaphragmatic irritation, associated with abdominal tenderness and peritoneal signs), emergency lab tests (hematocrit, base deficit and lactate, and liver enzymes), imaging (ultrasound +/− CT scan), and underlying medical conditions [14]. A neg-

---

A. Barcu
"Dan Setlacec" Center of General Surgery and Liver Transplantation, Fundeni Clinical Institute, Bucharest, Romania

F. Botea (✉) · I. Popescu
"Dan Setlacec" Center of General Surgery and Liver Transplantation, Fundeni Clinical Institute, Bucharest, Romania

"Titu Maiorescu" University, Bucharest, Romania

ative history and exam do not reliably exclude LI. Moreover, the consciousness is often altered by associated neurologic injury and/or intoxication, or due to sedation and intubation, and therefore medical history, symptoms and sign are impossible to be assessed in these cases [8].

High values of liver transaminase increase the likelihood of LI and may be an indicator of severity of the injury [15]. However, patients with comorbidities such as alcohol-induced liver disease or hepatitis may have elevated transaminase concentrations at baseline. A FAST ultrasound exam (Focused Assessment with Sonography for Trauma) is mandatory in all trauma patients. CT scan is the primary method for identifying all intra-abdominal injury [16], with high sensitivity and specificity (97–98% and 97–99%, respectively) [9]; in case of a negative CT scan, the rate of missed injury is extremely low (<0.06%) [9]. CT scan (multidetector helical computed tomography) is performed only in stabilized and cooperative (otherwise sedated) patients, (with particular care to potential spinal cord injuries), guiding the trauma management. Magnetic resonance imaging (MRI) may be useful in a subset of hemodynamically stable patients who cannot undergo CT scan (allergy to radiological contrast) or necessitate MRI cholangiography for extrahepatic biliary injury.

The American Association for the Surgery of Trauma (AAST) classification system is the most widely accepted injury grading scale based on CT scan (Table 60.1) [6, 17]. To correlate between AAST grade and patient's physiologic status, the World Society of Emergency Surgery (WSES) seems to be more useful, reflecting both the hemodynamic status and the anatomic grade of the LI [7, 18] (Table 60.2). Most LIs are of low-grade according to AAST classification, as 67% of LIs are AAST low grade I–III LI [6], when the success of NOM is most likely to occur. Higher grade LI (IV–V) may be managed by NOM or surgery, depending on the dynamics of the clinical status. Grade VI LI are always severely hemodynamically unstable (hemorrhagic shock) and therefore surgery is mandatory in this situation; however, due to the cataclysmic event, the patient often does not arrive in time for surgery [8]. However, there is no correlation between AAST grade and patient physiologic status, so AAST classification should be supplemented by hemodynamic status and associated injuries. Therefore, the LI grading system proposed by the World Society of Emergency Surgery (WSES) seems to be more useful, reflecting both the hemodynamic status and the anatomic grade of the LI [7, 18]. In our experience, World Society of Emergency Surgery (WSES) classification had more upfront relevancy, the hemodynamical instability being the main criteria for choosing surgery over NOM, LIs grade being of secondary importance.

Improved availability, rapidity and sensitivity of diagnostic imaging, most notably CT scan, alongside with the development of critical care monitoring, determined a shift from surgery to NOM for most hemodynamically stable patients with LI, leading to a significant decrease of both morbidity and mortality [19–21].

Table 60.1 The American Association for the Surgery of Trauma (AAST) classification system for liver injury (LI)

Grade	Type of Injury	Description of injury
I	Hematoma	Subcapsular hematoma <10% of the liver surface area;
	Laceration	<1 cm in depth
II	Hematoma	Subcapsular hematoma 10–50% of the liver surface area; intraparenchymal hematoma <10 cm in diameter;
	Laceration	1–3 cm in depth and ≤ 10 cm in length.
III	Hematoma	>50% surface area of ruptured subcapsular/parenchymal hematoma; intraparenchymal hematoma >10 cm/expanding
	Laceration	>3 cm in depth and >10 cm in length; liver vascular injury; active bleeding contained within the parenchyma.
IV	Laceration	Parenchymal disruption involving 25–75% of a hemiliver/1–3 Couinaud segments; active liver bleeding into the peritoneum.
V	Laceration	Parenchymal disruption involving >75% of a hemiliver/>3 Couinaud segments.
	Vascular	Juxtahepatic venous injury involving the retro hepatic vena cava/central major hepatic veins.
VI	Vascular	Hepatic avulsion

aAdvance one grade for multiple injuries up to grade III

Table 60.2 World Society of Emergency Surgery (WSES) classification and guidelines for blunt/penetrating (stab/gun) liver injury

Severity of LI	WSES grade	AAST grade	Hemodynamic	CT-scan	Treatment
Minor	I	I–II	Stable	Yes/No	NOM
Moderate	II	III	Stable	Yes + local exploration in penetrating LI	NOM
Severe	III	IV–V	Stable	Yes + local exploration in penetrating LI	NOM
	IV	I–VI	Unstable	No	Surgery

LI liver injury, NOM nonoperative management, AAST The American Association for the Surgery of Trauma

60.3 Treatment

Liver trauma had always represented a difficult challenge. Since the first documented liver resection performed in the XVII century by Hildanus for liver trauma, the significant developments in the last two decades in diagnosis, patient monitoring and interventional therapies, and the optimal results of non-operative approach in spleen trauma favor the non-operative management of liver trauma [22]. The current nonoperative and operative decisional algorithm in the management of liver trauma is depicted in Fig. 60.1.

Independently of the grade of LI, the management is determined by the hemodynamical status: surgery is mandatory in emergency in unstable patients, while non-operative approach, although still controversial in high-grade LI, may be used in stable cases. Even though surgery in high-grade

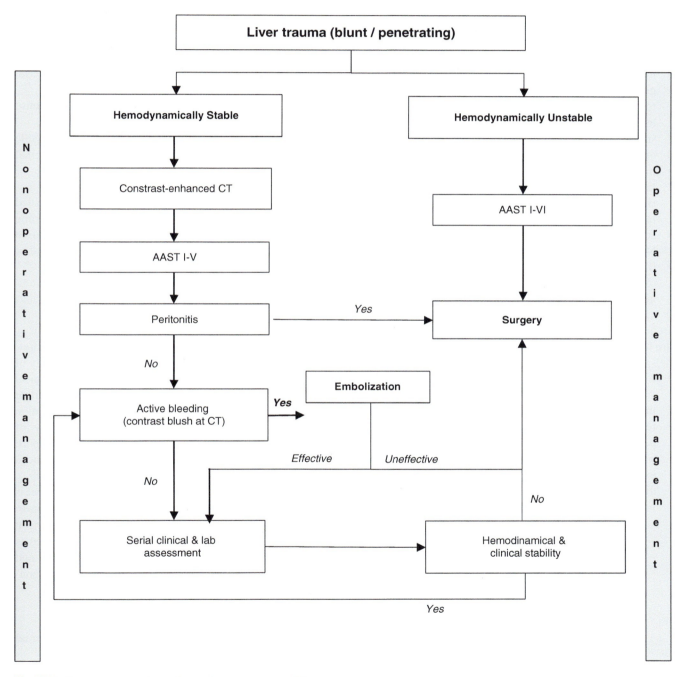

Fig. 60.1 Current nonoperative and operative management of liver trauma

injuries may result in high mortality as well [23, 24], there are no randomized studies to compare surgery versus NOM in stable patients [25].

Initial management of LI is aimed at rapid stabilization and identification of life-threatening injuries, as described in Advanced Trauma Life Support (ATLS) protocols. Primary assessment is carried out according to the ABCDE pattern: Airway, Breathing, Circulation, Disability (neurologic injuries), and Exposure.

Hemodynamic instability, not the grading of the injury, represents the main indication for operative approach (Fig. 60.2). Unstable patients are managed as follows:

- in case of positive FAST ultrasound exam—the patient goes directly to the operating room for emergency laparotomy. When available, resuscitative endovascular balloon occlusion of the aorta may provide hemodynamic support until definitive treatment with angioembolization or laparotomy.
- in case of unclear FAST exam, diagnostic peritoneal lavage with aspiration of 10 mL of gross blood indicates a significant bleeding, warranting the emergent laparotomy.
- subsequent hemodynamically instability after failed NOM warrants emergent surgery.
- if no evidence of intra-abdominal injury (negative FAST exam, and abdominal CT), other sites of bleeding or other non-hemorrhagic causes of shock are to be considered.

In hemodynamically stable patient, the following scenarios are to be considered:

- regular vital signs and lab tests (low risk)—clinical observation of <12 hours is usually enough to rule out occult intra-abdominal injury [5, 26, 27].
- regular vital signs but modified lab tests (hematocrit <30 percent, AST/ALT >130 units/L, microscopic hematuria >25 red blood cells per high power field) and/or high-risk examination findings (e.g. peritoneal signs, abdominal distension, seat belt sign)—CT scan is recommended, with the following scenario:
  - no LI at CT—clinical observation of <12 hours is recommended;
  - LI at CT, without active bleeding—NOM is recommended.
  - LI at CT with active bleeding—either NOM or immediate surgery is recommended, depending on hemodynamically stability:
    NOM is recommended in blunt or stab (but not gunshot) penetrating LI in hemodynamically stable patients, in I–V AAST grade injuries, in absence of other intra-abdominal injuries. Even though extra-abdominal lesions requiring surgery could be present (except severe head trauma), NOM of LI is still recommended.

emergent abdominal surgery must be offered to:

- hemodynamically unstable patient with a positive FAST ultrasound exam, independently of the AAST grade injury (I–VI).
- hemodynamically stable patients with associated intra-abdominal injuries leading to peritonitis (e.g. signs of peritoneal irritation, evidence of pneumoperitoneum) and/or diaphragmatic rupture, persistent and severe digestive bleeding.
- failure of NOM—patient becoming unstable despite aggressive conservative treatment, including blood transfusion +/− liver arterial embolization.
- persistent systemic inflammatory response (SIRS—ileus, fever, tachycardia, oliguria).
- unexplained signs of bleeding in an unstable patient with strongly suspected intra-abdominal trauma.

Fortunately, LI is usually minor and successfully treated by clinical observation, supportive treatment, and sometime arterial embolization [19] (NOM). Surgery is needed in <15% of cases, generally for unstable patients or in case of failed NOM [6].

60.3.1 Nonoperative Management

NOM is the treatment of choice for blunt and stab penetrating LI in hemodynamically stable patients, independently of injury grade. Failure of NOM leads to immediate surgical treatment. NOM comprises clinical observation, supportive care and, in selected cases, of liver arterial embolization [28], requiring optimal patient selection, availability of resources (intensive care unit beds, blood bank support, immediate operating room availability, and experienced interventional angiographers and surgeons).

NOM is deployed in over 80% of blunt LI with a success rate of over 90% [19, 21, 29, 30] (Fig. 60.3). NOM seems to be associated with improved overall survival in comparison with surgical treatment, while reducing the overall costs [31]. The improvements in intensive care management and use of interventional radiology appear to significantly contribute to the high successful rate of NOM [32].

NOM is contraindicated in case of [33]:

- hemodynamically unstable patient despite initial resuscitation.
- hemodynamically stable patients with:
  - other indication for abdominal surgery (e.g., peritonitis);

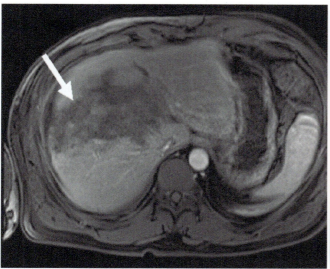 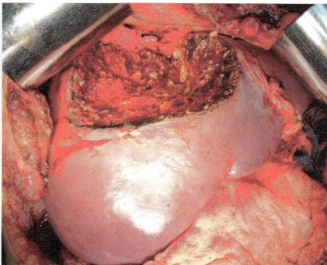

Fig. 60.2 Case presentation of an AAST IV grade liver injury (LI). 34-year old male with polytrauma by car accident, hemodynamically unstable; at CT-scan—rupture of segments 4, 5, and 8—parenchymal disruption involving 3 Couinaud's segments; previous surgery in other hospital (hepatorrhaphy and perihepatic packing); at admittance in our center: stable, ileus, fever, tachycardia, oliguria, high transaminase levels, leukocytosis (22.000 el/mm^3); relaparotomy after 36 hours (ultrasound guided nonanatomic liver resection of segments 4, 5 and 8), with no major complications (minor biliary fistula treated conservatively)

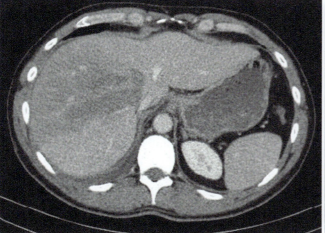 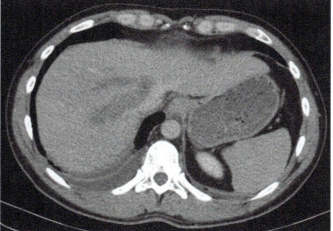

Fig. 60.3 Hemodynamically stable patient with AAST IV grade liver injury, with successful nonoperative management

- gunshot injury—relative contraindication because of high probability of NOM failure (up to 30% of cases) [34] and undetected associated intra-abdominal injuries;
- concomitant severe head injuries;
- absence of facilities and personnel for intensive care monitoring and treatment, for arterial embolization, and for urgent abdominal exploration in case of NOM failure.

Disadvantages of NOM are [35]:

- increased risk for biliary complications (biloma and/or persistent bile leak), occurring in up to 21% of cases, manifested as abdominal pain and/or a persistent SIRS (fever, tachycardia, and leukocytosis) [36];
- increased risk of missed intra-abdominal injury, particularly hollow organ injury;

- transfusion-related conditions: transfusion-associated circulatory overload (TACO), transfusion-related acute lung injury (TRALI), hypothermia, coagulopathy, immunologic and allergic reactions, and transfusion-related immune modulation (TRIM);
- risks associated with embolization techniques: ischemic complications (liver necrosis and abscess, biloma and bile leaks), arterial access site complications (hematoma or bleeding), inadvertent embolization of other organs (e.g., bowel, pancreas), contrast-induced nephropathy.

Failure of NOM, defined as the necessity for surgery, is associated with increased mortality [37, 38] and is usually due to [39, 40]:

- continuous or recurrent bleeding demonstrated by:
  - CT scan;
  - necessity of ongoing aggressive fluid resuscitation or transfusion of >3 units of blood (related to the LI)—independent risk factor for surgical intervention [38];
  - hemodynamic instability.
- associated intra-abdominal injuries [41].

60.3.2 Interventional Treatment

Angioembolization has become the gold standard for treating bleeding in LI in hemodynamically stable patients. Furthermore, interventional radiology has a paramount role in the management of posttraumatic complications, such as pseudoaneurysm, intrahepatic arterio-venous fistula, haemobilia (angioembolization), symptomatic biloma and abscesses (percutaneous guided drainage) [42]. Angioembolization can also be used adjunctively in case of ongoing liver bleeding or rebleeding after surgery [43] in 12–28% of operated patients [30]. The success rate of angioembolization in LI may be up to 93% [35], depending on the expertise and facilities. It appears to be most effective in hemodynamically stable patients with active bleeding at CT. When the source of bleeding is not seen at angiography, empiric embolization guided by the previous CT may be performed to reduce the risk of bleeding [44]. Therefore, up to 5% of NOM patients required embolization [30].

60.3.3 Surgery

Approximately 14% of patients with LI require surgical treatment [6]. In our experience, this rate was much higher (84.4%) because we addressed only high-grade LIs, IV and V grades LIs representing 82%, and most of our patients were transferred after prior surgery (67%). A base deficit less than −6 was associated with intra-abdominal hemorrhage and the need for laparotomy and blood transfusion [45].

The operative approach has also developed over the last two decades. Direct suture/ligation of the intra-parenchymal bleeding vessel, perihepatic packing, repair of venous injury under total vascular isolation, in association with preoperative and/or postoperative angioembolization are the methods initially preferred, while LR remain the main option in case of inefficiency of the above-mentioned methods [46, 47].

Surgical management of LIs is challenging even for experienced surgeons due to liver size, quality of parenchyma (such as steatosis, hepatitis), dual blood supply (portal, hepatic arterial), complex biliary drainage system, intricate and difficult-to-access venous drainage, and frequent anatomic variants of all these structures [48]. The operation is even more difficult due to impaired visibility due to presence of bulky clots and large quantity of blood into the peritoneum. Moreover, because the operation is carried out on a hemodynamically unstable patient, the surgical maneuvers must be swift in order to obtain rapid hemostasis, consisting in temporary bleeding control, to allow effective intensive resuscitation of the patient [48]. This is followed by definitive hemostasis using a variety of techniques, that can be deployed immediately in hemodynamically stable patients, or in a delayed manner, following intensive care resuscitation, in case of unstable patients [48].

The surgical approach is open. A large incision that offers best access is mandatory; in case of LI involving the right posterior section in patients with previous midline incision, a right transversal incision may be deployed, transforming the access in to a J-shaped incision. Good exposure by quickly and completely mobilizing the liver is usually useful. In absence of liver mobilization, the LI may not be accessible for treatment, it could be treated incompletely, or it may enlarge due to excessive traction used to expose the lesion.

Superficial liver lacerations may respond to conservative techniques such as manual compression with or without associated Pringle maneuver, electrosurgical techniques (mono- and bipolar cautery, argon beam coagulation, energy-device coagulation), topical hemostatic agents, and even perihepatic packing in case of failure of the other maneuvers (removed intraoperatively or during a second operation). Deep lacerations and voluminous parenchymal avulsions typically requires direct ligation of bleeding vessels, direct liver suturing, liver resection (resectional debridement or anatomic liver resection), selective hepatic artery ligation (right or left), with or without perihepatic packing; absorbable mesh-wrapping is also an option [49]. When bleeding originates from within a deep and narrow laceration of the liver (such as a penetrating wound), a balloon tamponade could control the bleeding. Whenever possible (in absence of sepsis or cancer), an autotransfusion procedure is recommended.

The use of perihepatic packing as maneuver for temporary bleeding control reduces the extent of subsequent surgical procedures. The more complex the LI, the better the chance for cure if the definitive treatment (LR) is performed during a second operation performed by an expert team in a tertiary center, after stabilizing the patient [48]. The timing of relaparotomy for removal of the perihepatic packs is controversial [50]. Removal after <24 hours has high risk of rebleeding, while >48 hours has a higher risk of sepsis. Therefore, the interval of 24–48 hours is generally excepted. If bleeding occurs after removing the packs, repacking should be considered, followed by relaparotomy after another 24–48 hours.

Nowadays, LR is considered to have minimal role in the management of hepatic injury because of the high morbidity and mortality in many reports. Nevertheless, it is known that high-volume centers and high-volume surgeons correlate with improved outcomes after LR [51, 52]. Indeed, in specialized liver surgery/transplant centers, the morbidity and the mortality after LR for severe LI are as low as 17–30%, and 2–9%, respectively [53, 54]. LR is reserved for severe injuries, the main policy being preservation of as much as possible of liver parenchyma. When LR is required, parenchymal transection is usually performed by clamp crushing method (Kelly-clasia), as it is usually faster. In order to reduce bleeding, vascular control consisting in Pringle maneuver and total vascular exclusion is recommended used.

Juxtahepatic injuries of vena cava and/or main hepatic veins (grade V) were very challenging to control due to the severe bleeding and the difficult surgical access to these veins, and total vascular exclusion is often used. In juxtahepatic injuries, packing sometime is effective in controlling such bleeding and should therefore be attempted first [55]; when ineffective, diversion of blood from the site of injury is mandatory (total vascular exclusion, venovenous bypass, or atriocaval shunting) [48]. Associated lesions of important juxtahepatic vessels (vena cava, main hepatic vein, portal vein, hepatic artery and main common bile duct) may involve various techniques for vascular and biliary reconstruction [48]. Coexistent injuries of other abdominal organs are to be explored and treated during surgery.

Liver transplantation is used when LI lead to acute liver failure due to extensive parenchymal necrosis, being the salvage option for a severe LI [56], including hepatic avulsion (grade V injury), resulting in acute liver failure. Good outcome in selected cases have been reported [57]. Compared with non-trauma recipients, post-trauma recipients experience a significantly higher retransplantation rate, but with similar long-term survival [58].

Persistent bile leak is recommended to be treated, as first line therapy, by endoscopic retrograde cholangiopancreatography with stent placement [59], or percutaneous transhepatic biliary drainage as an alternative. Failure of these interventional methods usually necessitates surgery with removal of the liver parenchyma feeding the bile leak or with biliary reconstruction. In case of significant choleperitoneum and failed interventional drainage, laparoscopy with abdominal irrigation and drainage is recommended. Similarly, in case of persistent large hemoperitoneum even in absence of active bleeding, surgical approach is recommended. Abscesses are usually successfully managed with antibiotics and percutaneous drainage techniques, but surgery may be needed if interventional techniques fail to provide adequate drainage [60]. In case of liver necrosis (following embolization or hepatorrhaphy) the treatment consists in surgical debridement for limited necrosis, upfront liver resection (rather than repeated debridement) in case of large necrosis [35, 61], and even LT in case of acute liver failure due to extensive necrosis.

60.3.4 Morbidity and Mortality

The morbidity is dependent on the AAST grade of LI [60], very low for grade I and II, 5% for grade III, and >50% for grade V [62]. Mortality increases in AAST high-grade LIs, and have decreased over time due to NOM and emergent perihepatic packing [63], especially in grade IV and V LIs [31, 62, 64]. Many of the high-grade LIs can be successfully managed by NOM with overall low mortality rates ranging from 0–8%. In our experience, the mortality after NOM was higher (16.6%), but the 1 case that died during NOM was not due to LI. Mortality rate is much higher (30–68%) for high-grade LI requiring surgery, regardless if it is deployed immediately or after failed NOM [30]; moreover, mortality increases significantly to up to 77% in case of injury of vena cava and liver hilum [65].

In conclusion, the management of liver injury must be based on both anatomy of injury and its physiopathological effects. The main approach is nonoperative, including angioembolization in selected cases, while surgery is reserved mainly for unstable patients. Continuous proactive monitoring off all trauma injuries is mandatory in order to be able to detect and treat immediately any complication related to the liver or other concomitant injured organs. Liver resections, vascular and biliary reconstructions are to be carried out in highly specialized tertiary centers, such as our center, minimizing the morbidity and mortality rates and having the liver transplantation as a salvage treatment. For optimal results, the emergency centers, emergency medical services transport and the tertiary centers must effectively cooperate.

References

1. Murray CJ, Lopez AD. Alternative projections of mortality and disability by cause 1990–2020: Global Burden of Disease Study. Lancet. 1997;349:1498–504.
2. Nishijima DK, Simel DL, Wisner DH, Holmes JF. Does this adult patient have a blunt intra-abdominal injury? JAMA. 2012;307:1517.
3. Isenhour JL, Marx J. Advances in abdominal trauma. Emerg Med Clin North Am. 2007;25:713.
4. Davis JJ, Cohn I Jr, Nance FC. Diagnosis and management of blunt abdominal trauma. Ann Surg. 1976;183:672.
5. Jones EL, Stovall RT, Jones TS, et al. Intra-abdominal injury following blunt trauma becomes clinically apparent within 9 hours. J Trauma Acute Care Surg. 2014;76:1020.
6. Tinkoff G, Esposito TJ, Reed J, et al. American Association for the Surgery of Trauma Organ Injury Scale I: spleen, liver, and kidney, validation based on the National Trauma Data Bank. J Am Coll Surg. 2008;207:646.
7. Coccolini F, Catena F, Moore EE, et al. WSES classification and guidelines for liver trauma. World J Emerg Surg. 2016;11:50.
8. Popescu I, Ciurea S. Traumatismele ficatului si cailor biliare. În "Tratat de chirurgie de urgenta" sub redactia lui Caloghera C., Editura Antib (Timisoara, Bucuresti, Cluj, Tg Mures) 2003, pag. 188–195.
9. Holmes JF, McGahan JP, Wisner DH. Rate of tra-abdominal injury after a normal abdominal computed tomographic scan in adults with blunt trauma. Am J Emerg Med. 2012;30:574.
10. Pachter HL, Hofstetter SR. The current status of nonoperative management of adult blunt hepatic injuries. Am J Surg. 1995;169:442–54.
11. Pachter HL, Knudson MM, Esrig B, Ross S, Hoyt D, Cogbill T, et al. Status of nonoperative management of blunt hepatic injuries in 1995: a multicenter experience with 404 patients. J Trauma. 1996;40:31–8.
12. Asensio JA, Demetriades D, Chahwan S, Gomez H, Hanpeter D, Velmahos G, et al. Approach to the management of complex hepatic injuries. J Trauma. 2000;48:66–9.
13. Carrillo EH, Platz A, Miller FB, Richardson JD, Polk HC Jr. Non-operative treatment of blunt hepatic trauma. Br J Surg. 1998;85:461–8.
14. Brasel KJ, Nirula R. What mechanism justifies abdominal evaluation in motor vehicle crashes? J Trauma. 2005;59:1057.
15. Koyama T, Hamada H, Nishida M, et al. Defining the optimal cut-off values for liver enzymes in diagnosing blunt liver injury. BMC Res Notes. 2016;9:41.
16. Soto JA, Anderson SW. Multidetector CT of blunt abdominal trauma. Radiology. 2012;265:678.
17. Gaarder C, Gaski IA, Næss PA. Spleen and liver injuries: when to operate? Curr Opin Crit Care. 2017;23(6):520–6.
18. Coccolini F, Montori G, Catena F, et al. Liver trauma: WSES position paper. World J Emerg Surg. 2015;10:39.
19. Croce MA, Fabian TC, Menke PG, et al. Nonoperative management of blunt hepatic trauma is the treatment of choice for hemodynamically stable patients. Results of a prospective trial. Ann Surg. 1995;221(744)
20. Sánchez-Bueno F, Fernández-Carrión J, Torres Salmerón G, et al. Changes in the diagnosis and therapeutic management of hepatic trauma. A retrospective study comparing 2 series of cases in different (1997–1984 vs. 2001–2008). Cir Esp. 2011;89:439.
21. Petrowsky H, Raeder S, Zuercher L, et al. A quarter century experience in liver trauma: a plea for early computed tomography and conservative management for all hemodynamically stable patients. World J Surg. 2012;36:247.
22. Popescu I (sub redactia). Chirurgia ficatului (2 vol)-ISBN: 973-7918-54-4. Editura Universitara "Carol Davila" Bucuresti, 2004.
23. Lamb CA. Rupture of the liver. N Engl J Med. 1939;221:855–9.
24. Gourgiotis S, Vougas V, Germanos S, Dimopoulos N, Bolanis I, Drakopoulos S, et al. Operative and nonoperative management of blunt hepatic trauma in adults: a single-center report. J Hepato-Biliary-Pancreat Surg. 2007;14:387–91.
25. Cirocchi R, Trastulli S, Pressi E, Farinella E, Avenia S, Morales Uribe CH, Botero AM, Barrera LM. Non-operative management versus operative management in high-grade blunt hepatic injury. Cochrane Database Syst Rev. 2015;8:CD010989.
26. Kozar RA, Moore FA, Moore EE, et al. Western Trauma Association critical decisions in trauma: nonoperative management of adult blunt hepatic trauma. J Trauma. 2009;67:1144.
27. Zafar SN, Rushing A, Haut ER, et al. Outcome of selective non-operative management of penetrating abdominal injuries from the North American National Trauma Database. Br J Surg. 2012;99(Suppl 1):155.
28. Stassen NA, Bhullar I, Cheng JD, et al. Nonoperative management of blunt hepatic injury: an Eastern Association for the Surgery of Trauma practice management guideline. J Trauma Acute Care Surg. 2012;73:S288.
29. Polanco PM, Brown JB, Puyana JC, et al. The swinging pendulum: a national perspective of nonoperative management in severe blunt liver injury. J Trauma Acute Care Surg. 2013;75:590.
30. Melloul E, Denys A, Demartines N. Management of severe blunt hepatic injury in the era of computed tomography and transarterial embolization: a systematic review and critical appraisal of the literature. J Trauma Acute Care Surg. 2015;79:468.
31. Pachter HL, Feliciano DV. Complex hepatic injuries. Surg Clin North Am. 1996;76:763.
32. Shrestha B, Holcomb JB, Camp EA, et al. Damage-control resuscitation increases successful nonoperative management rates and survival after severe blunt liver injury. J Trauma Acute Care Surg. 2015;78:336.
33. Badger SA, Barclay R, Campbell P, Mole DJ, Diamond T. Management of liver trauma. World J Surg. 2009;33:2522.
34. Richardson JD. Changes in the management of injuries to the liver and spleen. J Am Coll Surg. 2005;200:648.
35. Green CS, Bulger EM, Kwan SW. Outcomes and complications of angioembolization for hepatic trauma: a systematic review of the literature. J Trauma Acute Care Surg. 2016;80:529.
36. Hommes M, Nicol AJ, Navsaria PH, et al. Management of biliary complications in 412 patients with liver injuries. J Trauma Acute Care Surg. 2014;77:448.
37. van der Wilden GM, Velmahos GC, Emhoff T, et al. Successful nonoperative management of the most severe blunt liver injuries: a multicenter study of the research consortium of new England centers for trauma. Arch Surg. 2012;147:423.
38. Huang YC, Wu SC, Fu CY, et al. Tomographic findings are not always predictive of failed nonoperative management in blunt hepatic injury. Am J Surg. 2012;203:448.
39. Velmahos GC, Toutouzas KG, Radin R, Chan L, Demetriades D. Nonoperative treatment of blunt injury to solid abdominal organs: a prospective study. Arch Surg 2003;138:844–51.
40. Malhotra AK, Fabian TC, Croce MA, Gavin TJ, Kudsk KA, Minard G, et al. Blunt hepatic injury: a paradigm shift from operative to nonoperative management in the 1990s. Ann Surg. 2000;231:804–13.
41. Boese CK, Hackl M, Müller LP, et al. Nonoperative management of blunt hepatic trauma: a systematic review. J Trauma Acute Care Surg. 2015;79:654.
42. Goffette PP, Laterre PF. Traumatic injuries: Imaging and intervention in posttraumatic complication (delayed intervention). Eur Radiol. 2002;12:994–1021.
43. Letoublon C, Morra I, Chen Y, et al. Hepatic arterial embolization in the management of blunt hepatic trauma: indications and complications. J Trauma. 2011;70:1032.

44. Alarhayem AQ, Myers JG, Dent D, Lamus D, Lopera J, Liao L, et al. "Blush at first sight": significance of computed tomographic and angiographic discrepancy in patients with blunt abdominal trauma. Am J Surg. 2015;210:1104.
45. Mofidi M, Hasani A, Kianmehr N. Determining the accuracy of base deficit in diagnosis of intra-abdominal injury in patients with blunt abdominal trauma. Am J Emerg Med. 2010;28:933.
46. Fang JF, Chen RJ, Lin BC, Hsu YB, Kao JL, Chen MF. Blunt hepatic injury: minimal intervention is the policy of treatment. J Trauma. 2000;49:722–8.
47. Duane TM, Como JJ, Bochicchio GV, Scalea TM. Reevaluating the management and outcomes of severe blunt liver injury. J Trauma. 2004;57:494–500.
48. Popescu I (sub redactia). Tratat de chirurgie hepato-bilio-pancreatica si transplant hepatic. ISBN 978-973-27-2592-4, Editura Academiei Romane, 2016.
49. Søndenaa K, Tasdemir I, Andersen E, et al. Treatment of blunt injury of the spleen: is there a place for mesh wrapping? Eur J Surg. 1994;160:669.
50. Nicol AJ, Hommes M, Primrose R, et al. Packing for control of hemorrhage in major liver trauma. World J Surg. 2007;31:569.
51. Birkmeyer J, Siewers AE, Finlayson EV, Stukel TA, Lucas FL, Batista I, et al. High volume and surgical mortality in the United States. N Engl J Med. 2002;346:1128–37.
52. Eppsteiner R, Csikesz NG, Simons JP, Tseng JF, Shah SA. 217 high volume surgery and outcome after liver resection: Surgeon or center? J Gastroenterol Surg. 2008;134:1709–16.
53. Polanco P, Leon S, Pineda J, Puyana JC, Ochoa JB, Alarcon L, Harbrecht BG, Geller D, Peitzman AB. Hepatic resection in the management of complex injury to the liver. J Trauma. 2008;65(6):1264–1269; discussion 1269–70.
54. Li Petri S, Gruttadauria S, Pagano D, Echeverri GJ, Di Francesco F, Cintorino D, Spada M, Gridelli B. Surgical management of complex liver trauma: a single liver transplant center experience. Am Surg. 2012 Jan;78(1):20–5.
55. Liu PP, Chen CL, Cheng YF, et al. Use of a refined operative strategy in combination with the multidisciplinary approach to manage blunt juxtahepatic venous injuries. J Trauma. 2005;59:940.
56. Popescu I, Ionescu M, Braşoveanu V, Hrehoreţ D, Copca N, Lupaşcu C, Botea F, Dorobanţu B, Alexandrescu S, Grigorie M, Matei E, Zamfir R, Lungu V, et al. The Romanian National Program for Liver Transplantation – 852 Procedures in 815 Patients over 17 Years (2000–2017): a continuous evolution to success. Chirurgia (Bucur). 2017 May–Jun;112(3):229–243.
57. Heuer M, Kaiser GM, Lendemans S, et al. Transplantation after blunt trauma to the liver: a valuable option or just a "waste of organs"? Eur J Med Res. 2010;15:169.
58. Kaltenborn A, Reichert B, Bourg CM, et al. Long-term outcome analysis of liver transplantation for severe hepatic trauma. J Trauma Acute Care Surg. 2013;75:864.
59. Singh V, Narasimhan KL, Verma GR, Singh G. Endoscopic management of traumatic hepatobiliary injuries. J Gastroenterol Hepatol. 2007;22:1205.
60. Kozar RA, Moore JB, Niles SE, et al. Complications of nonoperative management of high-grade blunt hepatic injuries. J Trauma. 2005;59:1066.
61. Dabbs DN, Stein DM, Philosophe B, Scalea TM. Treatment of major hepatic necrosis: lobectomy versus serial debridement. J Trauma. 2010;69:562.
62. Kozar RA, Moore FA, Cothren CC, et al. Risk factors for hepatic morbidity following nonoperative management: multicenter study. Arch Surg. 2006;141:451.
63. Peitzman AB, Richardson JD. Surgical treatment of injuries to the solid abdominal organs: a 50-year perspective from the Journal of Trauma. J Trauma. 2010;69:1011.
64. Sivrikoz E, Teixeira PG, Resnick S, et al. Angiointervention: an independent predictor of survival in high-grade blunt liver injuries. Am J Surg. 2015;209:742.
65. Piper GL, Peitzman AB. Current management of hepatic trauma. Surg Clin North Am. 2010;90:775.

61. Indications for Liver Transplantation in Adults: Selection of Patients with End Stage Liver Diseases

Speranta Iacob and Liana Gheorghe

Abstract

Since it was first performed by Thomas Starlz in 1963, liver transplantation (LT) has become a well-established and overall accepted treatment with excellent long term outcomes for patients with end stage liver diseases and hepatocellular carcinoma. In the last years, there was a change in the main indications for LT, with increasing proportion of patients transplanted for alcoholic liver disease, NAFLD-related cirrhosis and hepatocellular carcinoma and a significant decrease in HCV- or HBV-related chronic liver failure. An overview of the indications and contraindications for LT is presented in this chapter. The selection of candidates, timing and organ allocation via a strict selection process that involves a multidisciplinary approach and complies with both urgency (individual needs) and utility (survival benefit), contribute to the optimal post-LT outcomes.

61.1 Historical Overview

Liver transplantation (LT) has made remarkable progress since his naissance on 1st March 1963. Thomas Starzl was the one that performed the first LT in the world and then contributed substantially to its actual success by continually developing procedures and principles governing LT to date. He was also the first one to report the use of tacrolimus in 1990 in LT recipients who suffered a rejection under cyclosporine/azathioprine/corticosteroids treatment. Nowadays, more than 55 years from the first LT, over 450,000 LTs have been performed in the world so far. Liver transplant patients' survival within the first year is over 80–90% due to improvement in surgical/technical problems, rejection treatment, infection risk control, intensive care management, as well as a better selection and preservation of the donors [1, 2]. However, this success has created difficulties. Ongoing challenges of LT include those concerning donor organ shortages, recipients with more advanced disease at transplant, growing need for retransplantation, toxicities and adverse effects associated with long-term immunosuppression, obesity and non-alcoholic steatohepatitis epidemics [3]. Although there was an immense expansion of the number of institutions performing this procedure, there is still need of better access for patients to transplantation centers, progresses in organization and improvements in transplantation system, filter in indications and prioritization and a better use of donations [4].

61.2 Referral for Liver Transplantation

The principle criteria for selection of candidates for LT are (1) risk of dying due to progression of liver diseases, (2) impact on quality of life, (3) benefit of survival and (4) some criteria applicable for special indications considered MELD exceptions.

For majority of patients (>90%) with decompensated liver cirrhosis and liver failure, selection for LT depends upon the risk of dying due to progression of liver disease compared to the mortality due to LT and associated immunosuppression. The severity of CLF is generally determined by the degree of synthetic failure (jaundice, coagulopathy, hypoalbuminemia) and portal hypertension. It is usually measured by two scoring systems, the Child-Turcotte-Pugh (CTP) and the model for end-stage liver disease (MELD) calculations. Admission of the patients with liver cirrhosis on the waiting list for LT is realized in accordance to the minimal selection criteria. These include patients with a CTP score ≥ 7 and/or a MELD score ≥ 10 or when an index complication of cirrhosis such as ascites or variceal hemorrhage

S. Iacob (✉) · L. Gheorghe
Digestive Diseases and Liver Transplantation Center, Fundeni Clinical Institute, Bucharest, Romania

"Carol Davila" University of Medicine and Pharmacy, Bucharest, Romania

occurs [5–7]. Patients with a MELD score ≥ 15 are most likely to benefit from LT. The MELD score does disadvantage a subset of patients who have severely decompensated liver disease but minimally abnormal laboratory results, those being listed as MELD exceptions. Recently, serum sodium has been incorporated into the MELD score (MELD-Na), hyponatremia being considered an independent predictor of mortality in patients with decompensated cirrhosis, and low serum sodium levels may be a surrogate marker of advanced portal hypertension [8].

LT has two major objectives: (1) increase considerably the survival and (2) restauration of the quality of life, social and professional functions as well as reproductive capacity for patients with advanced chronic liver diseases or fulminant liver failure.

61.2.1 Indications for LT

The indications for LT have slightly changed over the years. Overall, LT is indicated for acute liver failure, chronic liver failure leading to cirrhosis, hepatocellular carcinoma inherited metabolic liver diseases. It is also indicated for hepatocellular carcinoma (HCC) and other hepatic cancers, including hepatoblastoma, epithelioid haemangioendothelioma, and hilar cholangiocarcinoma (CCA). The main current indications for LT are listed in Table 61.1 [9–13].

61.2.1.1 Acute Liver Failure (ALF)

ALF is an uncommon (approximately 2000 cases/year), but a life-threatening critical illness, an important indication for LT. Although a significant proportion of patients with ALF may spontaneously recover (45%), its clinical course can be unpredictable (30% death) and early transfer to a LT center is recommended, regardless of the etiology. Patients with ALF have the highest priority for organ allocation if they meet specific criteria (United Network for Organ Sharing [UNOS] status 1A): rapidly progressively (<8 weeks usually) of altered mentation/encephalopathy, coagulopathy (INR > 2) and jaundice in patients with no prior history of chronic liver disease or cirrhosis [11, 14]. Wilson's disease is the single one to be considered ALF for listing purposes even with known history or cirrhosis. Most common etiology of ALF remains acetaminophen-induced hepatotoxicity (around 45%), followed by non-A-to-E hepatitis, other drug induced liver injuries (including recreational drugs or cocaine), viral hepatitis, mushroom intoxication, acute Budd Chiari syndrome or Wilson diasease, pregnancy related ALF. In 10–15% of cases, the cause of ALF remains unknown, despite intensive investigation; these cases often follow a subacute presentation, and rates of survival are poor without LT [15]. To note, autoimmune hepatitis may account for up to 30% of indeterminant cases, because 25–39% are ANA negative and with normal IgG. ALF due to Wilson disease is nearly always fatal without LT.

Table 61.2 shows clinical features in paracetamol and non-paracetamol ALF that correlate with poor outcome and mandate referral [16]. None of the parameters, such as intra-

Table 61.1 Indications for adult liver transplantation (LT)

Acute liver failure	Hepatitis A/B/E Intoxication (e.g., acetaminophen, halotan, Amanita phalloides) Wilson's disease Budd–Chiari syndrome
Chronic liver failure: Noncholestatic cirrhosis	Hepatitis B/C Autoimmune hepatitis Alcohol-induced cirrhosis
Chronic liver failure: Cholestatic cirrhosis	Primary biliary cirrhosis (PBC) Primary sclerosing cholangitis (PSC) Secondary biliary cirrhosis
Chronic liver failure: Metabolic	Wilson's disease Hemochromatosis a-1 Antitrypsin deficiency Familial amyloidosis Cystic fibrosis Tyrosinemia
Chronic liver failure: Vascular	Budd–Chiari syndrome
Other indications	Primary oxalosis Gycogen storage diseases Familial hyperlipidemia Polycystic liver disease
Malignant disease	Hepatocellular carcinoma (HCC) – T2 lesions (at least 2 cm in diameter) – Within Milan criteria (Eurotransplant) • Single tumor with a diameter ≤ 5 cm, or two or three tumors ≤3 cm each. • Absence of extrahepatic involvement, including the absence of portal vein invasion. – UNOS region 4 criteria (Texas and Oklahoma) • Single tumor with a diameter ≤ 6 cm, or no more than three tumors, none >5 cm, and a total diameter < 9 cm. • Absence of extrahepatic involvement, including the absence of portal vein invasion. – UCSF criteria (Australia and New Zealand) • One HCC ≤ 6.5 cm. • Up to three HCC ≤ 4.5 cm each. • Total HCC sum ≤8 cm. • No extra-hepatic disease. • No vascular invasion. –Outside Milan criteria according to each Transplant Center outside US that accepts this indication Fibrolamellar carcinoma Hepatoblastoma Epitheloid hemangioendothelioma Cholangiocellular adenocarcinoma Neuroendocrine liver metastases
Benign liver tumors	Adenomatosis

Table 61.2 Indications for LT referral for a patient with ALF

Paracetamol induced ALF	Non-paracetamol induced ALF
• Arterial pH <7.30 or HCO$_3$ < 18 mmol/l. • INR >3.0 on day two or >4.0 thereafter. • Oliguria and/or AKI. • Altered level of consciousness. • Hypoglycaemia. • Elevated arterial lactate (>4 mmol/L) unresponsive to fluid resuscitation.	• pH <7.30 or HCO$_3$ < 18 mmol/l, • INR >1.8. • Oliguria/renal failure or Na <130 mmol/L. • Encephalopathy, hypoglycaemia or metabolic acidosis. • Bilirubin >300 μmol/L (17.6 mg/dL).

AKI acute kidney injury, *ALF* acute liver failure, *CLF* chronic liver failure, *INR* international normalised ratio, *LT* liver transplantation

cranial pressure, age, grade of hepatic encephalopathy, APACHE score, has a discriminative value for exclusion of patients with ALF from LT. However, increased requirements for inotrope support, uncontrolled sepsis, and severe respiratory insufficiency are considered contraindications for LT [17]. The best survival after LT for ALF is encountered in Wilson disease and the lowest in idiosyncratic drug reactions.

61.2.1.2 Chronic Liver Failure

In the last years were noted important changes in the main indications for LT in liver cirrhosis. Alcohol-related liver disease (ALD), and chronic hepatitis B (CHB) and C (CHC) were the most common causes of cirrhosis and HCC [18] until recently, and this profile was also reflected in patients in need of an LT. Since the introduction of interferon-free antiviral regimens in 2013–2014, with excellent rates of cure, there was a sudden decline in the burden of CHC as a cause of chronic liver disease (CLD), cause of liver death and LT. With a worldwide **non-alcoholic steatohepatitis** (NASH) prevalence of 25%, this indication will took the first place as indication of LT in all countries. A recent study by Younoussi et al. [19] showed that NASH is the second most common non-HCC indication for LT in 2019 after ALD. In patients with CLD accompanied by HCC, the trends in subpopulations largely mirror those of the entire HCC sample where CHC remains the most common CLD aetiology despite a notable decline in the last 5 years. However, in Hispanic patients, NASH is now the most common indication for transplantation in the presence of HCC (32%) surpassing both CHC and ALD (26–28%), and in female patients it is close to that of CHC (33% vs. 37%). The same is also true for Europe where the percentage of LTs due to HCV-related liver disease decreased from 22.8% in the interferon/ribavirin era to 17.4% in the direct antiviral agents era, while those performed for NASH increased significantly (p < 0.0001). This decline was more evident in patients with HCV decompensated cirrhosis (−58.0%) than in those with HCC associated with HCV (−41.2%) [20]. Despite higher risk due to associated comorbidities, the outcome for NASH is likely comparable with other disease indication with HCC or without HCC (84% for NASH vs 86% for non-NASH; 98% for HCC-NASH vs 96% for HCC-non-NASH 1 year survival rate). Post-LT recipients with NASH have a high risk for metabolic diseases including diabetes, hypertension, hyperlipidemia, and also recurrent NAFLD/NASH (approximately 30%). Although post-LT NAFLD/NASH shows slow progression, and only a small population develop cirrhosis again, NASH related LT recipients have been reported as a higher risk for quick deterioration for fibrosis and close management may be required [21]. Compared to other etiologies, post-transplant cardiovascular events are higher in LT recipients with NASH cirrhosis, especially in the immediate postoperative period [22]. Therefore, several societies recommend comprehensive cardiovascular risk assessment (both structural and functional) and testing during the LT evaluation process. NASH patients experienced higher mortality due to cardiovascular disease (OR = 1.65; p = 0.05) and sepsis (OR = 1.71; p = 0.006), while graft failure was lower (OR = 0.21; p = 0.03) compared to non-NASH LT recipients [23]. The LT evaluation process should include a multidisciplinary team approach; including cardiology, cardiac anaesthesiology, nephrology; endocrinology and nutrition in addition to hepatology and transplant surgery, to appropriately risk stratify and optimize NASH patients to improve post-transplant outcomes [24].

In the last years, there is no appreciable clinical advance in the management of the **hepatitis B virus** in the LT field. In contrast, the management of patients with **hepatitis C virus** (HCV) infection has been dramatically changing after the emergence of direct-acting antivirals, as already stated. Due to the high efficacy in obtaining sustained virologic response, very good safety profile and improvement of liver function, even for patients with decompensated cirrhosis, a major decline was observed in the number of LT performed both in patients with HCV related decompensated cirrhosis and in those with HCV related HCC in the United States [25] and Europe [20]. In addition, the survival of LT recipients with HCV-related liver disease has clearly improved because of treatment for HCV recurrence, which used to be a common problem in clinical practice.

The improvement of liver function does not always reach the point of delisting and/or amelioration of complications from portal hypertension such as encephalopathy or refractory ascites. The patient with improved MELD score decreases the probability of receiving an LT under the MELD allocation systems (the so-called "MELD limbo or purgatory"), despite continuing to experience poor quality of life and severe complications of cirrhosis [26].

The debate about the optimal timing for treating HCV patients in LT waiting list is ongoing. Current recommendations by the International Liver Transplantation Society for management of HCV in LT candidates are summarized in Table 61.3 [27].

The persistent shortage of donor grafts along with robust data supporting the efficacy and safety of direct antivirals for treatment of recurrent HCV infection following LT has resulted in consideration of use of HCV-infected grafts for individuals with HCV infection listed for LT, but also from viral positive donors to negative recipients [28].

Alcohol-related liver disease (ALD) is also becoming a leading indication for LT in both United States and Europe. In 2016, ALD became the leading indication for LT waitlist additions in the United States by surpassing HCV [29]. Most organ allocation policies set some period (6–18 months) of abstinence to discriminate whether liver function could improve to avoid LT. However, this period certainly reflects ethical and social ideas based on the deeply ingrained view of alcohol-use disorder as simply self-inflicted behaviour. This period is often an unrealistic barrier because the prognosis of patients with acute onset alcoholic hepatitis shows 75–90% mortality within 2 months when they are not responsive for medical therapy except LT [28]. Lee et al. [30] showed the selective use of LT can be a lifesaving option for refractory alcoholic hepatitis, and the 3-year survival rate (84%) and frequency of alcohol use after LT (17%) appear to be acceptable without any abstinence period. Same authors also showed the early LT for selected severe alcoholic hepatitis increases survival periods of patients (a four-fold survival benefit over delayed LT) [31]. This is a result consistent with the landmark French study by Mathurin et al. [32]. The survival benefit was present across all UNOS regions and persisted irrespective of any estimated risk of sustained alcohol use post-LT [31]. However, life expectancy was significantly decreased (a 67% lower life expectancy) for early LT recipients who return to sustained alcohol use after transplant compared to recipients with post-LT abstinence.

The utility of the 6-month rule as a predictor of long-term sobriety is controversial. ALD patients with less than 6 months abstinence are more likely to drink after transplantation, but most data on drinking after LT come from studies that used the 6 month rule. Thus, the 6 month rule admits patients who will relapse after LT and excludes patients that will not drink after LT. This rule is not required by UNOS, nor advocated in the 2019 AASLD guidance [33], but it is mandatory in Eurotransplant [34]. Assessment by an addiction specialist that combines sobriety with assessment of other indicators of relapse risk is advisable. Main risk factors for relapse of alcohol use disorder are: lack of insight into addiction, social isolation (lack of employment, living alone, no spouse or companion), history of many failed rehabilitation attempts, psychiatric comorbid conditions. However, patients with decompensated alcohol-associated cirrhosis, Child-Pugh class C or MELD-Na ≥21 should be referred and considered for LT.

61.2.2 Cholestatic and Autoimmune Liver Diseases

The proportion of PBC decreased from 20% of LT in 1986 to 4% in 2015, as per the European Liver Transplantation Registry [35]. Current guidelines suggest using recent validated predictive models, such as the Toronto criteria or the GLOBE-PBC score to decide which patients may be considered at higher risk of liver-related complications. Prior to 2016, the only treatment was ursodeoxycholic acid (UDCA), but presently a second-line therapy has been approved called obeticholic acid (OCA). OCA is a potent farnesoid X receptor (FXR) agonist that has been shown in animal models to be anticholeretic, antifibrotic, and anti-inflammatory. OCA is not without adverse effects, such as pruritus, and its use in decompensated cirrhosis requires dose adjustment and close follow-up; however, in appropriately selected patients OCA is a safe and effective adjunct or alternative to UDCA that can prolong transplant-free survival [36]. However, LT remains the only radical treatment for PBC. Although the prognosis of PBC after LT is relatively good, the recurrence rates of PBC were in a range from 9% to 35% after LT [37].

Primary sclerosing cholangitis (PSC) is a rare disorder characterised by multi-focal bile duct strictures and progressive liver disease. There is currently no medical therapy proven to delay the development of liver cirrhosis in patients with PSC. There has been extensive debate as to the efficacy of UDCA, leading to inconsistent prescription practices worldwide from low dose 13–15 mg/kg/day to high dose 28–30 mg/kg/day UDCA [38, 39].

The indications for LT in PSC are similar to other liver diseases with the majority listed and transplanted with a qualifying MELD (or similar) score in a patient with cirrhosis. Overall <5% of transplants in the US are done on the basis of PSC, while about 15% of those in Scandinavia are

Table 61.3 International Liver Transplantation Society recommendations for management of hepatitis C in LT candidates

Patient population	Recommendation
Decompensated cirrhosis with MELD<20, without refractory portal hypertension or other conditions requiring more immediate LT	Treat HCV pre-LT
Decompensated cirrhosis with MELD ≥ 30 or LT expected within 3 months	Treat HCV post-LT
Compensated cirrhosis and HCC	Treat HCV pre-LT
Decompensated cirrhosis and HCC not expected to undergo LT within 3–6 months	Treat HCV pre-LT
Decompensated cirrhosis and HCC expected to undergo LT within 3–6 months	Treat HCV post-LT

HCC hepatocellular carcinoma, *HCV* hepatitis C virus, *LT* liver transplantation, *MELD* model for end-stage liver disease

undertaken for PSC, reflecting differences in practice and prevalence [40]. However, 5 year survival rates are ~85%, with disease recurrence of 20–25% in 5 to 10 years after LT.

Clinical indications for LT in patients with autoimmune hepatitis (AIH) are identical to those of patients with other chronic liver diseases that end in acute or semiacute liver failure, decompensated cirrhosis, or hepatocellular carcinoma. AIH accounts for ~6% of all LT in North America. Recurrent disease after LT has been reported in 10–50% of patients with AIH, with increasing frequency with time since LT; also the frequency of detection is influenced in part by the use of protocol or clinically indicated liver biopsy. Outcomes of patients with AIH are rather good with 5 and 10 year survival rates of 86% and 73%, respectively [41].

61.2.3 MELD Exceptions

The MELD exception system is in place to allow increased priority for those at higher risk for morbidity and mortality than that predicted by their MELD score.

Standardized MELD exceptions are those conditions for which there are sufficient data to warrant allocating automatic exception points to patients meeting formalized exception criteria (i.e., hepatocellular carcinoma).

Hepatocellular carcinoma (HCC) has become a leading indication for LT in the United States over the past 2 decades, accounting for approximately 25% of all LTs performed annually.

LT was a controversial treatment option for hepatocellular carcinoma (HCC) in the early years until Mazzaferro et al. described 75% 4-year survival in a cohort of patients with HCC limited to a single tumour lesion <5 cm or up to three tumour lesions, none greater than 3 cm [42]. These criteria, now known as the Milan criteria, have become the HCC listing criteria for LT. Since 1996, many studies were published aiming to expand the Milan criteria without impairing patient survival or recurrence-free survival. The most recent studies published lately, aiming to define predictors or new criteria for LT in patients with HCC are shown in Table 61.4.

In USA, expansion of the acceptable tumour burden is currently only permitted by UNOS in region 4 (Texas and Oklahoma). Treatment of one or more tumours with locoregional therapies may result in "down-staging" to within-acceptable tumour burden and permit LT [51]. In Europe, according to the ELTR study [53] vascular invasion is an important prognostic factor for patients transplanted for HCC. Patients without vascular invasion, regardless of size and number of nodules, had a survival comparable to that of patients within Milan and Up-to-seven criteria [43]. In addition, patients outside these criteria still had a fair prognosis in the absence of microvascular invasion. In near future, validation of better biomarkers of tumor biology through either direct sampling or non-invasive means (i.e. circulating tumor cells, cell-free DNA, DNA methylation patterns, etc.) may better guide transplant priority decision making.

Table 61.4 Prediction of HCC recurrence after liver transplantation

Author	Information
Mazzaferro [43]	For patients with HCC to have a 70% chance of HCC-specific survival 5 years after LT, their level of AFP should be <200 ng/mL and the sum of number and size of tumors should not exceed 7; if the level of AFP was 200–400 ng/mL, should be ≤5; if their level of AFP was 400–1000 ng/mL, should be ≤4. In the validation set, the model identified patients who survived 5 years after LT with 0.721 accuracy
Mehta [44]	RETREAT score predicts post LT HCC recurrence. Post-LT survival at 3 years; 91% for a score 0, 80% for a score of 3, and 58% for a score ≥ 5 ($P < 0.001$). Post-LT HCC recurrence probability within 3 years increased from 1.6% with RETREAT score of 0 to 29% for a score ≥ 5 ($P < 0.001$)
Mano [45]	A low Lymphocyte-to-Monocyte Ratio (LMR) was associated with poor prognosis and represented an independent prognostic factor, particularly among patients beyond Milan criteria. The ratio of CD3-positive to CD68-positive cells was significantly lower in the low-LMR group
Kornberg [46]	ALBI grade calculated using pre-LT serum albumin and bilirubin. Posttransplant HCC recurrence rates were 10.5%, 15.9%, and 68.2% in ALBI grade 1, 2, and 3, respectively. Along with AFP and CRP, ALBI grades 1 or 2 was identified as an independent predictor of RFS. ALBI grade 3 proved to be the strongest indicator of microvascular invasion
Shimamura [47]	The 5-5-500 rule (nodule size ≤5 cm in diameter, nodule number ≤ 5, and AFP value ≤500 ng/mL): 5-year recurrence rate of 7.3% and a 19% increase number in the eligible patients who are beyond Milan criteria
Firl [48]	The Hazard Associated with Liver Transplantation for Hepatocellular Carcinoma (HALTHCC) model is a continuous score calculated as follows; $(2.31*\ln(AFP)) + (1.33*\text{tumor burden score}) + (0.25*\text{MELD-Na}) - (5.57*\text{Asia})$. HALTHCC score predicted overall survival, recurrence rate, and vascular invasion, poorly differentiated components on explant pathology
Duvoux [49]	Tumor status is graded with the alfa-fetoprotein (AFP) model that includes tumor size, number of nodules, and AFP level. Only patients with HCC tumor-node metastasis (TNM) stage ≥2 (single nodule ≥2 cm in size or > 1 nodule) and AFP score ≤ 2 with or without downstaging are eligible for HCC score. Therefore, patients outside the Milan criteria may be eligible for transplantation provided the AFP score is ≤2
Meischl [50]	CRP >1 mg/dL was an independent risk factor for HCC recurrence with a 5-year recurrence rate of 27.4% vs 16.4%. Overall survival was similar in patients with normal vs elevated CRP levels

(continued)

Table 61.4 (continued)

Author	Information
Heimbach [51]	Patients initially outside the Milan criteria (or region 4 criteria if being listed in this region) are listed with their biological MELD score. Patients with AFP > 1000 ng/mL are not initially eligible for exception points, whereas those with AFP < 500 ng/mL after locoregional therapy do qualify for exception points. Locoregional therapy in all patients listed for LT for HCC is endorsed, as this intervention is associated with significant reductions of waitlist drop out
Halazun [52]	Independent predictors of worse recurrence-free survival (RFS) were: NLR ≥ 5 ($P < 0.0001$, HR: 6.2), AFP > 200 ng/mL ($P < 0.0001$, HR: 3.8), size >3 cm ($P < 0.001$, HR: 3.2). The Pre-MORAL score had a value between 0 points (no factors) to 13 points (all 3 factors). The highest risk patients in the Pre-MORAL had a 5-year RFS of 17.9% compared with 98.6% for the low risk group ($P < 0.0001$). The post-MORAL was constructed using grade 4 HCC's ($P < 0.0001$, HR: 5.6), vascular invasion ($P = 0.019$, HR: 2.0), size >3 cm ($P < 0.0001$, HR: 3.2) and number > 3 ($P = 0.048$, HR: 1.8). The pre- and post-MORAL were superior to Milan at predicting recurrence.

Table 61.5 Absolute contraindications to LT

- Uncontrolled sepsis
- Acquired immunodeficiency syndrome
- Active alcohol or substance abuse
- Advanced cardiac or pulmonary disease
- Intrahepatic cholangiocarcinoma
- Hepatic hemangiosarcoma
- HCC with metastasis
- Extrahepatic malignancy
- Anatomic abnormalities that preclude LT
- Lack of adequate social support
- Persistent non-adherence to medical care

61.2.4 Other Standardized MELD Exceptions

Besides HCC, there are several other conditions that are categorized as standardized MELD exceptions [11]: hepatopulmonary syndrome ($PaO_2 < 60$ mmHg on ambient air), cholangiocarcinoma (Stage I or II, transplant center must have a UNOS-approved protocol), familial amyloid polyneuropathy (FAP), cystic fibrosis (Forced expiratory volume in 1 s (FEV1) < 40%) or polycystic liver disease (PCLD), portopulmonary hypertension (PPH) (mean pulmonary arterial pressure < 35 mmHg with treatment), familial amyloid polyneuropathy, hepatic artery thrombosis (within 14 days of transplant, not meeting criteria for status 1a).

61.2.4.1 Non-Standardized MELD Exceptions

Non-standardized exceptions are those conditions which are clearly important by the transplant team, but for which the risk of mortality is not as clear-cut, and thus require review on a case-by-case basis. This category includes a broad range of conditions, such as hyponatremia, refractory ascites or variceal bleeding, hepatic encephalopathy, sarcopenia, recurrent cholangitis, intractable pruritus, along with many other less common conditions.

Exceptional MELD criteria and the awarded exceptional MELD scores for all Eurotransplant (ET) countries are listed in the ET liver allocation manual [54].

Patients who receive MELD exceptions are awarded an initial MELD score that ranges from an equivalent of a mortality of 10% at 3 months (20 points) for PCLD or cystic fibrosis to an equivalent of a mortality of 25% at 3 months (25 points) for PPH. Most MELD exceptions (HCC, familial amyloid polyneuropathy, hepatopulmonary syndrome, hereditary haemorrhagic telangiectasia, hepatic hemangio-endothelioma) initially receive an exceptional MELD score equivalent to a mortality of 15% at 3 months (22 points). Exceptional MELD scores for the above conditions increase by 2–3 points equivalent to an additional 10% of mortality every 3 months, as long as the defining condition persisted [55, 56].

61.2.5 Contraindications for LT

Contraindications to LT also evolved over time with different progress in surgical technique or management on the waiting list of complications. Relative contraindications are usually associated with suboptimal outcomes following LT and vary widely across different transplant centres. Absolute contraindications imply that a successful outcome following LT is unlikely, thus it should not be performed (Table 61.5) [10, 57].

61.3 Management of the Patients Included on the Waiting List

Patients meeting the minimal listing criteria undergo a comprehensive evaluation performed by a multidisciplinary team (hepatology/gastroenterology, cardiology, neurology, psychology/psychiatry, transplant surgery, radiology, anesthesiology) before being included on the waiting list. Patients already listed will be also periodically evaluated by multidisciplinary teams at the transplant center. Routine interventions recommended in this population are summarized in Table 61.6 [11, 57].

61.4 Allocation of Available Organs

The selection of candidates, timing and organ allocation via a strict selection process that involves a multidisciplinary approach and complies with both urgency (individual needs)

Table 61.6 Specific recommendations for patients listed for LT

Interventions	Specific recommendations
Surveillance for gastroesophageal varices	Upper endoscopy for gastroesophageal varices every 1–3 years; interval depends on the size of varices, CTP class, and ongoing vs. quiescent liver injury
Screening for hepatic malignancy	Liver ultrasound for HCC every 3–6 months + AFP; a contrast-enhanced multiphase CT or MRI at least once during follow-up
Age-appropriate screening for extrahepatic malignancies	Colon, breast, cervical cancer
Primary prophylaxis for SBP	Ascitic fluid protein <1.5 g/dL, and either impaired renal function (creatinine ≥1.2 mg/dL, BUN ≥25 mg/dL, or sodium ≤130 mEq/L) or severe hepatic dysfunction (CTP ≥ 9 and bilirubin ≥3 mg/dL); cirrhosis and gastrointestinal bleeding; patients with cirrhosis and ascitic fluid protein <1 g/dL hospitalized for other reasons
Secondary prophylaxis for SBP	Patients who have had one or more episodes of SBP, long-term antibiotic prophylaxis is recommended
Screen for bone mineral density disorders	DEXA scan
Nutritional assessment and support	Assessment and counselling by a dietician to identify and treat malnutrition, obesity, and/or specific nutritional deficiencies (i.e., fat-soluble vitamins in cholestatic diseases)
Immunizations	Hepatitis A and B vaccine if not immune; pneumococcal vaccine every 3–5 years, influenza vaccine on a yearly basis; diphtheria, pertussis, and tetanus vaccine booster every 10 years

AFP alpha feto-protein, *CT* computed tomography, *CTP* Child–Turcotte–Pugh, *DEXA* dual-energy X-ray absorptiometry, *MRI* magnetic resonance imaging, *SBP* spontaneous bacterial peritonitis

and utility (survival benefit), contribute to the optimal post-LT outcomes.

Transplant-related survival benefit is calculated as the difference between life expectancy with transplantation and life expectancy without transplantation. Determining eligibility and prioritization for LT based on the highest survival benefit is a superior strategy to prioritization based on the highest urgency (i.e., the highest wait-list mortality) or the highest utility (i.e., the highest post-transplant survival) because prioritization based on the highest survival benefit maximizes the overall life expectancy of all patients in need of LT [58].

As already known, the MELD score has been validated as a scoring tool to prioritize patients on LT waiting lists by predicting 3-month mortality risk with 83–87% accuracy. Wait-list mortality is directly proportional to the MELD score, where a MELD score of <9 is associated with a ~ mortality of 2% and a MELD score ≥ 40 is associated with a wait-list mortality of 71% [59]. It is imperative to establish, by a multidisciplinary team, a consensus of independently successful and futile predictors of transplant outcomes in patients with MELD scores ≥35, in order to optimize outcomes in these high-risk patients and prevent futile LT. The complexity of organ allocation systems in individual countries can further complicate organ allocation [60].

Although predictive models such as the MELD score and Milan criteria provide useful guidance for the selection of appropriate LT candidates, an individualized and comprehensive assessment of each patient's clinical, social, economic, and behavioural situation is necessary to continue improving outcomes in LT.

Selecting the most appropriate donor organ for the most appropriate recipient in order to provide the best postoperative survival is also challenging. However, this is probably the best way to provide the optimal post-LT outcome of the recipients.

References

1. Meirelles Júnior RF, Salvalaggio P, Rezende MB, et al. Liver transplantation: history, outcomes and perspectives. Einstein (Sao Paulo). 2015;13(1):149–52.
2. Bodzin A, Baker T. Liver transplantation today: where we are now and where we are going. Liver Transpl. 2018;24(10):1470–5.
3. Zarrinpar A, Busuttil RW. Liver transplantation: past, present and future. Nat Rev Gastroenterol Hepatol. 2013;10(7):434–40.
4. Song ATW, Avelino-Silva VI, Pecora RAA, et al. Liver transplantation: fifty years of experience. World J Gastroenterol. 2014;20(18):5363–74.
5. Lucey MR, Brown KA, Everson GT, et al. Minimal criteria for placement of adults on liver transplant waiting list: a report of a national conference organized by the American Society of Transplant Physicians and the American Association for the Study of Liver Disease. Liver Transpl Surg. 1997;3:628–37.
6. McCaughan GW, Crawford M, Sandroussi C, et al. Assessment of adult patients with chronic liver failure for liver transplantation in 2015: who and when? Intern Med J. 2016;46(4):404–12.
7. Devlin J, O'Grady J. Indications for referral and assessment in adult liver transplantation: a clinical guideline. Gut. 1999;45:1–22.
8. Kim WR, Biggins SW, Kremers WK, et al. Hyponatremia and mortality among patients on the liver-transplant waiting list. N Engl J Med. 2008;359(10):1018–26.
9. European liver transplant registry. Available: http://www.eltr.org
10. Ahmed A, Keeffe EB. Current indications and contraindications for liver transplantation. Clin Liver Dis. 2007;11:227–47.
11. Carrion A, Martin P. When to refer for liver transplantation? Am J Gastroenterol. 2019;114(1):7–10.
12. Millson C, Considine A, Cramp M, et al. Adult liver transplantation: a UK clinical guideline – Part 1: pre-operation. Frontl Gastroenterol. 2020;11:375–84.
13. Farkas S, Hackl C, Schlitt HJ. Overview of the indications and contraindications for liver transplantation. Cold Spring Harb Perspect Med. 2014;4(5):a015602.
14. Lee WM, Squires RH, Nyberg SL, Doo E, Hoofnagle J. Acute liver failure: summary of a workshop. Hepatology. 2008;47(4):1401–15.
15. Bernal W, Wendon J. Acute liver failure. N Engl J Med. 2013;369(26):2525–34.
16. Wendon J, Cordoba J, Dhawan A, et al. EASL clinical practical guidelines on the management of acute (fulminant) liver failure. J Hepatol. 2017;66:1047–81.

17. O'Grady JG. Acute liver failure. In: Arroyo V, Sanchez-Fueyo A, Fernandez-Gomez J, Forns X, Gines P, Rodes J, editors. Advances in the therapy of liver diseases. Barcelona: Ars Medica; 2007. p. 543–50.
18. Younossi ZM, Stepanova M, Younossi Y, et al. Epidemiology of chronic liver diseases in the USA in the past three decades. Gut. 2020;69(3):564–8.
19. Younossi ZM, Stepanova M, Ong J, et al. Nonalcoholic steatohepatitis is the most rapidly increasing indication for liver transplantation in the United States. Clin Gastroenterol Hepatol. 2020;S1542-3565(20):30775–8.
20. Belli LS, Perricone G, Adam R, et al. Impact of DAAs on liver transplantation: Major effects on the evolution of indications and results. An ELITA study based on the ELTR registry. J Hepatol. 2018;69(4):810–7.
21. Saeed N, Glass L, Sharma P, et al. Incidence and risks for nonalcoholic fatty liver disease and steatohepatitis post-liver transplant: systematic review and meta-analysis. Transplantation. 2019;103(11):e345–54.
22. Vanwagner LB, Bhave M, Te HS, et al. Patients transplanted for nonalcoholic steatohepatitis are at increased risk for postoperative cardiovascular events. Hepatology. 2012;56:1741–50.
23. Wang X, Li J, Riaz DR, et al. Outcomes of liver transplantation for nonalcoholic steatohepatitis: a systematic review and meta-analysis. Clin Gastroenterol Hepatol. 2014;12:394–402.
24. Gadiparthi G, Spatz M, Greenberg S, et al. NAFLD epidemiology, emerging pharmacotherapy, liver transplantation implications and the trends in the United States. J Clin Transl Hepatol. 2020;8(2):215–21.
25. Flemming JA, Kim WR, Brosgart CL, Terrault NA. Reduction in liver transplant wait-listing in the era of direct-acting antiviral therapy. Hepatology. 2017;65(3):804–12.
26. Carrion AF, Khaderi SA, Sussman NL. Model for end-stage liver disease limbo, model for end-stage liver disease purgatory, and the dilemma of treating hepatitis C in patients awaiting liver transplantation. Liver Transpl. 2016;22:279–80.
27. Terrault NA, McCaughan GW, Curry MP, et al. International liver transplantation society consensus statement on hepatitis C management in liver transplant candidates. Transplantation. 2017;101:945–55.
28. Ohira M, Tanimine N, Kobayashi T, Ohdan H. Essential updates 2018/2019: liver transplantation. Ann Gastroenterol Surg. 2020;4(3):195–207.
29. Cholankeril G, Ahmed A. Alcoholic liver disease replaces hepatitis C virus infection as the leading indication for liver transplantation in the United States. Clin Gastroenterol Hepatol. 2018;16(8):1356–135.
30. Lee BP, Mehta N, Platt L, et al. Outcomes of early liver transplantation for patients with severe alcoholic hepatitis. Gastroenterology. 2018;155(2):422–30.e1.
31. Lee BP, Samur S, Dalgic OO, et al. Model to calculate harms and benefits of early vs delayed liver transplantation for patients with alcohol-associated hepatitis. Gastroenterology. 2019;157(2):472–80.e5.
32. Mathurin P, Moreno C, Samuel D, et al. Early liver transplantation for severe alcoholic hepatitis. N Engl J Med. 2011;365(19):1790–800.
33. Crabb DW, Im GY, Szabo G, Mellinger JL, Lucey MR. Diagnosis and treatment of alcohol-associated liver diseases: 2019 practice guidance from the American association for the study of liver diseases. Hepatology. 2020;71(1):306–33.
34. Tacke F, Kroy DC, Barreiros AP, Neumann UP. Liver transplantation in Germany. Liver Transpl. 2016;22(8):1136–42.
35. Harms MH, Janssen QP, Adam R, et al. Trends in liver transplantation for primary biliary cholangitis in Europe over the past three decades. Aliment Pharmacol Ther. 2019;49(3):285–95.
36. Manne V, Kowdley K. Obeticholic acid in primary biliary cholangitis: where we stand. Curr Opin Gastroenterol. 2019;35:191–6.
37. Silveira MG, Talwalkar JA, Lindor KD, Wiesner RH. Recurrent primary biliary cirrhosis after liver transplantation. Am J Transplant. 2010;10(4):720–6.
38. European Association for the Study of the Liver. EASL Clinical Practice Guidelines: Management of cholestatic liver diseases. J Hepatol. 2009;51:237–67.
39. Chapman R, Fevery J, Kalloo A, et al. Diagnosis and management of primary sclerosing cholangitis. Hepatology. 2010;51:660–78.
40. Karlsen TH, Folseraas T, Thorburn D, Vesterhus M. Primary sclerosing cholangitis – a comprehensive review. J Hepatol. 2017;67(6):1298–323.
41. Stirnimann G, Ebadi M, Czaja AJ, Montano-Loza AJ. Recurrent and De Novo autoimmune hepatitis. Liver Transpl. 2019;25(1):152–66.
42. Mazzaferro V, Regalia E, Doci R, et al. Liver transplantation for the treatment of small hepatocellular carcinomas in patients with cirrhosis. N Engl J Med. 1996;334(11):693–9.
43. Mazzaferro V, Sposito C, Zhou J, et al. Metroticket 2.0 model for analysis of competing risks of death after liver transplantation for hepatocellular carcinoma. Gastroenterology. 2018;154(1):128–39.
44. Mehta N, Dodge JL, Roberts JP, Yao FY. Validation of the prognostic power of the RETREAT score for hepatocellular carcinoma recurrence using the UNOS database. Am J Transplant. 2018;18(5):1206–13.
45. Mano Y, Yoshizumi T, Yugawa K, et al. Lymphocyte-to-monocyte ratio is a predictor of survival after liver transplantation for hepatocellular carcinoma. Liver Transpl. 2018;24(11):1603–11.
46. Kornberg A, Witt U, Schernhammer M, Kornberg J, Müller K, Friess H, et al. The role of preoperative albumin-bilirubin grade for oncological risk stratification in liver transplant patients with hepatocellular carcinoma. J Surg Oncol. 2019;120(7):1126–36.
47. Shimamura T, Akamatsu N, Fujiyoshi M, et al. Expanded livingdonor liver transplantation criteria for patients with hepatocellular carcinoma based on the Japanese nationwide survey: the 5-5-500 rule—a retrospective study. Transpl Int. 2019;32(4):356–68.
48. Firl DJ, Sasaki K, Agopian VG, et al. Charting the path forward for risk prediction in liver transplant for hepatocellular carcinoma: international validation of HALTHCC among 4,089 patients. Hepatology. 2020;71(2):569–82.
49. Duvoux C, Roudot-Thoraval F, Decaens T, et al. for Liver Transplantation French Study Group. Liver transplantation for hepatocellular carcinoma: a model including alpha-fetoprotein improves the performance of Milan criteria. Gastroenterology. 2012;143:986–994.
50. Meischl T, Rasoul-Rockenschaub S, Györi G, et al. C-reactive protein is an independent predictor for hepatocellular carcinoma recurrence after liver transplantation. PLoS One. 2019;14(5):e0216677.
51. Heimbach JK, Kulik LM, Finn RS, et al. AASLD guidelines for the treatment of hepatocellular carcinoma. Hepatology. 2018;67:358–80.
52. Halazun KJ, Najjar M, Abdelmessih RM, et al. Recurrence after liver transplantation for hepatocellular carcinoma: a new MORAL to the story. Ann Surg. 2017;265(3):557–64.
53. Pommergaard HC, Rostved AA, Adam R, et al. Vascular invasion and survival after liver transplantation for hepatocellular carcinoma: a study from the European Liver Transplant Registry. HPB (Oxford). 2018;20(8):768–75.
54. Eurotransplant. Eurotransplant manual. Leiden, the Netherlands: Eurotransplant International Foundation; 2016. https://www.eurotransplant.org/cms/index.php?page5et_manual
55. Umgelter A, Hapfelmeier A, Kopp W, et al. Disparities in Eurotransplant liver transplantation wait-list outcome between patients with and without model for end-stage liver disease exceptions. Liver Transpl. 2017;23(10):1256–65.

56. Goldberg DS, Makar G, Bittermann T, French B. Center variation in the use of nonstandardized model for end-stage liver disease exception points. Liver Transpl. 2013;19(12):1330–42.
57. Martin P, DiMartini A, Feng S, et al. Evaluation for liver transplantation in adults: 2013 practice guideline by the American Association for the Study of Liver Diseases and the American Society of Transplantation. Hepatology. 2014;59:1144–65.
58. Ioannou G. Transplant-related survival benefit should influence prioritization for liver transplantation especially in patients with hepatocellular carcinoma. Liver Transpl. 2017;23:652–62.
59. Wiesner R, Edwards E, Freeman R, et al. Model for end-stage liver disease (MELD) and allocation of donor livers. Gastroenterology. 2003;124(1):91–6.
60. Bleszynski MS, Kim P. Liver transplantation. In: R. S. Rahimi (ed.), The critically Ill cirrhotic patient. Springer Nature Switzerland AG, 2020.

Indications for Liver Transplantation in Acute Liver Failure

Dana Tomescu and Mihai Popescu

Abstract

Acute liver failure (ALF) is a life-threatening condition characterised by abrupt onset of severe liver dysfunction and neurological impairment in patients without an underling chronic liver disease. Since ALF—associated mortality remains high, such patients need urgent assessment and advanced treatment to assure either spontaneous remission of liver failure or bridging them to liver transplantation (LT). To date, no universally accepted scoring systems exist to address the issue of LT in ALF and most experienced centres have developed their own criteria and indications for LT. However, due to the complexity of patient assessment and management, such decisions should be made on a case-by-case basis and by an experienced multidisciplinary team consisting of a transplant surgeon, anaesthesiologist and gastroenterologist in order to provide the best therapeutic option.

Recent studies have focused both on the general care of ALF patients and successfully bridging such patients to LT. However, despite a considerable improvement in patient care, LT remains the main therapeutic option associated with the highest survival rate in cases of severe ALF. This chapter will focus on recent evidence for assessment and early management of such patients, indication for LT, as well as recent advances in intensive care management.

62.1 Current Definition of ALF

ALF is mostly defined by a rapid deterioration of the liver function demonstrated by an international normalized ratio (INR) ≥ 1.5 and the development of hepatic encephalopathy within 26 weeks of jaundice in a patient with no previous history of liver disease [1]. Although, it is generally accepted that ALF presents in patients that previously had a normal liver function, patients with Wilson's disease, vertically-acquired hepatitis B virus (HBV), Budd-Chiari syndrome and autoimmune hepatitis may be included in this definition despite evidence of underlying cirrhosis due to acute presentation and similar clinical course and outcome as the general ALF population [2, 3].

The current definition of ALF has some important limitations that must be considered when the assessment of such a patient is performed. First, hepatic encephalopathy (HE) may be minimal in some patients despite a severely altered liver function. As most centres use West-Haven criteria (Table 62.1), a diagnostic of grade 1 HE may be overlooked, and the patient misdiagnosed as having no HE and hence no ALF. To avoid such situations, a thorough clinical examination should be performed in patients with acute liver dysfunction and expert help sought out. In some patients waiting for HE to occur may delay the initiation of an early treatment strategy that can decrease the chance for spontaneous recovery [5]. Secondarily, INR was not developed to assess patho-

D. Tomescu (✉) · M. Popescu
Department of Anaesthesia and Critical Care, "Carol Davila" University of Medicine and Pharmacy, Bucharest, Romania

Department of Anaesthesia and Critical Care, Fundeni Clinical Institute, Bucharest, Romania

Table 62.1 West-Haven criteria for hepatic encephalopathy [4]

Grade	Clinical manifestation	Neurologic examination
Grade 1	Mild lack of awareness Shortened attention span	Impaired addition or subtraction Mild asterixis or tremor
Grade 2	Lethargic Disoriented Inappropriate behaviour	Obvious asterixis Slurred speech
Grade 3	Somnolent but arousable Gross disorientation Bizarre behaviour	Muscular rigidity and clonus Hyperreflexia
Grade 4	Coma	Decerebrate posturing

Table 62.2 Differential diagnostic of Acute Liver Failure

Disease	Criteria for diagnostics
Acute-on-Chronic Liver Failure	Presence of a known chronic liver disease or radiological criteria of liver cirrhosis. An exception is represented by Wilson's disease, Budd-Chiari syndrome and autoimmune hepatitis.
Pre-eclampsia and eclampsia	Presence of a second or third trimester pregnancy associated with hypertension, proteinuria and grand-mal seizures
Sepsis	Presence of an underling infection and associated organ dysfunctions
Shock	Presence of an inadequate cardiac output or oxygen delivery to the tissues
Liver metastatic disease	Presence of liver metastases on abdominal imaging

physiology of coagulation, but to guide anticoagulant therapy. As a slight increase in INR may be seen in many other clinical situations and can physiologically be observed in children [6], borderline patients should be intensively monitored and considered as "pre-ALF" until ALF can be confirmed or excluded.

Based on the timespan between de development of jaundice and HE, ALF has been classified as: hyperacute (<7 days), acute (7–21 days) and subacute (>21 days and <26 weeks). However, this classification is no longer recommended as studies have failed to demonstrate a correlation between a more rapid onset of ALF and increased mortality. Patients with acetaminophen overdose, despite having a more severe presentation of the illness, have a higher rate of spontaneous recovery and rapidly evolve towards either clinical improvement or death [7]. A delay of more than 7 days between jaundice and HE is associated with a poorer outcome, especially in cases of indeterminate aetiology. A differential diagnosis should be performed early in the course of the illness, as other diseases can present with liver dysfunction and specific treatment should be started early (Table 62.2).

62.2 Aetiology of ALF

There is a great variability regarding both epidemiology and aetiology of ALF between geographic areas. The reported incidence varies between 11.3 per million person years in Germany, 5.5 per million population in the United States and 80.2 per million person-years in the Asian-Pacific region [8, 9]. The most common cause of ALF is represented by drug induced liver injury in the western world. However, viral hepatitis still remains an issue in some countries due to the low immunisation of the population through vaccination [10].

Acetaminophen overdose remains the main cause of ALF in the western world [11]. The development of ALF after acetaminophen administration has generally been reported for doses above 150 mg/kg body weight, but case reports have noted ALF after usual prescribed doses of 3–4 g/day [12]. Patients generally present after voluntary or accidentally ingested a high dose of acetaminophen. Clinically, symptoms may be minimal during the first 24 hours and mainly consist of nausea and vomiting. During the symptomatic phase, that usually lasts from 24–48 hours, general gastro-intestinal symptoms and fatigability are present. Clinical examination reveals right upper-quadrant pain and hepatomegaly and paraclinical tests demonstrate an increase in serum transaminases. Serum bilirubin and INR may be only slightly increased. ALF is generally seen between 72–96 hours are is characterised by a severe increase in serum transaminases, metabolic acidosis, coagulopathy and increase in bilirubin levels. Neurologic dysfunction may follow shortly. In severe cases, death usually occurs between the third and seventh day after ingestion. Spontaneous remission is noted in up to 70% of patients within two weeks [13].

Mushroom poisoning is frequently encountered in rural areas, especially during spring and autumn. After eating wild mushrooms the previous day, patients generally present with gastrointestinal symptoms: nausea, vomiting, diarrhoea and abdominal pain. Food poisoning is generally misdiagnosed if a careful patient history is not taken. After 24 hours, gastro-intestinal symptoms usually reside, and an apparent convalescence phase follows for 24–48 hours. ALF is noted 48–72 after mushroom ingestion and is characterised by a severe increase in serum transaminases and bilirubin levels, severe coagulopathy, HE, acute renal failure and metabolic acidosis. The main factors associated with poor survival are represented by a decrease in prothrombin index below or equal to 25% of normal values at any time between day 3 and day 10 associated with an increase in serum creatinine over 1.2 mg/dL [14].

Drug-induced liver injury (DILI) has become one of the most frequently encountered causes of ALF worldwide. Clinically, ALF has a subacute presentation with a latency between 30 and 90 days. The most commonly reported drugs are represented by antibiotics, including anti-tuberculous medication, non-steroidal anti-inflammatory agents and herbal and dietary supplements. Due to the relative long timespan between time of drug administration and symptoms, the diagnostic is challenging and requires a thorough medical history. Clinically, patients present with a mild increase in serum transaminases, low-grade HE, moderate jaundice and increased INR. Spontaneous recovery is noted in approximately 25% of patients and liver transplantation is indicated more frequently than after acetaminophen overdose [15]. A poorer outcome is seen in women, older patients, Asian ethnicity, thrombocytopenia and history of chronic liver disease.

Since the introduction of world-wide hepatitis B immunisation, the incidence of **acute viral hepatitis** has significantly decreased. Nowadays, hepatitis A and E account for the majority of cases globally, but high incidence of hepatitis B has been noted in Eastern Europe [16]. The clinical picture of hepatitis A (HAV) infection varies from asymptomatic patients to patients with a full picture of ALF. In most cases, patients present with anorexia, nausea, vomiting, low grade fever (38–39 °C), myalgia and light respiratory symptoms. Jaundice usually is seen between one to two weeks after the infection and is accompanied by upper right-quadrant abdominal pain. Extrahepatic involvement is rarely seen, and spontaneous recovery is noted in over 50% of patients. Hepatitis B virus (HBV) infection can present as either a *de novo* infection or a flair-up in patients chronically infected. Patients with *de novo* infection are usually asymptomatic but in rare cases they can progress to ALF characterised by gastro-intestinal symptoms, fatigability, low grade fever and jaundice. HE is frequently encounter and rapidly progresses to coma. Outside LT the prognosis is poor and transplant-free survival ranges from 25–53% [17]. Hepatitis E virus (HEV) has an incubation period of three to eight weeks, followed by a short prodromal phase and jaundice is shortly seen afterwards. The incidence of HE is low and transplant-free survival is one of the highest among all aetiologies of ALF.

Wilson's disease is an uncommon cause of ALF that mainly affects women between 5 and 35 years of age. Keiser-Fleischer rings represent one of the main diagnostic criteria and can be seen in over 90% of patients with neurological involvement and in almost half of patients without neurological involvement. Most frequently encountered neurological signs are represented by ataxia, tremor and dystonia. Clinical signs also include jaundice, abdominal pain and signs of chronic liver disease. Despite its low incidence, Wilson's disease accounts for more than 10% of liver transplantations for ALF [18].

Autoimmune hepatitis presents as a chronic necro-inflammatory liver disease, affecting mainly women, that can progress to ALF. Clinical presentation is typically subacute with non-specific symptoms including nausea, jaundice, fatigability and abdominal pain. The diagnosis is based mainly on histopathological results accompanied by clinical and paraclinical criteria, including abnormal serum globulin levels and the presence of autoantibodies.

HELLP syndrome is a life-threatening complication of pregnancy characterised by haemolysis, an increase in serum transaminases and thrombocytopenia. HELLP syndrome is observed in 0.5–0.9 of all pregnancies, but a higher incidence has been reported in patients with pre-eclampsia (10–20%) [19]. The majority of women present between 27 and 37 weeks of pregnancy with abdominal pain, nausea and vomiting. Haemolysis is generally secondary to microangiopathic haemolytic anaemia. Factors associated with a worst outcome are younger age, headache, bilirubin >2.0 mg/dL

Table 62.3 Diagnostic criteria for HELLP syndrome

Severity	Tennessee classification	Mississippi classification
1	Platelet count <100,000/mm^3 AST > 70 U/L LDH > 600 U/L	Platelet count <50,000/mm^3 AST or ALT >70 U/L LDH > 600 U/L
2		Platelet count: 50,000–100,000/mm^3 AST or ALT >70 U/L LDH > 600 U/L
3		Platelet count: 100,000–150,000/mm^3 AST or ALT >70 U/L LDH > 600 U/L

Legend: *AST* aspartate aminotransferase, *ALT* alanine aminotransferase, *LDH* lactate dehydrogenase

and low platelets (<50,000/mm^3) [20]. Two scoring systems are currently used for the diagnostic and classification of HELLP syndrome (Table 62.3).

Budd-Chiari syndrome is determined by an obstruction of the hepatic venous outflow due to either acute or chronic thrombosis of the hepatic veins. Pathophysiological consequences are represented by a decrease in hepatic blood flow and precapillary portal hypertension. In its chronic form, patients present with signs of decompensated chronic liver failure, ascites and porto-systemic collaterals. In acute presentations, due to the inability of the portal circulation to develop collaterals, patients present with ALF characterised by HE, jaundice and liver dysfunction. More than half the patients will require either transjugular intrahepatic porto-systemic shunt or LT [21].

62.3 Patient Assessment

After ALF is diagnosed, generally on the ward or in the emergency department, the patient needs to undergo a thorough clinical examination and paraclinical tests need to be closely monitored in order to assess the severity of liver dysfunction and associated organ failure, to promptly commence appropriate treatment and to assess the patient as a candidate for emergency LT. In general, such patients are best managed on a high-dependency gastroenterology ward or, as in the case of severe ALF, in the intensive care unit (ICU). Treating these patients in an ICU has some advantages, although with increased patient costs. Intensive care management can provide adequate communication between key players of the multidisciplinary ALF team, offers 24/7 advanced monitoring during standard therapy, sustains organ function and provide specialised care for either organ recovery or bridge to liver transplantation.

Initial evaluation should include a neurological examination to assess the degree of HE and patient history to diagnose aetiologies that require specific treatment, such as acetaminophen overdose. Alcoholic liver disease and malignant infiltration of the liver should be excluded as they represent general contraindications for emergency LT. Also, the presence of underling liver cirrhosis should also be actively sought out as acute-on-chronic liver failure represents the most common differential diagnostic of ALF.

Abdominal ultrasound examination is the initial imaging modality of choice in patients with ALF as is can assess liver anatomy and structure, identify liver cirrhosis and complications of liver disease, diagnose Budd-Chiari syndrome and is easily performed at the bedside. Computed tomography (CT) imaging, and especially contrast enhanced CT, can also be used if initial ultrasound examination is inconclusive, if there is a high suspicion of hepatic malignancy or to quantify the extent of hepatic vein thrombosis in Budd-Chiari syndrome. Other advanced imaginging techniques, like magnetic resonance imagining, may be required to assess liver anatomy if the patient is a candidate for living-donor LT.

Patients with a low cardiac output or in shock can present as ALF due to ischemic hepatitis and neurologic impairment secondary to decreased cerebral perfusion. A transthoracic echocardiography can demonstrate an impaired left ventricle function with decreased stroke volume and left ventricular failure. Transthoracic echocardiography should be routinely performed in patients with severe ALF as part of the differential diagnosis but also to assess fluid status and cardiovascular suitability for LT. As patients with Budd-Chiari syndrome can have a subacute course of the illness, inferior vena cava thrombosis must also be evaluated as it can extend in the right atrium with significant implications for vascular anastomoses in case of LT (Fig. 62.1).

In patients with severe HE, ultrasound examination of the optic nerve sheath diameter has been advocated to predict the severity of cerebral oedema. A bilateral increase in nerve sheath diameter above 5 mm correspond with elevations in intracranial pressure above 20 mmHg. However, because papillary and optic nerve oedema may take days to develop, a normal diameter of the optic nerve does not always exclude intracranial hypertension [22].

Paraclinical tests should focus to evaluate both the aetiology (Table 62.4) and the severity of liver failure as well as associated organ dysfunction (Table 62.5). Early testing should include a full blood count, coagulation parameters, routine biochemical assay, acid-base status, ammonia levels and specific tests to determine the trigger of ALF.

In patients with acetaminophen overdose, plasmatic concentrations are usually determined. However, a negative result does not exclude acetaminophen overdose since more than half of patients may have untraceable plasmatic amounts of paracetamol depending on the time and dose ingested [23]. A detailed patient history and an interview with friends or next of kin would generally identify a recent ingestion of acetaminophen. A complete toxicology screen should be

Table 62.4 Commonly recommended paraclinical tests for aetiologic diagnostic of ALF

Aetiology	Paraclinical tests	
Acetaminophen overdose	Acetaminophen level	
Viral hepatitis	HAV	IgM antibody to HAV
	HBV	Hepatitis B surface antigen (HBsAg); IgM antibody to hepatitis B Core (IgM anti-HBc); PCR for HBV DNA
	HEV	IgM antibody to HEV PCR for HEV RNA
Wilson's disease	Liver cupper, urinary cupper, ceruloplasmin levels	
	Ophthalmological examination (Keiser-Fleischer rings)	
DILI	Toxicology tests	
Autoimmune hepatitis	ANA, ASMA, Immunoglobulin levels	
HELLP syndrome	Platelet count, AST, LDH Liver biopsy	
Budd-Chiari syndrome	Abdominal ultrasound / contrast-enhanced computer tomography Thrombophilia assay	
Other rare hepatotropic viruses	Antibodies to HCV; PCR for hepatitis C virus RNA, IgM antibodies to herpes simplex1, IgM antibodies to varicella-zoster virus, IgM antibodies to cytomegalovirus, IgM antibodies to Epstein-Barr virus	

Legend: *HAV* hepatitis A virus, *HBV* hepatitis B virus, *HEV* hepatitis E virus, *IgM* Immunoglobulin M, *PCR* Polymerase Chain Reaction, *DNA* deoxyribonucleic acid, *RNA* ribonucleic acid, *ANA* antinuclear antibodies, *ASMA* anti-smooth muscle antibody, *AST* aspartate aminotransferase, *LDH* lactate dehydrogenase

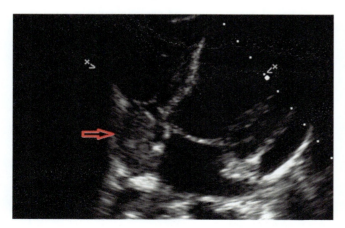

Fig. 62.1 Extensive right atrium thrombosis (red arrow) in a 18-year old patient with subacute Budd-Chiari syndrome

Table 62.5 Paraclinical tests at admission

Organ	Recommended tests
Liver	Serum transaminases, bilirubin (total and fractions), lactate dehydrogenase, creatine kinase, ammonia
Coagulation	Prothrombin time, INR, fibrinogen, coagulation factor V Thromboelastometry/thromboelastography
Blood count	White blood cells (including fractions), haemoglobin, haematocrit, platelet count
Renal	Urea, creatinine
Metabolic	Glycemia, lactate, triglycerides
Pancreas	Amylase, lipase
Acid-base status	pH, HCO_3^-, arterial partial pressure of CO_2 and O_2
Electrolyte	Na^+, K^+, Cl^-, anion gap

Legend: *INR* international normalized ratio

performed in patients suspected of voluntary or accidental ingestion of acetaminophen since overlap with other abuse substances like opioids, abuse drugs and alcohol is frequently encountered [24].

For decades, patients with ALF have been considered to have an acquired severe coagulopathy and increased risk for haemorrhagic complications. Current research has demonstrated a balanced haemostasis in such patients, although not to the extent of that of Acute-on-chronic liver failure. In a recent large observational study, only 11% of patients experience severe bleeding complications, both spontaneous and postprocedural blood loss, despite a profound alteration in standard coagulation tests [25]. It is now generally considered that, despite being a diagnostic criterion for ALF, standard coagulation tests overestimate de severity of coagulopathy in ALF and thrombotic complications may be as frequent as bleeding [26]. Routine correction of standard coagulation tests is no longer recommended and specific factors assays can guide targeted correction of specific factor deficits. Moreover, the use of viscoelastic testing, like thromboelastometry and thromboelastography, offer a better picture of the haemostatic process and specific protocols are currently available to guide coagulation management in patients with ALF.

Liver biopsy may be needed in cases in which commonly used paraclinical tests failed to determine the aetiological cause of ALF or when imaging results are unconclusive for a chronic liver disease. The transjugular route is usually preferred as it has been associated with the lowest complication rate. Liver biopsy may also be indicated in patients suspected of Wilson's disease, DILI or autoimmune hepatitis.

In up to 5% of patients no definitive aetiology for ALF can be identified. These patients may not have been completely evaluated or initial testing was not comprehensive enough. A superficial patient history may overlook prior medical treatments, including herbal medication, and the aetiology misdiagnosed as undetermined.

As ALF progression is usually rapid and hard to predict, all patients with a significant liver injury should be examined by an experienced ALF team to assess the potential benefit of emergency LT. As increased centre experience is associated with greater transplant free survival and reduced waitlist mortality for ALF, transfer to a dedicated liver ICU should be considered early in the disease course. Proposed criteria by the European Association for the Study of the Liver [27] are presented in Table 62.6.

Patient transfer should follow the same guidelines as any other critical ill patient and, when considered appropriate, an experienced retrieval team should be used. Careful patient assessment prior to transfer should be performed and appropriate fluid resuscitation, use of vasopressors to maintain stable haemodynamics and correction of metabolic and acid-base disturbances should be addressed. The fastest transfer route, usually air transport, is recommended and monitoring of neurological status and pupillary diameter (Fig. 62.2) as well as organ function should be frequently performed. In patients with HE a case-by-case decision should be made regarding tracheal intubation and commencement of mechanical ventilation considering the severity of HE and rapid progression to coma. A central venous line placed under ultrasound guidance to minimize complications, and invasive blood pressure monitoring are recommended for targeted vasopressor support and haemodynamic monitoring.

Table 62.6 EASL criteria for patient referral to a LT centre

Paracetamol and hyperacute aetiologies	Non-paracetamol
Arterial pH < 7.30 or HCO_3 < 18	Arterial pH < 7.30 or HCO_3 < 18
INR > 3 on day 2 or IRN > 4 thereafter	INR > 1.8
Oliguria and/or increased creatinine	Oliguria/renal failure or Na^+ < 130 mmol/L
Altered level of consciousness	Hepatic encephalopathy, hypoglycaemia or metabolic acidosis
Hypoglycaemia	Bilirubin>17.6 mg/dL
Increased lactate unresponsive to fluid resuscitation	Shrinking liver size

Legend: *INR* international normalized ratio

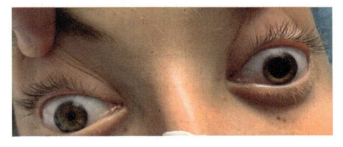

Fig. 62.2 Anisocoria developed during air transport in a patient with Acute Liver Failure

62.4 Prognostic Factors

For decades, medical research has focused on identifying factors associated with either decreased transplant free survival or unfavourable outcome after emergency LT. Most scoring systems are built around four determinants: aetiology, interval between jaundice and HE, age, and liver functional tests. Several prognostic criteria have been developed based on large cohorts of patients, but none have sufficient specificity and sensibility to be universally applied. Severity of EH is considered to be associated with a poorer outcome and patients should be routinely screened for irreversible brain damage before emergency LT is performed.

MELD is currently the most used scoring system for organ allocation in end-stage liver disease. Several studies have demonstrated its usefulness in mortality prediction for ALF. MELD scores over 30 are associated with a worse outcome [28]. However, the main disadvantage of MELD score is that it assesses only liver damage without taken into account associated organ dysfunction. Age is not only correlated with ALF mortality but also with mortality after LT. In a study performed by King's College [29] age above 45 years was associated with decreased survival after LT, especially in patients who received high dose vasopressors. However, age alone should not be considered a contraindication to LT. Other risk factors associated with a poorer outcome include time between jaundice to HE of over 7 days, presence of cerebral oedema, prothrombin time > 35 seconds and creatinine >1.5 mg/dL.

Specific prognostic factors of increased mortality have been identified in different aetiologies. Decreased survival in mushroom poisoned patients has been observed with increased prothrombin time and creatinine levels three to ten days after ingestion and a decrease in coagulation factor V under 20% has been proposed by some centres as an indication for emergency LT [30]. Patients with acute presentation of Wilson's disease and HE have almost 100% mortality. The main risk factors are represented by raised white blood cell count (WBC), bilirubin, INR, serum albumin and serum transaminases. A modified King's College score has been developed for early referral of patients with Wilson's disease to LT [31]. A cut-off value of 11 points was associated with 93% sensibility and 98% specificity (Table 62.7).

Patients with Acetaminophen overdose have a lower mortality compared with other aetiologies. However decreased survival has been observed in patients with high levels of acetaminophen. Early use of acetylcysteine has been associated with increased survival even in high dose intoxications. Viral hepatitis is generally associated with increased spontaneous remission, especially in patients with HAV and HEV.

Increased lactate has been proposed as a marker of severity in ALF. Patients presenting with high lactate levels, either due to decreased metabolism by the failing liver or tissue hypoperfusion have increased mortality rates. Lactate kinetics should be monitored closely especially in the perioperative period of LT. SOFA (Sequential Organ Failure Assessment) score and it's derivate the CLIF-SOFA score used in patients with Acute-on-chronic liver failure have been used to assess patient outcomes in patients with ALF. They may be superior to the classic MELD score as they offer a better picture of associated organ dysfunction. However, exact cut-off values to guide either proceed to liver transplantation or futility are treatment are still lacking.

The most used criteria for LT in ALF are represented by the Kings College Criteria and Clichy criteria (Table 62.8). Although validated in large cohorts of patients, their suboptimal sensibility and specificity deem careful utilisation and a case-by-case approach to either to proceed or not with LT should be considered.

The US-ALF Study Group Index has recently been described [32]. The authors identified HE grade, ALF aetiology, vasopressor support, log transformation of bilirubin and INR as significant prognostic factors associated with transplant-free survival. Based on these, they have constructed a predictive model. In the validation cohort, the US-ALF Study Group Index predicted 22-days transplant-free survival

Table 62.7 Modified King's College criteria for Wilson's disease

Score	Bilirubin (mg/dL)	INR	AST (U/L)	WBC (10^9/L)	Albumin (g/L)
0	0–5.8	0–1.29	0–100	0–6.7	>45
1	5.9–8.7	1.3–1.6	101–150	6.8–8.3	34–44
2	8.8–11.7	1.7–1.9	151–300	8.4–10.3	25–35
3	11.8–14.7	2.0–2.4	301–400	10.4–15.3	21–24
4	>14.8	>2.5	>401	>15.4	<20

Legend: *INR* international normalized ratio, *AST* aspartate aminotransferase, *WBC* white blood cell count

Table 62.8 King's College and Clichy criteria for LT in ALF

King's College criteria	
Acetaminophen overdose	Non-acetaminophen overdose
Arterial pH < 7.30 after fluid administration *Or* all of the following: • Prothrombin time > 100 s (INR > 6.5) • Serum creatinine>3.4 mg/dL • Grade 3 or 4 HE	Prothromin time > 100 sec (INR > 6.5) *Or* any 3 of the following: • Non-A, non-B viral hepatitis, DILI or indeterminate aetiology • Time from jaundice to HE >7 days • Age < 10 or > 40 • Prothrombin time > 50 sec (INR > 3.5) • - Serum bilirubin>17.4 mg/dL
Clichy Criteria	
Presence of HE **and** Factor V levels <20% in patients <30 years of age *Or* Factor V level < 30% in patients>30 years of age	

Legend: *INR* international normalized ratio, *DILI* drug induced liver injury, *HE* hepatic encephalopathy

with a c-statistic value of 0.84. However, this predictive model has to be validated by larger multicentre studies.

Other aetiology-specific scoring systems have also been investigated in the last years. The research team from King's College developed and validated a new statistical model to predict survival in patients with paracetamol-induced ALF [33]. In their two-day model, the authors included age, cardiovascular failure, Glasgow coma scale, arterial pH, creatinine, INR and arterial lactate as well as dynamic changes from day 1 to day 2 of arterial lactate and INR. This dynamic model predicted 30-days survival in 91% of patients. The ALFA (Hepatitis A-ALF) score [34] was developed in Korea to predict LT or 30-days death in patients with acute HVA hepatitis. The ALFA score contains paraclinical values acquired on the day of ALF diagnosis: age, INR, bilirubin, ammonia, creatinine, and haemoglobin. This score accurately predicted LT or death within 30 days in 87% of patients.

A recent international consensus of 35 experts in the field of LT defined threshold criteria for futility [35]. Severe frailty, and septic patients with persistent fever despite antibiotic treatment or less than 72 hours of appropriate antimicrobial therapy were considered reasonable criteria to delay LT. Most experts agreed that any of the following $PaO_2/FiO_2 < 150$, need for vasopressor support exceeding 1 µg/kg/min and a serum lactate level > 9 mmol/l were sufficient to contraindicate LT.

62.5 Bridging Patients to Liver Transplantation

Patients with ALF are best managed in the ICU. However, the exact criteria for ICU admission vary between centres depending on personal experience, availability of ICU beds and possibility of adequate treatment in the early stages on the general ward. However, patients should be frequently monitored for severity of HE, organ dysfunction or other life-threatening conditions. Advanced haemodynamic monitoring is usually recommended since most patients are volume depleted. Adequate fluid resuscitation should be performed but overzealous volemic therapy may aggravate cerebral oedema. Arterial and central venous lines may be placed in order to have an accurate beat-by-beat reading of arterial blood pressure and central venous pressure, but measures should be taken to avoid blood stream infections. Dynamic indices of fluid responsiveness are best used to guide fluid management and they should be frequently assessed. Hypotonic solutions, like Ringer lactate, should be avoided as they carry an increase risk of cerebral oedema and progression of HE. Lactate levels are hard to interpret in ALF patients as lactate may be high due to either tissue hypoperfusion or decreased metabolism by the liver. In low grade HE, the oral route is preferred, but if HE progresses patients may require urgent intubation and, in this situation, a nasogastric tube is preferred.

Enteral nutrition should be promptly initiated, if no contraindications (severe shock, gastro-intestinal dysfunction or ileus), as muscle wasting, and gastro-intestinal bacterial translocation are common findings in malnourished states associated with a worse outcome. Hypoglycaemia is a common in patients with severe ALF due to impaired gluconeogenesis, hyperinsulinemia and depleted glycogen stores. Glycaemia should frequently be monitored, and a continuous glucose infusion should be started if hypoglycaemia occurs. As hyperglycaemia increases intracranial pressure, a tight glucose control should be applied with a target blood glucose levels between 150–180 mg/dL [27].

Specific aetiological treatment should be promptly initiated to increase the likelihood of spontaneous remission (Table 62.9). N-acetylcysteine (NAC) was demonstrated to improve outcome in non-acetaminophen ALF. In a recently published trial [36], the use of an empirical therapy of 150 mg/kg in 100 ml 5% dextrose over 1 h, then 70 mg/kg over 20 h, followed by continuous infusion over 24 h of 150 mg/kg caused a reduction in mortality and need for transplantation. Also, early administration of NAC decreased the severity of HE, hospital stay, need for ICU admission and incidence of organ failure.

Hepatic encephalopathy represents one of the most severe organ dysfunctions associated with increased mortality in ALF patients. Although pathophysiological mechanisms are

Table 62.9 Aetiologic treatment of ALF

Aetiology	Specific therapy
Acetaminophen overdose	Gastric lavage and activated charcoal; NAC: loading dose of 150 mg/kg in 5% dextrose over 15 m; maintenance dose is 50 mg/kg given over 4 h followed by 6 mg/kg administered for up to 72 hours.
HVB	Antiviral therapy with entecavir or tenofovir
Autoimmune hepatits	Prednisone 40–60 mg/day
Wilson's disease	Continuous renal replacement therapy; Plasma-exchange
Budd-Chiari syndrome	Transjugular intrahepatic portosystemic shunt or surgical Porto-systemic shunt; Systemic anticoagulation
Mushroom poisoning	Gastric lavage and activated charcoal; High-dose Penicillin G 300,000–1,000,000 U/kg/day; Silymarin 30–40 mg/kg/day Albumin dialysis
HELLP syndrome	Delivery of the foetus
Herpes simplex virus	Acyclovir 5–10 mg/kg q 8 hours

Legend: *NAC* N-acetylcysteine, *HVB* hepatitis B virus, *HELLP* Hemolysis, Elevated Liver enzymes and Low Platelets

poorly understood, accumulation of liver toxins and systemic inflammation are key factors in the development of cerebral oedema and intracranial hypertension (ICH). Intracranial pressure (ICP) monitoring has been advocated to guide specific therapy, but its use is not universally accepted due to high complications rates including intracranial bleeding and infection. In an international survey [37] only 55% of centres used invasive ICP monitoring. The main indications were papillary abnormalities, renal failure, elevated ammonia levels and cardiovascular instability. New non-invasive techniques applying transcranial Doppler are becoming more popular, but their use is dependent on expertise. When measured, an ICP above 20 mmHg mandates urgent treatment. The aim is to decrease ICP and maintain a cerebral perfusion pressure above 50 mmHg in order to minimize cerebral ischemia. General measures taken to lower ICP include maintaining a neutral head position and raising the head at an angle of 20° to facilitate venous drainage. Prophylactic treatment of seizures is not recommended, but they should be promptly managed if diagnosed. Osmotic diuretics have long been used to lower cerebral oedema. Mannitol, in doses of 0.5–1 g/kg intravenously lowers ICP from >60 mmHg to 20 mmHg. However, its effects are short-lived and serious complications can occur. Plasma osmolarity should be closely monitored and mannitol administration stopped if it exceeds 320 mOsm/L. Common side-effects of mannitol therapy include hypernatremia, hyperosmolarity and fluid overload in patients with renal failure. Decreasing arterial pressure of carbon dioxide ($PaCO_2$) to levels between 25–30 mmHg is associated with a decrease in cerebral blood flow and ICP due to cerebral vasoconstriction. This can be obtained in mechanically ventilated and sedated patients by increasing the minute-volume. However, a low $PaCO_2$ for more than 72 hours has been associated with a worse neurological outcome [38]. Hypertonic saline, with a target of plasma sodium levels between 145–155 mEq/L, has been used to prevent and treat ICH. Sodium levels should be frequently monitored, and therapy guided as such that not to increase sodium by more than 16 mEq/L in 24 hours in order to avoid pontine demyelination. Hypothermia has historically been used to decrease cerebral metabolic rate. In patients with ALF at high risk of ICH, lowering the body core temperature to 33–34 °C did not confer a survival benefit or a lower incidence of ICH [39]. Routine hypothermia is not recommended, but temperature management should be applied to maintain normothermia and specially to avoid fever. Sedation has also been applied to decrease the cerebral metabolic rate or to facilitate mechanical ventilation in intubated patients. Propofol is frequently used due to its rapid onset, short context-sensitive half-life and effects in decreasing the risk of seizure activity. However, careful dose titration and short duration of therapy should be applied to avoid propofol infusion syndrome. Sedation breaks should be offered to allow for neurological examination in order to assess the severity of HE.

Cardiovascular changes associated with ALF are similar with those of sepsis. Patients have a hyperdynamic haemodynamic pattern characterised by an increased cardiac output and low systemic vascular resistance. Secondary to these changes, the mean arterial pressure is usually decreased, and this predisposes patients to tissue hypoperfusion. Cardiac arrhythmias are frequent and range from supraventricular tachycardia, premature supraventricular or ventricular beats to atrial fibrillation. These are mostly due to accumulation of bilirubin and bile salts, viral myocarditis or acid-base and electrolyte abnormalities. ST segment changes on the EKG may be encountered but are rarely of pathological significance. Patients should routinely be investigated for underlying cardiac disease, especially those who require cardiovascular support. Normovolemia should be maintained in the ICU and dynamic tests to assess fluid responsiveness (stroke volume variation, pulse pressure variation) should guide fluid management. Noradrenaline is the recommended vasopressor of choice and a mean blood pressure > 75 mmHg should be maintained to assure cerebral and renal perfusion.

Respiratory dysfunction may be encountered especially in patients with severe HE. Non-invasive ventilation is not recommended and endotracheal intubation to protect the airway from aspiration pneumonia is preferred. Mechanical ventilation should follow lung protective strategies, even in non-ARDS patients. Inspiratory pressures and respiratory rate should be titred to obtain a tidal volume of 6 ml/kg/ideal body weight and to maintain a normal arterial CO_2 and O_2 partial pressures. Hypercarbia should always be avoided as it increases cerebral blood flow and hypocarbia should only be applied for brief periods in severe ICH. Low levels of PEEP should be applied in non-ARDS patients as not to impair venous drainage through the superior vena cava. Care should be taken to prevent ventilator associated pneumonia and appropriate use of physiotherapy and patient positioning should be used.

Infections are common in ALF and patients are frequently at risk of developing sepsis and septic shock. Severe infections may contraindicate LT and so patients should undergo routinely bacteriological screening. As severe systemic inflammation is frequently encountered in these patients, the diagnosis of sepsis becomes difficult. Standard markers, such as a raised white blood cell count, are a common finding in non-infected ALF patients. C-reactive protein is synthetised by hepatocytes and may de decreased in infected patients with severe liver failure. A high grade of suspicion should be maintained, and cultures should be performed in patients with severely progressive HE [40]. Prophylactic antibiotics should not be routinely administered as they increase the risk of multi-drug resistant bacteria. Empirical antibiotherapy may be administered in patients with progressive grade III or IV HE, hypotension requiring vasopressor support and at least 2 SIRS criteria. Broad spectrum antibiotics are generally used to cover both Gram-positive and Gram-negative bacteria.

Acute kidney injury (AKI) is one of the most frequent extra-hepatic organ dysfunctions in patients with ALF and is associated with a worse outcome. In most cases renal hypoperfusion, direct drug-induced nephrotoxicity and systemic inflammation are responsible for the rapid decline in kidney function. Maintaining renal function is crucial in patients with ALF. This should be done my maintaining an adequate kidney perfusion pressure, early treatment of infections and avoidance of nephrotoxic medication. In AKI patients, urgent treatment and early initiation of renal replacement therapy should be considered as fluid overload, acid-base and electrolyte abnormalities may aggravate HE and ALF. Continuous renal replacement therapy is preferred to intermittent dialysis as it avoids the rapid metabolic and haemodynamic changes associated with intermittent dialysis. Outside AKI, the use of high-volume hemofiltration has been associated with an increased removal of ammonia and improvement in neurologic dysfunction and may be applied in patients with increased ICP where standard measures have failed [41].

Coagulation management in patients with liver disease has been extensively studied in the last years. Although standard coagulation tests are still used for the diagnosis of ALF, they do not accurately reflect haemostasis. Thromboelastometric studies have demonstrated that in general the haemostatic balance is maintained in ALF patients: the decreased synthesis of pro-coagulant factors is compensated by an increased in coagulation factor VIII and a decrease in anti-coagulant factors [26]. Fresh frozen plasma administration for correction of standard coagulation tests in the absence of clinical signs of bleeding is not recommended. However, specific factors deficits should be corrected if invasive procedures or surgery is planned and guided by thromboelastic tests. Factor concentrates, as fibrinogen and pro-thrombin complex are generally recommended as they avoid the complications of fresh frozen plasma administration like fluid overload and transfusion related acute lung injury. Platelet transfusion in recommended to maintain levels between 50,000–70,000/μL before invasive procedures. Although not universally accepted, in bleeding patients, platelet count should be maintained above 50.000/μL. Fibrinogen concentrate can be administered to maintain fibrinogen levels between 150–200 mg/dL [42].

62.6 Extracorporeal Liver Support Systems

Ideally, extracorporeal liver support systems (ECLS) should assist 3 major hepatic functions: detoxification, biosynthesis and regulation. To date, no system successfully

Table 62.10 Main indications for Extracorporeal liver support systems

Acute liver failure
Acute-on-chronic liver failure and one of the following:
Hepatic encephalopathy
Severe jaundice
Acute kidney injury
Severe pruritus
Acute intoxications (e.g. Mushroom poisoning, acetaminophen overdose)
Posthepatectomy liver failure
Primary graft non-function after liver transplantation

managed to accomplish this. Two types of ECLS have been introduced into clinical practice: artificial-ECLS and bioartificial-ECLS. Artificial-ECLS are based on the principles of adsorption and filtration and are aimed at removing circulating toxins by using membranes with different pore sizes and adsorbent columns. Bioartificial-ECLS are hybrid systems that incorporate hepatocytes, either human or porcine, in a bioactive platform. Their primary aim is to improve detoxification and support liver synthesis. ECLS have been used in different clinical situations with conflicting results (Table 62.10).

The most common used artificial-ECLS in clinical practice are MARS (Molecular Adsorbent Recirculation System) and Prometheus (Fractionated plasma separation and adsorption).

In MARS dialysis, blood is circulated against an albumin-contained solution. The filter contains a high-flux membrane with small porosities (<50 kDa). Toxins are cleared by diffusion and are bound by the albumin dialysate. Initial studies have demonstrated a significant removal capacity for bilirubin, bile acids, creatinine and urea [43] and an improvement in HE. A large multicentre study failed to demonstrate an improvement in survival in patients with ALF. However, patients on MARS had a higher change of receiving a liver transplant [44]. A meta-analysis that included 4 randomised trials comparing MARS with standard medical therapy has demonstrated a slight increase in survival in patients with ALF [45]. In the Prometheus system, plasma is fractionated through an albumin-permeable filter with a cut-off of 250 kDa. Albumin and plasma proteins cross the membrane and pass through two columns, an anion-exchanger and a neutral resin adsorber. The plasma is then returned to the blood circuit where it undergoes conventional high-flux haemodialysis. In clinical studies, the use of Prometheus was associated with an improvement in liver functional tests. However, a large multicentre study failed to demonstrate a survival benefit in patients with Acute-on-chronic liver failure [46]. Based on these evidence, current guidelines do not recommend the routine use of ESLD in patients with ALF [27].

The use of plasma-exchange (PE) in patients with ALF offers some theoretical benefits: higher removal of molecules compared to ESLD and substitutes plasma products including coagulation factors, improvement in haemodynamic parameters and related organ dysfunctions [47] and enhanced recovery in specific patient populations [48]. In a recent large open randomised controlled trial, the use of high-volume PE has been associated with increased transplant free survival. This was attributed to attenuation of innate immune activation and improvement of multi-organ dysfunction [49]. Current guidelines suggest that PE may be of greater benefit in patients if it is applied early in the disease course and in those patients who will benefit from emergency LT [27].

62.7 Timing of Liver Transplantation

The optimal timing for LT has long been debated without reaching an international consensus. In lack of evidence to guide the optimal timing for LT, the decision should be made by an experienced team on a case-by-case basis taken into account the severity of liver dysfunction and associated organ failures, progression of HE, severity scores, futility and co-existing disease as well as organ availability. As mentioned, such patients are best managed in a dedicated LT centre and early referral is useful in decision-making.

Patients fulfilling current transplant criteria should be listed for emergency LT and re-evaluated if a suitable organ graft becomes available. Based on existing criteria, an algorithmic approach to properly address the timing of LT in patients with ALF should soon follow. Patients who fulfil transplant criteria and have multiple factors associated with a poor prognosis, as well as patients in whom HE is rapidly progressing should undergo emergency LT. As previously mentioned, a clinical evaluation of co-morbidities, severity of ALF and extrahepatic organ failure and their prognosis should proceed the decision to continue with LT. The patient's family as well as a psychiatrist should also be involved in patients who ingested hepatotoxins in a suicidal attempt. A "wait and see" approach is more suitable in patients who exhibit signs of improvement under standard medical care and in patients with acetaminophen overdose without HE. A good liver graft is recommended in such patients, as well as living-donor LT and, outside severe ALF, incompatible ABO LT is seldom required. Patients with irreversible brain damage, sepsis, associated pancreatitis and rapidly increasing vasopressor support are rarely suitable candidates for LT.

Three type of LT have been described in patients with ALF: deceased—donor LT (DDLT), living—donor LT (LDLT) and auxiliary LT. Auxiliary LT has been used since more than 30 years ago based on the potential regeneration of the native liver if sufficient time is provided by by-passing it with a partial liver graft in an orthotopic position. The auxiliary liver should maintain partial hepatic function to assure survival until regeneration of the native liver is complete. When the native liver is regenerated, immunosuppression is progressively reduced, and this leads to graft atrophy. The surgical intervention is technically challenging and should be performed in well-experienced centres. Outcome data are limited to a low number of cases. A recent study reporting data from 13 preadolescents undergoing auxiliary-LT showed a 100% survival and with 10 patients being off immunosuppression therapy [50]. Older studies showed survival rates between 63% and 85% with different immunosuppression-free rates [51]. Patients considered suitable for auxiliary—LT are generally children and young adults because of their excellent regenerative potential. Also, auxiliary—LT should be the considered in aetiologies for associated with rapid liver regeneration such as acetaminophen overdose, HVA, HVE and mushroom poisoning.

A whole liver graft is preferred in ALF patients, especially in those with severe HE and associated organ dysfunction. However, due to urgency of LT and declining number of organ donors, as well as decreasing graft quality, many centres are performing more LDLT in detriment of DDLT. The use of marginal liver grafts from older donors and those with advanced hepatic steatosis has been associated with a negative impact on post-LT survival and perioperative complications [29]. The use of ABO-incompatible liver grafts has also been advocated. Such patients require extensive pre-transplant preparation and advanced protocols are in place [52]. However, data from the ELTR registry show a worse graft and recipient survival in patients with ABO-incompatible grafts [53], and hence, this option should be reserved for extreme cases that require emergency LT and no other liver grafts are available. As mentioned, LDLT is becoming extensively used outside Asia, in Europe and the Unitated States. However, this technique carries significant ethical issues, and a psychologist should always be involved since next of kin may experience emotional pressure to donate. Patient outcomes are good, are survival is similar to that reported for elective LDLT [54].

Changes in practice and early referral of such patients to dedicated liver ICU has significantly improved outcomes over the last years. A Scottish audit showed a constant improvement in spontaneous survival over time in ALF due to acetaminophen and non-paracetamol aetiologies [55]. This improvement was also observed even in the sickest patients meeting King's College criteria and in those undergoing LT. The main causes for mortality following LT for ALF are infection and sepsis, progressive organ failure and liver graft dysfunction or failure.

62.8 Conclusion

In conclusion, ALF is a rare but life-threatening organ dysfunction associated with increased mortality and morbidity if appropriate measures are not urgently applied. Such patients are best managed in dedicated liver intensive care units by experienced multidisciplinary teams and expert consult should be sought out early in the course of the disease. Early assessment is required in order to diagnose aetiology as well as associated organ dysfunction and initiate appropriate treatment. Management of ALF patients has significantly improved in the last years and spontaneous recovery without the need for LT is frequently encountered. However, criteria for indicating LT and the optimal time to perform it remain under debate and to date no scoring system can predict with sufficient accuracy and precision patient outcome. Patients should be listed for emergency LT early in the course of ALF and when a suitable liver graft is available the decision to proceed or not to LT should be made individually based on severity and progression of the disease.

References

1. Lee WM, Stravitz RT, Larson AM. Introduction to the revised American Association for the Study of Liver Diseases Position Paper on acute liver failure 2011. Hepatology. 2012;55:965–7.
2. European Association for the Study of the Liver. EASL clinical practice guidelines: Wilson's disease. J Hepatol. 2012;56(3):671–85.
3. Parekh J, Matei VM, Canas-Coto A, Friedman D, Lee WM. Acute Liver Failure Study Group. Budd-chiari syndrome causing acute liver failure: a multicenter case series. Liver Transpl. 2017;23(2):135–42.
4. Atterbury CE, Maddrey WC, Conn HO. Neomycin-sorbitol and lactulose in the treatment of acute portal-systemic encephalopathy. Am J Dig Dis. 1978;23(5):398–406.
5. Kakisaka K, Suzuki Y, Kataoka K, Okada Y, Miyamoto Y, Kuroda H, Takikawa Y. Predictive formula of coma onset and prothrombin time to distinguish patients who recover from acute liver injury. J Gastroenterol Hepatol. 2018;33(1):277–82.
6. Di Giorgio A, D'Antiga L. Acute liver failure in children: is it time to revise the diagnostic criteria? Liver Transpl. 2020;26(2):184–6.
7. MacDonald AJ, Speiser JL, Ganger DR, Nilles KM, Orandi BJ, Larson AM, Lee WM, Karvellas CJ, United States Acute Liver Failure Study Group. Clinical and neurological outcomes in acetaminophen-induced acute liver failure: a twenty-one-year multicenter cohort study. Clin Gastroenterol Hepatol. 2020; https://doi.org/10.1016/j.cgh.2020.09.016.
8. Weiler N, Schlotmann A, Schnitzbauer AA, Zeuzem S, Welker MW. The epidemiology of acute liver failure: results of a population-based study including 25 million state-insured individuals. Dtsch Ärztebl Int. 2020;117(4):43.
9. Bower WA, Johns M, Margolis HS, Williams IT, Bell BP. Population-based surveillance for acute liver failure. Am J Gastroenterol. 2007;102:2459–63.
10. Khuroo MS, Kamili S. Aetiology and prognostic factors in acute liver failure in India. J Viral Hepat. 2003;10:224–31.
11. Jayaraman T, Lee YY, Chan WK, Mahadeva S. Epidemiological differences of common liver conditions between Asia and the West. JGH Open. 2020;4(3):332–9.
12. Larson AM, Polson J, Fontana RJ, Davern TJ, Lalani E, Hynan LS, Reisch JS, Schiødt FV, Ostapowicz G, Shakil AO, Lee WM. Acetaminophen-induced acute liver failure: results of a United States multicenter, prospective study. Hepatology. 2005;42(6):1364–72.
13. Craig DG, Bates CM, Davidson JS, Martin KG, Hayes PC, Simpson KJ. Overdose pattern and outcome in paracetamol-induced acute severe hepatotoxicity. Br J Clin Pharmacol. 2011;71(2):273–82.
14. Ganzert M, Felgenhauer N, Zilker T. Indication of liver transplantation following amatoxin intoxication. J Hepatol. 2005;42(2):202–9.
15. Tujios SR, Lee WM. Acute liver failure induced by idiosyncratic reaction to drugs: challenges in diagnosis and therapy. Liver Int. 2018;38(1):6–14.
16. Bernal W, Wendon J. Acute liver failure. N Engl J Med. 2013;369:2525–34.
17. Manka P, Verheyen J, Gerken G, Canbay A. Liver failure due to acute viral hepatitis (AE). Visc Med. 2016;32(2):80–5.
18. Eisenbach C, Sieg O, Stremmel W, Encke J, Merle U. Diagnostic criteria for acute liver failure due to Wilson disease. World J Gastroenterol. 2007;13(11):1711.
19. Kongwattanakul K, Saksiriwuttho P, Chaiyarach S, Thepsuthammarat K. Incidence, characteristics, maternal complications, and perinatal outcomes associated with preeclampsia with severe features and HELLP syndrome. Int J Women's Health. 2018;10:371.
20. Erkılınç S, Eyi EG. Factors contributing to adverse maternal outcomes in patients with HELLP syndrome. J Matern Fetal Neonat Med. 2018;31(21):2870–6.
21. Parekh J, Matei VM, Canas-Coto A, Friedman D, Lee WM, Acute Liver Failure Study Group. Budd-chiari syndrome causing acute liver failure: a multicenter case series. Liver Transpl. 2017;23(2):135–42.
22. Rajajee V, Williamson CA, Fontana RJ, Courey AJ, Patil PG. Noninvasive intracranial pressure assessment in acute liver failure. Neurocrit Care. 2018;29(2):280–90.
23. Leventhal TM, Gottfried M, Olson JC, Subramanian RM, Hameed B, Lee WM, Acute Liver Failure Study Group. Acetaminophen is undetectable in plasma from more than half of patients believed to have acute liver failure due to overdose. Clin Gastroenterol Hepatol. 2019;17(10):2110–6.
24. Serper M, Wolf MS, Parikh NA, Tillman H, Lee WM, Ganger DR. Risk factors, clinical presentation, and outcomes in overdose with acetaminophen alone or with combination products: results from the acute liver failure study group. J Clin Gastroenterol. 2016;50(1):85.
25. Stravitz RT, Ellerbe C, Durkalski V, Schilsky M, Fontana RJ, Peterseim C, Lee WM, Acute Liver Failure Study Group. Bleeding complications in acute liver failure. Hepatology. 2018;67(5):1931–42.
26. Stravitz RT, Lisman T, Luketic VA, Sterling RK, Puri P, Fuchs M, Ibrahim A, Lee WM, Sanyal AJ. Minimal effects of acute liver injury/acute liver failure on hemostasis as assessed by thromboelastography. J Hepatol. 2012;56(1):129–36.
27. Wendon J, Cordoba J, Dhawan A, Larsen FS, Manns M, Nevens F, Samuel D, Simpson KJ, Yaron I, Bernardi M. EASL clinical practical guidelines on the management of acute (fulminant) liver failure. J Hepatol. 2017;66(5):1047–81.
28. Dhiman RK, Jain S, Maheshwari U, Bhalla A, Sharma N, Ahluwalia J, Duseja A, Chawla Y. Early indicators of prognosis in fulminant hepatic failure: an assessment of the Model for End-Stage Liver Disease (MELD) and King's College Hospital criteria. Liver Transpl. 2007;13(6):814–21.
29. Bernal W, Cross TJ, Auzinger G, Sizer E, Heneghan MA, Bowles M, Muiesan P, Rela M, Heaton N, Wendon J, O'Grady JG. Outcome after wait-listing for emergency liver transplantation in acute liver failure: a single centre experience. J Hepatol. 2009;50(2):306–13.
30. Enjalbert F, Rapior S, Nouguier-Soulé J, Guillon S, Amouroux N, Cabot C. Treatment of amatoxin poisoning: 20-year retrospective analysis. J Toxicol Clin Toxicol. 2002;40(6):715–57.
31. Dhawan A, Taylor RM, Cheeseman P, De Silva P, Katsiyiannakis L, Mieli-Vergani G. Wilson's disease in children: 37-year experience and revised King's score for liver transplantation. Liver Transpl. 2005;11(4):441–8.
32. Koch DG, Tillman H, Durkalski V, Lee WM, Reuben A. Development of a model to predict transplant-free survival

of patients with acute liver failure. Clin Gastroenterol Hepatol. 2016;14(8):1199–206.
33. Bernal W, Wang Y, Maggs J, Willars C, Sizer E, Auzinger G, Murphy N, Harding D, Elsharkawy A, Simpson K, Larsen FS. Development and validation of a dynamic outcome prediction model for paracetamol-induced acute liver failure: a cohort study. Lancet Gastroenterol Hepatol. 2016;1(3):217–25.
34. Kim JD, Cho EJ, Ahn C, Park SK, Choi JY, Lee HC, Kim DY, Choi MS, Wang HJ, Kim IH, Yeon JE. A model to predict 1-month risk of transplant or death in hepatitis a – related acute liver failure. Hepatology. 2019;70(2):621–9.
35. Weiss E, Saner F, Asrani SK, Biancofiore G, Blasi A, Lerut J, Durand F, Fernandez J, Findlay JY, Fondevila C, Francoz C. When is a critically ill cirrhotic patient too sick to transplant? Development of consensus criteria by a multidisciplinary panel of 35 international experts. Transplantation. 2020. https://doi.org/10.1097/TP.0000000000002858.
36. Darweesh SK, Ibrahim MF, El-Tahawy MA. Effect of N-acetylcysteine on mortality and liver transplantation rate in non-acetaminophen-induced acute liver failure: a multicenter study. Clin Drug Investig. 2017;37(5):473–82.
37. Rabinowich L, Wendon J, Bernal W, Shibolet O. Clinical management of acute liver failure: results of an international multi-center survey. W J Gastroenterol. 2016;22(33):7595.
38. Mohsenin V. Assessment and management of cerebral edema and intracranial hypertension in acute liver failure. J Crit Care. 2013;28(5):783–91.
39. Bernal W, Murphy N, Brown S, Whitehouse T, Bjerring PN, Hauerberg J, Frederiksen HJ, Auzinger G, Wendon J, Larsen FS. A multicentre randomized controlled trial of moderate hypothermia to prevent intracranial hypertension in acute liver failure. J Hepatol. 2016;65(2):273–9.
40. Donnelly MC, Hayes PC, Simpson KJ. Role of inflammation and infection in the pathogenesis of human acute liver failure: clinical implications for monitoring and therapy. W J Gastroenterol. 2016;22(26):5958.
41. Fujiwara K, Abe R, Yasui S, Yokosuka O, Kato N, Oda S. High recovery rate of consciousness by high-volume filtrate hemodiafiltration for fulminant hepatitis. Hepatol Res. 2019;49(2):224–31.
42. Kozek-Langenecker SA, Ahmed AB, Afshari A, Albaladejo P, Aldecoa C, Barauskas G, De Robertis E, Faraoni D, Filipescu DC, Fries D, Haas T. Management of severe perioperative bleeding: guidelines from the European Society of Anaesthesiology: first update 2016. Eur J Anaesthesiol. 2017;34(6):332–95.
43. Sponholz C, Matthes K, Rupp D, Backaus W, Klammt S, Karailieva D, Bauschke A, Settmacher U, Kohl M, Clemens MG, Mitzner S. Molecular adsorbent recirculating system and single-pass albumin dialysis in liver failure – a prospective, randomised crossover study. Crit Care. 2016;20(1):2.
44. Saliba F, Camus C, Durand F, Mathurin P, Letierce A, Delafosse B, Barange K, Perrigault PF, Belnard M, Ichaï P, Samuel D. Albumin dialysis with a noncell artificial liver support device in patients with acute liver failure: a randomized, controlled trial. Ann Intern Med. 2013;159(8):522–31.
45. He GL, Feng L, Duan CY, Hu X, Zhou CJ, Cheng Y, Pan MX, Gao Y. Meta-analysis of survival with the molecular adsorbent recirculating system for liver failure. Int J Clin Exp Med. 2015;8(10):17046.
46. Kribben A, Gerken G, Haag S, Herget-Rosenthal S, Treichel U, Betz C, Sarrazin C, Hoste E, Van Vlierberghe H, Escorsell À, Hafer C. Effects of fractionated plasma separation and adsorption on survival in patients with acute-on-chronic liver failure. Gastroenterology. 2012;142(4):782–9.
47. Stahl K, Hadem J, Schneider A, Manns MP, Wiesner O, Schmidt BM, Hoeper MM, Busch M, David S. Therapeutic plasma exchange in acute liver failure. J Clin Apher. 2019;34(5):589–97.
48. Kido J, Matsumoto S, Momosaki K, Sakamoto R, Mitsubuchi H, Inomata Y, Endo F, Nakamura K. Plasma exchange and chelator therapy rescues acute liver failure in Wilson disease without liver transplantation. Hepatol Res. 2017;47(4):359–63.
49. Larsen FS, Schmidt LE, Bernsmeier C, Rasmussen A, Isoniemi H, Patel VC, Triantafyllou E, Bernal W, Auzinger G, Shawcross D, Eefsen M. High-volume plasma exchange in patients with acute liver failure: an open randomised controlled trial. J Hepatol. 2016;64(1):69–78.
50. Weiner J, Griesemer A, Island E, Lobritto S, Martinez M, Selvaggi G, Lefkowitch J, Velasco M, Tryphonopoulos P, Emond J, Tzakis A. Longterm outcomes of auxiliary partial orthotopic liver transplantation in preadolescent children with fulminant hepatic failure. Liver Transpl. 2016;22(4):485–94.
51. Rela M, Kaliamoorthy I, Reddy MS. Current status of auxiliary partial orthotopic liver transplantation for acute liver failure. Liver Transpl. 2016;22(9):1265–74.
52. Kim SH, Lee EC, Shim JR, Park SJ. A simplified protocol using rituximab and immunoglobulin for ABO-incompatible low-titre living donor liver transplantation. Liver Int. 2018;38(5):932–9.
53. Germani G, Theocharidou E, Adam R, Karam V, Wendon J, O'Grady J, Burra P, Senzolo M, Mirza D, Castaing D, Klempnauer J. Liver transplantation for acute liver failure in Europe: outcomes over 20 years from the ELTR database. J Hepatol. 2012;57(2):288–96.
54. Pamecha V, Vagadiya A, Sinha PK, Sandhyav R, Parthasarathy K, Sasturkar S, Mohapatra N, Choudhury A, Maiwal R, Khanna R, Alam S. Living donor liver transplantation for acute liver failure: donor safety and recipient outcome. Liver Transpl. 2019;25(9):1408–21.
55. Donnelly MC, Davidson JS, Martin K, Baird A, Hayes PC, Simpson KJ. Acute liver failure in Scotland: changes in aetiology and outcomes over time (the Scottish Look-Back Study). Alim Pharmacol Ther. 2017;45(6):833–43.

Liver Graft Retrieval in Deceased Donors

Florin Botea, Genadyi Vatachki Roumenov, Radu Zamfir, Vladislav Brasoveanu, and Irinel Popescu

Abstract

Liver transplantation (LT) is the current curative treatment for end-stage liver disease and has become widespread due to advances in immune-suppression, standardized surgical techniques and strategies to expand the donor pool. However, assuring proper graft quality remains the primary goal in organ retrieval. This goal is achieved by proper organ perfusion to reduce reperfusion injury, and surgical regulations to minimize inadvertent graft injuries. Growing waiting lists have determined the transplant centers to expand the donor pool and reconsider the criteria for acceptable grafts. This has resulted in growing number LTs using extended criteria donors (ECD), living donors (LD), and, more recently and in few countries, donors after circulatory death (DCD). The donor pool was further extended by changing the national policies for donation to opt-out. However, donation after brain death (DBD) remains by far the primary source of organs for transplant. The key points of a successful retrieval are optimal retrieval technique, thorough flushing of the graft, and minimal warm and cold ischemia time.

63.1 Introduction

Liver transplantation (LT) is the current curative treatment for end-stage liver disease and has become widespread due to advances in immune-suppression, standardized surgical techniques and strategies to expand the donor pool. However, assuring proper graft quality remains the primary goal in organ retrieval. This goal is achieved by proper organ perfusion to reduce reperfusion injury, and surgical regulations to minimize inadvertent graft injuries [1].

Growing waiting lists have determined the transplant centers to expand the donor pool and reconsider the criteria for acceptable grafts. This has resulted in growing number LTs using extended criteria donors (ECD), living donors (LD), and, more recently and in few countries, donors after circulatory death (DCD). The donor pool was further extended by changing the national policies for donation to opt-out (Fig. 63.1). However, donation after brain death (DBD) remains by far the primary source of organs for transplant (Fig. 63.2) [4].

63.2 Donation After Brain Death

Donation after brain death (DBD) are patients with irreversible loss of all functions of the brain, including the brainstem. The three crucial elements that are compulsory in a DBD are coma, absence of brainstem reflexes, and apnea. The diagnosis consists of identifying an obvious cause of BD (brain death) in the medical history of the donor, excluding any condition that can mimic BD (hypothermia, barbiturate intoxication, etc.), and a thorough neurological examination [5].

Because of the increasing number of patients on the waiting lists, accepting extended criteria donors (ECD) (Table 63.1) [6, 7], so called "marginal donors", especially in emergency setting, has become current practice in many centers. Most frequently used ECD grafts are those with >30% hepatic steatosis, which have shown that in selected cases may have a low primary non-function rate and even reversed steatosis [8].

Expanded criteria donors are defined as the following [7]:

F. Botea (✉) · I. Popescu
"Dan Setlacec" Center of General Surgery and Liver Transplantation, Fundeni Clinical Institute, Bucharest, Romania

"Titu Maiorescu" University, Bucharest, Romania

G. V. Roumenov · R. Zamfir · V. Brasoveanu
"Dan Setlacec" Center of General Surgery and Liver Transplantation, Fundeni Clinical Institute, Bucharest, Romania

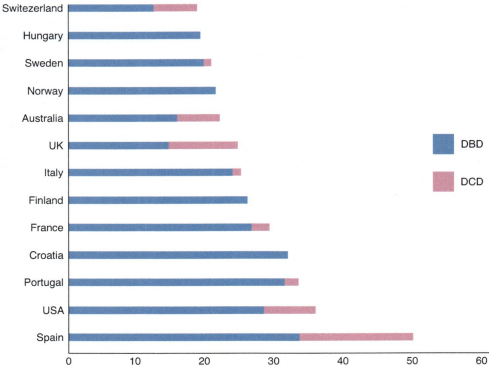

Fig. 63.1 Actual DBD and DCD organ donor rates for Europe, Australia and the USA in 2019 [2, 3]

*Actual deceased organ donor at least one organ has be en recovered for purpose of transplantation, n contrast to a utilised donor, who is an actual donor from whom at least one organ has been transplanted. The number of utilised donors is therefore lower of equal than the number of actual donors.

63.3 Donors after Circulatory Death

DCDs are defined by irreversible loss of heart and lung functions after cardiac arrest, from which one cannot or should not be resuscitated. The terminology of non-heart beating donor (NHBT) was abandoned. Also, the term "organ harvesting" was abandoned and replaced with "organ retrieval or procurement" [4]. DCD donors are classified in 4 categories, according to the Maastricht classification; the last two so called "controlled" groups are frequently used as liver graft donors, unlike the first two so called "uncontrolled categories in which grafts are frequently discarded due to excessively long ischemia periods (Fig. 63.3) [4].

DCD donors provide a lower quality graft and require a complex infrastructure and are therefore not a preferred source in many countries.

Because of longer ischemia time (when compared to DBD), the primary objective in DCD retrieval is organ perfusion, resulting in three techniques:

- rapid laparotomy and aortic cannulation—followed by organ dissection;
- femoral vessels cannulation with catheter followed by laparotomy and dissection;
- NRP—femoral vessel cannulation and regional perfusion, which may also improve liver graft quality according to recent studies [22];

The latter two can be performed in emergency by trained personnel and do not require an operating room. These methods may better bridge the time delay between diagnosis of DCD and arrival of the retrieval team, reducing the warm ischemia time by early organ perfusion.

Technically, there is no cross-clamping but an equivalent in which the aorta is cannulated, and the organs are flushed with preservation solution. The retrieval must be carried out in less than 35 minutes from cardiac arrest to provide proper results [23].

One of the retrieval techniques applied to cardiac arrest donors is done by in situ perfusion of the organs with preservation solution:

- a catheter is inserted into the aorta by femoral approach, through which the organs are infused with saline solution, followed by preservation solution. The two bal-

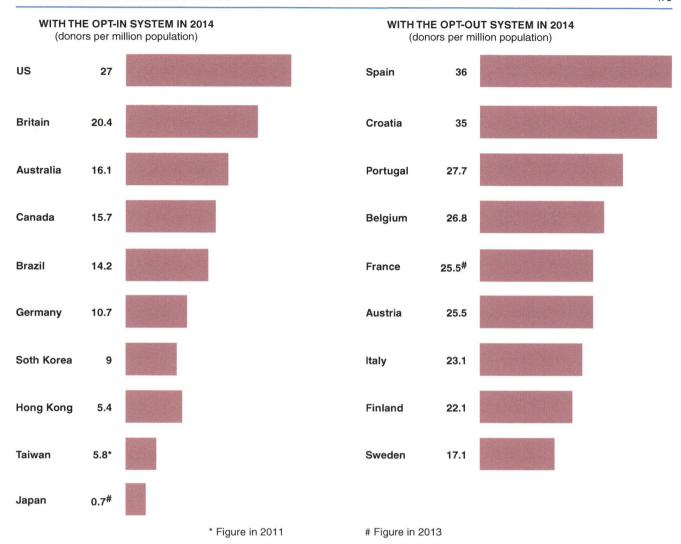

Fig. 63.2 DBD donation rate in different countries [3]

Table 63.1 The parameters for the extended criteria donors (ECD) [6, 7]

Donor-related features:	Age > 65 yrs BMI > 30 kg/m^2
Factors related to ICU:	ICU stay and ventilation support >7 days Hypotension and inotropic support (≥2 pressors at any time, high-dose dopamine or epinephrine) Resuscitated cardiac arrest
Liver steatosis:	Macrosteatosis (>30% but ≤60%)
Biochemical imbalances:	Hypernatremia (peak serum Na >165 mEq/L) Liver disfunction (AST/ALT>3X; BT > 3 mg/dl)
Cold ischemia time	> 12 hours
Viral infections:	Positive serology for HBV hepatitis • AgHBs (+) • AgHbc (+) Positive serology for HCV hepatitis
Sepsis-related factors:	Sepsis with positive blood culture Meningitis
Malignancy risk factors:	History of extrahepatic malignancy

Category I. Uncontrolled	Found dead IA. Out-of-hospital IB. In-hospital	Sudden unexpected CA without any attempt of resuscitation by a life-medical team; WIT to be considered according to National life-recommendations in place; refference to in- or out-of hopital life-(IH-OH) setting.
Category II. Uncontrolled	Witnessed cardiac arrest IIA. Out-of-hospital IIB. In-hospital	Sudden unexpected irreversible CA with unsuccessful resuscitation life-by a life-medical team; reference to in- or out-of- hospital life- (IH- OH) setting.
Category III. Controlled	Withdrawl of life-sustaining therapy	Planned withdrawl of life-sustainig therapy*; expected CA
Category IV. Uncontrolled Controlled	Cardiac arrest while life-brain dead	Sudden CA after brain death diagnosis during donor life-management but prior to planes organ retrieval

CA, circulatory arrest.
*This category mainly refers to the decision to withdraw life-sustaining therapies. Legislation in some countries allows euthanasia (medically assisted CA) and subsequent organ donation described as the fifth category.

Fig. 63.3 The modified Maastricht classification of DCD [4]

loons of the catheter are inflated in the supraceliac and infraceliac aorta to achieve isolated perfusion of the organs, which is the equivalent of in situ cross-clamping. Radiological guidance of the catheter position is recommended;
- another catheter is inserted into the inferior vena cava (IVC) via the femoral vein in order to achieve outflow of the perfusate;
- cooling of the peritoneal cavity by infusion of cold saline solution via a percutaneous catheter;
- retrieval is carried out as fast as possible, and the organs are perfused "ex-situ" with preservation solution [24].

An alternative to this technique is the rapid laparotomy only with aortic cannulation and clamping at infradiaphragmatic level, or at the aortic cross if a sternotomy is also performed.

The main concern about DCD is the systemic inflammation caused by prolonged warm ischemia time that has a major impact on graft quality. Unfortunately, this is difficult to control in DCDs [3], while easily controlled in DBD donors, making later the most frequent and unanimously accepted by most centers. However, nowadays DCD provides promising results in extending the donor pool as shown by recent comparative studies that recorded comparable results in terms of graft survival, postoperative complications, and readmission rate (Fig. 63.4) [26, 27].

The overall quality of DCD grafts can be improved by interposition of an oxygenation normothermic or hypothermic perfusion machine. This device acts like a bridging modality between the cardiac arrest and organ retrieval by perfusing and cooling of the organs using preservation solution.

63.4 Hypothermic Oxygenated Machine Perfusion

Recent studies regarding ex vivo machine oxygenating perfusion proved to significantly reduce the ischemia-reperfusion and biliary injury, in both DBD and DCD grafts, showing that up to 7 out of 10 otherwise rejected liver grafts are fit for transplantation, further expanding the donor pool [9]. Unlike renal grafts, where hypothermic oxygenated machine perfusion machine has become routine, for liver grafts, its use is still in early clinical experience phase (Fig. 63.5).

63.4.1 Surgical Technique

The most important maneuver of any retrieval procedure is the aortic clamping, followed by organ flushing with preservation fluid. Organ dissection may be performed before

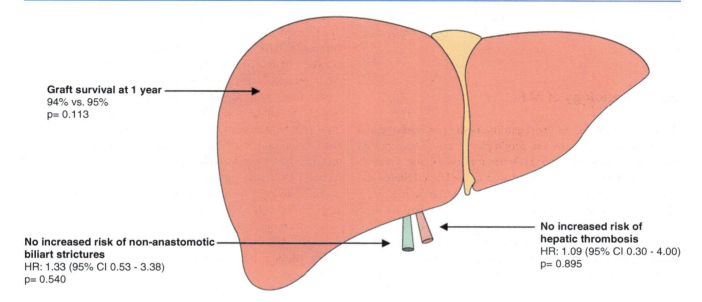

Fig. 63.4 DCD vs DBD liver transplantation in highly selected patients [25]

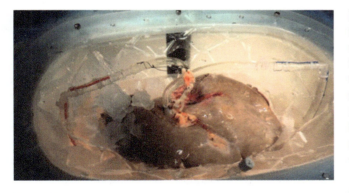

Fig. 63.5 Hypothermic oxygenated machine perfusion of both hepatic artery and portal vein (dual HOPE) for advanced steatosis (35%). The graft was successfully transplanted with no complications

and/or after, therefore the retrieval procedure may be described in two main phases: warm and cold phase dissections.

Initially, warm phase dissection was preferred because it decreased the risk of organ rewarming and allowed a more extensive dissection [10]. However, arterial injury during this phase might compromise the graft. This led to introducing a rapid technique, which aimed for early vascular control and cannulation followed by cold phase dissection, resulting in shorter operating times and less organ damage [11]. This technique requires high skills, as identifying vascular structures after perfusion may be more challenging and, therefore, it is paramount for the surgeon to balance dissection between the two phases according to his experience [12]. En-bloc retrieval may also be associated with reduced risk of organ injury, and is frequently used in pediatric donors, followed by organ separation on the back table. Regardless of the technique, the surgeon must ensure a rapid removal of the graft with minimal risk [10, 12].

After laparotomy, inspection and palpation of the liver are carried out, facilitated by the mobilization of the right hemiliver to expose the bare area. The main findings in terms of the appearance and consistency of the liver are:

- increased consistency because of over hydrating, frequently found in hypotensive patients who are aggressively perfused;
- fine, granular aspect could show diseased liver; if so, a biopsy with freeze section examination is required;
- a dark colored liver can show a hypotensive episode, or it can even predict an imminent cardiac arrest;
- yellow tint of the liver suggests liver steatosis (a biopsy with freeze section examination is required) (Fig. 63.6);

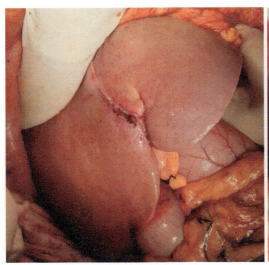
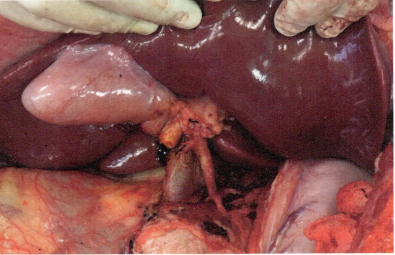

Fig. 63.6 Liver steatosis macroscopic aspect (left), normal (right) (from the photo collection of Genadyi Vatachki Roumenov)

- focal liver lesions (a biopsy with freeze section examination is required).

Fatty liver grafts carry an increased risk of primary nonfunction (PNF). Steatosis between 10% and 30% is acceptable as a marginal graft; some centers may even accept steatosis up to 60% [13].

Next, the colon, rectum, kidneys, and pelvic organs (in female donors) are inspected for malignancies. Any abnormal finding should be documented and reported to the transplant center, including biopsies.

Once the inspection is complete, the surgeon may proceed with the sternotomy. Then, the pericardium is opened for an appropriate exposure of the pericardial IVC; even if the heart is not procured, this step is also essential for keeping track of the heart movements and taking adequate measures in case cardiac arrest should occur.

The left lobe is mobilized, and the lesser sac is inspected for an aberrant left hepatic artery (ALHA) (Fig. 63.7a), then incised, preserving the artery if present. The right aspect of the porta hepatis is palpated for detecting an aberrant right hepatic artery (ARHA).

Possible arterial variations at this level are best classified by Varotti et al. [14]:

- Type 1—a single hepatic artery (HA) emerging from the celiac trunk;
- Type 2A—HA from the celiac trunk, giving both right and left HAs; left accessory HA emerging from the left gastric artery (LGA);
- Type 2B—HA from the celiac trunk, giving only a right HA; left HA from the LGA (replaced left HA);
- Type 3A—HA from the celiac trunk, giving both right and left HAs; right accessory HA from the superior mesenteric artery (SMA);
- Type 3B—right HA from SMA, and left HA from LGA;
- Type 4A—HA from the celiac trunk, and two accessory HAs: right accessory HA from SMA, and left accessory HA from LGA;
- Type 4B—HA from SMA, giving both right and left HAs; left accessory HA from LGA;
- Type 5—a single HA from SMA (Fig. 63.7b) [15].

According to a meta-analysis, classic branching of the common HA from the celiac trunk is seen in 55–60% of cases, while variations in hepatic arterial anatomy are observed in 40–45% of cases.

The liver hilum can be palpated from the left through the lesser sac. The presence of a posterior pulsation suggests a right HA originating from the SMA. Placed posterior to the duodenum, the right HAs stemming from the SMA come in several trajectory variations, in relation to the head of the pancreas: in the sagittal plane—posterior to the pancreatic head or through it, and in frontal plane—more lateral or medial in relation to the portal vein and splenomesenteric confluent, respectively. In this area, a HA originating from the celiac trunk or even from the aorta should be considered. (Fig. 63.7c and d).

Early proper identification of liver arterial anatomy is the key to a safe retrieval procedure. For example, a right HA coming from a low bifurcation of the proper HA may be confused with an aberrant right HA originating from the SMA. An aberrant right HA has a cranio-caudal trajectory, whereas in case of a low bifurcation, the right HA presents

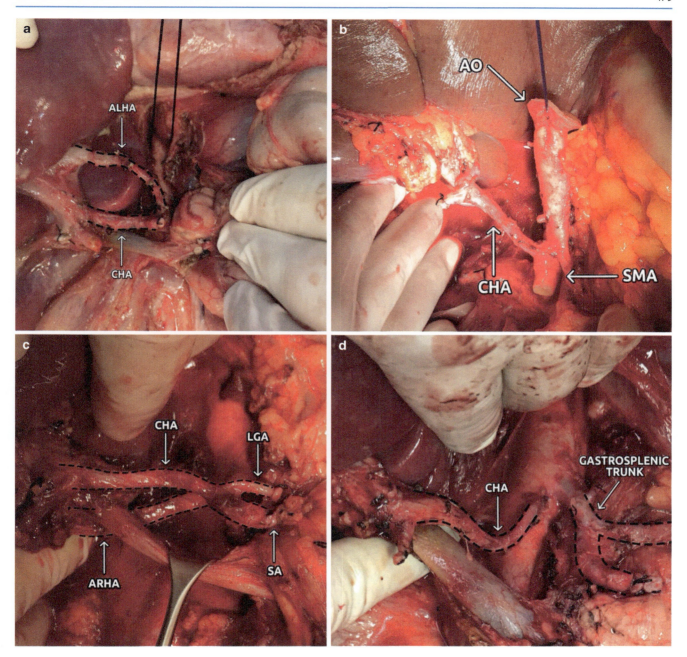

Fig. 63.7 (**a**) Aberrant left hepatic artery originating from left gastric artery. (**b**) Common hepatic artery originating from the superior mesenteric artery. (**c**) ARHA originating from celiac trunk. (**d**) Common hepatic artery originating directly from the aorta (from the photo collection of Genadyi Vatachki Roumenov)

an angulation from medial to lateral, followed by an ascending trajectory. The angulation spot is predisposed to accidental injury if the two variations are not identified correctly. A low bifurcation of the HA, below the emergence of the gastroduodenal artery, may be present in 6% of cases (Fig. 63.8).

By placing a fine bulldog clamp on a suspected aberrant artery, the surgeon can distinguish between an aberrant right HA and an artery of the common bile duct (CBD): clamping the aberrant artery may cause a visible ischemic delimitation on the liver parenchyma. The same method may identify an accessory left HA emerging from the LGA: the presence of a pulse distal to the bulldog placed on the aberrant HA indicates anastomotic arterial collaterals in the hilum.

The line of Told is incised to mobilize the colon and small bowel completely from the retroperitoneum (Cattell-Braasch maneuver), exposing the IVC, towards the left renal vein, and the aorta, up to the origin of the SMA (Fig. 63.9) [16]. Dissection continues cephalad from the right iliac

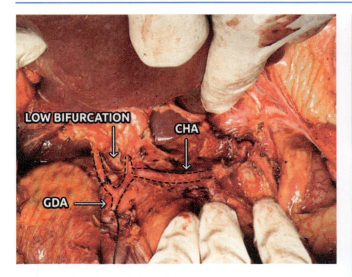

Fig. 63.8 Low bifurcation of common hepatic artery exposed after mobilization of the pancreatic head (from the photo collection of Genadyi Vatachki Roumenov)

artery towards the portal vein, and medially, to completely mobilize the head of the pancreas. Last, the surgeon places the index finger through the foramen of Winslow, posterior to the liver hilum, to expose and incise the connective tissue medially to the origin of the SMA, completing the mobilization maneuver [1].

If the donor is hemodynamically unstable, the surgeon may proceed with aortic cannulation at this point and complete dissection in the cold phase.

After cholecystostomy, the CBD is identified, ligated above the head of the pancreas, as distally as possible, sectioned, and flushed through the gallbladder followed by cholecystectomy. The pyloric and gastroduodenal arteries are identified and ligated; it is recommended to keep the gastroduodenal artery stump if possible, to facilitate blood flow assessment of the HA in the recipient, or even thrombectomy. Next the common HA is dissected along its axis, the LGA and splenic artery are identified and ligated preserving 5–10 mm stumps, followed by a good exposure of the celiac trunk. The extensive dissection of the celiac trunk must be done with utmost attention to avoid injuring the diaphragmatic arteries, which stem from its base. Exposure of the infra-diaphragmatic aorta is achieved by transversely sectioning the right diaphragmatic crus, and a vascular tie is passed around the aorta at this level (Fig. 63.10).

Alternatively, a tie may be passed around the aorta above the diaphragm by sectioning the inferior portion of the left pulmonary ligament, called the transpericardic transpleural approach. Circumferential dissection of the aorta at this level

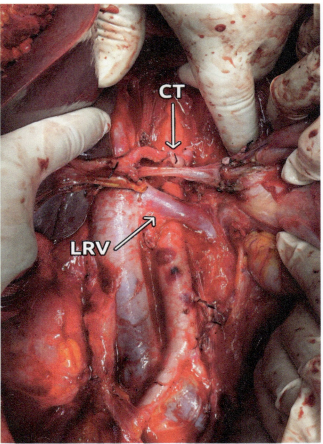

Fig. 63.9 Cattell-Braasch maneuver exposing the major vessels in the retroperitoneum (from the photo collection of Genadyi Vatachki Roumenov)

is preferably done under digital control, to prevent injuring any vertebral arteries.

The inferior mesenteric vein is then dissected at the Treitz's ligament and cannulated; after insertion, the portal cannula is placed in the PV. Alternatively, the cannula may be placed directly into the PV (Fig. 63.11). This maneuver should be followed by cross-clamping, to minimize the lack of portal blood flow. Alternatively, the cannula may be inserted directly into the PV (in the portion located posteriorly to the duodenum, or via the superior mesenteric vein. The patency of the portal cannula is confirmed by aspiration, followed by heparinized saline solution bolus infusion.

The dissection of the aorta is carried out above the iliac bifurcation by ligating and sectioning the inferior mesenteric artery. At this level, the aorta is ligated distally and cannulated (Fig. 63.11). The patency of the aortic cannula is checked by aspiration, followed by heparinized saline solution bolus infu-

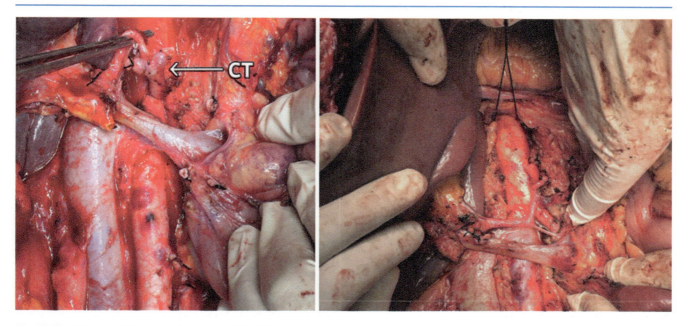

Fig. 63.10 Celiac trunk dissected circumferentially (left). Aortic ties positioned for cross-clamping (right) (from the photo collection of Genadyi Vatachki Roumenov)

sion. Bleeding from the aortic cannulation level may originate from a lumbar artery, which must be identified and sutured.

The IVC must also be identified and dissected at this level. A systemic heparin bolus is administered (300 UI/kg), followed by a 3-minute waiting time, allowing a full systemic circuit.

63.4.1.1 Cross-clamping

This maneuver consists of several steps that isolate the arterial and portal pathways of the abdominal organs in a closed circuit that is flushed with preservation solution and emptied through the IVC:

- clamping the infra-diaphragmatic aorta (by ligation);
- flushing the abdominal organs with cold preservation solution through the cannulas placed in the PV (1 ml/g of liver tissue, or 2 liters) and aorta (3 ml/g of liver tissue, or 5 liters);
- the IVC is sectioned inferior to the right atrium and above the iliac veins;
- topic cooling for the abdominal organs is applied by filling the abdomen with sterile ice;
- a clamp may also be placed on the mesentery root to exclude the intestines from the circuit.

After cross-clamping, the liver graft is detached en-bloc with a diaphragm patch. The retrohepatic IVC is dissected caudally and sectioned above the renal vein ostium. The PV is sectioned above the pancreas head, leaving a 1-cm stump distally if the pancreas is also retrieved. The aorta is sectioned above and below the celiac trunk, and completely dissected from its posterior attachments. The liver graft is now removed from the donor.

63.4.2 Technical Variants

63.4.2.1 Split Liver Retrieval

This type of retrieval is used to split the graft between 2 recipients. The split may be done between segments II-III and the rest of the liver (pediatric and adult split), or between segments II-III-IV and the rest of the liver (adult and adult split). Splitting may be difficult due to varying vascular and biliary anatomy. It is worth mentioning that certain arterial anatomical variants favor the splitting, such as types 2B and 3B according to Varotti's classification.

In-situ splitting requires separation of the liver before cross-clamping. The donor must meet the following criteria: optimal liver quality, medium-large size graft, and stable donor. The advantages of in-situ over ex-situ splitting are:

- optimal hemostasis of the liver cut surface, especially when transection is carried out with an ultrasound dissector,

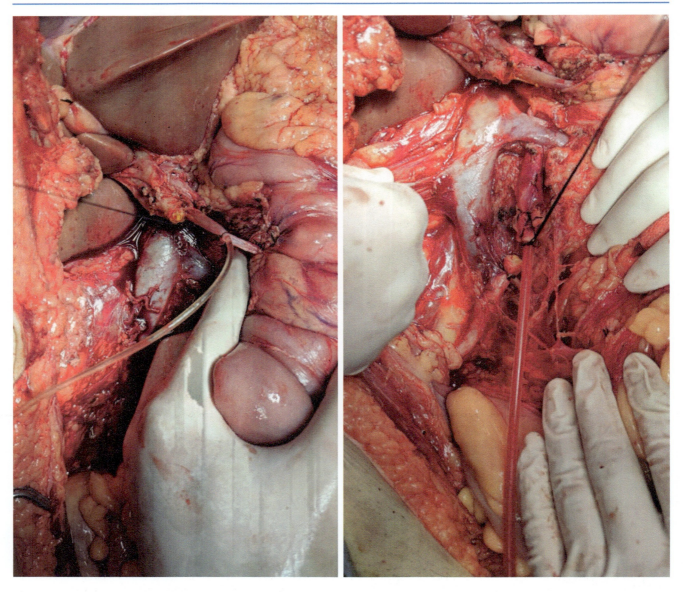

Fig. 63.11 Cannulation of the portal vein (left) and aorta (right) (from the photo collection of Genadyi Vatachki Roumenov)

- allows the assessment of the viability of both hepatic grafts.
- allows a meticulous transection facilitating the identification of veins with caliber larger than 5 mm (requiring reconstruction), and of aberrant vascular and biliary anatomy.

In ex-situ split liver retrieval, the liver graft is split after retrieval, on the "back-table". The advantages of ex-situ splitting are the reduced operating time and the diminished demand for resources.

63.4.2.2 En-bloc Liver-pancreas Retrieval

En-bloc retrieval of the two organs requires an aortic patch that includes the celiac trunk and SMA (Fig. 63.12). After mobilization of the organs and cross-clamping, the grafts are retrieved and separated on the back-table. For pancreas retrieval, the GDA and splenic artery are not ligated. The organs may be transplanted together, as a 'cluster' transplant, which has very few indications. During this type of retrieval, the 'no touch technique' is used for the pancreas, which is indirectly mobilized by using the spleen as "handle" (which is later removed on the back-table).

63.4.2.3 En-bloc Liver-bowel Retrieval

This type of retrieval involves bowel preparation and lavage through a nasojejunal tube with saline solution and antibiotics. The jejunum is sealed with stapler close to the angle of Treitz, marking the area with a suture thread for later orientation. The transvers mesocolon is sectioned and the right colon vascularization is ligated. The pancreas is separated from the portal and superior mesenteric vein and then transection at level of the pancreatic isthmus. In the event of an unstable donor, separation from the pancreas may also be done on the back-table. Stapling the ileum is performed as late as possible, to allow the complete evacuation of the intestinal content into the colon. The hepatic and intestinal grafts are lifted together with celiac trunk, SMA and aortic patch (Carell patch), which can be extended on the back-table using an iliac graft [17]. An "in-vivo" dissection of the liver hilum is recommended by some authors, to reduce the back-table organ separation time by early identification of anatomical variants [18].

63.4.3 Back-table

The graft is then moved to the back-table and positioned. The liver graft is perfused on the back-table with preservation solution through the PV and HA (Fig. 63.13). Flushing the CBD is also done in order to avoid autolysis of the biliary tree epithelium under the effect of the remnant bile during cold

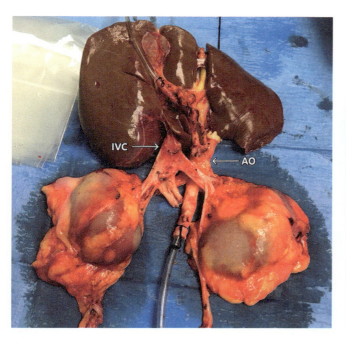

Fig. 63.12 En-bloc liver and kidney retrieval in pediatric donor (from the photo collection of Genadyi Vatachki Roumenov)

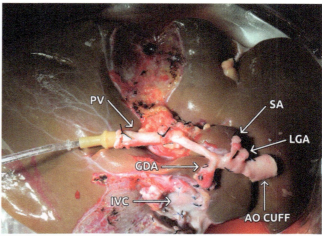

Fig. 63.13 Back-table dissection and perfusion (from the photo collection of Genadyi Vatachki Roumenov)

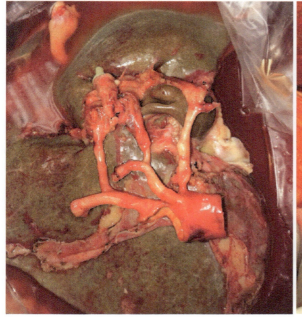
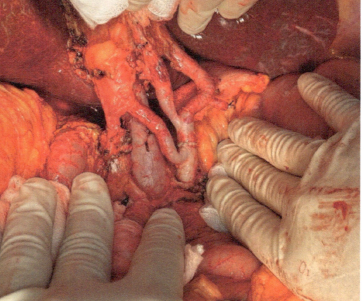

Fig. 63.14 Varotti 4A reconstruction on the back table and in recipient (from the photo collection of Genadyi Vatachki Roumenov)

ischemia time. Uniform discoloration of the liver and outflow of clear preservation fluid through the hepatic veins are proof of a proper flushing of the liver graft [17, 19]. The excess of connective tissue and the portion of diaphragm attached to the liver graft are also removed on the back-table.

The IVC is prepared for anastomosis depending on the technique used in the recipient: a termino-terminal (T-T) anastomosis between the recipient's and donor's and IVCs, a termino-lateral (T-L) anastomosis between the cranial extremity of the donor's IVC and the recipient's IVC anastomosis, after sealing both ends of the latter (the piggy back technique), a latero-lateral (L-L) anastomosis (the Belghiti technique), or a L-L anastomosis using the triangulation technique (the triangle is fashioned by an transversal incision on the anterior wall of the recipient's IVC, uniting the ostiums of the hepatic veins, combined with a longitudinal incision).

The hepatic pedicle elements are prepared for anastomosis. The portal vein and hepatic artery are checked again to assure all branches are properly sealed, by infusing sterile saline solution with a relative pressure.

If arterial variations are present, they are reconstructed and prepared for implantation (Fig. 63.14). The common practice in arterial anatomical variations is to reduce the anastomotic partner to a single arterial trajectory of convenient caliber. When a right HA originates from SMA, the celiac trunk and SMA aortic patches are sutured together. The distal portion of the SMA is connected to the recipient's HA. The right HA can also be T-T anastomosed to the GDA or splenic artery stumps; in this case, the anastomotic partner of the recipient's HA is the aortic patch corresponding to the celiac trunk. There is no need for arterial reconstruction in case of a left HA stemming from the LGA.

If the recipient's HA does not achieve an acceptable blood flow, the liver can be vascularized by an arterial graft interposition (donor's iliac artery) or implant the celiac trunk patch of the graft directly into the aorta distal to the origin of the renal veins.

After the preparation of the graft is completed, the liver is packed in three separate sterile bags with saline solution between each one for extra protection during transportation.

The recommended period of cold ischemia (the interval between cross-clamping and finishing the cavo-caval and porto-portal anastomoses with subsequent declamping) is less than 12 hours, since the liver graft quality declines after this period [19].

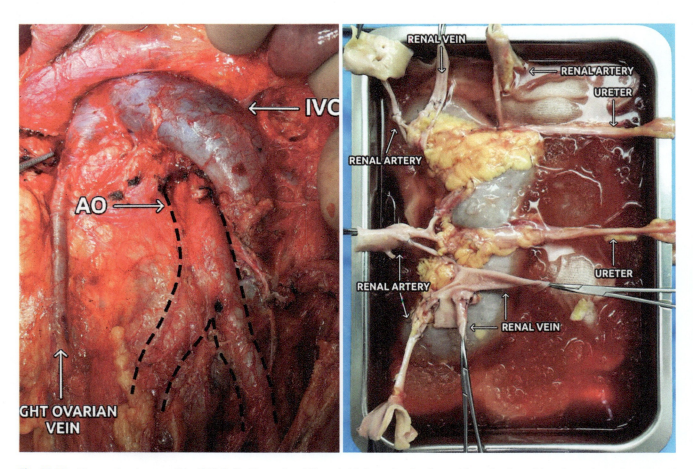

Fig. 63.15 Abnormal trajectory of the IVC (left). Horse-shoe kidney (with 4 arteries, 3 veins and 2 urethers), positioned anterior to the aorta and IVC; a surprising obstacle during Cattell-Braasch maneuver (right) (from the photo collection of Genadyi Vatachki Roumenov)

63.4.3.1 Incidents: Accidents

In a multiorgan retrieval, a wide array of unforeseen situations may arise due to donor instability, challenges generated by sharing the vascular capacity of the donor between retrieval teams, failure to recognize the anatomical vascular variants with consequent vascular injuries, or issues related to logistics (Fig. 63.15).

In case of an unstable donor or even cardiac arrest during retrieval, the next steps should be followed:

- systemic heparin administration—a bolus of 300 U/kg;
- aorta cannulation only (portal vein cannulation and perfusion are done on the "back-table")
- cross-clamping as fast as possible in order to avoid prolonged organ ischemia;
- cold phase dissection of the vessels followed by hepatic graft extraction [18, 20].

If cardiac arrest occurs, the donor status changes to a type IV cardiac arrest donor (according to the Maastricht classification). Cardiac arrest in a DBD donor is followed by sectioning of the IVC (venting), aortic cannulation and infusion with cold preservation solution, followed by clamping of the aorta, sterile ice cooling, portal vein cannulation, and liver graft extraction.

In case of a damaged or short IVC, the liver graft can be salvaged by reconstructive augmentation with venous grafts from the iliac veins.

During retrieval, if an accessory branch of right HA originating from SMA is injured, the management depends on when the injury was produced—before or after cross-clamping:

- before cross-clamping: proceeds with cross-clamping and separate infusion of the injured vessel through a thin catheter, to obtain a uniform flushing of the liver graft. After graft extraction, the injured branch will be re-attached to the GDA or splenic artery stump, on the back-table;
- after cross-clamping: the above-mentioned vascular reconstruction will be carried out on the back-table.

Sometimes, due to logistic or transportation reasons, the retrieval time must be cut short. For a shorter retrieval time, the surgeon may also exclude back-table time completely and carry it out at the transplantation center [12, 21].

The procedure must always be adapted to all contributing factors linked to the donor.

In conclusion, the key points of a successful retrieval are optimal retrieval technique, thorough flushing of the graft, and minimal warm and cold ischemia time.

References

1. Busuttil RW, Klintmalm GBG. Transplantation of the liver. 3rd ed. Philadelphia: Elsevier; 2013., ISBN978-1-4557-0268-8. https://doi.org/10.1016/C2010-0-66347-4.
2. Stewart C. Rate of deceased organ donors including both donation after brain death (DBD) and donation after cardiac death (DCD) in Europe from 2018 to 2019, by country(per million population). https://www.statista.com/statistics/537908/deceased-organ-donor-rate-in-europe/.
3. https://www.odt.nhs.uk/deceased-donation/best-practice-guidance/donation-after-circulatory-death/.
4. Thuong M, Ruiz A, Evrard P, et al. New classification of donation after circulatory death donors definitions and terminology. Transpl Int. 2016;29:749–59. https://doi.org/10.1111/tri.12776.
5. Goila AK, Pawar M. The diagnosis of brain death. Indian J Crit Care Med. 2009;13(1):7–11. https://doi.org/10.4103/0972-5229.53108.
6. Spitzer AL, Lao OB, Dick AA, et al. The biopsied donor liver: incorporating macrosteatosis into high-risk donor assessment. Liver Transpl. 2010;16:874–84.
7. Jiménez-Castro MB, Elias-Miró M, Peralta C. Expanding the donor pool in liver transplantation: influence of ischemia-reperfusion. In: Organ donation and organ donors. Hauppauge, NY., ISBN: 978-1-62618-853-2: Nova Science Publishers; 2013.
8. Nair A, Hashimoto K. Extended criteria donors in liver transplantation-from marginality to mainstream. Hepatobiliary Surg Nutr. 2018;7(5):386–8. https://doi.org/10.21037/hbsn.2018.06.08.
9. Mergental H, Laing RW, Kirkham AJ, et al. Transplantation of discarded livers following viability testing with normothermic machine perfusion. Nat Commun. 2020;11:2939. https://doi.org/10.1038/s41467-020-16251-3.
10. Imagawa DK, Olthoff KM, Yersiz H, et al. Rapid en bloc technique for pancreas-liver procurement. Improved early liver function. Transplantation. 1996;61(11):1605–9. https://doi.org/10.1097/00007890-199606150-00010.
11. Starzl TE, Miller C, Broznick B, Makowka L. An improved technique for multiple organ harvesting. Surg Gynecol Obstet. 1987;165(4):343–8.
12. Oniscu GC, Forsythe JL, Fung J, editors. Abdominal organ retrieval and transplantation bench surgery. Chichester: Wiley, First published:3 April 2013; Print ISBN: 9780470657867. Online ISBN:9781118513125. https://doi.org/10.1002/978111851312.
13. McCormack L, Petrowsky H, Jochum W, et al. Use of severely steatotic grafts in liver transplantation: a matched case-control study. Ann Surg. 2007;246(6):940–6.; discussion 946-8. https://doi.org/10.1097/SLA.0b013e31815c2a3f.
14. Varotti G, Gondolesi GE, Goldman J, et al. Anatomic variations in right liver living donors. J Am Coll Surg. 2004;198(4):577–82. https://doi.org/10.1016/j.jamcollsurg.2003.11.014.
15. Couinaud C. Controlled hepatectomies and exposure of the intrahepatic bile ducts – anatomical and technical study. Paris: C. Couinaud; 1981. p. 16–8.
16. Cattell RB, Braasch JW. A technique for the exposure of the third and fourth potions of the duodenum. Surg Gynecol Obstet. 1960;111:378–9.
17. Azoulay D, Samuel D, Adam R, et al. Paul Brousse liver transplantation: the first 1,500 cases. Clin Transpl. 2000;24:273–80.
18. Di BF, De RN, Masetti M, et al. Hepatic hilum management in 250 liver-multivisceral procurements. Transplant Proc. 2006;38(4):1068.

19. Jiménez-Romero C, Caso Maestro O, Cambra Molero F, et al. Using old liver grafts for liver transplantation: where are the limits? World J Gastroenterol. 2014;20(31):10691–702. https://doi.org/10.3748/wjg.v20.i31.10691.
20. Brockmann JG, Vaidya A, Reddy S, Friend PJ. Retrieval of abdominal organs for transplantation. Br J Surg. 2006;93(2):133–46.
21. Tector AJ, Mangus RS, Chestovich P, et al. Use of extended criteria livers decreases wait time for liver transplantation without adversely impacting posttransplant survival. Ann Surg. 2006;244(3):439–50.
22. Watson CJE, Hunt F, Messer S, et al. In situ normothermic perfusion of livers in controlled circulatory death donation may prevent ischemic cholangiopathy and improve graft survival. Am J Transplant. 2019;19(6):1745–58. https://doi.org/10.1111/ajt.15241.
23. Forsythe JLR. Transplantation. 4th ed. Edinburgh: Elsevier; 2009. p. 102–3.
24. Wigmore SJ. Similar liver transplantation survival with selected cardiac death donors and brain death donors (Br J Surg 2010; 97: 744-753). Br J Surg. 2010;97(5):753.
25. Trivedi PJ, Scalera I, Slaney E, et al. Clinical outcomes of donation after circulatory death liver transplantation in primary sclerosing cholangitis. J Hepatol. 2017;67(5):957–65. Epub 2017/07/12. https://doi.org/10.1016/j.jhep.2.
26. Eren EA, Latchana N, Beal E, et al. Donations after circulatory death in liver transplant. Exp Clin Transplant. 2016;14(5):463–70.
27. Kimura F, Miyazaki M, Suwa T, et al. Reduced hepatic acute-phase response after simultaneous resection for gastrointestinal cancer with synchronous liver metastases. Br J Surg. 1996;83(7):1002–6.

Deceased Donor Liver Transplantation: The Pendulum of Visions and Ideas

Jan Lerut and Quirino Lai

Abstract

During the second half of the twentieth-century, liver transplantation (LT) became a clinical reality. Many technical, medical, physiologic, and immunological hurdles needed to be taken to make this endeavour successful. Starzl stated already in 1989 that "the conceptual appeal of liver transplantation would become so great that the procedure should come to mind as a last resort for virtually every patient with lethal hepatic disease." Technical perfection and the introduction in the 80s of the selective immunosuppressive drugs cyclosporine A and tacrolimus transformed LT into a routine procedure. Since then, signs of progress have been spectacular. The number of procedures applied to more than 50 different benign and malignant liver diseases has grown exponentially, reaching the 400,000 marks nowadays.

This chapter deals with different aspects of this medical adventure, such as developed in the context of deceased donor LT experiences. The concept of this chapter is based on the "pendulum" of visions and ideas. Indeed, nearly all historical observations and descriptions made and written down by Starzl in his 1969 classical textbook, "Experience in Hepatic Transplantation," have been confirmed many decades later. This "closing circle concept" will be highlighted at the beginning of each section by recalling a visionary quote of Starzl followed by the current status of LT (Starzl, Experience in liver transplantation. WB Saunders Company, Philadelphia, 1969).

J. Lerut (✉)
Institute for Experimental and Clinical Research [IREC], Université catholique Louvain (UCL), Brussels, Belgium
e-mail: Jan.lerut@uclouvain.be

Q. Lai
General Surgery and Organ Transplantation Unit, Sapienza University of Rome, Rome, Italy

64.1 Introduction

There are clear signs that homotransplantation of the liver will be a valuable means in the future of treating patients who have otherwise hopeless prognosis from hepatic disease (Th. E. Starzl foreword book Experience in Hepatic Transplantation)

Liver transplantation (LT) has turned from a dream into a reality. The first attempts of canine LT covered a one-page short letter by St.Welch in 1955 in the 'Transplantation Bulletin,' a supplement of the Journal of Plastic and Reconstructive Surgery. At that time, a transplantation journal did even not exist! Later on, it was discovered that the Milanese surgeon V.Staudacher had realized the first experiments in 1952. Starzl's large animal experience resulted in the "first LT experiment in human" on March 26, 1963 [1]. Twenty years later, the National Institute of Health Consensus Development Conference based on only 540 LTs performed in Denver-Pittsburgh, Hannover, Cambridge, and Groningen, concluded that LT was "a promising alternative to current therapy in the management of late phase of several forms of severe liver diseases." Moreover, the Committee declared that LT had the potential to become a "clinical service" instead of an experimental procedure. This consensus conference's results represented the starting point for the high-speed implementation of LT as a curative treatment of many livers and liver-based diseases [1–4]. From 1960 to 1990, knowledge was almost exclusively based on deceased donor LT experiences. From 1990 onwards, living donor LT (LDLT) expanded further knowledge about surgical technique, physiology, and peri-operative care [5]. The LDLT experience will undoubtedly lead to the full development of all other technical LT variants, badly needed to overcome allograft shortage and optimize liver recipients' surgical and medical care [5].

64.2 The Pendulum of History

> At first, the results with the clinical trials of liver transplantation were disheartening. Instead of causing defeat and retreat, the consequence of the early failures was to evolve to solutions. (Foreword by W. R. Waddell, chair of the Department of Surgery in Denver, in "Experience in Hepatic Transplantation").

Starzl designed LT to treat unresectable primary as well as secondary hepatobiliary tumours. This idea was without doubt also influenced by his medical Colorado (nephrological) unfavourable environment, which was more than sceptical about the ethical justification of a procedure characterized by prohibitively high morbidity and mortality. The recipient either died after some days or weeks or the rare survivors had their kidneys destroyed by the nephrotoxic, calcineurin inhibiting based immunosuppression (IS). The Denver team embarked on a project full of uncertainties about surgical technique, organ preservation, allograft dysfunction, and use of IS. Moreover, organ procurement was very debated, still lacking a definition of brain death [6]. The tenth and first "successful" LT was done September 2, 1967, in a 1.5–year biliary atresia infant presenting a huge hepatocellular cancer (HCC). Substantial medical and surgical efforts (including seven major reinterventions!) allowed to obtain a 13-month "survival"; the child died of generalized tumour recurrence [7]. Although such therapeutic obstinacy would be condemned today by every Institutional Review Board, this "never, never give up" case paved the way for one of the most extraordinary modern medical developments. This remarkable event went along with another extraordinary expedition, namely the first moon landing! Twenty years and several hundreds of large animal experiments were necessary to refine and decipher surgical techniques of liver procurement and implantation, organ preservation, allograft dysfunction, and immunosuppression strategies. LT evolved from an 'unfinished' to a 'finished' product [1]. The most crucial progress was related to the identification of the different causes of allograft dysfunction. It became rapidly apparent that jaundice was no longer equal to rejection but also to benign cholestasis, (de novo or recurrent) viral hepatitis, allograft disease recurrence, graft quality, infection, and drug toxicity and biliary tract complications. Correct differential diagnosis allowed a more appropriate use of IS. As a corollary, lethal infections became less frequent, and the recipients' quality of life improved. These signs of surgical and medical progress paralleled the discovery in the '80s of the "miracle drugs" cyclosporine A and tacrolimus [8, 9]. Their introduction definitively transformed LT into a clinical service for liver-diseased patients, as exemplified by the rise of the one– and five-year survival rates to 90% and 75%. The 1983 Consensus Conference recognized the potential of LT on the condition to restrict the procedure to very selected patients complying with ten absolute and five relative contraindications (Table 64.1) [10]. Progresses in surgery, anaesthesiology, intensive care medicine, pathology, and infectious diseases management allowed taking down all but one (e.g., active sepsis outside the hepatobiliary system) of these contraindications, thereby bringing LT to the status of routine medicine!

Table 64.1 1983 National Institute of Health Consensus Conference and actual 2020 status: indications and contraindications for liver transplantation

Indications	Contra-indications Status 1983 Absolute	Relative	Contra-indications Status 2020
1) Young patient <50 years	1) Age > 55 years	1) Age > 50 years	NO
2) No viral infection	2) HBsAg-HBeAg positive status	2) HBsAg positive status	NO
3) No alcohol and drug abuse	3) Active alcoholism	3) Advanced alcoholic liver disease in an abstinent patient	NO
4) Ability to accept and understand the procedure	4) Inability to accept the procedure or understand its nature or costs		NO
5) Ability to accept costs	5) Severe hypoxemia (right to left shunts)		NO
6) Normal vessel status	6) Portal vein thrombosis		NO
7) No cardiopulmonary or renal disease	7) Advanced cardiopulmonary or renal disease		NO
8) No infection	8) Sepsis outside hepatobiliary system	4) Intrahepatic or biliary sepsis	**YES**
9) No (advanced) malignancy	9) Primary malignant disease outside hepatobiliary system		YES except haemangioendothelioma
10) No prior abdominal surgery	10) Metastatic hepatobiliary malignancy	5) Previous abdominal surgery	NO

64.3 The Pendulum of Indications

The unequivocal indication for the operation of liver replacement was originally considered to be primary malignancy which could not be treated with conventional techniques of *subtotal* liver resection (Th. E. Starzl)

This statement was written by the person who first performed extended right and left liver resections with or without removing the inferior vena cava! Although the indications for LT have been extensively dealt with in this textbook, some general, supplementary remarks, based on long-standing personal experience and recent developments, are put forward.

LT is indicated for four major liver disease groups: chronic parenchymatous and cholestatic (auto- immune) liver diseases (75%), benign and malignant hepatobiliary tumours (10 to 20%), acute liver failure (10%), and inherited liver-based metabolic diseases (5%).(Table 64.2). Recent signs of progress in hepatology, oncology, molecular biology, and societal behaviour drastically changed these indications' respective weights [11]. The original concept of LT as the treatment of unresectable liver cancers was abandoned because of the very early and high recurrence rates and the growing mortality on the waiting list of patients presenting end-stage failure due to benign, chronic liver diseases. In 1996, the Milan Criteria (MC) became the "gold standard" to allocate allografts to HCC patients because markedly improving five-year disease-free survival rates reaching 85% [12]. These criteria reduced these tumour patients' access to the waiting list from 50% to 10%. Recent studies, many based on LDLT experiences, revealed that up to 60% of HCC patients are unjustifiedly excluded from a potential curative LT when adhering to these restrictive MC [13]. Unexpected good results in some recipients outlying the MC started a movement to again broaden the inclusion criteria for LT in both Western and Eastern hemispheres without severely compromising oncologic outcome [14–16]. These extensions were merely driven by the application of sound oncologic principles combining "dynamic" tumour morphology (number and diameter with the evaluation of radiological response or downstaging to locoregional therapies based on m-RECIST criteria) [17] and biology (evolution of alpha-fetoprotein, descarboxy-prothrombin, neutrophil- or platelet-to-lymphocyte ratios) [18]. The use of reduced IS load, steroid-free and m-Tor inhibitor-based IS, will play an important role in the ongoing re-development of oncologic transplantation [19, 20]. The fact that unresectable hilar and intrahepatic cholangiocellular cancer (CCC) are nowadays also considered for LT if strict criteria and neoadjuvant radio-chemotherapy (Mayo Clinic protocol) are applied in line with this evolution [21]. Conversely, LT for mixed HCC-CCC, intrahepatic CCC or sarcomatoid HCC remains very questionnable seen their high recurrence rate.

Table 64.2 Indications for liver transplantation in 2020 (*questionable indications are mentioned in italic*)

Acute liver failure	*Familial homozygous*
Acetaminophen	*hypercholesterolemia*
Autoimmune hepatitis	*Galactosemia*
Budd-Chiari syndrome	*Glycogen storage disease I and*
Cryptogenic	*IV*
Fatty infiltration-acute fatty liver of pregnancy	*Haemophilia A and B*
HAV/HBV/HCV/HDV/HEV infection	*Hereditary haemochromatosis*
	Hereditary transthyretin amyloidosis (FAP)
Drug-induced liver injury	*Lysosomal storage diseases*
Post-operative	*Maple syrup urine disease*
Post-traumatic	*Methylmalonic acidemia*
Reye syndrome	*Other types of porphyria*
Wilson disease	*Primary hyperoxaluria*
Chronic liver failure	*Propionic acidemia*
Alcoholic liver disease	*Protoporphyria*
Autoimmune hepatitis	*Tyrosinemia*
Chronic HBV/HBV-HDV/HCV/HEV infection	*Urea cycle disease*
	Wilson disease
Cirrhosis drug-related	**Benign tumor liver diseases**
Cirrhosis virus-related (other viruses)	*Adenoma*
	Adenomatosis
Cryptogenic liver disease	*Focal nodular hyperplasia*
Non-alcoholic fatty liver disease (NAFLD)	*Giant haemangioma*
	Nodular regenerative hyperplasia
Cholestatic liver diseases	
Alagille syndrome	**Malignant tumor liver diseases**
Byler disease	CCC hilar
Caroli disease	*CCC intrahepatic*
Choledochal cyst	*Epithelioid haemangioendothelioma*
Congenital biliary fibrosis	
Extra-hepatic biliary atresia	HCC on cirrhosis
Primary biliary cholangitis	HCC in non cirrhotic/non-fibrotic liver
Primary sclerosing cholangitis	
Secondary biliary cirrhosis	Hepatoblastoma
Vascular liver diseases	Metastases neuro-endocrine
Budd-Chiari syndrome	*Metastaseis colorectal*
Hereditary haemorrhagic telangiectasia	*Mixed HCC-CCC*
	Sarcomatoid tumour
Veno-occlusive disease	**Miscellaneous**
Metabolic liver diseases	Alveolar echinococcosis
Alpha-1 antitrypsin deficiency	Cystic echinococcosis
Congenital disorder of glycosylation type Ib	Hepatic trauma
	Polycystic liver disease
Crigler-Najjar syndrome	Schistosomiasis
Cystic fibrosis	

Even in the case of primary hepatobiliary cancers, the remarkable successes obtained today triggered a renewed interest in LT as a treatment for unresectable secondary liver tumours [22]. The Milan group demonstrated that LT could cure patients with non–resectable gastrointestinal NET liver metastases when, again, adhering to strict inclusion criteria consisting of young age (<55 years), low proliferation index (Ki < 5%), the delay between R0 resection of the primary tumour and LT of more than six months, tumour location in the portal venous drainage system, avoidance of simultaneous major abdominal resection and administration of effective neo-adjuvant chemotherapy. Adapted IS, and adjuvant chemotherapy may further improve results [23]. Impressive improvements in chemotherapy, liver surgery (e.g., two-stage, repeated, and ALPPS procedures), and imaging all played a role in the renewed interest of the transplant community to treat unresectable colorectal metastases (CRLM) [24]. The historic Vienna series and the recent Oslo trials showed that good selection could generate 5-year actuarial overall survival rates of over 50% [24, 25]. Larger prospective, multicentre studies such as the ongoing European Transmet, the Toronto and Oslo trials will further finetune the place of LT in the treatment of CRLM [25, 26]. The observations that one-third of recurring patients can be made disease-free by aggressive post-LT (mainly thoracic) surgery; that the growth rate of extrahepatic metastases and tolerance of adjuvant chemotherapy are similar in non- and in immunosuppressed patients all indicate that LT will play a more prominent role in the treatment of CRLM [26, 27].

The pendulum of transplant indications for primary and secondary hepatobiliary cancers returned based on the application of sound oncologic principles combining surgery (e.g., R0 total hepatectomy) and neo- and adjuvant medical therapies.

A reversed pendulum has been observed concerning the indication of LT for decompensated cirrhosis. After a rise to 60% of all transplant procedures, indications drastically changed over time in different directions: alcoholic cirrhosis (from 25 to 40%), primary biliary cholangitis (PBC) (from 50 to <10%), and HBV/HCV-related cirrhosis (from 20 to 50%) [11]. During the last two decades, much fewer LTs are indeed performed for PBC and HBV/HCV-related cirrhosis due to the development of efficacious pharmacological treatments such as ursodeoxycholic acid [28, 29] and direct antiviral agents (DAAs) [30]. DAAs nowadays even allow to remove patients from the waiting list because of the improvement of their liver function. The HBV nucleos(t)ide analogues, lamivudine, adefovir, and tenofovir, allow to obtain excellent results of LT even in case of active viral replication. The efficacy of these drugs also challenge the dogma of life-long IV or IM administration of anti-HBs immunoglobulins (HBIg) to prevent allograft reinfection [31–33]. DAA almost eliminated the otherwise universal HCV graft reinfection, responsible for a rapid development towards allograft cirrhosis [34]. All these medications will also be of value to reduce allograft disease recurrence, thereby reducing the incidence of re-transplantation. Ironically enough, many transplant hepatologists, arguing before against LT for HCC, now favour LT for this indication due to the almost elimination of HBV/HCV patients from the(ir) waiting lists! Moreover this gap on the waiting list is now filled out with two "societal behaviour" diseases: alcoholic cirrhosis and non-alcoholic fatty liver disease. Alcoholic liver disease became the first and second most common LT indication throughout Europe and the United States. Non- alcoholic fatty liver disease (NAFLD) and non-alcoholic steatohepatitis (NASH), associated with obesity, metabolic syndrome, and HCC, is already the third leading indication for LT in the US (11% of recipients) and the second leading aetiology for HCC requiring LT [35, 36]. Overall 5-year survival rates are similar to other indications. However, these recipients have higher post-LT mortality due to cardiovascular events and infections [36]. To reduce these obesity-linked risks linked, bariatric surgery, during or after LT, has been introduced with a good safety and efficacy profile [37].

The role of LT in the treatment of (sub)acute liver failure (ALF) and inherited liver-based metabolic diseases has been reduced due to better, especially anti-infectious, care in specialized liver units and to developments in molecular biology. ALF is mainly due to drug-induced toxicity and acute viral infections. The revised King's College and Clichy criteria still stand the test of time concerning justification and timing of LT in case of paracetamol intoxication and viral hepatitis [38, 39]. Liver-assist devices, such as the albumin dialysis (Molecular Adsorbent Recirculating System (MARS) (Gambro, Lund, Sweden) and Fractionated Plasma Separation and Adsorption system (FPSA) (Prometheus, Fresenius Medical Care, Bad Homburg, Germany) unfortunately do not (yet) fulfil their promises, [40] and regenerative medicine is still in its developmental phase [41]. Auxiliary partial LT (APOLT) should be explored more widely in this context as the better solution for ALF patients because having the great advantage to allow gradual IS withdrawal after recovery of the diseased liver [42].

LT was for a long time the response to several inherited, liver-based, metabolic diseases, the most important ones being tyrosinemia, porphyria, propionic acidaemia (PA), methylmalonic acidaemia (MMA), primary hyperoxaluria (PH), hereditary transthyretin amyloidosis (ATTRv-amyloidosis (or familial amyloidotic polyneuropathy, FAP), congenital disorder of glycosylation type Ib, Wilson, urea cycle (UCD), maple syrup urine (MSUD), lysosomal, and glycogen storage (GSD) diseases (Table 64.2). Despite early dietetic measures, inhibition of tyrosine catabolism, copper chelation, enzyme replacement therapies and RNA interference (leading to robust gene silencing), LT remains indicated in UCD, GSD, PH, and PA/MMA and when end-stage chronic liver disease, HCC or CCC develops. In PH and PA/MMA, sequential or simultaneous liver-kidney transplantation is usually needed. LT considered as the reference treatment to halt or cure ATTRv (FAP)-related disabling neuropathy is also challenged by the very recent introduction of TTR kinetic stabilizers (slowing down the disease progression) and gene silencing drugs (inhibiting the production of the mutated TTR protein). Consequently, the number of listed ATTRv patients is markedly reduced thereby almost eliminating domino or sequential LT [43].

In the case of uncontrolled metabolic diseases, LT, APOLT, and LDLT should be timed adequately to avoid irreversible organ damage(s) related to the accumulation of the toxic molecules [44]. As portal hypertension is absent in most of these diseases, a small (left) living donor liver graft represents an excellent means to cope with these diseases [27].

64.4 The Pendulum of Liver Transplantation Technique

"There is an absolute necessity of having a technically perfect transplantation … this allows to have the benefits of better immunosuppression and improved quality of the homograft" and "In at least one important way an erroneous conclusion was reached from animal experimentation about the technical requisite for successful human transplantation, the use of external venous bypasses. The demonstration that bypasses are unnecessary in human recipients was a significant advance…" (Th. E. Starzl)

Recipient hepatectomy with the removal of the retro-hepatic inferior vena cava (IVC) and use of active, heparin-coated, veno-venous bypass (VVB) were the cornerstones of the recipient procedure for almost half a century. The IVC preserving hepatectomy, described initially by R.Calne in 1968, became accepted by most centres as the standard LT procedure since the '90s. The preservation of the IVC led to the development of piggy-back and cavo-caval implantation techniques. These techniques played also a seminal role in the development of split, domino, auxiliary full-size, and partial LT [45–48].

64.5 The Pendulum of Organ Procurement and Preservation

"The ultimate definition of death was the cessation of heartbeat…". "An alternative and a more complete measure in case there is no circulation is that of cadaveric perfusion with a heart-lung machine." "Several donors were aged…up to 79 years, in all there were histologic changes in the homografts…" (Th. E. Starzl)

The first 19 Denver cases were done using (almost!) cardiac death donors. During that period, the concept of brain death was first outlined and applied at the University of Louvain by G. Alexandre and later defined more precisely by the Harvard University Committee [49]. Terminal donor care did not compromise the allograft quality. Rapid cooling using balanced electrolyte solutions (such as developed by T.L. Marchioro in 1963 and P. Mikaeloff and P.J. Kestens in 1965 in Lyon and Louvain) further improved the quality of the allograft procured in "living cadavers." Brettschneider went a (logical) step further by developing in 1967 (!) a preservation unit using hypothermia, hyperbaric oxygenation, and perfusion with diluted, ABO-identical blood. Expanded criteria donor (e.g., aged up to 79 years!) and resuscitated (e.g., up to 18 times!) donors were frequent; three livers, perfused ex-vivo for 24 hours (!), were successfully transplanted. The advent of brain death donation, organ donor management and the University of Wisconsin (Belzer) solution rendered complex in-situ and ex-vivo organ perfusion "superfluous". Cardiac death donation faded away, and prolongation of ischaemia times transformed LT into a semi-urgent procedure. However, this policy did not pay off well, as shown by the high incidence of allograft loss due to non-function, severe dysfunction and ischaemic-type biliary lesions. The pendulum had gone too far, and liver donation had to comply with more and more restrictive criteria, a policy that resulted in a marked reduction of LT activity [50, 51].

The pendulum changed again following the renewed interest in extended brain death donor (DBD) criteria and more recently in donation after cardiac death (DCD) Maastricht 2 (uncontrolled) and 3 (controlled) DCD. Unfortunately these policies resulted in a very high incidence of graft loss and biliary tract complications [52]. Hypothermic, sub-normothermic, and normothermic perfusion strategies with or without blood were re-instituted recently to counteract these problems. Specialized "organ recovery" units explor the boundaries of the extended donor criteria and modulate liver grafts morphologically (e.g., defatting of steatotic livers or stimulating regeneration in fibrotic partial or full-sized liver grafts) and even immunologically will play an important in this evolution [53].

64.6 The Pendulum of Donor–Recipient Matching

Whether the undertaking of LT will become possible depends upon the procurement of the liver which is of proper size and antigenic structure and which has not been so badly damaged (e.g., by resuscitation) that it cannot support life in the new host. (Th. E. Starzl)

On top of a perfect technical intervention in both donor and recipient, good matching of the donor (D) and the recipient (R) is important to optimize results. Unfortunately, many mistakes are still repeated, although already described by the Starzl team in the '60s! Matching weight, age, gender, immunologic status (donor-specific antibodies), viral (CMV, HBV, and HCV) status, blood group, donor condition, recipient sickness status, and surgical history impact outcome. Some of them, such as donor weight, age, HBV/HCV infection status, and blood group, can be easily anticipated. Some others, such as CMV status, crossmatch, and gender, can't because of practical reasons [54, 55].

The "mechanical feasibility" of LT should be based on careful physical examination of D and R. D/R recipient *weight matching* remains an underestimated feature in LT. *Too large grafts* make the implantation difficult and even hazardous. Simultaneously, *too small grafts*, defined as a graft to body weight ratio ≤ of 0.5, lead to liver insufficiency or small for size syndrome resulting in severe cholestasis, coagulation disturbances, ascites formation, infection and eventually death. D/R weight differences should be within the 20% margin in favour of the recipient [56, 57].

In case of hepatomegaly, such as seen in cholestatic or polycystic liver disease and in large tumours this rule does not apply. The easy-to-use bedside calculation of the liver volume developed by Chaib et al. is a handy tool for evaluating liver volume... especially during mid-night and weekend calls [58]. The graft choice should also take into account the available right upper quadrant space, which can be (very) reduced in case of a shrunken, atrophic liver or conversely increased in case of severe ascites [56].

A good quality, DBD allograft should be allocated to recipients who present an *advanced sickness status* (e.g., very high Meld score or sarcopenic) recipients, a complex vascular situation (e.g., extended splanchnic venous thrombosis or arterial tree damage due to pre-LT locoregional chemotherapy) and especially to those patients presenting a biliary tract damage (e.g., primary sclerosing cholangitis or ischaemic-type biliary tract lesions). The combination of low graft quality (e.g., major macrosteatosis, long ischaemia time) and pronounced sickness state are equal to a poor outcome [59].

Adequate *timing* of donor and recipient operations is essential if problematic operative situations are to be expected (e.g., compromised vascular status, frozen abdomen, previous complex abdominal surgery, or delayed re-LT).

The role of donor *age* in determining allograft quality is unpredictable as the liver is the organ presenting the least senescence process [60]. Age mismatch plays a more important role in paediatric LT. Indeed, the more significant the age mismatch, the greater the impact on allograft survival [61].

In the case of *gender mismatch* (e.g., female to male grafting), a higher incidence of rejection has been reported [62, 63]. Mismatched but compatible blood group LT frequently leads to haemolytic graft versus host syndrome. This antigenic stimulus should be reduced by switching the blood product use to the blood group of the graft. ABO-incompatible LT evidently can only be done after specific recipient preparation, including plasmapheresis to reduce the natural antibody titer and B-cell therapy using anti-CD20 antibodies to neutralize antibody formation [64].

Viral status is another important D/R feature. Six to 9% of organ donors are HBc Ab positive; ideally, such allograft should be directed to an HBV positive recipient needing anyway HBV protection. If the recipient is HBV negative, antiviral HBV prophylaxis is necessary because of the 20% risk of viral transmission [33, 65]. If serum and biopsy of the donor are HBV DNA negative, this prophylactic antiviral therapy can be stopped later on.

HCV positive grafts should preferentially directed to HCV positive recipients because their need of DAA therapy [66–69]. CMV D/R matching is also essential; the risk for CMV transmission being around 60% in case of D positive/R negative status and 25% in case of D/R positivity. In such constellations prophylactic or pre-emptive (val)ganciclovir treatment is mandatory [54].

64.7 The Pendulum of Immunosuppression

"It is almost certain that the continuous presence of a transplanted organ in a host being treated with immunosuppressive therapy often leads to a selective loss of responsiveness to the antigens of the homograft (tolerance)." "Even minimal immunosuppression is too much immunosuppression". (Th. E. Starzl)

Unraveling the different causes of liver allograft dysfunction needed the study of rejection in unmodified and modified (e.g., immunosuppressed) large animals. The immunosuppression (IS) in the first Denver series consisted of the "secret cocktail BW322", containing prednisone and azathioprine. Later on heterologous antilymphocyte globulins (ALG) were added. Several of these patients survived for more than 20 years without any IS! Unfortunately, it became commonplace to take measures to prevent at any price the "repudiation" of the allograft [70]. This philosophy resulted in over-immunosuppression strategies, which in turn led to lethal infections, cardiovascular complications and de novo tumor formation. The introduction of the selective calcineurin inhibitors, cyclosporine A and tacrolimus, allowed the evolution towards the opposite concepts of minimization and tolerogenic IS protocols. Unfortunately, many lessons from the past were forgotten. Due to the multitude of, mostly industry-driven, studies still essentially looking at eliminating the physiologic process of allograft rejection or at renal function sparing. The discovery in 1993 by Starzl of cell migration and chimerism after whole-organ transplantation based on graft acceptance unequivocally confirmed Starzl's 1969 statement [9]. Graft acceptance is a dynamic process in which clonal deletion and exhaustion are the key players. Destroying this immunologic donor-recipient interaction at any price breaks the pathway to graft acceptance (under minimal or no IS at all) [71, 72]. The use of tacrolimus, the more efficacious calcineurin inhibitor, allows reaching such a state more easily [73]. Already from the beginning, it was observed that some large animals conserved a normal allograft function after a short-term low-dose IS only. Together with recent minimisation experiences, these seminal observations should incite the transplant community to design more investigator-driven, prospective studies concerning tolerogenic IS strategies [74] The reasons to do are multiple: reduction of lethal cardiovascular, infectious, and oncologic side effects, avoidance of metabolic syndrome and renal failure, improved quality of life and, last but not least, appropriate use of the immuno-privileged status of the liver graft (e.g., rejection and chimeric benefit). To be successful, such trials need to be built on solid immunologic and pathological ("the biopsy being the science of transplantation") grounds implying complete documentation of the recipient status from the start of IS withdrawal to long-term follow-up [75]. Recent multicentre studies indicate that IS can be reduced or even halted without (great) risk for graft loss [76].

64.8 The Pendulum of Post-transplant Follow-up

> As further experience accumulates, it is probably that other causative factors than rejection and tumor recurrence will be found to be important...such as viral hepatitis, drug toxicity, cholangitis... (Th. E. Starzl)

Organ transplantation is a complex undertaking involving all organ systems. The chronic use of IS drugs is responsible for severe (eventually lethal) side effects. Cardiovascular and de novo tumor formation occur in >10% of long-term survivors; incidence of (late) infectious complications is less well documented. Twenty and 40% of long-term survivors develop renal failure and metabolic syndrome. All these complications are the main reason of patient loss with a functioning grafts [77]. Multidisciplinary *but* centralized care and follow-up are necessary to continuously finetune the immunosuppressive load adapted to the evolution of both allograft and recipient condition. In patients transplanted for autoimmune (cholestatic) diseases, particular attention should be given to the evolution of extrahepatic disease manifestations, such as polyarthritis, colitis, sclerodermia, vasculitis and other thyroiditis. All of them may heavily compromise their quality of life. Unfortunately, many of these manifestations require a reinforcement of IS or introduction of steroids.

Clinical follow-up should be done in a well-structured way, ideally combined with a (regular) pathological follow-up. In the early (≤3 months) post-LT follow-up clinical judgment needs to go hand in hand with aggressive imaging (repeated doppler-ultrasound, scanning and interventional endoscopy and radiology), later on pathologic monitoring of the graft will play a more prominent role.

Early follow-up is dominated by graft loss due primary non-function (< 1%) or severe allograft dysfunction, technical problems (5–10%), acute cellular (5–30%) and antibody-mediated rejection (<1%). Thirty % of recipients will present biliary complications; these will be merely solved by interventional radiology but may also need redo biliary tract surgery. Hepatic artery and (portal and hepatic) venous complications are seen in respectively 1 to 5 and 1%, Hepatic artery thrombosis, the most feared complication, mostly leads to urgent re-transplantation. During late follow-up the picture is dominated by biliary complications (ranging from 10 to 30%, the incidence depending on diagnostic aggressivity), recurrent allograft disease and chronic rejection (5%) [78]. In the absence of prophylactic therapy, recurrent viral disease is almost universal. Luckily enough, this cause of allograft loss has almost been eliminated since the introduction of immune-prophylaxis and DAAs [30, 79]. The incidence of recurrent allograft disease in primary biliary cholangitis, primary sclerosing cholangitis, and autoimmune hepatitis is around 20, 40%, and 40%, respectively. Many of these recipients will need a delayed re-LT. A similar tendency is already observed in nonalcoholic steatohepatitis patients.

Although debated heavily, good follow-up should include histological documentation of the allograft [75, 80]. The now more frequent diagnoses of "de novo hepatitis" and (beginning) chronic rejection (also known as *vanishing* bile duct syndrome, merely due to non-compliance) illustrate well the importance of liver allograft biopsies. De novo hepatitis is possibly a form of chronic rejection [81]. If diagnosed, a biopsy-guided adaptation of the IS is required. Recent findings related to the impact of donor-specific antibodies (DSA) on outcome in LT have also to be interpreted in the context of delayed immunologic graft loss [82].

64.9 The Pendulum of Liver Transplantation Combined with Other Organs

> "Potentially there could be an occasional clinical use for a composite transplantation such as in case of intestinal infarction..." "the technical requirements of the procedure were no more difficult than with a standard hepatic transplantation since only three vascular anastomoses with large calibre vessels were involved". (Th. E. Starzl) [83]

Combined kidney–liver transplant (CKLT), combined liver–intestinal (CLIT) and multi-visceral transplantation. Up to 20% of diseased liver patients also present with renal dysfunction due to hepatorenal syndrome or to underlying morphologic kidney disorders [84]. The 2012 UNOS consensus meeting defined clear guidelines for CKLT in order to avoid futile kidney transplantation [85]. An essential aspect of CKLT relates to the liver allograft's immunologic protective capacity if both organs, especially if originating from a same donor, are transplanted simultaneously. The same observation has been made in combined liver -intestine transplantation. Liver and small bowel grafts can be transplanted as a composite or non–composite allograft. In case of a composite graft, donor pancreas and duodenum are transplanted together with the liver to preserve the biliary tract [86]. In the non-composite transplant, the liver and small bowel are transplanted separately. This approach allows adjusting significant donor-recipient size discrepancies and is valuable in case of a "troubled abdomen". It has been shown that combined liver–intestinal grafts do better than isolated IT [86]. Intestinal transplantation remains a challenging and costly endeavour. Outcomes improved during recent years by introducing less aggressive IS therapies, but there is still a long way to go to reach the results obtained in other types of organ transplantation.

Combined heart-liver transplantation (CHLT), combined lung-liver transplantation (CLuLT), and combined heart-lung-liver transplantation (CHLuLT). A liver disease may occasionally be responsible for heart failure. ATTRv (or familial amyloidotic polyneuropathy (FAP) and haemochromatosis are the most common indications for CHLT. Such recipients may reach 70–75% five years survival, similar to results obtained after isolated HT or LT [87].

CLuLT will expand due to improved care given to patients suffering from cystic fibrosis and α1–antitrypsin deficiency (leading to end-stage secondary liver cirrhosis) as well as patients presenting idiopathic pulmonary fibrosis and portopulmonary hypertension. CLuLT recipients reach a 50% five years survival rate [88].

Porto–pulmonary hypertension (POPH) and hepatopulmonary syndrome (HPS) merit particular attention; these diagnoses are made in 6% and 10% of patients presenting portal hypertension [89]. Typically, isolated LT results in the disappearance or major regression of HPS within six to twelve months. Conversely, results of isolated LT for POPH are poor, (5-year survival in some series reaching 28% only) [90]. Due to the prohibitive mortality of isolated LT in these patients, CLuLT, potentially including the heart, has been proposed [89]. Long-term patient survival rates reaching 85.7% have been reported in CLuLT. The management of HPS and especially POPH, has been improved recently by better understanding of the pathophysiology of these diseases, the implementation of aggressive medical therapies targeting endothelial receptors (using e.g. vasodilators) and finally the improved selection of potential recipients. Combined heart-lung–liver transplantation (CHLuLT) may be indicated in patients with end-stage respiratory failure complicated by advanced liver disease or end-stage liver failure complicated with advanced lung disease. The leading causes of this combined surgical approach are cystic fibrosis or POPH refractory to vasodilators [91].

64.10 The Pendulum of Ethics in Liver Transplantation

The period 1963–1980 was the period of *LT feasibility*. Not surprisingly, LT was merely done for advanced, primary, and secondary hepatobiliary tumours and very sick patients. Through relentless working and learning both from successes and failures, this impossible operation became finally possible. LT became rapidly the victim of its' success, so the gap between demand (sick patients) and offer (available allografts) progressively widened. Initially, patients were transplanted based on waiting time, later on the Child-Turcotte-Pugh (CTP) classification. Both parameters do however not allow to have an objective look at disease severity nor mortality on the waiting list. A scoring system based on parameters reflecting both severity and need for timely transplantation became necessary. The Meld (Model for End-stage Liver Disease) score, based on objective medical characteristics (bilirubin, creatinine, and INR values), was implemented in 2002 by UNOS in the USA and in 2003 in the Eurotransplant area. MELD ensured not only an equitable allocation of liver allografts (principle of justice and equity) and disease prognosis (estimation of 3-month mortality on the waiting list) but also introduced the concept of minimal listing criteria (principle of utility) [92]. Similarly, the PELD score was developed for the paediatric liver population. The MELD score needed to be adapted for HCC patients (usually) presenting a well-compensated chronic liver disease, hepatoblastoma, metabolic disorders, polycystic disease, and some particular indications such as hepatopulmonary syndrome, porto-pulmonary hypertension and hereditary haemorrhagic telangiectasia. Bonus points, added to the *lab-Meld score*, were needed to allow these patients a timely access to transplantation. The Meld-score was not only effective in ranking the patients on the waiting list by their disease severity but also by reducing the mortality on the waiting list. Some adaptations, such as e.g., sodium-Meld score, were proposed by different allocation organisms in order to further fine-tune the allograft allocation system. In the UK, the National Health Service further elaborated the utility concept by introducing a transplant benefit score. The future challenge will be to "mary" as good as possible the ethical principles of justice, equity and utility and to adapt the score continuously to the future progresses that will be made in hepatology and oncology [93].

A second ethical problem relates to the efforts aiming for expanding the organ pool by promoting all different forms of LT variants and by (re-)introducing more widely, again, the concept of cardiac death donation. Split, auxiliary and domino-LT represent less than 5% of all LT activities. Several studies revealed that 15% of liver grafts could be used as split grafts when adhering to simple, easily available, criteria such as normal liver tests, donor age ≤ 50 years and weight ≥ 50 kg. The benefits of a mandatory splitting policy as applied in Italy are clear. Results of split-LT and full-size LT are becoming similar in experienced centres and waiting time for children is almost inexistent (around three weeks) eliminating thereby even the need for living donor LT in this patient group. The underuse of split-LT is explained by technical, logistic, and also financial considerations. The LT community cannot go on to complain about allograft shortage when these problems are not tackled. The same applies to the insufficient implementation of DCD. The uniformization of legislations about DCD per se (e.g., legalized in Belgium and Netherlands but forbidden in Germany) or some types of DCD (e.g., Maastricht category V or donation after euthanasia) is needed to expand the liver allograft pool. The instauration of "organ hubs," allowing all different types of regional and machine perfusion modalities, should also become an "ethical obligation." Clearly, financial endorsement by the health authorities is necessary to foster and make successful split-LT, DCD-LT and, in-situ/ex-situ, machine perfusion, the latter being especially important in Maastricht categories I and II DCD [94–97].

A third ethical problem concerns the heavily debated indications for advanced hepatobiliary cancer and self-inflicted diseases due to (suicidal) drug or alcohol intoxication. Several studies have shown that the indication of LT for HCC can be widened without heavily compromising outcome (e.g., death due to tumour recurrence) when adhering to the combination of dynamic tumour "morphology and biology." [98].

Alcoholic liver disease is also a controversial indication in terms of public attitude towards the patient's responsibility for his/her self-inflicted hepatic disease. The discussion about this indication remains difficult because relapse after transplantation cannot be excluded despite adequate pre-LT psychological counceling and strict post-LT follow-up. The 6-month abstinence 'rule' considered as a 'safety belt' in most transplant centres is an unreliable selection criterion. The best selection parameter to justify LT remains the patient's integration in his/her familial, professional, and social environments. The "social debate" about LT and alcoholic liver disease has recently been fuelled by the Lille group, which proposed to perform LT even in case of severe alcoholic hepatitis not responding to medical therapy. Although LT represents the best therapy for decompensated alcoholic cirrhosis and hepatitis, alcohol abstinence represents a mandatory objective to be obtained, interconnecting patient compliance and public reassurance [99].

Finally, a fourth ethical problem concerns the justification of transplantation and re-LT in extremely sick patients. The organ availability being scarce, "futile LT" should be avoided at any price. The notion of the transplant benefit score (or utility) is here of utmost importance. Different studies taking into account pulmonary and renal function allowed developing scores to identify those patients who should be excluded from transplantation [59, 100, 101].

64.11 Conclusions

The history of medicine is that what was inconceivable yesterday and barely achievable today often becomes routine tomorrow. (Th. E. Starzl)

Transplantation revolutionized, without any doubt, modern medical practice of hepatology and hepatobiliary oncology. Progresses have been spectacular during the last four decades. Most contraindications have been, one after the other, eliminated, and today only extrahepatic active sepsis remains as an absolute contraindication to the procedure. Long-term survival rates are frequent, so the transplant community's attention need to be shifted to the long-term follow-up, ideally documented with allograft pathology and to the optimization of the recipient's quality of life. More clinical and immunologic research will be needed to make these long-term survivors "immunosuppression free," a condition necessary to face the more and more frequently diagnosed renal failure and, many times lethal, de novo tumour formation, cardiovascular and infectious events observed in an ever-aging transplant population. Recent developments in immunosuppressive handling and in combined organ failure care will lead to more frequent combined transplant procedures. Besides the further development of deceased donor LT, technical variants such as split and living liver donor LT will be necessary to cope with the ever-growing liver allograft shortage. The pendulum of liver transplantation will without any doubt further swing… !

References

1. Starzl TE. Experience in liver transplantation. Philadelphia: WB Saunders Company; 1969. p. 9.
2. Starzl TE, Marchioro TL, Vonkaulla KN, Hermann G, Brittain RS, Waddell WR. Homotransplantation of the liver in humans. Surg Gynecol Obstet. 1963;117:659–76.
3. Starzl TE, Demetris AJ. Liver transplantation: a 31-year perspective (current problems in surgery classic). Chicago, IL: Year Book Medical Publishers; 1990. p. 224.
4. http://www.transplant-observatory.org/ Accessed 25 Nov 2020.
5. Lee SG. A complete treatment of adult living donor liver transplantation: a review of surgical technique and current challenges to expand indication of patients. Am J Transplant. 2015;15:17–38.
6. Manara AR. All human death is brain death: the legacy of the Harvard criteria. Resuscitation. 2019;138:210–2.
7. Starzl TE, Groth CG, Brettschneider L, Penn I, Fulginiti VA, Moon JB, Blanchard H, Martin AJ Jr, Porter KA. Orthotopic homotransplantation of the human liver. Ann Surg. 1968;168:392–415.
8. Calne RY, Rolles K, White DJ, Thiru S, Evans DB, McMaster P, Dunn DC, Craddock GN, Henderson RG, Aziz S, Lewis P. Cyclosporin a initially as the only immunosuppressant in 34 recipients of cadaveric organs: 32 kidneys, 2 pancreases, and 2 livers. Lancet. 1979;2:1033–6.
9. Starzl TE, Todo S, Fung J, Demetris AJ, Venkataramman R, Jain A. FK 506 for liver, kidney, and pancreas transplantation. Lancet. 1989;2:1000–4.

10. National Institutes of Health Consensus Development Conference Statement: liver transplantation June 20–23, 1983. Hepatology 1983; Suppl: 107S–110S.
11. Adam R, Karam V, Cailliez VO, Grady JG, Mirza D, Cherqui D, Klempnauer J, Salizzoni M, Pratschke J, Jamieson N, Hidalgo E, Paul A, Andujar RL, Lerut J, Fisher L, Boudjema K, Fondevila C, Soubrane O, Bachellier P, Pinna AD, Berlakovich G, Bennet W, Pinzani M, Schemmer P, Zieniewicz K, Romero CJ, De Simone P, Ericzon BG, Schneeberger S, Wigmore SJ, Prous JF, Colledan M, Porte RJ, Yilmaz S, Azoulay D, Pirenne J, Line PD, Trunecka P, Navarro F, Lopez AV, De Carlis L, Pena SR, Kochs E, Duvoux C, all the other 126 contributing centers (www.eltr.org), the European Liver and Intestine Transplant Association (ELITA). Annual report of the European liver transplant registry (ELTR) - 50-year evolution of liver transplantation. Transpl Int. 2018;2018(31):1293–317.
12. Mazzaferro V, Regalia E, Doci R, Andreola S, Pulvirenti A, Bozzetti F, Montalto F, Ammatuna M, Morabito A, Gennari L. Liver transplantation for the treatment of small hepatocellular carcinomas in patients with cirrhosis. N Engl J Med. 1996;334:693–9.
13. Lerut J, Foguenne M, Lai Q. Hepatocellular cancer scores and liver transplantation: from the tower of babel to an ideal comprehensive score? A systematic review. Transpl Int. 2020; (submitted)
14. Yao FY, Ferrell L, Bass NM, Watson JJ, Bacchetti P, Venook A, Ascher NL, Roberts JP. Liver transplantation for hepatocellular carcinoma: expansion of the tumor size limits does not adversely impact survival. Hepatology. 2001;33:1394–403.
15. Mazzaferro V, Llovet JM, Miceli R, Bhoori S, Schiavo M, Mariani L, Camerini T, Roayaie S, Schwartz ME, Grazi GL, Adam R, Neuhaus P, Salizzoni M, Bruix J, Forner A, De Carlis L, Cillo U, Burroughs AK, Troisi R, Rossi M, Gerunda GE, Lerut J, Belghiti J, Boin I, Gugenheim J, Rochling F, Van Hoek B, Majno P. Metroticket investigator study group. Predicting survival after liver transplantation in patients with hepatocellular carcinoma beyond the Milan criteria: a retrospective, exploratory analysis. Lancet Oncol. 2009;10:35–43.
16. Mazzaferro V, Sposito C, Zhou J, Pinna AD, De Carlis L, Fan J, Cescon M, Di Sandro S, Yi-Feng H, Lauterio A, Bongini M, Cucchetti A. Metroticket 2.0 model for analysis of competing risks of death after liver transplantation for hepatocellular carcinoma. Gastroenterology. 2018;154:128–39.
17. Lai Q, Avolio AW, Graziadei I, Otto G, Rossi M, Tisone G, Goffette P, Vogel W, Pitton MB, Lerut J, European Hepatocellular Cancer Liver Transplant Study Group. Alpha-fetoprotein and modified response evaluation criteria in solid tumors progression after locoregional therapy as predictors of hepatocellular cancer recurrence and death after transplantation. Liver Transpl. 2013;19:1108–18.
18. Lai Q, Nicolini D, Inostroza Nunez M, Iesari S, Goffette P, Agostini A, Giovagnoni A, Vivarelli M, Lerut J. A novel prognostic index in patients with hepatocellular cancer waiting for liver transplantation: time-radiological-response-alpha-fetoprotein-INflammation (TRAIN) score. Ann Surg. 2016;264:787–96.
19. Vivarelli M, Dazzi A, Zanello M, Cucchetti A, Cescon M, Ravaioli M, Del Gaudio M, Lauro A, Grazi GL, Pinna AD. Effect of different immunosuppressive schedules on recurrence-free survival after liver transplantation for hepatocellular carcinoma. Transplantation. 2010;89:227–31.
20. Schnitzbauer AA, Filmann N, Adam R, Bachellier P, Bechstein WO, Becker T, Bhoori S, Bilbao I, Brockmann J, Burra P, Chazoullières O, Cillo U, Colledan M, Duvoux C, Ganten TM, Gugenheim J, Heise M, van Hoek B, Jamieson N, de Jong KP, Klein CG, Klempnauer J, Kneteman N, Lerut J, Mäkisalo H, Mazzaferro V, Mirza DF, Nadalin S, Neuhaus P, Pageaux GP, Pinna AD, Pirenne J, Pratschke J, Powel J, Rentsch M, Rizell M, Rossi G, Rostaing L, Roy A, Scholz T, Settmacher U, Soliman T, Strasser S, Söderdahl G, Troisi RI, Turrión VS, Schlitt HJ, Geissler EK. MTOR inhibition is most beneficial after liver transplantation for hepatocellular carcinoma in patients with active tumors. Ann Surg. 2020;272:855–62.
21. Azad AI, Rosen CB, Taner T, Heimbach JK, Gores GJ. Selected patients with unresectable perihilar cholangiocarcinoma (pCCA) derive long-term benefit from liver transplantation. Cancers (Basel). 2020;12:E 3157.
22. Le Treut YP, Grégoire E, Klempnauer J, Belghiti J, Jouve E, Lerut J, Castaing D, Soubrane O, Boillot O, Mantion G, Homayounfar K, Bustamante M, Azoulay D, Wolf P, Krawczyk M, Pascher A, Suc B, Chiche L, de Urbina JO, Mejzlik V, Pascual M, Lodge JP, Gruttadauria S, Paye F, Pruvot FR, Thorban S, Foss A, Adam R, For ELITA. Liver transplantation for neuroendocrine tumors in Europe-results and trends in patient selection: a 213-case European liver transplant registry study. Ann Surg. 2013;257:807–15.
23. Mazzaferro V, Pulvirenti A, Coppa J. Neuroendocrine tumors metastatic to the liver: how to select patients for liver transplantation? J Hepatol. 2007;47:460–6.
24. Hagness M, Foss A, Line PD, Scholz T, Jørgensen PF, Fosby B, Boberg KM, Mathisen O, Gladhaug IP, Egge TS, Solberg S, Hausken J, Dueland S. Liver transplantation for nonresectable liver metastases from colorectal cancer. Ann Surg. 2013;257:800–6.
25. Mühlbacher F, Huk I, Steininger R, Gnant M, Götzinger P, Wamser P, Banhegyi C, Piza F. Is orthotopic liver transplantation a feasible treatment for secondary cancer of the liver? Transplant Proc. 1991;23:1567–8.
26. Line PD, Dueland S. Liver transplantation for secondary liver tumours: the difficult balance between survival and recurrence. J Hepatol. 2020;73:1557–62.
27. Lerut J, Iesari S, Vandeplas G, Fabbrizio T, Ackenine K, Núñez MEI, Komuta M, Coubeau L, Ciccarelli O, Bonaccorsi-Riani E. Secondary non-resectable liver tumors: a single-center living-donor and deceased-donor liver transplantation case series. Hepatobiliary Pancreat Dis Int. 2019;18:412–22.
28. Montano-Loza AJ, Hansen BE, Corpechot C, Roccarina D, Thorburn D, Trivedi P, Hirschfield G, McDowell P, Poupon R, Dumortier J, Bosch A, Giostria E, Conti F, Parés A, Reig A, Floreani A, Russo FP, Goet JC, Harms MH, van Buuren H, Van den Ende N, Nevens F, Verhelst X, Donato MF, Malinverno F, Ebadi M, Mason AL, Global PBC Study Group. Factors associated with recurrence of primary biliary cholangitis after liver transplantation and effects on graft and patient survival. Gastroenterology. 2019;156:96–107.
29. Nevens F, Andreone P, Mazzella G, Strasser SI, Bowlus C, Invernizzi P, Drenth JP, Pockros PJ, Regula J, Beuers U, Trauner M, Jones DE, Floreani A, Hohenester S, Luketic V, Shiffman M, van Erpecum KJ, Vargas V, Vincent C, Hirschfield GM, Shah H, Hansen B, Lindor KD, Marschall HU, Kowdley KV, Hooshmand-Rad R, Marmon T, Sheeron S, Pencek R, Mac Conell L, Pruzanski M, Shapiro D, POISE Study Group. A placebo-controlled trial of Obeticholic acid in primary biliary cholangitis. N Engl J Med. 2016;375:631–43.
30. Belli LS, Perricone G, Adam R, Cortesi PA, Strazzabosco M, Facchetti R, Karam V, Salizzoni M, Andujar RL, Fondevila C, De Simone P, Morelli C, Fabregat-Prous J, Samuel D, Agarwaal K, Moreno Gonzales E, Charco R, Zieniewicz K, De Carlis L, Duvoux C, all the contributing centers (www.eltr.org), and the European Liver and Intestine Transplant Association (ELITA). Impact of DAAs on liver transplantation: major effects on the evolution of indications and results. An ELITA study based on the ELTR registry. J Hepatol. 2018;69:810–7.

31. Samuel D, Muller R, Alexander G, Fassati L, Ducot B, Benhamou JP, Bismuth H. Liver transplantation in European patients with the hepatitis B surface antigen. N Engl J Med. 1993;329:1842–7.
32. Lerut JP, Donataccio M, Ciccarelli O, Roggen F, Jamart J, Laterre PF, Cornu C, Mazza D, Hanique G, Rahier J, Geubel AP, Otte JB. Liver transplantation and HBsAg-positive postnecrotic cirrhosis: adequate immunoprophylaxis and delta virus co-infection as the significant determinants of long-term prognosis. J Hepatol. 1999;30:706–14.
33. Samuel D, Bismuth A, Mathieu D, Arulnaden JL, Reynes M, Benhamou JP, Brechot C, Bismuth H. Passive immunoprophylaxis after liver transplantation in HBsAg-positive patients. Lancet. 1991;337:813–5.
34. Curry MP, Forns X, Chung RT, Terrault NA, Brown R Jr, Fenkel JM, Gordon F, O'Leary J, Kuo A, Schiano T, Everson G, Schiff E, Befeler A, Gane E, Saab S, McHutchison JG, Subramanian GM, Symonds WT, Denning J, McNair L, Arterburn S, Svarovskaia E, Moonka D, Afdhal N. Sofosbuvir and ribavirin prevent recurrence of HCV infection after liver transplantation: an open-label study. Gastroenterology. 2015;148:100–7.
35. Shirazi F, Wang J, Wong RJ. Nonalcoholic steatohepatitis becomes the leading indication for liver transplant registrants among us adults born between 1945 and 1965. J Clin Exp Hepatol. 2020;10:30–6.
36. Wong RJ, Aguilar M, Cheung R, Perumpail RB, Harrison SA, Younossi ZM, Ahmed A. Nonalcoholic steatohepatitis is the second leading etiology of liver disease among adults awaiting liver transplantation in the United States. Gastroenterology. 2015;148:547–55.
37. Diwan TS, Lee TC, Nagai S, Benedetti E, Posselt A, Bumgardner G, Noria S, Whitson BA, Ratner L, Mason D, Friedman J, Woodside KJ, Heimbach J. Obesity, transplantation, and bariatric surgery: an evolving solution for a growing epidemic. Am J Transplant. 2020;20:2143–55.
38. Germani G, Theocharidou E, Adam R, Karam V, Wendon J, O'Grady J, Burra P, Senzolo M, Mirza D, Castaing D, Klempnauer J, Pollard S, Paul A, Belghiti J, Tsochatzis E, Burroughs AK. Liver transplantation for acute liver failure in Europe: outcomes over 20 years from the ELTR database. J Hepatol. 2012;57:288–96.
39. Renner EL. How to decide when to list a patient with acute liver failure for liver transplantation? Clichy or King's College criteria, or something else? J Hepatol. 2007;46:554–7.
40. Demetriou AA, Brown RS Jr, Busuttil RW, Fair J, McGuire BM, Rosenthal P, Am Esch JS 2nd, Lerut J, Nyberg SL, Salizzoni M, Fagan EA, de Hemptinne B, Broelsch CE, Muraca M, Salmeron JM, Rabkin JM, Metselaar HJ, Pratt D, De La Mata M, LP MC, Everson GT, Lavin PT, Stevens AC, Pitkin Z, Solomon BA. Prospective, randomized, multicenter, controlled trial of a bioartificial liver in treating acute liver failure. Ann Surg. 2004;239:660–7.
41. Edgar L, Pu T, Porter B, Aziz JM, La Pointe C, Asthana A, Orlando G. Regenerative medicine, organ bioengineering and transplantation. Br J Surg. 2020;107:793–800.
42. Shrivastav M, Rammohan A, Reddy MS, Rela M. Auxiliary partial orthotopic liver transplantation for acute liver failure. Ann R Coll Surg Engl. 2019;101:e71–2.
43. Suhr OB, Larsson M, Ericzon BG, Wilczek HE, FAPWTR's Investigators. Survival after transplantation in patients with mutations other than Val 30Met: extracts from the FAP world transplant registry. Transplantation. 2016;100:373–81.
44. Schielke A, Conti F, Goumarda C, Perdigaoa F, Calmus Y, Scatton O. Liver transplantation using grafts with rare metabolic disorders. Dig Liver Dis. 2015;47:261–70.
45. Calne RY, Williams R. Liver transplantation in man. BMJ. 1968;4:535–40.
46. Lerut J, Tzakis AG, Bron K, Gordon RD, Iwatsuki S, Esquivel CO, Makowka L, Todo S, Starzl TE. Complications of venous reconstruction in human orthotopic liver transplantation. Ann Surg. 1987;205:404–14.
47. Lerut J, Ciccarelli O, Roggen F, Laterre PF, Danse E, Goffette P, Aunac S, Carlier M, De Kock M, Van Obbergh L, Veyckemans F, Guerrieri C, Reding R, Otte JB. Cavocaval adult liver transplantation and retransplantation without venovenous bypass and without portocaval shunting: a prospective feasibility study in adult liver transplantation. Transplantation. 2003;75:1740–5.
48. Belghiti J, Noun R, Sauvanet A. Temporary portocaval anastomosis with preservation of caval flow during orthotopic liver transplantation. Am J Surg. 1995;169:277–9.
49. Machado C. The first organ transplant from a brain-dead donor. Neurology. 2005;64:1938–42.
50. Schlegel A, Muller X, Dutkowski P. Machine perfusion strategies in liver transplantation. Hepato Biliary Surg Nutr. 2019;8:490–50.
51. Ghinolfi D, Lai Q, Dondossola D, De Carlis R, Zanierato M, Patrono D, Baroni S, Bassi D, Ferla F, Lauterio A, Lazzeri C, Magistri P, Melandro F, Pagano D, Pezzati D, Ravaioli M, Rreka E, Toti L, Zanella A, Burra P, Petta S, Rossi M, Dutkowski P, Jassem W, Muiesan P, Quintini C, Selzner M, Cillo U. Machine perfusions in liver transplantation: the evidence-based position paper of the Italian society of organ and tissue transplantation. Liver Transpl. 2020;26:1298–315.
52. Croome KP, Taner CB. The changing landscapes in DCD liver transplantation. Curr Transplant Rep. 2020;13:1–11.
53. Yeung JC, Cypel M, Keshavjee S. Ex-vivo lung perfusion: the model for the organ reconditioning hub. Curr Opin Organ Transplant. 2017;22:287–9.
54. Fishman JA, Rubin RH. Infection in organ-transplant recipients. N Engl J Med. 1998;338:1741–51.
55. Starzl TE, Iwatsuki S, Shaw BW Jr, Gordon RD, Esquivel CO. Immunosuppression and other nonsurgical factors in the improved results of liver transplantation. Semin Liver Dis. 1985;5:334–43.
56. Adam R, Castaing D, Bismuth H. Transplantation of small donor livers in adult recipients. Transplant Proc. 1993;25:1105–6.
57. Croome KP, Lee DD, Saucedo-Crespo H, Burns JM, Nguyen JH, Perry DK, Taner CB. A novel objective method for deceased donor and recipient size matching in liver transplantation. Liver Transpl. 2015;21:1471–7.
58. Chaib E, Morales MM, Bordalo MB, Antonio LG, Feijo LF, Ishida RY, Lima Júnior J, Nunes PA. Predicting the donor liver lobe weight from body weight for split-liver transplantation. Braz J Med Biol Res. 1995;28:759–60.
59. Petrowsky H, Rana A, Kaldas FM, Sharma A, Hong JC, Agopian VG, Durazo F, Honda H, Gornbein J, Wu V, Farmer DG, Hiatt JR, Busuttil RW. Liver transplantation in highest acuity recipients: identifying factors to avoid futility. Ann Surg. 2014;259:1186–94.
60. Ghinolfi D, Lai Q, Pezzati D, De Simone P, Rreka E, Filipponi F. Use of elderly donors in liver transplantation: a paired-match analysis at a single center. Ann Surg. 2018;268:325–31.
61. Bittermann T, Goldberg DS. Quantifying the effect of transplanting older donor livers into younger recipients: the need for donor-recipient age matching. Transplantation. 2018;102:2033–7.
62. Brooks BK, Levy MF, Jennings LW, Abbasoglu O, Vodapally M, Goldstein RM, Husberg BS, Gonwa TA, Klintmalm GB. Influence of donor and recipient gender on the outcome of liver transplantation. Transplantation. 1996;62:1784–7.
63. Lai Q, Giovanardi F, Melandro F, Larghi Laureiro Z, Merli M, Lattanzi B, Hassan R, Rossi M, Mennini G. Donor-to-recipient gender match in liver transplantation: a systematic review and meta-analysis. World J Gastroenterol. 2018;24:2203–10.

64. Egawa H, Teramukai S, Haga H, Tanabe M, Fukushima M, Shimazu M. Present status of ABO-incompatible living donor liver transplantation in Japan. Hepatology. 2008;47:143–52.
65. Donataccio D, Roggen F, De Reyck C, Verbaandert C, Bodeus M, Lerut J. Use of anti-HBc positive allografts in adult liver transplantation: toward a safer way to expand the donor pool. Transpl Int. 2006;19:38–43.
66. Weinfurtner K, Reddy KR. Hepatitis C viremic organs in solid organ transplantation. J Hepatol. 2020;S0168-8278:33767–3.
67. Smith DM, Agura E, Netto G, Collins R, Levy M, Goldstein R, Christensen L, Baker J, Altrabulsi B, Osowski L, McCormack J, Fichtel L, Dawson DB, Domiati-Saad R, Stone M, Klintmalm G. Liver transplant-associated graft-versus-host disease. Transplantation. 2003;75:118–26.
68. Kwong AJ, Wall A, Melcher M, Wang U, Ahmed A, Subramanian A, Kwo PY. Liver transplantation for hepatitis C virus (HCV) nonviremic recipients with HCV viremic donors. Am J Transplant. 2019;19:1380–7.
69. Cotter TG, Paul S, Sandıkçı B, Couri T, Bodzin AS, Little EC, Sundaram V, Charlton M. Increasing utilization and excellent initial outcomes following liver transplant of Hepatitis C Virus (HCV)-viremic donors into HCV-negative recipients: outcomes following liver transplant of HCV-viremic donors. Hepatology. 2019;69:2381–95.
70. Starzl TE, Porter KA, Andres G, Halgrimson CG, Hurwitz R, Giles G, Terasaki PI, Penn I, Schroter GT, Lilly J, Starkie SJ, Putnam CW. Long-term survival after renal transplantation in humans: (with special reference to histocompatibility matching, thymectomy, homograft glomerulonephritis, heterologous ALG, and recipient malignancy). Ann Surg. 1970;172:437–72.
71. Starzl TE, Zinkernagel RM. Antigen localization and migration in immunity and tolerance. N Engl J Med. 1998;339:1905–13.
72. Iesari S, Ackenine K, Foguenne M, De Reyck C, Komuta M, Bonaccorsi Riani E, Ciccarelli O, Coubeau L, Lai Q, Gianello P, Lerut J. Tacrolimus and single intraoperative high-dose of anti-T-lymphocyte globulins versus tacrolimus monotherapy in adult liver transplantation: one-year results of an investigator-driven randomized controlled trial. Ann Surg. 2018;268:776–83.
73. O'Grady JG, Burroughs A, Hardy P, Elbourne D, Truesdale A, UK and Republic of Ireland Liver Transplant Study Group. Tacrolimus versus microemulsified ciclosporin in liver transplantation: the TMC randomised controlled trial. Lancet. 2002;360:1119–25.
74. Lerut JP, Pinheiro RS, Lai Q, Stouffs V, Orlando G, Rico Juri JM, Ciccarelli O, Sempoux C, Roggen FM, De Reyck C, Latinne D, Gianello P. Is minimal, [almost] steroid-free immunosuppression a safe approach in adult liver transplantation? Long-term outcome of a prospective, double blind, placebo-controlled, randomized, investigator-driven study. Ann Surg. 2014;260:886–91.
75. Demetris AJ. Longterm outcome of the liver graft: the pathologist's perspective. Liver Transpl. 2017;S1:S70–5.
76. Shaked A, Des Marais MR, Kopetskie H, Feng S, Punch JD, Levitsky J, Reyes J, Klintmalm GB, Demetris AJ, Burrell BE, Priore A, Bridges ND, Sayre PH. Outcomes of immunosuppression minimization and withdrawal early after liver transplantation. Am J Transplant. 2019;19:1397–409.
77. Watt KD. Keys to long-term care of the liver transplant recipient. Nat Rev Gastroenterol Hepatol. 2015;12:639–48.
78. Kotlyar DS, Campbell MS, Reddy KR. Recurrence of diseases following orthotopic liver transplantation. Am J Gastroenterol. 2006;101:1370–8.
79. Fung J, Wong T, Chok K, Chan A, Cheung TT, Dai JW, Sin SL, Ma KW, Ng K, Ng KT, Seto WK, Lai CL, Yuen MF, Lo CM. Long-term outcomes of entecavir monotherapy for chronic hepatitis B after liver transplantation: results up to 8 years. Hepatology. 2017;66:1036–44.
80. Berenguer M, Rayón JM, Prieto M, Aguilera V, Nicolás D, Ortiz V, Carrasco D, López-Andujar R, Mir J, Berenguer J. Are post-transplantation protocol liver biopsies useful in the long term? Liver Transpl. 2001;7:790–6.
81. Sebagh M, Castillo-Rama M, Azoulay D, Coilly A, Delvart V, Allard MA, Dos Santos A, Johanet C, Roque-Afonso AM, Saliba F, Duclos-Vallée JC, Samuel D, Demetris AJ. Histologic findings predictive of a diagnosis of de novo autoimmune hepatitis after liver transplantation in adults. Transplantation. 2013;96:670–8.
82. O'Leary JG, Demetris AJ, Friedman LS, Gebel HM, Halloran PF, Kirk AD, Knechtle SJ, McDiarmid SV, Shaked A, Terasaki PI, Tinckam KJ, Tomlanovich SJ, Wood KJ, Woodle ES, Zachary AA, Klintmalm GB. The role of donor-specific HLA alloantibodies in liver transplantation. Am J Transplant. 2014;14:779–87.
83. Starzl TE, Kaupp HA Jr. Mass homotransplantation of abdominal organs in dogs. Surg Forum. 1960;11:28–30.
84. Angeli P, Garcia-Tsao G, Nadim MK, Parikh CR. News in pathophysiology, definition and classification of hepatorenal syndrome: a step beyond the International Club of Ascites (ICA) consensus document. J Hepatol. 2019;71:811–22.
85. Nadim MK, Sung RS, Davis CL, Andreoni KA, Biggins SW, Danovitch GM, Feng S, Friedewald JJ, Hong JC, Kellum JA, Kim WR, Lake JR, Melton LB, Pomfret EA, Saab S, Genyk YS. Simultaneous liver-kidney transplantation summit: current state and future directions. Am J Transplant. 2012;12:2901–8.
86. Abu-Elmagd KM. Intestinal transplantation for short bowel syndrome and gastrointestinal failure: current consensus, rewarding outcomes, and practical guidelines. Gastroenterology. 2006;130:S132–7.
87. Cannon RM, Hughes MG, Jones CM, Eng M, Marvin MR. A review of the United States experience with combined heart-liver transplantation. Transpl Int. 2012;25:1223–8.
88. Corno V, Dezza MC, Lucianetti A, Codazzi D, Carrara B, Pinelli D, Parigi PC, Guizzetti M, Strazzabosco M, Melzi ML, Gaffuri G, Sonzogni V, Rossi A, Fagiuoli S, Colledan M. Combined double lung-liver transplantation for cystic fibrosis without cardio-pulmonary by-pass. Am J Transplant. 2007;7:2433–8.
89. Krowka MJ. Hepatopulmonary syndrome and portopulmonary hypertension: the pulmonary vascular enigmas of liver disease. Clin Liver Dis. 2020;15(Suppl 1):S13–24.
90. Aldenkortt F, Aldenkortt M, Caviezel L, Waeber JL, Weber A, Schiffer E. Portopulmonary hypertension and hepatopulmonary syndrome. World J Gastroenterol. 2014;20:8072–81.
91. Scouras NE, Matsusaki T, Boucek CD, Wells C, Cooper EA, Planinsic RM, Sullivan EA, Bermudez CA, Toyoda Y, Sakai T. Portopulmonary hypertension as an indication for combined heart, lung, and liver or lung and liver transplantation: literature review and case presentation. Liver Transpl. 2011;17:137–43.
92. Wiesner R, Edwards E, Freeman R, Harper A, Kim R, Kamath P, Kremers W, Lake J, Howard T, Merion RM, Wolfe RA, Krom R. United network for organ sharing liver disease severity score committee. Model for end-stage liver disease (MELD) and allocation of donor livers. Gastroenterology. 2003;124:91–6.
93. Malik AK, Masson S, Allen E, Akyol M, Bathgate A, Davies M, Hidalgo E, Hudson M, Powell J, Taylor R, Zarankaite A, Manas DM, UK Northern Liver Alliance. Impact of regional organ sharing and allocation in the UK northern liver alliance on waiting time to liver transplantation and waitlist survival. Transplantation. 2019;103:2304–11.
94. Broering DC, Schulte Am Esch J, Fischer L, Rogiers X. Split liver transplantation. HPB (Oxford). 2004;6:76–82.

95. Sebagh M, Yilmaz F, Karam V, Falissard B, Ichaï P, Roche B, Castaing D, Guettier C, Samuel D, Azoulay D. Cadaveric full-size liver transplantation and the graft alternatives in adults: a comparative study from a single Centre. J Hepatol. 2006;44:118–25.
96. Fondevila C, Hessheimer AJ, Flores E, Ruiz A, Mestres N, Calatayud D, Paredes D, Rodríguez C, Fuster J, Navasa M, Rimola A, Taurá P, García-Valdecasas JC. Applicability and results of Maastricht type 2 donation after cardiac death liver transplantation. Am J Transplant. 2012;12:162–70.
97. van Reeven M, Gilbo N, Monbaliu D, van Leeuwen OB, Porte RJ, Ysebaert D, van Hoek B, Alwayn IPJ, Meurisse N, Detry O, Coubeau L, Cicarelli O, Berrevoet F, Vanlander A, Ijzermans JNM, Polak WG. Evaluation of liver graft donation after euthanasia. JAMA Surg. 2020;155:917–24.
98. Lai Q, Vitale A, Iesari S, Finkenstedt A, Mennini G, Spoletini G, Hoppe-Lotichius M, Vennarecci G, Manzia TM, Nicolini D, Avolio AW, Frigo AC, Graziadei I, Rossi M, Tsochatzis E, Otto G, Ettorre GM, Tisone G, Vivarelli M, Agnes S, Cillo U, Lerut J, European Hepatocellular Cancer Liver Transplant Study Group. Intention-to-treat survival benefit of liver transplantation in patients with hepatocellular cancer. Hepatology. 2017;66:1910–9.
99. Louvet A, Wartel F, Castel H, Dharancy S, Hollebecque A, Canva-Delcambre V, Deltenre P, Mathurin P. Infection in patients with severe alcoholic hepatitis treated with steroids: early response to therapy is the key factor. Gastroenterology. 2009;137:541–8.
100. Linecker M, Krones T, Berg T, Niemann CU, Steadman RH, Dutkowski P, Clavien PA, Busuttil RW, Truog RD, Petrowsky H. Potentially inappropriate liver transplantation in the era of the "sickest first" policy - a search for the upper limits. J Hepatol. 2018;68:798–813.
101. Kim HJ, Larson JJ, Lim YS, Kim WR, Pedersen RA, Therneau TM, Rosen CB. Impact of MELD on waitlist outcome of retransplant candidates. Am J Transplant. 2010;10:2652–7.

Living Donor Liver Transplantation

Nobuhisa Akamatsu, Kiyoshi Hasegawa, Norihiro Kokudo, and Masatoshi Makuuchi

Abstract

Living donor liver transplantation (LDLT) has dramatically developed during the last three decades. Initially, left side liver graft had been mainly utilized, especially, in pediatric LDLT, however, right liver graft has become the most popular graft among adult LDLT. Variant graft type, such as right lateral sector graft, left trisector graft, right anterior graft, and dual graft, has been introduced to increase the donor pool. In addition, ABO blood-type incompatible LDLT has been established as a standard procedure. Expansion of the indication for hepatobiliary malignancies, especially, for the advanced hepatocellular carcinoma (HCC) has been a matter of debate in the last two decades. Various expanded criteria for HCC have been established, and recently the indication for colorectal cancer metastasis, neuroendocrine tumor metastasis, and cholangiocarcinoma has been aggressively investigated.

65.1 Introduction

Three decades have past since the initiation of living donor liver transplantation (LDLT) for pediatric patient with biliary atresia. In 1993, Makuuchi et al. reported the first successful LDLT for the adult patient with primary biliary cholangitis [1], and thereafter, LDLT has been flourished and established as a standard treatment for adult patients with end-stage liver disease, the outcome of which is now equal or even better to that of deceased donor whole liver transplantation [2]. Formerly, LDLT has evolved mainly in Asia where the number of deceased donor has been extremely scarce, however, it has become accepted as a treatment option in Western countries to cover the organ shortage of deceased donor liver transplantation (DDLT) [3].

In this chapter, we discussed the expansion of the donor pool in adult-to-adult LDLT, the technical refinements in LDLT, and LDLT for hepato-pancreato-biliary malignancies with special reference to the expansion of criteria for hepatocellular carcinoma patients.

65.2 Increasing the Donor Pool in Adult LDLT: Various Graft Types

In LDLT program, maintaining donor safety is the highest priority. Recent worldwide survey revealed that current morbidity and mortality rates following living liver donation were 24% and 0.2%, respectively [4]. Therefore, the risks imposed to the donor, although low, are still present, and when discussing increasing the donor pool in LDLT, strict donor selection according to structured protocols and center annual volume/experience are mandatory which determine donor safety.

65.2.1 Graft Size

Considering the expansion of the donor pool in LDLT, allowing the small graft is one of the major strategies, which in turn will decrease the donor risk. The lower limit of the partial liver graft in LDLT has been a matter of debate, and still is the unsolved problem in adult LDLT. There are two concepts in discussing the graft size, the graft to recipient weight ratio (GRWR) [5] and the graft ratio to standard liver volume (SLV) [6]. At the beginning of adult LDLT, the lower limit of

N. Akamatsu · K. Hasegawa (✉)
Artificial Organ and Transplantation Division, Department of Surgery, Graduate School of Medicine, The University of Tokyo, Tokyo, Japan
e-mail: hasegawa-2su@h.u-tokyo.ac.jp

N. Kokudo
Department of Surgery, National Center for Global Health and Medicine, Tokyo, Japan

M. Makuuchi
The University of Tokyo, Tokyo, Japan

the graft volume had been considered to be 1.0% in GRWR and 40% to SLV, however, with the advance in the operative techniques and the postoperative managements, these have been lowered, and nowadays some centers have gone down to 0.6% [7] and 30% [8], respectively. Adult LDLT has the intrinsic small sized graft problem, namely, small-for size graft syndrome (SFSS), characterized by the early graft dysfunction with prolonged cholestasis, prolonged prothrombin time, massive ascites, and sometimes encephalopathy. Actually, other factors such as preoperative recipient condition, donor age, graft quality (steatosis or fibrosis), portal flow modulation, and size of the outflow are complicatedly associated with the development of SFSS other than the size of the graft, and today it is well accepted that SFSS is not a simple problem of the graft size [9].

Left liver was the choice of graft at the beginning of adult LDLT, however, the right liver graft had soon replaced the major graft type since its introduction by Kyoto group in 1994 [10]. Hong Kong group proposed the safety and efficacy of the extended right liver graft including middle hepatic vein (MHV) [11]. In terms of the graft size, the right liver graft is undoubtedly preferable to left liver graft. The utilization of the right liver graft dramatically expanded the donor pool of LDLT and the indication for adult patients with various diseases of various degree of sickness. Now the right liver graft is widely used as a first choice in adult LDLT worldwide. In contrast, many Japanese centers are on the "left" side, using the left liver graft as a first choice if it satisfies the institutional lower limit of the graft size, considering that the smaller the graft size, the safer for the donor. Actually, most donor morality was reported in those with the right liver procurement [4], and the only donor mortality in Japan was of right liver case [12].

65.2.2 Left Liver Graft

As mentioned above, Makuuchi et al. reported the first successful left liver use in adult LDLT. Since then, we have proposed several technical tips to maximize the quality and quantity of the left liver graft. Miyagawa et al. reported the procurement of the left liver graft with the left caudate lobe, which increases the graft weight by about 8–12% [13]. Other technical innovations regarding left liver use were the reconstruction of the caudate hepatic vein and making the wide orifice of the left and middle hepatic vein with the aid of cryopreserved homologous veins [14]. Since the left liver is small in its nature, it is more vulnerable to portal hyperperfusion after reflow, meaning the risk of SFSS is higher than right liver graft. To overcome this drawback, we believe that making the outflow orifice as large as possible is utmost important especially in LDLT with left liver graft. Owing to these technical refinements, we can use the left liver graft safely in adult LDLT, demonstrating the similar functional/regenerative recovery and outcomes with the right liver graft 12 months after LDLT [15]. Figure 65.1 shows our venoplasty for the left live graft at bench surgery.

65.2.3 Right Liver Graft

Right liver graft is currently the most popular graft used in adult LDLT. For the donor safety, the left liver remnant should be over 30% of the total liver volume in the right liver procurement [16]. While Hong Kong group once proposed the extended right liver graft including MHV, considering the donor safety, a right lobe graft without MHV has become

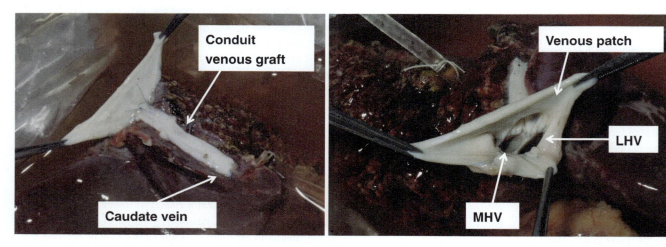

Fig. 65.1 Left liver graft. The orifice of left and middle hepatic vein was expanded with venous patch. Caudate vein was anastomosed to left and middle hepatic vein via venous conduit graft. *LHV* left hepatic vein, *MHV* middle hepatic vein

the most widely used graft type for adult LDLT [17]. However, when this type of graft is utilized, there has been debate about the necessity of reconstructing the segments 5 and 8 outflow to avoid right paramedian sector congestion, facilitate liver regeneration, and improve graft function. Although some centers are inclined to reconstruct these veins on a case-by-case basis, others suggest that all tributaries should be reconstructed if more than 5 mm in diameter [18]. We reported the importance of the reconstruction of MHV tributaries for the regeneration of the right paramedian sector, and proposed the reconstruction criteria to secure the uncongested graft volume over the lower limit of the graft for the recipient based on the preoperative volumetric analysis by computer simulation [19]. In addition to MHV tributaries, the reconstruction of inferior right hepatic vein (IRHV) is also important to secure the adequate venous drainage of the graft [20]. Figure 65.2 presents our venoplasty for MHV tributaries of the left live graft at bench surgery and the completion of venous reconstruction.

65.2.4 Right Lateral Sector Graft

Right lateral sector graft, which was firstly performed by us in 2000 [21], is another important option to increase donor pool in LDLT. Considering right lateral sector procurement becomes more valuable in donor whose right liver is larger than 70% of total liver volume, meaning both right and left liver grafts are not feasible. This type of graft can safely procured by the experienced hepatic surgeon with comparable recipients' outcomes with right liver graft, however, caution should be paid for the biliary anatomy in donor operation and the biliary complications in recipient [22]. Figure 65.3 shows the right lateral sector graft with IRHV.

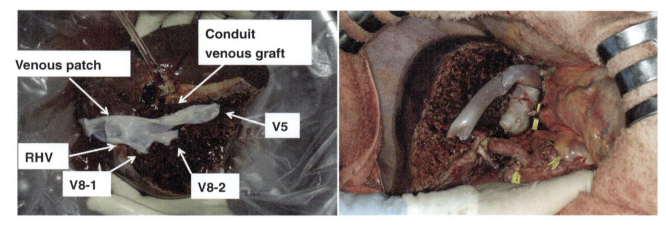

Fig. 65.2 Right liver graft. This right liver graft had three middle hepatic vein tributaries (namely, V5, V8-1, and V8-2), all of which were reconstructed to make one large orifice with right hepatic vein using venous grafts. *RHV* right hepatic vein, *V5* and *V8* middle hepatic venous tributary draining Segment 5 and 8 of the graft

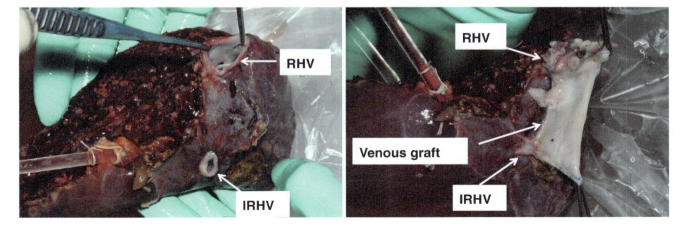

Fig. 65.3 Right lateral sector graft. There were right hepatic vein and inferior right hepatic vein in this graft. These were anastomosed to venous graft to make a new inferior vena cava at bench surgery. *RHV* right hepatic vein, *IRHV* inferior right hepatic vein

65.2.5 Dual Graft

Lee el al. of Asan medical center, South Korea, have successfully introduced dual graft adult LDLT, in which two grafts from different living donors are combined to provide a sufficient and safe graft volume to a single recipient [23]. Using this novel approach, the authors were able to expand the living donation pool by 12%, however, this technique is not popular in other areas than South Korea, may be due to the ethical consideration and the difference in social/cultural background.

65.2.6 ABO Blood Type Incompatible Graft

ABO incompatible (ABOi) graft is another important strategy to increase donor pool in LDLT. Initial experiences with ABOi grafts were complicated with increased rates of rejection, hepatic artery thrombosis, and diffuse intrahepatic biliary strictures resulting in poor outcome compared to outcomes in ABO compatible grafts, however, with the advances in rituximab based desensitization protocol in combination with plasmapheresis, local infusion of prostaglandins, intravenous immunoglobulin, or splenectomy, the results of LDLT with ABOi grafts have dramatically improved to the similar graft and patient survivals to those of ABO compatible LDLT [24, 25].

65.3 LDLT for HCC: Expanding the Indication

The dual composition of liver transplantation by donor and recipient makes its eligibility for HCC patients more complicated than other treatments for hepato-pancreato-biliary malignancies. Milan criteria, 5 cm in size or up to three HCCs no greater than 3 cm in size without vascular invasion or extrahepatic metastasis, have been the gold standard for the indication of liver transplantation for HCC patients in DDLT in Western countries [26]. It has become consensus that the Milan criteria is too strict in terms of recurrence rate and patient survival after liver transplantation, however, when expanding the criteria, we must consider the exceptional points for HCC patients which should be balanced with other liver transplant candidates. Expansion of the Milan criteria recruits more candidates with HCC who cannot be treated by locoregional therapy and are excluded from waiting list by conventional criteria due to the tumor burden. On the other hand, the increasing number of HCC patients on the waiting list for DDLT will certainly lower the chance of liver transplantation for those enlisted without malignant diagnosis under the limited donor pool. In contrast to DDLT, where the graft is public resource, the graft is private one in LDLT, and the expansion of the criteria may be easily adopted and accepted. Indeed, the downstaging and the bridging treatments for candidates with HCC to make and maintain them within the Milan criteria have been major strategies in DDLT setting, in contrast, the expansion of the criteria has been actively debated in LDLT [27, 28]. Table 65.1 summarizes various criteria utilized to select patients with HCC beyond Milan criteria for liver transplantation [27, 29–38]. Majority of criteria have achieved 5-year survival rate of over 70% or even 80%, indicating that these expansions are acceptable.

65.3.1 Size and Number Expansion

Expanding the Milan criteria was initially done by simple expansion of the maximal size and number of HCC nodules. University of California San Francisco (UCSF) criteria, in which patients with a solitary tumor ≤65 mm in diameter, or two or three tumors, each with a diameter ≤ 45 mm, and a total tumor diameter ≤ 80 mm, were the most famous expanded criteria [29]. "Tokyo criteria" from our group (tumors up to 5 nodules with maximum diameter) [27], "Asan criteria" from South Korea (tumor≤5 cm in diameter, ≤6 in nodule number) [30], and "Up-to-7 criteria" by Metroticket Investigator Study Group (the sum of tumor number and the size of largest tumor no larger than 7) were reported [31].

65.3.2 Expansion with Biomarkers

Recently, more and more authors have reported the importance of incorporation of biomarkers representing the tumor biological behavior into the selection criteria. Regarding the biomarkers incorporated into the expanded criteria, while the tumor markers such as alfa-fetoprotein (AFP) and des-gamma-carboxy prothrombin (DCP) have been investigated by many researchers, recently other markers such as the neutrophil-lymphocyte ratio (NLR) [39], the platelet-lymphocyte ratio (PLR), and fluorine-18-fluorodeoxyglucose positron emission tomography (FDG-PET) [40] were reported to be useful for the selection of the high risk group for the recurrence and for the prediction of the recurrence [41]. The Kyoto criteria expanded the number of tumors to 10 in addition to the largest diameter ≤ 5 cm and DCP level ≤ 400 mAU/ml

Table 65.1 Worldwide criteria for liver transplantation for hepatocellular carcinoma

Expanded criteria	Author (year)	Country	Eligibility	Outcomes
UCSF	Yao et al. (2001) [29]	US	Single tumor ≤6.5 cm or 3 tumors all ≤4.5 cm with TTD ≤8 cm	DFS: 90.9% (5 years), OS: 80.9% (5 years)
Asan medical center	Lee et al. (2008) [30]	Korea	Tumor size ≤5 cm, tumor number ≤ 6	DFS: 79.9% (2 years), OS: 73.2% (3 years)
Up-to seven	Mazzaferro et al. (2009) [31]	Italy	Sum of the number of nodules and diameter of the largest nodule (in cm) ≤7	DFS: 91% (5 years), OS: 71% (5 years)
Extended Toronto	Goldaracena et al. (2019) [32]	Canada	No limit in size and number, Biopsy of largest tumor not poorly differentiated	DFS: 78% (5 years), OS: 79% (5 years)
University of Hong Kong	Wong et al. (2019) [33]	China	No limit in size and number	DFS: 83.1% (5 years), OS: 80% (5 years)
French AFP model	Duvoux et al. (2012) [34]	France	No limit in size and number, Model combining log10 AFP, tumor size and number of tumors: Score > or ≤ 2	DFS: 86% (5 years), OS: 70% (5 years)
Hangzhou	Chen et al. (2014) [35]	China	TTD ≤8 cm; or TTD >8 cm with grade I or II histopathology and preoperative AFP ≤ 400 ng/ml	DFS: 80.3% (5 years), OS: 87.7% (5 years)
Tokyo	Akamatsu et al. (2014) [27]	Japan	Tumor size ≤5 cm, Tumor number ≤ 5	DFS: 86% (5 years), OS: 80% (5 years)
Kyoto	Kaido et al. (2013) [36]	Japan	Tumor size ≤5 cm, Tumor number ≤ 10, DCP ≤ 400 mAU/ml	DFS: 83% (5 years), OS: 82% (5 years)
Kyushu	Uchiyama et al. (2017) [37]	Japan	No limit in number, Tumor size≤5 cm, DCP ≤ 300 mAU/ml	DFS: 80.4% (5 years), OS: 82.1% (5 years)
5–5-500	Shimamura et al. (2019) [38]	Japan	Tumor size ≤5 cm, Tumor number ≤ 5, AFP ≤ 500 ng/ml	DFS: 73.2% (5 years), OS: 85.8% (5 years)

[36], and the Kyushu group further expanded the criteria by tumor with diameter ≤ 5 cm and serum DCP level < 300 mAU/ml without restricting tumor number [37]. Otherwise, AFP is the most popular biomarker used in the expanded criteria. Usefulness of AFP in predicting the recurrence after liver transplantation has been investigated by many researchers, and AFP is incorporated in some selection and prognostic models. The AFP model, developed by the Liver Transplantation French Study Group, combines serum AFP level, tumor size, and tumor number [34]. Another famous prognostic model is RETREAT score, which incorporated microvascular invasion, tumor diameter, tumor number, and AFP value as prognositic variables [42]. Another prognostic model, TRAIN score, incorporated AFP slope, which was defined as [(final-AFP)-(initial-AFP)]/time [43]. Toso et al. use the data from the Scientific Registry of Transplant Recipients with 6478 patients in USA to propose new criteria combining the total tumor volume ≤ 115 cm3 and AFP level ≤ 400 ng/ml [44]. Metroticket Investigator Study Group updated "Up-to-7 criteria" with the addition of AFP value [45]. A new prognostic model was developed in South Korea, i.e., MoRAL (Model to predict tumor Recurrence After LDLT) score using only serum levels of AFP and DCP, which was shown to be more effective than the Milan criteria in predicting the recurrence after liver transplantation [46]. In Japan, the 5–5-500 criteria (nodule size ≤5 cm in diameter, nodule number ≤ 5, and AFP value ≤500 ng/ml) were established based on a retrospective data analysis of the Japanese Liver Transplant Registry by our colleagues [38]. This expanded criterion was approved as the new national selection criteria for liver transplant candidates with HCC and started to be operated in August 2019. Now, the double eligibility criteria, Milan +5–5-500, is adopted as the Japanese new indication criteria for patients with HCC in both DDLT and LDLT.

65.3.3 LDLT Vs DDLT for HCC Recurrence

Initially some studies showed higher recurrence in patients transplanted with living donor and investigators hypothesized that rapid regeneration process of partial liver graft and cytokine released might induce the early recurrence of potential microscopic HCC. Another explanation was that the fast-track feature of LDLT and short observation period before liver transplantation may mask the aggressiveness of HCC which leads to higher recurrence [47]. However, more recent meta-analyses [48–50] and intention-to-treat analyses [32, 33, 51, 52] have revealed equal or even better outcomes of LDLT than DDLT in both patient survival and disease-free survival, and now it has become consensus that patients with HCC meeting the indication criteria and beyond the indication for locoregional treatments will be benefitted by LDLT if they have appropriate live donors. Recent studies support an expanded indication of LDLT for HCC beyond the standard Milan criteria with the advances of new knowledges that aid in predicting the long-term oncological outcomes with cautiously balancing the risks of harm to otherwise healthy donors. South Korean groups are challenging LDLT even for those with macrovascular invasion [53]. Expanding the indication for LDLT for HCC will provide a potential curable procedure to patients who otherwise have limited treatment options.

65.4 LDLT for Hepato-pancreato-biliary Malignancies Other than HCC

Liver transplantation for hepato-pancreato-biliary malignancies other than HCC had been contraindicated due to initial dismal outcomes, however, with the recent advances in chemo/radiotherapy, immunosuppressants, and transplant techniques, several researchers have published favorable outcomes of liver transplantation for colorectal liver metastases, neuroendocrine liver metastases, intrahepatic cholangiocarcinoma, and perihilar cholangiocarcinoma [54, 55]. Liver transplantation for these unresectable hepato-pancreato-biliary malignancies needs multiple disciplines of transplantation medicine and oncology, including transplantation and hepatobiliary surgeons, medical and radiation oncologists, hepatologists and gastroenterologists, immunologists, etc., to maximize the care and cure of cancer patients [56]. Considering the world shortage of donors and the clinical trial nature, LDLT practice will be of help in this multidisciplinary approach.

Regarding perihilar cholangiocarcinoma, Mayo clinic established the protocol for liver transplantation consisted of external beam radiation therapy with a target dose of 45 Gy combined with fluorouracil or oral capecitabine, followed by brachytherapy with iridium-192 with a target dose of 20–30 Gy, and final staging laparotomy [57]. Based on this protocol, 5-year disease free survival was reported to be 65% and 66.5% in US multicenter study [58] and 74 LDLT cases of Mayo clinic [59], respectively. The definition of "unresectable disease", however, is not universal, and some centers would potentially resect patients deemed unresectable in different institutions. In this sense, liver transplantation for perihilar cholangiocarcinoma should be argued in multidisciplinary approach among intergroups, balancing the risk/benefit of recipient and donor risk in LDLT, especially. The liver transplantation for intrahepatic cholangiocarcinoma should be limited for cirrhotic patients with very early stage (single tumor and up to 2 cm) [60]. With the advance in surgical techniques and highly-effective chemotherapy, the prognosis of patients with initially unresectable colorectal liver metastases has been improving. Norway group reported an approach, referred to as the RAPID concept (Resection And Partial Liver Segment 2/3 Transplantation With Delayed Total Hepatectomy), that combines the Associating Liver Partition and Portal Vein Ligation for Staged Hepatectomy (the so-called ALPPS procedure) with LDLT of segments 2 and 3, followed by total hepatectomy [61]. The same group recently reported 5-year survival rate of 83% among unresectable colorectal liver metastases with well-controlled disease under chemotherapy [62], however, at present liver transplantation for those with colorectal liver metastases should be very limited, provided the advanced resection strategies and the developing chemotherapy. Given the rarity and slow growing nature of disease, liver transplantation for neuroendocrine liver metastases is more controversial. Mazzaferro et al. developed the Milan criteria for neuroendocrine liver metastases: confirmed histology of G1 or G2 tumor, the primary tumor drained by the portal system, hepatic involvement of <50%, complete resection of primary tumor and all extrahepatic disease with stable disease or good response to therapies for at least 6 months, and age < 60 years. In their prospective study of 42 highly selected patients, 5- and 10-year survival rates of 97% and 89%, respectively, were achieved [63]. Finally, liver transplantation for these malignancies is still undergoing in clinical trial basis, and left to be argued with future evidences.

References

1. Hashikura Y, Makuuchi M, Kawasaki S, Matsunami H, Ikegami T, Nakazawa Y, et al. Successful living-related partial liver transplantation to an adult patient. Lancet. 1994;343(8907):1233–4.
2. Chen CL, Kabiling CS, Concejero AM. Why does living donor liver transplantation flourish in Asia? Nat Rev Gastroenterol Hepatol. 2013;10(12):746–51.
3. Humar A, Ganesh S, Jorgensen D, Tevar A, Ganoza A, Molinari M, et al. Adult living donor versus deceased donor liver transplant (LDLT versus DDLT) at a single center: time to change our paradigm for liver transplant. Ann Surg. 2019;270(3):444–51.
4. Cheah YL, Simpson MA, Pomposelli JJ, Pomfret EA. Incidence of death and potentially life-threatening near-miss events in living donor hepatic lobectomy: a world-wide survey. Liver Transpl. 2013;19(5):499–506.
5. Kiuchi T, Kasahara M, Uryuhara K, Inomata Y, Uemoto S, Asonuma K, et al. Impact of graft size mismatching on graft prognosis in liver transplantation from living donors. Transplantation. 1999;67(2):321–7.
6. Urata K, Kawasaki S, Matsunami H, Hashikura Y, Ikegami T, Ishizone S, et al. Calculation of child and adult standard liver volume for liver transplantation. Hepatology. 1995;21(5):1317–21.
7. Wong TC, Fung JYY, Cui TYS, Sin SL, Ma KW, She BWH, et al. The risk of going small: lowering GRWR and overcoming small-for-size syndrome in adult living donor liver transplantation. Ann Surg. 2020;274(6):e1260–8.
8. Ikegami T, Yoshizumi T, Sakata K, Uchiyama H, Harimoto N, Harada N, et al. Left lobe living donor liver transplantation in adults: what is the safety limit? Liver Transpl. 2016;22(12):1666–75.
9. Goldaracena N, Echeverri J, Selzner M. Small-for-size syndrome in live donor liver transplantation-pathways of injury and therapeutic strategies. Clin Transpl. 2017;31(2):e12885. https://doi.org/10.1111/ctr.12885.

10. Yamaoka Y, Washida M, Honda K, Tanaka K, Mori K, Shimahara Y, et al. Liver transplantation using a right lobe graft from a living related donor. Transplantation. 1994;57(7):1127–30.
11. Lo CM, Fan ST, Liu CL, Wei WI, Lo RJ, Lai CL, et al. Adult-to-adult living donor liver transplantation using extended right lobe grafts. Ann Surg. 1997;226(3):261–9. discussion 9-70
12. Akabayashi A, Slingsby BT, Fujita M. The first donor death after living-related liver transplantation in Japan. Transplantation. 2004;77(4):634.
13. Miyagawa S, Hashikura Y, Miwa S, Ikegami T, Urata K, Terada M, et al. Concomitant caudate lobe resection as an option for donor hepatectomy in adult living related liver transplantation. Transplantation. 1998;66(5):661–3.
14. Takemura N, Sugawara Y, Hashimoto T, Akamatsu N, Kishi Y, Tamura S, et al. New hepatic vein reconstruction in left liver graft. Liver Transpl. 2005;11(3):356–60.
15. Akamatsu N, Sugawara Y, Tamura S, Imamura H, Kokudo N, Makuuchi M. Regeneration and function of hemiliver graft: right versus left. Surgery. 2006;139(6):765–72.
16. Miller CM, Durand F, Heimbach JK, Kim-Schluger L, Lee SG, Lerut J, et al. The international liver transplant society guideline on living liver donation. Transplantation. 2016;100(6):1238–43.
17. Lee SG. A complete treatment of adult living donor liver transplantation: a review of surgical technique and current challenges to expand indication of patients. Am J Transplant. 2015;15(1):17–38.
18. Miller CM, Quintini C, Dhawan A, Durand F, Heimbach JK, Kim-Schluger HL, et al. The international liver transplantation society living donor liver transplant recipient guideline. Transplantation. 2017;101(5):938–44.
19. Akamatsu N, Sugawara Y, Nagata R, Kaneko J, Aoki T, Sakamoto Y, et al. Adult right living-donor liver transplantation with special reference to reconstruction of the middle hepatic vein. Am J Transplant. 2014;14(12):2777–87.
20. Ito K, Akamatsu N, Tani K, Ito D, Kaneko J, Arita J, et al. The reconstruction of hepatic venous tributary in right liver living-donor liver transplantation: the importance of the inferior right hepatic vein. Liver Transpl. 2015;22(4):410–9.
21. Sugawara Y, Makuuchi M, Takayama T, Imamura H, Kaneko J. Right lateral sector graft in adult living-related liver transplantation. Transplantation. 2002;73(1):111–4.
22. Kokudo T, Hasegawa K, Arita J, Yamamoto S, Kaneko J, Akamatsu N, et al. Use of a right lateral sector graft in living donor liver transplantation is feasible, but special caution is needed in respect of the liver anatomy. Am J Transplant. 2015;16(4):1258–65.
23. Song GW, Lee SG, Moon DB, Ahn CS, Hwang S, Kim KH, et al. Dual-graft adult living donor liver transplantation: an innovative surgical procedure for live liver donor pool expansion. Ann Surg. 2017;266(1):10–8.
24. Egawa H, Teramukai S, Haga H, Tanabe M, Mori A, Ikegami T, et al. Impact of rituximab desensitization on blood-type-incompatible adult living donor liver transplantation: a Japanese multicenter study. Am J Transplant. 2014;14(1):102–14.
25. Oh J, Kim JM. Immunologic strategies and outcomes in ABO-incompatible living donor liver transplantation. Clin Mol Hepatol. 2020;26(1):1–6.
26. Mazzaferro V, Regalia E, Doci R, Andreola S, Pulvirenti A, Bozzetti F, et al. Liver transplantation for the treatment of small hepatocellular carcinomas in patients with cirrhosis. N Engl J Med. 1996;334(11):693–9.
27. Akamatsu N, Sugawara Y, Kokudo N. Living donor liver transplantation for patients with hepatocellular carcinoma. Liver Cancer. 2014;3(2):108–18.
28. Mehta N, Bhangui P, Yao FY, Mazzaferro V, Toso C, Akamatsu N, et al. Liver transplantation for hepatocellular carcinoma. Working group report from the ILTS transplant oncology consensus conference. Transplantation. 2020;104(6):1136–42.
29. Yao FY, Ferrell L, Bass NM, Watson JJ, Bacchetti P, Venook A, et al. Liver transplantation for hepatocellular carcinoma: expansion of the tumor size limits does not adversely impact survival. Hepatology. 2001;33(6):1394–403.
30. Lee SG, Hwang S, Moon DB, Ahn CS, Kim KH, Sung KB, et al. Expanded indication criteria of living donor liver transplantation for hepatocellular carcinoma at one large-volume center. Liver Transpl. 2008;14(7):935–45.
31. Mazzaferro V, Llovet JM, Miceli R, Bhoori S, Schiavo M, Mariani L, et al. Predicting survival after liver transplantation in patients with hepatocellular carcinoma beyond the Milan criteria: a retrospective, exploratory analysis. Lancet Oncol. 2009;10(1):35–43.
32. Goldaracena N, Gorgen A, Doyle A, Hansen BE, Tomiyama K, Zhang W, et al. Live donor liver transplantation for patients with hepatocellular carcinoma offers increased survival vs. deceased donation. J Hepatol. 2019;70(4):666–73.
33. Wong TCL, Ng KKC, Fung JYY, Chan AAC, Cheung TT, Chok KSH, et al. Long-term survival outcome between living donor and deceased donor liver transplant for hepatocellular carcinoma: intention-to-treat and propensity score matching analyses. Ann Surg Oncol. 2019;26(5):1454–62.
34. Duvoux C, Roudot-Thoraval F, Decaens T, Pessione F, Badran H, Piardi T, et al. Liver transplantation for hepatocellular carcinoma: a model including alpha-fetoprotein improves the performance of Milan criteria. Gastroenterology. 2012;143(4):986–94.e3. quiz e14-5
35. Chen J, Xu X, Wu J, Ling Q, Wang K, Wang W, et al. The stratifying value of Hangzhou criteria in liver transplantation for hepatocellular carcinoma. PLoS One. 2014;9(3):e93128.
36. Kaido T, Ogawa K, Mori A, Fujimoto Y, Ito T, Tomiyama K, et al. Usefulness of the Kyoto criteria as expanded selection criteria for liver transplantation for hepatocellular carcinoma. Surgery. 2013;154(5):1053–60.
37. Uchiyama H, Itoh S, Yoshizumi T, Ikegami T, Harimoto N, Soejima Y, et al. Living donor liver transplantation for hepatocellular carcinoma: results of prospective patient selection by Kyushu University criteria in 7 years. HPB. 2017;19(12):1082–90.
38. Shimamura T, Akamatsu N, Fujiyoshi M, Kawaguchi A, Morita S, Kawasaki S, et al. Expanded living-donor liver transplantation criteria for patients with hepatocellular carcinoma based on the Japanese nationwide survey: the 5-5-500 rule - a retrospective study. Transpl Int. 2019;32(4):356–68.
39. Halazun KJ, Najjar M, Abdelmessih RM, Samstein B, Griesemer AD, Guarrera JV, et al. Recurrence after liver transplantation for hepatocellular carcinoma: a new MORAL to the story. Ann Surg. 2017;265(3):557–64.
40. Hong G, Suh KS, Suh SW, Yoo T, Kim H, Park MS, et al. Alpha-fetoprotein and (18) F-FDG positron emission tomography predict tumor recurrence better than Milan criteria in living donor liver transplantation. J Hepatol. 2016;64(4):852–9.
41. Citores MJ, Lucena JL, de la Fuente S, Cuervas-Mons V. Serum biomarkers and risk of hepatocellular carcinoma recurrence after liver transplantation. World J Hepatol. 2019;11(1):50–64.
42. Mehta N, Heimbach J, Harnois DM, Sapisochin G, Dodge JL, Lee D, et al. Validation of a risk estimation of tumor recurrence after transplant (RETREAT) score for hepatocellular carcinoma recurrence after liver transplant. JAMA Oncol. 2017;3(4):493–500.
43. Lai Q, Nicolini D, Inostroza Nunez M, Iesari S, Goffette P, Agostini A, et al. A novel prognostic index in patients with hepatocellular cancer waiting for liver transplantation: time-radiological-response-alpha-fetoprotein-INflammation (TRAIN) score. Ann Surg. 2016;264(5):787–96.

44. Toso C, Asthana S, Bigam DL, Shapiro AM, Kneteman NM. Reassessing selection criteria prior to liver transplantation for hepatocellular carcinoma utilizing the scientific registry of transplant recipients database. Hepatology. 2009;49(3):832–8.
45. Mazzaferro V, Sposito C, Zhou J, Pinna AD, De Carlis L, Fan J, et al. Metroticket 2.0 model for analysis of competing risks of death after liver transplantation for hepatocellular carcinoma. Gastroenterology. 2018;154(1):128–39.
46. Lee JH, Cho Y, Kim HY, Cho EJ, Lee DH, Yu SJ, et al. Serum tumor markers provide refined prognostication in selecting liver transplantation candidate for hepatocellular carcinoma patients beyond the Milan criteria. Ann Surg. 2016;263(5):842–50.
47. Akamatsu N, Kokudo N. Liver transplantation for hepatocellular carcinoma from living-donor vs. deceased donor. Hepatobiliary Surg Nutr. 2016;5(5):422–8.
48. Liang W, Wu L, Ling X, Schroder PM, Ju W, Wang D, et al. Living donor liver transplantation versus deceased donor liver transplantation for hepatocellular carcinoma: a meta-analysis. Liver Transpl. 2012;18(10):1226–36.
49. Grant RC, Sandhu L, Dixon PR, Greig PD, Grant DR, McGilvray ID. Living vs. deceased donor liver transplantation for hepatocellular carcinoma: a systematic review and meta-analysis. Clin Transpl. 2013;27(1):140–7.
50. Zhu B, Wang J, Li H, Chen X, Zeng Y. Living or deceased organ donors in liver transplantation for hepatocellular carcinoma: a systematic review and meta-analysis. HPB (Oxford). 2019;21(2):133–47.
51. Bhangui P, Vibert E, Majno P, Salloum C, Andreani P, Zocrato J, et al. Intention-to-treat analysis of liver transplantation for hepatocellular carcinoma: living versus deceased donor transplantation. Hepatology. 2011;53(5):1570–9.
52. Azoulay D, Audureau E, Bhangui P, Belghiti J, Boillot O, Andreani P, et al. Living or brain-dead donor liver transplantation for hepatocellular carcinoma: a Multicenter, Western, intent-to-treat cohort study. Ann Surg. 2017;266(6):1035–44.
53. Lee KW, Suh SW, Choi Y, Jeong J, Yi NJ, Kim H, et al. Macrovascular invasion is not an absolute contraindication for living donor liver transplantation. Liver Transpl. 2017;23(1):19–27.
54. Hibi T, Rela M, Eason JD, Line PD, Fung J, Sakamoto S, et al. Liver transplantation for colorectal and neuroendocrine liver metastases and hepatoblastoma. Working group report from the ILTS transplant oncology consensus conference. Transplantation. 2020;104(6):1131–5.
55. Sapisochin G, Javle M, Lerut J, Ohtsuka M, Ghobrial M, Hibi T, et al. Liver transplantation for cholangiocarcinoma and mixed hepatocellular cholangiocarcinoma: working group report from the ILTS transplant oncology consensus conference. Transplantation. 2020;104(6):1125–30.
56. Hibi T, Sapisochin G. What is transplant oncology? Surgery. 2019;165(2):281–5.
57. Rea DJ, Heimbach JK, Rosen CB, Haddock MG, Alberts SR, Kremers WK, et al. Liver transplantation with neoadjuvant chemoradiation is more effective than resection for hilar cholangiocarcinoma. Ann Surg. 2005;242(3):451–8. discussion 8-61
58. Darwish Murad S, Kim WR, Harnois DM, Douglas DD, Burton J, Kulik LM, et al. Efficacy of neoadjuvant chemoradiation, followed by liver transplantation, for perihilar cholangiocarcinoma at 12 US centers. Gastroenterology. 2012;143(1):88–98.e3. quiz e14
59. Tan EK, Rosen CB, Heimbach JK, Gores GJ, Zamora-Valdes D, Taner T. Living donor liver transplantation for perihilar cholangiocarcinoma: outcomes and complications. J Am Coll Surg. 2020;231(1):98–110.
60. Sapisochin G, Facciuto M, Rubbia-Brandt L, Marti J, Mehta N, Yao FY, et al. Liver transplantation for "very early" intrahepatic cholangiocarcinoma: international retrospective study supporting a prospective assessment. Hepatology. 2016;64(4):1178–88.
61. Line PD, Hagness M, Berstad AE, Foss A, Dueland S. A novel concept for partial liver transplantation in nonresectable colorectal liver metastases: the RAPID concept. Ann Surg. 2015;262(1):e5–9.
62. Dueland S, Syversveen T, Solheim JM, Solberg S, Grut H, Bjørnbeth BA, et al. Survival following liver transplantation for patients with nonresectable liver-only colorectal metastases. Ann Surg. 2020;271(2):212–8.
63. Mazzaferro V, Pulvirenti A, Coppa J. Neuroendocrine tumors metastatic to the liver: how to select patients for liver transplantation? J Hepatol. 2007;47(4):460–6.

Pyogenic Liver Abscess

Kai Siang Chan and Vishal Shelat

Abstract

Pyogenic liver abscess (PLA) is the most common type of liver abscess, accounting for up to 48% of all visceral abscesses and 13% of intra-abdominal abscesses with estimated mortality of 10–40% despite advances in healthcare. Risk factors for PLA include male gender, proton-pump inhibitors, hepatobiliary or pancreatic disease, diabetes mellitus, human immunodeficiency virus (HIV), immunosuppressant medications, and liver cirrhosis. Primary PLA is defined as direct seeding of pathogens into biliary system, such as hepatobiliary infection from biliary obstruction, or less commonly, from colonic source or haematogenous spread from systemic infections. Secondary PLA is defined as PLA due to complications from underlying pathology, such as hepatocellular carcinoma (HCC), or interventions, such as transarterial chemoembolization, radiofrequency ablation or endoscopic biliary procedures. Clinical presentation of PLA is with non-specific symptoms. Serum biochemistry findings of raised inflammatory markers and deranged liver enzymes is non-specific too. Diagnosis is often achieved via imaging. Ultrasound scan and Computerized tomography (CT) scan are widely used as first-line imaging modality. Principles of PLA management are in accordance with the Surviving Sepsis guidelines. Empirical antibiotics should be guided by local antibiogram. The common antibiotic regimes include combination of third-generation cephalosporin and metronidazole, or amoxicillin-clavulanic acid and once dose of gentamicin. Duration of antibiotics is guided by clinical and radiological response to source control. Drainage of PLA may be attempted percutaneously, endoscopically or surgically (open or laparoscopic). Percutaneous drainage (PD) has superior outcomes compared to antibiotics alone for abscess >4 cm. Giant PLA (size ≥10 cm), multiple loculations, gas formation, and patient co-morbidities predict poor outcomes and risk of failure of PD. In selected patients, surgical intervention is warranted. After treatment of acute PLA, it is prudent for follow-up with repeat imaging to rule out any abdominal pathology. A screening colonoscopy should be offered especially to patients with *Klebsiella pneumoniae* PLA. A PLA care bundle with integration of surgical and nursing care including drain care, interventional radiology and microbiology team (including transition to outpatient antibiotic therapy) is proposed to provide multimodal care and improved outcomes for PLA.

66.1 Background

A liver abscess is defined as a focal collection of suppurative material surrounded by a fibrous layer of tissue within the liver parenchyma [1]. It is commonly classified based on its etiology (amoebic or parasitic, and bacteria or pyogenic), number (solitary or multiple), size (small, large, or giant), or gas content (gas-forming or not gas-forming). A pyogenic liver abscess (PLA) is the most common type of liver abscess, accounting for up to 48% of all visceral abscesses and 13% of intra-abdominal abscesses [1]. Despite this, PLA remains relatively uncommon globally, with an incidence of 1.1 per 100,000 in Europe and a proportionately higher incidence of 17.6 per 100,000 in Asia [2]. Historically, PLA occurred mainly in young males due to pylephlebitis secondary to appendicitis [3]. Biliary tract diseases such as biliary stones, strictures, malignancy, or congenital anomalies now account

K. S. Chan
Ministry of Health Holdings Limited, Singapore, Singapore

Department of General Surgery, Tan Tock Seng Hospital, Singapore, Singapore

V. Shelat (✉)
Department of General Surgery, Tan Tock Seng Hospital, Singapore, Singapore

Lee Kong Chian School of Medicine, Nanyang Technological University, Singapore, Singapore
e-mail: Vishal_G_Shelat@ttsh.com.sg

for most PLA. In recent decades with advances in minimally invasive hepatobiliary interventions such as radiofrequency ablation (RFA), microwave ablation (MWA), and transarterial chemoembolization (TACE), these interventions have emerged as significant causes of PLA [4, 5]. Studies have shown that imaging biomarkers such as number, size, or gas presence in PLA allow for risk stratification [6], which subsequently allow for early intervention and improve clinical outcomes [7–10]. With advances in medical and surgical care, the traditionally high mortality of up to 80% in the 1900s has improved to 10–40% today, with a shift towards non-operative management [11]. This chapter provides an overview of evidence-based literature on PLA.

66.2 Risk Factors and Etiopathogenesis

Risk factors for PLA include male gender [3], proton-pump inhibitors [12], hepatobiliary or pancreatic disease [11], or compromised immune function, including diabetes mellitus [2], human immunodeficiency virus (HIV) [13], liver cirrhosis, and liver transplant [14–16].

Pathogenesis of PLA can be classified as primary or secondary. Primary PLA includes the direct seeding of pathogens into the biliary system. This includes biliary, colonic, hematogenous, or cryptogenic sepsis. The most common cause of primary PLA is hepatobiliary infection (incidence of 30–50%) [17]. Biliary stones, stricture, malignancy, or congenital biliary anomalies result in biliary obstruction, elevation in intrabiliary pressures, cholangiovenous reflux, resulting in endotoxemia commonly from gram-negative organisms. Figure 66.1 shows the computed tomography (CT) scan of a patient with acute cholecystitis with contiguous PLA. Portal venous system seeding is the second most common cause, accounting for 20% of primary PLA. Mucosal breach of bowel mucosa or infection of other intra-abdominal organs such as appendicitis leads to portal pylephlebitis with resulting PLA formation [18, 19]. Hematogenous spread, though less common, may occur from systemic infections, traumatic injuries, or intravenous drug usage [20]. Less commonly, hematogenous seeding from the severe periodontal disease has been reported during the Coronavirus Disease 2019 pandemic [21]. A diagnosis of cryptogenic PLA is made after excluding other PLA causes, where extensive workup fails to establish an etiology, including malignancy.

Secondary PLA is defined as PLA due to complications of underlying pathology or intervention. Malignancy such as hepatocellular carcinoma (HCC), though rare, has been reported to manifest initially as PLA [22]. Anecdotally, the senior author has performed liver resection on a patient with

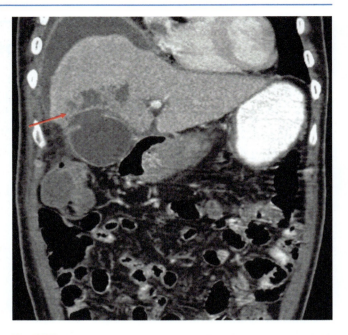

Fig. 66.1 Computed tomography scan of an 81-year-old male who presented with abdominal pain of a few days' duration: acute cholecystitis with contiguous pyogenic liver abscess (red arrow)

suspected HCC based on two imaging modalities, only to find an intra-operative diagnosis of PLA. It is postulated that spontaneous tumor necrosis and biliary obstruction caused by tumor thrombi with superimposed bacterial infection results in HCC presenting as PLA [23]. Minimally invasive therapeutic interventions such as RFA, MWA, and TACE are increasingly common causes of PLA due to their increasing use for the management of HCC with a reported incidence of 1.6% and 1.8% following MWA and RFA, respectively [24]. RFA, MWA, and TACE induce necrosis to reduce tumor burden but creates a nidus for infection [4, 5, 25, 26]. Figure 66.2 demonstrates the presence of PLA following MWA. Prophylactic antibiotics are administered for patients undergoing RFA and TACE. The use of prophylactic antibiotic monotherapy on the day of TACE reduces the incidence of PLA by 65% [27].

Endoscopic biliary procedures such as biliary stenting and sphincterotomy or surgical interventions such as pancreaticoduodenectomy may also cause PLA due to the disruption of the sphincter of Oddi, allowing bacterial colonization of the biliary tree and increased risk of PLA formation [28, 29]. Other rarer causes of PLA include PLA following cholecystectomy and liver transplantation [30, 31]. Figure 66.3 shows a patient who had an acute presentation of PLA 6 years following cholecystectomy, complicated by middle hepatic vein thrombosis.

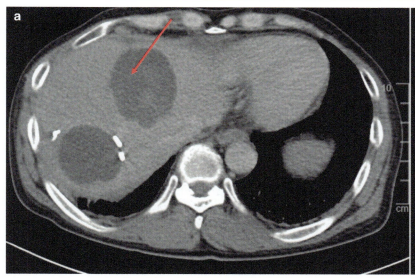
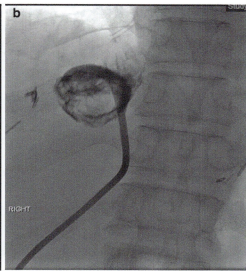

Fig. 66.2 Computed tomography scan of a 56-year-old male diagnosed with stage IV rectosigmoid adenocarcinoma with multiple bilobar liver metastases who underwent multiple liver wedge resections and intra-operative microwave ablation, with (**a**) resulting pyogenic liver abscess six weeks following the procedure (red arrow) and (**b**) percutaneous drainage showing a large cavity with 50 ml of pus drained, growing multi-drug resistant *Escherichia coli*

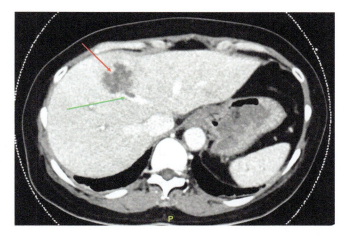

Fig. 66.3 Computed tomography (CT) scan of a 65-year-old female who presented with acute right upper quadrant pain who had cholecystectomy six years ago; CT scan shows a 3.5 cm pyogenic liver abscess (red arrow) with middle hepatic vein thrombosis (green arrow). Blood culture grew *Klebsiella variicola*

66.3 Clinical Presentation

The clinical presentation of PLA is non-specific; patients present with fever, right upper quadrant pain or discomfort, jaundice, nausea and vomiting, and constitutional symptoms such as malaise, loss of weight, anorexia, and lethargy [3, 11, 17, 32]. The classic triad of fever, right upper quadrant pain, and jaundice is seldom seen in patients with PLA [33]. Physical examination may demonstrate right upper quadrant tenderness (incidence of <40%), hepatomegaly, or jaundice but are similarly non-specific [34]. Differential diagnoses include cholecystitis, primary or secondary liver tumors, hepatic cysts, diverticulitis, and peptic ulcer disease. Rare though life-threatening, PLA may rupture and present as an acute abdomen with symptoms and signs suggestive of septic shock [35]. These patients require prompt resuscitation and imaging to identify the etiology of the abdominal pain to guide management.

66.4 Serum Biochemistry

Similar to the clinical presentation of PLA, the serum biochemistry of PLA is non-specific. These include leukocytosis with neutrophilia, raised C-reactive protein (CRP) and procalcitonin, hypoalbuminemia (<30 g/L), deranged liver enzymes, and hyperbilirubinemia [28, 36–39]. CRP is an acute-phase protein synthesized primarily in the liver and is stimulated by cytokine release, particularly interleukin-6, and is elevated in patients with PLA [40, 41]. CRP has also been examined to determine antibiotic treatment duration. About 70% of patients have derangement with liver enzymes but do not show a "hepatitic" nor "cholestatic" pattern [28, 36, 37, 40]. However, it has been observed that alkaline phosphatase (ALP) is commonly raised with normal serum bilirubin in two-thirds of patients with PLA [42, 43]. Tumor markers such as CA19-9 have no role in diagnosing PLA or differentiating PLA from malignant liver lesions [44].

66.5 Microbiology

PLA may be classified as monomicrobial or polymicrobial. Polymicrobial PLAs are common with mixed enteric facultative and anaerobic species [11]. Common organisms (in order of decreasing incidence) include *Klebsiella pneumoniae*, *Escherichia coli*, *Enterococcus spp*, *Streptococcus spp*, and *Staphylococcus spp*. There has been a gradual shift in microbiology from *Escherichia coli* to *Klebsiella pneumoniae* over the past three decades, especially in Asian countries [7, 8, 11]. *Klebsiella pneumoniae* has emerged to be an important cause of community and nosocomial-acquired infections globally. Isolation of monomicrobial *Klebsiella pneumoniae* should prompt evaluation for underlying colorectal malignancy [45–47]. Our policy is to recommend elective colonoscopy to all patients with PLA, and in our experience, the incidence of colorectal malignancy is low. The presence of *Staphylococcus spp* indicates hematogenous spread from skin or respiratory tract infections, which are more commonly found in immunocompromised patients [13]. Rarely, oral commensals such as *Fusobacterium nucleatum* may be present in PLA secondary to periodontal disease [21].

Negative blood cultures have been reported in 15–80% with sepsis secondary to PLA [48–51]. Cultures may be negative due to failure to adhere to sepsis guidelines, lack of advanced microbial detection techniques, and the avoidance of percutaneous aspiration or drainage in clinically improving patients (resulting in the absence of fluid cultures) [52]. In this subset of culture-negative PLA (CNPLA), empiric treatment with antibiotics and percutaneous drainage (PD) has similar outcomes to *Klebsiella pneumoniae* PLA [10]. In patients with a history of biliary interventions, polymicrobial or multi-drug resistant organisms can cause PLA, and treatment should be guided by local antibiogram and antibiotic stewardship guidance.

66.6 Radiological Imaging

There are three primary modalities of imaging for PLA: (1) ultrasonography (US), (2) CT, and (3) magnetic resonance imaging (MRI). Both US and CT imaging are sensitive in the diagnosis of PLA, with CT albeit more sensitive (US sensitivity 85% vs. CT sensitivity 95%) [53, 54]. Ultrasonographic features of PLA are variable; microabscesses (<2 cm) appear as hypoechoic nodules or ill-defined areas of distorted hepatic echogenicity [55]. Larger abscesses have variable echogenicity depending on thickened septa and debris [56, 57]. Gas-forming PLA (GFPLA) is characteristically hyperechoic [58]. The use of color doppler demonstrates the absence of central perfusion in PLA, distinguishing it from focal benign and malignant lesions. The use of contrast-enhanced US (CE-US) shows marginal wall enhancement in the arterial phase and progressive venous hypoenhancement in the portal and late phases. The most prominent feature of PLA is the lack of enhancement in liquefied necrotic areas [58, 59]. The US provides real-time imaging of the liver parenchyma and the biliary tree without radiation and is appropriate as initial abdominal imaging for patients presenting with right upper quadrant pain. An added benefit of US use is its superior sensitivity for diagnosing gallstones (US sensitivity 87% vs. CT sensitivity 60%) [60]. The use of US has been extended to the emergency department (ED), where emergency physicians utilize point-of-care US (POCUS) as first-line imaging modality to support early diagnosis of PLA due to its non-specific presentation, where the use of POCUS has been associated with a higher percentage of patients with PLA correctly diagnosed in the ED (34.4% with POCUS vs. 3.3% without POCUS) [61]. However, the accuracy of US is operator-dependent, and the diagnostic accuracy of POCUS has yet to be established.

CT scan is more widely used as the first-line radiological investigation for patients presenting with acute abdomen in our institution. It is available after office hours, provides a detailed evaluation for abdominal pain, and avoids potential delay in diagnosis and management. CT features include the typical finding of a well-defined, round lesion with peripheral rim enhancement and central hypoattenuation [55, 56]. Other features include the presence of internal septations, air-fluid levels, multiple loculations, or multifocal lesions. Characteristically but less commonly, a "double target" sign may be demonstrated, where there is an inner layer of hyperattenuation (pyogenic membrane) surrounded by an outer layer of hypoattenuation (edema of hepatic parenchyma) [56]. CT scan also aids in the diagnosis of underlying etiology. Both US and CT scans are essential for targeted percutaneous aspiration or drainage. MRI imaging is less commonly performed for the evaluation of an acute abdomen or specifically for PLA. However, MRI may be performed for further evaluation when CT imaging is equivocal for PLA versus liver malignancy. MRI features of PLA include central hypointensity on T1-weighted imaging and hyperintense signals on T2-weighted imaging [62, 63]. High-signal intensity is typically seen in diffuse-weighted imaging [64].

Other imaging forms include nuclear imaging such as technetium (^{99m}Tc) scintigraphy, and gallium scintigraphy has largely been replaced with modern-day CT and MRI imaging because of its low sensitivity of 50 to 80% [49, 65]. Nevertheless, imaging of PLA using ^{99m}Tc scintigraphy will demonstrate a focal area of decreased radiocolloid uptake, while gallium scintigraphy will demonstrate avid uptake in PLA [65, 66]. Imaging helps not only in diagnosis but also in guiding management. We consider PLA smaller than 4 cm as small and more than 10 cm as giant PLA [9].

66.7 Initial Management

The management of PLA involves supportive therapy to stabilize the patient and definitive management for sepsis and source control. In acute settings, patients should be managed as per the Surviving Sepsis guidelines [67]. Supportive measures such as fluid resuscitation, administration of oxygen, and analgesia should be administered. Empiric antibiotics should be administered after obtaining microbiology samples. There are three main methods of controlling the infection in PLA: (1) Antibiotics, (2) Percutaneous aspiration or drainage, and (3) Surgical drainage. Surgical drainage is usually reserved for patients who have failed both antibiotics and PD and giant PLAs [38, 68].

66.7.1 Antibiotics

Parenteral antibiotics are essential in the management of PLA [69]. The choice of antibiotic is guided by the microbiology of PLA and should cover *Streptococcus spp*, enteric gram-negative bacilli, and anaerobes. Typical regimens include the use of the third-generation cephalosporin (intravenous ceftriaxone 2 g once a day) and metronidazole (oral metronidazole 400 mg every 12 hours) [68]. The local policy is to administer intravenous amoxicillin-clavulanic acid and a stat dose of gentamicin based on the local antibiogram. This will be reviewed based on culture and sensitivity results. In patients with a history of anaphylaxis to penicillin, ciprofloxacin may be used as an alternative to cephalosporins.

Duration of parenteral antibiotics use, or the conversion from parenteral to oral antibiotics use is usually guided by the clinical and radiological response. It has been reported that the use of oral antibiotics upon discharge is an independent predictor of 30-day readmission (30-day readmission incidence 39.6% for oral antibiotics vs. 17.6% for parenteral antibiotics) [70]. Biomarkers have been used to guide antibiotic therapy in PLA. CRP serves as a useful biomarker in the diagnosis of PLA and a guide for response to treatment. Weekly trending of CRP may predict the response to antibiotic therapy trending [71]. The synthesis of CRP starts very rapidly after the onset of PLA, with serum concentration increasing beyond the normal range by about 6 hours and peaking around 48 hours if the septic process is under control. A CRP ratio (defined as the CRP value done at the particular week compared to the CRP value at week 1 of diagnosis) of ≤ 0.278 at week 3 is a marker of the adequacy of antibiotic therapy of 5 weeks or less (sensitivity 0.786; specificity 0.714) [72]. CRP ratio > 0.57 at week three may predict a higher risk of mortality or possibility of treatment failure. These results need to be validated. Locally, if the patient is hemodynamically stable and clinically improving, we switch to oral formulations early, and this helps reduce hospital length of stay. In exceptional situations, outpatient parenteral antibiotic therapy is considered after consultation with infectious disease specialty.

66.7.2 Percutaneous Aspiration

Locally, percutaneous aspiration, also known as needle aspiration, is rarely or never performed due to its inferior clinical outcomes to PD, high failure rate, and need for repeated percutaneous aspiration or eventual PD. A recent meta-analysis by Cai et al., which reviewed 306 patients in five randomized controlled trials, demonstrated a superior success rate of 96.1% (n = 147/153) in PD as compared to 77.8% (n = 119/153) in percutaneous aspiration (p = 0.041) [73]. However, multiple, intermittent percutaneous aspiration is worth consideration in settings with limited resources: a randomized trial by Yu et al. demonstrated comparable success rates between intermittent percutaneous aspiration and PD [74]. A small PLA may be managed with antibiotics and percutaneous aspiration.

66.7.3 Percutaneous Drainage (PD)

Percutaneous aspiration and drainage achieve source control and provides fluid for microbial isolation. PD is more inconvenient for patients but provides thorough source control, especially in large or multiseptated PLA patients. Studies have shown that combination therapy with PD may be superior to antibiotics alone for certain groups of patients [68]: (1) Size of abscess >4 cm (2) clinical and radiological features suggestive of impending perforation or (3) persistent fever after 48–72 hours of medical treatment. It is also recommended for elderly patients (≥ 55 years old) and patients with PLA based on an underlying malignancy to undergo early PD [75]. Prompt PD in other pathologies such as acute cholecystitis have also been shown to improve survival, with clinical resolution of sepsis within 48 hours of drainage [76]. There is debate on optimal size cut-off for considering PD. Using mathematical principles of the volume of a sphere, we have proposed a cut-off of 4 cm for drainage of PLA [8]. This is also validated in the drainage of appendix abscess [77].

Giant PLAs are less common, and surgical intervention may be considered first-line management in various institutions as size criteria are a predictor of PD failure. There is a paucity of studies comparing PD and surgical drainage in giant PLAs because of its low incidence (approximately 10%) [38]. It is essential to ensure PD's success as failure may result in uncontrolled sepsis, rupture, or eventual mortality. High-risk patients with multiple co-morbidities may require SD. Locally, we have demonstrated PD's safety in giant PLA with a reported success (defined as PD without needing secondary intervention) of 92.3% and an overall morbidity of 25% in 39 patients [9]. PD's high success is made possible by implementing a "liver abscess care bundle": integration of surgical and nursing care, interventional radiology, and microbiology teams in addition to standard treatment protocols such as initiation of broad-spectrum parenteral antibiotics, early imaging for diagnosis confirmation, obtaining tissue culture or blood culture [38]. Surgical and nursing care involves rigorous drain management with reinforcement of drain patency, flushing and negative pressure suction, good hepatobiliary nurse practitioner support, and caregiver training. Interventional radiology support involves the availability of services on a 24-hour basis, large-bore drains, and a policy of proactive drain review. Microbiology services involve infectious disease physician consults with appropriate local antibiotic stewardship program and ease of transition to outpatient antibiotic therapy.

66.7.4 Surgical Drainage (SD)

SD is traditionally reserved for PLAs refractory to medical therapy, multiloculated PLA, giant PLA, and free rupture of the abscess. It was initially shown to be superior to PD for larger PLAs. A study by Bertel et al. in 1986 on 39 patients with PLAs >5 cm demonstrated similar morbidity between both methods, but SD resulted in fewer secondary procedures and had higher resolution rates [78]. Another study by Tan et al., which reviewed 80 patients (36 patients PD, 44 patients SD) with PLA >5 cm demonstrated superior clinical outcomes for SD in terms of treatment success, need for secondary procedures, and length of hospitalization stay, with comparable morbidity and mortality [36]. A recent randomized controlled trial by Ali et al. in 2019 on 238 patients (119 with PD, 119 with SD) with PLA >5 cm demonstrated an 85% success rate in SD, while 70% success rate in PD [79]. A subgroup analysis of PLA >10 cm also demonstrated superior success of SD over PD (n = 78/89 (85.7%) vs n = 55/77 (71.4%), p = 0.0091). In all of the studies mentioned above, which demonstrate superior outcomes SD may confer, the multiloculated abscess was present in 80% of all the cases in both studies by Tan et al. and Ali et al. [36, 79]. Multiloculation is known to be a predictor of PD failure as compartmentalization of the abscess leads to suboptimal drainage and could have been a confounding factor for superior results observed in SD [80]. The study by Ahmed et al., which demonstrated a 92.3% success rate in giant PLAs, observed multiloculated abscesses in only 55% of the patients [9]. It is still unclear whether a size criterion of >10 cm alone is an absolute contraindication for PD. Locally, the only absolute indication for surgery is free rupture. SD, however, remains relevant despite the advantages conferred by PD. SD should still be considered first-line management for patients with concomitant intra-abdominal pathology, such as acute cholecystitis, which permits cholecystectomy and concomitant drainage of PLA for source control in sepsis. In special circumstances such as PLA following liver transplantation, the initial management stays the same: resuscitation, parenteral antibiotics, and PD. However, PLA, which does not respond to conservative measures, or those complicated by hepatic artery thrombosis and ischemic cholangiopathy, should undergo re-transplantation [31].

66.7.5 Laparoscopic Drainage (LD)

LD is an alternative to open surgical drainage. However, there is a paucity of evidence on its safety and efficacy. A review by Aydin et al. in 2010 demonstrated a mean success of 90.5% (range 85–100%) in 53 cases of laparoscopically treated abscess, with nil open conversion [81]. Benefits of LD compared to open drainage include shorter operating time, shorter length of hospitalization stay, and fewer surgical site infections [82]. A local study by Tan et al. in 2013 on 85 patients (67 PD, 18 LD) demonstrated higher failure rates in PD than LD (n = 27/67 (40.3%), n = 2/18 (11.1%), p = 0.020) with a mean abscess size of 7.6 ± 2.4 cm and 7.6 ± 3.3 cm in the PD and LD groups respectively [83]. However, multiloculation was present in >94% of the abscesses, which may have been a confounding factor for higher PD failure rates. Minimally-invasive video-assisted debridement has also been reported to be safe and feasible for persistent PLAs refractory to medical therapy and PD. A study by Klink et al. on ten patients with a median abscess size of 7.8 cm (range 4.0–11.5 cm) demonstrated no mortality or any significant complications [84].

66.7.6 Endoscopic Ultrasound (EUS)-guided Drainage

EUS-guided drainage is an alternative to traditional PD or surgery. Advances in EUS techniques in recent years place it in a more favorable position compared to surgical intervention. EUS-guided drainage of PLA was first described by Seewald et al. in 2005 [85]. It allows access to PLA within the left or central segments of the liver. EUS guidance also allows clear visualization of PLAs, minimizing inadvertent complications. The technical success and clinical success of EUS-guided drainage of PLA have been reported to be 88.9–100% and 71.4–100%, respectively [86]. EUS-guided drainage requires a high level of technical expertise, and the left liver lobe is challenging to access. Nevertheless, it is a promising technique that may be considered an alternative to SD or LD or where PD is contraindicated.

66.8 Subsequent Management

Management following the acute episode of PLA is primarily determined by underlying etiology. Patients with PLA secondary to cholelithiasis or acute cholecystitis who did not have index admission cholecystectomy should receive interval cholecystectomy to reduce the incidence of recurrent biliary events [87]. Elective screening colonoscopy should be offered to patients with PLA, especially in the subgroup of patients with KPPLA, cryptogenic PLA, or Eastern Asian origin, to rule out colorectal cancer. Colorectal cancer-related PLA is more commonly reported in Eastern Asia (80%), and *Klebsiella pneumoniae* is the most common pathogen [88]. Colonoscopy also detects diverticular disease and adenomatous polyps. Cryptogenic PLA is also associated with a seven-fold risk of having colorectal cancer [89]. Patients with PLA post-liver transplantation warrant rigorous follow-up; a one-year recurrence of up to 42.9% is reported following the initial episode [90]. Patients with recurrent PLA and ischemic cholangiopathy should consider early re-transplantation, with higher morbidity and mortality rates described in late re-transplantations [91].

66.9 Prognosis

Clinical outcomes of PLA are determined by an interplay of both disease factors and patient factors [75]. Disease factors include size, the distance of abscess to liver capsule [92], number of abscesses, presence of multiple loculations [93], and presence of gas formation [92, 94]. Patient factor includes concomitant pathologies and underlying co-morbidities. Studies have shown that underlying hypertension, hyperbilirubinemia, Eastern Cooperative Oncology Group (ECOG) performance status ≥ 2, and Acute Physiology and Chronic Health Evaluation (APACHE) II score ≥ 15 predicts the likelihood of failure of PD [75, 95, 96]. APACHE II ≥ 15 additionally predicts an increased risk of in-hospital mortality [97]. Major complications of PLA include free intraperitoneal rupture and invasion of adjacent structures. Risk factors for rupture include size more than 6 cm, liver cirrhosis, and gas presence [98].

66.9.1 Size of abscess

Size is a known imaging biomarker for prognostication of PLA. PLA can be classified by size into small, large, or giant. However, there is no clear consensus on the definition of a large or giant PLA, with the varying definition used in literature; for this review, a giant PLA is defined as >10 cm. A larger size is associated with a higher risk of failure of medical management and PD. A size of >6 cm also bears a higher risk of rupture (odds ratio 10.9) [98], while a size of >7.3 cm on CT scan has been reported to predict failure of PD (area under curve 0.72) [92].

66.9.2 Presence of Gas Formation

Gas formation occurs in 7–24% of PLA, which is traditionally associated with high mortality [99]. A qualitative review of retrospective studies conducted on PLA demonstrated a significantly higher mean mortality of 30.3% in GFPLA than 9% in non-GFPLA [94]. Gas formation is also associated with larger abscesses [100]. Integrating multimodal "liver abscess care bundle" in clinical practice, many authors have reported comparable morbidity and mortality regardless of the presence of gas formation [8, 9, 51, 94]. However, there is a paucity of evidence that compares clinical outcomes of PD versus SD based on gas formation alone.

66.9.3 Multiloculated abscess

Multiloculated abscess predicts failure of medical treatment and PD as it is not feasible to completely drain multiple locules with a single drain [42]. Multiloculated abscesses are usually managed by SD. However, multiloculated PLA is not an absolute contraindication for PD. Particular circumstances such as the presence of small and superficial abscesses may permit safe PD. A study by Liu et al. on 109 patients demonstrated no statistically significant difference in the success of PD and length of hospitalization stay between single and multiple abscesses, as well as single multiloculated and multiple multiloculated abscesses [101].

66.9.4 Microbiology

It is traditionally believed that PLAs secondary to *Escherichia coli* confers inferior outcomes compared to *Klebsiella pneumoniae* [102]. Locally, outcomes between *Escherichia coli* PLA and *Klebsiella pneumoniae* PLA (KPPLA) are reported to be comparable in morbidity and mortality with the implementation of multimodal "liver abscess care bundle" [8]. However, *Klebsiella pneumoniae* remains a significant cause of endophthalmitis, with an estimated incidence of 1 in 22 in a recent meta-analysis [103]. Endogenous endophthalmitis has also been reported in patients (n = 4/37, 16.3%) without *Klebsiella pneumoniae* bacteremia. Ophthalmological screening should be conducted in KPPLA with the timely institution of locally directed therapy to improve visual outcomes [103].

66.9.5 Unique Situation: Liver Transplantation

Liver transplantation complicated by PLA confers a poor prognosis with a high recurrence rate of up to 42.9% [90]. High mortality ranging from 10–40% has also been reported in various studies [104, 105]. It is therefore prudent for prompt diagnosis and management of PLA in this subgroup of patients. Failure of conservative management should warrant early surgical intervention with consideration of early re-transplantation [91].

66.10 Conclusion

PLA is a major hepatobiliary infection with an estimated 10–40% mortality despite advancements in healthcare. A high clinical index of suspicion and early imaging is required for prompt diagnosis of PLA, followed by the institution of resuscitation measures, initiation of parenteral antibiotics, and PD. Surgical drainage is usually reserved for patients who have failed both antibiotics and PD, free rupture, multiloculated abscess, or giant PLA. The prognosis of PLA is determined by an interplay of both disease factors and patient factors. Institutions should consider adopting the "liver abscess care bundle" and provide multimodal care to improve patient outcomes.

References

1. Altemeier W, Culbertson W, Fullen W, Shook CD. Intra-abdominal abscesses. Am J Surg. 1973;125(1):70–9.
2. Tian LT, Yao K, Zhang XY, Zhang ZD, Liang YJ, Yin DL, Lee L, Jiang HC, Liu LX. Liver abscesses in adult patients with and without diabetes mellitus: an analysis of the clinical characteristics, features of the causative pathogens, outcomes and predictors of fatality: a report based on a large population, retrospective study in China. Clin Microbiol Infect. 2012;18(9):E314–30. https://doi.org/10.1111/j.1469-0691.2012.03912.x.
3. Ochsner A, DeBakey M, Murray S. Pyogenic abscess of the liver: II. An analysis of forty-seven cases with review of the literature. Am J Surg. 1938;40(1):292–319.
4. Huang S-F, Ko C-W, Chang C-S, Chen G-H. Liver abscess formation after transarterial chemoembolization for malignant hepatic tumor. Hepato-Gastroenterology. 2003;50(52):1115–8.
5. Iida H, Aihara T, Ikuta S, Yamanaka N. Risk of abscess formation after liver tumor radiofrequency ablation: a review of 8 cases wtih a history of enterobiliary anastomosis. Hepato-Gastroenterology. 2014;61(135):1867–70.
6. Danson Y, Yuan TM, Shelat VG. Pyogenic liver abscess. Abdominal sepsis. Cham: Springer; 2018. p. 83–93.
7. Branum GD, Tyson GS, Branum MA, Meyers WC, Hepatic abscess. Changes in etiology, diagnosis, and management. Ann Surg. 1990;212(6):655.
8. Shelat VG, Chia CLK, Yeo CSW, Qiao W, Woon W, Junnarkar SP. Pyogenic liver abscess: does *Escherichia coli* cause more adverse outcomes than klebsiella pneumoniae? World J Surg. 2015;39(10):2535–42. https://doi.org/10.1007/s00268-015-3126-1.
9. Ahmed S, Chia CLK, Junnarkar SP, Woon W, Shelat VG. Percutaneous drainage for giant pyogenic liver abscess—is it safe and sufficient? Am J Surg. 2016;211(1):95–101. https://doi.org/10.1016/j.amjsurg.2015.03.002.
10. Shelat VG, Wang Q, Chia CL, Wang Z, Low JK, Woon WW. Patients with culture negative pyogenic liver abscess have the same outcomes compared to those with Klebsiella pneumoniae pyogenic liver abscess. Hepatobiliary Pancreat Dis Int. 2016;15(5):504–11. https://doi.org/10.1016/s1499-3872(16)60127-3.
11. Huang C-J, Pitt HA, Lipsett PA, Osterman FAJ, Lillemoe KD, Cameron JL, Zuidema GD. Pyogenic hepatic abscess: changing trends over 42 years. Ann Surg. 1996;223(5):600–9.
12. Wang YP, Liu CJ, Chen TJ, Lin YT, Fung CP. Proton pump inhibitor use significantly increases the risk of cryptogenic liver abscess: a population-based study. Aliment Pharmacol Ther. 2015;41(11):1175–81.
13. Zhang W, Yu H, Luo N, Hu Z. Clinical characteristics and treatment outcomes in human immunodeficiency virus (HIV)-infected patients with liver abscess: a retrospective study of 53 patients. Med Sci Monit. 2020;26:e923761.
14. Mølle I, Thulstrup A, Vilstrup H, Sørensen H. Increased risk and case fatality rate of pyogenic liver abscess in patients with liver cirrhosis: a nationwide study in Denmark. Gut. 2001;48(2):260–3.
15. Morii K, Kashihara A, Miura S, Okuhin H, Watanabe T, Sato S, Uesaka K, Yuasa S. Successful hepatectomy for intraperitoneal rupture of pyogenic liver abscess caused by Klebsiella pneumoniae. Clin J Gastroenterol. 2012;5(2):136–40.
16. Kaplan GG, Gregson DB, Laupland KB. Population-based study of the epidemiology of and the risk factors for pyogenic liver abscess. Clin Gastroenterol Hepatol. 2004;2(11):1032–8.
17. Lardière-Deguelte S, Ragot E, Amroun K, Piardi T, Dokmak S, Bruno O, Appere F, Sibert A, Hoeffel C, Sommacale D, Kianmanesh R. Hepatic abscess: diagnosis and management. J Visc Surg. 2015;152(4):231–43. https://doi.org/10.1016/j.jviscsurg.2015.01.013.
18. Murarka S, Pranav F, Dandavate V. Pyogenic liver abscess secondary to disseminated streptococcus anginosus from sigmoid diverticulitis. J Global Infect Dis. 2011;3(1):79.
19. Lim HE, Cheong HJ, Woo HJ, Kim WJ, Kim MJ, Lee CH, Park SC. Pylephlebitis associated with appendicitis. Korean J Intern Med. 1999;14(1):73.
20. Seeto RK, Rockey DC. Pyogenic liver abscess changes in etiology, management, and outcome. Medicine. 1996;75(2):99–113.
21. Collins L, Diamond T. Fusobacterium nucleatum causing a pyogenic liver abscess: a rare complication of periodontal disease that occurred during the COVID-19 pandemic. BMJ Case Reports CP. 2021;14(1):e240080.
22. Lin Y-T, Liu C-J, Chen T-J, Chen T-L, Yeh Y-C, Wu H-S, Tseng C-P, Wang F-D, Tzeng C-H, Fung C-P. Pyogenic liver abscess as the initial manifestation of underlying hepatocellular carcinoma. Am J Med. 2011;124(12):1158–64.
23. Yeh T-S, Jan Y-Y, Jeng L-B, Chen T-C, Hwang T-L, Chen M-F. Hepatocellular carcinoma presenting as pyogenic liver abscess: characteristics, diagnosis, and management. Rev Infect Dis. 1998;26(5):1224–6.

24. Su X-F, Li N, Chen X-F, Zhang L, Yan M. Incidence and risk factors for liver abscess after thermal ablation of liver neoplasm. Hepat Mon. 2016;16(7):e34588. https://doi.org/10.5812/hepatmon.34588.
25. Shin JU, Kim KM, Shin SW, Min SY, Park SU, Sinn DH, Gwak GY, Choi MS, Lee JH, Paik SW. A prediction model for liver abscess developing after transarterial chemoembolization in patients with hepatocellular carcinoma. Dig Liver Dis. 2014;46(9):813–7.
26. Elias D, Di Pietrantonio D, Gachot B, Menegon P, Hakime A, De Baere T. Liver abscess after radiofrequency ablation of tumors in patients with a biliary tract procedure. Gastroenterol Clin Biol. 2006;30(6–7):823–7.
27. Yoshihara S, Yamana H, Akahane M, Kishimoto M, Nishioka Y, Noda T, Matsui H, Fushimi K, Yasunaga H, Kasahara K, Imamura T. Association between prophylactic antibiotic use for transarterial chemoembolization and occurrence of liver abscess: a retrospective cohort study. Clin Microbiol Infect. 2021;27(10):1514.e5–1514.e10. https://doi.org/10.1016/j.cmi.2021.01.014.
28. Wong W-M, Wong BCY, Hui CK, Ng M, Lai KC, Tso WK, Lam SK, Lai CL. Pyogenic liver abscess: retrospective analysis of 80 cases over a 10-year period. J Gastroenterol Hepatol. 2002;17(9):1001–7. https://doi.org/10.1046/j.1440-1746.2002.02787.x.
29. Zhang KK, Mayody M, Shah RP, Vakiani E, Getrajdman GI, Brody LA, Solomon SB. Asymptomatic liver abscesses mimicking metastases in patients after Whipple surgery: infectious complications following percutaneous biopsy—a report of two cases. Case Rep Hepatol. 2012;2012:817314. https://doi.org/10.1155/2012/817314.
30. Ch'ng JK, Ng SY, Goh BKP. An unusual cause of sepsis after laparoscopic cholecystectomy. Gastroenterology. 2012;143(6):e1–2. https://doi.org/10.1053/j.gastro.2012.05.040.
31. Justo I, Jiménez-Romero C, Manrique A, Caso O, Calvo J, Cambra F, Marcacuzco A. Management and outcome of liver abscesses after liver transplantation. World J Surg. 2018;42(10):3341–9. https://doi.org/10.1007/s00268-018-4622-x.
32. Alkofer B, Dufay C, Parienti JJ, Lepennec V, Dargere S, Chiche L. Are pyogenic liver abscesses still a surgical concern? A Western experience. HPB Surg. 2012;2012:316013. https://doi.org/10.1155/2012/316013.
33. Berg GM, Vasquez DG, Hale LS, Nyberg SM, Moran DA. Evaluation of process variations in noncompliance in the implementation of evidence-based sepsis care. J Healthc Qual. 2013;35(1):60–9.
34. Rubin RH, Swartz MN, Malt R. Hepatic abscess: changes in clinical, bacteriologic and therapeutic aspects. Am J Med. 1974;57(4):601–10. https://doi.org/10.1016/0002-9343(74)90012-6.
35. Chou F-F, Sheen-Chen S-M, Lee T-Y. Rupture of pyogenic liver abscess. Am J Gastroenterol. 1995;90(5):767–70.
36. Tan Y-M, Chung AY-F, Chow PK-H, Cheow P-C, Wong W-K, Ooi LL, Soo K-C. An appraisal of surgical and percutaneous drainage for pyogenic liver abscesses larger than 5 cm. Ann Surg. 2005;241(3):485–90. https://doi.org/10.1097/01.sla.0000154265.14006.47.
37. Foo N-P, Chen K-T, Lin H-J, Guo H-R. Characteristics of pyogenic liver abscess patients with and without diabetes mellitus. Am J Gastroenterol. 2010;105(2):328.
38. Alvarez Pérez JA, González JJ, Baldonedo RF, Sanz L, Carreño G, Junco A, Rodríguez JI, Martínez MaD, Jorge JI. Clinical course, treatment, and multivariate analysis of risk factors for pyogenic liver abscess. Am J Surg. 2001;181(2):177–86. https://doi.org/10.1016/S0002-9610(00)00564-X.
39. Li W, Chen H, Wu S, Peng J. A comparison of pyogenic liver abscess in patients with or without diabetes: a retrospective study of 246 cases. BMC Gastroenterol. 2018;18(1):144. https://doi.org/10.1186/s12876-018-0875-y.
40. Pang TCY, Fung T, Samra J, Hugh TJ, Smith RC. Pyogenic liver abscess: an audit of 10 years' experience. World J Gastroenterol. 2011;17(12):1622–30. https://doi.org/10.3748/wjg.v17.i12.1622.
41. Chan KS, Chen CM, Cheng KC, Hou CC, Lin HJ, Yu WL. Pyogenic liver abscess: a retrospective analysis of 107 patients during a 3-year period. Jpn J Infect Dis. 2005;58(6):366–8.
42. Liew KV, Lau TC, Ho CH, Cheng TK, Ong YS, Chia SC, Tan CC. Pyogenic liver abscess - a tropical centre's experience in management with review of current literature. Singap Med J. 2000;41(10):489–92.
43. Stain SC, Yellin AE, Donovan AJ, Brien HW. Pyogenic liver abscess: modern treatment. Arch Surg. 1991;126(8):991–6. https://doi.org/10.1001/archsurg.1991.01410320077010.
44. Lee T, Teng TZJ, Shelat VG. Carbohydrate antigen 19-9 - tumor marker: past, present, and future. World J Gastrointest Surg. 2020;12(12):468–90. https://doi.org/10.4240/wjgs.v12.i12.468.
45. Kao WY, Hwang CY, Chang YT, Su CW, Hou MC, Lin HC, Lee FY, Lee SD, Wu JC. Cancer risk in patients with pyogenic liver abscess: a nationwide cohort study. Aliment Pharmacol Ther. 2012;36(5):467–76.
46. Huang WK, Chang JC, See LC, Tu HT, Chen JS, Liaw CC, Lin YC, Yang TS. Higher rate of colorectal cancer among patients with pyogenic liver abscess with Klebsiella pneumoniae than those without: an 11-year follow-up study. Color Dis. 2012;14(12):e794–801.
47. Lai HC, Lin CC, Cheng KS, Kao JT, Chou JW, Peng CY, Lai SW, Chen PC, Sung FC. Increased incidence of gastrointestinal cancers among patients with pyogenic liver abscess: a population-based cohort study. Gastroenterology. 2014;146(1):129–137.e121.
48. Meddings L, Myers RP, Hubbard J, Shaheen AA, Laupland KB, Dixon E, Coffin C, Kaplan GG. A population-based study of pyogenic liver abscesses in the United States: incidence, mortality, and temporal trends. Am J Gastroenterol. 2010;105(1):117.
49. Zibari GB, Maguire S, Aultman DF, McMillan RW, McDonald JC. Pyogenic liver abscess. Surg Infect. 2000;1(1):15–21.
50. Mangukiya DO, Darshan JR, Kanani VK, Gupta ST. A prospective series case study of pyogenic liver abscess: recent trends in etiology and management. Indian J Surg. 2012;74(5):385–90.
51. Chan KS, Thng CB, Chan Y-H, Shelat VG. Outcomes of gas-forming pyogenic liver abscess are comparable to non-gas-forming pyogenic liver abscess in the era of multimodal care: a propensity score matched study. Surg Infect. 2020;21(10):884–90.
52. Pletz MW, Wellinghausen N, Welte T. Will polymerase chain reaction (PCR)-based diagnostics improve outcome in septic patients? A clinical view. Intensive Care Med. 2011;37(7):1069–76.
53. Halvorsen RA, Korobkin M, Foster WL, Silverman PM, Thompson WM. The variable CT appearance of hepatic abscesses. AJR Am J Roentgenol. 1984;142(5):941–6. https://doi.org/10.2214/ajr.142.5.941.
54. Lin AC, Yeh D, Hsu Y, Wu C, Chang H, Jang T, Huang C. Diagnosis of pyogenic liver abscess by abdominal ultrasonography in the emergency department. Emerg Med J. 2009;26(4):273–5.
55. Mortelé KJ, Segatto E, Ros PR. The infected liver: radiologic-pathologic correlation. Radiographics. 2004;24(4):937–55.
56. Bächler P, Baladron MJ, Menias C, Beddings I, Loch R, Zalaquett E, Vargas M, Connolly S, Bhalla S, Huete Á. Multimodality imaging of liver infections: differential diagnosis and potential pitfalls. Radiographics. 2016;36(4):1001–23.
57. Benedetti NJ, Desser TS, Jeffrey RB. Imaging of Hepatic infections. Ultrasound Q. 2008;24(4):267–78. https://doi.org/10.1097/RUQ.0b013e31818e5981.

58. Kuligowska E, Connors SK, Shapiro JH. Liver abscess: sonography in diagnosis and treatment. Am J Roentgenol. 1982;138(2):253–7. https://doi.org/10.2214/ajr.138.2.253.
59. Chen L-D, Xu H-X, Xie X-Y, Xie X-H, Xu Z-F, Liu G-J, Wang Z, Lin M-X, Lu M-D. Intrahepatic cholangiocarcinoma and hepatocellular carcinoma: differential diagnosis with contrast-enhanced ultrasound. Eur Radiol. 2010;20(3):743–53.
60. Fagenholz PJ, Fuentes E, Kaafarani H, Cropano C, King D, de Moya M, Butler K, Velmahos G, Chang Y, Yeh DD. Computed tomography is more sensitive than ultrasound for the diagnosis of acute cholecystitis. Surg Infect. 2015;16(5):509–12.
61. Chia DWJ, Kuan WS, Ho WH, Sim TB, Chua MT. Early predictors for the diagnosis of liver abscess in the emergency department. Intern Emerg Med. 2019;14(5):783–91. https://doi.org/10.1007/s11739-019-02061-z.
62. Mendez RJ, Schiebler ML, Outwater EK, Kressel HY. Hepatic abscesses: MR imaging findings. Radiology. 1994;190(2):431–6.
63. Balci NC, Semelka RC, Noone TC, Siegelman ES, de Beeck BO, Brown JJ, Lee M-G. Pyogenic hepatic abscesses: MRI findings on T1- and T2-weighted and serial gadolinium-enhanced gradient-echo images. J Magn Reson Imaging. 1999;9(2):285–90. https://doi.org/10.1002/(SICI)1522-2586(199902)9:2<285::AID-JMRI20>3.0.CO;2-S.
64. Chan J, Tsui E, Luk S, Fung A, Yuen M, Szeto M, Cheung Y, Wong K. Diffusion-weighted MR imaging of the liver: distinguishing hepatic abscess from cystic or necrotic tumor. Abdom Imaging. 2001;26(2):161–5.
65. Rubinson HA, Isikoff M, Hill M. Diagnostic imaging of hepatic abscesses: a retrospective analysis. Am J Roentgenol. 1980;135(4):735–45.
66. Chauhan U, Prabhu SM, Shetty GS, Solanki RS, Udiya AK, Singh A. Emphysematous hepatitis – a fatal infection in diabetic patients: case report. Clin Res Hepatol Gastroenterol. 2012;36(6):e114–6. https://doi.org/10.1016/j.clinre.2012.05.018.
67. Singer M, Deutschman CS, Seymour CW, Shankar-Hari M, Annane D, Bauer M, Bellomo R, Bernard GR, Chiche J-D, Coopersmith CM, Hotchkiss RS, Levy MM, Marshall JC, Martin GS, Opal SM, Rubenfeld GD, van der Poll T, Vincent J-L, Angus DC. The third international consensus definitions for sepsis and septic shock (Sepsis-3). JAMA. 2016;315(8):801–10. https://doi.org/10.1001/jama.2016.0287.
68. Heneghan HM, Healy NA, Martin ST, Ryan RS, Nolan N, Traynor O, Waldron R. Modern management of pyogenic hepatic abscess: a case series and review of the literature. BMC Res Notes. 2011;4(1):80. https://doi.org/10.1186/1756-0500-4-80.
69. Sartelli M, Weber DG, Ruppé E, Bassetti M, Wright BJ, Ansaloni L, Catena F, Coccolini F, Abu-Zidan FM, Coimbra R, Moore EE, Moore FA, Maier RV, De Waele JJ, Kirkpatrick AW, Griffiths EA, Eckmann C, Brink AJ, Mazuski JE, May AK, Sawyer RG, Mertz D, Montravers P, Kumar A, Roberts JA, Vincent J-L, Watkins RR, Lowman W, Spellberg B, Abbott IJ, Adesunkanmi AK, Al-Dahir S, Al-Hasan MN, Agresta F, Althani AA, Ansari S, Ansumana R, Augustin G, Bala M, Balogh ZJ, Baraket O, Bhangu A, Beltrán MA, Bernhard M, Biffl WL, Boermeester MA, Brecher SM, Cherry-Bukowiec JR, Buyne OR, Cainzos MA, Cairns KA, Camacho-Ortiz A, Chandy SJ, Che Jusoh A, Chichom-Mefire A, Colijn C, Corcione F, Cui Y, Curcio D, Delibegovic S, Demetrashvili Z, De Simone B, Dhingra S, Diaz JJ, Di Carlo I, Dillip A, Di Saverio S, Doyle MP, Dorj G, Dogjani A, Dupont H, Eachempati SR, Enani MA, Egiev VN, Elmangory MM, Ferrada P, Fitchett JR, Fraga GP, Guessennd N, Giamarellou H, Ghnnam W, Gkiokas G, Goldberg SR, Gomes CA, Gomi H, Guzmán-Blanco M, Haque M, Hansen S, Hecker A, Heizmann WR, Herzog T, Hodonou AM, Hong S-K, Kafka-Ritsch R, Kaplan LJ, Kapoor G, Karamarkovic A, Kees MG, Kenig J, Kiguba R, Kim PK, Kluger Y, Khokha V, Koike K, Kok KYY, Kong V, Knox MC, Inaba K, Isik A, Iskandar K, Ivatury RR, Labbate M, Labricciosa FM, Laterre P-F, Latifi R, Lee JG, Lee YR, Leone M, Leppaniemi A, Li Y, Liang SY, Loho T, Maegele M, Malama S, Marei HE, Martin-Loeches I, Marwah S, Massele A, McFarlane M, Melo RB, Negoi I, Nicolau DP, Nord CE, Ofori-Asenso R, Omari AH, Ordonez CA, Ouadii M, Pereira Júnior GA, Piazza D, Pupelis G, Rawson TM, Rems M, Rizoli S, Rocha C, Sakakhushev B, Sanchez-Garcia M, Sato N, Segovia Lohse HA, Sganga G, Siribumrungwong B, Shelat VG, Soreide K, Soto R, Talving P, Tilsed JV, Timsit J-F, Trueba G, Trung NT, Ulrych J, van Goor H, Vereczkei A, Vohra RS, Wani I, Uhl W, Xiao Y, Yuan K-C, Zachariah SK, Zahar J-R, Zakrison TL, Corcione A, Melotti RM, Viscoli C, Viale P. Antimicrobials: a global alliance for optimizing their rational use in intra-abdominal infections (AGORA). World J Emerg Surg. 2016;11(1):33. https://doi.org/10.1186/s13017-016-0089-y.
70. Giangiuli SE, Mueller SW, Jeffres MN. Transition to oral versus continued intravenous antibiotics for patients with pyogenic liver abscesses: a retrospective analysis. Pharmacotherapy. 2019;39(7):734–40. https://doi.org/10.1002/phar.2296.
71. Cox ML, Rudd AG, Gallimore R, Hodkinson HM, Pepys MB. Real-time measurement of serum C-reactive protein in the management of infection in the elderly. Age Ageing. 1986;15(5):257–66. https://doi.org/10.1093/ageing/15.5.257.
72. Law S-T, Li KK. Role of C-reactive protein in response-guided therapy of pyogenic liver abscess. Eur J Gastroenterol Hepatol. 2014;26(2):179–86. https://doi.org/10.1097/MEG.0b013e328365a3b7.
73. Cai Y-L, Xiong X-Z, Lu J, Cheng Y, Yang C, Lin Y-X, Zhang J, Cheng N-S. Percutaneous needle aspiration versus catheter drainage in the management of liver abscess: a systematic review and meta-analysis. HPB. 2015;17(3):195–201. https://doi.org/10.1111/hpb.12332.
74. Yu SCH, Ho SSM, Lau WY, Yeung DTK, Yuen EHY, Lee PSF, Metreweli C. Treatment of pyogenic liver abscess: prospective randomized comparison of catheter drainage and needle aspiration. Hepatology. 2004;39(4):932–8. https://doi.org/10.1002/hep.20133.
75. Lo JZW, Leow JJJ, Ng PLF, Lee HQ, Mohd Noor NA, Low JK, Junnarkar SP, Woon WWL. Predictors of therapy failure in a series of 741 adult pyogenic liver abscesses. J Hepatobiliary Pancreat Sci. 2015;22(2):156–65. https://doi.org/10.1002/jhbp.174.
76. Yeo CSW, Tay VWY, Low JK, Woon WWL, Punamiya SJ, Shelat VG. Outcomes of percutaneous cholecystostomy and predictors of eventual cholecystectomy. J Hepatobiliary Pancreat Sci. 2016;23(1):65–73. https://doi.org/10.1002/jhbp.304.
77. Shelat VG. Letter regarding: "intra-abdominal abscess after appendectomy-are drains necessary in all patients?". J Surg Res. 2020;256:700. https://doi.org/10.1016/j.jss.2020.07.080.
78. Bertel CK, van Heerden JA, Sheedy PF II. Treatment of pyogenic hepatic abscesses: surgical vs percutaneous drainage. Arch Surg. 1986;121(5):554–8. https://doi.org/10.1001/archsurg.1986.01400050072009.
79. Ali M, Imran A, Ismail M, Khan S, Ibrahim M. Comparison of effectiveness of open drainage and percutaneous needle drainage of pyogenic liver abscess. Pak J Surg. 2019;35(2):125–31.
80. Chou FF, Sheen-Chen SM, Chen YS, Chen MC, Chen FC, Tai DI. Prognostic factors for pyogenic abscess of the liver. J Am Coll Surg. 1994;179(6):727–32.
81. Aydin C, Piskin T, Sumer F, Barut B, Kayaalp C. Laparoscopic drainage of pyogenic liver abscess. JSLS. 2010;14(3):418–20. https://doi.org/10.4293/108680810X12924466006567.
82. Wang W, Lee W-J, Wei P-L, Chen T-C, Huang M-T. Laparoscopic drainage of pyogenic liver abscesses. Surg Today. 2004;34(4):323–5. https://doi.org/10.1007/s00595-003-2709-x.

83. Tan L, Zhou HJ, Hartman M, Ganpathi IS, Madhavan K, Chang S. Laparoscopic drainage of cryptogenic liver abscess. Surg Endosc. 2013;27(9):3308–14. https://doi.org/10.1007/s00464-013-2910-y.

84. Klink CD, Binnebösel M, Schmeding M, van Dam RM, Dejong CH, Junge K, Neumann UP. Video-assisted hepatic abscess debridement. HPB. 2015;17(8):732–5. https://doi.org/10.1111/hpb.12445.

85. Seewald S, Imazu H, Omar S, Groth S, Seitz U, Brand B, Zhong Y, Sikka S, Thonke F, Soehendra N. EUS-guided drainage of hepatic abscess. Gastrointest Endosc. 2005;61(3):495–8. https://doi.org/10.1016/S0016-5107(04)02848-2.

86. Chin YK, Asokkumar R. Endoscopic ultrasound-guided drainage of difficult-to-access liver abscesses. SAGE Open Med. 2020;8:2050312120921273. https://doi.org/10.1177/2050312120921273.

87. Costi R, Le Bian A, Cauchy F, Diop PS, Carloni A, Catherine L, Smadja C. Synchronous pyogenic liver abscess and acute cholecystitis: how to recognize it and what to do (emergency cholecystostomy followed by delayed laparoscopic cholecystectomy). Surg Endosc. 2012;26(1):205–13. https://doi.org/10.1007/s00464-011-1856-1.

88. Qu K, Liu C, Wang Z-X, Tian F, Wei J-C, Tai M-H, Zhou L, Meng F-D, Wang R-T, Xu X-S. Pyogenic liver abscesses associated with nonmetastatic colorectal cancers: an increasing problem in eastern Asia. World J Gastroenterol. 2012;18(23):2948–55. https://doi.org/10.3748/wjg.v18.i23.2948.

89. Mohan BP, Meyyur Aravamudan V, Khan SR, Chandan S, Ponnada S, Asokkumar R, Navaneethan U, Adler DG. Prevalence of colorectal cancer in cryptogenic pyogenic liver abscess patients. Do they need screening colonoscopy? A systematic review and meta-analysis. Dig Liver Dis. 2019;51(12):1641–5. https://doi.org/10.1016/j.dld.2019.08.016.

90. Lafont E, Roux O, de Lastours V, Dokmak S, Leflon V, Fantin B, Lefort A. Pyogenic liver abscess in liver transplant recipient: a warning signal for the risk of recurrence and retransplantation. Transpl Infect Dis. 2020;22(6):e13360. https://doi.org/10.1111/tid.13360.

91. Dominguez Bastante M, Molina Raya A, Vilchez Rabelo A, Villar del Moral J, Exposito Ruiz M, Fundora Suarez Y. Analysis of ischemic cholangiopathy after treatment of arterial thrombosis in liver transplantation in our series. Transplant Proc. 2018;50(2):628–30. https://doi.org/10.1016/j.transproceed.2017.11.062.

92. Liao W-I, Tsai S-H, Yu C-Y, Huang G-S, Lin Y-Y, Hsu C-W, Hsu H-H, Chang W-C. Pyogenic liver abscess treated by percutaneous catheter drainage: MDCT measurement for treatment outcome. Eur J Radiol. 2012;81(4):609–15.

93. Barakate MS, Stephen MS, Waugh RC, Gallagher PJ, Solomon MJ, Storey DW, Sheldon DM. Pyogenic liver abscess: a review of 10 years' experience in management. Aust N Z J Surg. 1999;69(3):205–9. https://doi.org/10.1046/j.1440-1622.1999.01523.x.

94. Thng CB, Tan YP, Shelat VG. Gas-forming pyogenic liver abscess: a world review. Ann Hepatobiliary Pancreat Surg. 2018;22(1):11–8.

95. Hope WW, Vrochides DV, Newcomb WL, Mayo-Smith WW, Iannitti DA. Optimal treatment of hepatic abscess. Am Surg. 2008;74(2):178–82.

96. Hsieh H-F, Chen T-W, Yu C-Y, Wang N-C, Chu H-C, Shih M-L, Yu J-C, Hsieh C-B. Aggressive hepatic resection for patients with pyogenic liver abscess and APACHE II score ≥15. Am J Surg. 2008;196(3):346–50. https://doi.org/10.1016/j.amjsurg.2007.09.051.

97. Hsieh CB, Tzao C, Yu CY, Chen CJ, Chang WK, Chu CH, Chou SJ, Tung HJ, Yu JC. APACHE II score and primary liver cancer history had risk of hospital mortality in patients with pyogenic liver abscess. Dig Liver Dis. 2006;38(7):498–502. https://doi.org/10.1016/j.dld.2006.03.020.

98. Jun CH, Yoon JH, Wi JW, Park SY, Lee WS, Jung SI, Park CH, Joo YE, Kim HS, Choi SK, Rew JS. Risk factors and clinical outcomes for spontaneous rupture of pyogenic liver abscess. J Dig Dis. 2015;16(1):31–6. https://doi.org/10.1111/1751-2980.12209.

99. Lee H-L, Lee H-C, Guo H-R, Ko W-C, Chen K-W. Clinical significance and mechanism of gas formation of pyogenic liver abscess due to Klebsiella pneumoniae. J Clin Microbiol. 2004;42(6):2783–5.

100. Chou F-F, Sheen-Chen S-M, Chen Y-S, Lee T-Y. The comparison of clinical course and results of treatment between gas-forming and non–gas-forming pyogenic liver abscess. Arch Surg. 1995;130(4):401–5.

101. Liu C-H, Gervais DA, Hahn PF, Arellano RS, Uppot RN, Mueller PR. Percutaneous Hepatic abscess drainage: do multiple abscesses or multiloculated abscesses preclude drainage or affect outcome? J Vasc Interv Radiol. 2009;20(8):1059–65. https://doi.org/10.1016/j.jvir.2009.04.062.

102. Yang C-C, Yen C-H, Ho M-W, Wang J-H. Comparison of pyogenic liver abscess caused by non-Klebsiella pneumoniae and Klebsiella pneumoniae. J Microbiol Immunol Infect. 2004;37(3):176–84.

103. Hussain I, Ishrat S, Ho DCW, Khan SR, Veeraraghavan MA, Palraj BR, Molton JS, Abid MB. Endogenous endophthalmitis in Klebsiella pneumoniae pyogenic liver abscess: systematic review and meta-analysis. Int J Infect Dis. 2020;101:259–68. https://doi.org/10.1016/j.ijid.2020.09.1485.

104. Whiting JF, Rossi SJ, Hanto DW. Infectious complications after OKT3 induction in liver transplantation. Liver Transpl Surg. 1997;3(6):563–70. https://doi.org/10.1002/lt.500030602.

105. Tachopoulou OA, Vogt DP, Henderson JM, Baker M, Keys TF. Hepatic abscess after liver transplantation: 1990–2000. Transplantation. 2003;75(1):79–83.

Liver Transplantation for Colorectal and Neuroendocrine Liver Metastases and Hepatoblastoma

Taizo Hibi

Abstract

Liver transplantation was long considered an absolute contraindication for unresectable colorectal liver metastases because of the poor prognoses reported in the 1980s and 1990s. In 2013, the Oslo University group reported an outstanding 5-year survival of 60% after liver transplantation after ≥6 weeks of neoadjuvant chemotherapy for patients with unresectable liver-only disease and developed the Oslo score based on 4 prognostic factors (SECA-I trial). For unresectable neuroendocrine tumor liver metastases, Mazzaferro et al. described in 2016 that the Milan criteria to purse a curative intent by liver transplantation accomplished excellent 5- and 10-year survival rates of 97% and 89%, respectively. These criteria formed the basis of guidelines adopted in the U.S. and Europe. For unresectable and borderline-resectable hepatoblastoma, liver transplantation is the treatment of choice even in patients with extrahepatic disease if the lesions are controlled. The principles of transplant oncology form the basis of safe institution of liver transplantation for hepatobiliary malignancies and are expected to redefine cancer care and research. "Resectability" is no longer an exclusive technical argument; instead, "oncological eliminability," regardless of resection or transplantation, should be discussed in a multidisciplinary setting to achieve the care and cure of patients in their desperate need of help.

67.1 Introduction

In 1967, Starzl et al. reported the first successful liver transplantation (LT) for a 19-month-old girl with a hepatocellular carcinoma [1]. The concept of brain death became widely accepted since 1968 [2], which apparently increased the availability of high-quality liver grafts. Calne et al. introduced cyclosporine (calcineurin inhibitor) in 1979 [3]. Owing to these iconic events, along with the groundbreaking improvements in surgical techniques and recipient perioperative management, LT was recognized as the last resort for end-stage liver disease [4]. The indications for LT for unresectable hepatocellular carcinoma known as the Milan criteria were proposed by Mazzaferro et al. in 1996 and have become the gold standard [5]. For other unresectable hepatobiliary malignancies, the indications for LT have been carefully expanded, giving rise to the new era of "transplant oncology" [6]. Transplant oncology is composed of four pillars (the 4 E's) as follows: *evolution* of multidisciplinary cancer treatment by incorporating LT, *extension* of the limit of conventional surgical resection by adopting LT techniques, *elucidation* of self- and non-self-recognition systems by linking tumor immunology and transplant immunology, and *exploration* of the disease mechanism by applying cancer genomics to surgical specimens that were unavailable if not for LT techniques [7, 8]. More than a half century after the first successful LT, the first international consensus conference on transplant oncology was held in 2019 and the evolving new oncological indications were discussed [9, 10].

67.2 Colorectal Liver Metastases

Aggressive liver resection using portal vein embolization, two-stage hepatectomy, or associating liver partition and portal vein ligation for staged hepatectomy (ALPPS) has significantly improved the prognoses of patients with resectable colorectal liver metastases (CRLM), and the 5-year survival rates after resection range from 40% to 50% [11–13]. However, approximately 80% of patients with CRLM have unresectable diseases at the time of diagnoses, and their 5-year survival rates are likely to range from 5% to 20%. The vigorous efforts to introduce LT for unresectable CRLM were all in vain because of the poor outcomes (5-year sur-

T. Hibi (✉)
Department of Pediatric Surgery and Transplantation, Kumamoto University Graduate School of Medical Sciences, Kumamoto, Japan

vival <20%) in the early experiences [14]. Nevertheless, the SECA-I (Secondary Cancer) trial was launched in 2006 at Oslo University Hospital, in the privileged situation of Norway, which has excellent access to deceased organs, accomplishing a median waiting time of 6 weeks for LT. The landmark results of the SECA-I trial were published in 2013: A 5-year overall survival of 60% was reached for 21 patients with liver-only, unresectable CRLM who underwent LT after receiving at least 6 weeks of neoadjuvant chemotherapy [15]. Tumor diameters >5.5 cm, carcinoembryonic antigen levels >80 μg/L, time interval < 2 years from the resection of the primary tumor to LT, and progression of the metastatic disease during the course of chemotherapy were identified as poor prognostic indicators. The Oslo score (number of risk factors) effectively stratified the prognoses of the patients into 3 groups (0–1, 2–3, and 4), and none of the patients with all 4 factors survived for 5 years. The study was criticized because of the high recurrence rate (19/21 patients had a disease recurrence); however, the authors found that lung-only metastases were associated with favorable prognoses as compared with multiple metastatic sites, including the liver graft [16]. The SECA-I trial provided a reappraisal of the role of LT in the treatment of unresectable CRLM. The same group conducted the SECA-II trial and attained a 5-year survival rate exceeding 80% after LT for 15 patients by applying more stringent patient criteria for unresectable liver-only CRLM (a minimum of 10% response to chemotherapy, a time interval of at least 1 year between the diagnosis of CRLM to LT listing, no lesions >10 cm in size before chemotherapy, and for patients with more than 30 tumors, all lesions should be <5 cm with at least 30% response to chemotherapy) [17]. The group also reported that 13 patients with an Oslo score of 0–2 in the SECA-I and SECA-II trials had better 5-year overall survival than 6 patients with an Oslo score of 3–4 (67% vs. 17%, $P = 0.004$) during a median follow-up of 85 months [18]. The group claimed that disease-free survival is not an appropriate indicator of treatment success because pulmonary recurrence alone has a modest impact on survival outcomes [18]. On the contrary, the Compagnons Hépato-Biliaires demonstrated that long-term disease-free survival can be achieved if LT was performed as a deliberate procedure after patients had undergone a combination of oncological/surgical management (5 of 12 patients were alive and free of cancer 7, 43, 47, 48, and 108 months after LT) [19]. More recently, the "RAPID concept" (resection and partial liver segment 2–3 transplantation with delayed total hepatectomy) incorporated accelerated remnant liver hypertrophy induced by ALPPS to both deceased and living donor LT with successful outcomes [20, 21]. Fourteen prospective studies from nine countries have been registered at ClinicalTrials.gov as of 2021 (Table 67.1). Five randomized controlled trials are currently underway. The first international consensus conference on transplant oncology made a "moderate recommendation" that "LT can be a viable option in highly selected patients with unresectable CRLM with only liver involvement" [10]. The significantly improved outcomes after LT for unresectable CRLM is mainly attributable to highly effective chemotherapy. However, the unsolved questions include, but not limited to, standardized imaging protocols, use of a mammalian target of rapamycin inhibitors as post-transplant immunosuppression agents and the optimal adjuvant therapy, definition of unresectability [22], and genomic profile (e.g., KRAS and BRAF mutations) [23]. LT for unresectable CRLM should only be performed in the context of a multidisciplinary team approach. The results of ongoing trials are awaited to establish universal indications for LT for CRLM. In addition, creating an international registry should be a critical step to accumulate worldwide experience and evidence on LT for CRLM [10].

Table 67.1 Ongoing studies of liver transplantation for colorectal liver metastases registered on ClinicalTrials.gov

Year	ClinicalTrials.gov identifier Status	Institution (Country)	Title	Number of participants and study design	Primary outcome measures
2012	NCT01479608 Recruiting	Oslo University Hospital (Norway)	A Randomized Controlled Clinical Trial to Evaluate the Benefit and Efficacy of Liver Transplantation as Treatment for Selected Patients With Liver Metastases From ColoRectal Carcinoma (SECA-II)	25 (RCT): liver resection vs. LT (for resectable CRLM); NACTx (≥6 weeks) required	10-year OS
2014	NCT02215889 Recruiting	Oslo University Hospital (Norway)	A Phase I/II Clinical Trial to Evaluate the Benefit and Efficacy of Liver Resection And Partial Liver Segment 2/3 Transplantation With Delayed Total Hepatectomy as Treatment for Selected Patients With Liver Metastases From ColoRectal Carcinoma (RAPID)	20 (single arm): NACTx (≥8 weeks) + liver resection + LT (segment 2/3) followed by delayed total hepatectomy	Percent of transplanted patients receiving 2nd stage hepatectomy within 4 weeks of segment 2/3 LT
2015	NCT02597348 Recruiting	Paul Brousse Hospital, multicenter (France)	Curative Potential of Liver Transplantation in Patients With Definitively Unresectable Colorectal Liver Metastases (CLM) Treated by Chemotherapy: a Prospective Multicentric Randomized Trial (TRANSMET)	90 (RCT): NACTx (≥3 months) + LT vs. standard chemotherapy	5-year OS

Table 67.1 (continued)

Year	ClinicalTrials.gov identifier Status	Institution (Country)	Title	Number of participants and study design	Primary outcome measures
2016	NCT02864485 Recruiting	University Health Network, Toronto (Canada)	Assessment of a Protocol Using a Combination of Neo-adjuvant Chemotherapy Plus Living Donor Liver Transplantation for Non-Resectable Liver Metastases From Colorectal Cancer	20 (single arm): NACTx (≥3 months)+ LDLT	5-year OS and RFS
2016	NCT03494946 Recruiting	Oslo University Hospital (Norway)	A Randomized Clinical Trial Comparing Overall Survival in Selected Patients With ColoRectal Carcinoma Treated by Liver Transplantation or Chemotherapy (SECA-III)	30 (RCT): NACTx (progressive disease or intolerance to first line CTx) + LT vs. standard CTx	2-year OS
2018	NCT03488953 Recruiting	Jena University Hospital, University Hospital Tübingen (Germany)	Living Donor Liver Transplantation With Two Stage Hepatectomy for Patients With Isolated, Irresectable Colorectal Liver Metastases (LIVER-T(W)O-HEAL)	40 (single arm): Neoadjuvant chemo Tx (≥8 weeks) + LDLT (left lobe) + two-stage hepatectomy	3-year OS
2019	NCT03803436 Recruiting	Fondazione IRCCS Istituto Nazionale dei Tumori, Milano, Italy (multicenter)	Improving Outcome of Selected Patients With Non-resectable Hepatic Metastases From Colo-rectal Cancer With Liver Transplantation: a Prospective Parallel Trial (COLT)	22 (non-randomized comparison): NACTx (≥4 months) + LT vs. triplet CTx + anti EGFR	5-year OS
2019	NCT04161092 Recruiting	Sahlgrenska University Hospital and Karolinska University Hospital, Sweden	A Randomized Controlled, Open-label, Multicentre Study Evaluating if Liver Transplantation With Liver Grafts From Extended Criteria Donors Not Utilised for Approved Indications Increases Overall Survival in Patients With Non-resectable Isolated Liver Metastases From Colorectal Metastases, in Comparison With Best Alternative Care (SOULMATE)	45 (RCT): NACTx (≥2 months) + LT vs. best alternative care	5-year OS
2020	NCT04616495 Recruiting	Hospital Universitario La Fe, Spain	Liver Transplantation in Patients With Unresectable Colorectal Liver Metastases (TRASMETIR)	30 (single arm): neoadjuvant chemotherapy + LDLT	5-year OS
2021	NCT04874259 Not yet recruiting	Seoul National University Hospital (South Korea)	Effectiveness of Liver Transplantation for Unresectable Colorectal Liver Metastasis; Pilot Study	20 (single arm): LDLT for treatment-naïve patients	1-year OS
2021	NCT04865471 Recruiting	Azienda Ospedaliera di Padova (Italy)	Resection And Partial Liver Segmental Transplantation With Delayed Total Hepatectomy as Treatment for Selected Patients With Unresectable Liver Metastases From Colorectal Carcinoma (RAPID-Padova)	18 (single arm): NACTx (≥3 months) + LT (segment 2/3) followed by delayed total hepatectomy	Percentage of transplanted patients receiving 2nd stage hepatectomy within 4 weeks of segment 2/3 LT
2021	NCT04870879 Recruiting	Azienda Ospedaliera di Padova (Italy)	Colorectal Metastasis and Liver Transplantation With Organs From Deceased Donors (MELODIC)	18 (non-randomized, parallel assignment): NACTx (≥3 months) + DDLT vs. CTx alone	3-year OS
2021	NCT04898504 Recruiting	Oslo University Hospital (Norway)	HAI-Floxuridine, or Liver-Tx, Combined With 2nd Line Chemotherapy Versus 2nd Line Chemotherapy Alone for Patients With Colorectal Liver Metastases and Heavy Tumour Burden (EXCALIBUR 1+2)	45 (RCT): 2nd line CTx + HAI-floxuridine vs. 2nd line CTx + LT vs. 2nd line CTx alone	2-year OS
2021	NCT04742621 Recruiting	Weill Medical College of Cornell University (U.S.)	Liver Transplantation for Unresectable Liver Limited Colorectal Metastases	20 (single arm): NACTx (≥6 months) + LDLT	To develop a registry

LT liver transplantation, *CRLM* colorectal liver metastases, *NACTx* neoadjuvant chemotherapy, *RFS* recurrence-free survival, *OS* overall survival, *LDLT* living donor liver transplantation, *EGFR* epidermal growth factor receptor, *DDLT* deceased donor liver transplantation, *HAI* hepatic artery infusion

67.3 Neuroendocrine Tumor Liver Metastases

An estimated 50%–90% of patients with neuroendocrine tumor (NET) may develop neuroendocrine tumor liver metastases (NETLM) with heterogeneous presentation ranging from classical carcinoid syndromes associated with small tumors to no symptoms with nearly total replacement of the liver by metastatic lesions [24]. Although the treatment of choice for NETLM is liver resection [24–26] with acceptable 5-year overall survival rates within the 60%–70% range, less than half of patients with NETLM are eligible for resection [14]. For unresectable NETLM, systemic chemotherapy, transcatheter arterial chemoembolization, and so on are viable options with varying success rates. Since the 1980s, LT has been performed for highly selected patients. Two systematic reviews reported that the 5-year survival rates after LT for unresectable NELTM from pancreatic primaries (n = 89) and from pancreatic, gastrointestinal, bronchial, and other primaries combined (n = 1120) were 44% [27] and 63% [28], respectively. In the largest systematic review on LT for NETLM, the recurrence rate ranged from 31.3% to 56.8%, and several prognostic factors, including >50% liver involvement, high Ki67 index, and a pancreatic rather than a gastrointestinal NET tumor location, were associated with worse long-term survival [28]. Mazzaferro et al. claimed in 2007 that LT for NETLM should be "reconsidered not only as a bare palliation but also as a therapy with high potential of not just prolonging survival but of pursuing a curative intent" [29]. Eligibility for LT (the Milan criteria for NETLM) was defined as follows: 1. a confirmed histology of low-grade NET with or without syndrome, 2. a primary tumor drained by the portal system (pancreas and intermediate gut: from the distal stomach to the sigmoid colon) that was removed with a curative resection (pretransplant removal of all extrahepatic tumor deposits) through surgical procedures different and separate from transplantation, 3. metastatic diffusion occupying ≤50% of the liver parenchyma, 4. good response or stable disease for at least 6 months during the pretransplantation period, and 5. age ≤ 55 years (modified later to <60 years). Of the 88 consecutive patients who met these criteria in the prospective study between 1995 and 2010, 42 underwent LT and achieved outstanding 5- and 10-year survival rates of 97% and 89%, respectively [30]. The remaining 46 patients with similar tumor burdens were unable to receive LT because of non-compliance, patient refusal, and transplant list unavailability, and their 5- and 10-year survival rates were 51% and 22% respectively, significantly worse than those of the patients who underwent LT ($P < 0.001$). The adjusted survival benefit of LT over non-LT was 6.8 and 38.4 months at 5 and 10 years, respectively. On the basis of these excellent outcomes, the United Network for Organ Sharing in the US adopted these criteria for the Model for End-stage Disease exception listing of patients with unresectable NETLM [31]. The aforementioned international consensus conference made a "strong recommendation" that "LT should be considered as a potentially curable treatment option for selected patients with unresectable NETLM" [10]. The areas of controversy and future research include, but not limited to, the following: (a) how to combine LT with nonoperative modalities such as peptide receptor radionuclide therapy and molecular-targeted agents; (b) standardized imaging protocols for evaluating LT candidates; (c) use of a mammalian target of rapamycin inhibitors as post-transplant immunosuppression agents and/or adjuvant therapy; and (d) definition of unresectability. LT candidacy for unresectable NETLM should be thoroughly discussed in a multidisciplinary setting on a case-to-case basis by convening experts involved in transplantation medicine and oncology [7, 8, 14].

67.4 Hepatoblastoma

Hepatoblastoma (HB) is the most common primary liver cancer in children and its incidence has continued to increase over the last several decades. Surgical resection with a curative intent combined with chemotherapy is the treatment of choice. LT is reserved for unresectable HB and achieves an overall 5-year survival of 60% to >80%. Significant improvements in chemotherapy have made patients even with extrahepatic disease eligible for LT when lesions are controlled by either chemotherapy or surgical resection [32, 33]. Patients with borderline-resectable HB are also LT candidates because the outcomes of salvage LT are unsatisfactory [32, 34, 35]. The pre- and post-treatment extent of disease (PRETEXT and POST-TEXT, respectively) systems are used to determine the treatment strategy [36, 37]. Indocyanine green was effective in identifying primary and metastatic disease [38] and re-LT for recurrent HB might be justified in highly selected patients by achieving complete tumor removal under indocyanine green navigation [39]. Longer time on the waiting list was demonstrated as a risk factor of recurrence after LT and patients undergoing chemotherapy should be prioritized for deceased donor allocation to optimize the timing of LT [40]. Living donors are a precious source of liver grafts, as they enable prompt LT between chemotherapy sessions [10, 34]. The ongoing Children's Oncology Group international study of pediatric liver cancer AHEP-1531: Pediatric Hepatic Malignancy International Therapeutic Trial (NCT03533582) is a partially randomized phase II/III trial designed to evaluate the efficacy of cisplatin-based chemotherapy in combination with surgery in the treatment of HB and hepatocellular carcinoma of children and young adults. This study employed a novel risk stratification algorithm that was defined by the efforts of the Children's Hepatic tumors International Collaboration [35, 37]. The risk stratification is based on the presence of positive annotation factors: tumor ingrowth into vena cava or all 3 hepatic veins (V), right/left portal veins or bifurcation (P), contiguous organ (E); multifocal tumor (F); or pre-diagnosis tumor rupture (R), age (<8 or ≥ 8 years for PRETEXT III and < 3 or ≥ 3 years for PRETEXT IV), and alpha fetoprotein levels [37]. The aforementioned international consensus conference

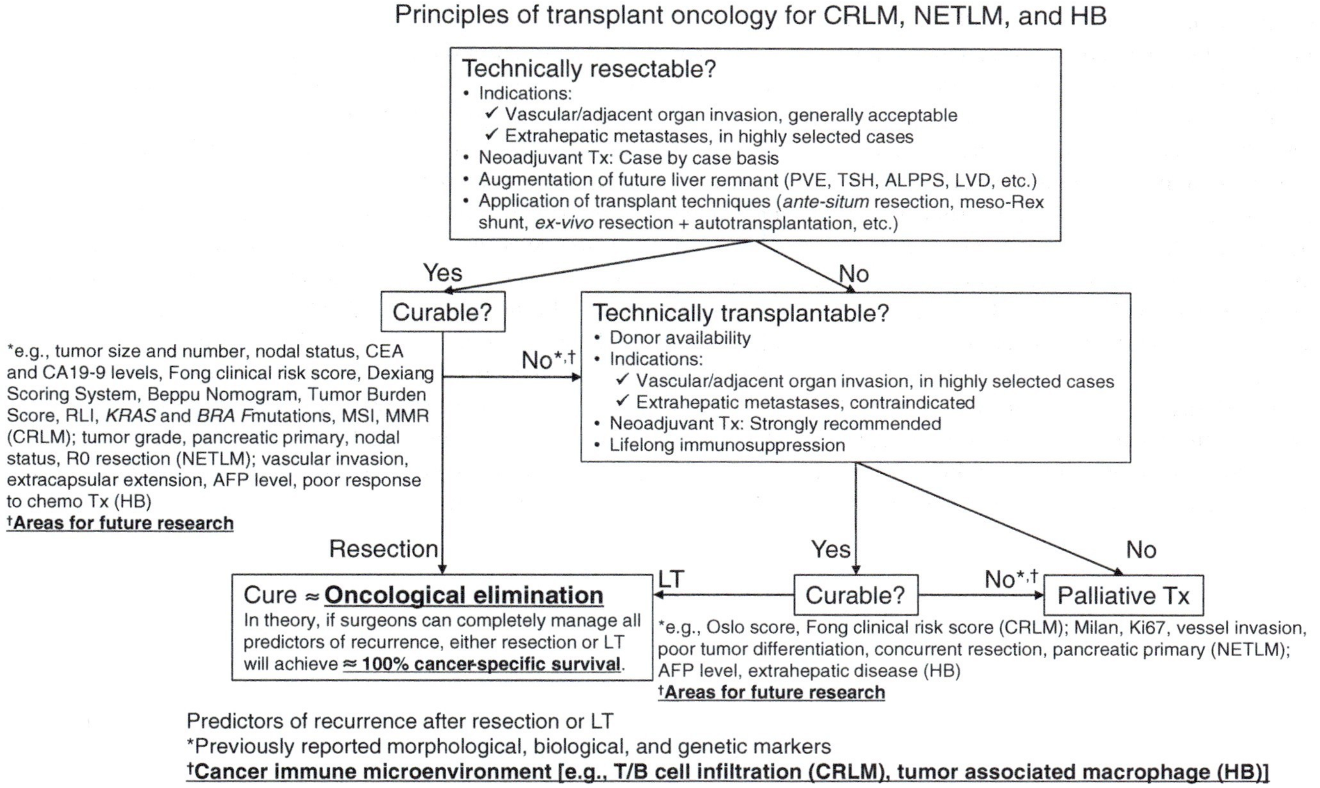

Principles of transplant oncology for CRLM, NETLM, and HB

Technically resectable?
- Indications:
  - ✓ Vascular/adjacent organ invasion, generally acceptable
  - ✓ Extrahepatic metastases, in highly selected cases
- Neoadjuvant Tx: Case by case basis
- Augmentation of future liver remnant (PVE, TSH, ALPPS, LVD, etc.)
- Application of transplant techniques (*ante-situm* resection, meso-Rex shunt, *ex-vivo* resection + autotransplantation, etc.)

Yes → Curable?

*e.g., tumor size and number, nodal status, CEA and CA19-9 levels, Fong clinical risk score, Dexiang Scoring System, Beppu Nomogram, Tumor Burden Score, RLI, KRAS and BRAF mutations, MSI, MMR (CRLM); tumor grade, pancreatic primary, nodal status, R0 resection (NETLM); vascular invasion, extracapsular extension, AFP level, poor response to chemo Tx (HB)
†**Areas for future research**

No → Technically transplantable?
- Donor availability
- Indications:
  - ✓ Vascular/adjacent organ invasion, in highly selected cases
  - ✓ Extrahepatic metastases, contraindicated
- Neoadjuvant Tx: Strongly recommended
- Lifelong immunosuppression

Resection → Cure ≈ Oncological elimination
In theory, if surgeons can completely manage all predictors of recurrence, either resection or LT will achieve ≈ **100% cancer-specific survival**.

LT ← Yes — Curable? — No*,† → Palliative Tx

*e.g., Oslo score, Fong clinical risk score (CRLM); Milan, Ki67, vessel invasion, poor tumor differentiation, concurrent resection, pancreatic primary (NETLM); AFP level, extrahepatic disease (HB)
†**Areas for future research**

Predictors of recurrence after resection or LT
*Previously reported morphological, biological, and genetic markers
†Cancer immune microenvironment [e.g., T/B cell infiltration (CRLM), tumor associated macrophage (HB)]

Fig. 67.1 A conceptual flow chart that demonstrates the principles of transplant oncology for CRLM, NETLM, and HB. If we have perfect control of factors that determine disease recurrence, either resection or LT would achieve oncological elimination, resulting in ≈100% cancer-specific survival. Abbreviations: *CRLM* colorectal liver metastases, *NETLM* neuroendocrine tumor liver metastases, *HB* hepatoblastoma, *Tx* treatment, *PVE* portal vein embolization, *TSH* two-stage hepatectomy, *ALPPS* associating liver partition and portal vein ligation for staged hepatectomy, *LVD* liver venous deprivation, *CEA* carcinoembryonic antigen, *CA19-9* carbohydrate antigen 19-9, *RLI* remnant liver ischemia, MSI microsatellite instability, *MMR* mismatch repair, *AFP* alpha fetoprotein, *LT* liver transplantation

has made strong recommendations that "Unifocal POST-TEXT IV tumors and/or POST-TEXT III or IV with persistent widespread multifocality or major vessel involvement are clear indications for LT" [10]. The guidelines also strongly recommended that "PRETEXT IV, age > 3 years, extrahepatic metastases, alpha-fetoprotein level < 100 ng/mL, and major bilobar vascular involvement" should be considered as high-risk factors, and patients with these risk factors should be referred early to specialized centers with abundant experience in complex liver surgery or LT [10]. Recently, aggressive liver resections including ante situm liver resection, ALPPS, and ex vivo liver resection with autotransplantation of the liver have been reported in the pediatric population [41–44]; therefore, the definition of unresectability is not universal. Moreover, further investigations on cancer genomics in HB (e.g., Wnt/β-catenin signaling pathway) are expected to establish precision medicine [45].

67.5 Conclusions

Transplant oncology has brought about a paradigm shift in the management of CRLM, NETLM, and HB. Whether the approach is surgical resection or LT, we should determine the oncological eliminability of the disease. Rapidly evolving cancer immunogenomics is expected to dramatically improve the predictability of disease recurrence. As its accuracy approximates 100%, either resection or LT is likely to accomplish oncological elimination, i.e., ≈100% cancer-specific survival (Fig. 67.1). This is the ultimate goal of transplant oncology.

References

1. Starzl TE, Groth CG, Brettschneider L, et al. Orthotopic homotransplantation of the human liver. Ann Surg. 1968;168(3):392–415.
2. Beecher HK. Ethical problems created by the hopelessly unconscious patient. N Engl J Med. 1968;278(26):1425–30.
3. Calne RY, Rolles K, White DJ, et al. Cyclosporin A initially as the only immunosuppressant in 34 recipients of cadaveric organs: 32 kidneys, 2 pancreases, and 2 livers. Lancet. 1979;2(8151):1033–6.
4. National Institutes of Health Consensus Development Conference Statement: liver transplantation-June 20–23, 1983. Hepatology 1984;4(1 Suppl):107S–110S.
5. Mazzaferro V, Regalia E, Doci R, et al. Liver transplantation for the treatment of small hepatocellular carcinomas in patients with cirrhosis. N Engl J Med. 1996;334(11):693–9.
6. Hibi T, Itano O, Shinoda M, et al. Liver transplantation for hepatobiliary malignancies: a new era of "transplant oncology" has begun. Surg Today. 2017;47(4):403–15.
7. Hibi T, Sapisochin G. What is transplant oncology? Surgery. 2019;165(2):281–5.

8. Sapisochin G, Hibi T, Toso C, et al. Transplant oncology in primary and metastatic liver tumor: principles, evidence and opportunities. Ann Surg. 2020; https://doi.org/10.1097/SLA.0000000000004071. Epub ahead of print
9. Sapisochin G, Hibi T, Ghobrial M, et al. The ILTS consensus conference on transplant oncology: setting the stage. Transplantation. 2020;104(6):1119–20.
10. Hibi T, Rela M, Eason JD, et al. Liver transplantation for colorectal and neuroendocrine liver metastases and hepatoblastoma. Working Group Report from the ILTS Transplant Oncology Consensus Conference. Transplantation. 2020;104(6):1131–5.
11. Shindoh J, Tzeng CW, Aloia TA, et al. Portal vein embolization improves rate of resection of extensive colorectal liver metastases without worsening survival. Br J Surg. 2013;100(13):1777–83.
12. Wicherts DA, Miller R, de Haas RJ, et al. Long-term results of two-stage hepatectomy for irresectable colorectal cancer liver metastases. Ann Surg. 2008;248(6):994–1005.
13. Petrowsky H, Linecker M, Raptis DA, et al. First long-term oncologic results of the ALPPS procedure in a large cohort of patients with colorectal liver metastases. Ann Surg. 2020;272(5):793–800.
14. Moeckli B, Ivanics T, Claasen M, et al. Recent developments and ongoing trials in transplant oncology. Liver Int. 2020;40(10):2326–44.
15. Hagness M, Foss A, Line PD, et al. Liver transplantation for nonresectable liver metastases from colorectal cancer. Ann Surg. 2013;257:800–6.
16. Hagness M, Foss A, Egge TS, et al. Patterns of recurrence after liver transplantation for nonresectable liver metastases from colorectal cancer. Ann Surg Oncol. 2014;21:1323–9.
17. Dueland S, Syversveen T, Solheim JM, et al. Survival following liver transplantation for patients with nonresectable liver-only colorectal metastases. Ann Surg. 2020;271(2):212–8.
18. Dueland S, Grut H, Syversveen T, et al. Selection criteria related to long term survival following liver transplantation for colorectal liver metastasis. Am J Transplant. 2020;20(2):530–7.
19. Toso C, Pinto Marques H, Andres A, Compagnons Hépato-Biliaires Group, et al. Liver transplantation for colorectal liver metastasis: survival without recurrence can be achieved. Liver Transpl. 2017;23:1073–6.
20. Line PD, Hagness M, Berstad AE, et al. A novel concept for partial liver transplantation in nonresectable colorectal liver metastases: the RAPID concept. Ann Surg. 2015;262(1):e5–9.
21. Königsrainer A, Templin S, Capobianco I, et al. Paradigm shift in the management of irresectable colorectal liver metastases: living donor auxiliary partial orthotopic liver transplantation in combination with two-stage hepatectomy (LD-RAPID). Ann Surg. 2019;270(2):327–32.
22. Imai K, Adam R, Baba H. How to increase the resectability of initially unresectable colorectal liver metastases: a surgical perspective. Ann Gastroenterol Surg. 2019;3:476–86.
23. Line PD, Dueland S. Liver transplantation for secondary liver tumours: the difficult balance between survival and recurrence. J Hepatol. 2020;73(6):1557–62.
24. Hibi T, Sano T, Sakamoto Y, et al. Surgery for hepatic neuroendocrine tumors: a single institutional experience in Japan. Jpn J Clin Oncol. 2007;37(2):102–7.
25. Wakabayashi T, Hibi T, Yoneda G, et al. Predictive model for survival after liver resection for noncolorectal liver metastases in the modern era: a Japanese multicenter analysis. J Hepatobiliary Pancreat Sci. 2019;26(10):441–8.
26. Yamamoto M, Yoshida M, Furuse J, et al. Clinical practice guidelines for the management of liver metastases from extrahepatic primary cancers 2021. J Hepatobiliary Pancreat Sci. 2020; https://doi.org/10.1002/jhbp.868. Epub ahead of print
27. Máthé Z, Tagkalos E, Paul A, et al. Liver transplantation for hepatic metastases of neuroendocrine pancreatic tumors: a survival-based analysis. Transplantation. 2011;91(5):575–82.
28. Moris D, Tsilimigras DI, Ntanasis-Stathopoulos I, et al. Liver transplantation in patients with liver metastases from neuroendocrine tumors: a systematic review. Surgery. 2017;162(3):525–36.
29. Mazzaferro V, Pulvirenti A, Coppa J. Neuroendocrine tumors metastatic to the liver: how to select patients for liver transplantation? J Hepatol. 2007;47:460–6.
30. Mazzaferro V, Sposito C, Coppa J, et al. The long-term benefit of liver transplantation for hepatic metastases from neuroendocrine tumors. Am J Transplant. 2016;16:2892–902.
31. US Department of Health & Human Service Web site. Guidance to Liver Transplant Programs and the National Liver Review Board for: Adult MELD Exception Review. https://optnpilot.unos.org/media/2847/liver_guidance_adult_meld_201706.pdf. Accessed 20 Dec 2020.
32. Cruz RJ Jr, Ranganathan S, Mazariegos G, et al. Analysis of national and single-center incidence and survival after liver transplantation for hepatoblastoma: new trends and future opportunities. Surgery. 2013;153:150–9.
33. O'Neill AF, Towbin AJ, Krailo MD, et al. Characterization of pulmonary metastases in children with hepatoblastoma treated on Children's Oncology Group protocol AHEP0731 (the treatment of children with all stages of hepatoblastoma): a report from the Children's Oncology Group. J Clin Oncol. 2017;35:3465–73.
34. Sakamoto S, Kasahara M, Mizuta K, Japanese Liver Transplantation Society, et al. Nationwide survey of the outcomes of living donor liver transplantation for hepatoblastoma in Japan. Liver Transpl. 2014;20:333–46.
35. Lim IIP, Bondoc AJ, Geller JI, et al. Hepatoblastoma-the evolution of biology, surgery, and transplantation. Children (Basel). 2018;6(1):1.
36. Towbin AJ, Meyers RL, Woodley H, et al. 2017 PRETEXT: radiologic staging system for primary hepatic malignancies of childhood revised for the paediatric hepatic international tumour trial (PHITT). Pediatr Radiol. 2018;48:536–54.
37. Meyers RL, Maibach R, Hiyama E, et al. Risk-stratified staging in paediatric hepatoblastoma: a unified analysis from the children's hepatic tumors international collaboration. Lancet Oncol. 2017;18(1):122–31.
38. Souzaki R, Kawakubo N, Matsuura T, et al. Navigation surgery using indocyanine green fluorescent imaging for hepatoblastoma patients. Pediatr Surg Int. 2019;35(5):551–7.
39. Takahashi N, Yamada Y, Hoshino K, et al. Living donor liver retransplantation for recurrent hepatoblastoma in the liver graft following complete eradication of peritoneal metastases under Indocyanine green fluorescence imaging. Cancers (Basel). 2019;11(5):730.
40. Pham TA, Gallo AM, Concepcion W, et al. Effect of liver transplant on long-term disease-free survival in children with hepatoblastoma and hepatocellular cancer. JAMA Surg. 2015;150:1150–8.
41. Fuchs J, Cavdar S, Blumenstock G, et al. POST-TEXT III and IV hepatoblastoma: extended hepatic resection avoids liver transplantation in selected cases. Ann Surg. 2017;266(2):318–23.
42. Angelico R, Passariello A, Pilato M, et al. Ante situm liver resection with inferior vena cava replacement under hypothermic cardiopulmonary bypass for hepatoblastoma: report of a case and review of the literature. Int J Surg Case Rep. 2017;37:90–6.
43. Hong JC, Kim J, Browning M, et al. Modified associating liver partition and portal vein ligation for staged hepatectomy for hepatoblastoma in a small infant: how far can we push the envelope? Ann Surg. 2017;266(2):e16–7.
44. Shi SJ, Wang DL, Hu W, et al. Ex vivo liver resection and autotransplantation with cardiopulmonary bypass for hepatoblastoma in children: a case report. Pediatr Transplant. 2018;22(7):e13268.
45. Mavila N, Thundimadathil J. The emerging roles of cancer stem cells and Wnt/Beta-catenin signaling in hepatoblastoma. Cancers (Basel). 2019;11(10):1406.

Technical Variant Liver Transplantation: Split, Dual Graft, and Auxiliary Transplantation

Vladislav Brasoveanu, Doina Hrehoret, Florin Botea, Florin Ichim, and Irinel Popescu

Abstract

Because of the shortage of cadaveric donors, other techniques of partial liver grafting have been developed. These techniques are placed in perspective in relation to the organ shortage. Reduced size liver transplantation (RSLT) was used and had results comparable to those from whole liver grafting. However, this technique, while benefitting pediatric patients, reduces the adult donor liver pool. It also makes inefficient use of an available adult donor liver. In split liver transplantation (SPLTx), the whole liver is used after bipartition for two recipients. The results are comparable to those of RSLTx. The problem with SPLTx is that it is a very demanding technique applied only in centers with extensive experience with liver resection and reduction. Living related liver transplantation (LRLTx) yields excellent results; however, it places an otherwise healthy person at risk. Domino liver transplantation (DLT) has emerged as a strategy for increasing the number of liver grafts available: morphologically normal livers from donors with metabolic diseases can be used for select recipients with hepatocellular carcinoma (usually outside the Milan criteria). Familial amyloidotic polyneuropathy (FAP) is the most common indication for DLT. In patients with acute liver failure (ALF) who fulfill criteria, liver transplantation is the only effective treatment which can substitute metabolic and excretory function of the liver. Auxiliary liver transplantation (APOLT) was developed because a significant minority of patients with ALF who fulfill transplant criteria can have a complete morphological and functional recovery of their liver.

V. Brasoveanu · F. Botea · I. Popescu (✉)
"Dan Setlacec" Center of General Surgery and Liver Transplantation, Fundeni Clinical Institute, Bucharest, Romania

"Titu Maiorescu" University, Bucharest, Romania

D. Hrehoret · F. Ichim
"Dan Setlacec" Center of General Surgery and Liver Transplantation, Fundeni Clinical Institute, Bucharest, Romania

The first technical variant liver transplantation (TVLT) was the split technique performed by Pichlmayer et al., and Bismuth et al. in the late 80′ [1, 2]. The next technique was the use of reduced-size graft in pediatric LT, consisting in reducing a whole graft to a left hemiliver (LH) or to a left lateral section (LLS) [3]. In this way, pediatric small sized recipients (body weight below 10 kg) could be transplanted; however, this procedure reduced the number of grafts available for adult recipients. This led to the development of living donation in the late 80 [4, 5], that brought an alternative source of grafts, and the boost of split LT (SLT), that addressed the deceased donor organ shortage by providing grafts to two recipients from a single deceased donor [6]. Initially, the SLT with the right hemiliver (RH) had a much worse outcome compared to the LH or the LLS in pediatric patients (that provided the best outcome). This was overcome by the expertise gained from living donor LT (LDLT) that led to the use of in situ and ex-situ SLT, improving the results of this procedure [7, 8]. Nowadays, SLT may have similar results as LDLT [9]. Using monosegmental grafts in recipients with a body weight below 5 kg needs further validation. Another TVLT that was more recently introduced is the transplant of an auxiliary partial orthotopic liver graft after partial hepatectomy (APOLT) [10].

In high-volume centers (with over 40 transplants per year), the survival after LDLT, SLT, reduced or full-size graft were similar in the pediatric population. However, in series such as the SPLIT [7], UNOS [11] and ELTR [8] reports, where also data from less experienced centers were included, LDLT or deceased donor LT had superior results when compared to SLT.

68.1 Split Liver Transplantation

One type of TVLT that increases the number of liver transplants, while reducing the mortality on the waiting list. is to split the liver from a deceased donor into two grafts which are then transplanted into two recipients (split LT). In this way, a whole adult liver can be divided into two functioning grafts. Split-liver transplantation (SLT) is an attractive alternative to living donation. However, it involves a complex mechanism, being technically demanding and requiring additional logistic and personnel support.

Surgical complications are more common in SLT (vs. whole graft) recipients, related to the cut surface of the liver, smaller vessels for anastomosis, and more complicated biliary reconstruction.

In a large series of 106 SLT, adults recipients had 1-, 5-, and 10-year survival rates of 93, 77, and 73%, respectively, with graft survival rates of 89, 76, and 65%, respectively. For pediatric recipients, 1-, 5-, and 10-year survival rates were 84, 75, and 69 percent, respectively, with graft survival rates of 77, 63, and 57%, respectively [12].

68.1.1 Donor Recipient Matching

Careful donor and recipient selection is of paramount importance for the success of this procedure. Donors should be carefully selected in order to minimize the risks of primary nonfunction, especially for LH recipients. Young, hemodynamically stable donors with normal liver function and with a relatively short period of hospitalization should be selected. In this way, primary nonfunction for the recipients should be uncommon.

The suitable donors for SLT are only hemodynamically stable who meet the following criteria: age under 55 years, liver steatosis below 30%, ICU stay less than 5 days, Na <160 mmol/L, serum glutamic pyruvic transaminase <60 U/L, gamma-glutamyl transpeptidase <50 U/L. Organs from donors with body weight over 70 kg may be suitable for a full right/full left split, resulting in grafts for two adult recipients. In this situation, the requirements of organ quality are stricter: age under 40 years, liver steatosis under 10%, ICU stay less than 3 days [13]. The final decision on whether the graft quality is fit for splitting is made on macroscopic assessment of the graft and, ideally, based on liver biopsy, which performed routinely would help to undertake an external split graft with more confidence.

A study on a large series of 407 deceased donors determined that approximately 15% of donors fulfil such conditions for a split liver procedure, and about 9% could be eligible as donors for two adults. More optimistic calculations estimate up to 13% of donors being eligible for splitting for two adults [13]. It is difficult to estimate how much impact adult SLTs have on the donor pool. About 25% of all deceased donors in the United States are between 15 and 35 years of age. If many of these livers could be used for splits, the number of liver transplants could potentially increase with 20–25%. Moreover, with better preservation techniques, more livers may be amenable to splitting.

Proper recipient selection is also crucial in ensuring a good outcome. Administrative actions in the current methods of organ allocation to ensure optimal combinations of graft and recipient will be needed if SLT in adults is to succeed. A GW/RW ratio of close to 0.8% should likely be the minimum when selecting appropriate recipients. Moreover, due to the high risk of complications, one important aspect of the recipient selection process is adequately informing the potential recipient on the splitting procedure and obtaining informed consent.

More data are needed to better define donor and recipient selection criteria, which are crucial to success.

68.1.2 Graft Harvesting

The SLT is commonly applied at outside facilities during routine donor procurements without specialized equipment and simultaneous with additional organ (heart, lung, kidney) procurements. Additional time is required for the procedure but this has not been an excessive burden provided adequate communication has occurred between donor teams. The current challenge within the transplant community is the implementation of public policy that will facilitate its great potential to enlarge a critically limited donor pool.

Prior to the performance of SLT, the standard procedures of abdominal organ procurement including supraceliac and infrarenal aortic dissection as well as cannulation of the inferior mesenteric vein should be completed such that if the donor were to become unstable, the SLT could be aborted with rapid progression to aortic cannulation, cross-clamping, and organ cold perfusion.

68.1.2.1 In-situ Versus Ex-situ Splitting
Cold ischemic time should be minimized as much as possible in all SLT donors. For this reason, it is preferable to do the actual transection of the parenchyma in-situ (in the donor), as doing the split on the back table (ex-situ) could add up to 2 to 3 hours of cold ischemia and more likely to be some warming of the liver, even if the split is being performed in a cold ice bath of University of Wisconsin solution. Performing the split in-situ also has other advantages. Significantly less bleeding occurs when the organs are reperfused. Additionally, the two liver grafts can be assessed in the donor immediately after parenchymal transection and before vascular interruption, to ensure adequate perfusion and viability. Despite the fact that in situ splitting seems to have certain advantages concerning graft quality and subsequent recipient operation and course, logistical circumstances may favour ex situ splitting in selected cases.

68.1.3 Adult and Pediatric Recipients

The vast majority of SLTs have been performed between an adult and a pediatric recipient. The benefits for pediatric recipients have been tremendous, with a significant decrease in waiting times and mortality rates. Splitting an adult liver for pediatric recipients has no negative impact on the adult donor pool, but it does not increase it either.

68.1.3.1 Technical Features

The technique creates a LLS graft of about 250 cc, for pediatric recipients, and a right trisection graft (Couinaud segment I, IV–VIII) of about 1000 cc, for adult recipients. The in-situ procedure is described below (Fig. 68.1).

Preparation of the LLS graft begins with hilar dissection at the base of the round ligament with isolation of the left hepatic artery (HA) and left portal vein (PV) branch. The left HA is encircled and dissection is carried along its entire length. Particular attention is dedicated to the preservation of segment IV penetrating arteries. PV branches to segment IV are ligated and divided lateral to the umbilical fissure to isolate the entire left PV however, PV branches to segment I are preserved as they originate from the main, not left PV. After total vascular control of the LLS is achieved, parenchymal transection is carried out between the LLS and segment IV, 1 cm above the left hepatic duct (HD) in the umbilical fissure. Small penetrating vessels and biliary radicles are suture ligated. The remaining left hilar plate and HD are sharply transected with scissors close to the surface so as to preserve biliary drainage of segment IV. Intraoperative cholangiogram can be performed to better define the biliary anatomy. Upon completion of the dissection, the LLS is separated from the remaining parenchyma with its own vascular pedicle and venous drainage. Organ procurement continues with perfusion and cooling of the donor organs. Following perfusion, the left HA, the left PV, and the left HVs are divided and the left HD is flushed with preservation solution prior to storage of the graft in cold solution. The right trisection graft is removed in the usual fashion and stored in cold preservative solution.

Transplantation of the LLS graft involves preservation of the native inferior vena cava (IVC). The right hepatic vein (HV) entrance to the IVC and the smaller accessory HVs are suture ligated. The septum dividing the left, middle, and right HV openings to the IVC is divided to form a large common trunk for left HV anastomosis. Anastomosis of the left PV is achieved either in an end-to-end or end-to-side fashion, while the left HA is anastomosed to the common HA or

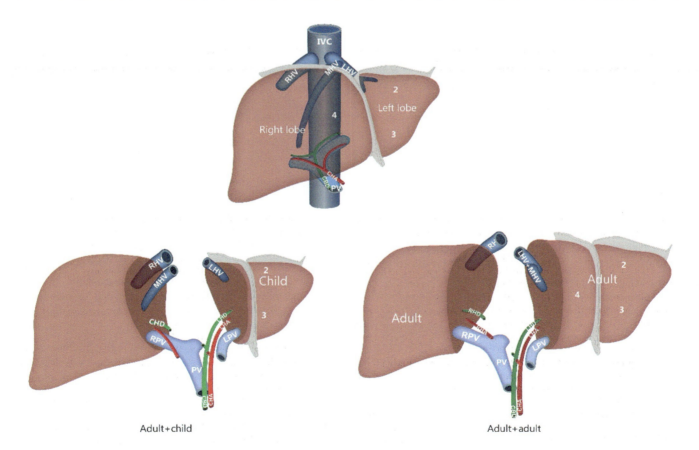

Fig. 68.1 Adult and child, and adult and adult SLT

infrarenal aorta by an iliac artery interposition graft. Biliary drainage is achieved by a duct-to-duct or Roux-en-Y hepaticojejunostomy.

Transplantation of the extended right graft is done by standard techniques.

68.1.4 Adult and Adult Recipients

The most important advantage of SLT with adult and adult recipients is the increase of the adult donor pool. Adults account nowadays for 96% of patients dying on the waiting list, while in 1988, they represented only 70%.

Transection in the midplane of the liver divides the whole graft into the anatomic right (60% of the liver) and LH (40% of the liver), commonly generating grafts with sufficient size for two adult recipients. The minimum amount of liver mass needed to sustain life after SLT is unclear. Experience with LDLT suggests that a graft weight to recipient weight (GW/RW) ratio of 0.8% is the minimal requirement. However, in deceased donors, the minimum amount of liver mass is also influenced by factors as donor hemodynamic stability and cold ischemic time, so this amount may be sometimes insufficient.

68.1.4.1 Technical Features

Several technical points need to be discussed about the operation in donor, which is very similar to a LH procurement from a living donor. The middle HV should be preserved with the LH to ensure that there is no congestion of Segment IV. Loss of the middle HV usually does not significantly affect drainage of segment V and VIII in the LH graft, as these segments usually drain adequately via the right HV. Hence, the transection plane is placed to the right of the middle HV, vein that is retained with the LH graft. Regarding the hilum dissection, our preference has been to leave the full length of the hilar structures intact with the LH graft, because the right-sided hilar structures are usually larger than the left-sided ones. Therefore, leaving the main vessels intact with the LH graft makes the transplant easier.

One crucial technical point for the recipient operation is ensuring adequate venous outflow of the grafts to prevent congestion. Preserving the IVC with the LH graft helps to maximize outflow by preserving inferior HVs (Fig. 68.2). This also allows for back-table reconstruction of large segment V and VIII veins (>5 mm in diameter) draining from the LH to the middle HV (Fig. 68.3).

The liver is mobilized by division of the falciform and left ligaments. The common trunk of the left and middle HV is encircled with an umbilical tape. The LH including the caudate lobe is completely mobilized from the IVC. The right HA and right PV are dissected free and mobilized (after removing the gallbladder). The left hilar plate is taken down and the left HD in its extrahepatic portion is encircled. The

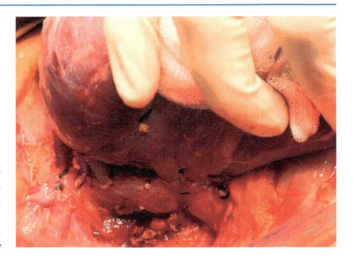

Fig. 68.2 The right hemiliver graft is harvested with the IVC preserving the inferior HVs

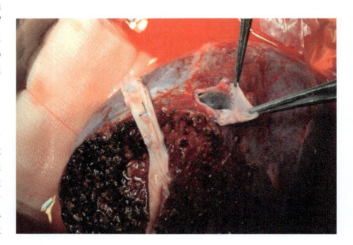

Fig. 68.3 Reconstruction of large segment V and VIII veins

line of planned transection through the hilum is through the origin of the right PV and right HA, and at the junction of the left HD with the common HD. A line for parenchymal transection is drawn just to the right of the estimated course of the middle HV. The umbilical tape is passed around the LH to suspend it upward. Liver transection is then performed in situ, and, when completed, the two halves of the liver are inspected to make sure there is no significant vascular injuries. Organs are flushed with cold preservation solution in the usual manner.

Final separation of the grafts is done on the back table. The following structures are divided to completely separate the LH and RH: the common junction of the middle and left HV, the left HD at the junction with the right, the right HA, and the right PV close to its origin. In the LH graft, the vascular stumps of the right PV and the right HA are oversewn; the outflow of the graft is represented by the combined orifices of the middle and left HVs.

68.2 Dual Graft Liver Transplantation

Living donor liver transplantation (LDLT) rate is increasing due to the shortage of deceased liver donations. However, small for size syndrome and small donor liver remnant are two uncommon but potentially lethal complications of LDLT.

68.2.1 Small for Size Syndrome

Previous studies show that at least 50% of the recipient's liver volume is mandatory for adequate liver function [14]. Small for size syndrome (SFSS) occurs when the graft recipient weight ratio (GRWR) is less than 0.8. There is an unbalance between increased metabolic demand and liver regeneration, which leads to a severe graft dysfunction. Clinically, SFSS presents with intractable ascites, coagulopathy, and jaundice. The most accepted pathophysiological mechanism is the graft over-perfusion [15]. Recently, the number of morbidly obese patients undergoing LT is raising because of the high incidence of non-alcoholic steatohepatitis related end stage liver disease, a fact that further increases the risk of SFSS.

68.2.2 Rationale

To overcome the risk of SFSS, the first successful dual graft LT, using LH and LLS grafts, was performed in 2000 by Lee SG et al. [16] (Fig. 68.4). In 2017, Lee SG et al. reported 400 such procedures [17]. To date, cases of dual liver transplantation have been reported worldwide, including from our center [18]. Little is known about the indications and contraindications of dual graft LT, and there are no selection standard selection criteria of the donors and recipient for dual graft LT.

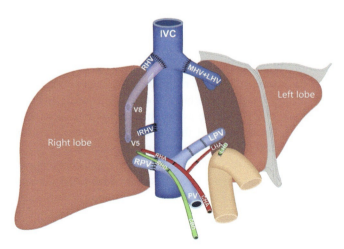

Fig. 68.4 Dual graft liver transplantation

The metabolic demands of a larger recipient will not be satisfied by a LH from a relatively small donor. The alternatives are to harvesting the RH, which accounts for 60–70% of the total liver volume, or to transplant dual grafts into one recipient. Harvesting the RH of the donor is not always safe, depending primarily on the volume of the remaining LH [19]. When the remaining LH would be insufficient after a RH harvesting, a possible and safe alternative is the dual graft LT with LH or LLS from two donors, that can avoid the SFSS while maximizing donor safety [16]. If the recipient requires a larger liver volume than the combined volume of the two potential LH grafts, a dual graft LT using a RH and a LH is the best option to avoid a SFSS, provided that the RH harvest is safe [17].

Another indication for dual graft LT may be in case of marginal grafts. It is common knowledge that the remaining liver in the donor should be over 35% of the standard liver volume of the donor; however, if the donor is of marginal quality, the size should be increased. Unfortunately, there are no available criteria for marginal liver donor. Moon et al. [20] extended the indications for dual liver transplantation to using marginal grafts such as fatty liver grafts; rapid improvement in the graft steatosis within two weeks after dual graft LT was proven. Therefore, increased volume of the marginal donor is recommended and feasible by performing dual graft LDLT.

Balancing the safety of the two donors with a good outcome in recipient is a crucial issue in the process of living donation. The ethical issue of putting two donors at risk simultaneously for one recipient is debatable. The overall mortality in donors is about 0.15–0.20% [21], while for LSS harvesting is estimated to be around 0.1% [22], and for RH harvesting from 0.4–0.5% [23]. Therefore, the donor risk in dual graft LDLT when using LH and LLS grafts, even though involves two donors, is relatively low. Although there will be constant ethical concerns about placing two donors at risk for one patient, we believe that dual graft LDLT can offer an effective and safe therapeutic option for a family who hopes to save one of their own family members.

The immune microenvironment may be more complicated when two grafts become the target of rejection. There is a risk of rejection not only between two grafts and recipient but also between grafts. Lee SG et al. reported that acute rejection was found by biopsy in both orthotopic and heterotopic grafts simultaneously [24].

68.2.3 Technical Features

In case of dual graft LDLT with two LHs or one LH and LLS [16], the second liver graft needs to be rotated 180° and heterotopically positioned in the right upper quadrant after the

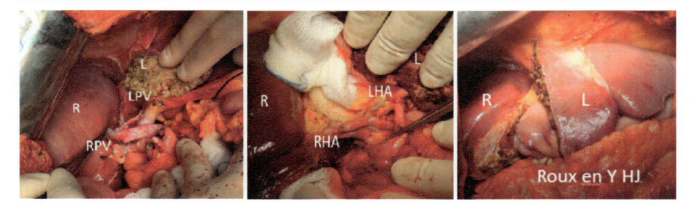

Fig. 68.5 Dual graft living donor liver transplantation using right and left hemiliver. R-right hemiliver, L-left hemiliver, LPV-left portal vein, RPV- right portal vein, RHA-right hepatic artery

first liver graft is orthotopically implanted. The HD is reconstructed by duct-to-duct anastomosis before PV and HV anastomoses, because it is placed behind the PV and the HA. This makes the hepaticojejunostomy of the second liver graft difficult with poor access once the PV anastomosis is made. An interposition vein graft obtained from cadaveric iliac vein is frequently necessary to bridge the gap between the recipient's right HV and the hepatic venous end of the liver graft.

The LH or LLS implanted heterotopicaly in the right side display particular haemodynamic properties, and there can be some competition in blood supply between the two grafts. Lee et al. reported two right-sided heterotopic grafts undergoing atrophy, which was considered to be the result of portal venous blood flow favoring the left-sided orthotopic graft [24].

Regarding the grafts of RH and LH (Fig. 68.5), the match of the grafts and recipient in spatial position makes the operation relatively easy. With regard to technical aspects, a combination of RH and LH grafts is probably the ideal option in dual graft LT.

68.3 Auxiliary Partial Orthotopic Liver Transplantation

The main causes of acute liver failure (ALF) leading to consideration of patients for liver transplantation (LT) are acute viral hepatitis, including HBV infection, and drug- or toxin-induced hepatic injury, including paracetamol overdose. In the majority of cases, patients with previously healthy livers can recover from ALF without sequelae. However, some patients develop severe forms that progress to multisystem failure, including cerebral oedema, leading to death within a few hours or days. In these patients, LT is the only effective treatment that can substitute liver function. LT is indicated in cases with severe encephalopathy (confusion or coma) associated with important impairment of the coagulation factors (factor V < 20%), with 1-year survival rates of about 60–70%.

68.3.1 Rationale

Nevertheless, a significant subset of patients with ALF who fulfil transplant criteria would have had complete morphological and functional recovery of their native liver if they would had not undergone LT. These considerations have led to the concept of auxiliary partial orthotopic LT (APOLT), based on the potential for spontaneous regeneration of the native liver and eventual withdrawal of immunosuppressive drugs for the auxiliary graft [25].

In selected young recipients (under 40 years) and hemodynamically stable, the use of ABO-compatible, the use of non-steatotic auxiliary partial grafts harvested from young donors (living or deceased), with normal liver function, can restore liver function and prevent the occurrence of irreversible brain damage [26]. The size of the graft has to be adapted to the severity of the recipient's encephalopathy. When a graft from a deceased donor is used, an important decision is whether the other partial graft not used for APOLT is discarded or used in another recipient as SLT; due to the scarcity of donor organs, the latter option is obviously the best. However, one should be aware that the splitting procedure increases the duration of the back table procedure in comparison with the reduced-size technique, and this may be detrimental for the recipient in case of severe encephalopathy that involves emergent transplantation. Moreover, the split procedure decreases the size and the length of both portal and arterial vessels, making the APOLT more technically demanding, leading to longer operative time and increased risk of complication. Thus, the perspective of transplanting another recipient should not put the APOLT recipient at increased risk [26].

After standard post-LT immunosuppression, the recovery of the native liver is assessed by biopsies, hepatobiliary scintigraphy and computed tomography. In more than 50% of the recipients, the histology, scintigraphy and morphological data show sufficient regeneration of the native liver, and the patients can be withdrawn from immunosuppression [27]. Therefore, in selected patients, the advantages of APOLT seem to surpass its drawbacks [26].

68.3.2 Technical Features

Auxiliary LT consists of implanting a healthy partial liver graft placed either heterotopically or orthotopically, after partial hepatectomy, leaving part of the native liver in place. Early experience with heterotopic placement of the graft below the native liver has been disappointing with a high rate of technical failure, probably due to inadequate portal perfusion of the graft and insufficient drainage of hepatic blood flow in an area of low pressure. The favorable outcome reported in European series using auxiliary partial orthotopic liver transplantation after partial hepatectomy (APOLT) and the expertise gained from SLT and LDLT have revived interest in this approach (Fig. 68.6).

APOLT requires that both the graft and the recipient's liver are reduced in volume, so that, after transplantation, the patient has an approximately normal overall liver volume. A frozen section biopsy of the native liver is usually sampled to assess the absence of fibrosis (that would otherwise suggest that poor regeneration of the native liver is expected) and the presence of viable hepatocytes. A right or a left hepatectomy/left lateral sectionectomy of the native liver is performed in order to prepare a space large enough to accommodate the right or left liver graft, respectively [26, 28]. In the majority of cases the auxiliary graft is a right graft which is placed orthotopically after a right hepatectomy in the recipient. The parenchymal transection tends to be easier in patients with fulminant liver failure because the liver is usually atrophic; however, this can be performed under intermittent clamping.

The partial liver graft is prepared and its size has to fit the implantation site created after partial hepatectomy of the diseased liver in recipient. Two types of auxiliary grafts can be used for APOLT: a right liver (segments V–VIII) or a left liver (segments I–IV).

Afterwards, the partial liver graft is implanted orthotopically so that both cut surfaces of the graft and of the native liver are face-to-face. The graft is slightly rolled to allow completion of an end-to-side anastomosis between the HV stump of the graft and the recipient's IVC. The corresponding side of the recipient's PV is clamped laterally just above the head of the pancreas and opened. An end-to-side is performed between the graft's and the recipient's PVs, and the graft is subsequently revascularized. The graft's coeliac axis is anastomosed end-to-side to the recipient's splenic artery or infrarenal aorta. Bile flow is restored through a Roux-en-Y hepaticojejunostomy. Intraoperative ultrasound is mandatory to assess the patency of all vascular anastomoses. A primary abdominal closure is almost always possible. However, in case of graft compression, only the skin is closed after placing an absorbable mesh sutured to the musculofascial walls; full abdominal closure is performed some days or weeks later. One should be aware that the risk of parenchymal or vascular compression at the time of abdominal closure is greater with these left grafts. A biliary drain may be placed in the recipient's cystic duct, to allow monitoring of the native liver's bile. With the proper expertise, the APOLT may provide comparable short- and long-term results with conventional LT [29, 30].

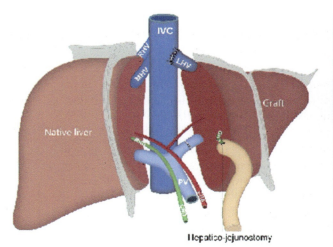
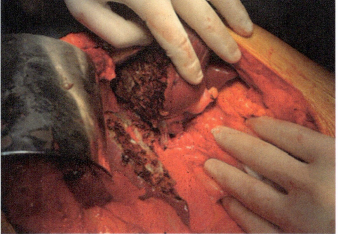

Fig. 68.6 Auxiliary partial orthotopic liver transplantation

In conclusion, improvements of surgical techniques make possible to use the technical variant liver grafts with results comparable to those of conventional LT, contributing to the increase of the donor pool, the decrease of mortality on the waiting list or to providing therapeutic option for emergent LT. Further studies are needed in order to validate their indications, donor-recipient matching and further increase the number of such procedures.

References

1. Pichlmayr R, Ringe B, Gubernatis G, Hauss J, Bunzendahl H. Transplantation einer Spenderleber auf zwei Empfänger: Eine neue Methode in der Weiterentwicklung der Lebersegmenttransplantation. Langembecks Arch Chir. 1988;373:127–30.
2. Bismuth H, Morino M, Castaing D, et al. Emergency orthotopic liver transplantation of two patients using one donor liver. Br J Surg. 1989;76:722–4.
3. Otte JB, Ville de Goyet JH, Sokal E. Size reduction of the donor liver as a safe way to allieviate the shortage of donor organs in pediatric liver transplantation. Ann Surg. 1990;211:146–57.
4. Broelsch CE, Emond JC, Whitington PF, et al. Application of reduced-size liver transplants as split grafts, auxiliary orthotopic grafts and livingrelated segmental transplants. Ann Surg. 1990;214:368–74.
5. Broelsch CE, Burdelski M, Rogiers X, et al. Living donor for liver transplantation. Hepatology. 1994;20:49S–555.
6. Emond JC, Whitington PF, Thistlethwaite JR, et al. Transplantation of two patients with one liver: analysis of a preliminary experience with 'split-liver' grafting. Ann Surg. 1990;212:14–9.
7. The SPLIT Research Group, Martin SR, Atkinson P, Lindblad AS. Studies of pediatric liver transplantation 2002: patient and graft survival and rejection in pediatric recipients of a first transplant in the United States and Canada. Pediatr Transplant. 2004;8:273–83.
8. ELTR. ELTR report, 2002 including data until 12.2002.
9. Lee WC, Chan KM, Chou HS, et al. Feasibility of split liver transplantation for 2 adults in the model of end-stage liver disease era. Ann Surg. 2013;258(2):306–11. https://doi.org/10.1097/SLA.0b013e3182754b8e.
10. Belghiti J, Zinzindohoue F, Durand F, et al. Auxiliary liver transplantation for fulminant liver failure: limits of an attractive concept. Hepatology. 1995;22:153a.
11. Sindhi R, Rosendale J, Mundy D, et al. Impact of segmental grafts on pediatric liver transplantation: review of the united network for organ sharing scientific registry data (1990–1996). J Pediatr Surg. 1999;34:107–10.
12. Vagefi PA, Parekh J, Ascher NL, et al. Outcomes with split liver transplantation in 106 recipients: the University of California, San Francisco, experience from 1993 to 2010. Arch Surg. 2011;146(9):1052–9.
13. Toso C, Ris F, Mentha G, Oberholzer J, et al. Potential impact of in situ liver splitting on the number of available grafts. Transplantation. 2002;74(2):222–6. https://doi.org/10.1097/00007890-200207270-00013.
14. Fan ST, Lo CM, Liu CL, et al. Safety of donors in live donor liver transplantation using right lobe grafts. Arch Surg. 2000;135(3):336–40. https://doi.org/10.1001/archsurg.135.3.336.
15. Kiuchi T, Kasahara M, Uryuhara K, et al. Impact of graft size mismatching on graft prognosis in liver transplantation from living donors. Transplantation. 1999;67(2):321–7.
16. Lee S, Hwang S, Park K, et al. An adult-to-adult living donor liver transplant using dual left lobe grafts. Surgery. 2001;129(5):647–50. https://doi.org/10.1067/msy.2001.114218.
17. Song GW, Lee SG, Moon DB, et al. Dual-graft adult living donor liver transplantation: an innovative surgical procedure for live liver donor pool expansion. Ann Surg. 2017;266(1):10–8.
18. Botea F, Braşoveanu V, Constantinescu A, Ionescu M, Matei E, Popescu I. Living donor liver transplantation with dual grafts -- a case report. Chirurgia (Bucur). 2013;108(4):547–52.
19. Kawasaki S, Makuuchi M, Matsunami H, et al. Living related liver transplantation in adults. Ann Surg. 1998;227(2):269–74. https://doi.org/10.1097/00000658-199802000-00017.
20. Moon D, Lee S, Hwang S, et al. Resolution of severe graft steatosis following dual-graft living donor liver transplantation. Liver Transpl. 2006;12(7):1156–60. https://doi.org/10.1002/lt.20814.
21. Trotter JF, Adam R, Lo CM, Kenison J. Documented deaths of hepatic lobe donors for living donor liver transplantation. Liver Transpl. 2006;12(10):1485–8. https://doi.org/10.1002/lt.20875.
22. Otte JB. Donor complications and outcomes in live-liver transplantation. Transplantation. 2003;75(10):1625–6. https://doi.org/10.1097/01.tp.0000065020.55959.4a.
23. Hwang S, Lee SG, Lee YJ, et al. Lessons learned from 1,000 living donor liver transplantations in a single center: how to make living donations safe. Liver Transpl. 2006;12(6):920–7. https://doi.org/10.1002/lt.20734.
24. Lee SG, Hwang S, Park KM, et al. Seventeen adult-to-adult living donor liver transplantations using dual grafts. Transplant Proc. 2001;33(7–8):3461–3.
25. Chenard-Neu MP, Boudjema K, Bernuau J, et al. Auxiliary liver transplantation: regeneration of the native liver and outcome in 30 patients with fulminant hepatic failure--a multicenter European study. Hepatology. 1996;23(5):1119–27. https://doi.org/10.1002/hep.510230528.
26. Belghiti J, Sommacale D, Dondéro F, et al. Auxiliary liver transplantation for acute liver failure. HPB (Oxford). 2004;6(2):83–7. https://doi.org/10.1080/13651820310020783.
27. Buyck D, Bonnin F, Bernuau J, Belghiti J, Bok B. Auxiliary liver transplantation in patients with fulminant hepatic failure: hepatobiliary scintigraphic follow-up. Eur J Nucl Med. 1997;24(2):138–42. https://doi.org/10.1007/BF02439545.
28. Boudjema K, Cherqui D, Jaeck D, et al. Auxiliary liver transplantation for fulminant and subfulminant hepatic failure. Transplantation. 1995;59:218–23.
29. Azoulay D, Samuel D, Ichai P, et al. Auxiliary partial orthotopic versus standard orthotopic whole liver transplantation for acute liver failure: a reappraisal from a single center by a case-control study. Ann Surg. 2001;234(6):723–31. https://doi.org/10.1097/00000658-200112000-00003.
30. Weiner J, Griesemer A, Island E, et al. Longterm outcomes of auxiliary partial orthotopic liver transplantation in preadolescent children with fulminant hepatic failure. Liver Transpl. 2016;22(4):485–94. https://doi.org/10.1002/lt.24361.

Domino Liver Transplantation

Irinel Popescu, Vladislav Brasoveanu, Doina Hrehoret, Florin Botea, Simona Dima, and Florin Ichim

Abstract

Domino Liver transplant (DLT) is a surgical strategy to expand the liver donor pool, addressing the organ shortage, in selected patients who would otherwise not have the opportunity to benefit from liver transplantation. In this sense, DLT uses morphologically normal livers from donors with certain metabolic disorders (familial amyloidotic polyneuropathy, primary hyperoxaluria, acute intermittent porphyria, maple syrup urine disease, and homozygous familial hypercholesterolemia) in selected recipients, usually with hepatocellular carcinoma (generally outside the Milan criteria). However, the benefit of expanding the donor pool must be balanced against the risk of metabolic disease transmission. Despite some typical technical challenges, DLT appears to be a safe and reasonable transplant option.

69.1 Background

Liver transplantation (LT) is an established therapeutic option for patients in a series of acute and chronic liver disorders. However, the donor pool does not meet the continuously increasing demand for patients on the waiting list.

Limited organ availability and the significant percentage of drop-outs from the waiting list because of cirrhosis and/or tumor progression still represent major drawbacks for transplantation strategies. Because of these drawbacks, not all patients initially eligible for transplantation eventually benefit from it [1]. As a result, novel strategies, such as increased use of marginal donors, living donor liver grafts, split liver grafts from deceased donors, and so-called domino liver grafts from patients with metabolic liver disease, have been explored to address the organ shortage.

In this context, domino liver transplant (DLT) has emerged as a strategy for expanding the donor pool for LT [2], based on the fact that certain metabolic disorders, such as familial amyloidotic polyneuropathy, primary hyperoxaluria, acute intermittent porphyria, maple syrup urine disease, and homozygous familial hypercholesterolemia, may be amended by LT while the explant is a well-functioning liver that can be used in another recipient [3, 4].

DLT, that consists in transplanting a patient that in turn donates his liver to another recipient, was introduced in 1995 by Furtado A et al. [5]. DLT uses morphologically normal livers from donors with metabolic disorders generally, that is in the same time recipient (domino donor), for selected recipients (domino recipients) generally with hepatocellular carcinoma (usually outside the Milan criteria). Grafts from these donors are usually received by patients with advanced stage hepatocellular carcinoma [6], with low priority on the waiting list and/or unlikely to survive until standard LR, or by tumor free cirrhotic domino recipients, sporadic cases of metabolic fulminant liver failure [3], and retransplants [7, 8].

This procedure raises ethical and surgical issues. The most important ethical principle concerns the informed consent of both the domino recipient and the donor, emphasizing that the recipient may develop the domino donor's genetic disease. Additionally, the domino donors must be assured that the technical demands of the hepatectomy for this procedure will not expose to any additional risks.

In order to gather as much information as possible about DLT, an international registry (the Domino Liver Transplant Registry) was created in 1999 as an extension of the already existing Familial Amyloidotic Polyneuropathy World Transplant Registry.

I. Popescu (✉) · V. Brasoveanu · F. Botea
"Dan Setlacec" Center of General Surgery and Liver Transplantation, Fundeni Clinical Institute, Bucharest, Romania

"Titu Maiorescu" University, Bucharest, Romania

D. Hrehoret · S. Dima · F. Ichim
"Dan Setlacec" Center of General Surgery and Liver Transplantation, Fundeni Clinical Institute, Bucharest, Romania

69.2 Indications in Domino Donor

In the last decades, DLT have been validated in more than 1000 patients, mainly using domino livers procured from patients with familial amyloid polyneuropathy (FAP). Other, less common, indications for domino liver graft are: fibrinogen A α-chain amyloidosis, homozygous familial hypercholesterolemia (HFHC), maple syrup urine disease (MSUD), acute intermittent porphyria (AIP), primary hyperoxaluria (PH); very rare indications are hemochromatosis, Wilson's disease, methylmalonic acidemia, hyperhomocysteinemia, and ornithine transcarbamylase deficiency, [9]. However, insufficient data about the use of livers from patients with these rare metabolic disorders are available. PH is not a good indication for DLT because recipients of PH livers develop hyperoxaluria and early acute renal failure. AIP also seems to be a debatable indication for DLT because of the rapid development of neurotoxicity in AIP liver recipients. However, the outcomes of DLT with HFHC and MSUD liver grafts (which include the risk of the de novo development of these genetic disorders) are promising. For these rare metabolic liver disorders to be established as indications for DLT, more reports and studies are needed.

Except for the production of an abnormal protein or enzyme, the livers of the domino donors are morphologically normal and fully functional. Additionally, the metabolic disorders of the donors usually should not produce symptoms in the DLT recipients for many years. LT is an increasingly popular therapeutic option for many liver-based inborn errors of metabolism. These explanted, metabolically dysfunctional livers create new categories of potential donors and recipients.

69.2.1 Familial Amyloidotic Polyneuropathy

FAP is an autosomal dominant disease that is associated with a mutation of the transthyretin (TTR) gene, characterized by the extracellular deposition of TTR amyloid fibrils, especially in the peripheral nervous system. The clinical symptoms of FAP take 20 to 30 years to appear and another 10 to 14 years to become fatal. Because more than 95% of the circulating TTR is produced in the liver, LT represents a curative treatment for this disease [10]. Mutations in the fibrinogen Aα-chain (Afib) gene are the main causes of hereditary renal amyloidosis. Combined liver-kidney transplantation has been performed in such patients with kidney impairment. Stangou et al. reported DLT with grafts from Afib patients [11].

Domino FAP grafts are structurally and functionally normal livers (except producing variant transthyritin protein), from usually young donors. FAP is the most common indication for DLT, although de novo FAP development within various periods of time has been described in the domino recipients. DLT with a liver from a patient with FAP was first performed in October 1995 in Portugal by Furtado et al. [5], shortly followed by others [12–14]. By the end of 2017, a total of 1254 domino transplantations were registered in FAP World Transplant Registry (http://www.fapwtr.org). FAP is the most common indication for DLT, and DLT is performed more frequently in areas in which the incidence of this disease is higher (Portugal, Sweden, and Japan). Worldwide, many centers have reported successful DLT with FAP liver grafts.

One reason for expanding the indications for DLT is that this procedure is associated with decreased graft dysfunction and perioperative bleeding, possibly because of the protective role of the short ischemia time in DLT and the younger age of the donors. However, the de novo development of FAP within various periods of time (2–9 years) has been described in DLT recipients of FAP livers [15].

69.2.2 Familial Hypercholesterolemia

Familial hypercholesterolemia is an autosomal codominant metabolic disorder due to a mutation in the low-density lipoprotein gene; this mutation causes a reduced number of functional low-density lipoprotein receptors (LDLRs) on the cell membrane. Defects in the genes for apolipoprotein B and proprotein convertase subtilisin/kexin type 9 have also been identified in patients with FHC. In homozygous cases of familial hypercholesterolemia (HFHC), there are no or few LDLRs; the disease is present from birth, and the serum cholesterol levels often exceed 1000 mg/dL. Consequently, the patient develops severe systemic atherosclerosis and dies from myocardial infarction before the age of 20 years [16].

HFHC patients must undergo either portocaval shunting or LT. Low-density lipoprotein apheresis is another option for these patients, but it is marked by multiple complications (eg, difficulties with the long-term maintenance of vascular access and poor quality of life due to repeated procedures).

LT, which was introduced as a curative procedure for HFHC by Starzl et al. in 1984, is based on the large proportion (50%–75%) of LDLRs in the liver. LT must be performed as early as possible for HFHC before the development of severe atherosclerosis and coronary heart disease; otherwise, combined heart and liver transplantation must be performed [16]. Maiorana et al. showed that preemptive LT performed before the onset of cardiovascular disease may the only definitive therapy for this disease [17].

The indications for DLT with a graft from a patient with HFHC are rare, the first being performed in our center by Popescu I. et al. [18] and the second in Taiwan by Liu C. et al.

[19]; in fact, there are few published such cases. There have been at least 4 additional cases in Turkey (Y. Tokat, unpublished data, 2011). The first reported procedure was performed at our center by Popescu et al.: a liver from a 25-year-old patient with HFHC was transplanted into a 46-year-old patient with HCC (a 5-cm-diameter nodule, with a high alpha fetoprotein value of 500 ng/mL, unresponsive to repeated chemoembolization), and hepatitis B virus (HBV)–related liver cirrhosis in 2001 (Fig. 69.1). The immediate postoperative course was uneventful. Three years after transplantation, an autologous CD34 cell transplant was performed for better control over the patient's hypercholesterolemia [16]. To-date, 20 years after DLT, the patient is still free of disease with no HCC recurrence or complications related to HFHC (I. Popescu, unpublished data).

The positive outcomes of these patients can be explained by the activity of extrahepatic LDLRs. Therefore, each recipient candidate should ideally be screened for extrahepatic receptor activity; in reality, however, this is difficult and impractical. It is also important to use medications (eg, a 3-hydroxy-3-methylglutaryl-coenzyme A reductase inhibitor and a cholesterol absorption inhibitor) and to modify the diet appropriately after DLT [16].

69.2.3 Maple Syrup Urine Disease

Maple syrup urine disease (MSUD) is an autosomal recessive metabolic disorder that is characterized by impaired activity of the branched-chain a-keto acid dehydrogenase complex, which results in an accumulation of branched-chain L-amino acids (BCAAs) and a-keto acids. The clinical course is marked by episodes of ketoacidosis with neurotoxic effects. The treatment consists of supplementation with thiamine and, in most patients, a strict diet with a reduced intake of protein and branched amino acids. However, even under these conditions, subsequent complications such as brain damage and death are often reported. The serum marker of MSUD is alloisoleucine, which is also used for treatment control.

LT has been performed for some patients with MSUD. LT corrects the BCAA levels, eliminates the metabolic crisis, and improves the long-term outcomes of patients with MSUD. The recipients maintained nearly normal levels of plasma amino acids, demonstrating absence of the disorder. This phenomenon can be explained by the fact that they maintained their normal extrahepatic oxidation of leucine. Because branched chain a-keto acid dehydrogenase is

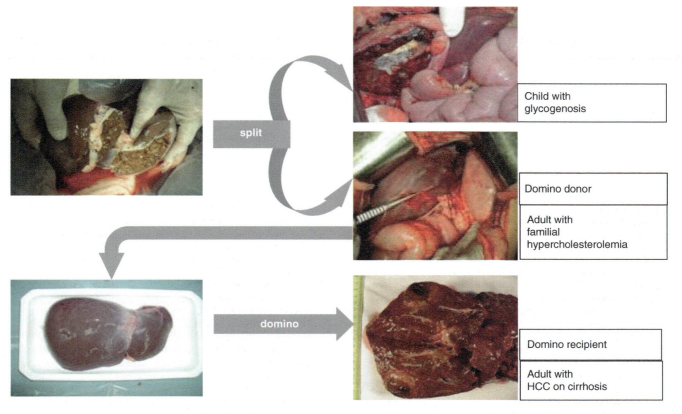

Fig. 69.1 DLT with a liver from a 25-year-old patient with HFHC (domino donor) that was transplanted into a 46-year-old patient with HCC and hepatitis B virus–related liver cirrhosis (domino recipient). The domino donor received a split graft (segments 4–8) from a deceased donor

expressed in extrahepatic tissues, DLT with livers explanted from patients with MSUD is feasible, but more studies are required [20].

69.2.4 Primary Hyperoxaluria

Primary hyperoxaluria (PH) is a rare autosomal recessive metabolic disorder that is characterized by a defect in alanine-glyoxylate aminotransferase (AGT), which is encoded by a gene that is expressed only in the liver. This deficiency results in liver oxalate overproduction, hyperoxaluria, calcium oxalate deposition, nephrocalcinosis, and end-stage renal failure. Fifty percent of all patients reach end-stage renal disease by 25 years of age, and in these patients, conventional dialysis is ineffective because it does not clear sufficient amounts of oxalate. The treatment for these patients is usually combined liver-kidney transplantation. PH is a Model for End-Stage Liver Disease exception for organ allocation in Eurotransplant. Saner et al. published a small series (5 cases) of DLT with PH livers in the Eurotransplant region, all domino recipients developing dialysis-dependent kidney failure despite good liver function [21]. Hyperoxaluria in the donor should also be carefully considered because extrahepatic AGT in the domino recipient would be inadequate for detoxifying the de novo generated glyoxylate from a PH type 1 liver [21]. Due to these disadvantages, the indication remains controversial.

69.2.5 Acute Intermittent Porphyria

Acute intermittent porphyria (AIP) is the most common hepatic porphyria. AIP is an autosomal dominant disorder of the third enzyme in the heme biosynthetic pathway and results from a partial deficiency of hydroxy-methylbilane synthase/porphobilinogen deaminase. The liver is the source of the heme precursor aminolevulinic acid, which is the major cause of neurological attack during AIP.

LT represents a potentially effective treatment for severely affected patients with recurrent life-threatening neurovisceral attacks despite optimal medical therapy with human hemin. The outcomes showed that livers from donors with AIP are neurotoxic when they are transplanted into recipients without porphyria, and acute attacks can result from the production of neurotoxins by the liver [22], therefore this indication is practically abandoned.

69.3 Indications in Domino Recipient

When DLT first began to be used, the domino recipient indications were primary hepatocellular carcinoma and, rarely, cholangiocarcinoma or even secondary liver metastases. As experience with transplantation accumulated, HCC has remained the main liver malignancy in DLT recipients, especially in those recipients who are beyond the Milan criteria [22]. Nowadays, domino donor grafts are used also for patients with alcohol- and virus-related liver cirrhosis. The typical candidate is a patient whose condition will ensure a long time on the waiting list, elderly patients (55–60 years old) with a life expectancy shorter than the time needed to develop the symptoms of the domino donor's disorder. There is also a tendency to use these grafts (similarly to split grafts) as a bridging therapy for neonates; this allows them to grow until they can receive a normal and size-compatible liver.

Indications for the recipient in DLT vary between countries and must take into account factors including age, potential hazards, probability of recurrence, prognosis and priorities in the transplant waiting lists. Many centers select older and more marginal transplant candidates for DLT [23]. Main indications for the domino recipients included: primary hepatic malignancy (41.4%), alcoholic cirrhosis (19%), cirrhosis secondary to hepatitis B and/or C (17%), metastatic hepatic malignancy (2.3%) and retransplantation (5.3%) (http://www.fapwtr.org).

69.4 Technical Considerations

The hepatectomy in the domino recipient is particularly demanding, as it is not a regular hepatectomy for LT, but a graft harvesting for subsequent implantation in the domino recipient. In case of FAP domino donor, if the resection of the inferior vena cava (IVC) along with the liver is decided, venovenous bypass is required because FAP patients are particularly sensitive to hemodynamic changes after caval clamping. The "double piggy-back" technique described by Marques et al. [24], that allows preservation of the donor's IVC may be used in order to eliminate the need of caval clamping or bypass.

Moreover, in the FAP domino donor, unnecessary mobilizations that may contribute to small periods of warm ischemia are to be avoided. The hilum is minimally dissected, and the common bile duct is divided at its mid length. Accessory hepatic veins greater than 5 mm in diameter are preserved if clamping results in congestion of part of the liver. The right hepatic vein (RHV) and the cuff of middle (MHV) and left hepatic (LHV) veins are isolated. After dissection, the proper hepatic artery is divided at the bifurcation of gastroduodenal and common hepatic arteries and the portal vein is divided 1 cm below its bifurcation. The RHV is transected close to the liver parenchyma using a vascular stapler. The isolated M-LHV cuff is double clamped and hepatic veins are then divided close to the liver surface, completing total hepatectomy. The harvested graft is perfused with preservation solution through the portal vein and the hepatic artery [24].

To overcome the problem of short vascular stumps, many techniques of outflow reconstruction of the domino graft have been reported. Graft options to create a "neo" suprahepatic IVC include the use of a cadaveric IVC with or without renal vein, iliac veins, and pulmonary artery, among others. The reconstruction will allow the surgeon to perform the domino liver transplant in a standard piggyback fashion [22, 25, 26].

The domino donor receives a whole or split graft from a deceased donor, or a partial graft from a living donor, using the standard techniques.

The domino recipient receives the whole graft harvested from the domino donor, graft that may require more technically demanding vascular reconstructions, mainly for the venous anastomosis and, but also for the arterial and portal anastomoses, especially in case of anatomical variants.

69.5 Long-term Results

DLT should not expose the recipients or the donors to any significant additional operative risks when compared with deceased donor liver transplantation (DDLT). The survival of the domino recipients should be as good as it would be with DDLT, and the morbidity and mortality of the domino donors must be kept to a minimum.

DLT is not associated with a higher morbidity or mortality rate in the donor. While the risks of DLT are unique, several studies show a similar survival rates when compared to DDLT. In the Domino Liver World Transplant Register, the overall 1-year, 5-year, and 8-year graft survival in DLT recipients was 79.9%, 65.3%, and 61.6%, respectively. Also, several studies found no difference in the rates of acute rejection, perioperative bleeding, vascular complications or biliary complications [27, 28].

However, the recipient carries the risk of developing "de novo" FAP disorder in case of FAP domino donors [10]. It was assumed that this disorder disease would only become clinically apparent 25 or 30 years after DLT. However, there were concerns about the impact of the recipient's age and immunosuppression on the underlying biological mechanisms and their possible contribution on the earlier onset of symptoms in the domino recipient [29], concerns that were confirmed as FAP symptoms appear earlier than anticipated, that is after only 5 years after DLT [30–32]. Domino recipients should follow a permanent follow-up, and, when iatrogenic amyloid neuropathy and systemic amyloidosis are diagnosed, treatment options are limited and retransplantation with a non-domino liver should be considered. However, retransplantation is a high-risk procedure due to the comorbidities of patients [30].

In conclusion, outcome of DLT depend on the underlying disorders of the domino donors. The risk of each metabolic disorder must be assessed in the context of each recipient. DLT is feasible but requires proper selection of recipients and careful planning for the surgical procedures used for the liver explants.

Given the known risk of FAP disease transmission, the selection of domino recipients must take into account the status of the patient 7–8 years after LT, in the event that a retransplant is necessary. Although the use of DLT is limited so far, grafts from HFHC patients can offer satisfactory results to the appropriate recipients. The outcomes of DLT with HFHC and MSUD liver grafts (which include the risk of the de novo development of these genetic disorders) are promising. The results with livers from PH and AIP patients are still debatable, and it has been suggested that PH livers be used only as a bridge to LT or for selected recipients who are excluded from regular allocation. The reason for this restriction is the onset of metabolic disease in DLT patients with PH or AIP liver grafts; this occurs much sooner in these patients versus those with HFHC or MSUD liver grafts. For rare metabolic liver disorders to be established as indications for DLT, larger numbers of patients with long-term follow-up must be studied. Until then, the decision to use this method will remain individualized and center-oriented.

References

1. Sotiropoulos GC, Paul A, Molmenti E, et al. Liver transplantation for hepatocellular carcinoma in cirrhosis within the Eurotransplant area: an additional option with "livers that nobody wants". Transplantation. 2005;7:897.
2. Carrera MT, Bogue EH, Schiano TD. Domino liver transplantation: a practical option in the face of the organ shortage. Prog Transplant. 2003;13(2):151–3. https://doi.org/10.7182/prtr.13.2.y7750570q8t50891.
3. Wilczek HE, Larsson M, Yamamoto S, et al. Domino liver transplantation. J Hepato-Biliary-Pancreat Surg. 2008;2:139.
4. Celik N, Squires JE, Soltys K, et al. Domino liver transplantation for select metabolic disorders: expanding the living donor pool. JIMD Rep. 2019;48(1):83–9. https://doi.org/10.1002/jmd2.12053.
5. Furtado A, Tome L, Oliveira FJ, et al. Sequential liver transplantation. Transplant Proc. 1997;2:467.
6. Nishizaki T, Kishikawa K, Yoshizumi T, et al. Domino liver transplantation from a living related donor. Transplantation. 2000;8:1236.
7. Ericzon BG, Larsson M, Wilczek HE. Domino liver transplantation: risks and benefits. Transplant Proc. 2008;4:1130.
8. Nunes F, Valente M, Pereira R, et al. Domino liver transplant: influence on the number of donors and transplant coordination. Transplant Proc. 2004;4:916.
9. Marques HP, Barros I, Li J, Murad SD, di Benedetto F. Current update in domino liver transplantation. Int J Surg. 2020;82S:163–8. https://doi.org/10.1016/j.ijsu.2020.03.017.
10. Ericzon BG. Domino transplantation using livers from patients with familial amyloidotic polyneuropathy: should we halt? Liver Transpl. 2007;13(2):185–7. https://doi.org/10.1002/lt.21073.
11. Stangou AJ, Banner NR, Hendry BM, Benson MD, et al. Hereditary fibrinogen a alpha-chain amyloidosis: phenotypic characterization of a systemic disease and the role of liver transplan-

tation. Blood. 2010;115(15):2998–3007. https://doi.org/10.1182/blood-2009-06-223792.
12. Hesse UJ, Troisi R, Mortier E, et al. Die sequentielle orthotope Lebertransplantation--Dominotransplantation [sequential orthotopic liver transplantation--domino transplantation]. Chirurg. 1997;68(10):1011–3.
13. Stangou AJ, Heaton ND, Rela M, et al. Domino hepatic transplantation using the liver from a patient with familial amyloid polyneuropathy. Transplantation. 1998;65(11):1496–8. https://doi.org/10.1097/00007890-199806150-00016.
14. Ando Y, Ericzon BG, Suhr OB, Tashima K, Ando M. Reuse of a Japanese familial amyloidotic polyneuropathy patient's liver for a cancer patient: the domino liver transplantation procedure. Intern Med. 1997;36(11):847. https://doi.org/10.2169/internalmedicine.36.847.
15. Stangou AJ, Heaton ND, Hawkins PN. Transmission of systemic transthyretin amyloidosis by means of domino liver transplantation. N Engl J Med. 2005;352(22):2356. https://doi.org/10.1056/NEJM200506023522219.
16. Popescu I, Habib N, Dima S, et al. Domino liver transplantation using a graft from a donor with familial hypercholesterolemia: seven-yr follow-up. Clin Transpl. 2009;23(4):565–70.
17. Maiorana A, Nobili V, Calandra S, et al. Preemptive liver transplantation in a child with familial hypercholesterolemia. Pediatr Transplant. 2011;15(2):E25–9.
18. Popescu I, Simionescu M, Tulbure D, et al. Homozygous familial hypercholesterolemia: specific indication for domino liver transplantation. Transplantation. 2003;76(9):1345–50.
19. Liu C, Niu DM, Loong CC, et al. Domino liver graft from a patient with homozygous familial hypercholesterolemia. Pediatr Transplant. 2010;14(3):E30–3. https://doi.org/10.1111/j.1399-3046.2009.01133.x.
20. Spada M, Angelico R, Dionisi-Vici C. Maple syrup urine disease and domino liver transplantation: when and how? Liver Transpl. 2019;25(6):827–8. https://doi.org/10.1002/lt.25481.
21. Saner FH, Treckmann J, Pratschke J, et al. Early renal failure after domino liver transplantation using organs from donors with primary hyperoxaluria type 1. Transplantation. 2010;90(7):782–5.
22. Popescu I, Dima SO. Domino liver transplantation: how far can we push the paradigm? Liver Transpl. 2012;18(1):22–8. https://doi.org/10.1002/lt.22443.
23. Kitchens WH. Domino liver transplantation: indications, techniques, and outcomes. Transplant Rev (Orlando). 2011;25(4):167–77. https://doi.org/10.1016/j.trre.2011.04.002. Epub 2011 Jul 30
24. Marques HP, Ribeiro V, Almeida T, et al. Long-term results of domino liver transplantation for hepatocellular carcinoma using the "double piggy-back" technique: a 13-year experience. Ann Surg. 2015;262(5):749–56.; discussion 756. https://doi.org/10.1097/SLA.0000000000001446.
25. Qu W, Zhu ZJ, Wei L, et al. Reconstruction of the outflow tract in cross-auxiliary double-domino donor liver transplantation. Transplant Proc. 2016;48(8):2738–41. https://doi.org/10.1016/j.transproceed.2016.07.031.
26. Cepeda-Franco C, Marín-Gómez LM, Bernal-Bellido C, et al. Alternative outflow reconstruction in domino liver transplantation. Liver Transpl. 2017;23(9):1226–8. https://doi.org/10.1002/lt.24816.
27. Bispo M, Marcelino P, Marques HP, et al. Domino versus deceased donor liver transplantation: association with early graft function and perioperative bleeding. Liver Transpl. 2011;17(3):270–8.
28. Geyer ED, Burrier C, Tumin D, et al. Outcomes of domino liver transplantation compared to deceased donor liver transplantation: a propensity-matching approach. Transpl Int. 2018;31(11):1200–6.
29. Banerjee D, Roeker LE, Grogan M, et al. Outcomes of patients with familial transthyretin amyloidosis after liver transplantation. Prog Transplant. 2017;27(3):246–50. https://doi.org/10.1177/1526924817715463.
30. Yamamoto S, Wilczek HE, Iwata T, et al. Long-term consequences of domino liver transplantation using familial amyloidotic polyneuropathy grafts. Transpl Int. 2007;20(11):926–33.
31. Adams D, Lacroix C, Antonini T, et al. Symptomatic and proven de novo amyloid polyneuropathy in familial amyloid polyneuropathy domino liver recipients. Amyloid. 2011;18(Suppl 1):174–7.
32. Lladó L, Baliellas C, Casasnovas C, et al. Risk of transmission of systemic transthyretin amyloidosis after domino liver transplantation. Liver Transpl. 2010;16(12):1386–92.

Cell Transplantation

Allogeneic and Autologous Pancreatic Islet Cell Transplantation

Takayuki Anazawa, Takashi Ito, Koichiro Hata, Toshihiko Masui, and Kojiro Taura

Abstract

In hepato-pancreato-biliary disease treatment, pancreatic islet transplantation (PIT) is the most clinically successful cell transplantation. Allogeneic PIT can effectively treat patients with type 1 diabetes with intractable impaired awareness of hypoglycemia and severe hypoglycemic events. The indication of this treatment has been widely investigated through several clinical trials, and further development is expected. Patients with painful chronic pancreatitis undergoing total pancreatectomy may receive total pancreatectomy with islet autotransplantation to prevent surgical diabetes. This treatment has been increasingly applied; thus, evaluations of its indication and usefulness should be determined. In this chapter, we provide an outline on allogeneic and autologous PIT and introduce the refinement that might improve the clinical outcome.

70.1 Introduction

In the field of hepato-pancreato-biliary disease treatment, several cell transplantation procedures, including pancreatic islet transplantation (PIT) [1] and hepatocyte transplantation [2], have been currently developed to make procedure less invasive. Among these procedures, PIT is widely clinically applied with two treatment methods, namely, allogeneic PIT as a radical treatment for type 1 diabetes and total pancreatectomy with islet autotransplantation (TPIAT) as a pain-relieving treatment for painful chronic pancreatitis (CP).

Allogeneic PIT is a cell transplantation method that transplants only the islets isolated from the pancreas donated by donors after brain death or cardiac death, thereby restoring blood glucose stability while preventing severe hypoglycemia events (SHEs). Meanwhile, pancreas transplantation, which is performed for similar patients, has a high therapeutic effect, but it is highly invasive, placing the patient highly at risk of complications. Conversely, allogeneic PIT, wherein a pancreatic islet is simply infused into the portal vein under local anesthesia, is minimally invasive and safe.

As islet transplantation continues to evolve and improve in terms of insulin independence, immunosuppression, cost, and availability, solid organ transplantation may eventually shift to islet transplantation. Likewise, with continuous development in allogeneic PIT, pancreas transplantation may shift to allogeneic PIT, considering the improved insulin independent rates associated with the enhanced immunosuppressive therapy. As an example, Table 70.1 shows the current indication criteria for allogeneic PIT in Japan.

TPIAT is another treatment method that can relieve incapacitating pain and preserve β cell mass and insulin secretory capacity as much as possible to prevent or minimize the inevitable post-pancreatectcomy diabetes [3]. In this procedure, the pancreas is completely resected to remove the visceral source of pain; then, the islets are transplanted back into the patient, most typically via infusion into the portal vein. In North America, Europe, and Australia, TPIAT is increasingly being used to treat patients with painful CP. However, the islet yield can be varied from case to case; hence, they must still accept the possibility of acquiring diabetes for the relief of pain. TPIAT initially had no established guideline as to who is a suitable candidate, when to intervene, or what the therapeutic effect is, but with the increase in the number of cases conducted in recent years, a certain consensus has been attained.

In this chapter, we provide an outline on allogeneic PIT and TPIAT and introduce the refinement that has been attempted to improve the clinical outcome.

T. Anazawa (✉) · T. Ito · K. Hata · T. Masui · K. Taura
Division of Hepato-Biliary-Pancreatic Surgery and Transplantation, Department of Surgery, Graduate School of Medicine, Kyoto University, Kyoto, Japan
e-mail: anazawa@kuhp.kyoto-u.ac.jp

Table 70.1 Indications for allogeneic pancreatic islet transplantation in Japan

Patients suffering from diabetes with absent endogenous insulin secretory capacity, highly unstable glycemic fluctuations even with intensive diabetic management, and inability of achieving good glycemic control caused by severe hypoglycemia event.

Inclusion criteria
1. Type 1 diabetes mellitus, duration >5 years
2. Age: 20–75 years
3. Refractory hypoglycemia despite the following:
    a. Optimal intensive insulin or insulin pump with appropriate monitoring
    b. Supervision of a diabetologist or endocrinologist
4. Fasting c-peptide levels <0.2 ng/mL

Exclusion criteria
1. Body mass index (BMI) > 30 kg/m^2
2. Severe coexisting cardiac disease
3. Severe liver dysfunction
4. Estimated glomerular filtration rate < 30 mL/min/1.73 m^2 (individually evaluated after kidney transplantation)
5. Untreated proliferative diabetic retinopathy
6. Known active alcohol or substance abuse
7. Active and latent infections that may be exacerbated under posttransplant immunosuppression
8. Active foot ulcer/gangrene
9. Recent history of malignancy
10. Any medical condition that, according to the physician, will interfere with safe transplantation

70.2 Allogeneic PIT

To achieve better graft function on allogeneic PIT, surgeons need to transplant a sufficient mass of viable islets. Prior to PIT, the following brief islet isolation methods (Fig. 70.1) should be performed. Initially, the procured and cold-preserved pancreas is distended with cold collagenase and protease solution through the pancreatic duct. The distended pancreas is digested using the semiautomated method [4]. The pancreatic digest is purified by continuous density gradient under cold conditions. If the releasing criteria (islet mass ≥ 5000 IE/kg [recipient body weight], islet purity ≥30%, membrane-integrity viability ≥70%, packed-tissue volume < 10 mL, negative Gram stain, and content ≤5 endotoxin U/kg [recipient body weight]) are met, the isolated islets will be transplanted. In this islet isolation procedure, the islet must be damaged by hypoxia, warm ischemia, and activated proteolytic enzymes released from the acinar cells. Consequently, the pancreas' cellular and noncellular components are seriously damaged. Hence, a method that can alleviate these damaging factors should be established [5].

With the success of the "Edmonton Protocol" reported by the University of Alberta in Edmonton, Canada in 2000 [6],

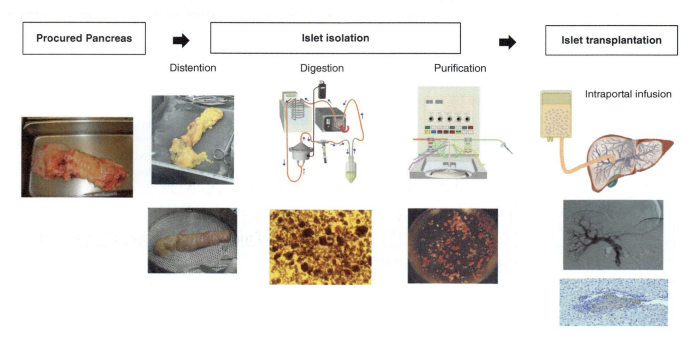

Fig. 70.1 Schematic representation of the islet isolation and transplantation. After procurement, the donor pancreas is transported to the islet-processing facility where the pancreatic duct is cannulated and then distended with cold islet isolation enzymes using a pressure-controlled pump system. The distended pancreas is placed in a Ricordi chamber and digested using the semiautomated method. When most of the islets are free from exocrine tissues, the digestion phase is switched to dilution phase. All diluted and centrifuged pellets are recombined in a cold preservation solution. Then, the digested tissue is purified by continuous iodixanol density gradient on a COBE 2991 cell separator. The final islet preparation is placed in culture media before it is released for clinical transplantation through percutaneous transhepatic intraportal infusion

allogeneic PIT has been recognized as a clinically meaningful treatment. Through the advances in immunosuppressive therapy, clinical results are improving. According to a report based on islet transplant cases registered in the Collaborative Islet Transplant Registry (CITR: https://citregistry.org/), which is an international islet transplant registry group, the insulin independence rate at 3 years after transplant improved from 27% in the early era (1999–2002) to 37% in the mid era (2003–2006) and to 44% in the recent era (2007–2010) [7]. In addition, SHEs were continuously prevented even in cases where insulin independence was not preserved. This improvement in insulin independence rate was mainly contributed by the initial T cell-depleting therapy and tumor necrosis factor-α (TNF-α) inhibition. These findings are progressing forward in phase 3 trials to obtain Biological Licensure Application for an islet product from the FDA (CIT-07: Islet Alone Licensure Study). In the immunosuppressive therapy of this trial, the T cell-depleting therapy and TNF-α inhibition were induced, combined with the maintenance of calcineurin inhibitor with mTOR inhibitor or mycophenolate mofetil. The primary endpoint included the achievement of HbA1c < 7.0% (53 mmol/mol) at day 365 and freedom from SHEs from day 28 to day 365 after the first PIT; both were achieved by 87.5% of patients at 1 year and 71% at 2 years. At both 1 and 2 years, the median HbA1c level was 5.6% (38 mmol/mol). This trial concluded that allogeneic PIT should be considered for patients with type 1 diabetes in whom other less invasive current treatments would have been ineffective in preventing SHEs [8]. Furthermore, another phase 3 trial was conducted in patients with type 1 diabetes after undergoing kidney transplantation sponsored by National Institutes of Health (CIT06). Likewise, allogeneic PIT was effective, with 62.5% of patients achieving the primary endpoint of freedom from SHEs and HbA1c ≤ 6.5% or reduced by ≥1 percentage point at 1 year after the transplant. These trial results further support the indication of allogeneic PIT in the post-renal transplant setting [9]. Moreover, the TRIMECO trial, which was the first randomized controlled trial in the field of PIT, showed that compared with insulin therapy, allogeneic PIT effectively obtained optimal glycemic control in patients with unstable type 1 diabetes or in patients with type 1 diabetes after kidney transplantation [10]. Although the importance of PIT versus new medical technologies, such as insulin pump therapy, requires further confirmation, allogeneic PIT is being established as an effective treatment for type 1 diabetes with glycemic instability. Figure 70.2 shows a continuous glucose monitoring

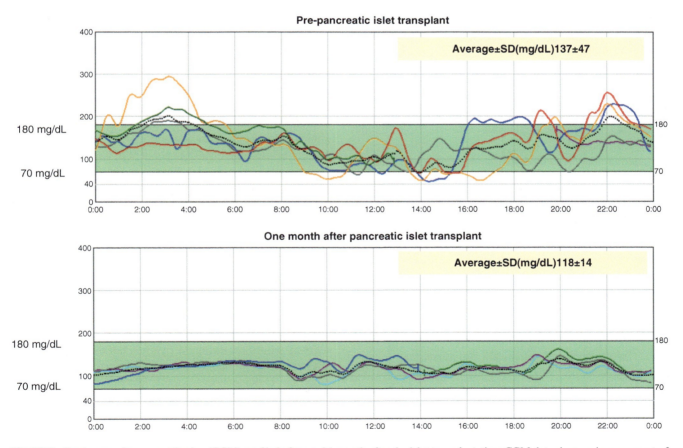

Fig. 70.2 Continuous glucose monitoring (CGM) profile before and 1 month after the islet transplantation. CGM data show an improvement of glycemic control and glycemic fluctuation: 137 ± 47 mg/dL at 8 months before the PIT, 118 ± 14 mg/dL at 1 month after the PIT

(CGM) profile before and 1 month after the islet transplantation, and it shows an improvement of glycemic control and glycemic fluctuation.

70.3 Problems and Solutions to Allogeneic PIT

Insulin independence by allogeneic PIT often requires multiple transplants because isolating all islets is difficult. Many islets are also lost because of instant blood-mediated inflammatory reaction (IBMIR), which is characterized by platelet activation, coagulation, and complement systems that are triggered when islets are exposed to ABO-compatible blood during islet transplantation into the portal vein [11]. Although several approaches, including low-molecular weight-dextran sulfate [12] and islet surface heparinization [13], are valuable in preventing IBMIR, suboptimal engraftment into the liver remains limitation to PIT. Nonetheless, alternative transplant sites are currently explored to establish a more efficient engraftment. Several clinical trials have been conducted to verify the efficacy of alternative transplant sites such as the omentum (ClinicalTrials.gov id NCT02213003, NCT02803905), subcutaneous space (NCT01652911), and gastric submucosa (NCT02402439). Furthermore, numerous studies, including animal studies, have investigated many extrahepatic sites, but the intraportal route remains superior in clinical settings.

Another approach that seemingly improves PIT engraftment is the identification of pathways that regulate posttransplant detrimental inflammatory events. Inflammatory cytokines, including TNF-α and interleukin (IL) 1 (IL-1), are considered therapeutic targets for improving islet engraftment. Currently, the TNF-α receptor antibody etanercept is included in many islet transplant protocols [7, 14]. Anakinra, which is an IL-1 receptor antagonist, has also been applied; the combination of etanercept and anakinra improved islet engraftment using a marginal-dose transplantation model [15]. The CXCL1–CXCR1/2 axis is also a therapeutic target for improving engraftment. Posttransplant recruitment of polymorphonuclear leukocytes and NKT cells is significantly reduced by using CXCR1/2 chemokine receptor inhibitor [16]. A phase 3, multicenter, randomized, double-blind study was conducted in allogeneic PIT recipients randomly selected for reparixin, which is an inhibitor of CXCR1/2 chemokine receptor, or placebo therapy in addition to immunosuppression. Unfortunately, no significant difference was found in C-peptide AUC after PIT, and reparixin did not prevent islet inflammation-mediated damage [17]. However, high-quality clinical trials focusing on islet transplantation are currently conducted, and treatment results are expected to improve in the future as the evidence accumulates.

Immune tolerance to allografts has been pursued in the field of transplantation. In nonhuman primate (NHP) models, inducing apoptotic donor leukocytes leads to long-term tolerance of islet allografts. Peritransplant infusions of apoptotic donor leukocytes under short-term immunotherapy with antagonistic anti-CD40 antibody, rapamycin, soluble TNF receptor and anti–IL-6 receptor antibody induce more than 1-year tolerance to islet allografts in nonsensitized, MHC class I-disparate and one MHC class II DRB allele-matched rhesus macaques. Apoptotic donor leukocyte infusions are an important approach as a cellular, nonchimeric, and translatable method for inducing antigen-specific tolerance [18].

70.4 TPIAT

CP is a progressive inflammatory disease that irreversibly destructs the pancreatic tissue, causing a decline in pancreatic exocrine and endocrine function. Patients suffer from refractory abdominal pain, which can be relieved by pancreatic duct drainage procedures, currently usually done endoscopically, or partial resection; however, these procedures are ineffective in some patients [19], leading to a significantly decreased quality of life (QOL). Total pancreatectomy is the only way to control pain in the long-term, but unfortunately, it inevitably leads to the development of surgical insulin-dependent diabetes postoperatively. Such development has a significant effect on disease prognosis; at least approximately 20% of patients have diabetic vascular complications [20]. In TPIAT, the patient's own islets are isolated from the totally resected pancreas and infused into the liver without any immunosuppressive agents. TPIAT primarily aims to relieve incapacitating pain caused by CP and then to prevent brittle-type insulin-dependent diabetes through islet autotransplantation (IAT). First performed in 1977 [21], TPIAT has been applied to alleviate debilitating pain in patients suffering from CP with favorable outcomes of decreased opioid requirements and improved QOL [22, 23]. Although advanced technique is required for the implementation, TPIAT has been increasingly performed in North America, Europe, and Australia; according to the 2017 report of CITR, 819 patients received TPIAT by July 2015 (https://citregistry.org/system/files/1st_AR_Auto.pdf).

The technique of total pancreatectomy before IAT generally involves the removal of the pancreas with a duodenal segment while preserving the pylorus. For the reconstruction after resection, duodenoduodenostomy or duodenojejunostomy and choledochoenterstomy just proximal or distal to the enteroenterostomy were performed. Blood supply to the pancreas is preserved as much as possible to minimize the warm ischemia time; thus, ligation and division of the splenic artery at its origin and the splenic vein at its termination are the final steps of pancreatectomy. The resected pancreas is added with a cold preservation solution and then transported to the cell-processing laboratory. In performing a brief islet isolation procedure before IAT [24], first, the pancreas is distended with cold enzyme solution through the pancreatic duct. Then, the distended pancreas is placed in a Ricordi chamber and is subsequently digested. Next, the digested tissue is purified by continuous iodixanol density gradient on a COBE 2991 cell separator when the pellet volume exceeds 15–20 mL [25]. Thereafter, the islets are collected in a transplant bag, delivered to the operative room, and infused to the liver through the splenic vein or portal vein.

Judgment of TAIAT indication is extremely difficult and requires multifaceted examination, considering the numerous surgery-associated risks, such as bleeding, wound and intra-abdominal infections, anastomotic leaks, delayed gastric emptying, and portal vein thrombosis [26, 27]. After the TPIAT, patients have lifelong exocrine insufficiency, and most of them require some exogenous insulin permanently even with IAT. In some patients undergoing TPIAT, pain even persists [28].

Global recommendations for assessing the utility of TPIAT are required. Hence, the TPIAT working group, which is part of the International Consensus Guidelines for Chronic Pancreatitis, formed a joint effort with the American Pancreatic Association, International Association of Pancreatology, European Pancreatic Club, and Japan Pancreas Society [29]. Although the evidence is inadequate, several recommendations on TPIAT indications and outcomes have been reported through this working group. Table 70.2 summarizes the questions and statements agreed by this working group. Below are some of the agreed statements. Through TPIAT implementation, reducing opioid use and intractable pain is possible, and strong recommendations for improving QOL are obtained. After TPIAT, the average opioid doses reduced by 71%, 69%, and 67% at 1, 2, and 5 years, respectively [30]. As demonstrated in several studies, the health-related QOL of patients with CP has improved after undergoing TPIAT. Most studies utilized the validated SF36 and SF12, and individual subscale scores increased at 1 and 2 years post-TPIAT, and sustained at 5 years [30, 31]. TPIAT is mainly indicated for pancreatitis-related debilitating pain that reduces the patient's QOL. Conversely, its major contraindications include active alcoholism, pancreatic cancer, end-stage systemic illness, and a psychiatric or socioeconomic status that precludes the safe performance of the surgery and postoperative care [29]. Moreover, TPIAT can offer better glycemic control than TP alone [29]. In the study of 97 patients at a single center, TPIAT obtained a higher insulin independence rate (18% insulin independent vs. 0%) and a lower insulin dosing (22 units/day vs. 35 units/day) than TP alone, but both had similar pain improvement

Table 70.2 Summary of consensus statements from the TPIAT workgroup [29]

Q1: What are the outcomes of TPIAT for patients with CP? **Statements:**
1.1 Improvement in the quality of life is attained in patients with CP following TPIAT.
1.2 Pancreatic pain and opioid use are significantly reduced in patients with CP following TPIAT.
1.3 TPIAT may be associated with reduced medical utilization after the surgery; however, evidence is currently limited for healthcare utilization following TPIAT.
Q2: When should TPIAT be considered for CP versus other therapy forms (e.g., continued medical care, endoscopic therapies, other surgeries including head resection or drainage)? **Statement:**
2.1 The true standing of TPIAT among all forms of CP therapy remains unidentified. Studies including the head-to-head comparisons of TPIAT with other therapy options, such as medical, endoscopic or other surgery forms, are also unavailable.
Q3: What are the unique benefits of TPIAT over TP alone? **Statement:**
3.1 TPIAT offers the possibility of insulin independence and seems to be superior to TP alone in glycemic control and long-term diabetes outcome. TPIAT should be considered as an option and offered to patients with CP requiring TP.
Q4: What are the indications and contraindications for TPIAT? **Statement:**
4.1. TPIAT is mainly indicated for debilitating pain from CP or recurrent pancreatitis that limits the subject's quality of life.
4.2. The major contraindications include but are not limited to the following: active alcoholism, pancreatic cancer, end-stage systemic illness, and a psychiatric or socioeconomic status that precludes the safe performance of the surgery and postoperative care.
Q5: What factors are associated with favorable or poor pain outcomes after TPIAT for CP? **Statement:**
5.1 TPIAT might be considered for the effective management of well-defined, selected cohorts of patients with CP. Early surgery, i.e., at a young age, before multiple endoscopic attempts and before the activation of neuropathic pain circuits is likely to achieve better pain outcomes.
Q6: What factors are associated with favorable or poor diabetes outcomes? **Statement:**
6.1 The transplanted islet mass is the factor that is most consistently predictive of islet graft function and insulin independence across multiple studies. Previous pancreatic surgery, advanced pancreatic disease including calcifications, alcoholic pancreatitis, and possibly prolonged disease might adversely impact islet mass or chance of insulin independence.

Abbreviations: *TPIAT* Total pancreatectomy with islet autotransplantation, *TP* Total pancreatectomy, *CP* Chronic pancreatitis

[32]. The most consistently predictive value of islet graft function and insulin independence is the transplanted islet mass. The ability to achieve insulin independence after TPIAT correlates with the transplanted islet yield [3, 33]. Previous pancreatic surgery [34], alcoholic pancreatitis [35], and advanced pancreatic disease including atrophy and calcifications [36, 37] might adversely impact islet yield. When to perform TPIAT is also important because prolonged illness can have a negative impact on islet yield. Conditional agree-

ment was reached; unfortunately, the role of TPIAT for all forms of CP remains unidentified. Hence, studies including the head-to-head comparisons of TPIAT with other therapy options, such as medical, endoscopic, or other surgery forms, are needed. TPIAT might be considered for the effective management of well-defined, selected cohorts of patients with CP. Early surgery before multiple endoscopic attempts and before the activation of neuropathic pain circuits is likely to achieve better pain outcomes [29].

70.5 Future Directions of Allogeneic PIT and TPIAT

70.5.1 Alternative Cell Sources for Islet Transplantation

Donor shortage is a major problem in allogeneic PIT because this procedure requires two or three transplants to achieve insulin independence. Nonetheless, utilization of xenogeneic (porcine) islet transplantation and stem cell-derived β cells likely overcomes donor shortage and achieves on-demand cell supply.

Porcine islets have several advantages, such as unlimited and on-demand supply and ethical acceptance [38]. For the clinical application of xenogeneic islet transplantation, the major obstacles include the difficulty in controlling xenogeneic immune responses, such as hyperacute rejection and the possibility of zoonotic infection of porcine endogenous retrovirus (PERV). Thus, several solutions have been proposed; one is the administration of multiple immunosuppressive agents, which were given to NHPs in a previous study [39]. Other methods, including genetic engineering [40], and encapsulating devices [41], have been studied. Clinical trials have been conducted in Oceania and South America for intraperitoneal porcine islet transplantation using microencapsulation technique and showed that xenograft is relatively beneficial for treating type 1 diabetes [42]. PERV transmission has been a major safety concern, but it may be resolved through recent advances in genomic-editing technology in the future [43].

Embryonic stem (ES)/iPS cell-derived pancreatic β cell (insulin-producing cells) transplantation possibly cures diabetes at the small animal level [44, 45]. The approach of producing ES/iPS cell-derived pancreatic β cell for type 1 diabetes treatment has already reached the stage of clinical trials in North America. Phase 2 or 3 trial has already been undertaken (NCT 02239354) wherein human ESC is implanted at the differentiation stage of endocrine progenitors. Researchers conducting the trial adopted a method of subcutaneous implantation using a macroencapsulation device to mitigate the risk of tumor formation and protect cells from allogeneic immunity and autoimmunity [46].

Furthermore, novel devices that enable angiogenesis to encapsulated ESC-derived β cells have been developed and started to be used in clinical trials (NCT 03162926). These devices are safe because it can be removed after transplantation; however, its clinical efficacy is unknown, and clinical trial results must be awaited. If the problems on safety, cost, and therapeutic effect are solved, the ES/iPS cell-derived pancreatic β cell can be already clinically applied.

70.5.2 Expanding Indication for TPIAT

Improvements in allogeneic PIT technology, especially islet isolation technology and islet engraftment methods, will directly lead to IAT development. In the future development of IAT, expanding its indications seems important. Some centers have advocated the expansion of IAT indications to include patients undergoing pancreatectomy for reasons other than CP. Among the nonneoplastic conditions are pancreatic arteriovenous malformation [47] and pancreatic trauma [48]. However, considering the small number of cases being studied, further investigation is needed, but if these diseases require extensive pancreatic resection, IAT may be considered as an option.

Meanwhile, expanding indications for neoplastic diseases must be done cautiously. Generally, neoplasms are a contraindication to IAT because of the fear of disseminating malignant cells through the infusion of islets, which still contain some acinar cells and pancreatic ductal cells even after purification. Pancreatic resection with IAT for neoplasms with no or low malignant potential, such as a pancreatic neuroendocrine tumor, had been reported [49]. Therefore, low malignant potential tumors, which include intraductal papillary mucinous neoplasm, serous cystic neoplasms, pancreatic neuroendocrine tumors, metastatic tumors, and mucinous cystic neoplasms, may be applicable to IAT in the future. If the methods of detecting contamination of malignant cells or new circulating tumor markers in islet preparations are established, the indication of IAT for neoplasms may be expanded.

70.6 Conclusions

This review outlines the current status and prospects of cell transplantation therapy in the treatment of insulin-dependent diabetes. In recent years, insulin treatment has made a remarkable progress, as well as the development of regenerative medicine approaches. Thus, the role played by transplantation medicine may change. In the future, new treatment strategies for insulin-dependent diabetes will be established while taking advantage of the strengths of various treatments and complementing each other's weaknesses.

References

1. Shapiro AM, Pokrywczynska M, Ricordi C. Clinical pancreatic islet transplantation. Nat Rev Endocrinol. 2017;13(5):268–77.
2. Iansante V, Mitry RR, Filippi C, Fitzpatrick E, Dhawan A. Human hepatocyte transplantation for liver disease: current status and future perspectives. Pediatr Res. 2018;83(1–2):232–40.
3. Wahoff D, Papalois B, Najarian J, Kendall D, Farney A, Leone J, et al. Autologous islet transplantation to prevent diabetes after pancreatic resection. Ann Surg. 1995;222(4):562–75. discussion 75-9
4. Ricordi C, Lacy P, Scharp D. Automated islet isolation from human pancreas. Diabetes. 1989;38(Suppl 1):140–2.
5. Anazawa T, Okajima H, Masui T, Uemoto S. Current state and future evolution of pancreatic islet transplantation. Ann Gastroenterol Surg. 2019;3(1):34–42.
6. Shapiro AM, Lakey JR, Ryan EA, Korbutt GS, Toth E, Warnock GL, et al. Islet transplantation in seven patients with type 1 diabetes mellitus using a glucocorticoid-free immunosuppressive regimen. N Engl J Med. 2000;343(4):230–8.
7. Barton FB, Rickels MR, Alejandro R, Hering BJ, Wease S, Naziruddin B, et al. Improvement in outcomes of clinical islet transplantation: 1999-2010. Diabetes Care. 2012;35(7):1436–45.
8. Hering BJ, Clarke WR, Bridges ND, Eggerman TL, Alejandro R, Bellin MD, et al. Phase 3 trial of transplantation of human islets in type 1 diabetes complicated by severe hypoglycemia. Diabetes Care. 2016;39(7):1230–40.
9. Markmann JF, Rickels MR, Eggerman TL, Bridges ND, Lafontant DE, Qidwai J, et al. Phase 3 trial of human islet-after-kidney transplantation in type 1 diabetes. Am J Transplant. 2020;21(4):1477–92.
10. Lablanche S, Vantyghem MC, Kessler L, Wojtusciszyn A, Borot S, Thivolet C, et al. Islet transplantation versus insulin therapy in patients with type 1 diabetes with severe hypoglycaemia or poorly controlled glycaemia after kidney transplantation (TRIMECO): a multicentre, randomised controlled trial. Lancet Diabetes Endocrinol. 2018;6(7):527–37.
11. Bennet W, Groth CG, Larsson R, Nilsson B, Korsgren O. Isolated human islets trigger an instant blood mediated inflammatory reaction: implications for intraportal islet transplantation as a treatment for patients with type 1 diabetes. Ups J Med Sci. 2000;105(2):125–33.
12. Johansson H, Goto M, Dufrane D, Siegbahn A, Elgue G, Gianello P, et al. Low molecular weight dextran sulfate: a strong candidate drug to block IBMIR in clinical islet transplantation. Am J Transplant. 2006;6(2):305–12.
13. Cabric S, Sanchez J, Lundgren T, Foss A, Felldin M, Källen R, et al. Islet surface heparinization prevents the instant blood-mediated inflammatory reaction in islet transplantation. Diabetes. 2007;56(8):2008–15.
14. Hering B, Kandaswamy R, Ansite J, Eckman P, Nakano M, Sawada T, et al. Single-donor, marginal-dose islet transplantation in patients with type 1 diabetes. JAMA. 2005;293(7):830–5.
15. McCall M, Pawlick R, Kin T, Shapiro AM. Anakinra potentiates the protective effects of etanercept in transplantation of marginal mass human islets in immunodeficient mice. Am J Transplant. 2012;12(2):322–9.
16. Citro A, Cantarelli E, Maffi P, Nano R, Melzi R, Mercalli A, et al. CXCR1/2 inhibition enhances pancreatic islet survival after transplantation. J Clin Invest. 2012;122(10):3647–51.
17. Maffi P, Lundgren T, Tufveson G, Rafael E, Shaw JAM, Liew A, et al. Targeting CXCR1/2 does not improve insulin secretion after pancreatic islet transplantation: a phase 3, double-blind, randomized, placebo-controlled trial in type 1 diabetes. Diabetes Care. 2020;43(4):710–8.
18. Singh A, Ramachandran S, Graham ML, Daneshmandi S, Heller D, Suarez-Pinzon WL, et al. Long-term tolerance of islet allografts in nonhuman primates induced by apoptotic donor leukocytes. Nat Commun. 2019;10(1):3495.
19. Schnelldorfer T, Lewin D, Adams D. Operative management of chronic pancreatitis: longterm results in 372 patients. J Am Coll Surg. 2007;204(5):1039–45. discussion 45-7
20. Gruessner R, Sutherland D, Dunn D, Najarian J, Jie T, Hering B, et al. Transplant options for patients undergoing total pancreatectomy for chronic pancreatitis. J Am Coll Surg. 2004;198(4):559–67. discussion 68-9
21. Sutherland D, Matas A, Najarian J. Pancreatic islet cell transplantation. Surg Clin North Am. 1978;58(2):365–82.
22. Ahmad S, Lowy A, Wray C, D'Alessio D, Choe K, James L, et al. Factors associated with insulin and narcotic independence after islet autotransplantation in patients with severe chronic pancreatitis. J Am Coll Surg. 2005;201(5):680–7.
23. Blondet J, Carlson A, Kobayashi T, Jie T, Bellin M, Hering B, et al. The role of total pancreatectomy and islet autotransplantation for chronic pancreatitis. Surg Clin North Am. 2007;87(6):1477–501. x
24. Anazawa T, Balamurugan A, Bellin M, Zhang H, Matsumoto S, Yonekawa Y, et al. Human islet isolation for autologous transplantation: comparison of yield and function using SERVA/Nordmark versus Roche enzymes. Am J Transplant. 2009;9(10):2383–91.
25. Anazawa T, Matsumoto S, Yonekawa Y, Loganathan G, Wilhelm JJ, Soltani SM, et al. Prediction of pancreatic tissue densities by an analytical test gradient system before purification maximizes human islet recovery for islet autotransplantation/allotransplantation. Transplantation. 2011;91(5):508–14.
26. John GK, Singh VK, Pasricha PJ, Sinha A, Afghani E, Warren D, et al. Delayed gastric emptying (DGE) following total pancreatectomy with islet auto transplantation in patients with chronic pancreatitis. J Gastrointest Surg. 2015;19(7):1256–61.
27. Shahbazov R, Naziruddin B, Salam O, Saracino G, Levy MF, Beecherl E, et al. The impact of surgical complications on the outcome of total pancreatectomy with islet autotransplantation. Am J Surg. 2020;219(1):99–105.
28. Bellin MD, Freeman ML, Gelrud A, Slivka A, Clavel A, Humar A, et al. Total pancreatectomy and islet autotransplantation in chronic pancreatitis: recommendations from pancreas fest. Pancreatology. 2014;14(1):27–35.
29. Abu-El-Haija M, Anazawa T, Beilman GJ, Besselink MG, Del Chiaro M, Demir IE, et al. The role of total pancreatectomy with islet autotransplantation in the treatment of chronic pancreatitis: a report from the international consensus guidelines in chronic pancreatitis. Pancreatology. 2020;20(4):762–71.
30. Morgan KA, Lancaster WP, Owczarski SM, Wang H, Borckardt J, Adams DB. Patient selection for total pancreatectomy with islet autotransplantation in the surgical management of chronic pancreatitis. J Am Coll Surg. 2018;226(4):446–51.
31. Wilson GC, Sutton JM, Abbott DE, Smith MT, Lowy AM, Matthews JB, et al. Long-term outcomes after total pancreatectomy and islet cell autotransplantation: is it a durable operation? Ann Surg. 2014;260(4):659–65. discussion 65-7
32. Garcea G, Pollard CA, Illouz S, Webb M, Metcalfe MS, Dennison AR. Patient satisfaction and cost-effectiveness following total pancreatectomy with islet cell transplantation for chronic pancreatitis. Pancreas. 2013;42(2):322–8.
33. Sutherland D, Gruessner A, Carlson A, Blondet J, Balamurugan A, Reigstad K, et al. Islet autotransplant outcomes after total pancreatectomy: a contrast to islet allograft outcomes. Transplantation. 2008;86(12):1799–802.
34. Sutherland DE, Radosevich DM, Bellin MD, Hering BJ, Beilman GJ, Dunn TB, et al. Total pancreatectomy and islet autotransplantation for chronic pancreatitis. J Am Coll Surg. 2012;214(4):409–24. discussion 24-6

35. Dunderdale J, McAuliffe JC, McNeal SF, Bryant SM, Yancey BD, Flowers G, et al. Should pancreatectomy with islet cell autotransplantation in patients with chronic alcoholic pancreatitis be abandoned? J Am Coll Surg. 2013;216(4):591–6. discussion 6-8
36. Johnston PC, Lin YK, Walsh RM, Bottino R, Stevens TK, Trucco M, et al. Factors associated with islet yield and insulin independence after total pancreatectomy and islet cell autotransplantation in patients with chronic pancreatitis utilizing off-site islet isolation: Cleveland Clinic experience. J Clin Endocrinol Metab. 2015;100(5):1765–70.
37. Khan KM, Desai CS, Kalb B, Patel C, Grigsby BM, Jie T, et al. MRI prediction of islet yield for autologous transplantation after total pancreatectomy for chronic pancreatitis. Dig Dis Sci. 2013;58(4):1116–24.
38. Schuetz C, Anazawa T, Cross SE, Labriola L, Meier RPH, Redfield RR, et al. β cell replacement therapy: the next 10 years. Transplantation. 2018;102(2):215–29.
39. Hering B, Wijkstrom M, Graham M, Hårdstedt M, Aasheim T, Jie T, et al. Prolonged diabetes reversal after intraportal xenotransplantation of wild-type porcine islets in immunosuppressed nonhuman primates. Nat Med. 2006;12(3):301–3.
40. Bottino R, Wijkstrom M, van der Windt DJ, Hara H, Ezzelarab M, Murase N, et al. Pig-to-monkey islet xenotransplantation using multi-transgenic pigs. Am J Transplant. 2014;14(10):2275–87.
41. Dufrane D, Goebbels RM, Gianello P. Alginate macroencapsulation of pig islets allows correction of streptozotocin-induced diabetes in primates up to 6 months without immunosuppression. Transplantation. 2010;90(10):1054–62.
42. Matsumoto S, Abalovich A, Wechsler C, Wynyard S, Elliott RB. Clinical benefit of islet xenotransplantation for the treatment of type 1 diabetes. EBioMedicine. 2016;12:255–62.
43. Yang L, Güell M, Niu D, George H, Lesha E, Grishin D, et al. Genome-wide inactivation of porcine endogenous retroviruses (PERVs). Science. 2015;350(6264):1101–4.
44. Pagliuca FW, Millman JR, Gürtler M, Segel M, Van Dervort A, Ryu JH, et al. Generation of functional human pancreatic β cells in vitro. Cell. 2014.159(2):428–39.
45. Rezania A, Bruin JE, Arora P, Rubin A, Batushansky I, Asadi A, et al. Reversal of diabetes with insulin-producing cells derived in vitro from human pluripotent stem cells. Nat Biotechnol. 2014;32(11):1121–33.
46. Agulnick AD, Ambruzs DM, Moorman MA, Bhoumik A, Cesario RM, Payne JK, et al. Insulin-producing endocrine cells differentiated in vitro from human embryonic stem cells function in macroencapsulation devices in vivo. Stem Cells Transl Med. 2015;4(10):1214–22.
47. Sakata N, Goto M, Motoi F, Hayashi H, Nakagawa K, Mizuma M, et al. Clinical experiences in the treatment of pancreatic arteriovenous malformation by total pancreatectomy with islet autotransplantation. Transplantation. 2013;96(5):e38–40.
48. Jindal RM, Ricordi C, Shriver CD. Autologous pancreatic islet transplantation for severe trauma. N Engl J Med. 2010;362(16):1550.
49. Oberholzer J, Mathe Z, Bucher P, Triponez F, Bosco D, Fournier B, et al. Islet autotransplantation after left pancreatectomy for non-enucleable insulinoma. Am J Transplant. 2003;3(10):1302–7.

Printed by Printforce, the Netherlands